VOLUME ONE

DIAGNOSTIC ULTRASOUND

SECOND EDITION

VOLUME ONE

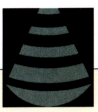

DIAGNOSTIC ULTRASOUND

SECOND EDITION

Carol M. Rumack, M.D.

Professor of Radiology and Pediatrics
University of Colorado Health Sciences Center
Denver, Colorado

Stephanie R. Wilson, M.D.

Professor of Radiology and Obstetrics and Gynecology
University of Toronto
Head, Division of Ultrasound
The Toronto Hospital
Toronto, Ontario, Canada

J. William Charboneau, M.D.

Professor of Radiology
Mayo Clinic
Rochester, Minnesota

with 3698 illustrations, including 461 in color

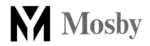

St. Louis Baltimore Boston Carlsbad Chicago Minneapolis New York Philadelphia Portland
London Milan Sydney Tokyo Toronto

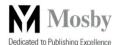

Dedicated to Publishing Excellence

A Times Mirror
Company

Executive Editor: Robert A. Hurley
Managing Editor: Elizabeth Corra
Associate Developmental Editor: Mia Cariño
Project Manager: Christopher J. Baumle
Project Specialist: David Orzechowski
Manufacturing Manager: William A. Winneberger, Jr.
Designer: Carolyn O' Brien

Composition by Accu-Color Inc.
Printing/binding by Von Hoffman Press, Inc.
Printed in the United States of America

Mosby–Year Book, Inc.
11830 Westline Industrial Drive
St. Louis, Missouri 63146

Library of Congress Cataloging-in-Publication Data

Diagnostic ultrasound / [edited by] Carol M. Rumack, Stephanie R.
    Wilson, J. William Charboneau. — 2nd ed.
        p.   cm.
    Includes bibliographical references and index.
    ISBN 0-8151-8683-5
    1. Diagnosis, Ultrasonic.   I. Rumack, Carol M.   II. Wilson,
Stephanie R.   III. Charboneau, J. William.
        [DNLM: 1. Ultrasonography.   WN 208 D5357 1997]
RC78.7.U4D514   1997
616.07'543—dc21
DNLM/DLC   97-41915
for Library of Congress   CIP

98 99 00 01 02 / 9 8 7 6 5 4 3 2

EDITORS

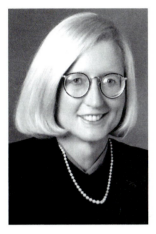

CAROL M. RUMACK, M.D., is Professor of Radiology and Pediatrics at the University of Colorado School of Medicine in Denver, Colorado. Her clinical practice is based at The Children's Hospital and University Hospital in Denver. Her main research focus has been on neonatal sonography in the high-risk perinatal nursery and in newborns referred for complex imaging. Dr. Rumack has published widely in this field and has lectured frequently on pediatric ultrasound. She was the Founding President of the American Association for Women Radiologists and has been a member of the Board of Directors of the American Institute of Ultrasound in Medicine and the Society for Pediatric Radiology. She and her husband, Barry, have two children, Becky and Marc.

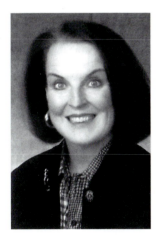

STEPHANIE R. WILSON, M.D., is Professor of Radiology and Obstetrics and Gynecology at the University of Toronto and Head of the Division of Ultrasound at The Toronto Hospital. Her current research endeavors with Dr. Peter N. Burns are focused on oral and intravascular ultrasound contrast agents. An authority on ultrasound of the gastrointestinal tract and abdominal and pelvic viscera, she is the recipient of many university awards and is a frequent international speaker and author. Dr. Wilson also was the first woman President of the Canadian Association of Radiologists and a past Vice President of the Radiological Society of North America. A golf enthusiast, she and her husband, Ken, have two children, Jessica and Jordan.

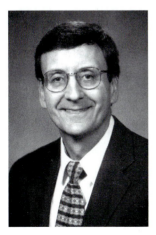

J. WILLIAM CHARBONEAU, M.D., is Professor of Radiology at the Mayo Clinic at Rochester, Minnesota. His current research interests are in small-parts imaging and ultrasound-guided interventional procedures. He is a coauthor of approximately 100 publications, assistant editor of the *Mayo Clinic Family Health Book*, and an active lecturer nationally and internationally. He and his wife, Cathy, have three children, Nick, Ben, and Laurie.

CONTRIBUTORS

Mostafa Atri, M.D., F.R.C.P.(C)
Associate Professor of Radiology
McGill University
Director, Division of Ultrasound
Montreal General Hospital
Montreal, Quebec, Canada

E. Michel Azouz, M.D., F.R.C.P.C.
Professor of Radiology
McGill University
Assistant Director, Department of Medical Imaging
Montreal Children's Hospital
Montreal, Quebec, Canada

Diane S. Babcock, M.D., F.A.C.R.
Professor of Radiology and Pediatrics
University of Cincinnati College of Medicine
University Hospital
Children's Hospital Medical Center
Cincinnati, Ohio

Carol B. Benson, M.D.
Associate Professor of Radiology
Harvard Medical School
Co-Director of Ultrasound
Brigham & Women's Hospital
Boston, Massachusetts

William E. Brant, M.D.
Associate Professor of Radiology
University of California, Davis, School of Medicine
Department of Radiology
University of California, Davis, Medical Center
Sacramento, California

Robert L. Bree, M.D.
Professor of Radiology
University of Michigan Medical School
University of Michigan Medical Center
Ann Arbor, Michigan

Linda K. Brown, M.D.
Staff Radiologist
Quantum Radiology Northwest
Atlanta, Georgia

Peter N. Burns, Ph.D.
Professor of Medical Biophysics and Radiology
University of Toronto
Senior Scientist, Imaging Research
Sunnybrook Health Science Centre
Toronto, Ontario, Canada

Barbara A. Carroll, M.D.
Professor of Radiology
Chief, Section of Ultrasound
Duke University Medical Center
Durham, North Carolina

John M. Caspers, M.D.
Abdominal Imaging Fellow
Mayo Clinic
Rochester, Minnesota
Staff Radiologist
St. Paul Radiology
United Hospital
St. Paul, Minnesota

**Daniel E. Challis, M.B., B.S.,
F.R.A.C.O.G., D.D.U.**
Clinical Fellow
University of Toronto
Mount Sinai Hospital
Toronto, Ontario, Canada

William F. Chandler, M.D.
Professor of Neurosurgery
University of Michigan Medical Center
Ann Arbor, Michigan

J. William Charboneau, M.D.
Professor of Radiology
Mayo Clinic
Rochester, Minnesota

**David Chitayat, M.D., F.C.C.M.G.,
F.A.B.M.G., F.R.C.P.C.**
Associate Professor
University of Toronto
Head, Prenatal Diagnosis Program
The Toronto Hospital General Division
Toronto, Ontario, Canada

Christine H. Comstock, M.D.
Assistant Professor
Wayne State University
Detroit, Michigan
Director, Fetal Imaging
William Beaumont Hospital
Royal Oak, Michigan

Peter L. Cooperberg, M.D., F.R.C.P.C.
Professor and Vice Chairman of Radiology
University of British Columbia
Chairman of Radiology
St. Paul's Hospital
Vancouver, British Columbia, Canada

Jeanne A. Cullinan, M.D.
Assistant Professor of Radiology
and Radiological Sciences
Assistant Professor of Obstetrics and Gynecology
Vanderbilt University Medical Center
Nashville, Tennessee

Timothy J. Dambro, M.D.
Hospital of the University of Pennsylvania
Philadelphia, Pennsylvania

Sidney M. Dashefsky, M.D., F.R.C.P.
Assistant Professor of Radiology
University of Manitoba
Radiologist
Health Sciences Centre
Winnipeg, Manitoba, Canada

Michael A. DiPietro, M.D.
Associate Professor of Radiology
University of Michigan
Pediatric Radiologist
C.S. Mott Children's Hospital
Ann Arbor, Michigan

Peter M. Doubilet, M.D., Ph.D.
Associate Professor of Radiology
Harvard Medical School
Co-Director of Ultrasound
Brigham & Women's Hospital
Boston, Massachusetts

Dónal B. Downey, M.B., B.Ch., F.R.C.P.C.
Assistant Professor, Department of Diagnostic
Radiology and Nuclear Medicine
Associate Scientist, The John P. Robarts
Research Institute
University of Western Ontario
Director of Diagnostic Ultrasound
London Health Sciences Centre
London, Ontario, Canada

Julia A. Drose, B.A., R.D.M.S., R.D.C.S.
Senior Instructor
University of Colorado School of Medicine
Chief Diagnostic Medical Sonographer
University of Colorado Health Sciences Center
Denver, Colorado

Steven Falcone, M.D.
Assistant Professor of Clinical Radiology and
Neurological Surgery
University of Miami School of Medicine
University of Miami/Jackson Memorial
Medical Center
Attending Neuroradiologist
MRI Center
Miami, Florida

Dan Farine, M.D., F.R.C.S.C.
Associate Professor, Department of Obstetrics
and Gynecology
University of Toronto
Staff Perinatologist and Director of Obstetrics
Mount Sinai Hospital
Toronto, Ontario, Canada

Paul W. Finnegan, M.D., C.M., F.R.C.P.(C)
MBA Program
University of Chicago, Graduate School of Business
Chicago, Illinois
Private Practice
Toronto, Ontario, Canada, and Chicago, Illinois

Katherine W. Fong, M.B., B.S., F.R.C.P.(C)
Assistant Professor of Medical Imaging
University of Toronto
Head, Division of Ultrasound
Women's College Hospital
Toronto, Ontario, Canada

Bruno D. Fornage, M.D.
Professor of Radiology
Chief, Section of Ultrasound
University of Texas, M.D. Anderson Cancer Center
Houston, Texas

J. Brian Fowlkes, Ph.D.
Assistant Research Scientist
University of Michigan Medical Center
Ann Arbor, Michigan

Margaret A. Fraser-Hill, M.D., F.R.C.P.C.
Assistant Professor
Faculty of Medicine
McGill University
Department of Radiology
Montreal General Hospital
Montreal, Quebec, Canada

Kelly S. Freed, M.D.
Clinical Associate
Duke University Medical Center
Durham, North Carolina

Phyllis Glanc, M.D., F.R.C.P.C.
Assistant Professor
University of Toronto
Women's College Hospital
Toronto, Ontario, Canada

Charles M. Glasier, M.D.
Professor of Radiology and Pediatrics
University of Arkansas for Medical Sciences
Chief, Magnetic Resonance Imaging
Arkansas Children's Hospital
Little Rock, Arkansas

Lawrence P. Gordon, M.D.
Associate Pathologist
Crouse Hospital
Associate Professor of Pathology
State University of New York Health Science Center
Syracuse, New York

Calvin A. Greene, M.D., F.R.S.C.(C)
Assistant Clinical Professor
University of Calgary
Division Chief, Reproductive Endocrinology
and Infertility
Director, Regional Fertility Program
Foothills Hospital
Calgary, Alberta, Canada

Leslie E. Grissom, M.D.
Assistant Professor of Radiology and Pediatrics
Jefferson Medical College
Philadelphia, Pennsylvania
Attending Radiologist
Chief of Diagnostic Imaging
Alfred I. duPont Institute
Wilmington, Delaware

H. Theodore Harcke, M.D.
Professor of Radiology and Pediatrics
Jefferson Medical College
Philadelphia, Pennsylvania
Attending Radiologist
Chief of Imaging Research
Alfred I. duPont Institute
Wilmington, Delaware

Curtis L. Harlow, M.D.
Assistant Clinical Professor
University of Colorado
Chief of Radiology
St. Thomas More Hospital
Cañon City, Colorado

Christopher R. Harman, M.D., F.R.C.S.C.
Associate Professor, Department of Obstetrics
and Gynecology
University of Manitoba
Director, Fetal Assessment Unit
Women's Hospital
Winnipeg, Manitoba, Canada

**Ian D. Hay, M.B., Ph.D., F.A.C.E.,
F.A.C.P., F.R.C.P.**
Professor of Medicine
Mayo Medical School
Consultant in Endocrinology and Internal Medicine
Mayo Clinic
Rochester, Minnesota

Christy K. Holland, Ph.D.
Associate Professor, Department of Radiology
University of Cincinnati College of Medicine
Cincinnati, Ohio

Susan C. Holt, M.D., F.R.C.P.(C)
Assistant Professor, Department of Radiology
Health Sciences Centre
Winnipeg, Manitoba, Canada

C. Richard Hopkins, M.D.
Associate in Radiology
Ogden Regional Medical Center
Ogden, Utah
Davis North Hospital
Layton, Utah

E. Meredith James, M.D., F.A.C.R.
Associate Professor of Radiology
Mayo Clinic
Rochester, Minnesota

Ann Jefferies, M.D., F.R.C.P.C.
Assistant Professor
University of Toronto
Neonatologist
Mount Sinai Hospital
Toronto, Ontario, Canada

Susan D. John, M.D.
Associate Professor of Radiology and Pediatrics
University of Texas Medical Branch
Galveston, Texas

Jo-Ann M. Johnson, M.D., F.R.C.S.C.
Assistant Professor
University of Toronto
Division of Maternal Fetal Medicine
The Toronto Hospital
Toronto, Ontario, Canada

Neil D. Johnson, M.B., B.S., F.R.A.C.R., M.Med.
Assistant Professor
University of Cincinnati
Associate Director, Department of Radiology
Children's Hospital Medical Center
Cincinnati, Ohio

Robert A. Kane, M.D., F.A.C.R.
Vice Chairman, Department of Radiological Sciences
Director, Ultrasonography
Associate Professor of Radiology
Harvard Medical School
Beth Israel Deaconess Medical Center
Boston, Massachusetts

Terese I. Kaske, M.D.
Radiology Resident
University of Colorado Health Sciences Center
Denver, Colorado

Bernard F. King, Jr., M.D.
Associate Professor, Department of
Diagnostic Radiology
Mayo Graduate School
Mayo Clinic and Affiliated Hospitals
Rochester, Minnesota

Cheryl L. Kirby, M.D.
Assistant Professor of Diagnostic Imaging
Temple University School of Medicine
Attending Radiologist
Albert Einstein Medical Center
Philadelphia, Pennsylvania

Janet S. Kirk, M.D.
Assistant Director, Fetal Imaging
William Beaumont Hospital
Royal Oak, Michigan

Faye C. Laing, M.D.
Professor of Radiology
Harvard University
Director, Resident Education and Training
Brigham & Women's Hospital
Boston, Massachusetts

Eric J. Lantz, M.D.
Assistant Professor
Mayo Medical School
Staff Radiologist
Mayo Clinic
Rochester, Minnesota

Robert A. Lee, M.D.
Assistant Professor of Radiology
Consultant in Diagnostic Radiology
Mayo Foundation
Rochester, Minnesota

Richard E. Leithiser, Jr., M.D.
Associate Professor of Radiology
University of Arkansas for Medical Sciences
Arkansas Children's Hospital
Little Rock, Arkansas

Clifford S. Levi, M.D., F.R.C.P.(C)
Professor of Radiology
University of Manitoba
Section Head, Diagnostic Ultrasound
Health Sciences Centre
Winnipeg, Manitoba, Canada

Bernard J. Lewandowski, M.D., C.M., R.V.T., M.B.A.
Clinical Associate Professor
University of Ottawa
Head, Ultrasound (Radiology)
Ottawa Civic Hospital
Ottawa, Ontario, Canada

Bradley D. Lewis, M.D.
Assistant Professor
Mayo Medical School
Mayo Graduate School of Medicine
Consultant in Diagnostic Imaging
Mayo Clinic
Rochester, Minnesota

Edward A. Lyons, M.D., F.R.C.P.(C), F.A.C.R.
Professor of Radiology and Obstetrics
and Gynecology
University of Manitoba
Health Sciences Centre
Winnipeg, Manitoba, Canada

†Laurence A. Mack, M.D.
Professor of Radiology, Obstetrics and Gynecology,
and Orthopaedics
Director of Ultrasound
University of Washington School of Medicine
Seattle, Washington

Marie-Jocelyne Martel, M.D.
Fellow, Maternal Fetal Medicine
University of Manitoba
Winnipeg, Manitoba, Canada

John R. Mathieson, M.D., F.R.C.P.C.
Head, Section of Radiology
Department of Medical Imaging
Capital Health Region
Royal Jubilee Hospital
Victoria, British Columbia, Canada

Frederick A. Matsen, III, M.D.
Professor and Chairman, Department
of Orthopaedics
University of Washington Medical Center
Seattle, Washington

John P. McGahan, M.D.
Professor of Radiology
Professor and Director of Abdominal Imaging
University of California, Davis, Medical Center
Sacramento, California

Ellen B. Mendelson, M.D.
Clinical Associate Professor of Diagnostic Radiology
University of Pittsburgh School of Medicine
Director, Mammography and Women's Imaging
Western Pennsylvania Hospital
Pittsburgh, Pennsylvania

Christopher R.B. Merritt, M.D.
Chairman, Department of Radiology
Ochsner Clinic and the Alton Ochsner
Medical Foundation
New Orleans, Louisiana

Berta Maria Montalvo, M.D.
Associate Professor of Radiology
University of Miami School of Medicine
Medical Director, Vascular Diagnostic Center
University of Miami Hospitals and Clinics
University of Miami/Jackson Memorial Medical Center
Miami, Florida

Khanh T. Nguyen, M.Sc., M.D., F.R.C.P.C.
Associate Professor
Queen's University
Kingston General Hospital
Hotel Dieu Hospital
Kingston, Ontario, Canada

Stuart F. Nicholson, M.D., F.R.C.P.C.
Clinical Associate Professor
University of Calgary
Foothills Hospital
Calgary, Alberta, Canada

Carl A. Nimrod, M.B., F.R.C.S.C.
Professor of Obstetrics and Gynecology
and Radiology
University of Ottawa
Chief of Obstetrics and Gynecology
Ottawa General Hospital
Ottawa, Ontario, Canada

---

† Deceased

Robert L. Nolan, B.Sc., M.D., F.R.C.P.C.
Professor and Head, Department of
Diagnostic Radiology
Queen's University
Head, Imaging Services
Kingston General Hospital
Hotel Dieu Hospital
St. Mary's of the Lake Hospital
Kingston, Ontario, Canada

David A. Nyberg, M.D.
Associate Clinical Professor of Radiology and
Obstetrics and Gynecology
University of Washington Medical Center
Co-Director of Obstetric Ultrasound
Swedish Medical Center
Seattle, Washington

Heidi B. Patriquin, M.D., F.R.C.P.(C)
Clinical Professor of Radiology
University of Montreal
Hopital Ste. Justine
Montreal, Quebec, Canada

Roger A. Pierson, M.S., Ph.D.
Professor, Department of Obstetrics and Gynecology
University of Saskatchewan College of Medicine
Royal University Hospital
Saskatoon, Saskatchewan, Canada

Joseph F. Polak, M.D., M.P.H.
Associate Professor of Radiology
Harvard Medical School
Director of Noninvasive Vascular Imaging
Brigham & Women's Hospital
Boston, Massachusetts

Carl C. Reading, M.D.
Professor of Diagnostic Radiology
Mayo Medical School
Consultant, Diagnostic Radiology
Mayo Clinic
Rochester, Minnesota

**Henrietta Kotlus Rosenberg, M.D.,
F.A.C.R., F.A.A.P.**
Professor of Diagnostic Imaging
Temple University School of Medicine
Chairman, Department of Radiology
Albert Einstein Medical Center
Philadelphia, Pennsylvania

Jonathan M. Rubin, M.D., Ph.D.
Professor of Radiology
University of Michigan
Ann Arbor, Michigan

Carol M. Rumack, M.D., F.A.C.R.
Professor of Radiology and Pediatrics
University of Colorado School of Medicine
Denver, Colorado

**Greg Ryan, M.B., M.R.C.O.G.,
F.R.C.S.C.**
Assistant Professor, Department of Obstetrics
and Gynecology
Faculty of Medicine
University of Toronto
Director of the Fetal Assessment Unit
Staff Perinatologist
Mount Sinai Hospital
Toronto, Ontario, Canada

Shia Salem, M.D., F.R.C.P.C.
Associate Professor, Medical Imaging
University of Toronto
Head, Division of Ultrasound
Mount Sinai Hospital
Toronto, Ontario, Canada

**Eric E. Sauerbrei, B.Sc., M.Sc., M.D.,
F.R.C.P.C.**
Professor of Radiology
Queen's University
Director of Ultrasound
Kingston General Hospital
Hotel Dieu Hospital
Kingston, Ontario, Canada

Joanna J. Seibert, M.D.
Professor of Radiology and Pediatrics
University of Arkansas for Medical Sciences
Director of Radiology
Arkansas Children's Hospital
Little Rock, Arkansas

Robert W. Seibert, M.D.
Professor, Department of Otolaryngology-Head and
Neck Surgery
University of Arkansas for Medical Sciences
Chief, Pediatric Otolaryngology
Arkansas Children's Hospital
Little Rock, Arkansas

†Nancy H. Sherman, M.D.
Assistant Professor of Radiology
Jefferson Medical College
Philadelphia, Pennsylvania
Director of Ultrasound
Alfred I. duPont Institute
Wilmington, Delaware

Luigi Solbiati, M.D.
Vice Chairman and Radiologist
Department of Radiology
General Hospital
Busto Arsizio, Varese, Italy

Beverly A. Spirt, M.D., F.A.C.R.
Professor of Radiology and Obstetrics
and Gynecology
Chief of Women's Imaging Section
State University of New York Health Science Center
Syracuse, New York

Elizabeth R. Stamm, M.D.
Associate Professor
University of Colorado Health Sciences Center
Administrative Co-Director of Body CT
University Hospital
Denver, Colorado

Rhonda R. Stewart, M.D.
Diagnostic Radiologist
Director of CT
Alexandria Hospital
Alexandria, Virginia

Leonard E. Swischuk, M.D.
Professor of Radiology and Pediatrics
University of Texas Medical Branch
Director of Pediatric Radiology
Children's Hospital
Galveston, Texas

George A. Taylor, M.D.
Associate Professor of Radiology and Pediatrics
Harvard Medical School
Director, Body Imaging Division
Children's Hospital
Boston, Massachusetts

Wendy Thurston, M.D., B.Sc., F.R.C.P.C.
Assistant Professor
Division Head, Genitourinary Radiology
University of Toronto
Staff Radiologist
The Toronto Hospital
Toronto, Ontario, Canada

Ants Toi, M.D., F.R.C.P.C.
Associate Professor
University of Toronto
Radiologist
The Toronto Hospital
Toronto, Ontario, Canada

Marnix T. van Holsbeeck, M.D.
Associate Professor of Radiology
Case Western Reserve University
Director, Musculoskeletal and ER Radiology
Henry Ford Hospital
Detroit, Michigan

Keith Y. Wang, Ph.D., M.D.
Clinical Assistant Professor, Department
of Radiology
University of Washington
Swedish Medical Center
Seattle, Washington

Stephanie R. Wilson, M.D., F.R.C.P.C.
Professor of Radiology and Obstetrics and
Gynecology
University of Toronto
Head, Division of Ultrasound
The Toronto Hospital
Toronto, Ontario, Canada

David A. Wiseman, M.D., F.R.C.P.(C)
Associate Professor
Faculty of Medicine
University of Calgary School of Medicine
Radiologist
Foothills Hospital
Calgary, Alberta, Canada

Cynthia E. Withers, M.D., F.R.C.P.C.
Staff Radiologist
Sansum Medical Clinic
Santa Barbara, California

† Deceased

To Barry, Becky, and Marc, for their love and wonderful support through an extremely intense year. To my parents, for their love and their belief in me. And to all my students, for responding to the challenge and joy of studying medicine, in particular ultrasound.

CMR

To Ken, Jessica, and Jordan, who generously lived without me for the many months required for this endeavor. Your independence and continuous encouragement were my inspiration.

SRW

To Cathy, Nicholas, Ben, and Laurie, for all the love and joy you bring to my life. You are all I could ever hope for.

JWC

PREFACE
TO THE SECOND EDITION

The First Edition of *Diagnostic Ultrasound*, released at the RSNA in 1991, has become the most commonly used reference textbook at ultrasound practices worldwide. Because sonography has so expanded its frontiers in the past 6 years, we believed that a major revision was required for *Diagnostic Ultrasound* to remain the definitive reference work for this specialty. In particular, greater use of color and power Doppler imaging and improved high-resolution transducers have required the introduction of new chapters and new authors, as well as the expansion and enhancement of the First Edition's original material.

Approximately 100 outstanding authors, all recognized experts in the field of ultrasound, bring you the latest state-of-the-art concepts on ultrasound performance, imaging, diagnosis, and expanded applications, including hysterosonography, laparoscopic sonography, and ultrasound-guided biopsy and drainage techniques.

There has been a 25% increase in the size of the two volumes, the major space reallocation applied to obstetrics and gynecology. Thousands of the original images have been replaced, and new images have been added. The Second Edition also includes more than 450 images in full color. The layout has been exhaustively revamped and now includes multiple-picture "Key Feature Collages." These reflect the spectrum of sonographic changes that may occur in a given disease instead of just the most common manifestation.

Many improvements in the book's format have been designed to facilitate reading and review. Color-enhanced boxes highlight the important or critical features of sonographic diagnoses. Key terms and concepts are emphasized in boldface type. To direct the reader to other research and literature of interest, the comprehensive reference lists are well organized by topic.

The book is again divided into two volumes. Volume I consists of Parts I–IV. Part I contains chapters on physics and biologic effects of ultrasound, as well as the latest developments in ultrasound contrast agents. Part II covers abdominal, pelvic, and thoracic sonography, including interventional procedures. Part III presents intraoperative and laparoscopic sonography. Part IV contains many chapters on small-parts imaging, including carotid and peripheral artery and vein evaluation. Volume II begins with Part V, a greatly expanded section on obstetric and fetal sonography. Part VI comprehensively covers pediatric sonography. Two new chapters on pediatric brain Doppler and pediatric interventional sonography have been added to Part VI.

This book is for practicing physicians, residents, medical students, sonographers, and others interested in understanding the vast applications of diagnostic sonography in patient care. As with the First Edition, *it is our goal to present to you the most comprehensive reference book available on diagnostic ultrasound.*

PREFACE
TO THE FIRST EDITION

Sonography has expanded rapidly over the last two decades on a world-wide basis. Despite the explosive growth of this field and the extensive applications of sonographic techniques, few comprehensive reference texts are available. To this end, we undertook the task of producing a state-of-the-art text on ultrasonography.

The authors who have contributed chapters to this book are recognized experts in their fields. We believe that they have provided the most up-to-date information available, making the book current and comprehensive. We hope that it will become a trusted primary reference for all who are interested in this exciting field of medical imaging.

This book is intended for practicing physicians, residents, medical students, and sonographers. It is organized into six parts, covering all aspects of sonography except cardiac and opthalmologic applications. The information in Volume One, Part I, covers the physics of sonography; Part II, abdominal, pelvic, and thoracic imaging; Part III, intraoperative imaging; and Part IV, small parts imaging, including carotid and peripheral vessels. The contents of Volume Two include Part V, obstetric and fetal topics and Part VI, pediatric applications. Every effort was made to cover the broad scope of ultrasound practice without redundancy.

We greatly appreciate the efforts of the contributing authors. Without their experience, expertise, and commitment, we could not have achieved the goal of a comprehensive and authoritative textbook. We are indebted to them.

The high-quality images are the product of many talented sonographers, and to them we offer our sincere thanks. Their dedication to sonography has contributed substantially to its rapid growth and acceptance.

We also thank Janine Jacobson, our talented manuscript coordinator, whose patience and care with multiple manuscript revisions has led to a first-class product. Further, we acknowledge the support of Elaine Steinborn, Jo Salway, Jim Ryan, and Anne Patterson of Mosby–Year Book for encouraging us in this endeavor.

ACKNOWLEDGMENTS

Our deepest appreciation and sincerest gratitude:

To all of our outstanding authors who have contributed extensive, newly updated, and authoritative text and images. We cannot thank them enough for their efforts on this project.

To Lisa Wolfe in Denver, Colorado, whose outstanding secretarial skills and smooth coordination supported the review and final revision of the entire manuscript between editors and authors. Her speed and organization are greatly appreciated.

To Mark Sawyer of Science Imaging Group in Toronto, Canada for excellent photographic assistance, and Jenny Tomash, also in Toronto, for her beautiful illustrations.

To Nick Charboneau, our digital image editor, for his outstanding work in the production of the "Key Image Collages" and other image enhancements.

To Rose Baldwin and Lori Kulas, our secretaries, for their expert and energetic assistance in the preparation of the manuscripts.

To Mia Cariño and Dave Orzechowski at Mosby who have been dedicated and enthusiastic coordinators of the project through development and production.

To Liz Corra at Mosby, an outstanding managing editor, who has guided the project with patient and untiring encouragement.

To Anne Patterson at Mosby who guided this project through its First Edition and has encouraged us to climb this steep mountain of effort again.

CONTENTS

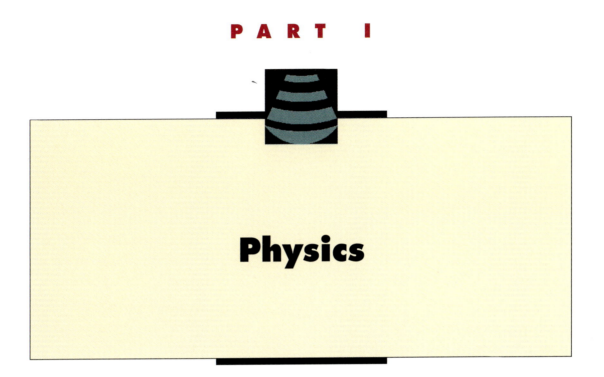

PART I

Physics

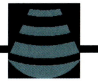

Physics of Ultrasound

•

Christopher R. B. Merritt, M.D.

The bases of all diagnostic ultrasound applications are the detection and display of acoustic energy reflected from interfaces within the body. These interactions provide the information needed to generate high-resolution, two-dimensional, gray-scale images of the body as well as display flow parameters. The unique imaging attributes of ultrasound have made it an important and versatile medical imaging tool.

Unfortunately, the use of expensive, state-of-the-art ultrasound instrumentation does not guarantee the production of high-quality studies of diagnostic value. Gaining maximum benefit from this complex technology requires a combination of skills, including knowledge of the physical principles that empower ultrasound with its unique diagnostic capabilities. The user must understand the fundamentals of the interactions of acoustic energy with tissue and the methods and instruments used to produce and optimize the ultrasound display. With this knowledge the user can collect the maximum information from each examination, avoiding pitfalls and errors in diagnosis that may result from the omission of information or the misinterpretation of artifacts.

Both ultrasound imaging and Doppler ultrasound are based on the scattering of sound energy by interfaces formed of materials of different properties through interactions governed by acoustic physics. The amplitude of reflected energy is used to generate ultrasound images, and frequency shifts in the backscattered ultrasound provide information relating to blood flow. To produce, detect, and process ultrasound data, numerous variables, many under direct user control, must be managed. To do this the user must understand the methods used to generate ultrasound data and the theory and operation of the instruments that detect, display, and store the acoustic information generated in clinical examinations. This chapter will provide an overview of the fundamentals of acoustics, the physics of ultrasound imaging and flow detection, and ultrasound instrumentation with emphasis on points most relevant to clinical practice.

BASIC ACOUSTICS

Wavelength and Frequency

Sound is the result of mechanical energy traveling through matter as a wave producing alternating compression and rarefaction. Pressure waves are propagated by limited physical displacement of the material through which the sound is being transmitted. A plot of these changes in pressure is a sinusoidal waveform (Fig. 1-1) in which the Y axis indicates the pressure at a given point while the X axis indicates time. **Changes in pressure with time define the basic units of measurement for sound.** The distance between corresponding points on the time-pressure curve is defined as the **wavelength,** λ, and the time, T, to complete a single cycle is called the **period.** The number of complete cycles in a unit of time is the **frequency,** f, of the sound. Frequency and period are inversely related. If the period, T, is expressed in seconds, then $f = 1/T$ or $f = T \times \sec^{-1}$. The unit of **acoustic frequency** is the **hertz** (Hz) where 1 Hz = 1 cycle per second. High frequencies are expressed in kilohertz (kHz; 1 kHz = 1000 Hz) or megahertz (MHz; 1 MHz = 1,000,000 Hz).

In nature, acoustic frequencies span a range from less than 1 Hz to more than 100,000 Hz (100 kHz). Human hearing is limited to the lower part of this range, extending from 20 to 20,000 Hz. Ultrasound differs from audible sound only in its frequency, and

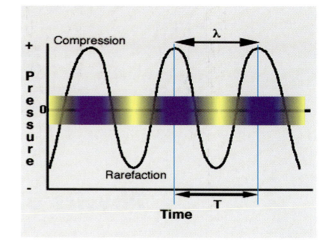

FIG. 1-1. Sound waves. Sound is transmitted as a series of alternating pressure waves producing compression and rarefaction of the conducting medium. The time for a pressure wave to pass a given point is the period, T. The frequency of the wave is l/T. The wavelength, λ, is the distance between corresponding points on the time-pressure curve.

is 500 to 1000 times higher than the sound we normally hear. Sound frequencies used for diagnostic applications typically range from 2 to 15 MHz, although frequencies as high as 50 to 60 MHz are under investigation for certain specialized imaging applications. In general, the frequencies used for ultrasound imaging are higher than those used for Doppler. Regardless of the frequency, the same basic principles of acoustics apply.

Propagation of Sound

Most clinical applications of ultrasound use brief bursts or pulses of energy that are transmitted into the body where they are propagated through tissue. It is possible for acoustic pressure waves to travel in a direction perpendicular to the direction of the particles being displaced (transverse waves), but in tissue and fluids, sound propagation is along the direction of particle movement (longitudinal waves). The speed at which the pressure wave moves through tissue varies greatly and is affected by the physical properties of the tissue. Propagation velocity is largely determined by the resistance of the medium to compression. This, in turn, is influenced by the density of the medium and its stiffness or elasticity. Propagation velocity is increased by increasing stiffness and reduced by increasing density. In the body, propagation velocity may be regarded as constant for a given tissue and is not affected by the frequency or wavelength of the sound. Fig. 1-2 shows **typical propagation velocities** for a variety of materials. In the body the propa-

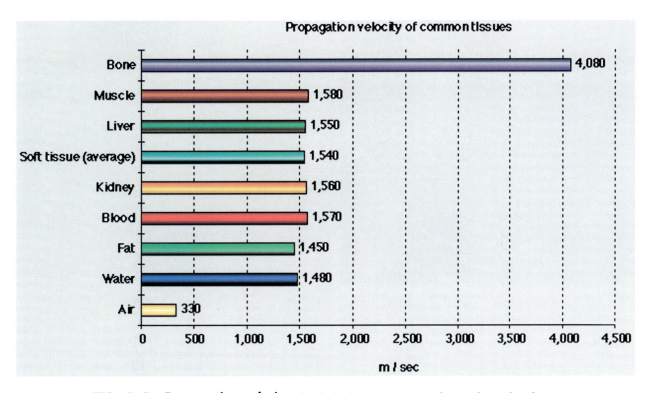

FIG. 1-2. Propagation velocity. In the body, propagation velocity of sound is determined by the physical properties of tissue. As shown, this varies considerably. Medical ultrasound devices base their measurements on an assumed average propagation velocity of 1540 m/sec.

gation velocity of sound is assumed to be 1540 m/sec. This value is the average of measurements obtained from normal tissues.[1,2] Although this is a value representative of most soft tissues, some tissues such as aerated lung and fat have propagation velocities significantly less than 1540 m/sec, and others such as bone have greater velocities. Because a few normal tissues have propagation values significantly different from the average value assumed by the ultrasound scanner, the display of such tissues may be subject to measurement errors or artifacts (Fig. 1-3).

The propagation velocity of sound, c, is related to frequency and wavelength by the following simple equation:

$$c = f\lambda \qquad (1)$$

Thus a frequency of 5 MHz can be shown to have a wavelength of 0.308 mm in tissue:

$$\lambda = c/f = 1540 \text{ m sec}^{-1}/5{,}000{,}000 \text{ sec}^{-1}$$
$$= 0.000308 \text{ m} = 0.308 \text{ mm}$$

Distance Measurement

Propagation velocity is a particularly important value in clinical ultrasound and is critical in deter-

mining the distance of a reflecting interface from the transducer. Much of the information used to generate an ultrasound scan is based on the precise measurement of time. If an ultrasound pulse is transmitted into the body and the time until an echo returns is measured, it is simple to calculate the depth of the interface that generated the echo, provided the propagation velocity of sound for the tissue is known. For example, if the time interval from the transmission of a pulse until the return of an echo is 0.05 ms (0.00005 sec) and the velocity of sound is 1540 m/sec, the distance that the sound has traveled must be 7.7 cm (1540 m/sec × 100 cm/m × 0.00005 sec = 7.7 cm). Since the time measured includes the time for sound to travel to the interface and then return along the same path to the transducer, the distance from the transducer to the reflecting interface is 7.7 cm ÷ z = 3.85 cm (Fig. 1-4). The accuracy of this measurement is therefore highly influenced by how closely the presumed velocity of sound corresponds to the true velocity in the tissue being observed (see Figs. 1-2 and 1-3).

Acoustic Impedance

Current diagnostic ultrasound scanners rely on the detection and display of **reflected sound or**

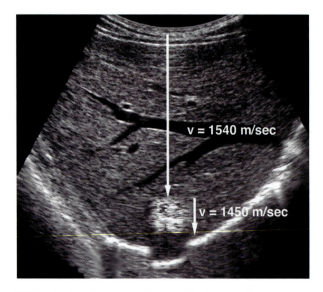

FIG. 1-3. Propagation velocity artifact. When sound passes through a lesion containing fat, echo return is delayed because fat has a propagation velocity of 1450 m/sec, which is less than the liver. Since the ultrasound scanner assumes that sound is being propagated at the average velocity of 1540 m/sec, the delay in echo return is interpreted as indicating a deeper target. Therefore the final image shows a misregistration artifact in which the diaphragm and other structures deep to the fatty lesion are shown in a deeper position than expected (simulated image).

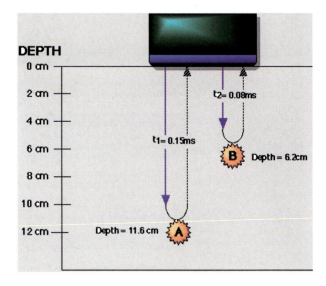

FIG. 1-4. Ultrasound ranging. The information used to position an echo for display is based on the precise measurement of time. Here the time for an echo to travel from the transducer to object A and return to the transducer is 0.15 ms. For object B, this time is 0.08 ms. Multiplying the velocity of sound in tissue by these times shows that the sound returning from object A has traveled 23.2 cm. Object A therefore lies half this distance, or 11.6 cm, from the transducer. Similar calculations indicate that object B lies at a depth of 6.2 cm.

echoes. (Imaging based on transmission of ultrasound is also possible, but is not used clinically at the present time.) To produce an echo, a reflecting interface must be present. Sound passing through a **totally homogeneous medium** encounters no interfaces to reflect sound, and the medium appears anechoic or cystic. At the junction of tissues or materials with different physical properties, **acoustic interfaces** are present. These interfaces are responsible for the reflection of variable amounts of the incident sound energy. Thus when ultrasound passes from one tissue to another or encounters a vessel wall or circulating blood cells, some of the incident sound energy is reflected.

The amount of reflection or backscatter is determined by the difference in the acoustic impedances of the materials forming the interface. **Acoustic impedance,** Z, is determined by product of the density, p, of the medium propagating the sound and the propagation velocity, c, of sound in that medium ($Z = pc$). Interfaces with large acoustic impedance differences, such as interfaces of tissue with air or bone, reflect almost all of the incident energy; interfaces composed of substances with smaller differences in acoustic impedance, such as a muscle and fat interface, reflect only part of the incident energy, permitting the remainder to continue on. Like propagation

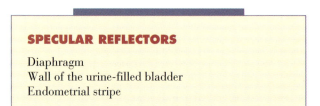

SPECULAR REFLECTORS

Diaphragm
Wall of the urine-filled bladder
Endometrial stripe

velocity, acoustic impedance is determined by the properties of the tissues involved, and is independent of frequency.

Reflection

The way ultrasound is reflected when it strikes an acoustic interface is determined by the size and surface features of the interface (Fig. 1-5). If the interface is large and relatively smooth, it reflects sound much as a mirror reflects light. Such interfaces are called **specular reflectors** because they behave like mirrors for sound. Examples of specular reflectors include the diaphragm, the wall of the urine-filled bladder, and the endometrial stripe. The amount of energy reflected by an acoustic interface can be expressed as a fraction of the incident energy. This is termed the reflection coefficient, R. If a specular reflector is perpendicular to the

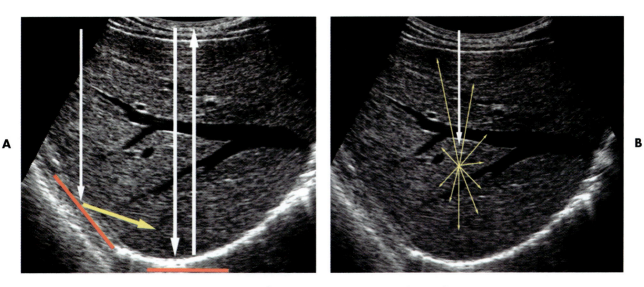

FIG. 1-5. Specular and diffuse reflectors. Specular reflector. A, The diaphragm is a large and relatively smooth surface that reflects sound like a mirror reflects light. Thus, sound striking the diaphragm at nearly a 90-degree angle is reflected directly back to the transducer, resulting in a strong echo. Sound striking the diaphragm obliquely is reflected away from the transducer, and an echo is not displayed *(yellow arrow)*. **Diffuse reflector. B,** In contrast to the diaphragm, the liver parenchyma consists of acoustic interfaces that are small in comparison to the wavelength of sound used for imaging. These interfaces scatter sound in all directions, and only a portion of the energy returns to the transducer to produce the image.

incident sound beam, the amount of energy reflected is determined by the following relationship:

$$R = (Z_2 - Z_1)^2 / (Z_2 + Z_1)^2 \qquad (2)$$

where Z_1 and Z_2 are the acoustic impedances of the media forming the interface.

Since ultrasound scanners detect only those reflections that return to the transducer, the **display of specular interfaces is highly dependent on the angle of insonation.** Specular reflectors will return echoes to the transducer only if the sound beam is perpendicular to the interface. If the interface is not at a 90-degree angle to the sound beam, it will be reflected away from the transducer, and therefore the echo will not be detected (see Fig. 1-5, *A*).

Most echoes in the body do not arise from specular reflectors, but come from much smaller interfaces within solid organs. In this case the acoustic interfaces involve structures with individual dimensions much smaller than the wavelength of the incident sound. The echoes from these interfaces are scattered in all directions. Such reflectors are called **diffuse reflectors** and account for the echoes that form the characteristic echo patterns seen in solid organs and tissues (see Fig. 1-5, *B*). For some diagnostic applications the nature of the reflecting structures creates important conflicts. For example, most vessel walls behave as specular reflectors that require insonation at a 90-

degree angle for best imaging, while Doppler imaging requires an angle of less than 90 degrees between the sound beam and the vessel.

Refraction

Another event that can occur when sound passes from a tissue with one acoustic propagation velocity to a tissue with a higher or lower sound velocity is a change in the direction of the sound wave. This change in direction of propagation is called **refraction** and is governed by Snell's law:

$$\sin\Theta_1/\sin\Theta_2 = c_1/c_2 \qquad (3)$$

where Θ_1 is the angle of incidence of the sound approaching the interface, Θ_2 is the angle of refraction, and c_1 and c_2 are the propagation velocities of sound in the media forming the interface (Fig. 1-6). Refraction is important because it is one of the **causes of misregistration** of a structure in an ultrasound image (Fig. 1-7). When an ultrasound scanner detects an echo, it assumes that the source of the echo is along a fixed line of sight from the transducer. If the sound has been refracted, the echo detected and displayed in the image may, in fact, be coming from a different depth or location than is shown in the display. If this is suspected, **increasing the scan angle so that it is perpendicular to the interface** causes the refraction to minimize the artifact.

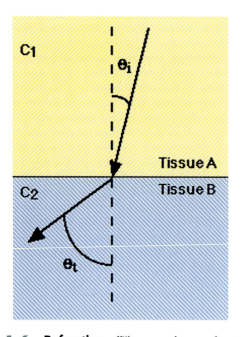

FIG. 1-6. Refraction. When sound passes from tissue A with one acoustic propagation velocity, c_1, to tissue B, which transmits sound at a different velocity, c_2, there is a change in the direction of the sound wave due to refraction. The degree of change is related to the ratio of the propagating velocities of the media forming the interface $(\sin\Theta_i/\sin\Theta_t = c_1/c_2)$.

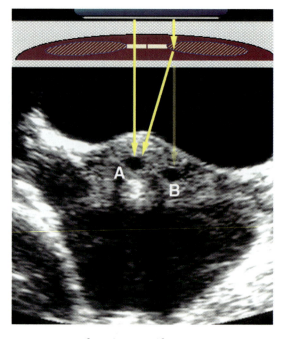

FIG. 1-7. Refraction artifact. Axial transabdominal image of the uterus shows a small gestational sac, A, and what appears to be a second sac, B. In this case the artifact, B, is caused by refraction at the edge of the rectus abdominis muscle. The bending of the path of the sound results in the creation of a duplicate of the image of the sac in an unexpected and misleading location (simulated image).

Attenuation

As the acoustic energy moves through a uniform medium, work is performed and energy is ultimately transferred to the transmitting medium as heat. The capacity to perform work is determined by the quantity of acoustic energy produced. **Acoustic power,** expressed in watts (w) or milliwatts (mW), describes the amount of acoustic energy produced in a unit of time. Although measurement of power provides an indication of the energy as it relates to time, it does not take into account the spatial distribution of the energy. **Intensity** is used to describe the spatial distribution of power. Intensity, I, is calculated by dividing the power by the area over which the power is distributed:

$$I(w/cm^2) = Power(w)/Area(cm^2) \qquad (4)$$

The attenuation of sound energy as it passes through tissue is of great clinical importance because it influences the depth in tissue from which useful information can be obtained. This in turn affects transducer selection and a number of operator-controlled instrument settings, including time (or depth) gain compensation, power output attenuation, and system gain levels.

Attenuation is measured in relative rather than absolute units. The decibel (dB) notation is generally used to compare different levels of ultrasound power or intensity. This value is 10 times the $\log_{10}$ of the ratio of the power or intensity values being compared. For example, if the intensity measured at one point in tissues is 10 mW/cm^2 and at a deeper point is 0.1 mW/cm^2, the difference in intensity is

$$(10)(\log_{10} 0.01/10) = (10)(\log_{10} 0.001) =$$
$$(10)(-\log_{10} 1000) = (10)(-3) = -30 \text{ dB}$$

As sound passes through tissue it loses energy, and the pressure waves decrease in amplitude as they travel further from their source. Contributing to the attenuation of sound are the transfer of energy to tissue, resulting in heating (absorption), and the removal of energy by reflection and scattering. **Attenuation** is therefore the result of the **combined effects of absorption, scattering, and reflection.** Attenuation depends on the insonating frequency as well as the nature of the attenuating medium. High frequencies are attenuated more rapidly than lower frequencies, and transducer frequency is a major determinant of the useful depth from which information can be obtained with ultrasound. Attenuation determines the efficiency with which ultrasound penetrates a specific tissue and varies considerably in normal tissues (Fig. 1-8).

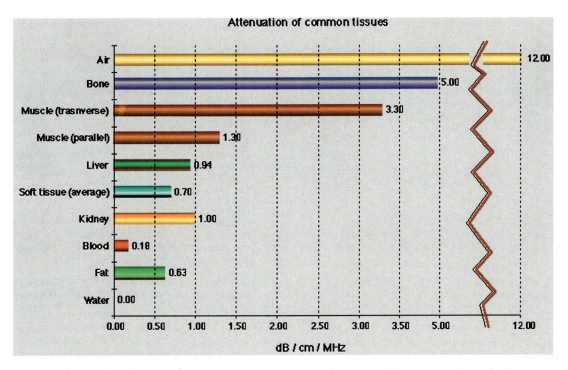

FIG. 1-8. Attenuation. As sound passes through tissue, it loses energy through the transfer of energy to tissue by heating, reflection, and scattering. Attenuation is determined by the insonating frequency and the nature of the attenuating medium. Attenuation values for normal tissues show considerable variation. Attenuation also increases in proportion to an increase in insonating frequency, resulting in less penetration at higher frequencies.

INSTRUMENTATION

Ultrasound scanners are among the most complex and sophisticated imaging devices currently in use. Despite their complexity, all scanners consist of similar basic components to perform key functions—a transmitter or pulser to energize the transducer, the ultrasound transducer itself, a receiver and processor to detect and amplify the backscattered energy and manipulate the reflected signals for display, a display that presents the ultrasound image or data in a form suitable for analysis and interpretation, and, finally, a method to record or store the ultrasound image.

Transmitter

Most clinical applications use pulsed ultrasound in which brief bursts of acoustic energy are transmitted into the body. The ultrasound transducer that is the source of these pulses is energized by application of precisely timed, high-amplitude voltage. The maximum voltage that may be applied to the transducer is limited by federal regulations that restrict the acoustic output of diagnostic scanners. Most scanners provide a control that permits attenuation of the output voltage. Since the use of **maximum output** results in higher exposure of the patient to ultrasound energy,

prudent use dictates use of the output attenuation controls to reduce power levels to the lowest levels consistent with the diagnostic problem.[3]

The transmitter also controls the rate of pulses emitted by the transducer or the **pulse repetition frequency** (PRF). The PRF determines the time interval between ultrasound pulses and is important in determining the depth from which unambiguous data can be obtained both in imaging and Doppler modes. The ultrasound pulses must be spaced with enough time between the pulses to permit the sound to travel to the depth of interest and return before the next pulse is sent. For imaging, PRFs from 1 to 10 kHz are used, resulting in an interval of from 0.1 to 1 ms between pulses. Thus a PRF of 5 kHz permits an echo to travel and return from a depth of 15.4 cm before the next pulse is sent.

Transducers

A transducer is any device that converts one form of energy to another. In the case of ultrasound, the transducer converts electric energy to mechanical energy and vice versa. In diagnostic ultrasound systems, the transducer serves two functions. It **converts the electric energy** provided by the transmitter to the **acoustic pulses** directed into the patient. The transducer also serves as the **receiver of reflected echoes**, converting weak pressure changes into electric signals for processing. Ultrasound transducers use **piezo-electricity,** a principle discovered by Pierre Curie in 1880. Piezoelectric materials have the unique ability to respond to the action of an electric field by changing shape. They also have the property of generating electric potentials when compressed. Changing the polarity of a voltage applied to the transducer changes the thickness of the transducer, which expands and contracts as the polarity changes. This results in the generation of mechanical pressure waves that can be transmitted into the body. The piezoelectric effect also results in the generation of small potentials across the transducer when the transducer is struck by returning echoes. Positive pressures cause a small polarity to develop across the transducer; negative pressure during the rarefaction portion of the acoustic wave produces the opposite polarity across the transducer. These tiny polarity changes and the voltages associated with them are the source of all of the information processed to generate an ultrasound image or Doppler display.

When stimulated by the application of a voltage difference across its thickness, the transducer vibrates. The frequency of vibration is determined by the transducer material. When the transducer is electrically stimulated, a range or band of frequencies results. The preferential frequency produced by a transducer is determined by the propagation speed of the transducer material and its thickness. In the pulsed operating modes used for most clinical ultrasound applications, the ultrasound pulses contain additional frequencies both higher and lower than the preferential frequency. The **range of frequencies** produced by a given transducer is termed its **bandwidth**. Generally the shorter the pulse of ultrasound produced by the transducer, the greater the bandwidth.

The length of an ultrasound pulse is determined by the number of alternating voltage changes applied to the transducer. For **continuous wave (CW) ultrasound devices**, a constant alternating current is applied to the transducer, the alternating polarity producing a continuous ultrasound wave. For imaging, a single, brief voltage change is applied to the transducer, causing it to vibrate at its preferential frequency. Since the transducer continues to vibrate or "ring" for a short time after it is stimulated by the voltage change, the ultrasound pulse will be several cycles long. The number of cycles of sound in each pulse determines the **pulse length**. For imaging, short pulse lengths are desirable, since longer pulses result in poorer axial resolution. To reduce the pulse length to no more than two or three cycles, damping materials are used in the construction of the transducer. In clinical imaging applications, very short pulses are applied to the transducer, and the transducers have highly efficient damping. This results in very short pulses of ultrasound, generally consisting of only two or three cycles of sound.

The ultrasound pulse generated by a transducer must be propagated in tissue to provide clinical information. Special transducer coatings and ultrasound coupling gels are necessary to allow efficient transfer of energy from the transducer to the body. Once in the body, the ultrasound pulses are propagated, reflected, refracted, and absorbed, in accordance with the basic acoustic principles summarized earlier.

The ultrasound pulses produced by the transducer result in a series of wavefronts that form a three-dimensional beam of ultrasound. The features of this beam are influenced by constructive and destructive interference of the pressure waves, the curvature of the transducer, and acoustic lenses used to shape the beam. Interference of pressure waves results in an area near the transducer in which the pressure amplitude varies greatly. This region is termed the **near field** or Fresnel zone. Further from the transducer at a distance determined by the radius of the transducer and the frequency, the sound field begins to diverge and the pressure amplitude decreases at a steady rate with increasing distance from the transducer. This region is called the **far field** or Frauenhofer zone. In modern multielement transducer arrays, precise timing of the firing of elements allows correction of this divergence of the ultrasound beam and **focusing** at selected depths.

Only reflections of pulses that make their way back to the transducer are capable of stimulating the transducer with small pressure changes, which are converted into the voltage changes that are detected, amplified, and processed to build an image based on the echo information.

Receiver

When returning echoes strike the transducer face, minute voltages are produced across the piezoelectric elements. The receiver detects and amplifies these weak signals. The receiver also provides a means for compensating for the differences in echo strength, which result from attenuation by different tissue thickness by control of time depth compensation or **time gain compensation** (TGC).

Sound is attenuated as it passes into the body, and additional energy is removed as echoes return through tissue to the transducer. The attenuation of sound is proportional to the frequency and is constant for specific tissues. Since echoes returning from deeper tissues are weaker than those returning from more superficial structures, they must be amplified more by the receiver to produce a uniform tissue echo appearance. This adjustment is accomplished by TGC controls that permit the user to selectively amplify the signals from deeper structures or suppress the signals from superficial tissues, compensating for tissue attenuation. Although many newer machines provide for some means of automatic TGC, the manual adjustment of this control by the user is one of the most important user controls and may have a profound effect on the quality of the ultrasound image provided for interpretation.

Another important function of the receiver is the compression of the wide range of amplitudes returning to the transducer into a range that can be displayed to the user. The ratio of the highest to the lowest amplitudes that can be displayed may be expressed in decibels and is referred to as the **dynamic range**. In a typical clinical application, the range of reflected signals may vary by a factor of as much as $1:10^{12}$, resulting in a dynamic range of up to 120 dB. Although the amplifiers used in ultrasound machines are capable of handling this range of voltages, grayscale displays are limited to display a signal intensity range of only 35 to 40 dB. **Compression and remapping of the data** are required to adapt the dynamic range of the backscattered signal intensity to the dynamic range of the display (Fig. 1-9). Compression is performed in the receiver by selective amplification of weaker signals. Additional manual postprocessing controls permit the user to selectively map the returning signal to the display. These controls affect the brightness of different echo levels in the image and therefore determine the image contrast.

Image Display

Ultrasound signals may be displayed in several ways.[4] Over the years, imaging has evolved from simple A-mode and bistable display to high-resolution, realtime, gray-scale imaging. The earliest **A-mode devices** displayed the voltage produced across the transducer by the backscattered echo as a vertical deflection on the face of an oscilloscope. The horizontal sweep of the oscilloscope was calibrated to indicate the distance from the transducer to the reflecting surface. In this form of display, the strength or amplitude of the reflected sound is indicated by the height of the vertical deflection displayed on the oscilloscope. With A-mode ultrasound, only the position and strength of a reflecting structure are recorded.

Another simple form of imaging, **M-mode ultrasound**, displays echo amplitude and shows the position of moving reflectors (Fig. 1-10). M-mode imaging uses the brightness of the display to indicate the intensity of the reflected signal. The time base of the display can be adjusted to allow for varying degrees of temporal resolution, as dictated by clinical application. M-mode ultrasound is interpreted by assessing motion patterns of specific reflectors and determining anatomic relationships from characteristic

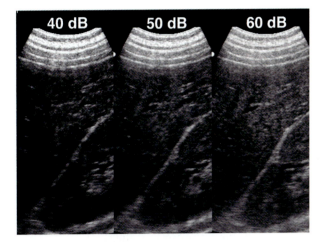

FIG. 1-9. Dynamic range. The ultrasound receiver must compress the wide range of amplitudes returning to the transducer into a range that can be displayed to the user. Here compression and remapping of the data to display dynamic ranges of 40 dB, 50 dB, and 60 dB are shown. The widest dynamic range shown (60 dB) permits the best differentiation of subtle differences in echo intensity and is preferred for most imaging applications. The narrower ranges increase conspicuity of larger echo differences.

patterns of motion. Today the major application of M-mode display is in the evaluation of the rapid motion of cardiac valves and of cardiac chamber and vessel walls. M-mode imaging may play a future role in measurement of subtle changes in vessel wall elasticity accompanying atherogenesis.

The mainstay of imaging with ultrasound is provided by **real-time, gray-scale, B-mode display** in which variations in display intensity or brightness are used to indicate reflected signals of differing amplitude. To generate a two-dimensional (2D) image, multiple ultrasound pulses are sent down a series of successive scan lines (Fig. 1-11), building a 2D representation of echoes arising from the object being scanned. When an ultrasound image is displayed on a black background, signals of greatest intensity appear as white, absence of signal is shown as black, and signals of intermediate intensity appear as shades of gray. If the ultrasound beam is moved with respect to the object being examined and the position of the reflected signal is stored, a 2D image results, with the brightest portions of the display indicating structures reflecting more of the transmitted sound energy back to the transducer.

In most modern instruments a digital memory of 512×512 or 512×640 pixels is used to store values that correspond to the echo intensities originating from corresponding positions in the patient. At least 2^8 or 256 shades of gray are possible for each pixel, in accord with the amplitude of the echo being repre-

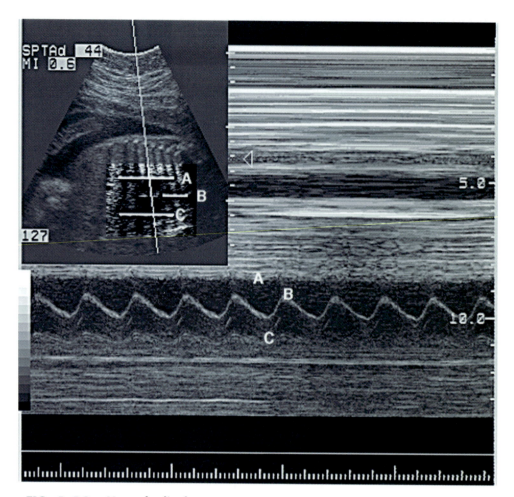

FIG. 1-10. M-mode display. M-mode ultrasound displays changes of echo amplitude and position with time. Display of changes in echo position is useful in the evaluation of rapidly moving structures such as cardiac valves and chamber walls. Here the three major moving structures in an M-mode image of the fetal heart correspond to the near ventricular wall, *A*, the interventricular septum, *B*, and the far ventricular wall, *C*. The baseline is a time scale and permits the calculation of heart rate from the M-mode data.

sented. The image stored in memory in this fashion can then be sent to a video monitor for display. Since B-mode display relates the strength of a backscattered signal to a brightness level on the display device (usually a video display monitor), it is important that the operator understand how the amplitude information in the ultrasound signal is translated into a brightness scale in the image display. Each ultrasound manufacturer offers several options for the way the dynamic range of the target is compressed for display as well as the transfer function that assigns a given signal amplitude to a shade of gray. Although these technical details vary from one machine to another, the way they are used by the operator of the scanner may have a profound impact on the clinical value of the final image. In general, it is desirable to **display as wide a dynamic range as possible** in order to identify subtle differences in tissue echogenicity (see Fig. 1-9).

Real-time ultrasound produces the impression of motion by generating a series of individual 2D images at rates of from 15 to 60 frames per second. Real-time, 2D, B-mode ultrasound is now the major method for ultrasound imaging throughout the body and is the most common form of B-mode display. Real-time ultrasound permits assessment of both anatomy and motion. When images are acquired and displayed at rates of several times per second, the effect is dynamic, and since the image reflects the state and motion of the organ at the time it is examined, the information is regarded as being shown in real time. In cardiac applications, the terms "2D echocardiography" and "2D echo" are used to describe real-time, B-mode imaging: in most other applications, the term "real-time" ultrasound is used.

Transducers used for real-time imaging may be classified by the method used to steer the beam to

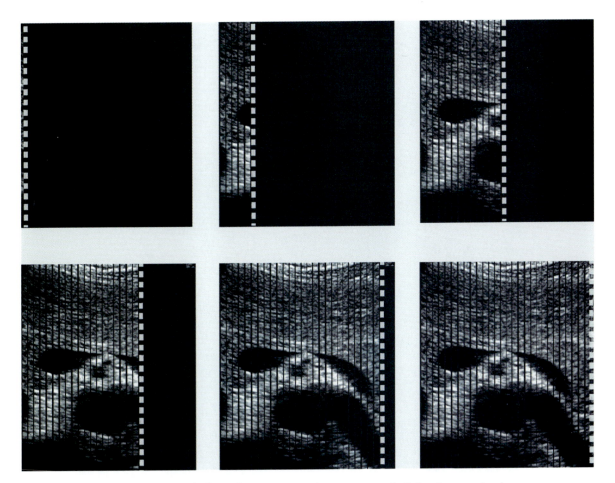

FIG. 1-11. B-mode imaging. A 2D, real-time image is built by ultrasound pulses sent down a series of successive scan lines. Each scan line adds to the image, building a 2D representation of echoes from the object being scanned. In real-time imaging, an entire image is created 15 to 60 times per second.

rapidly generate each individual image, keeping in mind that as many as 30 to 60 complete images must be generated per second for real-time applications. Beam steering may be by **mechanical rotation** or **oscillation** of the transducer, or the beam may be **steered electronically** (Fig. 1-12). Electronic beam steering is used in linear array and phased array transducers and permits a variety of image display formats. Most electronically steered transducers currently in use also provide electronic focusing adjustable for depth. Mechanically steered transducers may use single-element transducers with a fixed focus or may use annular arrays of elements with electronically controlled focusing. For real-time imaging, transducers using mechanical or electronic beam steering generate display in a rectangular or pie-shaped format. For obstetric, small parts, and peripheral vascular examinations, **linear array transducers** with a rectangular image format are often used. The rectangular image display has the advantage of a larger field of view near the surface but requires a large surface area for transducer contact. **Sector scanners** with either mechanical or electronic steering require only a small surface area for contact and are better suited for examinations in which access is limited.

Mechanical Sector Scanners

Early ultrasound scanners used transducers consisting of a single piezoelectric element. To generate real-time images with these transducers, mechanical devices were required to move the transducer in a linear or circular motion. Mechanical sector scanners using one or more single-element transducers do not allow variable focusing. This problem is overcome by using annular array transducers. Although important in the

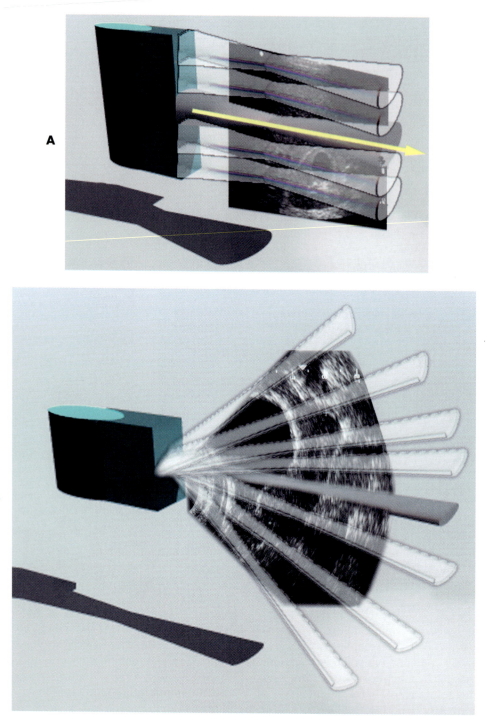

FIG. 1-12. Beam steering. A, Linear array. In a linear array transducer, individual elements or groups of elements are fired in sequence. This generates a series of parallel ultrasound beams, each perpendicular to the transducer face. As these beams move across the transducer face, they generate the lines of sight that combine to form the final image. Depending on the number of transducer elements and the sequence in which they are fired, focusing at selected depths from the surface can be achieved. **B, Phased array.** A phased array transducer produces a sector field of view by firing multiple transducer elements in precise sequence to generate interference of acoustic wavefronts. The ultrasound beam that results generates a series of lines of sight at varying angles from one side of the transducer to the other, producing a sector image format.

early days of real-time imaging, mechanical sector scanners with fixed-focus, single-element transducers are not in common use today.

Arrays

Current technology uses a transducer composed of multiple elements, usually produced by precise slicing of a piece of piezoelectric material into numerous small units, each with its own electrodes. Such transducer arrays may be formed in a variety of configurations. Most commonly these are linear, curved, phased, or annular arrays. By precise timing of the firing of combinations of elements in these arrays, interference of the wavefronts generated by the individual elements can be exploited to change the direction of the ultrasound beam, and this can be used to provide a steerable beam for the generation of real-time images in a linear or sector format.

Linear Arrays. Linear array transducers are commonly used for small parts, vascular, and obstetric applications, since the rectangular image format produced by these transducers is well suited for these applications. In these transducers, individual elements are arranged in a linear fashion. By firing the transducer elements in sequence, either individually or in groups, a series of parallel pulses is generated, each forming a line of sight perpendicular to the transducer face. These individual lines of sight combine to form the image field of view (see Fig. 1-12, *A*). Depending on the number of transducer elements and the sequence in which they are fired, focusing at selected depths from the surface can be achieved.

Curved Arrays. Linear arrays that have been shaped into convex curves produce an image that combines a relatively large surface field of view with a sector display format. Curved array transducers are used for a variety of applications, the larger versions serving for general abdominal, obstetric, and transabdominal pelvic scanning. Small, high-frequency, curved array scanners are often used in transvaginal and transrectal probes and for pediatric imaging.

Phased Arrays. In contrast to mechanical sector scanners, phased array scanners have no moving parts. A sector field of view is produced by multiple transducer elements fired in precise sequence under electronic control. By controlling the time and sequence in which the individual transducer elements are fired, the ultrasound wave that results can be steered in different directions as well as focused at different depths (see Fig. 1-12, *B*). By rapidly steering the beam to generate a series of lines of sight at varying angles from one side of the transducer to the other, a sector image format is produced. This allows the fabrication of transducers of relatively small size but with large fields of view at depth. These transducers are particularly useful for intercostal scanning to evaluate the heart, liver, or spleen, and for examinations in other areas where access is limited.

Annular Arrays. Transducer arrays can be formed by slicing a rectangular piece of transducer material perpendicular to its long axis to produce a number of small rectangular elements or by creating a series of concentric elements nested within one another in a circular piece of piezoelectric material to produce an annular array. The use of multiple concentric elements permits precise focusing. A particular advantage of annular array construction is that the beam can be focused both in elevation and lateral planes, and a uniform and highly focused beam can be produced. Unlike linear arrays, in which delays in the firing of the individual elements may be used to steer the beam, annular arrays do not permit beam steering, and to be used for real-time imaging they must be steered mechanically.

Transducer Selection

Practical considerations in the selection of the optimal transducer for a given application include not only the requirements for spatial resolution but the distance of the target object from the transducer, since penetration of ultrasound diminishes as frequency increases. In general, the **highest ultrasound frequency permitting penetration to the depth of interest should be selected.** For superficial vessels and organs such as the thyroid, breast, or testicle lying within 1 to 3 cm of the surface, imaging frequencies of from 7.5 to 10 MHz are usually used. These high frequencies are also ideal for intraoperative applications. For evaluation of deeper structures in the abdomen or pelvis more than 12 to 15 cm from the surface, frequencies as low as 2.25 to 3.5 MHz may be required. When maximal resolution is needed, a high-frequency transducer with excellent lateral and elevation resolution at the depth of interest is required.

Image Storage

With real-time ultrasound, user feedback is immediate and is provided by video display. The brightness and contrast of the image on this display are determined by the brightness and contrast settings of the video monitor, by the system gain setting, and the TGC adjustment. Probably the single greatest factor affecting image quality in many ultrasound departments is improper adjustment of the video display and lack of appreciation of the relationship of the video display settings to the appearance of hard copy. Because of the importance of the real-time video display in providing feedback to the user, it is essential that the display and lighting conditions under which the display is viewed are standardized and matched to the hard copy device.

Permanent storage of images for review and archiving may be in the form of transparencies printed on film by optical or laser cameras and printers, as well as on videotape. Increasingly, digital storage is being used for archiving of ultrasound images.

IMAGE QUALITY

The key determinants of the quality of an ultrasound image include its spatial, contrast, and temporal resolution, and freedom from certain artifacts.

Spatial Resolution

The ability to differentiate two closely situated objects as distinct structures is determined by the spatial resolution of the ultrasound device. Spatial resolution must be considered in three planes, and there are different determinants of resolution in each of these. Simplest is the resolution along the axis of the ultrasound beam—**axial resolution.** With pulsed wave ultrasound, the transducer introduces a series of brief bursts of sound into the body. Each ultrasound pulse typically consists of two or three cycles of sound. The pulse length is the product of the wavelength and the number of cycles in the pulse. Axial resolution, the maximum resolution along the beam axis, is determined by the pulse length (Fig. 1-13). Since ultrasound frequency and wavelength are inversely related, the pulse length decreases as the imaging frequency increases. Since the pulse length determines the maximum resolution along the axis of the ultrasound beam, higher transducer frequencies provide higher image resolution. For example, a transducer operating at 5 MHz produces sound with a wavelength of 0.308 mm. If each pulse consists of three cycles of sound, the pulse length is slightly less than 1 mm, and this becomes the maximum resolution along the beam axis. If the transducer frequency is increased to 10 MHz, the pulse length is less than 0.5 mm, permitting resolution of smaller details.

In addition to axial resolution, resolution in the planes perpendicular to the beam axis must also be considered. **Lateral resolution** refers to resolution in the plane perpendicular to the beam and parallel to the transducer. **Azimuth or elevation resolution** refers to the slice thickness in the plane perpendicular to the beam and to the transducer (Fig. 1-14). Lateral resolution is determined by the width of the ultrasound beam. Ultrasound is a tomographic method of imaging producing thin slices of information from the body, and the width and thickness of the ultrasound beam are important determinants of image quality. Excessive beam width and thickness limit the ability to delineate small features such as the tiny cystic areas in atheromatous plaque associated with intraplaque

hemorrhage. The width and thickness of the ultrasound beam determine lateral resolution and elevation resolution, respectively. Lateral and elevation resolution are significantly poorer than the axial resolution of the beam. Lateral resolution is controlled by focusing the beam, usually by electronic phasing, to alter the beam width at a selected depth of interest. Elevation resolution is determined by the construction of the transducer and generally cannot be controlled by the user.

IMAGING PITFALLS

In ultrasound, perhaps more than in any other imaging method, the quality of the information obtained is determined by the ability of the operator to recognize and avoid artifacts and pitfalls.[5] Many imaging artifacts are induced by errors in scanning technique or improper use of the instrument and are preventable. Artifacts may suggest the presence of structures that are not present, causing misdiagnosis, or they may cause important findings to be obscured. Because an understanding of artifacts is essential for correct interpretation of ultrasound examinations, several of the most important artifacts deserve discussion.

Many artifacts suggest the presence of structures not actually present. These include reverberation, refraction, and side lobes. **Reverberation artifacts** arise when the ultrasound signal reflects repeatedly between highly reflective interfaces that are usually but not always near the transducer (Fig. 1-15). Reverberations may also give the false impression of solid structures in areas where only fluid is present. Certain types of reverberation may be helpful because they allow the identification of a specific type of reflector, such as a surgical clip. Reverberation artifacts can usually be reduced or eliminated by changing the scanning angle or transducer placement to avoid the parallel interfaces that contribute to the artifact.

Refraction causes bending of the sound beam so that targets not along the axis of the transducer are insonated. Their reflections are then detected and displayed in the image. This may cause structures that actually lie outside the volume the investigator assumes is being examined to appear in the image (see Fig. 1-7). Similarly, **side lobes** may produce confusing echoes that arise from sound beams that lie outside the main ultrasound beam (Fig. 1-16). These artifacts are of clinical importance because they may create the impression of structures or debris in fluid-filled structures (Fig. 1-17). Side lobes may also result in errors of measurement by reducing lateral resolution. As with most other artifacts, repositioning the transducer and its focal zone or using a different transducer will usually allow the differentiation of

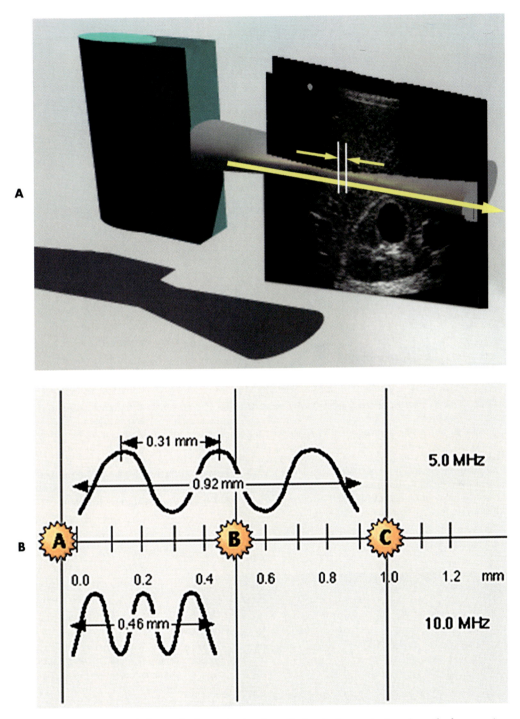

FIG. 1-13. Axial resolution. A, Axial resolution is the resolution along the beam axis and, **B,** is determined by the pulse length. The pulse length is the product of the wavelength (which decreases with increasing frequency) and the number of waves (usually two to three). Since the pulse length determines axial resolution, higher transducer frequencies provide higher image resolution. For example, a transducer operating at 5 MHz produces sound with a wavelength of 0.31 mm. If each pulse consists of three cycles of sound, the pulse length is slightly less than 1 mm, and objects *A* and *B,* which are 0.5 mm apart, cannot be resolved as separate structures. If the transducer frequency is increased to 10 MHz, the pulse length is less than 0.46 mm, permitting *A* and *B* to be identified as separate structures.

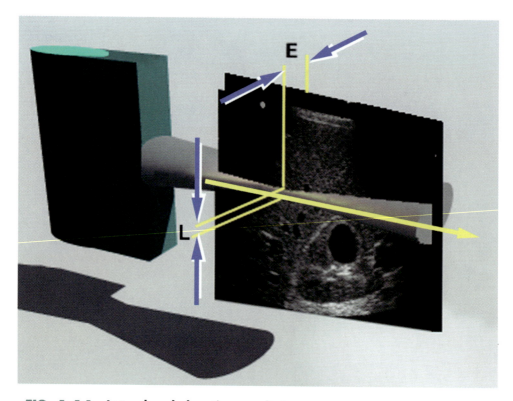

FIG. 1-14. Lateral and elevation resolution. Resolution in the planes perpendicular to the beam axis is an important determinant of image quality. Lateral resolution, *L*, is resolution in the plane perpendicular to the beam and parallel to the transducer, and is determined by the width of the ultrasound beam. Lateral resolution is controlled by focusing the beam, usually by electronic phasing to alter the beam width at a selected depth of interest. Azimuth or elevation resolution, *E*, is determined by the slice thickness in the plane perpendicular to the beam and the transducer and is determined by the height of the beam. Elevation resolution is controlled by the construction of the transducer. Both lateral and elevation resolution are less than the axial resolution.

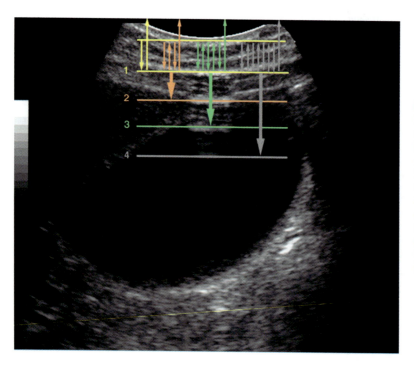

FIG. 1-15. Reverberation artifact. Reverberation artifacts arise when the ultrasound signal reflects repeatedly between highly reflective interfaces near the transducer, resulting in delayed echo return to the transducer. This appears in the image as a series of regularly spaced echoes at increasing depth. The echo at depth 1 is produced by simple reflection from a strong interface. Echoes at levels 2 through 4 are produced by multiple reflections between this interface and the surface (simulated image).

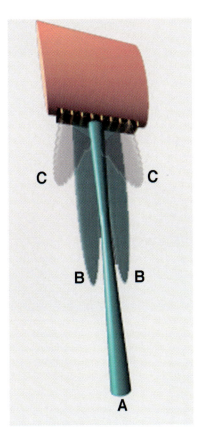

FIG. 1-16. **Side lobes.** Although most of the energy generated by a transducer is emitted in a beam along the central axis of the transducer, *A*, some energy is also emitted from the sides of the primary beam, *B* and *C*. These are called side lobes and are lower in intensity than the primary beam. Side lobes may interact with strong reflectors that lie outside of the scan plane and produce artifacts that are displayed in the ultrasound image (see also Fig. 1-17).

artifactual from true echoes. Artifacts may also remove real echoes from the display or obscure information, and important pathology may be missed. **Shadowing** results when there is a marked reduction in the intensity of ultrasound deep to a strong reflector or attenuator. Shadowing causes partial or complete loss of information due to attenuation of the sound by superficial structures. Another common cause of loss of image information is improper adjustment of system gain and TGC settings. Many low-level echoes are near the noise levels of the equipment, and considerable skill and experience are needed to adjust instrument settings to display the maximum information with the minimum noise. **Poor scanning angles, inadequate penetration,** and **poor resolution** may also result in loss of significant information. Careless selection of transducer frequency and lack of attention to the focal characteristics of the beam will cause loss of clinically important information from deep, low-amplitude reflectors and small targets. Finally, ultrasound artifacts may alter the size, shape, and position of structures. For example, a **multipath artifact** is created when the path of the returning echo is not the one expected, resulting in display of the echo at an improper location in the image (Fig. 1-18).[6]

DOPPLER SONOGRAPHY

Conventional B-mode ultrasound imaging uses pulse-echo transmission, detection, and display techniques. Brief pulses of ultrasound energy emitted by the transducer are reflected from acoustic interfaces within the

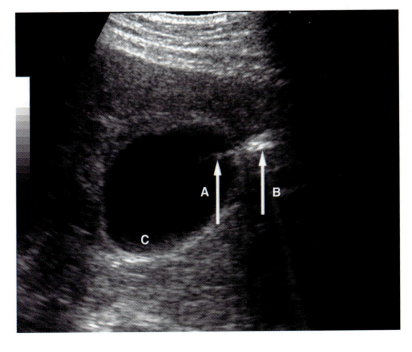

FIG. 1-17. **Side lobe artifact.** Transverse image of the gallbladder reveals a bright internal echo, *A*, that suggests a band or septum within the gallbladder. This is a side lobe artifact related to the presence of a strong out-of-plane reflector, *B*, medial to the gallbladder. The low-level echoes in the dependent portion of the gallbladder, *C*, are also artifactual and are caused by the same phenomenon. Side lobe and slice thickness artifacts are of clinical importance because they may create the impression of debris in fluid-filled structures. As with most other artifacts, repositioning the transducer and its focal zone or using a different transducer will usually allow the differentiation of artifactual from true echoes.

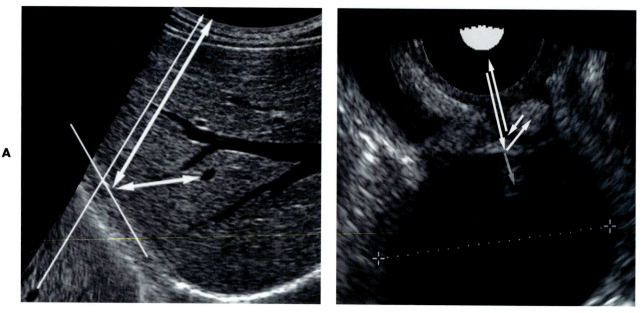

A
B

FIG. 1-18. Multipath artifact. Echoes reflected from the **diaphragm, A,** and the wall of an **ovarian cyst, B,** create complex echo paths that delay return of echoes to the transducer. This results in the display of these echoes at a greater depth than they should normally appear. In **A,** this results in an artifactual image of the liver appearing above the diaphragm (simulated image). In **B,** the effect is more subtle and more likely to cause misdiagnosis, as the artifact suggests a mural nodule in what is actually a simple ovarian cyst.

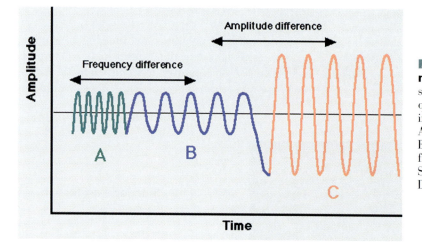

FIG. 1-19. Backscattered information. The backscattered ultrasound signal contains amplitude, phase, and frequency information. Signals *B* and *C* differ in amplitude but have the same frequency. Amplitude differences are used to generate B-mode images. Signals *A* and *B* differ in frequency but have similar amplitudes. Such frequency differences are the basis of Doppler ultrasound.

body. Precise timing allows determination of the depth from which the echo originates. When pulsed wave ultrasound is reflected from an interface, the backscattered (reflected) signal contains amplitude, phase, and frequency information (Fig. 1-19). This information permits inference of the position, nature, and motion of the interface reflecting the pulse. B-mode ultrasound imaging uses only the amplitude information in the backscattered signal to generate the image, with differences in the strength of reflectors

displayed in the image in varying shades of gray. Rapidly moving targets, such as red cells within the blood stream, produce echoes of low amplitude that are not commonly displayed, resulting in a relatively anechoic pattern within the lumens of large vessels.

Although gray-scale display relies on the amplitude of the backscattered ultrasound signal, additional information is present in the returning echoes, which can be used to evaluate the motion of moving targets. When high-frequency sound impinges on a stationary

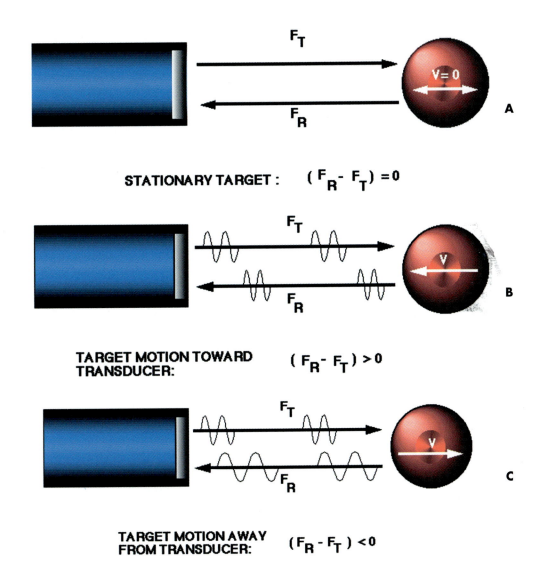

STATIONARY TARGET : $(F_R - F_T) = 0$

TARGET MOTION TOWARD
TRANSDUCER: $(F_R - F_T) > 0$

TARGET MOTION AWAY
FROM TRANSDUCER: $(F_R - F_T) < 0$

FIG. 1-20. Doppler effect. A, Stationary target. If the reflecting interface is stationary, the backscattered ultrasound has the same frequency or wavelength as the transmitted sound, and there is no difference in the transmitted, F_T, and reflected, F_R, frequencies. **B and C, Moving targets.** If the reflecting interface is moving with respect to the sound beam emitted from the transducer, there is a change in the frequency of the sound scattered by the moving object. When the interface moves toward the transducer, B, the difference in reflected and transmitted frequencies is greater than zero. When the target is moving away from the transducer, C, this difference is less than zero. The Doppler equation is used to relate this change in frequency to the velocity of the moving object. (Adapted from Merritt CRB. Doppler US: the basics. *RadioGraphics* 1991;11:109-119.)

interface, the reflected ultrasound has essentially the same frequency or wavelength as the transmitted sound (Fig. 1-20, A). If, however, the reflecting interface is moving with respect to the sound beam emitted from the transducer, there is a change in the frequency of the sound scattered by the moving object (Fig. 1-20, B and C). This change in frequency is directly proportional to the velocity of the reflecting interface relative to the transducer, and is a result of the Doppler effect. The relationship of the returning ul-

trasound frequency to the velocity of the reflector is described by the Doppler equation:

$$\Delta F = (F_R - F_T) = 2F_T \, v/c \qquad (5)$$

The Doppler frequency shift is ΔF; F_R is the frequency of sound reflected from the moving target; F_T is the frequency of sound emitted from the transducer; v is the velocity of the target toward the transducer; and c is the velocity of sound in the medium. The Doppler frequency shift ΔF, as described above, applies only if

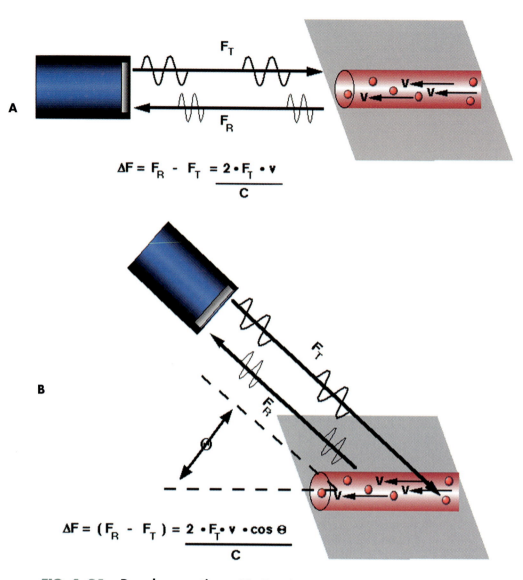

FIG. 1-21. **Doppler equations.** The Doppler equation describes the relationship of the Doppler frequency shift to target velocity. **A,** In its simplest form, it is assumed that the direction of the ultrasound beam is parallel to the direction of movement of the target. This situation is unusual in clinical practice. More often the ultrasound impinges on the vessel at an angle, Θ. **B,** In this case the Doppler frequency shift detected is reduced in proportion to the cosine of Θ. (Adapted from Merritt CRB. Doppler US: the basics. *RadioGraphics* 1991;11:109-119.)

the target is moving directly toward or away from the transducer as is shown in Fig. 1-21, *A*. In most clinical settings, the direction of the ultrasound beam is seldom directly toward or away from the direction of flow, and the ultrasound beam usually approaches the moving target at an angle designated as the Doppler angle (Fig. 1-21, *B*). In this case the frequency shift ΔF is reduced in proportion to the cosine of this angle. Therefore

$$\Delta F = (F_R - F_T) = (2F_T \, v/c)\cos\Theta \qquad (6)$$

where Θ is the angle between the axis of flow and the incident ultrasound beam. If the Doppler angle can be

measured, estimation of flow velocity is possible. Accurate estimation of target velocity requires precise measurement of both the Doppler frequency shift and the angle of insonation to the direction of target movement. As the Doppler angle, Θ, approaches 90 degrees the cosine of Θ approaches 0. **At an angle of 90 degrees** there is no relative movement of the target toward or away from the transducer, and **no Doppler frequency shift is detected** (Fig. 1-22). Since the cosine of the Doppler angle changes rapidly for angles more than 60 degrees, accurate angle correction requires that Doppler measurements be made at angles of less than 60 degrees. Above 60 degrees, relatively

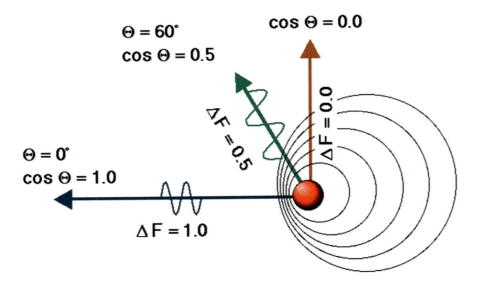

FIG. 1-22. The effect of the Doppler angle on the frequency shift detected by the transducer is illustrated. At an angle of 60 degrees, the detected frequency shift is only 50% of the shift detected at an angle of 0 degrees. At 90 degrees, there is no relative movement of the target toward or away from the transducer, and no frequency shift is detected. The detected Doppler frequency shift is reduced in proportion to the cosine of the Doppler angle. Because the cosine of the angle changes rapidly at angles above 60 degrees, the use of Doppler angles of less than 60 degrees is recommended in making velocity estimates. (Adapted from Merritt CRB. Doppler US: the basics. *RadioGraphics* 1991;11:109-119.)

small changes in the Doppler angle are associated with large changes in cosΘ, and therefore a small error in estimation of the Doppler angle may result in a large error in the estimation of velocity. These considerations are important in using both duplex and color flow instruments, as optimal imaging of the vessel wall is obtained when the axis of the transducer is perpendicular to the wall whereas maximal Doppler frequency differences are obtained when the transducer axis and the direction of flow are at a relatively small angle. In peripheral vascular applications it is highly desirable that Doppler frequencies measured be corrected for the Doppler angle to provide velocity measurement. This allows data from systems using different Doppler frequencies to be compared and eliminates error in interpretation of frequency data obtained at different Doppler angles. For abdominal applications, **angle-corrected velocity measurements** are encouraged, although qualitative assessments of flow are often made using only the Doppler frequency shift data.

The interrelation of transducer frequency, F_T, and the Doppler angle, Θ, to the Doppler frequency shift and target velocity described by the Doppler equation are important in proper clinical use of Doppler equipment.

Doppler Signal Processing and Display

Several options exist for the processing of ΔF, the Doppler frequency shift, to provide useful information regarding the direction and velocity of blood. Doppler frequency shifts encountered clinically fall in the audible range. This audible signal may be analyzed by ear and, with training, the operator can identify many flow characteristics. More commonly, the Doppler shift data are displayed in graphic form as a time-varying plot of the frequency spectrum of the returning signal. A fast Fourier transformation is used to perform the frequency analysis. The resulting Doppler frequency spectrum displays the variation with time of the Doppler frequencies present in the volume sampled, the envelope of the spectrum representing the maximum frequencies present at any given point in time, and the width of the spectrum at any point indicating the range of frequencies present (Fig. 1-23, *A*). In many instruments the amplitude of each frequency component is displayed in gray scale. The presence of a large number of different frequencies at a given point in the cardiac cycle results in so-called **spectral broadening.**

In color flow Doppler imaging systems, velocity information determined from Doppler measurements is displayed as a feature of the image itself (Fig. 1-23, *B*).

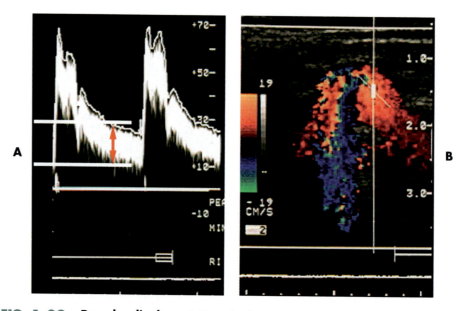

FIG. 1-23. **Doppler display.** **A, Doppler frequency spectrum** shows changes in flow velocity and direction by vertical deflections of the waveform above and below the baseline. The width of the spectral waveform (spectral broadening) is determined by the range of frequencies present at any instant in time *(red arrow)*. A brightness (gray) scale is used to indicate the amplitude of each frequency component. **B, Color flow Doppler imaging.** Amplitude data from stationary targets provide the basis for the B-mode image. Signal phase provides information about the presence and direction of motion, and changes in frequency relate to the velocity of the target. Backscattered signals from red blood cells are displayed in color as a function of their motion toward or away from the transducer, and the degree of the saturation of the color is used to indicate the frequency shift from moving red cells.

In addition to the detection of Doppler frequency shift data from each pixel in the image, these systems may also provide range-gated pulsed wave Doppler with spectral analysis for display of Doppler data.

Doppler Instrumentation

In contrast to A-mode, M-mode, and B-mode grayscale ultrasonography, which display the information from tissue interfaces, Doppler ultrasound instruments are optimized to display flow information. The simplest Doppler devices use continuous wave rather than pulsed wave ultrasound, using two transducers that transmit and receive ultrasound continuously (**continuous wave or CW Doppler**). The transmit and receive beams overlap in a sensitive volume at some distance from the transducer face (Fig. 1-24, *A*). Although direction of flow can be determined with CW Doppler, these devices do not allow discrimination of motion coming from various depths, and the source of the signal being detected is difficult if not impossible to ascertain with certainty. Inexpensive and portable, CW Doppler instruments are used primarily at the bedside or intraoperatively to confirm the presence of flow in superficial vessels.

Because of the limitations of CW systems, most applications use range-gated, pulsed wave Doppler. Rather than a continuous wave of ultrasound emission, pulsed wave Doppler devices emit brief pulses of ultrasound energy (Fig. 1-24, *B*). Using pulses of sound permits use of the time interval between the transmission of a pulse and the return of the echo as a means of determining the depth from which the Doppler shift arises. In a pulsed wave Doppler system, the sensitive volume from which flow data are sampled can be controlled in terms of shape, depth, and position. When combined with a 2D, real-time, B-mode imager in the form of a duplex scanner, the position of the Doppler sample can be precisely controlled and monitored.

The most common form of Doppler ultrasound to be used for radiology applications is **color flow Doppler imaging** (Fig. 1-25, *A*).[7] In color flow imaging systems, flow information determined from Doppler measurements is displayed as a feature of the image itself. Stationary or slowly moving targets provide the basis for the B-mode image. Signal phase provides information about the presence and direction of motion, and changes in echo signal frequency relate to

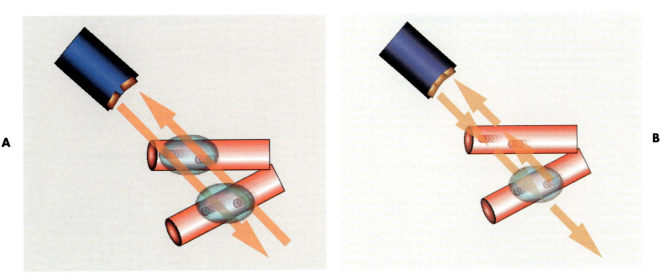

FIG. 1-24. Continuous wave Doppler and pulsed wave doppler. A, Continuous wave Doppler uses separate transmit and receive crystals that continuously transmit and receive ultrasound. Although able to detect the presence and direction of flow, continuous wave devices are unable to distinguish signals arising from vessels at different depths *(shaded areas)*. **B, Pulsed wave Doppler** permits the sampling of flow data from selected depths by processing only the signals that return to the transducer after precisely timed intervals *(shaded area in the deeper vessel)*. The operator is able to control the position of the sample volume and, in duplex systems, to view the location from which the Doppler data are obtained.

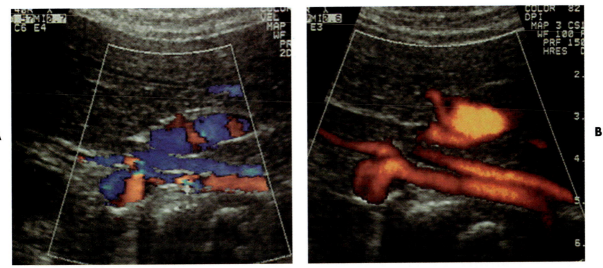

FIG. 1-25. Color flow and power mode Doppler. A, Color flow Doppler **imaging** uses a color map to display information based on the detection of frequency shifts from moving targets. Noise in this form of display appears across the entire frequency spectrum and limits sensitivity. **B, Power mode Doppler** uses a color map to show the distribution of the power or amplitude of the Doppler signal. Flow direction and velocity information are not provided in power mode Doppler display, but noise is reduced, allowing higher gain settings and improved sensitivity for flow detection.

the velocity of the target. Backscattered signals from red blood cells are displayed in color as a function of their motion toward or away from the transducer, and the degree of the saturation of the color is used to indicate the relative velocity of the moving red cells. Color flow Doppler imaging expands conventional duplex sonography by providing additional capabilities. The use of color saturation to display variations in Doppler shift frequency allows a **semiquantitative estimate of flow** to be made from the image alone, provided that variations in the Doppler angle are noted. The display of flow throughout the image field allows the position and orientation of the vessel of interest to be observed at all times. The display of spatial information with respect to velocity is ideal for display of small, localized areas of turbulence within a vessel, which provide clues to stenosis or irregularity of the vessel wall caused by atheroma, trauma, or other disease. Flow within the vessel is observed at all points, and **stenotic jets and focal areas of turbulence** are displayed that might be overlooked with duplex instrumentation. The contrast of flow within the vessel lumen (1) permits visualization of small vessels that are invisible when using conventional imagers and (2) enhances the visibility of wall irregularity Color flow Doppler imaging aids in precise determination of the direction of flow and measurement of the Doppler angle. Limitations of color flow Doppler imaging include angle dependence, aliasing, inability to display the entire Doppler spectrum in the image, and artifacts caused by noise.

Power Mode Doppler

An alternative to the display of frequency information with color flow Doppler imaging is to use a color map that displays the integrated power of the Doppler signal instead of its mean frequency shift (Fig. 1-25, B).[8] Since frequency shift data are not displayed, there is no aliasing. The image does not provide any information related to flow direction or velocity, and power mode Doppler imaging is much less angle dependent than frequency-based color flow Doppler display. In contrast to color flow Doppler, where noise may appear in the image as any color, power mode

Doppler permits noise to be assigned to a homogeneous background color that does not greatly interfere with the image. This results in a significant increase in the usable dynamic range of the scanner, permitting higher effective gain settings for flow detection and increased sensitivity for flow detection (Fig. 1-26).

Interpretation of the Doppler Signal

Doppler data components that must be evaluated both in spectral display and in color flow imaging include the Doppler shift frequency and amplitude, the Doppler angle, the spatial distribution of frequencies across the vessel, and the temporal variation of the signal. Because the Doppler signal itself has no anatomic significance, the examiner must interpret the Doppler signal and then determine its relevance in the context of the image.

The detection of a Doppler frequency shift indicates movement of the target, which in most applications is related to the presence of flow. The sign of the frequency shift (positive or negative) indicates the direction of flow relative to the transducer. **Vessel stenosis** is typically associated with large Doppler frequency shifts in both systole and diastole at the site of greatest narrowing, with turbulent flow in post-stenotic regions. In peripheral vessels, analysis of the Doppler changes allows accurate prediction of the degree of vessel narrowing. In addition, information related to the resistance to flow in the distal vascular tree can be obtained by analysis of changes of blood velocity with time shown in the Doppler spectral display. Fig. 1-27 provides a graphic example of the changes in the Doppler spectral waveform resulting from physiologic changes in the resistance of the vascular bed supplied by a **normal brachial artery**. In Fig. 1-27, A, a blood pressure cuff has been inflated to above systolic pressure to occlude the distal branches supplied by the brachial artery. This causes reduced systolic amplitude and cessation of diastolic flow, resulting in a waveform different than is found in the normal resting state. Fig. 1-27, B, shows the waveform in the brachial artery immediately after release of 3 minutes of occluding pressure. During the **period of ischemia** induced by pressure cuff occlu-

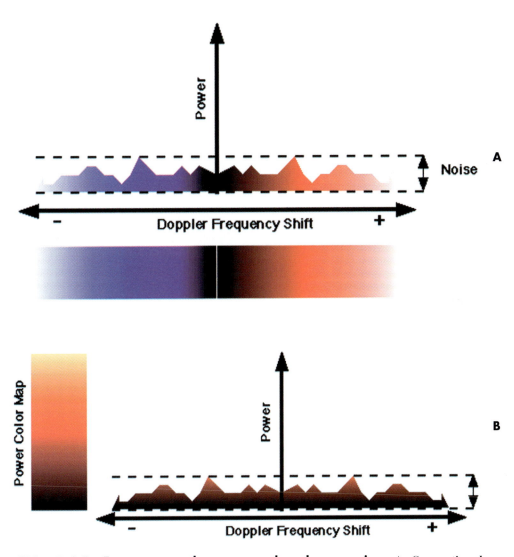

FIG. 1-26. Frequency and power mode color mapping. A, Conventional color flow Doppler uses the color map to show differences in flow direction and Doppler frequency shift. Since noise appears over the entire frequency spectrum, gain levels are limited to those that do not introduce excessive noise. **B, Power mode Doppler color map,** in contrast, indicates the amplitude of the Doppler signal. Since most noise is of low amplitude, it is possible to map this to colors near the background. This permits the use of high gain settings that offer significant improvements over conventional color flow Doppler in flow detection.

sion of the forearm vessels, vasodilitation has occurred. The Doppler waveform now reflects a low-resistance peripheral vascular bed with increased systolic amplitude and rapid flow throughout diastole. Doppler indices such as the systolic/diastolic ratio, resistive index, and pulsatility index, which compare the flow in systole and diastole, provide an indication of the resistance in the peripheral vascular bed and are used to aid in evaluation of perfusion of renal transplants, the placenta, and uterus. With Doppler ultrasound it is therefore possible to identify vessels, determine the direction of blood flow, evaluate narrowing or occlusion, and characterize flow to organs

and tumors. Analysis of the Doppler shift frequency with time can be used to infer both proximal stenosis and changes in distal vascular impedance. Most work using pulsed wave Doppler imaging has emphasized the detection of stenosis, thrombosis, and flow disturbances in major peripheral arteries and veins. In these applications, measurements of peak systolic and end diastolic frequency or velocity, analysis of the Doppler spectrum, and calculation of certain frequency or velocity ratios have been the basis of analysis. Changes in the spectral waveform measured by indices comparing flow in systole and diastole provide insight into the resistance of the vascular bed

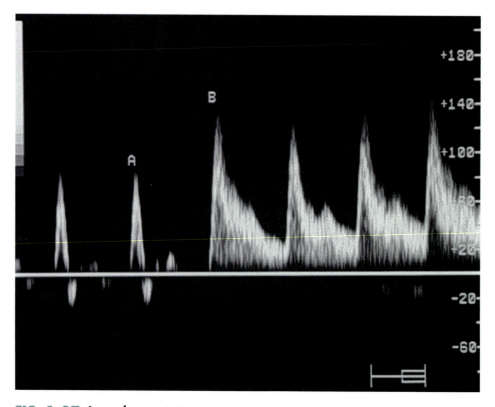

FIG. 1-27. Impedance. *A*, **High-resistance waveform in the brachial artery** produced by inflating blood pressure cuff applied to the forearm to a pressure above the systolic blood pressure. As a result of high peripheral resistance, there is low systolic amplitude and reversed diastolic flow. *B*, **Low resistance** in the peripheral vascular bed due to vasodilatation stimulated by the prior ischemia. Immediately after release of 3 minutes of occluding pressure, the Doppler waveform shows increased amplitude and rapid antegrade flow throughout diastole.

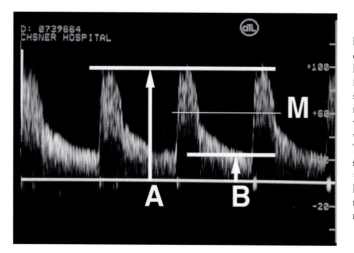

FIG. 1-28. **Doppler indices.** Doppler imaging is capable of providing information about flow in both large and small vessels. Small vessel impedance is reflected in the Doppler spectral waveform of afferent vessels. Doppler flow indices used to characterize peripheral resistance are based on the **peak systolic frequency or velocity**, *A*, the minimum or **end diastolic frequency** or velocity, *B*, and the **mean frequency or velocity**, *M*. The most commonly used indices are: the **systolic/diastolic ratio** (S/D ratio = A/B); the **resistive index** [RI = (A−B)/A]; and the **pulsatility index** [PI = (A−B)/M]. In calculation of the pulsatility index, the minimum diastolic velocity or frequency is used; calculation of the S/D ratio and resistive index use the end diastolic value.

supplied by the vessel and indicate changes resulting from a variety of pathologies (Fig. 1-28). Changes of these indices from normal may be important in the early identification of rejection of transplanted organs, parenchymal dysfunction, and malignancy. Although these indices are useful, it is important to keep in mind that these measurements are influenced not only by the resistance to flow in peripheral vessels but by many other factors, including heart rate, blood pressure, vessel wall length and elasticity, and extrinsic organ compression. Interpretation must therefore always take into account all of these variables.

MAJOR SOURCES OF DOPPLER IMAGING ARTIFACTS

Doppler frequency
Higher frequencies lead to more tissue attenuation

Wall filters
Remove signals from low-velocity blood flow

Spectral broadening
Excessive system gain or changes in dynamic range of the gray-scale display can increase it
Excessively large sample volume increases it
Sample volume too near the vessel wall increases it

Aliasing
Decreased PRF increases aliasing
Decreasing the Doppler angle will increase aliasing
Higher Doppler frequency transducer will increase aliasing

Doppler angle
Relatively inaccurate above 60 degrees

Sample volume size
Increases vessel wall noise if large sample volumes

Although the more graphic presentation of color flow Doppler imaging suggests that interpretation is made easier, the complexity of the color flow Doppler image actually makes this a more demanding image to evaluate than the simple Doppler spectrum. Nevertheless, color flow Doppler imaging has important advantages over pulsed wave duplex Doppler imaging in which flow data are obtained only from a small portion of the area being imaged. To be confident that a conventional Doppler study has achieved reasonable sensitivity and specificity in detection of flow disturbances, a methodical search and sampling of multiple sites within the field of interest must be performed. Color flow Doppler imaging devices permit simultaneous sampling of multiple sites and are less susceptible to this error.

Other Technical Considerations

Although many of the problems and artifacts associated with B-mode imaging, such as shadowing, are encountered with Doppler ultrasonography, the detection and display of frequency information related to moving targets add a group of special technical considerations that are not encountered with other forms of ultrasonography. An understanding of the source of these artifacts and their influence on the interpretation of the flow measurements obtained in clinical

practice is important. Major sources of Doppler artifacts include the following.

Doppler Frequency. A primary objective of the Doppler examination is the accurate measurement of characteristics of flow within a vascular structure. The moving red blood cells that serve as the primary source of the Doppler signal act as point scatterers of ultrasound rather than specular reflectors. This interaction results in the intensity of the scattered sound varying in proportion to the fourth power of the frequency. This has an important implication with respect to the selection of the Doppler frequency to be used for a given examination. As the transducer frequency increases, Doppler sensitivity improves, but attenuation by tissue also increases, resulting in diminished penetration. Careful balancing of the requirements for sensitivity and penetration is an important responsibility of the operator during a Doppler examination. Because many abdominal vessels lie several centimeters beneath the surface, Doppler frequencies in the range of 3 to 3.5 MHz are usually required to permit adequate penetration.

Wall Filters. Doppler instruments detect motion not only from blood flow but also from adjacent structures. To eliminate these low-frequency signals from the display, most instruments use high pass filters or "wall" filters, which remove signals that fall below a given frequency limit. Although effective in **eliminating low-frequency noise**, these filters may also **remove signals from low-velocity blood flow** (Fig. 1-29). In certain clinical situations, the measurement of these slower flow velocities is of clinical importance, and the improper selection of the wall filter may result in serious errors of interpretation. For example, low-velocity venous flow may not be detected if an improper filter is used, and low-velocity diastolic flow in certain arteries may also be eliminated from the display, resulting in errors in the calculation of Doppler indices such as the systolic-diastolic ratio or resistive index. In general, the filter should be kept at the lowest practical level, usually in the range of 50 to 100 Hz.

Spectral broadening refers to the presence of a large range of flow velocities at a given point in the pulse cycle and is an important criterion of high-grade vessel narrowing. Excessive system gain or changes in the dynamic range of the gray-scale display of the Doppler spectrum may suggest spectral broadening; opposite settings may mask broadening of the Doppler spectrum, causing diagnostic inaccuracy. Spectral broadening may also be produced by the selection of an excessively large sample volume or by the placement of the sample volume too near the vessel wall where slower velocities are present (Fig. 1-30).

Aliasing. Aliasing is an artifact arising from ambiguity in the measurement of high Doppler frequency shifts. To ensure that samples originate only from a se-

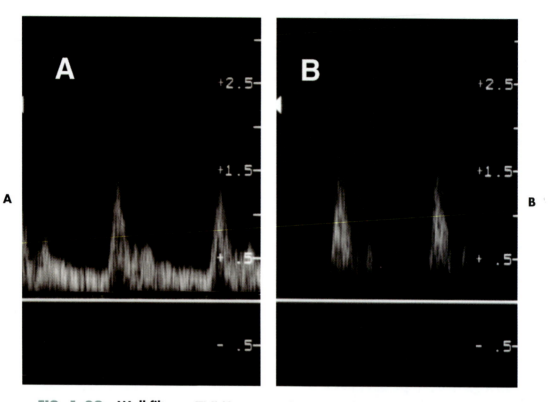

FIG. 1-29. Wall filters. Wall filters are used to eliminate low frequency noise from the Doppler display. Here the effect on the display of low velocity flow is shown with wall filter settings of **A,** 100 Hz, and **B,** 400 Hz. High wall filter settings remove signal from low velocity blood flow and may result in interpretation errors. In general, wall filters should be kept at the lowest practical level, usually in the range of 50 to 100 Hz.

lected depth when using a pulsed wave Doppler system, it is necessary to wait for the echo from the area of interest before transmitting the next pulse. This limits the rate with which pulses can be generated, a lower PRF being required for greater depth. The PRF also determines the maximum depth from which unambiguous data can be obtained. If the PRF is less than twice the maximum frequency shift produced by movement of the target (the Nyquist limit), aliasing results. Fig. 1-31 illustrates the origin of aliasing. When the PRF is less than twice the frequency shift being detected, lower frequency shifts than are actually present are displayed. Because of the need for lower PRFs to reach deep vessels, signals from deep abdominal arteries are prone to aliasing if high velocities are present. In practice, aliasing is usually readily recognized (Fig. 1-31, C and D). Aliasing can be reduced by increasing the PRF, by increasing the Doppler angle (Fig. 1-31, D) (thereby decreasing the frequency shift), or by using a lower-frequency Doppler transducer.

Doppler Angle. When making Doppler measurements, it is desirable to correct for the Doppler angle and display the measurements in terms of velocity. These measurements are independent of the Doppler frequency. The accuracy of a velocity estimate obtained with Doppler is only as great as the accuracy of the measurement of the Doppler angle. This is particularly true as the Doppler angle exceeds 60 degrees. In general, the Doppler angle is best kept at 60 degrees or less because small changes in the Doppler angle above 60 degrees result in significant changes in the calculated velocity, and therefore measurement inaccuracies result in much greater errors in velocity estimates than similar errors at lower Doppler angles.

Sample Volume Size. With pulsed wave Doppler systems, the length of the Doppler sample volume can be controlled by the operator, and the width is determined by the beam profile. Analysis of Doppler signals requires that the sample volume be adjusted to exclude as much of the unwanted clutter from near the vessel walls as possible.

OPERATING MODES: CLINICAL IMPLICATIONS

Ultrasound devices may operate in several modes, including real-time, color flow Doppler, spectral Doppler, and M-mode imaging. Imaging is produced

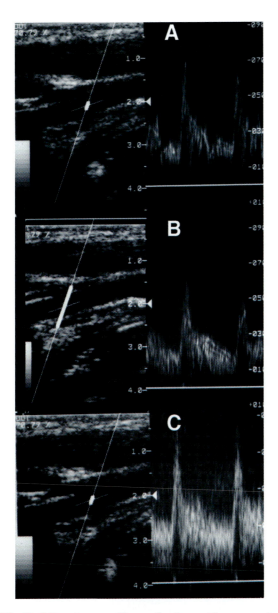

FIG. 1-30. Spectral broadening. The range of velocities detected at a given time in the pulse cycle is reflected in the Doppler spectrum as spectral broadening. **A, Normal spectrum.** Spectral broadening may arise from turbulent flow in association with vessel stenosis. **Artifactual spectral broadening** may be produced by improper positioning of the sample volume near the vessel wall or, **B,** use of an excessively large sample volume or, **C,** excessive system gain.

in a scanned mode of operation. In scanned modes, pulses of ultrasound from the transducer are directed down lines of sight that are moved or steered in sequence to generate the image. This means that the number of ultrasound pulses arriving at a given point in the patient over a given interval of time is relatively small, and relatively little energy is deposited at any given location. In contrast, **spectral Doppler** imaging is an unscanned mode of operation in which mul-

tiple ultrasound pulses are sent in repetition along a line to collect the Doppler data. In this mode the beam is stationary, resulting in **considerably greater potential for heating** than in imaging modes. For imaging, PRFs are usually a few thousand hertz with very short pulses. Longer pulse durations are used with Doppler than with other imaging modes. In addition, to avoid aliasing and other artifacts with Doppler imaging, it is often necessary to use higher PRFs than with other imaging applications. Longer pulse duration and higher PRF result in higher duty factors for Doppler modes of operation and increase the amount of energy introduced in scanning. Color flow Doppler, although a scanned mode, produces exposure conditions between those of real-time and Doppler imaging because color flow Doppler devices tend to send more pulses down each scan line and may use longer pulse durations than imaging devices. Clearly every user needs to be aware of the fact that switching from an imaging to a Doppler mode changes the exposure conditions and potential for bioeffects.

With current devices operating in imaging modes, bioeffects concerns are minimal as intensities sufficient to produce measurable heating are seldom used. With Doppler ultrasound the potential for thermal effects is greater. Preliminary measurements on commercially available instruments suggest that at least some of these are capable of producing temperature rises of greater than $1°$ C at soft tissue/bone interfaces if the focal zone of the transducer is held stationary. Care is therefore warranted when Doppler measurements are obtained at or near soft tissue/bone interfaces as may be the case in the second and third trimester of pregnancy. In these applications, thoughtful application of the principle of ALARA (as low as reasonably achievable) is required. Under the principle of ALARA, the user should use the lowest possible acoustic exposure to obtain the necessary diagnostic information.

ARE BIOEFFECTS THE REAL ISSUE?

Although there is clearly a need for users of ultrasound to be aware of bioeffects concerns, it is equally important to place bioeffects concerns in perspective by considering another key element in the safe use of ultrasound—the user. The knowledge and skill of the user are major determinants of the risk-to-benefit implications of the use of ultrasound in a specific clinical situation. For example, an unrealistic emphasis on risks may discourage an appropriate use of ultrasound, resulting in harm to the patient by preventing the acquisition of useful information or by subjecting the patient to another more hazardous examination. The skill and experience of the individual performing

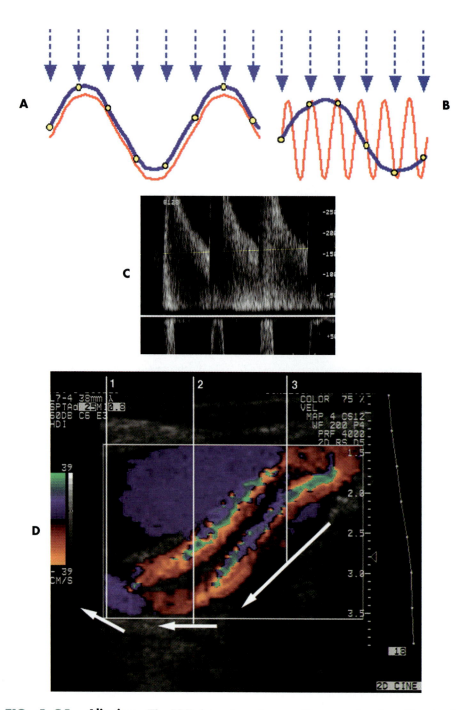

FIG. 1-31. Aliasing. The PRF determines the sampling rate of a given Doppler frequency shift. **A,** If the PRF is sufficient, the sampled waveform (*blue curve*) will **accurately** estimate the frequency being sampled (*red curve*). **B,** If the PRF is less than half the frequency being measured, **undersampling** will result in a lower frequency shift being displayed *(blue curve)*. **C,** In a clinical setting, **aliasing** appears in the spectral display as a "wrap around" of the higher frequencies to display below the baseline. **D,** In color flow Doppler display, **aliasing** results in a "wrap around" of the frequency color map from one flow direction to the opposite direction, passing through a transition of unsaturated color. In **D,** the velocity throughout the vessel is constant, but **aliasing appears only in portions of the vessel.** This is because of the effect of the Doppler angle on the Doppler frequency shift. As the angle increases, the Doppler frequency shift decreases and aliasing is no longer seen.

and interpreting the examination are likely to have a major impact on the overall benefit of the examination. In view of the rapid growth of ultrasound and its proliferation into the hands of minimally trained clinicians, it is likely that far more patients are likely to be harmed by misdiagnosis resulting from improper indications, poor examination technique, and errors in interpretation than from biologic effects. The failure to diagnose a significant anomaly or misdiagnosis of an ectopic pregnancy are real dangers, and poorly trained users may, in fact, turn out to be the greatest current hazard of diagnostic ultrasound.

In conclusion, an understanding of bioeffects is essential for the prudent use of diagnostic ultrasound and is important in ensuring that the excellent risk-to-benefit performance of diagnostic ultrasound is preserved. All users of ultrasound should be prudent, understanding as fully as possible the potential risks and obvious benefits of ultrasound examinations as well as those of alternate diagnostic methods. With this information, users can monitor exposure conditions and implement the principle of ALARA to keep patient and fetal exposure as low as possible in keeping with diagnostic objectives.

REFERENCES
Basic Acoustics
1. Chivers RC, Parry RJ. Ultrasonic velocity and attenuation in mammalian tissues. *J Acoust Soc Am* 1978;63:940-953.
2. Goss SA, Johnston RL, Dunn F. Comprehensive compilation of empirical properties of mammalian tissues. *J Acoust Soc Am* 1978;64:423-457.
3. Merritt CRB, Kremkau FW, Hobbins JC. *Diagnostic Ultrasound: Bioeffects and Safety. Ultrasound in Obstetrics and Gynecology.* 1992;2:366-374.
4. Merritt CRB, Hykes DL, Hedrick WR et al. Medical diagnostic ultrasound instrumentation and clinical interpretation. Topics in Radiology/Council Report. *JAMA* 1991;265:1155-1159.

Instrumentation
5. Merritt CRB. Doppler US: The basics. *RadioGraphics* 1991;11: 109-119.

Imaging Pitfalls
6. Burns PN. Interpretation and analysis of Doppler signals. In: Taylor KJW, Burns PN, Wells PNT, eds. *Clinical Applications of Doppler Ultrasound.* New York: Raven Press; 1988:77.

Doppler Ultrasonography
7. Merritt CRB. Doppler color flow imaging. *J Clin Ultrasound* 1987;15:591-597.
8. Rubin JM, Bude RO, Carson PL et al. Power Doppler US: a potentially useful alternative to mean frequency-based color Doppler US. *Radiology* 1994;190:853-856.

CHAPTER 2

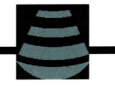

Biologic Effects and Safety

•

J. Brian Fowlkes, Ph.D.
Christy K. Holland, Ph.D.

CHAPTER OUTLINE

OVERVIEW

Widespread Use of Ultrasound

Ultrasound has provided an incredible wealth of knowledge in diagnostic medicine. Few would be willing to deny the impact this imaging modality has had on medical practice, particularly in obstetrics. It is estimated that millions of sonographic examinations are performed each year, and ultrasound remains one of the fastest-growing imaging modalities. This growth is due to many factors, including its low cost, real-time interactions, and, to no lesser extent, its apparent lack of bioeffects. Despite the large number of sonographic exams performed to date, there have been very few indications that clinical applications of diagnostic ultrasound have caused biologic effects on the patient or operator.

Regulation of Ultrasound Output

At present the U.S. Food and Drug Administration (FDA) regulates the maximum output of ultrasound devices to an established level through a marketing approval process that requires devices to be equivalent in efficacy and output to those produced prior to 1976. This historic regulation of sonography has provided a safety margin for ultrasound while allowing clinically useful performance. The mechanism has restricted ultrasound exposure to levels that apparently produce few if any obvious bioeffects based on the epidemiologic evidence, although there has been some evidence indicating the potential for bioeffects in animal studies.

Increasing Role for the Operator

Recent proposals concerning the regulation of acoustic output from medical ultrasound systems have suggested greatly increasing the role the physician and/or sonographer play in limiting the potential for ultrasound bioeffects. Because the maximum output limit was arbitrarily dictated by the FDA, and because it might be diagnostically advantageous to increase this limit (e.g., patients with large amounts of subcutaneous fat are difficult to scan), ultrasound devices might produce higher outputs in the near future. Therefore an informed decision concerning the possible adverse effects of ultrasound in comparison to desired diagnostic information will probably become more important over the next few years. As currently envisioned, information would be provided to the operator concerning the relative potential for bioeffects but would allow physicians the discretion to increase acoustic output beyond a level that might induce a biologic response.

Need for Informed Operators

Although the choices made during sonographic examinations may not be equivalent to the risk versus benefit decisions associated with imaging modalities using ionizing radiation, there will be an increasing reliance on the operator to determine the amount of ultrasound exposure that is diagnostically required. For these reasons an operator should know the potential bioeffects associated with ultrasound exposure. Patients also need to be reassured about the safety of a diagnostic ultrasound scan. The scientific community has identified some potential bioeffects from sonography, and although no causal relation has been established, it does not mean that no effects exist. Therefore it is important to understand the interaction of ultrasound with biologic systems.

PHYSICAL EFFECTS OF SOUND

The physical effects of sound can be divided into two principal groups: **thermal** and **nonthermal.** The thermal effects are within the common experience of most medical professionals. The effect of elevated temperature on tissue can be recognized, and the effects due to ultrasound are not substantially different from those of any other localized heat source. In this case the heating is principally due to the attenuation of the sound field as it propagates through tissue. However, "nonthermal" mechanisms can generate heat as well.

Many nonthermal mechanisms for biologic effects exist. Acoustic fields can apply **radiation forces** (not ionizing radiation) on the structures within the body both at the macroscopic and microscopic levels, resulting in exerted pressure and torque. The time average pressure in an acoustic field is different than the hydrostatic pressure of the fluid, and any object in the field is subject to this change in pressure. The effect is typically considered smaller than many others because it relies on less significant factors in the formulation of the acoustic field. Acoustic fields can also cause motion of fluids. Such acoustically induced flow is called **streaming.**

A topic of great interest is the effect of **acoustic cavitation.** Acoustic cavitation is the action of acoustic fields within a fluid to generate bubbles and/or cause their volume pulsation and even collapse in response to the acoustic field. The result of this activity can be heat generation and associated free radical generation, microstreaming of fluid around the bubble, radiation forces generated by the scattered acoustic field from the bubble, and mechanical actions resulting from bubble collapse. The interaction of acoustic fields with bubbles or "gas bodies" (as they are generally called) has been a significant area of bioeffects research in recent years.

THERMAL EFFECTS

Ultrasound Produces Heat

As ultrasound propagates through the body, energy is lost through **attenuation.** Attenuation causes loss in penetration and the inability to image deeper tissues. Attenuation is the result of two processes. **Scattering** of the ultrasound results from the redirection of the acoustic energy by tissue encountered during propagation. In the case of diagnostic ultrasound, some of the acoustic energy transmitted into the tissue is scattered back in the direction of the transducer (termed **backscatter**), which allows a signal to be detected. Energy also is lost along the propagation path of the ultrasound by absorption. **Absorption** is the conversion of the ultrasound energy into heat. This heating provides a mechanism for ultrasound-induced bioeffects.

Factors Controlling Tissue Heating

The rate at which temperature will increase in tissues exposed to ultrasound depends on a number of factors. These include spatial focusing, ultrasound frequency, exposure duration, and tissue type.

Spatial Focusing

Ultrasound systems use various techniques to concentrate or **focus** ultrasound energy in order to improve the quality of measured signals. The analog is that of a magnifying glass. The glass collects all of the light striking its surface and concentrates it into a small region. In sonography and acoustics in general, the term **intensity** is used to describe the spatial distribution of ultrasonic **power** (energy per unit time) where **Intensity = Power/Area** and the area refers to the cross-sectional area of the ultrasound beam. Another beam dimension that is often quoted is the **beam width** at a specified location of the field. If the same ultrasonic power is concentrated into a smaller area, then the intensity will increase. Focusing in an ultrasound system can be used to improve the spatial resolution of the images. The side effect is an increased potential for bioeffects due to heating and cavitation. In general the greatest heating potential will lie somewhere between the scanhead and the focus, but the exact position will depend on the focal distance, tissue properties, and heat generated within the scanhead itself.

Returning to the magnifying glass analogy, most children learn at an early age that the secret to incineration is a steady hand. Movement distributes the power of the light beam over a larger area, thereby re-

ducing its intensity. The same is true in ultrasound imaging. Thus imaging systems that scan a beam through tissue reduce the average intensity. **Spectral Doppler** and **M-mode** imaging maintain the ultrasound beam in a stationary position (both considered **unscanned modes**) and therefore provide no opportunity to spatially distribute the ultrasonic power whereas **color flow Doppler, power mode Doppler,** and **B-scale** (often called **gray-scale**) imaging require that the beam be moved to new locations (**scanned**) at a rate sufficient to produce the real-time nature of these imaging modes.

Temporal Considerations

The ultrasound power is the temporal rate at which ultrasound energy is produced; therefore it seems reasonable that controlling how ultrasound is produced in time is a method for limiting its effects. Ultrasound can be produced in bursts rather than continuously. Ultrasound imaging systems operate on the principle of **pulse-echo** in which a burst of ultrasound is emitted followed by a quiescent period listening for echoes to return. This **pulsed** ultrasound sequence is repeated numerous times during an imaging sequence. On the other hand, ultrasound may be transmitted in a **continuous wave** (CW) mode in which the ultrasound transmission is not interrupted. The **temporal peak intensity** refers to the largest intensity at any time during ultrasound exposure (Fig. 2-1). The **pulse average intensity** is the average value over the entire ultrasound burst. And the **temporal average** is the average over the pulse repetition period (the elapsed time between the onset of ultrasound bursts). The **duty factor** is defined as the fraction of time the ultrasound field is on. Given significant time off between pulses (small duty factor), the temporal average value will be significantly smaller. For example, a duty factor of 10% will reduce the temporal average intensity by a factor of 10 compared to the pulse average. It is the time averaged quantities that are most related to the potential for thermal bioeffects. When combined with spatial information, some common terms are produced such as the spatial peak temporal average intensity, I_{SPTA}, or the spatial average temporal average intensity, I_{SATA}. Finally, the overall duration, or **dwell time,** of the ultrasound exposure to a particular tissue is important because the longer the tissue is exposed, the greater the risk of bioeffect. The motion of the scanhead during an examination reduces the dwell time within a particular region of the body and minimizes the potential for bioeffects of ultrasound. Therefore performing an efficient scan, spending only the time required for diagnosis, is a simple way to reduce exposure.

Tissue Type

Numerous physical and biologic parameters control heating of tissues. Absorption is normally the domi-

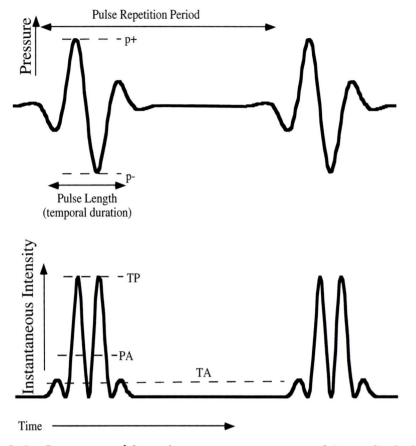

FIG. 2-1. Pressure and intensity parameters measured in medical ultrasound. The variables are defined as follows: p+ = peak positive pressure in waveform; p− = peak negative pressure in waveform; TP = temporal peak; PA = pulse average; TA = temporal average.

nant contribution to attenuation in soft tissue. The attenuation coefficient is the attenuation per unit length of sound travel and is usually given in units of dB/cm-MHz. The attenuation typically increases with increasing ultrasound frequency. The attenuation ranges from a negligible amount for fluids like amniotic fluid, blood, and urine to the highest value for bone with some variation among different soft tissue types (Fig. 2-2).

Another important factor is the body's ability to cool tissue via blood perfusion. Well-perfused tissue will more effectively regulate its temperature by carrying away the excess heat produced by ultrasound. The exception to this is when heat is deposited too rapidly as in thermal ablation used for therapy.[1]

From the tissue considerations noted above, there are two specific areas of interest based on the differences in the nature of heating phenomena. First is **bone,** which is of interest because of its high attenuation of incident acoustic energy. The second is the attenuation of ultrasound by **soft tissue.** In the case of bone, it is common in examinations during pregnan-

cies for calcified bone to be subjected to ultrasound. A case in point is the measurement of the biparietal diameter (BPD) of the skull. Fetal bone contains increasing degrees of mineralization as gestation progresses, thereby increasing risk of localized heating. Special heating situations may also occur in soft tissue, which are relevant to obstetric and gynecologic examinations.

Bone Heating. Carstensen et al. combined an analytical approach and experimental measurements of the temperature rise in mouse skull exposed to continuous wave ultrasound to estimate the temperature increments in bone exposures.[2] Because bone has a large absorption coefficient, the incident ultrasonic energy is assumed to be absorbed in a thin planar sheet at the bone surface. The temperature rise of mouse skull has been studied in a 3.6-MHz focused beam with a beam width of 2.75 mm (Fig. 2-3). The temporal average intensity in the focal region was 1.5 W/cm^2. One of two models (shown as the highest curve) in common use[3] predicts values for the temperature rise about 20% greater than that actually mea-

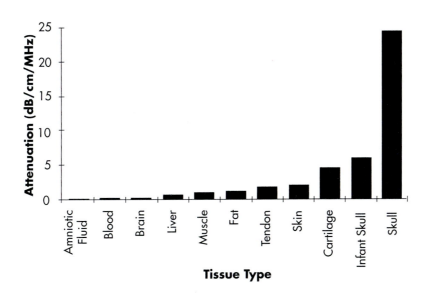

FIG. 2-2. Tissue attenuation. Values for types of human tissue at body temperature. (Data from Duck FA, Starritt HC, Anderson SP. A survey of the acoustic output of ultrasonic Doppler equipment. *Clin Phys Physiol Meas* 1987;8:39-49.)

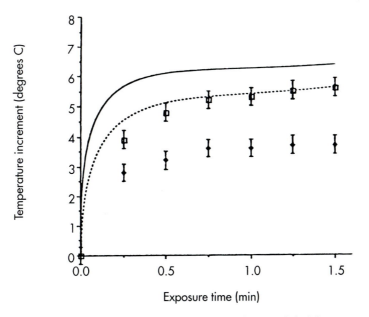

FIG. 2-3. Heating of mouse skull in a focused sound field. For these experiments the frequency was 3.6 MHz and the temporal average focal intensity was 1.5 W/cm². *Lower curve:* young (< 17 week) mice (N = 7); *middle curve:* old (> 6 month) mice (N = 4); *vertical bars:* two standard errors in height; *top curve:* theoretical estimation of the temperature increase by Nyborg.[3] (From Carstensen EL, Child SZ, Norton S et al. Ultrasonic heating of the skull. *J Acoust Soc Am* 1990;87:1310-1317.)

TABLE 2-1

FETAL FEMUR TEMPERATURE INCREMENTS AT 1 W/CM²

Gestational Age (days)	Diameter (mm)	Temperature Increments (°C)
59	0.5	0.10
78	1.2	0.69
108	3.3	2.92

Temperature increments in human fetal femur exposed for 20 seconds were found to be approximately proportional to incident intensity.[4]

sured in this experiment.[1] Thus the theoretical model is conservative in nature.

Similarly for the fetal femur, Drewniak et al.[4] indicated that the size and calcification state of the bone contributed to the *ex vivo* heating of bone (Table 2-1). To put this in perspective and to give an awareness of the role the operator can play in controlling potential heating, consider the following scenario. By reducing the output power of an ultrasound scanner by 10 dB, the predicted temperature rise would be reduced by a factor of 10, making the 3°C rise seen by these researchers (see Table 2-1) virtually nonexistent. **This strongly suggests the use of maximum gain and reduction in output power during ultrasound exams** (see section below on controlling ultrasound output). In the case of fetal examinations, a clear attempt should be made to maximize amplifier gain since this comes at no cost to the patient in terms of exposure. Distinctions are often made between bone positioned deep to the skin at the focal plane of the transducer and bone near the skin surface as would be

the case in transcranial applications. This distinction is discussed further in the thermal index.

Soft Tissue Heating. Two special scenarios for ultrasound exposure in soft tissue are particularly relevant to obstetric/gynecologic applications. First is the common condition of **scanning through a full bladder.** In this case the urine is a fluid with a relatively low ultrasound attenuation coefficient. The reduced attenuation will allow larger acoustic amplitudes to be applied deeper within the body. In addition, it is possible for the propagating wave to experience **finite amplitude distortion,** resulting in energy being shifted by a nonlinear process from lower to higher frequencies. The result is a gradual wave steepening (Fig. 2-4) where the steep edge is composed of higher frequency components. Since attenuation increases with increasing frequency, the absorption of a large portion of the energy in such a wave occurs over a much shorter distance, concentrating the energy deposition in the tissue encountered. This range may include the fetus. These nonlinear effects are also under extensive consideration as part of the thermal modeling for fetal exposure.

Another common situation worth noting is **transvaginal ultrasound.** This procedure is mentioned in particular because of the proximity of the transducer to sensitive tissues such as the ovaries. As will be discussed later, temperature increases near the transducer may provide a heat source at sites other than the focal plane of the transducer. In addition, the transducer face itself may be a significant heat source because of inefficiencies in its conversion of electrical to acoustic energy. Therefore such considerations must be made in the estimation of potential thermal effects in transvaginal ultrasound or any other endocavitary application.

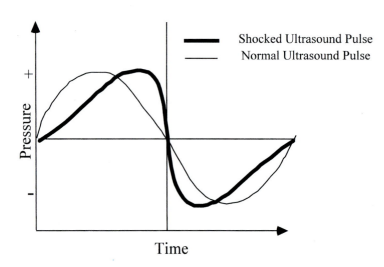

Shocked Ultrasound Pulse
Normal Ultrasound Pulse

FIG. 2-4. Effect of finite amplitude distortion on a propagating ultrasound pulse. Note the increasing steepness in the pulse, which contains higher frequency components.

Hyperthermia and Ultrasound Safety

Our knowledge of the bioeffects for ultrasound heating is based on the experience available from other more common forms of hyperthermia that serve as a basis for safety criteria. There is an extensive body of knowledge concerning the effects of short-term and extended temperature increases, or **hyperthermia.** Teratologic effects due to hyperthermia have been demonstrated in birds, all the common laboratory animals, farm animals, and nonhuman primates.[5] The wide range of observed bioeffects, from subcellular chemical alterations to gross congenital abnormalities and fetal death, is an indication of the effectiveness or universality of hyperthermic conditions for perturbing living systems.[6] The National Council on Radiation Protection and Measurements (NCRP) Scientific Committee on Biological Effects of Ultrasound has compiled a comprehensive list of the lowest reported thermal exposures producing teratogenic effects.[7] An examination of this data (Fig. 2-5) shows known hyperthermia bioeffects endpoints that have been plotted for a given temperature rise and as a function of exposure-induced time. The *dotted line* indicates a lower boundary for observed thermally induced bioeffects. This line has been used as a benchmark for thermal effects of ultrasound in a recommendation by the NCRP, which states that a diagnostic exam need not be withheld as long as exposure conditions do not exceed this level of temperature rise and duration.[7] Therefore if a method to indicate ultrasonic conditions that might exceed this line is devised, then this might provide meaningful feedback to the operator.

The Thermal Index

In keeping with this criterion, a general statement has been proposed by the NCRP concerning the safety of exams in which no temperature rise greater than 1°C is expected. In an afebrile patient within this limit, there is no basis for expecting an adverse effect. In those cases where the temperature rise might be greater, the operator would weigh the benefit versus potential risks. To assist in this decision given the range of different imaging conditions seen in practice, a **thermal index (TI)** has been approved as part of the *Standard for Real-Time Display of Thermal and Mechanical Acoustical Output Indices on Diagnostic Ultrasound Equipment*, which gives the operator an indication of the proximity to a thermal threshold[8] (see box on p. 42). In this standard, a series of calculations is made based on the present imaging conditions, and an on-screen display of the thermal index is provided to the operator.

The NCRP Scientific Committee on Biological Effects of Ultrasound introduced the concept of a thermal index **(TI).**[7] The goal of the TI is to provide an indication of the relative potential for increasing tissue

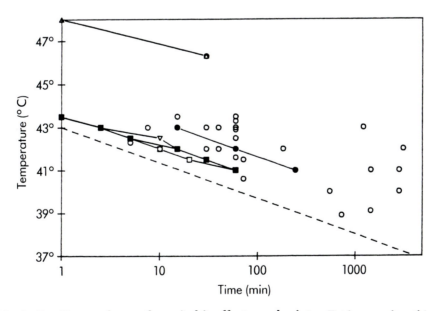

FIG. 2-5. **Known hyperthermia bioeffects endpoints.** Evidence such as this was used to support the conclusion that an ultrasound examination need not be withheld because of concern for thermally mediated adverse effects if the duration of the exposure (*t*, in minutes) and the maximum anticipated temperature (*T*, in degrees Celsius) satisfy the inequality $t \le 4^{<43 - T>}$. This is based on short exposures to an elevated temperature of 39°C. Discussions of these results were used in the development of the thermal index. (From Miller MW, Ziskin MC. Biological consequences of hyperthermia. *Ultrasound Med Biol* 1989;15:707-722. Adapted from the NCRP.)

temperature, but it is not meant to provide the actual temperature rise. Two tissue models were recommended by the NCRP to aid in the calculation of the ultrasound power that could raise the temperature in tissue by 1°C: (1) a homogeneous model in which the attenuation coefficient is uniform throughout the region of interest and (2) a fixed-attenuation model in which the minimum attenuation along the path from transducer to a distant anatomic structure is independent of the distance because of a low-attenuation fluid path (such as amniotic fluid).[7,9,10] Because of concern for the patient, it was recommended that "reasonable worst-case" assumptions be made with respect to estimation of temperature elevations *in vivo*. The American Institute of Ultrasound in Medicine (AIUM), the National Electrical Manufacturers Association (NEMA), and the FDA have adopted the thermal index as an output display standard. They advocate estimating the effect of attenuation in the body by reducing the acoustic power/output of the scanner (W_0) by derating factor equal to 0.3 dB/cm-MHz for the homogeneous, or soft tissue, case.[8]

Thermal Index Models

Three tissue models were considered by the AIUM thermal index working group: a homogeneous tissue or soft tissue model, a tissue model with bone at the focus, and a tissue model with bone at the surface, or transcranial model.[8] The thermal index takes on three different forms for these tissue models.

Homogeneous Tissue Model (Soft Tissue).

The assumption of homogeneity allows for simplification in determining the effects of acoustic propagation and attenuation as well as the heat transfer characteristics of the tissue. This is one of the most common cases for ultrasound imaging and applies to those circumstances where bone is not present and can generally be used for fetal examinations during the first trimester (low calcification in bone). Considerable ef-

fort went into the estimation of potential heating, and many assumptions and compromises had to be made in order to calculate a single quantity that would guide the operator. Calculations of the temperature rise along the axis of a focused beam are shown for a simple spherically curved single element transducer (Fig. 2-6). Note the existence of two thermal peaks. The first is in the near field (between the transducer and the focus), and the second appears close to the focal region.[11,12] The **first thermal peak** actually occurs in a region with low ultrasound intensity and wide beam width. When the beam width is large, cooling will occur mainly because of perfusion. In the near field, the magnitude of the local intensity will be the chief determinant of the degree of heating. The **second thermal peak** occurs at the location of high intensity *(I)* and narrow beam width *(w)* at or near the focal plane. Here the cooling will be dominated by conduction, and the total acoustic power will be the chief determinant of the degree of heating.

Given the thermal "twin peaks" dilemma, the AIUM thermal index working group compromised in creating a thermal index that included contributions from both heating domains.[8] Their rationale was based on the need to minimize the acoustic measurement load for manufacturers of ultrasound systems. In addition, adjustments had to be made to compensate for effects of the large range of potential apertures. The result is a complicated series of calculations and measurements that must be performed, and to the credit of the many manufacturers, there has been considerable effort in implementing a display standard to provide user feedback.

Tissue Model with Bone at the Focus (Fetal Applications).

Applications of ultrasound in which the acoustic beam travels through soft tissue for a fixed distance and impinges on bone occur most often in obstetric scanning during the second and third trimesters. Carson et al. have made sonographic measurements of the maternal abdominal wall thickness in various stages of pregnancy.[10] Based on their results, the NCRP recommends that the attenuation coefficients for the first, second, and third trimesters be 1.0, 0.75, and 0.5 dB/MHz, respectively.[7] These values represent "worst case" estimates. In addition, Siddiqi et al. determined the average tissue attenuation coefficient for transabdominal insonification in a patient population of nonpregnant, healthy volunteers was 2.98 dB/MHz.[13] This value represents an average measured value and is obviously very different than the worst case estimates listed above. This leads to considerable debate on how such parameters should be included in an index.

In addition, bone is a complex hard connective tissue with a calcified collagenous intercellular substance. Its absorption coefficient for longitudinal

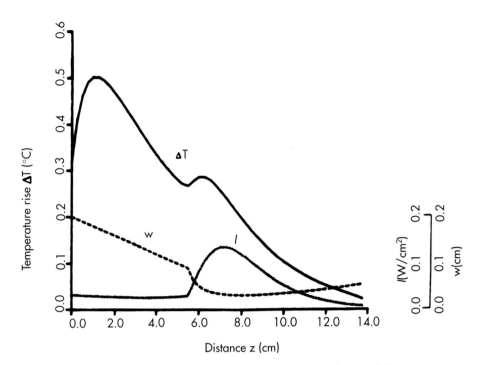

FIG. 2-6. Thermal peaks of a single spherically focused beam. Plots of beamwidth *(w)*, intensity *(I)*, and temperature rise *(ΔT)* along the axis of the beam. With aperture = 2 cm, focal length = 10 cm, and center frequency = 3 MHz. The absorption coefficient and attenuation coefficient are both equal and near that of soft tissue (0.15 nepers/cm). The perfusion time is a quantity that prescribes the heat dissipation due to blood flow and was set at 1000 seconds, and the ultrasonic source power is 0.1 W.[7] (From *Exposure criteria for medical diagnostic ultrasound: I. Criteria based on thermal mechanisms.* Bethesda, MD: National Council on Radiation Protection and Measurements; 1992. NCRP report no. 113.)

waves is a factor of 10 greater than that for most soft tissues (see Fig. 2-2). Shear waves are also created in bone as sound waves strike bone at oblique incidence. The absorption coefficients for shear waves are even greater than those for longitudinal waves.[14-16]

Based on the data of Carstensen et al. described earlier,[2] the NCRP proposed a thermal model for bone heating. Using this model, the thermal index for bone (**TIB**) is estimated for those conditions in which the focus of the beam is at or near bone. Once again a number of assumptions and compromises had to be made to develop a functional thermal index (TI) for the case of bone exposure.

- For **unscanned mode** transducers (operating in a fixed position) with bone in the focal region, the location of the maximum temperature increase is at the surface of the bone. Therefore the thermal index for bone (TIB) is calculated at an axial distance that maximizes TIB, a worst case assumption.
- For **scanned modes,** the thermal index for soft tissue is used because the temperature increase at the surface is either greater than or approximately equal to the temperature increase with bone in the focus.

Tissue Model with Bone at the Surface (Transcranial Applications). For adult cranial applications, the same model is used to estimate the temperature distribution *in situ* as in the focal bone case. However, because the bone is located at the surface, immediately after the acoustic beam enters the body, attenuation of the acoustic power output is not included.[8] Here the equivalent beam diameter at the surface is used to calculate the acoustic power.

Thermal Index Estimates
Thermal Effects

There are a number of points to keep in mind when referring to the thermal index as a means of estimating the potential for thermal effects. First, the TI is not synonymous with temperature rise. A TI equal to 1 does not mean the temperature will rise 1°C. An increased potential for thermal effects can be expected as the index increases. Second, a high index does not mean that bioeffects are occurring but only that the potential exists. Several factors may reduce the actual temperature rise generated, and these may not be taken into account by the thermal models employed for TI calculation. However, the index should be monitored during exams and minimized when possible. Finally, there is no consideration in the TI for the duration of the scan, so minimizing examination time will reduce the potential for effects.

Summary Statement on Thermal Effects

The AIUM statement concerning thermal effects[17] (see box on p. 45) includes several conclusions that can be summarized as follows:

- Exams resulting in a 2°C temperature rise or less are not expected to cause bioeffects. (Many ultrasound examinations fall within these parameters.)
- A significant number of factors control heat production by diagnostic ultrasound.
- Ossified bone is a particularly important concern for ultrasound exposure.
- A labeling standard now provides information concerning potential heating in soft tissue and bone.
- Even though an FDA limit exists for fetal exposures, predicted temperature rises can exceed 2°C.
- Thermal indices are expected to track temperature increases better than any single ultrasonic field parameter.

EFFECTS OF ACOUSTIC CAVITATION

Potential Sources for Bioeffects

Our knowledge concerning the interaction of ultrasound with gas bodies (which many term "cavitation") has significantly increased recently, although our knowledge base is not as extensive as that for ultrasound thermal effects and other sources of hyperthermia. **Acoustic cavitation inception** is demarcated by a specific threshold value: the minimum acoustic pressure necessary to initiate the growth of a cavity in a fluid during the rarefaction phase of the cycle. A number of parameters affect this threshold, including initial bubble or **cavitation nucleus** size, acoustic pulse characteristics (such as center frequency, pulse repetition frequency, and pulse duration), ambient hydrostatic pressure, and host fluid parameters (such as density, viscosity, compressibility, heat conductivity, and surface tension). **Inertial cavitation** refers to bubbles that undergo large variations from their equilibrium sizes in a few acoustic cycles. Specifically during contraction, the surrounding fluid inertia controls the bubble motion.[18] Large acoustic pressures are necessary to generate inertial cavitation, and the collapse of these cavities is often violent.

The effect of **preexisting cavitation nuclei** may be one of the principal controlling factors in mechanical effects that result in biologic effects. The body is such an excellent filter that these nucleation sites may only be found in small numbers and only at selected

sites. For instance, if water is filtered down to 2 μm, the cavitation threshold doubles.[19] Theoretically, the tensile strength of water that is devoid of cavitation nuclei is about 100 megapascals (MPa).[20] Various models have been suggested to explain bubble formation in animals,[21,22] and these models have been used extensively in cavitation threshold determination. One model[23] is used in the prediction of SCUBA diving tables and may also have applicability to patients. It remains to be seen how well such models will predict the nucleation of bubbles from diagnostic ultrasound in the body.

A photograph of a 1-MHz therapeutic ultrasound unit generating bubbles in gas-saturated water is shown in Fig. 2-7. This particular medium and ultrasound parameters were chosen to optimize the conditions for cavitation. Using continuous wave ultrasound and plenty of preexisting gas pockets in the water set the stage for the production of cavitation. Even though these acoustic pulses are longer than those typically used in diagnostic ultrasound, cavitation effects have also been observed with diagnostic pulses in fluids.[24]

Sonochemistry. Free radical generation and detection provides a means to observe cavitation and to gauge its strength and potential for damage. The sonochemistry of free radicals is the result of very high temperatures and pressures within the rapidly collapsing bubble. These conditions can even generate light, or **sonoluminescence**.[25] With the addition of the correct compounds, chemical luminescence can also be used for free radical detection.[26] **Chemiluminescence** can be generated by a therapeutic ultrasound device (Fig. 2-8). The setup is backlighted (in red) to show the bubbles and experimental apparatus. The chemiluminescence emissions are the blue bands seen through the middle of the liquid sample holder. The light emitted is sufficient to be seen by simply adapting one's eyes to darkness. Electron spin resonance can also be used with molecules that trap free radicals to detect cavitation activity capable of free radical production.[27] A number of other chemical detection schemes are presently employed to detect cavitation from diagnostic devices *in vitro*.

Evidence of Cavitation from Lithotripters. It is possible to generate bubbles *in vivo* using short pulses with high amplitudes of an extracorporeal shock wave lithotripter (ESWL). The peak positive pressure for lithotripsy pulses can be as much as 50 MPa and the negative pressure around 20 MPa. **Finite amplitude distortion** causes high frequencies to appear in high-amplitude ultrasound fields. Although ESWL pulses have significant energy at high frequencies due to finite amplitude distortion, a large portion of the energy is actually in the 100-kHz range, much lower than

THERMAL BIOEFFECTS: CONCLUSIONS REGARDING HEAT

1. Excessive temperature increase can result in toxic effects in mammalian systems. The biological effects observed depend on many factors, such as the exposure duration, the type of tissue exposed, its cellular proliferation rate, and its potential for regeneration. These are important factors when considering fetal and neonatal safety. Temperature increases of several degrees Celsius above the normal core range can occur naturally; there have been no significant biological effects observed resulting from such temperature increases except when they were sustained for extended time periods.

a. For exposure durations up to 50 hours, there have been no significant biological effects observed due to temperature increases less than or equal to 2°C above normal.

b. For temperature increases greater than 2°C above normal, there have been no significant biological effects observed due to temperature increases less than or equal to

$$6 - \frac{\log_{10}(t)}{0.6}$$

where t is the exposure duration ranging from 1 to 250 min. For example, for temperature increases of 4°C and 6°C, the corresponding limits for the exposure duration t are 16 min. and 1. min., respectively.

c. In general adult tissues are more tolerant of temperature increases than fetal and neonatal tissues. Therefore higher temperatures and/or longer exposure durations would be required for thermal damage.

2. The temperature increase during exposure of tissues to diagnostic ultrasound fields is dependent upon (a) output characteristics of the acoustical source such as frequency, source dimensions, scan rate, power, pulse repetition frequency, pulse duration, transducer self heating, exposure time and wave shape, and (b) tissue properties such as attenuation, absorption, speed of sound, acoustic impedance, perfusion, thermal conductivity, thermal diffusivity, anatomical structure, and nonlinear parameter.

3. For similar exposure conditions, the expected temperature increase in bone is significantly greater than in soft tissues. For this reason, conditions where an acoustic beam impinges on ossifying fetal bone deserve special attention due to its close proximity to other developing tissues.

4. Calculations of the maximum temperature increase resulting from ultrasound exposure *in vivo* should not be assumed to be exact because of the uncertainties and approximations associated with the thermal, acoustic, and structural characteristics of the tissues involved. However, experimental evidence shows that calculations are capable of predicting measured values within a factor of two. Thus, it appears reasonable to use calculations to obtain safety guidelines for clinical exposures where temperature measurements are not feasible. To provide a display of real-time estimates of tissue temperature increases as part of a diagnostic system, simplifying approximations are used to yield values called Thermal Indices.* Under most clinically relevant conditions, the soft-tissue thermal index, TIS, and the bone thermal index, TIB, either overestimate or closely approximate the best available estimate of the maximum temperature increase (ΔT_{max}). For example, if TIS = 2, then $\Delta T_{max} \leq 2$°C.

5. The current FDA regulatory limit for $I_{SPTA.3}$ is 720 mW/cm^2. For this, and lesser intensities, the best available estimate of the maximum temperature increase in the conceptus can exceed 2°C.

6. The soft-tissue thermal index, TIS, and the bone thermal index, TIB, are useful for estimating the temperature increase *in vivo*. For this purpose, these thermal indices are superior to any single ultrasonic field quantity such as the derated spatial-peak, temporal-average intensity, $I_{SPTA.3}$. That is, TIS and TIB track changes in the maximum temperature increases, $\Delta Tmax$, thus allowing for implementation of the ALARA principle, whereas $I_{SPTA.3}$ does not. For example,

a. At a constant value of $I_{SPTA.3}$, TIS increases with increasing frequency and with increasing source diameter.

b. At a constant value of $I_{SPTA.3}$, TIB increases with increasing focal beam diameter.

*The Thermal Indices are the nondimensional ratios of the estimated temperature increases to 1°C for specific tissue models.[8]
From American Institute of Ultrasound in Medicine. *Bioeffects and Safety of Diagnostic Ultrasound*. Laurel, Md: American Institute of Ultrasound in Medicine; 1993.

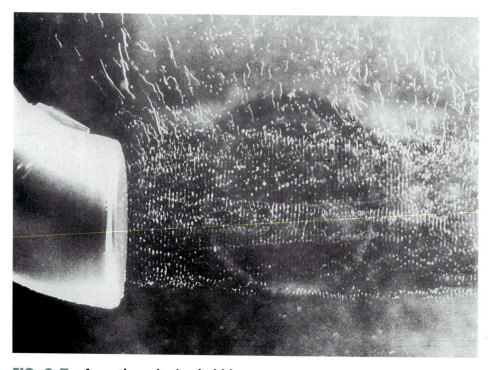

FIG. 2-7. Acoustic cavitation bubbles. This cavitation activity is being generated in water using a common therapeutic ultrasound device. (Courtesy National Center for Physical Acoustics, University of Mississippi.)

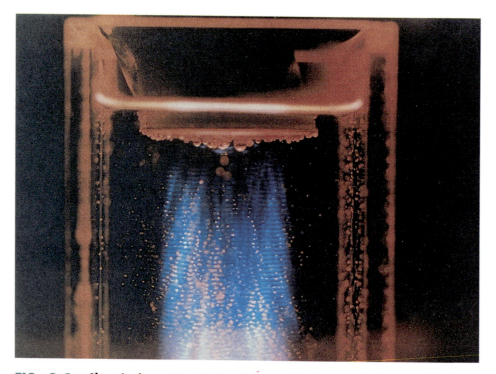

FIG. 2-8. Chemical reaction induced by cavitation producing visible light. The reaction is the result of free radical production. (Courtesy National Center for Physical Acoustics, University of Mississippi.)

frequencies in diagnostic scanners. The lower frequency makes cavitation more likely. As an example of the effect, Aymé and Carstensen have shown that the higher frequency components in nonlinearly distorted pulses contribute little to the killing of *Drosophila* larvae.[28] Interestingly enough, there is now evidence to indicate that collapsing bubbles may play a role in stone disruption.[29-31] A bubble collapsing near a surface may form a liquid jet through its center, which strikes the surface (Fig. 2-9). If a sheet of aluminum foil is placed at the focus of a lithotripter, small pinholes will be generated.[32] The impact is even sufficient to pit solid brass and aluminum plates. Clearly, lithotripsy and diagnostic ultrasound differ in the acoustic power generated and are not at all comparable in the bioeffects produced. Yet some diagnostic devices produce peak rarefactional pressures greater than 3 MPa, which is in the lower range of lithotripter outputs.[33-35] Interestingly, lung damage and surface petechiae have been noted as side effects of ESWL in clinical cases.[36] Inertial cavitation was suspected as the cause of this damage and has prompted several researchers to study the effects of diagnostic ultrasound exposure on the lung parenchyma.

Bioeffects in Lung. Lung tissue has proven to be an interesting location to examine for bioeffects of diagnostic ultrasound. The presence of air in the alveolar spaces constitutes a significant source of gas bodies. Child et al. measured threshold pressures for hemorrhage in mouse lung exposed to 1- to 4-MHz short-pulse diagnostic ultrasound (i.e., 10 microsecond and 1 microsecond pulse durations).[37] The threshold of damage in murine lung at these frequencies was established to be 1.4 MPa. Pathologic features of this damage included extravasation of blood cells into the alveolar spaces.[38] It was hypothesized that cavitation, originating from gas-filled alveoli, was

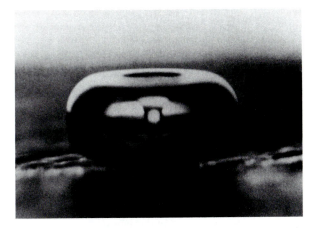

FIG. 2-9. Collapsing bubble near a boundary. When cavitation is produced near boundaries, a liquid jet may form through the center of a bubble and strike the boundary surface. (Courtesy of Lawrence A. Crum.)

responsible for the damage. Their data are the first to provide direct evidence that clinically relevant, pulsed ultrasound exposures produce deleterious effects in mammalian tissue in the absence of significant heating. Hemorrhagic foci induced by 4-MHz pulsed Doppler have also been reported in the monkey.[39] Damage in the monkey lung was of a significantly lesser degree than that in the mouse. In these studies it was impossible to show categorically that these effects were induced by bubbles because the cavitation-induced bubbles were themselves not observed. Further studies are required to determine the relevance of these findings to humans.

The gross organization and cellular composition of the lung are similar in mammals, although there are significant physiologic and anatomic differences related to organization of the distal airways, alveolar morphology, and blood supply.[40] Morphologic studies demonstrate that capillaries within the alveolar septa of most mammals are arranged as a single layer separated from the air spaces by a thin cellular barrier (100 nm). Because of this anatomic configuration, Tarantal and Canfield[39] hypothesized that these regions are more susceptible to conditions where bubble oscillation and rupture may occur. They also noted that an important factor specific to the lung may be the monolayer of surfactant within the alveoli. Surfactant, the alveolar lining fluid, is responsible for modifying surface tension in order to promote lung expansion and prevent lung collapse. It is possible that, during exposure to ultrasound, small microbubbles are created within edges of the surfactant-rich alveolus. These microbubbles may oscillate and collapse, causing localized disruption of the epithelial/endothelial barrier and subsequent extravasation of red blood cells into the alveolar space. Holland and Apfel have previously shown a direct correlation between a reduction in the cavitation threshold and reduced host fluid surface tension.[41,42]

Although a proven phenomenon *in vitro*,[43] the occurrence of cavitation *in vivo* due to diagnostic ultrasound has been difficult to document in mammalian systems primarily because of the transient nature of its occurrence (i.e., microseconds) and the localized character of the resultant effects (i.e., <10 microns). To explore the hypothesis of cavitation-based bioeffects from diagnostic ultrasound, research has been performed on the thresholds of damage in rat lungs exposed to 4-MHz pulsed Doppler and color Doppler ultrasound.[44] A 30-MHz active detection scheme developed by Roy et al[45] was used to provide the first direct evidence of cavitation from diagnostic ultrasound pulses. Damage was observed with histologic features consistent with those seen in mice and monkeys because of diagnostic ultrasound exposures. However, in this limited study, bubble activity was not correlated with histologic damage.

Mechanical Index

Calculations for cavitation prediction have yielded a rough trade-off between peak rarefactional pressure and frequency.[46] This predicted trade-off assumes short-pulse (a few acoustic cycles) and low-duty cycle ultrasound (<1%). This relatively simple result can be used to gauge the potential for the onset of cavitation from diagnostic ultrasound. The **mechanical index,** or **MI** (see box below), was adopted by the FDA, AIUM, and NEMA as a real-time output display to estimate the potential for bubble formation *in vivo*, in analogy to the thermal index. As indicated before, the collapse temperature for inertial cavitation is very high. For this index, a collapse temperature of 5000 K was chosen based on the potential for free radical generation, and the frequency dependence of the pressure required to generate this thermal threshold takes a relatively simple form. The MI is a kind of "mechanical energy index" because the square of the MI is roughly proportional to mechanical work that can be performed on a bubble in the acoustic rarefaction phase.

THE MECHANICAL INDEX

The index is designed to indicate acoustic outputs that have the potential for producing cavitation based on the existence of free bubbles with a broad size distribution. It is defined as

$$MI = \frac{P^*}{f^{*a}}$$

where the normalized pressure is $P^* = P/(1\ MPa)$, P is the peak negative pressure in the acoustic field, which is derated according to 0.3 dB/cm-MHz to allow for *in vivo* attenuation, $f^* = f/(1\ MHz)$, f is the center frequency of the transducer, and a is 0.5 for physiologically relevant fluids.[46]

Overview of Observed Bioeffects

A summary of results from several investigators (Fig. 2-10) indicates the mechanical index above which bioeffects associated with cavitation have been observed in animals and insects.[17] The dotted lines are calculations for several values of the mechanical index where all of the effects appear to occur at or above an MI value of 0.3. However, it should be noted that in many of these cases stable pockets of gas (gas bodies) are known to exist in the exposed tissues. It is further suggested that other areas in the body containing gas bodies might also be particularly susceptible to ultrasound damage. These might include the intestinal lining, for example.[47]

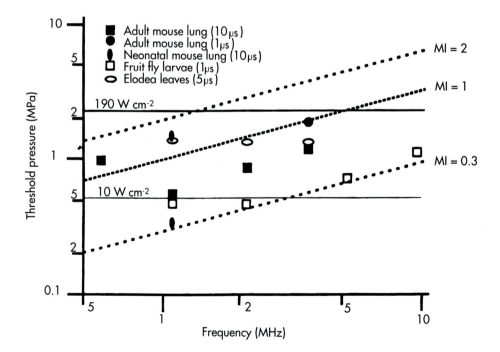

FIG. 2-10. Threshold for bioeffects from low temporal-average-intensity, pulsed ultrasound. Data shown are the threshold for effects measured in peak rarefactional pressures (p− in Fig. 2-1) as a function of ultrasound frequency used in the exposure. Pulse durations are shown in parentheses in the legend. Also shown for reference purposes are the values for the mechanical index and the local spatial peak, pulse average intensity I_{SPPA}. (From American Institute of Ultrasound in Medicine. *Bioeffects and Safety of Diagnostic Ultrasound.* Rockville, Md: American Institute of Ultrasound in Medicine; 1993.)

Experimentation continues, and it remains to be seen if such damage occurs in human tissue.

Additional Comments on the Mechanical Index

Inherent in the formulation of the MI are the conditions only for the onset of inertial cavitation. The degree to which the threshold is exceeded, however, relates to the degree of bubble activity that may occur, and the amount of bubble activity may correlate with the probability of an undesirable bioeffect. Note that given our present knowledge, exceeding the cavitation threshold does *not* mean there will be a bioeffect. Below an MI of 0.7, the physical conditions probably do not exist to promote bubble growth even in the presence of a broad bubble nuclei distribution in the body. Moreover, whereas the thermal index is a *time averaged* measure of the interaction of ultrasound with tissue, the MI is a *peak* measure of this interaction. Thus there is a desirable parallel between these two measures, one thermal and one mechanical, for informing the user of the extent to which the diagnostic tool can produce undesirable changes in the body.

Summary Statement on Gas Bodies Bioeffects

The AIUM statement concerning bioeffects in locations where gas bodies exist[17] (see box) includes several conclusions that can be summarized as follows:

- Current ultrasound systems can produce cavitation *in vitro* and *in vivo* and can cause blood extravasation in animal tissues.
- A mechanical index can gauge the likelihood for cavitation and apparently works better than other field parameters in predicting cavitation.
- Several interesting results have been observed concerning animal models for lung damage, which indicate a very low threshold for damage, but the implications for human exposure are not yet determined.
- In the absence of gas bodies, the threshold for damage is much higher. (This last point is significant because ultrasound examinations may be performed predominantly in tissues with no identifiable gas bodies.)

OUTPUT DISPLAY STANDARD

Several groups, including the FDA, AIUM, and NEMA, have developed the *Standard for Real-Time Display of Thermal and Mechanical Acoustical Output Indices on Diagnostic Ultrasound Equipment*, which introduces a method to provide the user with information concerning the thermal and mechanical

GAS BODIES BIOEFFECTS: CONCLUSIONS REGARDING GAS BODIES

1. The temporal peak outputs of some currently available diagnostic ultrasound devices can exceed the threshold for cavitation in vitro and can generate levels that produce extravasation of blood cells in the lungs of laboratory animals.

2. A mechanical index (MI)* has been formulated to assist users in evaluating the likelihood of cavitation-related adverse biological effects for diagnostically relevant exposures. The MI is a better indicator than derated spatial peak, pulse average intensity ($I_{SPPA.3}$), or derated peak rarefactional pressure ($_{Pr.3}$) for known adverse nonthermal biological effects of ultrasound.

3. Thresholds for adverse nonthermal effects depend on tissue characteristics and ultrasound parameters such as pressure amplitude, pulse duration, and frequency. Thus far, biologically significant, adverse, nonthermal effects have only been identified with certainty for diagnostically relevant exposures in tissues that have well-defined populations of stabilized gas bodies. For extravasation of blood cells in postnatal mouse lung, the threshold values of MI increase with decreasing pulse duration in the 1 to 100 µs range, increase with decreasing exposure time, and are weakly dependent on pulse repetition frequency. The threshold value of MI for extravasation of blood cells in mouse lung is approximately 0.3. The implications of these observations for human exposure are yet to be determined.

4. No extravasation of blood cells was found in mouse kidneys exposed to peak pressures in situ corresponding to an MI of 4. Furthermore, for diagnostically relevant exposures, no independently confirmed, biologically significant adverse nonthermal effects have been reported in mammalian tissues that do not contain well-defined gas bodies.

*The MI is equal to the derated peak rarefactional pressure (in MPa) at the point of the maximum pulse intensity integral divided by the square root of the ultrasonic center frequency (in MHz).[8]

From American Institute of Ultrasound in Medicine. *Bioeffects and Safety of Diagnostic Ultrasound.* Laurel, Md: American Institute of Ultrasound in Medicine; 1993.

indices. Real-time display of the MI and TI will allow a more informed decision on the potential for bioeffects during exams. The standard requires dynamic updates of the indices as instrument output is modified and provides the opportunity for the operator to learn how controls will affect these indices. Fig. 2-11 shows an example of an ultrasound system displaying

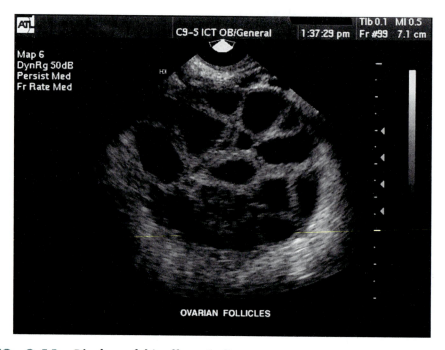

FIG. 2-11. Display of bioeffects indices. Typical appearance of an ultrasound scanner display showing the TI and MI *(right upper corner)* for an endocavitary transducer.

the mechanical index. There are a few important things to remember about this display standard:

- It should be clearly visible on the screen and should begin to appear when the instrument exceeds an index value of 0.4. An exception is made for those instruments incapable of exceeding index values of 1. Those instruments are not required to display the bioeffects indices.
- Sometimes only one index will be displayed at a time. The choice is often based on whether a given output condition is more likely to produce an effect by either mechanism.
- The standard also requires that appropriate default output settings be in effect at power-up, new patient entry, or when changing to a fetal examination. After that time the operator can adjust the instrument output as necessary to acquire clinically useful information while attempting to minimize the index values.
- As indicated previously, the bioeffects indices do not include any factors associated with the time taken to perform the scan. Efficient scanning is still an important component in limiting potential bioeffects.

The AIUM document entitled *Medical Ultrasound Safety*[48] suggests that the operator ask four questions to effectively use the output display.

1. Which index should be used for the exam being performed?

2. Are there factors present that might cause the reading to be too high or low?
3. Can the index value be reduced further even when it is already low?
4. How can the ultrasound exposure be minimized without compromising the diagnostic quality of the exam?

Clinicians are being presented with real-time data on acoustic output of diagnostic scanners and are being asked not only to understand the manner in which ultrasound propagates through and interacts with tissue, but also to gauge the potential for adverse bioeffects. The output display is a tool that can be used to guide an ultrasound exam and control for potential adverse effects. The thermal and mechanical indices provide the user with more information and more responsibility in limiting outputs.

GENERAL AIUM SAFETY STATEMENTS

It is important to consider some official positions concerning the status of bioeffects resulting from ultrasound. The most important item to note is the high level of confidence in the safety of ultrasound in official statements. For example, in 1993 the AIUM reiterated its earlier statement concerning the clinical use of diagnostic ultrasound (see box in left column on next page) by stating that no known bioeffects have

AIUM SAFETY STATEMENTS

American Institute of Ultrasound in Medicine Official Statement on Clinical Safety. Approved October 1983; revised and approved March 1988; reapproved March 1993 by AIUM.[49]

Diagnostic ultrasound has been in use since the late 1950s. Given its known benefits and recognized efficacy for medical diagnosis, including use during human pregnancy, the American Institute of Ultrasound in Medicine herein addresses the clinical safety of such use:

> No confirmed biological effects on patients or instrument operators caused by exposure at intensities typical of present diagnostic ultrasound instruments have ever been reported. Although the possibility exists that such biological effects may be identified in the future, current data indicate that the benefits to patients of the prudent use of diagnostic ultrasound outweigh the risks, if any, that may be present.

American Institute of Ultrasound in Medicine Official Statement on Safety in Training and Research. Approved March 1983; revised and approved March 1988; reapproved March 1993 by AIUM.[49]

Diagnostic ultrasound has been in use since the late 1950s. No confirmed adverse biological effects on patients resulting from this usage have ever been reported. Although no hazard has been identified that would preclude the prudent and conservative use of diagnostic ultrasound in education and research, experience from normal diagnostic practice may or may not be relevant to extended exposure times and altered exposure conditions. It is therefore considered appropriate to make the following recommendation:

> In those special situations in which examinations are to be carried out for purposes other than direct medical benefit to the individual being examined, the subject should be informed of the anticipated exposure conditions and of how these compare with conditions for normal diagnostic practice.

Reprinted with permission.

MAMMALIAN *IN VIVO* ULTRASONIC BIOLOGICAL EFFECTS

American Institute of Ultrasound in Medicine Statement on Mammalian *In Vivo* Ultrasonic Bioeffects. Approved August 1976; Reapproved October 1992 by AIUM.[49]

Information from experiments utilizing laboratory mammals has contributed significantly to our understanding of ultrasonically induced biological effects and the mechanisms that are most likely responsible. The following statement summarizes observations relative to specific ultrasound parameters and indices. The history and rationale for this statement are provided in *Bioeffects and Safety of Diagnostic Ultrasound* (AIUM, 1993).[17]

In the low megahertz frequency range there have been no adverse biological effects in mammalian tissues exposed *in vivo* under experimental ultrasound conditions, as follows.

a. When a thermal mechanism is involved, these conditions are unfocused beam-intensities* below 100 mW/cm^2, focused†-beam intensities below 1 W/cm^2, or thermal index values less than 2. Furthermore, such effects have not been reported for higher values of thermal index when it is less than

$$6 - \frac{\log_{10}(t)}{0.6}$$

where t is exposure time ranging from 1 to 250 minutes, including off time for pulsed exposure.

b. When a nonthermal mechanism is involved‡ in tissues that contain well-defined gas bodies, these conditions are in situ peak rarefactional pressures below approximately 0.3 MPa or mechanical index values less than approximately 0.3. Furthermore, for other tissues no such effects have been reported.

*Free-field spatial peak, temporal average (SPTA) for continuous wave and pulsed exposures.
†Quarter-power (−6 dB) beam width smaller than four wavelengths or 4 mm, whichever is less at the exposure frequency.
‡For diagnostically relevant ultrasound exposures.
Reprinted with permission.

been confirmed for the use of *present diagnostic equipment* and although it remains a possibility, the patient benefits for prudent use outweigh the risks if any that exist. In a similar fashion, the AIUM commented on the use of diagnostic ultrasound in research by recommending that in the case of exposure for other than direct medical benefit, the person be informed concerning the exposure conditions and how

these relate to normal exposures. For the most part, examinations even for research purposes are comparable to normal diagnostic exams and pose no additional risk. In fact, many research exams can be performed in conjunction with routine exams.

The effects based on *in vivo* animal models can be summarized by the AIUM conclusion statement shown in the box above.[17] No independently confirmed experimental evidence indicates damage in animal models below certain prescribed levels (TI<2 and MI<0.3). The level for the MI is strict because tissues containing gas bodies exhibit damage at much lower levels than tissues devoid of gas bodies. Biological effects have not been detected even at an MI of 4 in the absence of gas bodies (see box on p. 49).

EPIDEMIOLOGY

With all of the potential causes for bioeffects, one must now examine the epidemiologic evidence that has been used in part to justify the apparent safety of ultrasound. Many studies of an epidemiologic nature have been conducted over the last three decades. Ziskin and Petitti, who reviewed these studies in 1988, concluded, "epidemiologic studies and surveys in widespread clinical usage over 25 years have yielded no evidence of any adverse effect from diagnostic ultrasound."[50]

Epidemiologic studies are difficult to conduct, and data analysis and interpretation of results are perhaps even more difficult. Several epidemiologic studies of fetal exposure to ultrasound have claimed to detect certain bioeffects and have also been a subject of criticism. Only one indication of an unspecified effect was reported in a general survey involving an estimated 1.2 million examinations in Canada.[51] However, this is an extremely low rate of incidence of an unspecified effect. In addition, an earlier study that included 121,000 fetal exams reported no effect.[52] Moore et al. reported an increased incidence of low birth weight.[53] However, Stark et al. examined the same data using a different statistical treatment and found no significant increase.[54] Abnormal grasp and tonic neck reflexes were noted by Scheidt et al.[55]; however, these results are difficult to interpret given the statistical treatment of the data. Increased incidence of dyslexia was de-

tected in a study by Stark et al.,[54] yet the same children exhibited below average birth weights. As with these studies, there are a number of general problems that plague the epidemiologic studies. These include the lack of clearly stated exposure conditions and gestational age, problems in statistical sampling, which applies to both positive *and negative* results, and use of less than current scanning systems particularly with regard to use of fetal Doppler.

Ziskin and Petitti also provided a summary and discussion of the factors involved in the evaluation of epidemiologic evidence.[50] It is important to recognize that epidemiologic evidence can be used to identify an association between exposures and biologic effects, but this does not prove that the exposure caused that bioeffect. The strength of the association is established by the statistical significance of the relationship. Hill,[56] Salvesen,[57] and Ziskin[58] have developed seven criteria for judging **causality:**

- Strength of the association;
- Consistency in reproducibility and with previous related research;
- Specificity to a particular bioeffect or exposure site;
- Classical time relationship of cause followed by effect;
- Existence of a dose response;
- Plausibility of the effect; and
- Supporting evidence from laboratory studies.

When considering these factors, there seems not to be a clear causal relationship between an adverse biologic response and ultrasound exposure of a diagnostic nature.

Recent experiments have raised the question of potential associations. The first is the Newnham et al. study, which reported the observation of higher intrauterine growth restriction during a study designed to determine the efficacy of ultrasound in reducing the number of neonatal days and prematurity rate.[59] Therefore the study was not designed to detect an adverse bioeffect, but a statistically significant one was observed as a result of subsequent data analysis. Several other deficiencies in methodology are evident in the selection and exposure of their experimental groups, but in general some association might be inferred from the results of this well-conducted, randomized clinical trial. In a case-control study, Campbell et al. reported a statistically significant higher rate of delayed speech in those children who were insonified *in utero.*[60] Case-control studies do not provide as strong evidence of association as prospective studies, and measures of delayed speech are difficult. Follow-up prospective studies will be necessary to confirm these findings.

In 1995 the AIUM revised and approved a statement regarding the epidemiology of diagnostic ultrasound safety (see box on opposite page).[49] This state-

AIUM EPIDEMIOLOGY STATEMENT

Conclusions Regarding Epidemiology. Approved March 1995 by AIUM.[49]

Based on the epidemiologic evidence to date and on current knowledge of interaction mechanisms, there is insufficient justification to warrant a conclusion that there is a causal relationship between diagnostic ultrasound and adverse effects.

Reprinted with permission.

ment differs only slightly from that approved in 1987 in which the statement was made that no confirmed effects associated with ultrasound exposure existed at that time. The distinction being made is that although some effects may have been detected now, one cannot justify a conclusion of a causal relationship based on this evidence.

CONTROLLING ULTRASOUND OUTPUT: KNOBOLOGY

Perhaps the most important aspect of a discussion of potential bioeffects is what the physician or sonographer can do to minimize these effects. It is essential that operators understand the risks involved in the process, but without some ability to control the output of the ultrasound system, this knowledge has limited use. Some specific methods can be used to limit ultrasound exposure while maintaining diagnostically relevant images.

Controls for the ultrasound system can be divided into two groups for the purposes of this discussion. These are **direct controls** and **indirect controls.** The direct controls are the **application types** and **output intensity.** Application types are those broad system controls that allow convenient selection of a particular examination type. These often come in the form of icons that are selected by the user. These default settings help to minimize the time required to optimize the imaging parameters for the myriad of applications for diagnostic ultrasound. These settings should only be used as indicated; for example, do not use the cardiac settings for a fetal exam. Output intensity (which may be called "power," "output," or "transmit") controls the overall ultrasonic power emitted by the transducer. This control will generally affect the intensity at all points in the image to varying degrees, depending on the focusing. The lowest output intensity that produces a good image should be used to minimize the exposure intensity. Focusing of the system is controlled by the operator and can be used to improve image quality in order to limit required acoustic intensity. Focusing at the correct depth can improve the image without requiring increased intensity.

The **indirect controls** are numerous but greatly affect the ultrasound exposure by dictating how the ultrasonic energy is distributed temporally and spatially. By choosing the mode of ultrasound used (e.g., B-mode, pulsed Doppler, color Doppler), the operator controls whether the beam is scanned. Unscanned modes deposit energy along a single path and increase the potential for heating. The pulse repetition frequency (PRF) indicates how often the transducer is excited. Increasing the number of ultrasound bursts per second will increase the time average intensity. Control of the PRF is usually carried out by changing the maximum image depth in B-mode, or the velocity range in Doppler modes. **Burst length** (or "pulse length" or "pulse duration") controls the duration of on-time for each ultrasonic burst transmitted. Increasing the burst length while maintaining the same PRF will increase the time average intensity. The control of burst length may not be obvious. For example, in pulsed Doppler, increasing the Doppler sample volume length will increase the burst length.

The selection of the **appropriate transducer** will also limit the need for high acoustic power. Even though higher frequencies provide better spatial resolution, the attenuation of tissue increases with increasing ultrasound frequency, so penetration may be lost. Perhaps most important are the **receiver gain controls.** The receiver gain control does not affect the amplitude of the acoustic output in any way. Therefore before turning up the acoustic output intensity, try increasing receiver gain first. It should be noted that some system controls actually interact with the acoustic output intensity without direct control. Check to see whether the manufacturer provides separate controls for receiver gain, **time gain compensation (TGC),** and acoustic output intensity. The time gain compensation (TGC) can improve image quality without increasing the output.

There is really no substitute for a well-instructed operator. The indices and requirement of output display standards will help only those willing to use and understand them. Real-time display of the mechanical and thermal indices on diagnostic scanners will help clinicians evaluate and minimize potential risks in the use of such instrumentation. Physicians and sonographers are encouraged to learn more about the role they can play in minimizing the potential effects.

METHODS TO DECREASE ULTRASOUND EXPOSURE

- Use specific application per body part (set for safe power level)
- Keep power low
- Focus at specific depth (improves image with increased intensity)
- Choose scanned modes over unscanned modes (sector B-mode less intensity than M-mode)
- Use fewer ultrasound pulses per second (PRF)
- Decrease pulse length
- Use appropriate transducer
- Increase receiver gain rather than power

REFERENCES
Thermal Effects

1. Hynynen K. Ultrasound therapy. In: Goldman LE, Fowlkes JB, eds. *Medical CT and Ultrasound: Current Technology and Applications.* Madison, Wis: Advanced Medical Publishing; 1995:249-265.

2. Carstensen EL, Child SZ, Norton S et al. Ultrasonic heating of the skull. *J Acoust Soc Am* 1990;87:1310-1317.

3. Nyborg WL. Solutions of the bio-heat transfer equation. *Phys Med Biol* 1988;33(7):785-792.

4. Drewniak JL, Carnes KI, Dunn F. In vitro ultrasonic heating of fetal bone. *J Acoust Soc Am* 1989;86:1254-1258.

5. Edwards MJ. Hyperthermia as a teratogen: a review of experimental studies and their clinical significance. *Teratogenesis Carcinog Mutagen* 1986;6:563-582.

6. Miller MW, Ziskin MC. Biological consequences of hyperthermia. *Ultrasound Med Biol* 1989;15:707-722.

7. Scientific Committee on Biological Effects of Ultrasound. *Exposure Criteria for Medical Diagnostic Ultrasound. I. Criteria Based on Thermal Mechanisms.* Bethesda, Md: National Council on Radiation Protection and Measurements; 1992. Report no. 113.

8. American Institute of Ultrasound in Medicine and National Electrical Manufacturers Association. *Standard for Real-Time Display of Thermal and Mechanical Acoustical Output Indices on Diagnostic Ultrasound Equipment,* Rockville, Md: American Institute of Ultrasound in Medicine and National Electrical Manufacturers Association; 1992.

9. Carson PL. Medical ultrasound fields and exposure measurements. In: *Nonionizing Electromagnetic Radiations and Ultrasound.* Bethesda, Md: National Council on Radiation Protection and Measurements; 1988:287-307. NCRP Proceedings no. 8.

10. Carson PL, Rubin JM, Chiang EH. Fetal depth and ultrasound path lengths through overlying tissues. *Ultrasound Med Biol* 1989;15:629-663.

11. Thomenius KE. Scientific rationale for the TIS index model. Presented at the National Electrical Manufacturers Association Output Display Standard Seminar; 1993; Rockville, Md.

12. Thomenius KE. Estimation of the potential for bioeffects. In: Ziskin MC, Lewin PA, eds. *Ultrasonic Exposimetry.* Ann Arbor, Mich: CRC Press; 1993.

13. Siddiqi T, O'Brien WD, Meyer RA et al. In situ exposimetry: the ovarian ultrasound examination. *Ultrasound Med Biol* 1991;17:257-263.

14. Chan AK, Sigelman RA, Guy AW et al. Calculation by the method of finite differences of the temperature distribution in layered tissues. *IEEE Trans Biomed Eng* 1973;BME-20:86-90.

15. Chan AK, Sigelman RA, Guy AW. Calculations of therapeutic heat generated by ultrasound in fat-muscle-bone layers. *IEEE Trans Biomed Eng* 1974;BME-21:280-284.

16. Frizzell LA. *Ultrasonic Heating of Tissues.* Rochester, NY: University of Rochester; 1975. Dissertation.

17. American Institute of Ultrasound in Medicine. *Bioeffects and Safety of Diagnostic Ultrasound.* Rockville, Md: American Institute of Ultrasound in Medicine; 1993.

Effects of Acoustic Cavitation

18. Flynn HG. Cavitation dynamics. I. A mathematical formulation. *J Acoust Soc Am* 1975;57:1379-1396.

19. Roy RA, Atchley AA, Crum LA et al. A precise technique for measurement of acoustic cavitation thresholds and some preliminary results. *J Acoust Soc Am* 1985;78(5):1799-1805.

20. Kwak H-Y, Panton RL. Tensile strength of simple liquids predicted by a model of molecular interactions. *J Phys D* 1985;18:647.

21. Harvey EN, Barnes DK, McElroy WD et al. Bubble formation in animals. I. Physical factors. *J Cell Compar Phys* 1944;24:1-22.

22. Harvey EN, Barnes DK, McElroy WD et al. Bubble formation in animals. II. Gas nuclei and their distribution in blood and tissues. *J Cell Compar Phys* 1944;24:23-34.

23. Yount DE. Skins of varying permeability: a stabilization mechanism for gas cavitation nuclei. *J Acoust Soc Am* 1978;65:1429-1439.

24. Holland CK, Roy RA, Apfel RE et al. In vitro detection of cavitation induced by a diagnostic ultrasound system. *IEEE Trans UFFC* 1992;39:95-101.

25. Walton AJ, Reynolds GT. Sonoluminescence. *Adv Physics* 1984;33:595-660.

26. Crum LA, Fowlkes JB. Acoustic cavitation generated by microsecond pulses of ultrasound. *Nature* 1986;319(6048):52-54.

27. Carmichael AJ, Mossoba MM, Riesz P et al. Free radical production in aqueous solutions exposed to simulated ultrasonic diagnostic conditions. *IEEE Trans UFFC* 33:148-155.

28. Aymé E, Carstensen EL. Occurrence of transient cavitation in pulsed sawtooth ultrasonic fields. *J Acoust Soc Am* 1988;84:1598-1605.

29. Coleman AJ, Saunders JE, Crum LA et al. Acoustic cavitation generated by an extracorporeal shockwave lithotripter. *Ultrasound Med Biol* 1987;15:213-227.

30. Delius M, Brendel W, Heine G. A mechanism of gallstone destruction by extracorporeal shock wave. *Naturwissenschaften* 1988;75:200-201.

31. Williams AR, Delius M, Miller DL et al. Investigation of cavitation in flowing media by lithotripter shock waves both in vitro and in vivo. *Ultrasound Med Biol* 1989;15:53-60.

32. Coleman AJ, Saunders JE, Crum LA et al. Acoustic cavitation generated by an extracorporeal shockwave lithotripter. *Ultrasound Med Biol* 1987;13(2):69-76.

33. Duck FA, Starritt HC, Aindow JD et al. The output of pulse-echo ultrasound equipment: a survey of powers, pressures and intensities. *Br J Rad* 1985;58:989-1001.

34. Duck FA, Starritt HC, Anderson SP. A survey of the acoustic output of ultrasonic Doppler equipment. *Clin Phys Physiol Meas* 1987;8:39-49.

35. Patton CA, Harris GR, Phillips RA. Output levels and bioeffects indices from diagnostic ultrasound exposure data reported to the FDA. *IEEE Trans Ultrason Ferroelec Freq Contr* 1994;41:353-359.

36. Chaussy C, Schmiedt E, Jocham D et al. *Extracorporeal Shock Wave Lithotripsy* Basel: Karger; 1986.

37. Child SZ, Hartman CL, Schery LA et al. Lung damage from exposure to pulse ultrasound. *Ultrasound Med Biol* 1990;16:817-825.

38. Penney DP, Schenk EA, Maltby K et al. Morphological effects of pulsed ultrasound in the lung. *Ultrasound Med Biol* 1993;19:127-135.

39. Tarantal AF, Canfield DR. Ultrasound-induced lung hemorrhage in the monkey. *Ultrasound Med Biol* 1994;20:65-72.

40. Tyler WS, Julian WD. Gross and subgross anatomy of lungs, pleura, connective tissue septa, distal airways, and structural units. In: Parent RA, ed. *Treatise on Pulmonary Toxicology. Vol. I. Comparative Biology of the Normal Lung.* Boca Raton, Fla: CRC Press; 1992:35-58.

41. Holland CK, Apfel RE. An improved theory for the prediction of microcavitation thresholds. *IEEE Trans Ultrason Ferroelec Freq Contr* 1989;36:204-208.

42. Holland CK, Apfel RE. Thresholds for transient cavitation produced by pulsed ultrasound in a controlled nuclei environment. *J Acoust Soc Am* 1990;88:2059-2069.

43. Holland CK, Roy RA, Apfel RE et al. In vitro detection of cavitation induced by a diagnostic ultrasound system. *IEEE Trans Ultrason Ferroelec Freq Contr* 1992;39:95-101.

44. Holland CK, Zheng X, Apfel RE et al. Direct evidence of cavitation in vivo from diagnostic ultrasound. *Ultrasound Med Biol* accepted for publication, 1996.

45. Roy RA, Madanshetty S, Apfel RE. An acoustic backscattering technique for the detection of transient cavitation produced by microsecond pulses of ultrasound. *J Acoust Soc Am* 1990;87:2451-2455.

46. Apfel RE, Holland CK. Gauging the likelihood of cavitation from short-pulse, low-duty cycle diagnostic ultrasound. *Ultrasound Med Biol* 1991;17:179-185.

47. Dalecki D, Raeman CH, Child SZ et al. A test for cavitation as a mechanism for intestinal hemorrhage in mice exposed to a piezoelectric lithotripter. *Ultrasound Med Biol* 1996;22:493-496.

48. American Institute of Ultrasound in Medicine. *Medical Ultrasound Safety*. Rockville, Md: American Institute of Ultrasound in Medicine; 1994.

49. AIUM Safety Statement. Approved March 1995. Current versions are available to the public upon request.

50. Ziskin MC, Petitti DB. Epidemiology of human exposure to ultrasound: a critical review. *Ultrasound Med Biol* 1988;14:91-96.

Epidemiology

51. EDH Environment Health Directorate. *Canada-Wide Survey of Nonionizing Radiation Emitting Medical Devices. II. Ultrasound Devices*. 1980. Report 80-EDH-53.

52. Ziskin MC. Survey of patient exposure to diagnostic ultrasound. In: Reid, Sikov, eds. *Interaction of Ultrasound and Biological Tissues*. 1972. US Dept of Health, Education, and Welfare publication FDA 78-8008:203.

53. Moore RM Jr, Barrick KM, Hamilton TM. Ultrasound exposure during gestation and birthweight. Presented at the Meeting of the Society for Epidemiological Research; June 16-18, 1982; Cincinnati, Ohio.

54. Stark CR, Orleans M, Haverkamp AD et al. Short- and long-term risks after exposure to diagnostic ultrasound in utero. *Obstet Gynecol* 1984;63:194-200.

55. Scheidt PC, Stanley F, Bryla DA. One-year follow-up of infants exposed to ultrasound in utero. *Am J Obstet Gynecol* 1978;131:743-748.

56. Hill AB. The environment and disease: association or causation? *Proceed Royal Soc Med* 1965;58:295-300.

57. Salveser KA, Eik-Nes SH. Is ultrasound unsound? A review of epidemiological studies of human exposure to ultrasound. *Ultrasound Obstet Gynecol* 1995;6(4):293-298.

58. Ziskin MC. Epidemiology of ultrasound exposure. *Ultrasound Med Biol* submitted for publication, 1996.

59. Newnham B, Evans SF, Michael CA. Effects of frequent ultrasound during pregnancy: a randomized controlled trial. *Lancet* 1993;342:887-891.

60. Campbell S, Elford RW, Brant RF. Case-control study of prenatal ultrasonography exposure in children with delayed speech. *Can Med Assoc J* 1993;149:1435-1440.

61. Nyborg WL, Steele RB. Temperature elevation in a beam of ultrasound. *Ultrasound Med Biol* 1983;9:611-620.

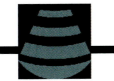

C H A P T E R   3

Contrast Agents for Ultrasound Imaging and Doppler

•

Peter N. Burns, Ph.D.

Contrast agents are a routine part of clinical x-ray, CT, MR, and radionuclide imaging. Yet in spite of the importance of the vascular component of an ultrasound examination, the modality has yet to exploit the potential benefit of contrast enhancement. Why? A common response from ultrasonographers is that in-travascular injections would detract from one of ultrasound's major attractions—that it is noninvasive. But this is a sentimental point of view. If it could be shown that the additional diagnostic information obtained with contrast enhancement would spare the patient from a more invasive procedure, we would be doing them no favor to deny them a painless intravenous injection. Another response appeals to the ultrasound image itself. When we look at an image of a blood vessel, we can see that there is a naturally high contrast between blood and solid tissue. It could be argued that we do not need a subtraction method to see blood. Furthermore, if we are interested in seeing where the blood flows, the Doppler shift associated with blood's rather weak echoes can be used to add to this contrast, as evidenced routinely by color Doppler imaging. Doppler also provides quantitative information about, for example, the direction and velocity of flow. In the early days of echocardiography, a B-mode image could be used to see blood in a cardiac chamber but not to see whether it was flowing across a septal defect. Bubbles were injected into the cavity and their trajectory imaged. That was really the first use of a contrast agent in ultrasound.[1] Yet this invasive procedure, which required catheterization, is no longer necessary; color Doppler imaging has largely supplanted the intra-arterial injection of bubbles in cardiac diagnosis. In spite of this, the most recent developments in ultrasound contrast for cardiac diagnosis are redefining the capabilities of echocardiography and, we argue here, are likely to do the same for ultrasound imaging and Doppler in radiology.

THE NEED FOR CONTRAST AGENTS IN ULTRASOUND

The major motivation for the current rapid rate of development of contrast agents for ultrasound lies in the nature of the current performance limits of ultrasound imaging and Doppler. Consider the bifurcation structure of the vascular system: as ultrasound is used to investigate more peripheral vessels, the spatial resolution of imaging and the sensitivity of Doppler systems impose limits on the minimum size of detectable vessels. At present, most duplex and color Doppler imaging systems are capable of detecting flow from vessels whose lumina lie below the resolution of the image. The detection of such "unresolved" flow using Doppler systems can be demonstrated simply by using a duplex scanner to create a power Doppler image of the kidney, in which vessels that are not seen on the gray scale image become visible using the Doppler mode. These vessels are the arcuate and intralobular branches of the renal artery; their diameter is known to be less than 100 μm and therefore below the resolution limit of the image. However, as we progress distally in the arterial system, the blood flows more slowly as the rate of bifurcation increases, giving lower Doppler shift frequencies, and the quantity of blood in a given volume of tissue also decreases, weakening the backscattered echo. Eventually, a point is reached at which the vessel cannot be visualized and the Doppler signals cannot be detected.

Two factors determine where that point will lie: Doppler shift frequency and echo strength. First, the velocity of blood must be sufficient to produce a Doppler shift frequency that is distinguishable from that produced by the normal motion of tissue, and second, the received intensity of the backscattered ultrasound must provide adequate signal strength for detection by the transducer, above the acoustic and electrical noise of the system. Using a higher ultrasound frequency helps in both respects: the Doppler shift corresponding to a given flow velocity increases in proportion to the transmitted sound's frequency and the backscattered intensity increases with the fourth power of transmitted frequency, as predicted by the Rayleigh relationship.[2] In practice, of course, the penetration of the sound through tissue places an upper limit on the ultrasound frequency that can be used. For the deeper vessels of the abdomen, ultrasound frequencies above 5 MHz produce blood echoes whose amplitude at the skin surface is too small for detection by most current systems. In this and many other applications involving small vessels, it is the strength of the backscattered echo, rather than the Doppler shift frequency, that defines the smallest vessels from which Doppler signals can be detected. This limit of echo strength presents a barrier to the Doppler detection of flow in the vessels and organ parenchyma of the abdomen and pelvis as well as in the breast, testes, and extremities. It also defines the scale of the vasculature it is possible to detect in a neovascularized mass or a collateral vessel to a vascular occlusion. For the Doppler detection of blood flow in larger vessels, the effect of increasing the echo from blood is to enhance the signal-to-noise ratio, which again determines detectability in such vessels as the renal artery or the middle cerebral arteries when approached transcranially. There is, then, clear clinical potential for a method capable of enhancing the echo of moving blood, especially in the systemic arterial system.

CONTRAST AGENTS FOR ULTRASOUND

The principal requirements for an ultrasound contrast agent are that it be easily introducible into the vascular system, be stable for the duration of the diagnostic examination, have low toxicity, and modify one or more of the acoustic properties of tissues that determine the ultrasound imaging process. Although it is conceivable that applications may be found for ultrasound contrast agents that will justify their injection directly into arteries, the clinical context for contrast ultrasonography requires that they be capable of administration intravenously. As we shall see, these constitute demanding specifications for a drug—specifications that have only recently been met.

MODE OF ACTION

Contrast agents might act by their presence in the vascular system, from where they are ultimately metabolized (blood pool agents), or by their selective uptake in tissue after a vascular phase. Of the properties of tissue that influence the ultrasound image, the most important are backscatter coefficient, attenuation, and acoustic propagation velocity.[3] Most agents seek to enhance the echo by increasing as much as possible the backscatter of the tissue that bears them, while increasing as little as possible the attenuation in the tissue.

Blood Pool Agents

The concept of using an ultrasound contrast agent to enhance the blood pool echo was first introduced by Gramiak and Shah in 1968.[1] These investigators injected **saline** into the ascending aorta during echocardiographic recording. The saline gave rise to strong echoes within the normally echo-free lumen of the aorta and the chambers of the heart. Subsequent work showed that these reflections were the result of **free bubbles of air** that came out of solution either by agitation or by cavitation during the injection itself.

Many other solutions were found to produce a contrast effect when similarly injected.[4,5] The intensity of the echoes produced varied with the type of solution used; the more viscous the solution, the more microbubbles were trapped in a bolus for a sufficient length of time to be appreciated on the image. Agitated solutions of compounds such as **indocyanine green** and **Renografin** were also used. Most of the subsequent research into the application of these bubbles as ultrasound contrast agents focused on the heart, including evaluation of valvular insufficiency,[6,7] intracardiac shunts,[8] and cavity dimensions.[9] The fundamental limitation of bubbles produced in this way is that they are large, so they are effectively filtered by the lungs, and that they are unstable, so they go back into solution within a second or so. Hence, this procedure is invasive and, except by direct injection, unsuitable for the imaging of left-sided cardiac chambers, abdominal organs, or the systemic arterial tree.

To tackle the natural instability of free gas bubbles, various attempts have been made to encapsulate gas within a shell so as to create a more stable particle. In 1980 Carroll et al.[10] **encapsulated nitrogen bubbles in gelatin** and injected them into the femoral artery of rabbits with VX2 tumors in the thigh. Ultrasound enhancement of the tumor rim was identified. However, the large size of the particles (80 μm) precluded intravenous administration. The challenge to produce a stable, encapsulated microbubble of a size comparable to that of a red blood cell, one that could survive passage through the heart and the pulmonary capillary network, was first met by Feinstein et al. in 1984.[11] They produced microbubbles by sonication of a solution of **human serum albumin** and showed that it could be visualized in the left heart after a peripheral venous injection.

A burgeoning number of manufacturers have since produced forms of **stabilized microbubbles** that are currently being assessed for use as intravenous contrast agents for ultrasound. Several have passed through phase 3 clinical trials and gained regulatory approval in both Europe and North America. *Albunex*® (Molecular Biosystems Inc., San Diego, CA) is composed of air-filled human albumin microspheres produced by sonication having a mean size of approximately 3.5 microns (μm), ranging from 1 to 8 μm. The microparticles are stable ex vivo, with acoustic properties lasting 8 to 12 minutes in an albumin solution.[12] Albunex has been shown to pass successfully through the pulmonary capillary circulation of the lungs[13] and can produce left ventricular cavity opacification.[14] Additionally, Albunex® is stable enough following injection to produce consistent, dose-related Doppler signal enhancement in large and small arteries within the abdomen of small animals. However, transpulmonary survival of the agent in humans in sufficient concentration to provide diagnostic enhancement of images or Doppler studies of small vessels has yet to be demonstrated. Imaging studies of small, experimental hepatic tumors demonstrate the dramatic impact intravenous contrast injections can have on the detection of small vessels.[15] Note that in these studies, visible alterations to the gray level of the parenchymal ultrasound image were not detected, nor have they been reported elsewhere in the literature.

Levovist® (SHU508A, Schering AG, Berlin, Germany) is a stable mixture consisting of 99.9% specially manufactured microcrystalline galactose microparticles and 0.1% palmitic acid. Upon dissolution and agitation in sterile water for injection, the galactose disaggregates into microparticles that provide an irregular surface for the adherence of microbubbles 3 to 4 μm in size. Stabilization of the microbubbles takes place as they become coated with palmitic acid, which separates the gas-to-liquid interface and slows their dissolution.[16] These microbubbles are highly echogenic and are sufficiently stable for transit through the pulmonary circuit. The estimated median particle size is 1.8 μm and the median bubble diameter approximately 2 μm, with the 97th percentile approximately 6 μm.[17] The agent is chemically related to *Echovist*® (SHU454, Schering AG, Berlin, Germany), a galactose agent that forms larger bubbles and has been used extensively without any suggestion of toxicity.[30] Both preclinical[18] and clinical[19] studies with Levovist demonstrate its capacity to traverse the pulmonary bed in sufficient concentrations to enhance both color Doppler and, in some instances, the B-mode image itself.

The shells that stabilize the microbubbles are extremely thin so they allow a gas such as air to diffuse out and go back into solution in the blood. How fast this happens depends on a number of factors that have been seen to vary not only from agent to agent but also from patient to patient. After venous introduction, however, the effective duration of the two agents described above is on the order of a few minutes. Because they are introduced as a bolus and the maximum effect of the agent is in the first pass, the useful imaging time is usually considerably less than that. Newer agents, sometimes referred to as second-generation agents, designed both to increase backscatter enhancement further and to last longer in the bloodstream, are currently under experimental investigation. Instead of air, many of these agents take advantage of low-solubility gases such as **perfluorocarbons**; the consequent lower diffusion rate increases the longevity of the agent in the blood. *FS069* (Mallinckrodt Inc.) is a perfluoropropane-filled albumin shell with a size distribution similar to that of Albunex. The stability of the smaller bubbles in its population is the probable cause of the greater enhancement observed with this agent. *Echogen*® (Sonus Inc., Bothell, WA) is an emulsion of dodecafluoropentane droplets that undergo a phase change in the blood, literally boiling at body temperature. Recent reports suggest that this agent produces visible enhancement of the renal parenchyma on conventional gray scale imaging.[20] Yet another agent (*DMP115*, DuPont Merck Inc., Boston, MA) is a perfluoropropane microbubble coated with a bilipid shell; it also shows improved stability and high enhancements at low doses.[21]

Selective Uptake Agents

In addition to exploring free or encapsulated gas bubbles as contrast agents, investigators have devised other approaches to the enhancement of ultrasound images. They include **colloidal suspensions, emulsions,** and **aqueous solutions.** Of these, colloidal suspensions appear to hold the most promise for clinical application. Perfluorocarbons developed primarily as plasma volume expanders have been used as ultrasound contrast agents for parenchymal enhancement of organs such as the liver and spleen. **Perfluorooctlybromide** (PFOB) is a colloidal suspension with a density significantly higher (~1.9 g/ml) and a speed of sound significantly lower (~600 m/s) than that of tissue, yielding an acoustic impedance difference of about 30%. Although the particles of liquid responsible for the scattering are much less efficient than bubbles of gas, they are somewhat more stable, and they have the potential advantage of remaining intact while phagocytosis takes place. After PFOB is administered intravenously in emulsion form, it remains within the intravascular space for a relatively long period, after which it is taken up by the reticuloendothelial system and finally breathed out by the lungs and secreted in the bile. Echo enhancement of the liver or spleen is noticeable about 6 hours after administration.[22] Production of an echogenic "rim" around liver tumors in the delayed phase has also been reported with PFOB.[23] A major limitation of PFOB to date is its long half-life in the body. Another particulate agent is made of **iodipimide ethyl ester** (IDE) formulated as biocompatible, micron-sized, spherical particles.[24] When IDE particles are injected intravenously, the Kupffer cells of the hepatic sinusoids accumulate particles within 10 to 20 minutes, after which clearance and excretion take place. During the uptake phase, the scattering increases the echogenicity of normal liver tissue. In comparison, tumors and other lesions that lack Kupffer cells remain at preinjection echogenicity, thus providing a new potential way of identifying liver masses.[25] That these particles need to be present within liver cells in sufficient concentration to produce

visible enhancement of the liver parenchyma on B-mode scanning raises the potential problem of toxicity, one that might be overcome if a more sensitive method of detecting particles in solid tissue could be devised. One potential approach is discussed later.

THE IMPACT OF CONTRAST ENHANCEMENT

In a Doppler examination, the arrival of the contrast agent, some seconds after peripheral venous injection, in the portion of the systemic vasculature under interrogation is marked by a dramatic increase in signal strength. In spectral Doppler this is seen as an intensifying of the gray scale of the spectrum. For a given vessel, this enhancement is related to dose (Fig. 3-1). For spectral Doppler examinations that fail because of lack of signal strength, the effect of the contrast agent is to rescue the examination.

In color Doppler, it should be remembered that the parameter mapped to color is the estimated Doppler shift frequency, which corresponds to the relative blood flow velocity; color should therefore remain unaltered by contrast enhancement. What does change, however, is the range of locations from which color signals are detected. To avoid the display of color noise, most ultrasound systems do not display color in a given pixel unless a Doppler signal is detected above a certain threshold level. The effect of a contrast agent is to raise the signal from small vessels above that threshold to the point at which they are effectively detectable on a color image. Thus, more vessels appear in a contrast-enhanced ultrasound image. Fig. 3-2 illustrates small-vessel detection in the neovasculature of naturally occurring hepatocellular carcinomas in a small animal. The spectral display (Fig. 3-2, *A* and 3-2, *B*) of vessels at the periphery of one tumor shows enhancement of the signal, while color imaging of another 1-cm tumor (Fig. 3-2, *C* and 3-2, *D*) demonstrates the vascular rim around the lesion (which is isoechoic) only after administration of the agent. Fig. 3-2, *E* shows the same vessels angiographically.

In the past few years, many studies have been carried out in which the sole indication for contrast agents has been a nondiagnostic Doppler examination. These have demonstrated the capacity of contrast agents to increase the technical success rate of Doppler ultrasound. For example, in clinical transcranial Doppler studies of the middle cerebral artery, administration of 10 ml of Levovist® in concentrations of 200, 300, and 400 mg/ml resulted in dose-dependent increases in both signal intensity and duration of enhancement.[26] At a concentration of 400 mg/ml, Levovist® increased the Doppler signal by approximately 25 dB. The time to peak enhancement was be-

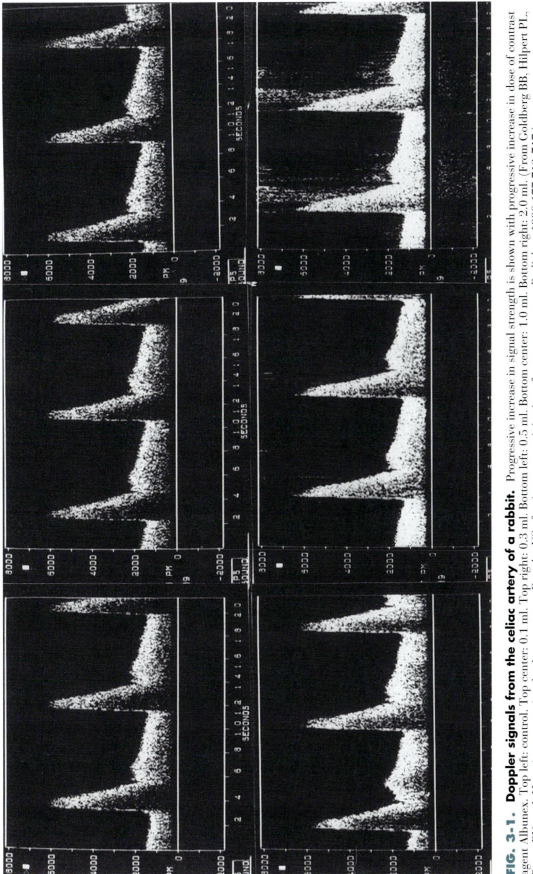

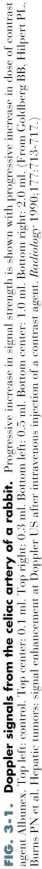

FIG. 3-1. Doppler signals from the celiac artery of a rabbit. Progressive increase in signal strength is shown with progressive increase in dose of contrast agent Albunex. Top left: control. Top center: 0.1 ml. Top right: 0.3 ml. Bottom left: 0.5 ml. Bottom center: 1.0 ml. Bottom right: 2.0 ml. (From Goldberg BB, Hilpert PL, Burns PN et al. Hepatic tumors: signal enhancement at Doppler US after intravenous injection of a contrast agent. *Radiology* 1990;177:713-717.)

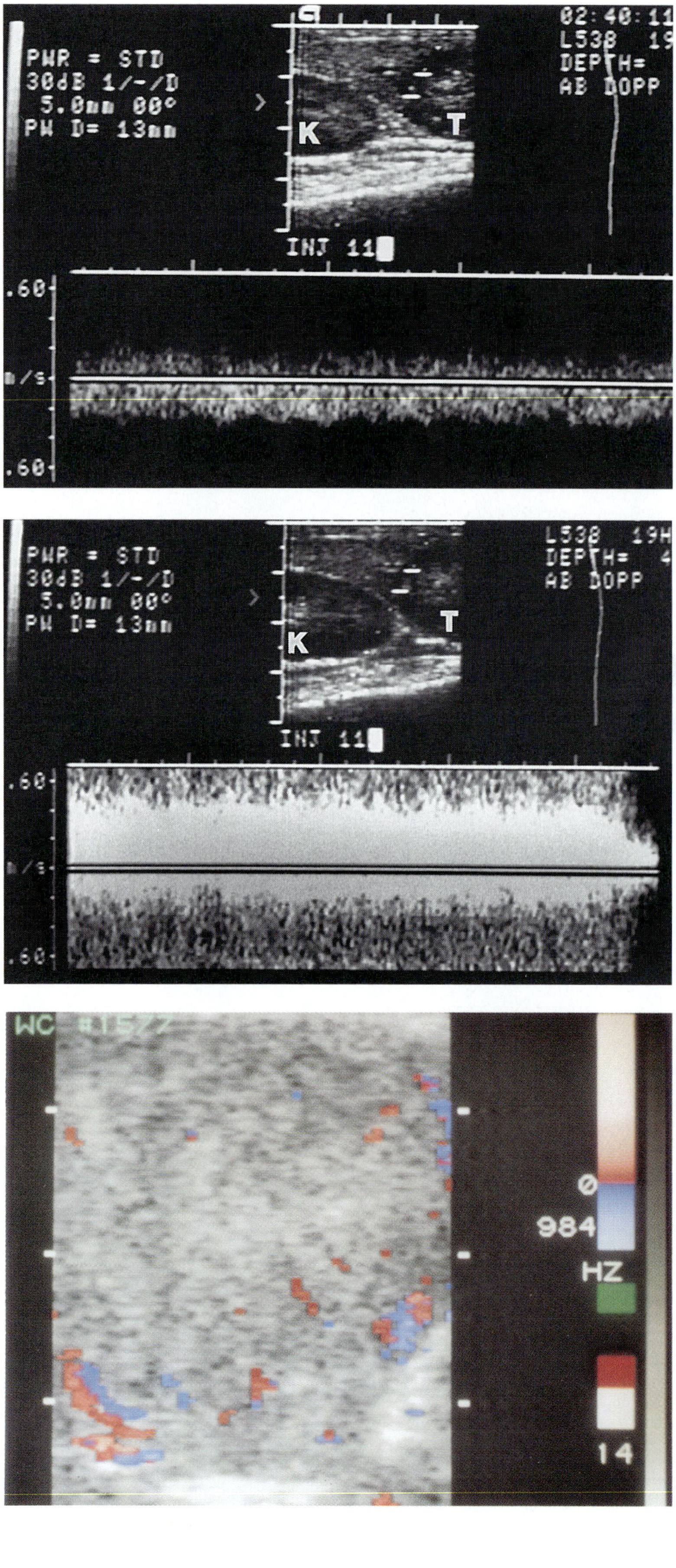

FIG. 3-2. Albunex® in hepatocellular carcinomas of a woodchuck. Duplex Doppler study in two 4 kg animals, with intravenous injection. **A,** 5 MHz sample volume situated in tumor (T), preinjection. Note inferior pole of right kidney (K). **B,** After 1 ml Albunex® administered in jugular vein. Note that enhancement of this signal exceeds the dynamic range of the spectral display. **C,** Color imaging of a 1 cm tumor, preinjection.

Continued.

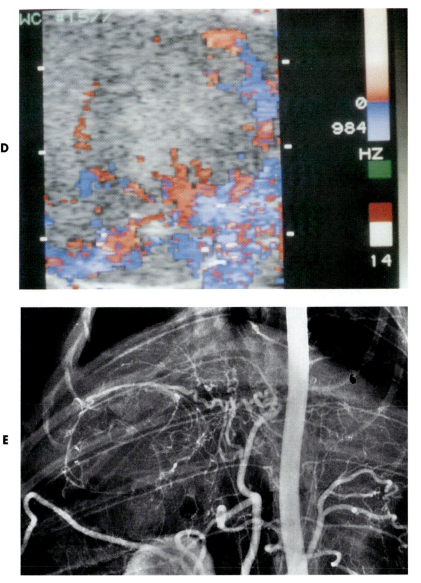

FIG. 3-2, cont'd. D, Postperipheral venous injection of 1 ml. The gray level of the tumor parenchyma has not changed, but the enhancement of the detected Doppler signals demarcates the tumor margin. The ultrasound frequency is 7.5 MHz. Note that the criterion for the detection of the contrast agent using conventional color Doppler systems is the extent of the detected Doppler signal, not the color itself. Note also that in the postinjection image, gray levels are not detectably changed by the contrast agent. E, Arteriogram showing detected vasculature at tumor rim. (From Goldberg BB, Hilpert PL, Burns PN et al. Hepatic tumors: signal enhancement at Doppler US after intravenous injection of a contrast agent. *Radiology* 1990;177:713-717.)

tween 30 and 60 seconds and the duration of enhancement was reported to be sufficiently long to be clinically useful. In another transcranial study, the agent reduced the technical failure rate by 80%.[27,28] In cardiac diagnosis, the agent Levovist® also improved the technical success rate in quantitative Doppler assessment of aortic stenosis, mitral regurgitation, and pulmonary venous flow, in which case it rose 27% to 80%.[29]

In radiologic studies, the enhanced detection of small-vessel flow by spectral and color Doppler flow with contrast agents has been demonstrated in a number of clinical studies, including observation of flow in the renal parenchyma[30] and in tumors of the breast,[31,32] prostate,[33] and liver.[34] In the liver, for example, otherwise undetectable flow was seen in 54 of 74 solid lesions.[35] Another study demonstrated that

these findings correlated well with angiographic findings.[36] If the target vessel is large and the flow detectable, the impact of the agent may be to shorten the examination time; in one study, Levovist® halved the examination time for the duplex investigation of renal artery stenosis.[37] Yet, another study suggested improved accuracy in measuring peripheral vascular velocity when contrast is used.[38] The effect of the agent may be considered in other ways, too. For example, given a satisfactory color Doppler study of the abdomen, one use of the agent might simply be to enable a higher ultrasound frequency to be used, exploiting the agent to counter the higher tissue attenuation. In such a case, the contrast enhancement translates into higher spatial resolution. Alternatively, the color system may be set to use fewer pulses per scan line (that is, a lower ensemble length) while still achieving

LATERAL BLOOMING

AXIAL BLOOMING

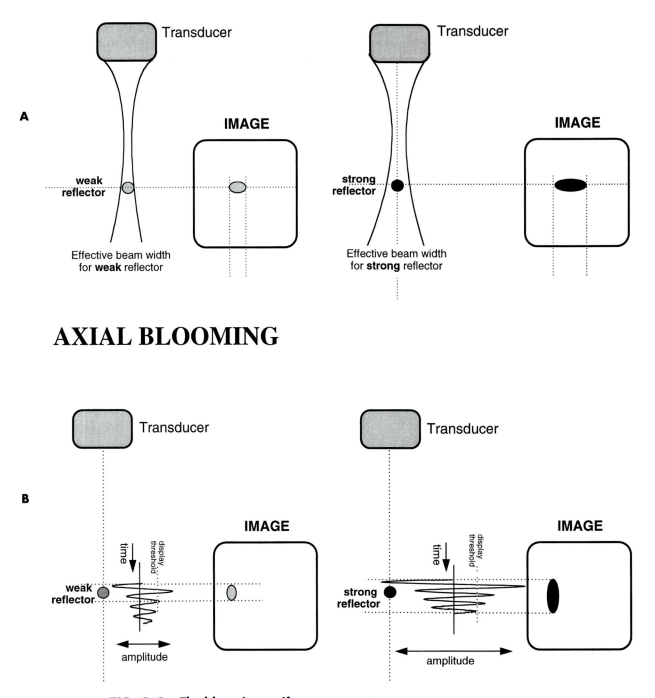

FIG. 3-3. The blooming artifact. A, Lateral blooming: the beam does not have a perfectly sharp boundary, but has tapered sensitivity in a lateral direction. Stronger targets such as the contrast-enhanced vessel are therefore artifactually imaged to extend in a lateral direction. **B,** Axial blooming: in a similar way, the ultrasound pulse does not have a uniform amplitude over its duration. Axial blooming is generally less severe than lateral blooming.

Continued.

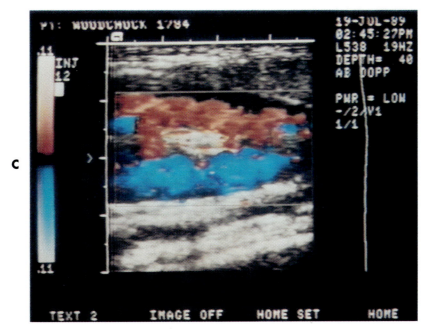

FIG. 3-3, cont'd. C, An example of blooming in a contrast-enhanced image.

the same sensitivity to blood flow by means of the contrast enhancement. The agent will then provide the user with a higher frame rate.

With these agents, enhancement is not usually seen on the gray scale image of the blood vessel lumen or in the vascular parenchyma of organs such as the liver and kidney, even though the agent is present and enhancing the Doppler signal. This is because blood is a very weak scatterer of ultrasound and provides an echo whose power is some 30 to 40 dB (1000 to 10,000 times) lower than the echo from solid tissue such as the vessel wall. The contrast agent can boost this by 10 to 20 dB (100 to 1000 times) without bringing the echo up to a level at which it can be seen on the gray scale image. In order to enhance the visible gray level, either higher concentrations of bubbles must be achieved or specific, new imaging strategies must be employed.

ARTIFACTS IN CONTRAST STUDIES

Contrast-enhanced studies subject the ultrasound system to signals that, on the whole, it was not designed to encounter. As with all ultrasound images, appreciation of potential artifacts helps in their interpretation.[39]

Color Blooming
The ultrasound beam used to form an image is not of a precise width like that of a laser light beam, but ta-

pers in intensity at its edges more like a flashlight beam. Just as when the intensity of a flashlight beam is increased, the illuminated spot it creates appears to get bigger, so when an ultrasound beam encounters a strong scatterer, it detects it near the edge of the beam and so interprets it to be bigger than its actual size (Fig. 3-3). Because of the threshold criterion for color Doppler images previously described, this effect is especially noticeable in a color image, where vessels already detected on color will appear to "bloom" when the agent arrives. A comparable effect occurs in the axial direction (Fig. 3-3, B), again because the axial sensitivity of the pulsed Doppler resolution cell is not sharp but tapers at its proximal and distal boundaries. The effect can be to smother the image with color, destroying its spatial resolution (Fig. 3-3, C). It is important that this effect not be misinterpreted as enhanced detection of flow in small vessels. One way of resolving the problem is to reduce the effective sensitivity of the color system by decreasing the receiver gain or, more constructively perhaps, by decreasing the ensemble length of the color detection scheme so that more lines can be made in a shorter time, potentially increasing both the spatial and temporal resolution.

Artifactually Increased Spectral Peak Frequencies
In a spectral Doppler system, the arrival of the agent has the effect of increasing the gray level intensity of the display. The peak Doppler shift frequency, which corresponds to the maximum flow velocity in the

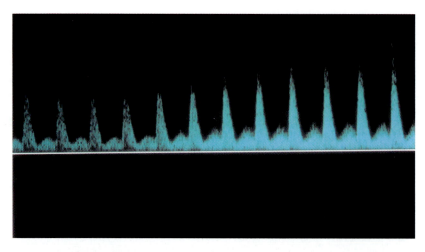

FIG. 3-4. Artifactual increase in peak systolic velocity on spectral Doppler. As the contrast agent arrives, the power of the Doppler signal increases and Doppler-shifted echoes, which were outside the dynamic range of the system, are now detected and displayed. Because the Doppler spectrum tapers steadily to zero with increasing frequency, the effect on the spectral display is to show a higher peak systolic Doppler shift frequency. The contrast agent does not affect the real blood flow velocity.

sample volume, remains unaffected. If, however, the power of the Doppler signal tapers steadily to zero at high Doppler shift frequencies, as is commonly the case,[40] another form of the blooming artifact occurs. In Fig. 3-4 one can see that the arrival of the contrast agent is accompanied by an apparent increase in the peak systolic frequency. The blood is not, in fact, flowing any faster; it is simply that the enhanced sensitivity of the detection is causing the weaker signals at the higher Doppler shift frequencies to be displayed. Put more concisely, if the dynamic range of the display is not as great as the dynamic range of the signal, the agent will cause the weaker echoes to be displayed preferentially. In most spectral Doppler systems, the same effect can be obtained simply by increasing the Doppler receiver gain setting. The clear conclusion here is that contrast agents should be used to bring undetectable signals into the dynamic range of the display, not to push detectable signals beyond the dynamic range of the display!

Large-Bubble Noise

Small bubbles enhance the Doppler signal without affecting the echo statistics to the point where a change in the character of the spectral Doppler sounds can be appreciated. Larger bubbles, on the other hand, pass the sensitive volume as single, highly reflective scatterers and create transient larger bubbles that are readily heard as popping sounds. In the spectral display, they give rise to the familiar bidirectional spike that has been described in relation to, for example, air bubbles in the portal vein.[41] Some contrast agents, as

they disintegrate in the blood stream, appear to aggregate into larger collections of gas that are capable of producing this artifactual echo appearance. Good examples are provided by Albunex, which can break up quite easily as a result of its passage through the heart and lungs (Fig. 3-5).

QUANTITATIVE MEASURES OF ENHANCEMENT

In order to use an agent clinically, certain fundamental questions must be answered about its behavior in tissue. How do the dose concentration and injected volume relate to the effect on the echo? How long does the agent last? Does it recirculate? Is it affected by the heart and lungs or the mesentric vasculature? Does absence of agent in a vessel mean absence of flow? Quantitative measurement of the effect of an agent is not only of practical importance; as will be seen, it also provides important insight into the mechanism of bubble contrast.

To date, ultrasound contrast agents have been detected by using conventional B-scan imaging and Doppler methods. Quantitation relies on video presentation of the echo data and, in general, has borrowed methods of video densitometric analysis.[42-45] The relationship between video level on a B-scan display and received echo intensity is, however, complicated by technical factors such as dynamic range compression and nonlinear processing, so that quantitative interpretation of these images is unreliable or even mis-

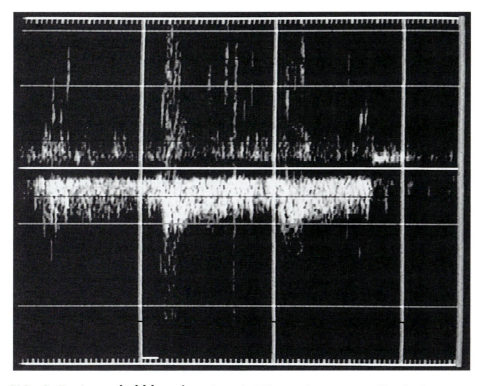

FIG. 3-5. Large-bubble noise. Large bubbles, in this case caused by the destruction of Albunex® as it passes through the heart and lungs, cause transient high amplitude signals as they pass through the sample volume. The spectrum shows artifactual spikes in both directions.

leading. Similarly, color Doppler imaging systems provide video data that bear nonlinear relationships to the backscattered power of moving targets and to video level as well as to different Doppler shift frequencies and to machine settings such as the receiver gain and the filter.[46,47] By relying on such methods, one can obtain only a qualitative assessment of the agents' effects. By exploiting the Doppler signal itself, however, one can use a quantitative method to measure the relative backscatter intensity of the RF signal and, hence, the amount of enhancement due to the agent. The outline is shown in Fig. 3-6 and described more completely elsewhere.[48] The principle relies on the fact that, for sufficiently small Doppler sample volumes, the power of the Doppler signal is proportional to the power of the echo that gives rise to the Doppler shift. By frequency-domain filtering of the Doppler signal, the large power components resulting from the movement of solid structures (the clutter) can be eliminated, and the contribution to the echo for which the contrast agent is responsible can be measured. This method allows both the degree of enhancement and the time course of the enhancement to be quantified, thus opening the way to the measurement of dose response in different vessels and to indicator-dilution applications of ultrasound contrast.[49]

These measurements can be carried out using a Doppler probe positioned on, say, the femoral artery of a patient. For the most precise measurements, one can use the invasive technique of placing a cuff around the blood vessel of interest. The cuff houses a miniature 10 MHz pulsed Doppler transducer; the sample volume is 0.5 mm in axial extent and is positioned in the center stream of the vessel. The Albunex dose-response curves for both the celiac artery and the vasculature of the tumor are shown in Fig. 3-7. The 25 dB peak response in the vessel and the 14 dB peak response in the tumor correspond to a large and clinically significant increase in the signal-to-noise ratio and, hence, in vessel detectability. Fig. 3-8 shows how Levovist®, even in very small doses, recirculates in the rabbit, producing detectable enhancement for more than two minutes. In Fig. 3-9 on page 70, outstanding enhancement of Doppler signals from the parenchyma of the 5 mm diameter testis of the rabbit is shown 10 minutes after an intravenous injection.

In the future, it is likely that data will be collected for analysis at the radio frequency level of the receiver and processed separately from the imaging and color Doppler detection procedure. The results of such analysis could embrace both backscatter, texture, and Doppler shift phenomena and be displayed along with

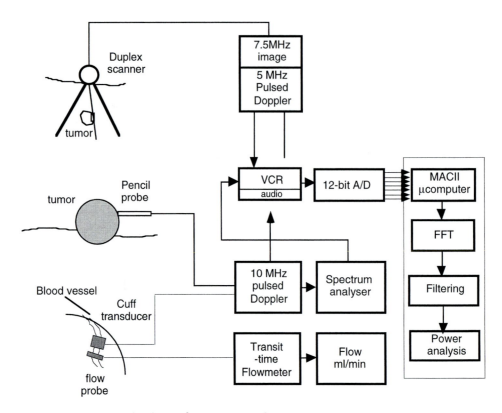

FIG. 3-6. Quantitation of contrast enhancement in blood vessels. Experimental setup for in vivo acquisition, recording, and analysis of Doppler signals. The signals are digitized from the quadrature outputs of either a duplex clinical scanner or an experimental invasive cuff-probe-pulsed Doppler flowmeter. Power is then calculated in the frequency domain.

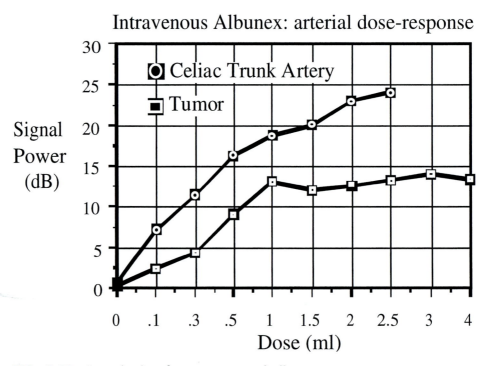

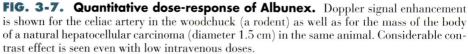

FIG. 3-7. Quantitative dose-response of Albunex. Doppler signal enhancement is shown for the celiac artery in the woodchuck (a rodent) as well as for the mass of the body of a natural hepatocellular carcinoma (diameter 1.5 cm) in the same animal. Considerable contrast effect is seen even with low intravenous doses.

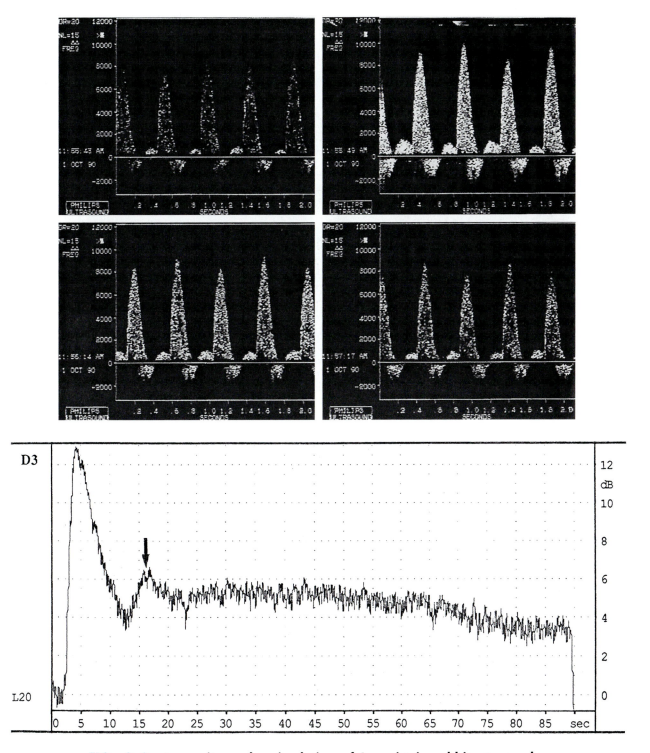

FIG. 3-8. **Longevity and recirculation of Levovist in rabbit at very low doses.** Above: 0.125 ml/kg venous injection, signal from celiac artery. The Doppler spectra are produced using a 10 MHz cuff transducer stabilized on the vessel surface. Top left: Before injection. Top right: Injection +5s. Bottom left: Injection +40s. Bottom right: Injection +100s. Note persistent enhancement of signal strength. Below: Calculated mean spectral power plotted against time in seconds, showing second pass enhancement of about 6 dB *(arrow)*.

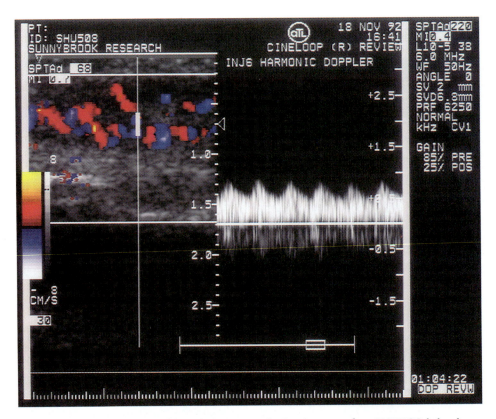

FIG. 3-9. Flow in the rabbit testis imaged 10 minutes after SHU508 injection.

the video image, perhaps as a video overlay comparable to that of the color Doppler image, thus allowing a separate **Doppler contrast mode of ultrasound imaging** in suitably modified machines. This will certainly allow measurement of the wash-in and wash-out of the contrast agent and assessment of its behavior as a blood pool indicator. However, it is possible to deduce that such a method, of itself, will not necessarily solve the problem of detecting flow in the microcirculation. For that, the ultrasound instrumentation itself must be adapted to the contrast agent and a mode that is capable of imaging the agent selectively must be developed.

CONTRAST-AGENT-SPECIFIC IMAGING

The Problem

One of the major diagnostic objectives of using an ultrasound contrast agent is the detection of flow in the circulation at a level that is lower than would otherwise be possible. The echoes from blood associated with such flow—at the arteriolar level, for example—exist in the midst of echoes from the surrounding solid structures of the organ parenchyma, echoes that are almost always

stronger than even the contrast-enhanced blood echo. In fact, Fig. 3-10 shows that the effect of the contrast agent in the blood vessel is to *lower* the contrast between blood and the surrounding tissue, making the lumen of the blood vessel less visible. Thus, in order to be able to image flow in, for example, the liver, a contrast agent must enhance the blood echo to a level that is substantially higher than that of the surrounding tissue or must be able to be used with a means of suppressing the echo from non–contrast-bearing structures. X-ray angiography, which is faced with a similar problem, deals with the clutter components of the image by simple subtraction of a preinjection image. What is left behind might reveal flow in individual vessels, or the blush of perfusion at the tissue level. If, however, we subtract two consecutive ultrasound images of an organ such as a kidney, we get a third ultrasound image, one produced by the decorrelation of the speckle pattern between acquisitions. In order to show parenchymal enhancement due to the agent, speckle variance must first be reduced by filtering, which results in a consequent loss of spatial or temporal resolution. Even if the speckle problem could be overcome, subtraction would still be poorly suited to the dynamic and interactive nature of ultrasound imaging.

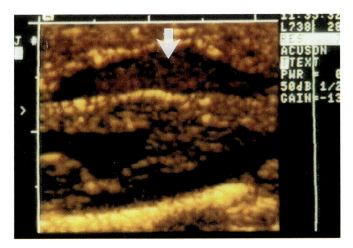

FIG. 3-10. Levovist in rabbit portal vein. Post peripheral venous injection of 0.15 ml/kg, the B-scan image shows the agent in portal vein. This agent has successfully traversed the heart as well as the pulmonary and mesenteric capillary beds.

Doppler is an alternative and effective method for separating echoes from blood and tissue. It relies on the relatively high velocity of the flowing blood as compared to the velocity of the surrounding tissue. Although this distinction (which allows the use of a highpass, or wall, filter to separate the Doppler signals due to bloodflow from those due to clutter) is valid for flow in large vessels, it is not valid for flow at the organ-parenchymal level, where the tissue is moving at the same speed as or faster than the blood that flows in its vasculature. Thus, the Doppler shift frequency from the moving solid tissue is comparable to or higher than that of the moving blood itself. Furthermore, the power of the solid tissue echo is about 1000 times higher than that of the blood echo. Because the wall filter cannot be used without eliminating both the flow and the clutter echoes, the use of Doppler in such circumstances is defeated by the overwhelming signal caused by tissue movement: the **flash artifact in color** or the **thump artifact in spectral Doppler**. Thus, true parenchymal flow cannot be imaged with conventional Doppler, with or without intravenous contrast agents.

How then might contrast agents be used to improve the visibility of small vascular structures within tissue? Clearly, a method that could identify the echo coming from the contrast agent and thereby suppress the echo coming from solid tissue would provide both a real-time subtraction mode for contrast-enhanced B-mode imaging and a means of suppressing Doppler clutter without the use of a velocity-dependent filter in spectral and color modes. Harmonic imaging aims to provide such a method and, thereby, the means of detecting flow in smaller vessels than is currently possible.

HARMONIC IMAGING

Examining the behavior of contrast-enhanced ultrasound reveals two important pieces of evidence. First, the size of the echo enhancement at very high dilution following a small peripheral injection (7 dB at a dose of 0.01 ml/kg of Levovist®, for example[50]) is much larger than would be expected from such sparse scatterers of this size in blood. Second, investigations of the acoustic characteristics of several agents[12] have demonstrated an approximately linear dependence of the backscattered coefficient on the numerical density of the agent at low concentrations, as expected, but they have also demonstrated a dependence of attenuation on ultrasound frequency different from that predicted by the Rayleigh law, which describes how the echogenicity of normal tissue changes with frequency. Instead, peaks exist that are dependent on both the ultrasound frequency and on the size of the microbubbles, which suggests resonance phenomena. This important observation indicates that the bubbles resonate in the ultrasound field—the bubbles get bigger and smaller in sympathy with the oscillations of pressure caused by the incident sound. Like vibrations in other structures, these radial oscillations have a natural, or **resonant,** frequency of oscillation at which they will both absorb and scatter ultrasound with a peculiarly high efficiency. Considering the linear oscillation of a free bubble of air in water, one can use a simple theory[3] to predict the resonant frequency of radial oscillation of a bubble 3 μm in diameter, the median diameter of a typical transpulmonary microbubble agent. As Fig. 3-11 shows, it is about 3 MHz, approximately the middle of the frequencies used in a typical abdominal scan. This extraordinary and fortunate coincidence explains why ultrasound

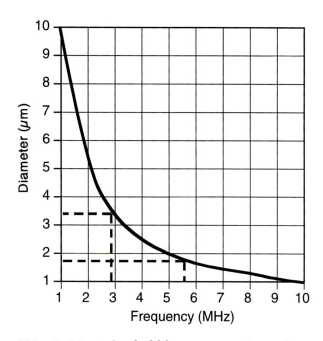

FIG. 3-11. Microbubbles resonate in a diagnostic ultrasound field. This graph shows that the resonant, or natural, frequency of oscillation of a bubble of air in an ultrasound field depends on its size. For a 3.5 μm diameter, the size needed for an intravenously injectible contrast agent, the resonant frequency is about 3 MHz.

contrast agents are so efficient and can be administered in such small quantities. It also predicts that bubbles undergoing resonant oscillation in an ultrasound field could be prodded into nonlinear motion, the basis of harmonic imaging.

Bubbles oscillating in an ultrasound field can, indeed, be induced to move nonlinearly. It has long been recognized[51] that if bubbles are driven by the ultrasound field at sufficiently high acoustic pressures, the oscillatory excursions of the bubbles reach a point where their alternate expansions and contractions are not equal. Lord Rayleigh, the originator of the theoretical understanding of sound upon which ultrasound imaging is based, was first led to investigate this, in 1917, by his curiosity about the creaking noises his tea kettle made as the water came to the boil. The consequence of such nonlinear motion is that the sound emitted by the bubble and detected by the transducer contains harmonics, just as the resonant strings of a musical instrument, if plucked too vigorously, produce a harsh timbre containing overtones. Fig. 3-12 shows the frequency spectrum of an echo produced by a microbubble contrast agent following a 3.75 MHz burst. This particular agent is Levovist, but many microbubble agents behave in a similar way. Ultrasound frequency is on the horizontal axis, with the relative amplitude on the vertical axis. A strong echo, at 13 dB with respect to the fun-

damental, is seen at twice the transmitted frequency; this is known as the **second harmonic**. Peaks in the echo spectrum at sub- and ultraharmonics are also seen. Key factors in the harmonic response of an agent, which varies from material to material, are the incident pressure of the ultrasound field, the frequency and size distribution of the bubbles, and the mechanical properties of the bubble capsule (a stiff capsule, for example, will dampen the oscillations and attenuate the nonlinear response).

We have developed a new real-time imaging and Doppler method based on this principle, which we call **harmonic imaging**.[52] The system transmits normally at one frequency, but when in harmonic mode, it receives only echoes at double that frequency. A commercially available digital color flow system (UM9 HDI and HDI3000, ATL Inc., Bothell, WA) has been modified to transmit at between 1.5 and 4.0 MHz and to receive at the second harmonic, between 3.0 and 8.0 MHz (Fig. 3-13). Harmonic imaging uses the same array transducers as conventional imaging and only software changes are needed for this particular ultrasound system. In harmonic mode, echoes from the contrast agent are received preferentially by means of a bandpass filter whose center frequency is at the second harmonic. Echoes from solid tissue, as well as from red blood cells themselves, are suppressed. Real-time harmonic imaging, Doppler, and color Doppler modes have now been implemented experimentally on a number of commercially available systems. Clearly, an exceptional transducer bandwidth is needed to operate over such a large range of frequencies, so it is fortunate that much effort has been directed in recent years toward increasing the bandwidth of transducer arrays because of its significant bearing on conventional imaging performance.

Results

In harmonic images, the echo from tissue-mimicking material is reduced but not eliminated, **reversing the contrast** between the agent and its surroundings (Fig. 3-14). The value of this effect is that it increases the detectability of the agent when it is in blood vessels normally hidden by the strong echoes from tissue. In spectral Doppler, one would expect the suppression of the tissue echo to reduce the thump due to tissue motion that is familiar to all echocardiographers. Fig. 3-15 on page 76 shows spectral Doppler being applied to a region of the aorta in which there is wall motion as well as blood flow within the sample volume. The conventional Doppler image of Fig. 3-15, *A* shows the thump artifact due to clutter, which is almost completely absent in the harmonic Doppler image in Fig. 3-15, *B*. All instrument settings, including the filters, are identical in these images; we have merely switched between modes. In vivo measurements from spectral

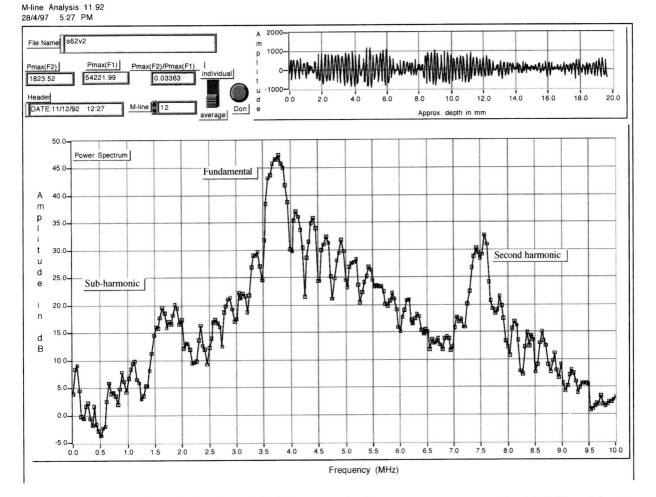

FIG. 3-12. **Harmonic emission from SHU508.** A sample of a contrast agent is insonated at 3.75 MHz and the echo analyzed for its frequency content. It is seen that most of the energy in the echo is at 3.75 MHz, but that there is a clear second peak in the spectrum at 7.5 MHz, as well as a third at 1.875 MHz. The second harmonic echo is only 13 dB lower than that of the main, or fundamental, echo. Harmonic imaging and Doppler aim to separate and process this signal alone.

Doppler show that the signal-to-clutter ratio is improved, through the combination of harmonic imaging and a contrast agent, by as much as 35 dB.[53] Fig. 3-16, *A* on page 77 shows harmonic color images of an aorta with a flash artifact from respiratory motion. The harmonic image in Fig. 3-16, *B* demonstrates the flow without the flash artifact. The particular potential application of this entirely new diagnostic method is the detection of blood flow in small vessels surrounded by tissue that is moving—in the branches of the coronary arteries[54] or in the myocardium itself[55] as well as in the parenchyma of abdominal organs.[56]

Harmonic Power Imaging

In color Doppler studies using a contrast agent, the effect of the arrival of the agent in a color region of interest is often to produce a **blooming** of the color image, whereby signals from major vascular targets spread out to occupy the entire region. Thus, although flow from smaller vessels might be detectable, the color images can be swamped by artifactual flow signals. The origin of this artifact is the amplitude thresholding that governs most color displays in conventional, or **velocity**, mode imaging. Increasing the backscattered signal power has the effect of merely displaying the velocity estimate, at full intensity, over a wider range of pixels around the detected location. A display in which the parameter mapped to color is related directly to the backscattered signal power, on the other hand, has the advantage of making such thresholding unnecessary and of displaying lower-amplitude Doppler shifts (such as those that result from side-lobe interference) at a lower visual amplitude, rendering them less conspicuous. Echo-enhanced flow signals, in contrast, are

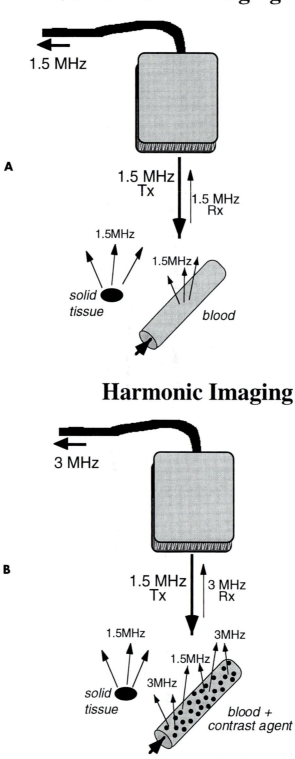

FIG. 3-13. The principle of harmonic imaging and Doppler. A conventional linear array is used, with the receiver tuned to double the transmitting frequency. The tissue and blood give an echo at the fundamental frequency (**A**), but the contrast agent undergoing nonlinear oscillation in the sound field emits the harmonic which is detected by the harmonic system (**B**).

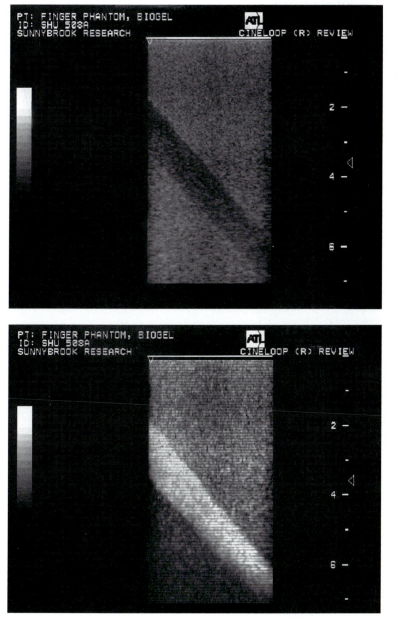

FIG. 3-14. Harmonic imaging. An in vitro phantom shows a finger-like void in tissue-equivalent material filled with dilute contrast agent, barely visible in **A,** conventional mode. **B,** Harmonic imaging is seen to reverse the contrast between the microbubble agent and the surrounding material.

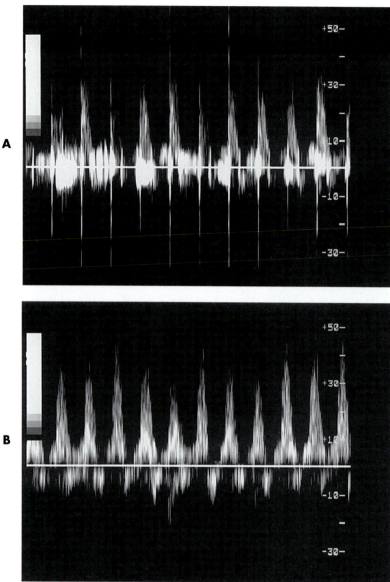

FIG. 3-15. Clutter rejection with harmonic spectral Doppler. A, The abdominal aorta of an animal is examined with harmonic spectral Doppler. In conventional mode, clutter from the moving wall causes the familiar artifact which also obscures diastolic flow. **B,** In harmonic mode, the clutter is almost completely suppressed, so that flow can be resolved. The settings of the filter and other relevant instrument parameters are identical.

displayed at a higher level. This is the basis of the power imaging map (also known as color power angiography, or color Doppler energy mapping). Power Doppler can help eliminate some other limitations of small-vessel flow detection with color Doppler. Low-velocity detection requires lowering the Doppler pulse repetition frequency (PRF), which results in multiple aliasing and loss of directional resolution. A display method that does not use the velocity estimate is not prone to the aliasing artifact and therefore allows the PRF to be lowered, thus increasing the likelihood of detecting the lower-velocity flow in smaller vessels.

Because it maps a parameter directly related to the acoustic quantity that is enhanced by the contrast agent, the power map is a natural choice for contrast-enhanced color Doppler studies. However, the advantages of the power map for contrast-enhanced detection of small-vessel flow are balanced by a po-

tentially devastating shortcoming: its increased susceptibility to interference from clutter. **Clutter** is both detected more readily, because of the power mode's increased sensitivity, and displayed more prominently, because of the high-intensity display of high-amplitude signals. Furthermore, frame averaging has the additional effect of sustaining and blurring the flash over the cardiac cycle, thus exacerbating its effect on the image.

At the small expense of some sensitivity, amply compensated for by the enhancement caused by the agent, harmonic mode effectively overcomes this clutter problem (Fig. 3-17). Combining the harmonic method with power Doppler produces an especially effective tool for the detection of flow in the small vessels of the organs of the abdomen which may be moving with cardiac pulsation or respiration (Fig. 3-18). In a study in which flow imaged on con-

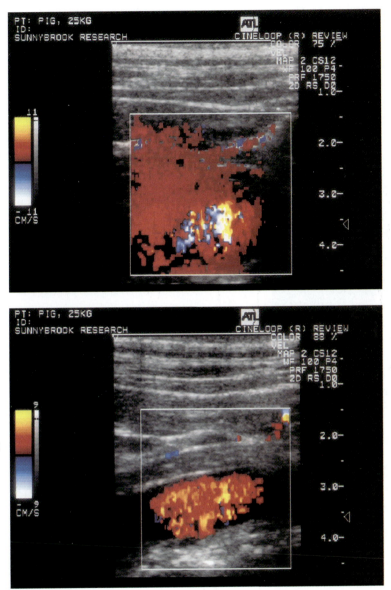

FIG. 3-16. Clutter rejection with harmonic color Doppler. A, Flow in the abdominal aorta is superimposed on respiratory motion, producing severe flash artifact. **B,** In harmonic mode at the same point in the respiratory cycle, the flash artifact disappears. Flow from a smaller vessel (the cranial mesenteric artery) is visualized. All instrument settings are the same.

trast-enhanced power harmonic images was compared with histologically sized arterioles in the corresponding regions on the renal cortex,[50] it was concluded that the method is capable of demonstrating flow in vessels of less than 40 μm in diameter—about ten times smaller than the corresponding imaging resolution limit, even as the organ was moving with normal respiration. Recent studies of this power mode method in the heart[57] show that flow can be imaged in the myocardium even with a first-generation agent such as Levovist®.[58]

Discussion

Harmonic imaging is a method that succeeds in identifying a microbubble contrast agent in the tissue vasculature by means of its **echo signature.** In doing so, it helps tackle some old problems in ultrasound such as the rejection of the tissue echo in Doppler modes designed to image moving blood, and it creates a **subtraction mode** without sacrificing the real-time nature of the examination. Fig. 3-19 summarizes graphically the effect on the Doppler process of contrast agents and harmonic detection. In conventional Doppler, the signal from blood is stronger than the clutter signal from tissue. In contrast-enhanced Doppler, the signal from blood is raised, sometimes nearly to that of tissue (as in Fig. 3-10). In the harmonic mode, the signal from blood is raised but the signal from the tissue is reduced, thus reversing the contrast between tissue and blood. Another way of perceiving the harmonic method is to say that because of its greater sensitivity to small quantities of agent, a given level of enhancement due to a bolus will last longer (Fig. 3-20). This is the reason that a number of investigators have found that cardiac contrast imaging of small vessels such as

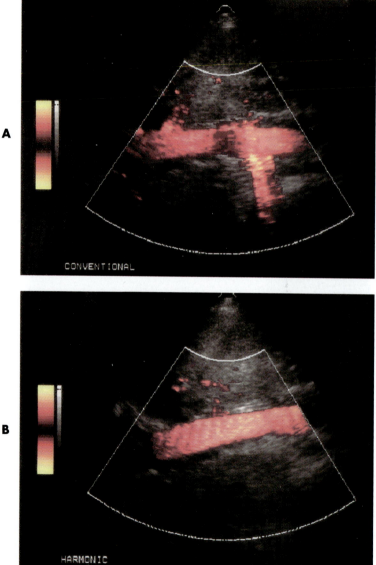

FIG. 3-17. **Reduction of the flash artifact in harmonic power Doppler.** The harmonic contrast method helps overcome one of the principal shortcomings of power Doppler, its increased susceptibility to tissue motion. **A,** Aortic flow in power mode with flash artifact from cardiac motion of wall. **B,** In harmonic mode at the same point in the cardiac cycle, the flash is largely suppressed. All instrument settings are the same.

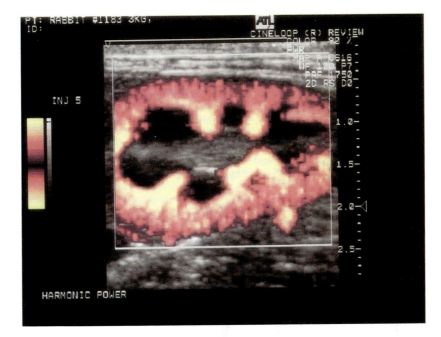

FIG. 3-18. Harmonic power mode imaging of a rabbit kidney. In this moving organ with only a 3 cm diameter, flow is detected beyond the cortico-medullary junction, to within 2 mm of the capsule.

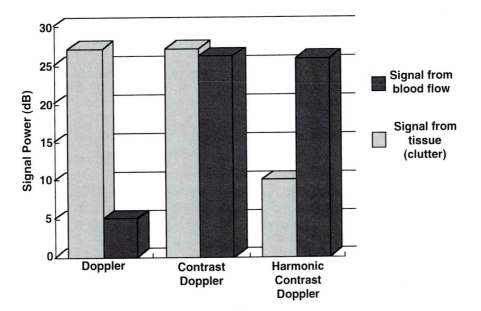

FIG. 3-19. Quantitating the impact of harmonic Doppler. Clutter and spectral Doppler signal levels measured in conventional, contrast-enhanced, and harmonic contrast-enhanced modes.[50]

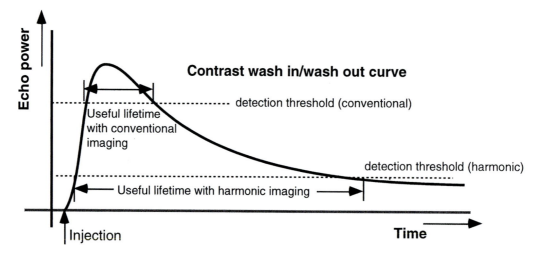

FIG. 3-20. **The improved sensitivity of the harmonic method translates into increased useful imaging time from a contrast agent bolus.** Time-enhancement curve caused by circulation of contrast-agent bolus shows how harmonic imaging, by reducing the detection threshold, increases the imaging lifetime of the agent.

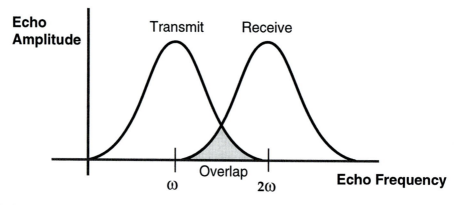

FIG. 3-21. **Harmonic imaging is a compromise between image resolution and contrast.** The transmit/receive frequency response in harmonic mode shows an area of overlap between transmit and receive frequencies, resulting in residual tissue image. Narrowing the bandwidth on transmit or receive provides better separation of the contrast-agent echo from those of normal tissue, but at the expense of axial resolution.

those in the myocardium is more effective when using harmonic mode.[54,55]

Harmonic imaging demands exceptional performance from the transducer array and system beamformer. Its implementation forces implicit compromises between, for example, image resolution and rejection of the non–contrast-agent echo (Fig. 3-21). It places unusual demands on the bandwidth performance of transducers as well as on the flexibility of the architecture of the imaging system. The ease with which it has been developed on modern instruments, however, reflects this flexibility and augers well for the future of the method. More significantly, contrast agents are now being developed specifically with nonlinear response as a design criterion. Entirely new agents present opportunities for entirely new detection strategies.[59] Our laboratory measurements show that some new contrast

agents are capable of creating an echo with more energy in the second harmonic than in the fundamental; that is, they are more efficient in harmonic than in conventional mode. With such agents, nonlinear imaging could become the preferred clinical method.

NEW DEVELOPMENTS IN CONTRAST IMAGING

Imaging Methods

Adapting ultrasound imaging systems to these new targets in the body is a field in its infancy. For example, it was recently discovered that by pressing the freeze button on a scanner for a few moments, hence interrupting the acquisition of ultrasound images during a contrast study, it is possible to increase the effectiveness of a contrast agent. So dramatic is this effect that it can raise the visibility of a contrast agent in the myocardial circulation to the point where it can be seen on a B-mode image above the echo level of the normal heart muscle.[60] It is now understood that the ultrasound field, if its peak pressure is sufficiently high, is capable of disrupting a bubble shell and destroying it.[61,62] By pausing between acquisitions, one allows new agent to wash in and fill the organ's vascular bed. The next imaging pulse results in a strong transient echo, one that is substantially stronger than the normal echo from the agent, which causes further destruction of the bubbles. This imaging strategy is sometimes referred to as **intermittent**, or **transient, imaging**. We[57] and others[55] have found that with harmonic imaging, this single-acquisition imaging provides even more contrast. By combining intermittent harmonic imaging with power Doppler, we can assemble the most sensitive imaging mode available to date for contrast agents, and with it, we have been able to demonstrate the first Doppler images of myocardial perfusion.[57,58]

Future imaging strategies are likely to be based on an improved understanding of the way in which a microbubble oscillates in an ultrasound field. They may result in contrast-specific modes that improve sensitivity to the agent over normal tissue but without the sacrifice in image quality currently experienced in harmonic mode.

CONTRAST AGENTS

As manufacturers of the agents gain more control over the rather difficult process of producing stable microbubbles, the possibilities of tailoring their behavior in the body increase. One of the most significant efforts is focused on targeting agents to specific sites in the body. Agents have been developed that adhere to thrombus, for example.[63] Initial in vitro studies show a 6 dB enhancement of clot by the agent when imaged with intravascular ultrasound.[64] The potential for such materials is clear, although questions remain about the proportion of injected material that will reach the desired target and the dose needed to attain the desired contrast.

This dose can be minimized if the targeted agent itself contains gas. As described above, agents that are phagocytized and remain intact in the Kupffer cells offer the prospect of a new kind of ultrasound liver imaging. However, until recently only particles have successfully performed this function. Now a gas-based agent (**Sonovist®**, SHU 563, Schering AG, Berlin Germany) has been developed; it is a polymer particle with a gas-filled interior and a mean particle size of approximately 1 μm. It acts as an efficient ultrasound contrast agent in its blood pool phase and has extremely strong harmonic emission.[65] After 15 to 20 minutes, the agent is taken up, largely intact, into the reticuloendothelial system. When imaged with color Doppler at high peak pressures, the bubbles are disrupted in the liver. The large change in signal level between two consecutive pulses is interpreted by the Doppler system as a random change in phase, and a random Doppler shift is assigned to this strong signal. The result is that the liver, though stationary, can be imaged with color Doppler (Fig. 3-22). Once again, defects in the Kupffer cells brought about by, for example, a cancer, show as an absence of these Doppler signals. The method is so sensitive that we have shown that individual bubbles can be detected in this way; thus, only extremely low doses (10 μl/kg, for example) are necessary. Using this technique, an isoechoic VX2

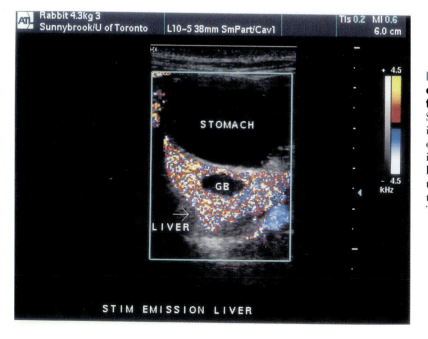

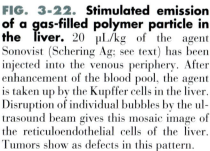

FIG. 3-22. Stimulated emission of a gas-filled polymer particle in the liver. 20 μL/kg of the agent Sonovist (Schering Ag; see text) has been injected into the venous periphery. After enhancement of the blood pool, the agent is taken up by the Kupffer cells in the liver. Disruption of individual bubbles by the ultrasound beam gives this mosaic image of the reticuloendothelial cells of the liver. Tumors show as defects in this pattern.

cancer with a diameter of less than 2 mm has been imaged in an animal liver.[59]

Future development of targeted agents can yield even more exciting prospects. By combining the targeting of an agent with the ability of diagnostic ultrasound to disrupt bubbles in a selected region in the body, a new method of drug delivery might become possible.[66] Drugs may be delivered so that they attain toxic levels only in desired volumes of tissue. Genetic material itself might be transported within a microbubble into a cell and released by acoustic means.

Modern agents for the production of ultrasound contrast offer the prospect that extremely small, harmless injections of a solution into a peripheral vein will produce spectacular improvements in the detection of blood-filled structures and blood flow velocity in the vascular system. New uses are likely to include the detection of smaller vessels, the detection of flow in moving parenchyma such as that of the kidney, liver, and myocardium, the detection and mapping of neovascular flow associated with tumors, and possibly the measurement of relative blood flow rates by indicator dilution methods. Harmonic imaging will give new capabilities to imaging and Doppler systems, effectively allowing **real-time subtraction imaging** of flowing blood with ultrasound and allowing the detection of flow in smaller vessels than hitherto possible.

ACKNOWLEDGMENTS

This work was supported by the National Cancer Institute of Canada and by the Medical Research Council.

REFERENCES

1. Gramiak R, Shah, PM. Echocardiography of the aortic root. *Invest Radiol* 1968;3:356-366.

The Need for Contrast Agents in Ultrasound

2. Burns PN. Interpreting and analyzing the Doppler examination. In: Taylor KJW, Burns PN, Wells PNT, eds. New York: Raven Press; 1995:55-99.

Mode of Action

3. Ophir J, Parker, KJ. Contrast agents in diagnostic ultrasound [published erratum appears in Ultrasound Med Biol 1990; 16:209]. *Ultrasound Med Biol* 1990;15:319-333.
4. Ziskin MC, Bonakdapour A, Weinstein DP, Lynch PR. Contrast agents for diagnostic ultrasound. *Invest Radiol* 1972;6:500-505.
5. Kremkau FW, and Carstensen EL. Ultrasonic detection of cavitation at catheter tips. *Am J Roentgenol* 1968;3:159-167.
6. Kerber RE, Kioschos JM, Lauer RM. Use of an ultrasonic contrast method in the diagnosis of valvular regurgitation and intracardiac shunts. *Am J Cardiol* 1974;34:722-727.

7. Reid CL, Kawanishi DT, McKay CR. Accuracy of evaluation of the presence and severity of aortic and mitral regurgitation by contrast 2-dimensional echocardiography. *Am J Cardiol* 1983;52:519-524.
8. Sahn DJ, Valdex-Cruz LM. Ultrasonic contrast studies for the detection of cardiac shunts. *J Am Coll Cardiol* 1983;3:978-985.
9. Roelandt J. Contrast echocardiography. *Ultrasound Med Biol* 1982;8:471.
10. Carroll BA, Turner RJ, Tickner EG, Boyle DB, Young SW. Gelatin-encapsulated nitrogen microbubbles as ultrasonic contrast agents. *Invest Radiol* 1980;15:260-266.
11. Feinstein SB, Shah PM, Bing RJ, Meerbaum S, Corday E, Chang BL, Santillan G, Fujibayashi Y. Microbubble dynamics visualized in the intact capillary circulation. *J Am Coll Cardiol* 1984;4:595-600.
12. Bleeker H, Shung K, Barnhart J. On the application of ultrasonic contrast agents for blood flowmetry and assessment of cardiac perfusion. *J Ultrasound Med* 1990;9:461-471.
13. Tencate FJ, et al. Two-dimensional contrast echocardiography. II. Transpulmonary studies. *J Am Coll Cardiol* 1984;3:21.
14. Keller MW, Glasheen W, Kaul S. Albunex: a safe and effective commercially produced agent for myocardial contrast echocardiography. *J Am Soc Echocardiogr* 1989;2:48-52.
15. Goldberg BB, Hilpert PL, Burns PN, Liu JB, Newman LM, Merton DA, Witlin LA. Hepatic tumors: signal enhancement at Doppler US after intravenous injection of a contrast agent. *Radiology* 1990;177:713-717.
16. Schlief R. Echo enhancement: agents and techniques—basic principles. *Adv Echo-Contrast* 1994;4:5-19.
17. Fritzsch T, Schartl M, Siegert J. Preclinical and clinical results with an ultrasonic contrast agent. *Invest Radiol* 1988;23:5.
18. Goldberg BB, Liu JB, Burns PN, Merton DA, Forsberg F. Galactose-based intravenous sonographic contrast agent: experimental studies. *J Ultrasound Med.* 1993;12:463-470.
19. Fobbe F, Ohnesorge O, Reichel M, Ernst O, Schuermann R, Wolf K. Transpulmonary contrast agent and color-coded duplex sonography: first clinical experience. *Radiology* 1992; 185(P):142.
20. Albrecht T, Cosgrove DO, Correas JM, Rallidis L, Nihoyanopoulos P, Patel N. Renal, hepatic, and cardiac enhancement on Doppler and gray-scale sonograms obtained with EchoGen. *Academ Radiol* 1996;3:S198-200.
21. Unger E, Shen D, Fritz T, Kulik B, Lund P, Wu G-L, Yellowhair D, Ramaswami R, Matsunaga T. Gas-filled lipid bilayers as ultrasound contrast agents. *Invest Radiol* 1994; 29:134-136.
22. Mattrey RF, Scheible FW, Gosink BB, Leopold GR, Long DM, Higgins CB. Perfluoroctylbromide: a liver/spleen-specific and tumor-imaging ultrasound contrast material. *Radiology* 1982;145:759-762.
23. Mattrey RF, Leopold GR, vanSonnenberg E, Gosink BB, Scheible FW, Long DM. Perfluorochemicals as liver- and spleen-seeking ultrasound contrast agents. *J Ultrasound Med* 1983;2:173-176.
24. Violante MR, Parker KJ, Fischer HW. Particulate suspensions as ultrasonic contrast agents for liver and spleen. *Invest Radiol* 1988;23:7.
25. Parker KJ, Baggs RB, Lerner RM, Tuthill TA, Violante MR. Ultrasound contrast for hepatic tumors using IDE particles. *Invest Radiol* 1990;25:1135-1139.

The Impact of Contrast Enhancement

26. Ries F, Honisch C, Lambertz M, Hillekamp J, Schlief R. A transpulmonary contrast medium enhances the transcranial Doppler signal in humans. *Stroke* 1993;24:1903-1909.
27. Rosenkrantz K, Zendel W, Langer RD, Felix R, Schuermann R, Schlief R. Transcranial color-coded duplex sonography with an intravenous US contrast agent. *Radiology* 1992; 185(P):143.

28. Bauer A, Becker G, Krone A, Frohlich T, Bogdahn U. Transcranial duplex sonography using ultrasound contrast enhancers. *Clin Radiol* 1996;51:19-23.

29. Von Bibra H, Sutherland G, Becher H, Neudert J, Nihoyannopoulos P. Clinical evaluation of left heart Doppler contrast enhancement by a saccharide-based transpulmonary contrast agent. The Levovist Cardiac Working Group. *J Am Coll Cardiol* 1995;25:500-508.

30. Fobbe F, Siegert J, Fritzsch T, Koch HC, Wolf KJ. Color-coded duplex sonography and ultrasound contrast media—detection of renal perfusion defects in experimental animals. *Rofo Fortschr Geb Rontgenstr Neuen Bildgeb Verfahr* 1991; 154:242-245.

31. Kedar RP, Cosgrove D, McCready VR, Bamber JC, Carter ER. Microbubble contrast agent for color Doppler US: effect on breast masses: work in progress. *Radiology* 1996;198:679-686.

32. Cosgrove D. Ultrasound contrast enhancement of tumours. *Clin Radiol* 1996;51:44-49.

33. Balen FG, Allen CM, Lees WR. Ultrasound contrast agents. *Clin Radiol* 1994;49:77-82.

34. Campani R, Bozzini A, Calliada F, Bottinelli O, Anguissola R, Conti MP, Corsi G. Impiego di un mezzo di contrasto per ecografia SH U 508A (Levovist) Schering nello studio delle metastasi epatiche con color-Doppler. *Radiol Med* 1994; 87:32-40.

35. Maresca G, Barbaro B, Summaria V, De Gaetano AM, Salcuni M, Mirk P, Marano P. Color Doppler ultrasonography in the differential diagnosis of focal hepatic lesions: the SH U 508 A (Levovist) experience. *Radiologia Medica* 1994;87:41-49.

36. Fujimoto M, Moriyasu F, Nishikawa K, Nada T, Okuma M. Color Doppler sonography of hepatic tumors with a galactose-based contrast agent: correlation with angiographic findings. *Am J Roentgenol* 1994;163:1099-104.

37. Missouris CG, Allen CM, Balen FG, Buckenham T, Lees WR, MacGregor GA. Non-invasive screening for renal artery stenosis with ultrasound contrast enhancement. *J Hyperten* 1996;14:519-524.

38. Tschammler A, Viesr G, Schindler R, Schuermann R, Wolf K. Ultrasound contrast media: in vitro studies. *J Ultrasound Med* 1993;12:S33.

Artifacts in Contrast Studies

39. Forsberg F, Liu JB, Burns PN, Merton DA, Goldberg BB. Artifacts in ultrasonic contrast agent studies. *J Ultrasound Med* 1994;13:357-365.

40. Burns PN. Hemodynamics. In: Taylor KJW, Burns PN, Wells NT, eds. *Clinical Applications of Doppler Ultrasound.* New York: Raven Press; 1995:35-55.

41. Lafortune ML, Trinh BC, Burns PN, Breton G, Burke M, Dery R, Gianfelice D, Philie M, Cote J. Sonographic and Doppler manifestations of air in the portal vein. *Radiology* 1991;180:667-670.

Quantitative Measures of Enhancement

42. Vandernberg B, Kieslo R. Quantitation of myocardial perfusion by contrast echocardiography: analysis of contrast gray level appearance variables and intracyclic variability. *J Am Coll Cardiol* 1989;13:200-206.

43. Rovai D, Nissen S. Contrast echo washout curves from the left ventricle: application of basic principles of indicated dilution theory and calculation of ejection fraction. *J Am Coll Cardiol* 1987;10:125-134.

44. Smith MD, Kwan OL, Reiser HJ, DeMaria AN. Superior intensity and reproducibility of SHU-454, a new right heart contrast agent. *J Am Coll Cardiol* 1984;3:992-998.

45. Cheirif J, Zoghbi W. Assessment of myocardial perfusion in humans by contrast echocardiography. I: evaluation of regional coronary reserve by peak contrast intensity. *J Am Coll Cardiol* 1988;11:735-743.

46. Burns PN, Needleman L, Merton D, Goldberg BB. Criteria for the detection of tumor blood flow with Doppler US (RSNA presentation). *Radiology* 1989;173:180.

47. Burns PN, Hilpert P, Goldberg BB. Intravenous contrast agent for ultrasound Doppler: in vivo measurement of small vessel dose-response. *IEEE Eng Med Biol Soc* 1990;1:322-324.

48. Burns PN, Liu J-B, Hilpert P, Goldberg BB. Intravenous US contrast agent for tumor diagnosis: quantitative studies. *Radiology* 1990;177(P):140.

49. Shung KK, Bleeker H. Contrast ultrasonic blood flowmetry. In: *IEEE Ultrasonics Symposium.*

Harmonic Imaging

50. Burns PN, Powers JE, Hope-Simpson D, Brezina A, Kolin A, Chin CT, Uhlendorf V, Fritzsch T. Harmonic power mode Doppler using microbubble contrast agents: an improved method for small vessel flow imaging. *Proc IEEE UFFC* 1994;1547-1550.

51. Neppiras EA, Nyborg WL, Miller PL. Nonlinear behavior and stability of trapped micron-sized cylindrical gas bubbles in an ultrasound field. *Ultrasonics* 1983;21:109-115.

52. Burns PN, Powers JE, Fritzsch T. Harmonic imaging: a new imaging and Doppler method for contrast-enhanced ultrasound (abstract.) *Radiology* 1992;185(P):142.

53. Burns PN, Powers JE, Hope-Simpson D, Uhlendorf V, Fritzsch T. Harmonic contrast enhanced Doppler as a method for the elimination of clutter: in vivo duplex and color studies. *Radiology* 1993;189:285.

54. Mulvagh SL, Foley DA, Aeschbacher BC, Klarich KK, Seward JB. Second harmonic imaging of an intravenously administered echocardiographic contrast agent: visualization of coronary arteries and measurement of coronary blood flow. *J Am Coll Cardiol* 1996;27:1519-1525.

55. Porter TR, Xie F, Kricsfeld D, Armbruster RW. Improved myocardial contrast with second harmonic transient ultrasound response imaging in humans using intravenous perfluorocarbon-exposed sonicated dextrose albumin. *J Am Coll Cardiol* 1996;27:1497-1501.

56. Kono Y, Moriyasu F, Yamada K, Nada T, Matsumura T. Conventional and harmonic gray scale enhancement of the liver with sonication activation of a US contrast agent. *Radiology* 1996;201.

57. Burns PN, Wilson SR, Muradali D, Powers JE, Fritzsch T. Intermittent US harmonic contrast-enhanced imaging and Doppler improves sensitivity and longevity of small vessel detection. *Radiology* 1996;201:159.

58. Becher H. Second harmonic imaging with Levovist: initial clinical experience. In: Cate FT, deJong N, eds. *Second European Symposium on Ultrasound Contrast Imaging: Book of Abstracts.* Rotterdam: Erasmus University Press; 1997.

59. Fritzsch T, Hauff P, Heldmann F, Luders F, Uhlendorf V, Weitschies W. Preliminary results with a new liver-specific ultrasound contrast agent. *Ultrasound Med Biol* 1994;20:137.

New Developments in Contrast Imaging

60. Porter TR, Xie F. Transient myocardial contrast after initial exposure to diagnostic ultrasound pressures with minute doses of intravenously injected microbubbles: demonstration and potential mechanisms. *Circulation* 1995;92:2391-2395.

61. Uhlendorf V, Scholle F-D. Imaging of spatial distribution and flow of microbubbles using nonlinear acoustic properties. *Acoust Imag* 1996;22:233-238.

62. Burns PN, Wilson SR, Muradali D, Powers JE, Greener Y. Microbubble destruction is the origin of harmonic signals from FS069. *Radiology* 1996;201:158.

Contrast Agents

63. Lanza GM, Wallace KD, Scott MJ, Sheehan CK, Cacheris WM, Christy DH, Sharkey AM, Miller JG, Wickline SA. Initial description and validation of a novel site-targeted ultrasonic contrast agent. *Circulation* 1995;92:260.

64. Christy DH, Wallace KD, Lanza GM, Holland MR, Hall CS, Scott MJ, Cacheris WP, Gaffney PJ, Miller JG, Wickline SA. Quantitative intravascular ultrasound: demonstration using a novel site-targeted acoustic contrast agent. *Proc IEEE Ultrason Symp* 1995;1125-1128.

65. Uhlendorf V, Hoffmann C. Nonlinear acoustical response of coated microbubbles in diagnostic ultrasound. *Proc IEEE Ultrason Symp* 1994;1559-1562.

66. Unger EC. Drug delivery applications of ultrasound contrast agents. In: Cate FT, deJong N, eds. *Second European Symposium on Ultrasound Contrast Imaging: Book of Abstracts*. Rotterdam: Erasmus University Press: 1997.

PART II

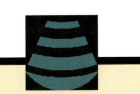

Abdominal, Pelvic, and Thoracic Sonography

CHAPTER 4

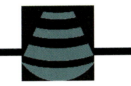

The Liver

•

Cynthia E. Withers, M.D., F.R.C.P.C.
Stephanie R. Wilson, M.D., F.R.C.P.C.

The liver is the largest organ in the human body, weighing approximately 1500 g in the adult. Because it is frequently involved in systemic and local disease, sonographic examination is often requested to assess hepatic abnormality.

TECHNIQUE

The liver is best examined with real-time sonography, ideally, following a 6-hour fast so that bowel gas is limited and the gallbladder is not contracted. Both supine and right anterior oblique views should be obtained if the patient can move or be moved. Because many patients have livers that are tucked beneath the lower right ribs, a transducer with a small scanning face, allowing an intercostal approach, is invaluable. Suspended inspiration enables examination of the dome of the liver, frequently an ultrasound "blind spot." Sagittal, transverse, coronal, and subcostal oblique views are required for a complete survey.

NORMAL ANATOMY

The liver lies in the right upper quadrant of the abdomen, suspended from the right hemidiaphragm. Functionally, it can be divided into **three lobes**—the right, left, and caudate lobes. The **right lobe** of the liver is separated from the left by the main lobar fissure, which passes through the gallbladder fossa to the inferior vena cava (Fig. 4-1). The right lobe of the liver can be further divided into anterior and posterior segments by the right intersegmental fissure. The left intersegmental fissure divides the **left lobe** into medial and lateral segments. The **caudate lobe** is situated on the posterior aspect of the liver, having as its posterior border the inferior vena cava and as its anterior border the fissure for the ligamentum venosum (Fig. 4-2, A). The papillary process is the anteromedial extension of the caudate lobe, which may appear separate from the liver and mimic lymphadenopathy (Fig. 4-2, B).

Understanding the vascular anatomy of the liver is essential to an appreciation of the relative positions of the hepatic segments. The major **hepatic veins** course **between** the lobes and segments (**interlobar and intersegmental**). They are ideal segmental boundaries but are visualized only when scanning the superior liver (Fig. 4-3). The middle hepatic vein courses

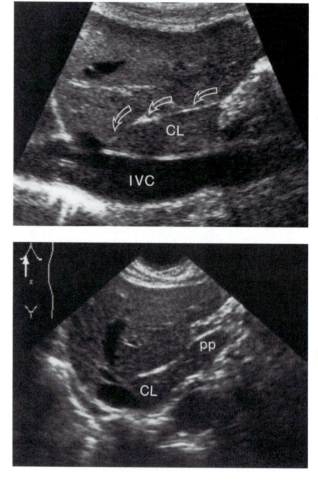

A

B

FIG. 4-2. Caudate lobe. A, The caudate lobe (CL) is separated from the left lobe by the fissure for the ligamentum venosum (arrows) anteriorly and inferior vena cava (IVC) posteriorly. **B,** The papillary process (pp) is a tonguelike projection of the caudate lobe (CL).

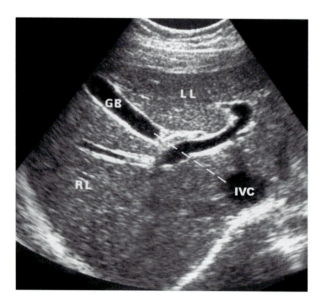

FIG. 4-1. Normal lobar anatomy. The right lobe of the liver (RL) can be separated from the left lobe of the liver (LL) by the main lobar fissure which passes through the gallbladder fossa (GB) and the inferior vena cava (IVC).

within the main lobar fissure and separates the anterior segment of the right lobe from the medial segment of the left. The right hepatic vein runs within the right intersegmental fissure and divides the right lobe into anterior and posterior segments. In more caudal sections of the liver, the right hepatic vein is no longer identified, therefore the segmental boundary becomes a more ill-defined division between the anterior and posterior branches of the right portal vein. The major branches of the right and left **portal veins** run centrally **within** the segments (**intrasegmental**), with the exception of the ascending portion of the left portal vein, which runs in the left intersegmental fissure. The **left intersegmental fissure,** which separates the medial segment of the left lobe from the lateral segment, can be divided into cranial, middle, and caudal sections. The left hepatic vein forms the boundary of the cranial third, the ascending branch of the left portal vein represents the middle third, and the fissure for the ligamentum teres acts as the most caudal division of the left lobe (Table 4-1).[1]

Couinaud's Anatomy

Because sonography allows evaluation of liver anatomy in multiple planes, the radiologist can precisely localize a lesion to a given segment for the surgeons. Couinaud's anatomy, widely used in Europe and French Canada, is now becoming the universal nomenclature for hepatic lesion localization (Table 4-2).[2] This description is based on portal segments and is of both functional and pathologic importance. Each segment has its own blood supply (arterial, portal, hepatic venous), lymphatics, and biliary drainage. Thus, the surgeon may resect a segment of an hepatic lobe, providing the vascular supply to the remaining lobe is left intact. Each segment has a branch or branches of the portal vein at its center, bounded by an hepatic vein. There are eight segments. **The right, middle, and left hepatic veins divide the liver longitudinally into four sections.** Each of these sections is further **divided transversely** by an imaginary plane through the right main and left main portal pedicles. Segment I is the caudate lobe, II and III are the left superior and inferior lateral segments, respectively, and segment IV, which is further divided into IVa and IVb, is the medial segment of the left lobe. The right lobe consists of segments V and VI, located caudal to the transverse plane, and segments VII and VIII, which are cephalad (Fig. 4-4).[3,4,5] The caudate lobe (segment I) may receive branches of both the right and left portal veins. In contrast to the other segments, it has one or several hepatic veins which drain directly into the inferior vena cava.

The **portal venous supply for the left lobe** can be visualized using an oblique, cranially-angled subxiphoid view (recurrent subcostal oblique projection).

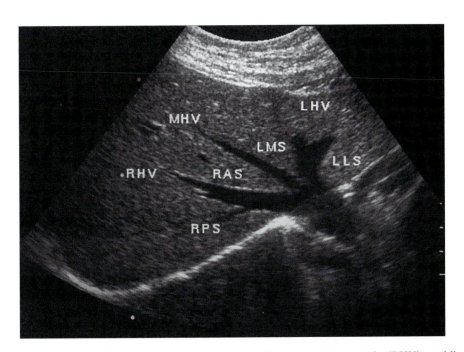

FIG. 4-3. **Hepatic venous anatomy.** The three hepatic veins, right (RHV); middle, (MHV); and left (LHV), are interlobar and intersegmental separating the lobes and segments. The right hepatic vein separates the right posterior segment (RPS) from the right anterior segment (RAS). The left hepatic vein separates the left medial segment (LMS) from the left lateral segment (LLS). The middle hepatic vein separates the right and left lobes.

TABLE 4-1
NORMAL HEPATIC ANATOMY:
ANATOMIC STRUCTURES USEFUL FOR IDENTIFYING THE HEPATIC SEGMENTS

Structure	Location	Usefulness
RHV	Right intersegmental fissure	Divides cephalic aspect of anterior and posterior segments of right lobe
MHV	Main lobar fissure	Separates right and left lobes
LHV	Left intersegmental fissure	Divides cephalic aspect of medial and lateral segments of left lobe
RPV (anterior branch)	Intrasegmental in anterior segment of right lobe	Courses centrally in anterior segment of right lobe
RPV (posterior branch)	Intrasegmental in posterior segment of right lobe	Courses centrally in posterior segment of right lobe
LPV (horizontal segment)	Anterior to caudate lobe	Separates caudate lobe posteriorly from medial segment of left lobe anteriorly
LPV (ascending segment)	Left intersegmental fissure	Divides medial from lateral segment of left lobe
GB fossa	Main lobar fissure	Separates right and left lobes
Fissure for the ligamentum teres	Left intersegmental fissure	Divides caudal aspect of left lobe into medial and lateral segments
Fissure for the ligamentum venosum	Left anterior margin of the caudate lobe	Separates caudate lobe posteriorly from left lobe anteriorly

RHV indicates right hepatic vein; *MHV*, middle hepatic vein; *LHV*, left hepatic vein; *RPV*, right portal vein; *LPV*, left portal vein; *GB*, gallbladder.
Modified from Marks WM, Filly RA, Callen PW. Ultrasonic anatomy of the liver: a review with new applications. *J Clin Ultrasound* 1979;7:137-146.

TABLE 4-2
HEPATIC ANATOMY

Couinaud	Traditional
Segment I	Caudate lobe
Segment II	Lateral segment left lobe (superior)
Segment III	Lateral segment left lobe (inferior)
Segment IV	Medial segment left lobe
Segment V	Anterior segment right lobe (inferior)
Segment VI	Posterior segment right lobe (inferior)
Segment VII	Posterior segment right lobe (superior)
Segment VIII	Anterior segment right lobe (superior)

A **"recumbent H"** is formed by the main left portal vein, the ascending branch of the left portal vein and the branches to segments, II, III, and IV (Fig. 4-5).[6] Segments II and III are separated from segment IV by the left hepatic vein as well as by the ascending branch of the left portal vein and the falciform ligament. Segment IV is separated from segments V and VIII by the middle hepatic vein and the main hepatic fissure.

The **portal venous supply to the right lobe** of the liver can also be seen as a **"recumbent H."**[6] The main right portal vein gives rise to branches which supply segments V and VI (inferiorly) and VII and VIII (superiorly). They are seen best in a sagittal or oblique-sagittal plane (Fig. 4-6).[6]

With the oblique subxiphoid view, the right portal vein is seen in cross-section and enables identification of the more superiorly located segment VIII (which is closer to the confluence of hepatic veins) from segment V (Fig. 4-6). Segments V and VIII are separated from segments VI and VII by the right hepatic vein.[6]

Ligaments

The liver is covered by a thin connective tissue layer called **Glisson's capsule.** The capsule surrounds the entire liver and is thickest around the inferior vena cava and the porta hepatis. At the porta hepatis the main portal vein, the proper hepatic artery, and the common bile duct are contained within investing peritoneal folds known as the **hepatoduodenal ligament** (Fig. 4-7). The **falciform ligament** conducts the umbilical vein to the liver during fetal development (Fig. 4-8). After birth, the umbilical vein atrophies, forming the **ligamentum teres.** As it reaches the liver, the leaves of the falciform ligament separate. The right layer forms the upper layer of the **coronary ligament;** the left layer forms the upper layer of the **left triangular ligament.** The most lateral portion of the coronary ligament is known as the **right triangular ligament** (Fig. 4-9). The peritoneal layers that form the coronary ligament are widely separated, leaving an

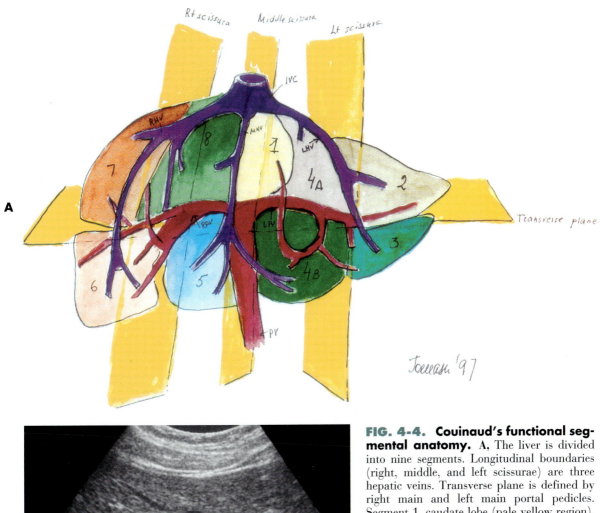

FIG. 4-4. Couinaud's functional segmental anatomy. A, The liver is divided into nine segments. Longitudinal boundaries (right, middle, and left scissurae) are three hepatic veins. Transverse plane is defined by right main and left main portal pedicles. Segment 1, caudate lobe (pale yellow region), is situated posteriorly. RHV—indicates right hepatic vein; MHV—middle hepatic vein; LHV—left hepatic vein; RPV—right portal vein; LPV—left portal vein; GB—gallbladder. **B,** Subcostal oblique sonogram at level of major branches of right (RPV) and left (LPV) portal veins. Cephalad to this level lie segments II, IVa, VII, and VIII. Caudally located are segments III, IVb, V, and VI. (**A,** Modified from Sugarbaker PH: Toward a standard of nomenclature for surgical anatomy of the liver. *Neth J Surg* 1988, PO:100.)

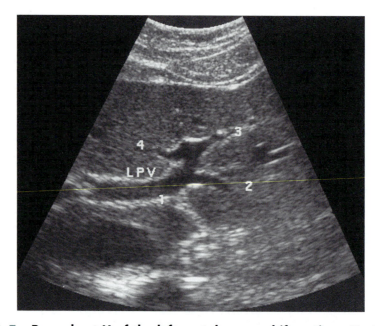

FIG. 4-5. **Recumbent H of the left portal venous bifurcation.** The left portal vein (LPV), the ascending branch of the LPV, and the branches to segments 2, 3, and 4 create an appearance suggesting a recumbent H. 1 is on the caudate lobe which does not have visible branches from the portal vein.

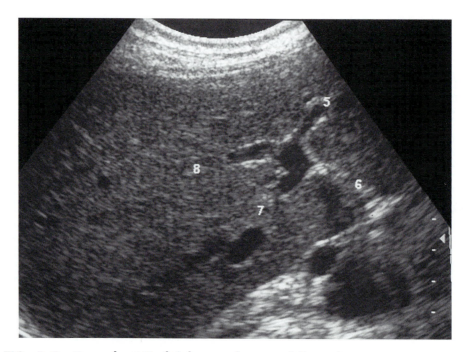

FIG. 4-6. **Recumbent H of right portal venous bifurcation** is more difficult to visualize, and is best seen with an intercostal view. Right portal venous bifurcation shows the branches to the anterior segments, 5 and 8, and the posterior segments 6 and 7.

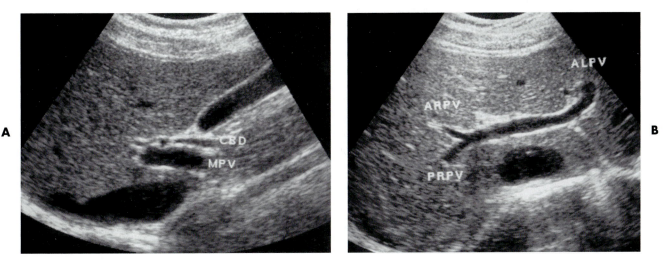

FIG. 4-7. Porta hepatis. **A,** Sagittal image of the porta hepatis shows the common bile duct (CBD) and main portal vein (MPV), which are enclosed within the hepatoduodenal ligament. **B,** Transverse image of the porta hepatis shows the portal vein, which bifurcates into right and left branches. Anterior right portal vein (ARPV), posterior right portal vein (PRPV), ascending left portal vein (ALPV).

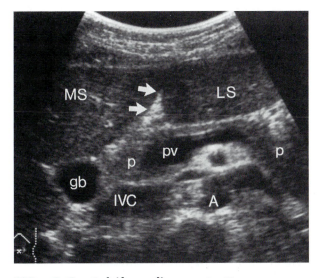

FIG. 4-8. Falciform ligament. Transverse scan through midabdomen shows echogenic falciform ligament (*arrows*), which separates lateral segment (LS) of left lobe from medial segment (MS). IVC—inferior vena cava; A—aorta; gb—gallbladder, p—pancreas; pv—portal vein.

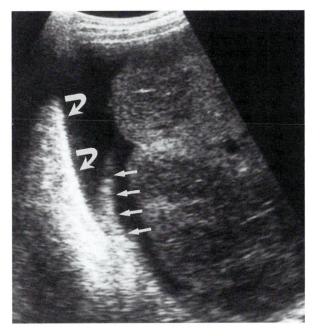

FIG. 4-9. Right triangular ligament. Subcostal oblique scan near dome of right hemidiaphragm (*curved, arrows*). Note lobulated contour and inhomogeneity of liver in this patient with cirrhosis. Right triangular ligament (*straight arrows*) is visualized because of ascites.

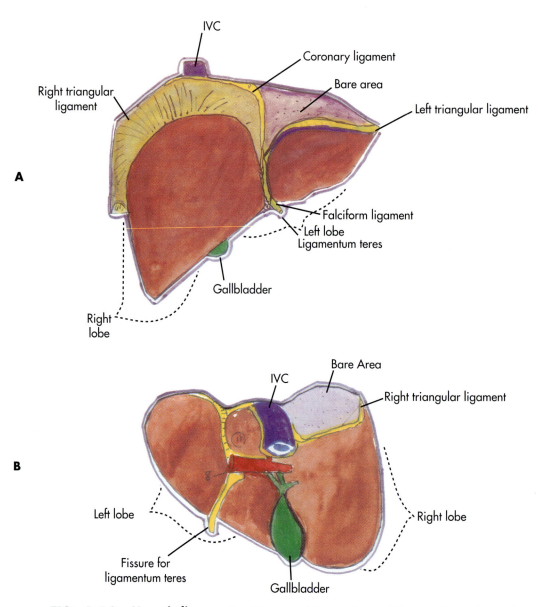

FIG. 4-10. **Hepatic ligaments.** Diagram of **A,** anterior, and **B,** posterior surfaces of the liver.

area of the liver not covered by peritoneum. This posterosuperior region is known as the "bare area" of the liver. The ligamentum venosum carries the obliterated ductus venosus, which until birth shunts blood from the umbilical vein to the inferior vena cava (Fig. 4-10).

HEPATIC CIRCULATION

Portal Veins

The liver receives a dual blood supply from both the portal vein and the hepatic artery. Although the portal vein carries incompletely oxygenated (80%) venous blood from the intestines and spleen, it supplies up to half the oxygen requirements of the hepatocytes be-

cause of its greater flow. This dual blood supply explains the low incidence of hepatic infarction.

The **portal triad** contains a branch of the portal vein, hepatic artery, and bile duct. These are contained within a connective tissue sheath that gives the portal vein an echogenic wall on sonography and allows for its distinction from the hepatic veins, which have an almost imperceptible wall. The main portal vein divides into right and left branches. The right portal vein has an anterior branch that lies centrally within the anterior segment of the right lobe and a posterior branch that lies centrally within the posterior segment of the right lobe. The left portal vein initially courses anterior to the caudate lobe (Fig. 4-11). The ascending branch of the left portal vein then travels anteriorly in the left

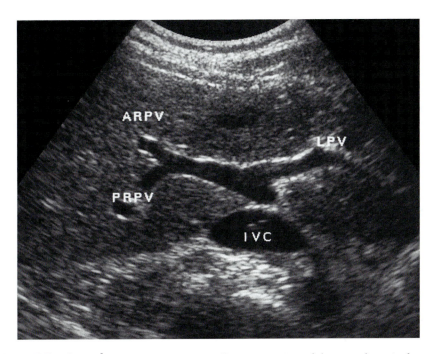

FIG. 4-11. **Portal venous anatomy.** Transverse view of the porta hepatis shows the main portal vein dividing into its right and left branches. Anterior right portal vein (ARPV), posterior right portal vein (PRPV), left portal vein (LPV), inferior vena cava (IVC). The anterior and posterior right portal venous branches lie centrally within the right anterior and posterior segments. The visualized portion of the left portal vein courses anterior to the caudate lobe.

intersegmental fissure to divide the medial and lateral segments of the left lobe.

Arterial Circulation

The branches of the hepatic artery accompany the portal veins. The terminal branches of the portal vein and their accompanying hepatic arterioles and bile ducts are known as the acinus.

Hepatic Venous System

Blood perfuses the liver parenchyma through the sinusoids and then enters the terminal hepatic venules. These terminal branches unite to form sequentially larger veins. The hepatic veins vary in number and position. However, in the general population, there are three major veins: the right, middle, and left hepatic veins (Fig. 4-12). All drain into the inferior vena cava and, like the portal veins, are without valves. The right hepatic vein is usually single and runs in the right intersegmental fissure, separating the anterior and posterior segments of the right lobe. The middle hepatic vein, which courses in the main lobar fissure, forms a common trunk with the left hepatic vein in the majority of individuals. The left hepatic vein forms the most cephalad boundary between the medial and lateral segments of the left lobe.

NORMAL LIVER SIZE AND ECHOGENICITY

The upper border of the liver lies approximately at the level of the fifth intercostal space at the midclavicular line. The lower border extends to or slightly below the costal margin. An accurate assessment of liver size is difficult with real-time ultrasound equipment because of the limited field of view. Gosink[7] proposed measuring the liver length in the midhepatic line. In 75% of patients with a liver length of greater than 15.5 cm, hepatomegaly is present. Niederau et al.[8] measured the liver in a longitudinal and anteroposterior diameter in both the midclavicular line and midline and correlated these findings with gender, age, height, weight, and body surface area. They found that organ size increases with height and body surface area and decreases with age. The mean longitudinal diameter of the liver in the midclavicular line in this study was 10.5 with 1.5 (standard deviation) cm and the mean midclavicular anteroposterior diameter was 8.1 with 1.9 (standard deviation) cm. In most patients, measurement of the liver length suffices to measure liver size. In heavy or asthenic individuals, the anteroposterior diameter should be added to avoid underestimations or overestimations, respectively. **Reidel's**

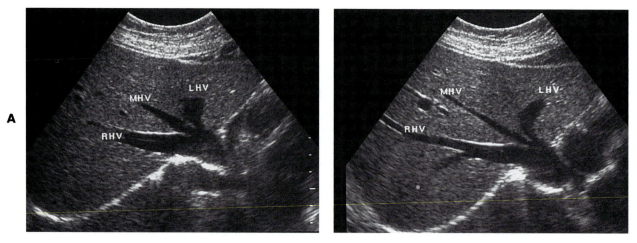

FIG. 4-12. Hepatic venous anatomy, best seen on subcostal oblique view, A, The three hepatic veins, right (RHV), middle (MHV), and left (LHV), drain into the most cephalad aspect of the inferior vena cava. **B,** Increasing the obliquity of the transducer shows a longer length of the three veins.

lobe is a tonguelike extension of the inferior tip of the right lobe of the liver, which is frequently found in asthenic women.

The normal liver is homogeneous, contains fine-level echoes, and is either minimally hyperechoic or isoechoic compared to the normal renal cortex (Fig. 4-13, *A*). The liver is hypoechoic compared to the spleen. This relationship is evident when the lateral segment of the left lobe is elongated and wraps around the spleen (Fig. 4-13, *B*).

DEVELOPMENTAL ANOMALIES

Agenesis
Agenesis of the liver is incompatible with life. Agenesis of both the right and left lobes has been reported.[9,10] In three of five reported cases of agenesis of the right lobe, the caudate lobe was also absent.[10] Compensatory hypertrophy of the remaining lobes normally occurs, and liver function tests are normal.

Anomalies of Position
In situs inversus totalis, the liver is found in the left hypochondrium. In congenital diaphragmatic hernia or omphalocele, varying amounts of liver may herniate into the thorax or outside the abdominal cavity.

Accessory Fissures
Although invaginations of the dome of the diaphragm have been called accessory fissures, strictly speaking, these are not fissures but rather diaphragmatic slips. They are a cause of pseudomasses on sonography if

the liver is not carefully examined in both sagittal and transverse planes (Fig. 4-14). True accessory fissures are uncommon and are caused by an infolding of peritoneum. The inferior accessory hepatic fissure is a true accessory fissure that stretches inferiorly from the right portal vein to the inferior surface of the right lobe of the liver.[11]

Vascular Anomalies
The **common hepatic artery** arises from the celiac axis and divides into right and left branches at the porta hepatis. This classic textbook description of the hepatic arterial anatomy occurs in only 55% of the population. The remaining 45% have some variation of this anatomy, of which the main patterns are: (1) replaced left hepatic artery originating from the left gastric artery (10%); (2) replaced right hepatic artery originating from the superior mesenteric artery (11%); and (3) replaced common hepatic artery (2.5%) originating from the superior mesenteric artery.

Congenital anomalies of the **portal vein** include atresias, strictures and obstructing valves—all of which are uncommon. Sonographic variations include absence of the right portal vein with anomalies of branching from the main and left portal veins and absence of the horizontal segment of the left portal vein.[12]

In contrast, variations in the branching of the hepatic veins and accessory hepatic veins are relatively common. The most common accessory vein drains the superoanterior segment of the right lobe (segment VIII) and is seen in approximately one third of the population. It usually empties into the middle hepatic vein, although occasionally it joins the right hepatic

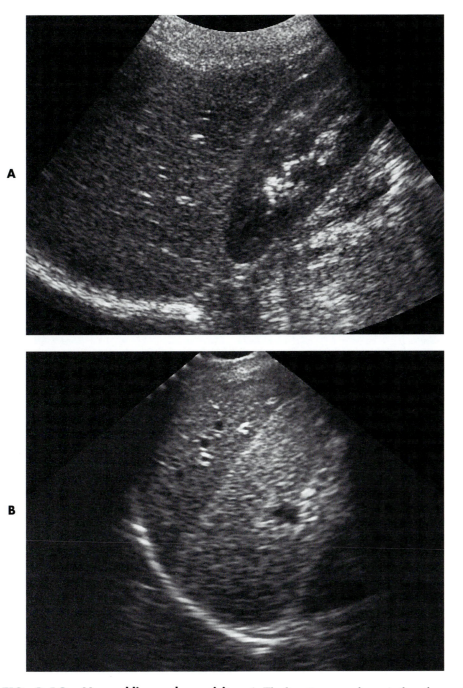

FIG. 4-13. **Normal liver echogenicity.** **A,** The liver is more echogenic than the renal cortex. **B,** The liver is less echogenic than the spleen as can be seen in many thin women whose left lobe of the liver wraps around the spleen.

vein.[13] An inferior right hepatic vein, which drains the inferoposterior portion of the liver (segment VI), is observed in 10% of individuals. This inferior right hepatic vein drains directly into the inferior vena cava and may be as large as or larger than the right hepatic vein.[14] Left and right marginal veins, which drain into the left and right hepatic veins, occur in approxi-

mately 12% and 3% of individuals, respectively. Absence of the main hepatic veins is relatively less common, occurring in approximately 8% of people.[14] Awareness of the normal variations of the hepatic venous system is helpful in accurately defining the location of focal liver lesions and aids the surgeon in segmental liver resection.

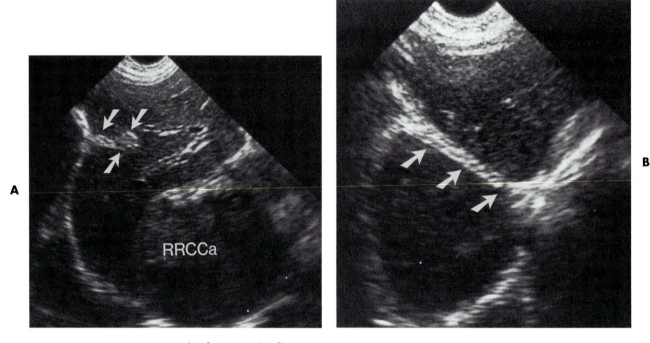

FIG. 4-14. Diaphragmatic slip. A, Sagittal sonogram shows echogenic "mass" (*arrows*) adjacent to right hemidiaphragm in this patient with right renal cell carcinoma (RRCCa). **B,** Subcostal oblique image reveals "mass" is diaphragmatic slip (*arrows*).

CONGENITAL ABNORMALITIES

Liver Cyst

A liver cyst is defined as a fluid-filled space having an epithelial lining. Abscesses, parasitic cysts, and post-traumatic cysts are therefore not true cysts. The frequent presence of columnar epithelium within simple hepatic cysts suggests they have a ductal origin, although their precise cause is unclear. Nor is it clear why these lesions do not appear until middle age. Although thought at one time to be relatively uncommon, ultrasound examination has shown that liver cysts occur in 2.5% of the general population, increasing to 7% in the population older than 80 years of age.[15]

On sonographic examination, benign hepatic cysts are anechoic with a well-demarcated, thin wall and posterior acoustic enhancement. Occasionally, the patient may develop pain and fever secondary to cyst hemorrhage or infection. In this situation, the cyst may contain internal echoes (Fig. 4-15) and septations, a thickened wall, or may appear solid (Fig. 4-16). Active intervention is recommended only in the symptomatic patient. Although aspiration will yield fluid for evaluation, the cyst with an epithelial lining will recur. Cyst ablation with alcohol can be performed using ultrasound guidance.[16] Alternatively, surgical excision is indicated. The appearances of liver cysts may mimic biliary cystadenoma (Fig. 4-17) and

necrotic or cystic metastases. If thick septae or nodules are seen within liver cysts, computed tomography (CT) is recommended.

Peribiliary Cysts

Peribiliary cysts have been described in patients with severe liver disease.[17] These cysts are small, ranging in size from 0.2 to 2.5 cm and are usually located centrally within the porta hepatis or at the junction of the main right and left hepatic ducts. They generally are asymptomatic although may rarely cause biliary obstruction.[17] Pathologically, they are believed to represent obstructed small periductal glands. **Sonographically,** the peribiliary cysts may be seen as discrete, clustered cysts, or as tubular-appearing structures having thin septae, paralleling the bile ducts and portal veins.

Adult Polycystic Disease

The adult form of polycystic kidney disease is inherited in an autosomal dominant pattern. The frequency of liver cysts in association with this condition varies between 57% to 74%.[18] No correlation exists between the severity of the renal disease and the extent of liver involvement. Liver function tests are usually normal and, unlike the infantile autosomal recessive form of polycystic kidney disease, there is no association with hepatic fibrosis and portal hypertension. Indeed, if liver function tests are abnormal, complications of

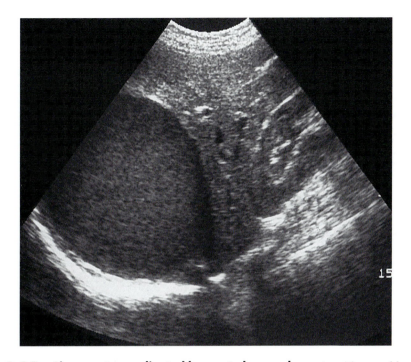

FIG. 4-15. **Liver cyst complicated by acute hemorrhage** in a 46-year-old woman with acute right upper-quadrant pain. Sagittal right lobe sonogram shows a very well-defined subdiaphragmatic mass with uniform low-level internal echoes. This appearance could be misinterpreted as a solid mass.

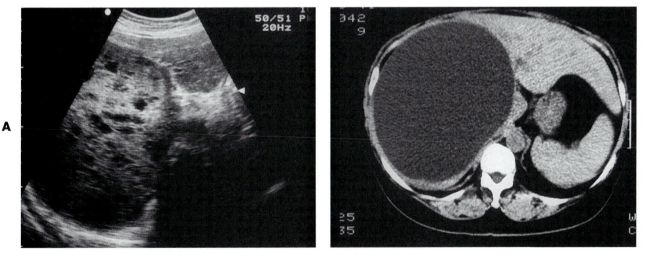

A   B

FIG. 4-16. **Hemorrhagic cyst,** surgically confirmed. **A,** Transverse sonogram shows a large, well-defined mass with a complex but predominantly solid internal character. **B,** Enhanced computed tomography (CT) scan shows a nonenhancing low-density mass consistent with a cyst. Ultrasound is superior to CT scan at characterization of the mass.

polycystic liver disease such as tumor, cyst infection, or biliary obstruction should be excluded.[18]

Biliary Hamartomas (von Meyenburg Complexes)

Bile duct hamartomas, first described by von Meyenburg in 1918,[19] are small, focal developmental lesions of the liver composed of groups of dilated intrahepatic bile ducts set within a dense collagenous stroma.[20] They are benign liver malformations that are detected incidentally in 0.6 to 5.6% of reported autopsy series.[21]

Imaging features of von Meyenburg complexes (VMC) are described in the literature in isolated case

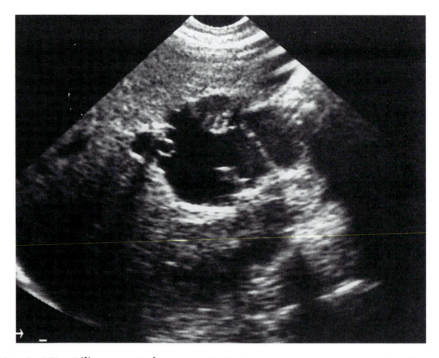

FIG. 4-17. Biliary cystadenoma. Sagittal sonogram shows an irregular liver cyst with thick septae and mural nodules.

reports and a few small series including sonographic, CT, and magnetic resonance imaging (MRI) appearances.[22] VMC are often confused with metastatic cancer and reports describe single, multiple, or most often innumerable well-defined solid nodules usually less than 1 cm in diameter. Nodules are usually uniformly hypoechoic[22] (Fig. 4-18) and less commonly hyperechoic on sonography[23,24] and hypodense on contrast-enhanced CT scan. Bright echogenic foci in the liver with distal ringdown artifact without obvious mass effect are also documented on sonograms related to the presence of cholesterol crystals in the dilated tubules of the VMC (Fig. 4-19).[25]

Although VMC are usually isolated and insignificant observations, some patients with the cholesterol crystals may have repeated episodes of recurrent cholangitis responsive to antibiotic therapy.[25] VMC may occur with other congenital disorders such as congenital hepatic fibrosis or polycystic kidney or liver disease.[21] Association of VMC with cholangiocarcinoma has been suggested.[26]

INFECTIOUS DISEASES

Viral

Viral hepatitis is a common disease that occurs worldwide. It is responsible for millions of deaths secondary to acute hepatic necrosis or chronic hepatitis, which in turn may lead to portal hypertension, cirrhosis, and

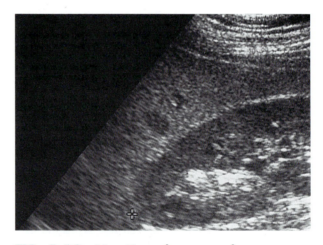

FIG. 4-18. Von Meyenburg complex in a patient with breast cancer. Sagittal sonogram of the right lobe shows a single small hypoechoic liver mass just anterior to the kidney. As there was no other evidence of metastatic disease, a biopsy was performed and proved the benign insignificant nature of this lesion.

hepatocellular carcinoma. Recent medical advances have identified at least six distinct hepatitis viruses: hepatitis A through E and G.[27]

Hepatitis. Hepatitis A occurs throughout the world and can be diagnosed using serosurveys with the antibody to Hepatitis A (anti-HAV) as the marker. The primary mode of spread is via the fecal-oral route. In developing countries, the disease is endemic and in-

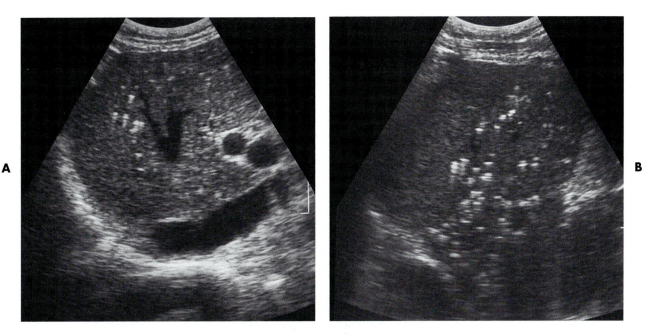

FIG. 4-19. **Von Meyenburg complexes (VMC)** in a 47-year-old man with multiple episodes of cholangitis responsive to antibiotic therapy. **A,** Sagittal and **B,** transverse images of the left lobe of the liver show multiple bright echogenic foci in the liver with ringdown artifact. Biopsy showed VMC with cholesterol crystals.

fection occurs early in life. In the United States, transmission occurs in crowded quarters, i.e., the Army, day-care centers, institutions; where there is fecal contamination of water or food; and among homosexual men and susceptible travellers. Hepatitis A is an acute infection leading to either complete recovery or death from acute liver failure.

Hepatitis B is transmitted parenterally, for example via blood transfusions and needle punctures as well as by nonpercutaneous exposure through sexual contact. Hepatitis B, unlike A, has a carrier state, which is estimated worldwide at 300 million. The regions of highest carrier rates (5% to 20%) are Southeast Asia, China, sub-Saharan Africa and Greenland. The interpretation of tests for hepatitis B markers is complex and beyond the scope of this book. The two most useful markers for acute infection are hepatitis B surface antigen (HBs Ag) and antibody to hepatitis B core antigen (anti-HBc).

Non-A, Non-B (NANB) (predominantly C) hepatitis was first recognized in 1974-1975. Investigators in the United States were surprised to learn that the majority of cases of post-transfusion hepatitis were not secondary to hepatitis B but to an unknown virus or viruses. Since then, it has been realized that many cases are not the result of percutaneous transmission and that in almost 50%, no source could be identified. Acutely infected individuals have a much greater risk of chronic infection, with up to 85% progressing to chronic liver disease. Chronic hepatitis C is

diagnosed by the presence in blood of the antibody to HCV (anti-HCV).

Hepatitis D or hepatitis delta virus is entirely dependent upon the hepatitis B virus for its infectivity, requiring the HBsAg to provide an envelope coat for the hepatitis D virus. Its geographic distribution is therefore similar to that of hepatitis B. It is an uncommon infection in North America, occurring primarily in intravenous (IV) drug users.

Hepatitis E has the clinical characteristics of hepatitis A infection and is transmitted via the fecal-oral route. It is responsible for the vast majority of waterborne epidemics in India and may soon surpass hepatitis B as the world's most common cause of hepatitis.

Clinical Manifestations of Hepatitis. **Uncomplicated acute hepatitis** implies clinical recovery within four months. It is the outcome of 99% of cases of hepatitis A.

Subfulminant and fulminant hepatic failure occur following the onset of jaundice and include worsening jaundice, coagulopathy, and hepatic encephalopathy. Most cases are due to hepatitis B or drug toxicity. This condition is characterized by hepatic necrosis. Death occurs if the loss of hepatic parenchyma is greater than 40%.[28]

Chronic hepatitis is defined as the persistence of biochemical abnormalities beyond six months. It has many etiologies other than viral, i.e., metabolic (Wilson's disease, alpha-1 antitrypsin deficiency, hemochromatosis), autoimmune, and drug induced. The prog-

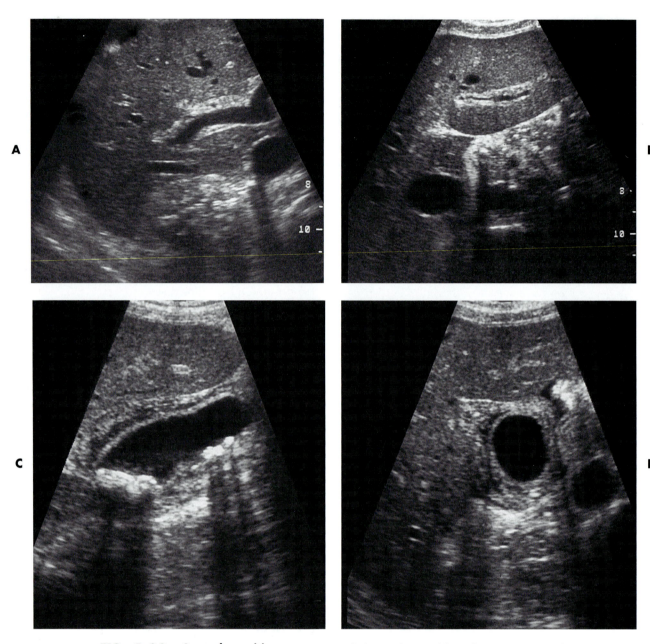

FIG. 4-20. **Acute hepatitis** in a patient with fever, abnormal liver function tests, and incidental gallstones. **A,** Transverse view of porta hepatis and **B,** transverse view of left lobe of liver both show prominent thick echogenic bands surrounding the portal veins in the portal triads, referred to as "periportal cuffing." **C,** Sagittal and **D,** transverse views of the gallbladder show moderate edema and thickening of the gallbladder wall. The gallbladder is not large or tense and the patient does not have acute cholecystitis. Incidental cholelithiasis, as in this case, may be confusing.

nosis and treatment of the disease depend upon the specific etiology.[29]

In acute hepatitis, there is diffuse swelling of the hepatocytes, proliferation of Kupffer cells lining the sinusoids and infiltration of the portal areas by lymphocytes and monocytes. **The sonographic features** parallel the histologic findings. The liver parenchyma may have a diffusely decreased echogenicity, with accentu-ated brightness of the portal triads, periportal cuffing (Fig. 4-20, *A* and *B*). Hepatomegaly and thickening of the gallbladder wall are associated findings (Fig. 4-20, *C* and *D*). In most cases the liver appears normal.[30] Most cases of chronic hepatitis are also sonographically normal. When cirrhosis develops, sonography may demonstrate a coarsened echotexture and other morphologic changes of cirrhosis (Fig. 4-21).

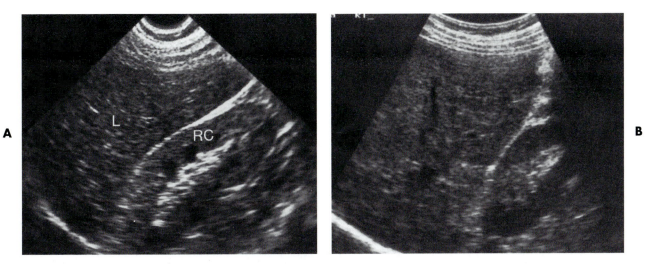

FIG. 4-21. Chronic active hepatitis. A, At presentation, liver (L) is minimally hypo-echoic compared with normal renal cortex (RC). **B,** Eight months later, clinical deterioration. Liver texture is inhomogeneous and coarse. Repeat liver biopsy confirmed worsening disease.

Bacterial

Pyogenic bacteria reach the liver by several routes, the most common being direct extension from the biliary tract in patients with suppurative cholangitis and cholecystitis. Other routes are through the portal venous system in patients with diverticulitis or appendicitis and through the hepatic artery in patients with osteomyelitis and subacute bacterial endocarditis. Pyogenic bacteria may also be present in the liver as a result of blunt or penetrating trauma. No cause can be found in approximately 50% of the cases of hepatic abscesses. Most of this latter group are caused by anaerobic infection. Diagnosis of bacterial liver infection is often delayed. The most common presenting features of pyogenic liver abscess are fever, malaise, anorexia, and right upper quadrant pain. Jaundice may be present in approximately 25% of these patients.

Sonography has proved to be extremely helpful in the detection of abdominal abscesses. The ultrasound features of pyogenic liver abscesses are varied. Frankly purulent abscesses appear cystic, with the fluid ranging from echo-free to highly echogenic (Fig. 4-22). Regions of early suppuration may appear solid with altered echogenicity, usually hypoechoic, related to the presence of necrotic hepatocytes (Fig. 4-23).[31] Occasionally gas-producing organisms give rise to echogenic foci with a posterior reverberation artifact (Fig. 4-24). Fluid-fluid interfaces, internal septations, and debris have all been observed (Fig. 4-25). The abscess wall can vary from well-defined to irregular and thick (Fig. 4-22).

The **differential diagnosis** of pyogenic liver abscess includes amoebic or echinococcal infection, simple cyst with hemorrhage, hematoma, and necrotic

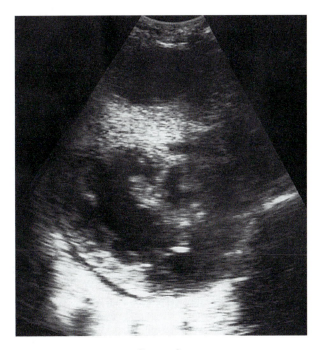

FIG. 4-22. Mature liver abscess. Transverse sonogram shows two focal hypoechoic masses. The large lesion has a thick, shaggy wall with extensive internal necrotic debris and increased through transmission.

or cystic neoplasm. Ultrasound-guided liver aspiration is an expeditious means to confirm the diagnosis. Specimens should be sent for both aerobic and anaerobic culture. Fifty percent of abscesses in the past were considered sterile. This was almost certainly caused by failure to transport the specimen in an oxygen-free container, and thus anaerobic organisms were not identified.[32] Once the diagnosis of liver ab-

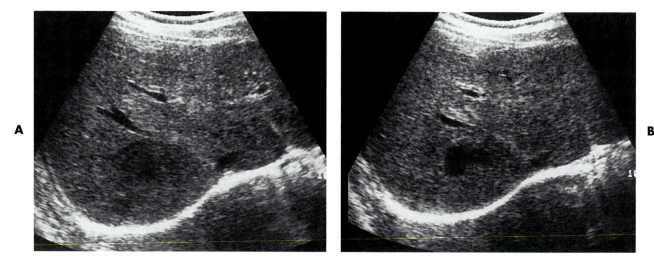

FIG. 4-23. **Pyogenic liver abscess—rapid evolution from phlegmon to liquefaction.** **A,** Transverse sonogram of right lobe shows a subtle hypoechoic poorly defined "mass effect" in segment 7 deep to the right hepatic vein. **B,** Twenty-four hours later, there is liquefaction in the central area of the abscess.

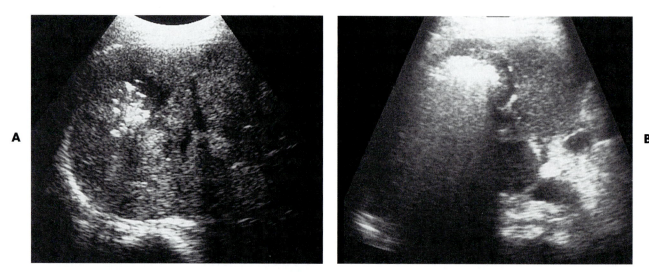

FIG. 4-24. **Liver abscess with gas bubbles** in two different patients. **A,** Multiple gas bubbles are seen as innumerable tiny bright echogenic foci within a poorly defined hypoechoic liver mass. The gas bubbles have a highly suggestive appearance and assist with the diagnosis of abscess secondary to gas-forming organisms. **B,** A large pocket of gas within a hypoechoic mass shows as an amorphous area of bright echogenicity with distal dirty shadowing totally obscuring the deep area of the liver. This gross abnormality may be easily overlooked or mistaken for bowel gas if its visceral origin is not appreciated.

scess is made by the presence of pus or a positive gram stain and culture, the collection can be drained percutaneously using ultrasound or CT guidance.

Fungal

Candidiasis. The liver is frequently involved secondary to hematogenous spread of mycotic infections in other organs, most commonly the lungs. Patients are generally immunocompromised, al-

though systemic candidiasis may occur in pregnancy or following hyperalimentation. The clinical characteristics include persistent fever in a neutropenic patient whose leukocyte count is returning to normal.[33]

The **ultrasound features** of hepatic candidiasis include:[34]

• **"Wheel within a wheel"**—Peripheral hypoechoic zone with an inner echogenic wheel and central hypoechoic nidus. The central nidus represents focal

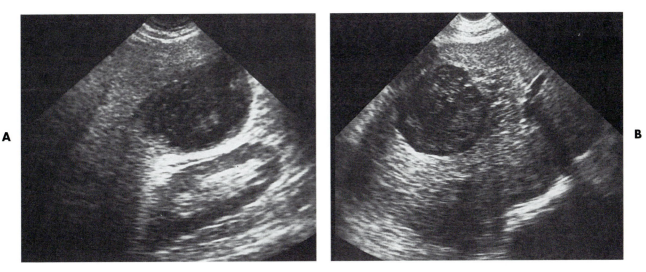

FIG. 4-25. Pyogenic liver abscess—classic morphology in two patients. **A,** Sagittal sonogram shows a poorly marginated hypoechoic mass bulging the liver capsule. There are internal echoes and debris. **B,** Transverse sonogram shows a well-defined hypoechoic mass with increased through transmission which supports a cystic nature. There is extensive internal echogenicity associated with the necrotic contents of the abscess cavity.

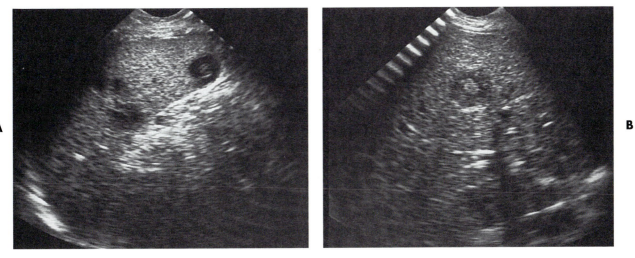

FIG. 4-26. Fungal infection, "bulls eye" morphology, in a 24-year-old man with ALL and fever. **A,** Sagittal sonogram through the spleen shows focal hypoechoic target lesions. **B,** The liver showed multiple masses. This magnified view shows a thick echogenic rim and a thin hypoechoic inner rim with a dense echogenic nidus. Biopsy revealed pseudohyphae.

necrosis in which fungal elements are found. This is seen early in the disease.

- **"Bull's eye"**—1- to 4-cm lesion having a hyperechoic center and a hypoechoic rim. It is present when neutrophil counts return to normal. The echogenic center contains inflammatory cells (Fig. 4-26).
- **"Uniformly hypoechoic"**—Most common. This corresponds to progressive fibrosis (Fig. 4-27, *A*).

- **"Echogenic"**—Variable calcification representing scar formation (Fig. 4-27, *B*).

It is interesting to note that, although percutaneous liver aspiration is of great benefit in obtaining the organism in pyogenic liver abscesses, it frequently yields falsely negative results for the presence of *Candida* organisms.[34] This may be caused by failure to sample the central necrotic portion of the lesion where the pseudohyphae are found.[33]

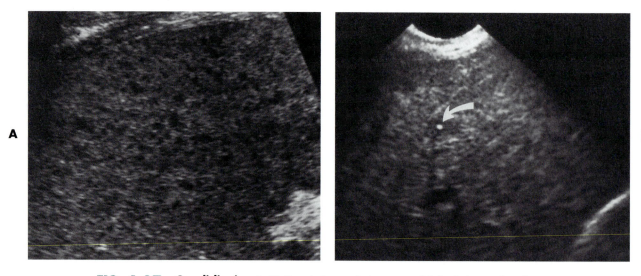

FIG. 4-27. **Candidiasis.** A, Uniformly hypoechoic pattern. Multiple hypoechoic hepatic lesions are present in this young patient with acute myelogenous leukemia. **B,** Echogenic pattern, following medical therapy. Small calcified lesion (*arrow*) is visualized in a second immunocompromised patient.

ULTRASOUND FEATURES OF HEPATIC CANDIDIASIS

"Wheel within a wheel"
Peripheral hypoechoic zone
Inner echogenic wheel
Central hypoechoic nidus

"Bull's eye"
Hyperechoic center
Hypoechoic rim

"Uniformly hypoechoic"
Progressive fibrosis

"Echogenic"
Calcification representing scar formation

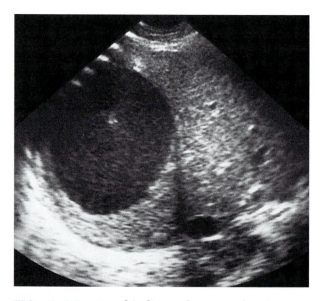

FIG. 4-28. **Amebic liver abscess—classic morphology.** Transverse sonogram shows a well-defined oval subdiaphragmatic mass with increased through transmission. There are uniform low-level internal echoes and absence of a well-defined abscess wall.

Parasitic

Amebiasis. Hepatic infection by the parasite *Entamoeba histolytica* is the most common extraintestinal manifestation of amebiasis. Transmission is by the fecal-oral route. The protozoan reaches the liver by penetrating through the colon, invading the mesenteric venules, and entering the portal vein. However, in more than one half of patients with amebic abscesses of the liver, the colon appears normal and stool culture results are negative, thus delaying diagnosis. The most common presenting symptom in patients with amoebic abscess is pain, which occurs in 99% of patients. Approximately 15% of patients have diarrhea at the time of diagnosis.

Sonographic features include a round or oval-shaped lesion, absence of a prominent abscess wall,

hypoechogenicity compared to normal liver, fine low-level internal echoes, distal sonic enhancement, and contiguity with the diaphragm (Fig. 4-28).[35,36] These features, however, can all be found in pyogenic abscesses.

In a review of 112 amebic lesions by Ralls et al. two sonographic patterns were significantly more prevalent in amebic abscesses: (1) round or oval shapes in 82% versus 60% of pyogenic abscess and (2) hypoechoic appearance with fine internal echoes at high

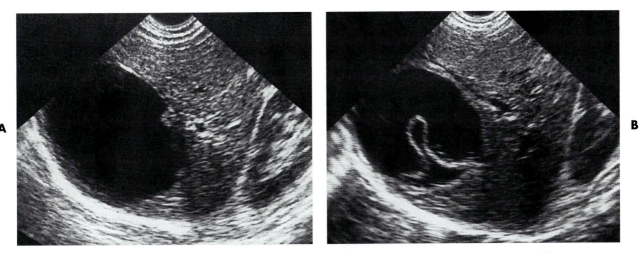

FIG. 4-29. Hydatid cyst. A, Baseline sonogram shows a fairly simple cyst in the right lobe with a small mural nodule and a fleck of peripheral calcium anteriorly. **B,** Three weeks later, the patient presented with right upper-quadrant pain and eosinophilia. The detached endocyst is floating within the lesion.

gain in 58% versus 36% of pyogenic abscesses.[37] Most amebic abscesses occur in the right lobe of the liver. Practically speaking, the **diagnosis** of amebic liver abscess is made using a combination of the clinical features, the ultrasound findings and results of serologic testing. The indirect hemagglutination test is positive in 94% to 100% of patients.

Amebicidal drugs are effective therapy. Patient's symptoms improve by 24 to 48 hours and most are afebrile in four days on medical therapy. Those who exhibit clinical deterioration may also benefit from catheter drainage. This is unusual however. The majority of hepatic amebic abscesses disappear with adequate medical therapy.[38] The time from termination of therapy to resolution varies from 1.5 to 23 months (median 7 months).[39] A minority of patients have residual hepatic cysts and focal regions of increased or decreased echogenicity.

Hydatid Disease. The most common cause of hydatid disease in humans is infestation by the parasite *Echinococcus granulosus*. *E. granulosus* has a worldwide distribution. It is most prevalent in sheep- and cattle-raising countries, notably in the Middle East, Australia, and the Mediterranean. Endemic regions are also present in the United States (the central valley in California, the lower Mississippi valley, Utah, and Arizona) and northern Canada. *E. granulosus* is a tapeworm, 3 to 6 mm in length, which lives in the intestine of the definitive host, usually the dog. Its eggs are excreted in the dog's feces and swallowed by the intermediate hosts—sheep, cattle, goats, or humans. The embryos are freed in the duodenum and pass through the mucosa to reach the liver through the portal venous system. Most of the embryos remain

trapped in the liver, although the lungs, kidneys, spleen, central nervous system, and bone may become secondarily involved. In the liver, the right lobe is more frequently involved. The surviving embryos form slow-growing cysts. The cyst wall consists of an external membrane that is approximately 1 mm thick, which may calcify (the **ectocyst**). The host forms a dense connective tissue capsule around the cyst (the **pericyst**). The inner germinal layer (the **endocyst**) gives rise to brood capsules that enlarge to form protoscolices. The brood capsules may separate from the wall and form a fine sediment called hydatid sand. When hydatid cysts within the organs of a herbivore are eaten, the scolices attach to the intestine and grow to adult tapeworms, thus completing the life cycle.

Several reports describe the **sonographic features** of hepatic hydatid disease (Fig. 4-29).[40-42] Lewall proposed four groups:[41]

- Simple cysts containing no internal architecture except sand (Fig. 4-29, *A*)
- Cysts with detached endocyst secondary to rupture (Fig. 4-29, *B*)
- Cysts with daughter cysts (Fig. 4-30), matrix (echogenic material between the daughter cysts), or both
- Densely calcified masses (Fig. 4-31)

Surgery is the conventional **treatment** in echinococcal disease, although recent reports describe success with percutaneous drainage.[43-45] Although anaphylaxis from hydatid cyst rupture has been reported, its occurrence is rare. Ultrasound has been used to monitor the course of medical therapy in patients with abdominal hydatid disease.[46] Changes noted in the res-

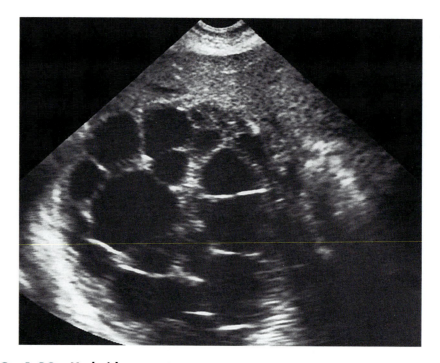

FIG. 4-30. Hydatid cyst. Classic appearance on sonography of a hydatid cyst with multiple daughter cysts.

SONOGRAPHIC FEATURES OF HEPATIC HYDATID DISEASE

Simple cysts
Cysts with detached endocyst secondary to rupture
Cysts with daughter cysts
Densely calcified masses

---

olution of the disease were a gradual reduction in cyst size (43%), membrane detachment (30%), progressive increase in echogenicity of the cyst cavity (12%), and wall calcification (6%). No change was identified in 26% of patients. A reappearance or persistence of fluid within the cavity may signify inadequate therapy and viability of the parasites (Fig. 4-32).[47]

Hepatic alveolar echinococcus is a rare parasitic infestation by the larvae of *E. multilocularis*. The fox is the main host. The **sonographic features** include echogenic lesions, which may be single or multiple; necrotic, irregular lesions without a well-defined wall; clusters of calcification within lesions; and dilated bile ducts.[48] The differential diagnosis is that of primary or metastatic tumors. Diagnosis is made using immunologic tests or percutaneous biopsy.[48]

Schistosomiasis. Schistosomiasis is one of the most common parasitic infections in humans, estimated to affect 200 million people worldwide.[49] Hepatic schistosomiasis is caused by *Schistosoma mansoni, S. japonicum, S. mekongi,* and *S. intercalatum*. Hepatic involvement by *S. mansoni* is particularly severe. *S. mansoni* is prevalent in Africa, Egypt, and South America, particularly in Venezuela and Brazil. The ova reach the liver through the portal vein and incite a chronic granulomatous reaction first described by Symmers as clay-pipestem fibrosis.[50] The terminal portal vein branches become occluded, leading to presinusoidal portal hypertension, splenomegaly, varices, and ascites.

The **sonographic features** of schistosomiasis are widened echogenic portal tracts, sometimes reaching a thickness of 2 cm.[51,52] The porta hepatis is the region most often affected. Initially the liver size is enlarged; however, as the periportal fibrosis progresses, the liver becomes contracted and the features of portal hypertension prevail.

Pneumocystis carinii. *Pneumocystis carinii* is the most common organism causing opportunistic infection in patients with acquired immunodeficiency syndrome (AIDS). Pneumocystis pneumonia is the most common cause of life-threatening infection in patients with human immunodeficiency virus (HIV). *P. carinii* also affects patients undergoing bone marrow and organ transplantation as well as those receiving

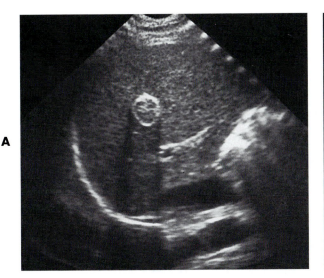

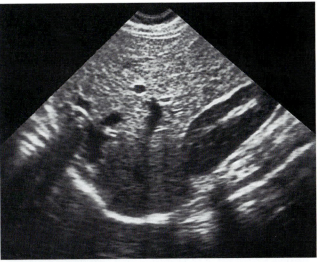

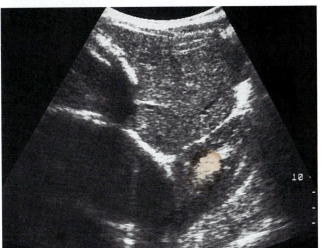

FIG. 4-31. Hydatid disease—liver calcification, in three different patients. **A,** A rim calcification is seen as a continuous, bright, echogenic rim surrounding a small isoechoic mass. **B,** A sagittal right lobe sonogram shows a complex, cystic and solid, subdiaphragmatic mass. Calcification within the mass shows as a bright echogenic focus with shadowing. **C,** Sagittal sonogram shows dense peripheral calcification of two right subdiaphragmatic cysts. As in this case, visualization of the areas deep to the dense calcification may be obscured with a potential for misdiagnosis.

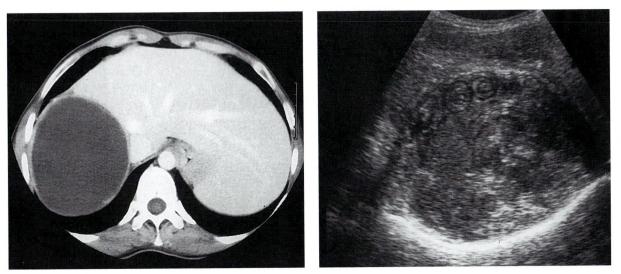

FIG. 4-32. Hydatid cyst in a young woman with episodic severe upper-quadrant pain and jaundice. **A,** Enhanced computed tomography scan shows a low density nonenhancing liver mass suggestive of a cyst. **B,** Sonogram through mass shows a complex internal character with multiple tight ringlike structures anteriorly. At surgery, the cyst contained liters of thick debris with scolices.

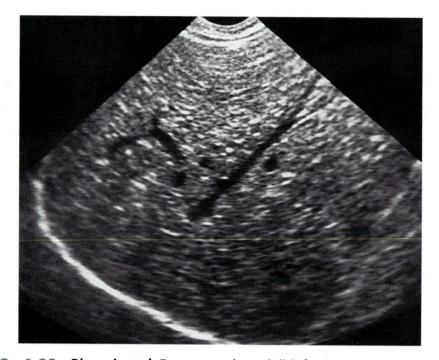

FIG. 4-33. Disseminated *Pneumocystis carinii* infection in an AIDS patient who had previously used a pentamidine inhaler. Sonogram shows innumerable tiny bright echogenic foci without shadowing throughout the liver parenchyma.

corticosteroids or chemotherapy.[53] Extrapulmonic *P. carinii* infection is being reported with increasing frequency.[54-57] It is postulated that the use of maintenance aerosolized pentamidine achieves lower systemic levels than the intravenous form, allowing subclinical pulmonary infections and systemic dissemination of the protozoa. Extrapulmonary *P. carinii* infection has been documented in the liver, spleen, renal cortex, thyroid gland, pancreas, and lymph nodes. The **sonographic findings** of *P. carinii* involvement of the liver (Fig. 4-33) range from diffuse, tiny, nonshadowing echogenic foci to extensive replacement of the normal hepatic parenchyma by echogenic clumps representing dense calcification. A similar sonographic pattern has been identified with hepatic infection by *Mycobacterium avium intracellulare* and cytomegalovirus.[58]

DISORDERS OF METABOLISM

Fatty Liver

Fatty liver is an acquired, reversible disorder of metabolism, resulting in an accumulation of triglycerides within the hepatocytes. Probably the most common **cause** of a fatty liver is obesity. Excessive alcohol intake produces a fatty liver by stimulating lipolysis, as does starvation. Other causes of fatty infiltration include poorly controlled hyperlipidemia, diabetes, excess exogenous or endogenous corticosteroids, pregnancy, total parenteral hyperalimenta-

tion, severe hepatitis, glycogen storage disease, jejunoileal bypass procedures for obesity, cystic fibrosis, congenital generalized lipodystrophy, several chemotherapeutic agents including methotrexate, and toxins such as carbon tetrachloride and yellow phosphorus.[59] Correction of the primary abnormality will reverse the process.

Sonography of fatty infiltration may be varied depending on the amount of fat and whether deposits are diffuse or focal (Fig. 4-34).[60] **Diffuse steatosis** may be:

- **Mild**—Minimal diffuse increase in hepatic echogenicity; normal visualization of diaphragm and intrahepatic vessel borders (Fig. 4-34, *A*)
- **Moderate**—Moderate diffuse increase in hepatic echogenicity; slightly impaired visualization of intrahepatic vessels and diaphragm (Fig. 4-34, *B*)
- **Severe**—Marked increase in echogenicity; poor penetration of the posterior segment of the right lobe of the liver and poor or nonvisualization of the hepatic vessels and diaphragm.

Focal fatty infiltration and **focal fatty sparing** may mimic neoplastic involvement.[61] In focal fatty infiltration, regions of increased echogenicity are present within a background of normal liver parenchyma. Conversely, islands of normal liver parenchyma may appear as hypoechoic masses within a dense, fatty infiltrated liver. Features of **focal fatty change** include:

- Focal fatty sparing and focal fatty liver both most commonly involve the periportal region of the

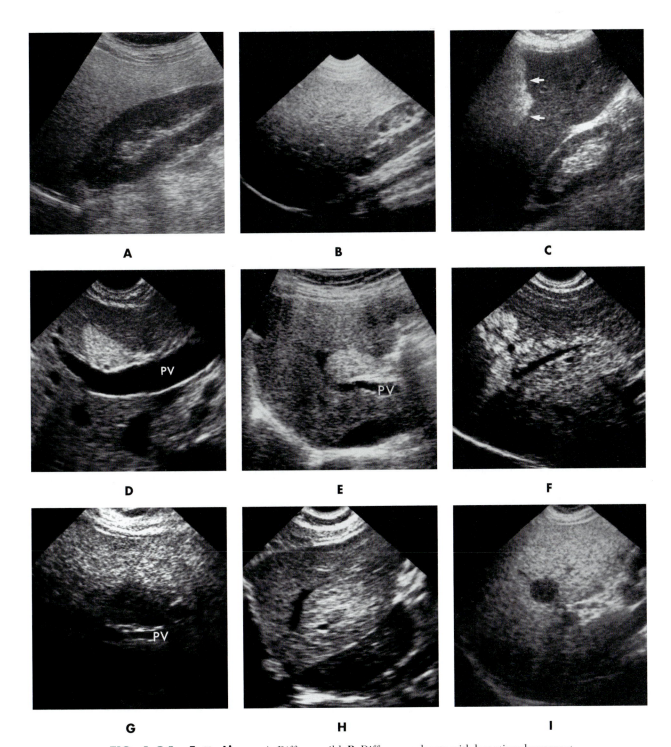

FIG. 4-34. **Fatty Liver.** **A,** Diffuse, mild. **B,** Diffuse, moderate with hepatic enlargement and beam attenuation. **C,** Geographic. The fatty liver looks white (*arrows*). The boundary is "maplike." **D,** Focal fat, segment 4, seen as an echogenic "mass effect" anterior to the portal vein (PV), the classic location. **E,** Focal fat in diabetes mellitus without sugar control. An irregular margined mass is seen anterior to but not altering the right PV. **F,** Focal fat of pregnancy. An ill-defined area of increased echogenicity in the right lobe does not alter regional vessels. **G,** Focal sparing, segment 4, seen as a hypoechoic mass anterior to the PV, the classic site. **H,** Focal sparing, caudate lobe. **I,** Focal sparing mimicking a hypoechoic mass. Normal liver on biopsy and follow-up.

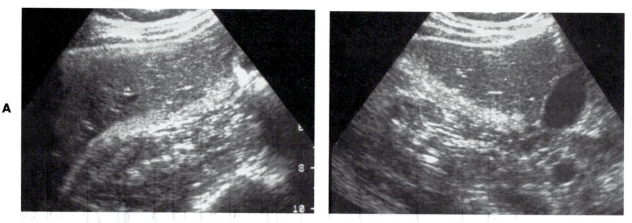

FIG. 4-35. **Steatonecrosis** in diabetic renal failure patient with insulin delivery in peritoneal dialysate. **A,** Sagittal and **B,** transverse sonograms of the right lobe show focal increased echogenicity in a subcapsular location.

SONOGRAPHY OF DIFFUSE STEATOSIS

Mild
  Minimal diffuse increase in hepatic echogenicity
Moderate
  Moderate diffuse increase in hepatic echogenicity
  Slightly impaired visualization of intrahepatic
    vessels and diaphragm
Severe
  Marked increase in echogenicity
  Poor penetration of the posterior liver
  Poor or nonvisualization of the hepatic vessels and
    diaphragm

SONOGRAPHIC FEATURES OF FOCAL FATTY CHANGE

May show rapid change with time, both in
  appearance and resolution
Does not alter course or caliber of regional vessels
Does not produce contour abnormalities
Preferred site for **focal sparing**
  Anterior to portal vein at porto hepatis
  Gallbladder fossa
  Liver margins
Preferred site for **focal fat**
  Anterior to portal vein at porta hepatis
Geographic fat—maplike boundaries

---

medial segment of the left lobe (segment IV) (Fig. 4-34, *D, E, G*).[62,63]

• Sparing also occurs commonly by the gallbladder fossa and along the liver margins

• Focal subcapsular fat may occur in diabetics receiving insulin in peritoneal dialysate (Fig. 4-35)[64]

• Lack of mass (Fig. 4-34, *F*) effect: Hepatic vessels as a rule are not displaced. A recent report, however, has demonstrated the presence of traversing vessels in metastases[65]

• Geometric margins are present, although focal fat may appear round, nodular, or interdigitated with normal tissue (Fig. 4-34, *C*)[66]

• Rapid change with time: Fatty infiltration may resolve as early as within 6 days

• CT scans of the liver will demonstrate corresponding regions of low attenuation

Chemical shift MRI techniques are useful in distinguishing diffuse or focal fatty infiltration. Radio-nuclide liver and spleen scintigraphic examination will yield normal results, indicating adequate numbers of Kupffer cells within the fatty regions.[60] It has been postulated that these focal spared areas are caused by a regional decrease in portal blood flow as demonstrated by CT scans during arterial porto-graphic examinations.[67] Knowledge of typical patterns and use of CT scans, MRI, or nuclear medicine scintigraphy will avoid the necessity for biopsy in the majority of cases of focal fatty alteration.

Glycogen Storage Disease (Glycogenosis)

Recognition of glycogen storage disease (GSD) affecting the kidneys and liver was first made by von Gierke in 1929. Type 1 GSD (von Gierke's disease, glucose 6-phosphatase deficiency) is manifested in the neonatal period by hepatomegaly, nephromegaly, and hypoglycemic convulsions. Because of the enzyme deficiency, large quantities of glycogen are deposited in the hepatocytes and proximal convoluted tubules of the kidney.[68] With dietary management and supportive therapy, more patients currently are surviving to childhood and young adulthood. As a result, several patients have developed benign adenomas or, less commonly, hepatocellular carcinoma.[69] **Sonographically**, type 1 GSD appears indistinguishable from other causes of diffuse fatty infiltration. Secondary hepatic adenomas are well-demarcated, solid masses of variable echogenicity. Malignant transformation can be recognized by rapid growth of the lesions, which may become more poorly defined.[69]

Cirrhosis

Cirrhosis is defined by the World Health Organization (WHO) as a diffuse process characterized by fibrosis and the conversion of normal liver architecture into structurally abnormal nodules.[70] There are three major **pathologic** mechanisms which, in combination, create cirrhosis: cell death, fibrosis, and regeneration. Cirrhosis has been classified as **micronodular,** in which nodules are 0.1 to 1 cm in diameter, and **macronodular,** characterized by nodules of varying size, up to 5 cm in diameter. Alcohol consumption is the most common cause of micronodular cirrhosis, and chronic viral hepatitis is the most frequent cause of the macronodular form.[71] Patients who continue to drink may go on to end-stage liver disease, which is indistinguishable from cirrhosis of other causes. Other etiologies are biliary cirrhosis (primary and secondary), Wilson's disease, primary sclerosing cholangitis, and hemochromatosis. The classic **clinical presentation** of cirrhosis is hepatomegaly, jaundice, and ascites. However, serious liver injury may be present without any clinical clues. In fact, only 60% of patients with cirrhosis have signs and symptoms of liver disease.

As liver biopsy is invasive, there has been great clinical interest in the ability to detect cirrhosis by noninvasive means, such as sonography. The **sonographic patterns** associated with cirrhosis include (Fig. 4-36):

- **Volume redistribution**—In the early stages of cirrhosis the liver may be enlarged, whereas in the advanced states the liver is often small (Fig. 4-36, C and D), with relative enlargement of the caudate, left lobe, or both in comparison with the right lobe (Fig. 4-36, E). Several studies have evaluated the ratio of the caudate lobe width to the right lobe width (C/RL) as an indicator of cirrhosis.[72] A C/RL value of 0.65 is considered indicative of cirrhosis. The specificity is high (100%) but the sensitivity is low (ranging from 43% to 84%), indicating that the C/RL ratio is a useful measurement if it is ab-

normal.[72] It should be noted, however, that there were no patients in these studies with Budd-Chiari syndrome, which may also cause caudate lobe enlargement.

- **Coarse echotexture**—Increased echogenicity and coarse echotexture are frequent observations in diffuse liver disease (Fig. 4-36, A and B). These are subjective findings, however, and may be confounded by inappropriate TGC settings and overall gain. Liver attenuation is correlated with the presence of fat and not fibrosis.[73] Cirrhotic livers without fatty infiltration had attenuation values similar to those of controls. This accounts for the relatively low accuracy in distinguishing diffuse liver disease[74] and for the conflicting reports regarding attenuation values in cirrhosis.

- **Nodular surface**—Irregularity of the liver surface during routine scanning has been appreciated as a sign of cirrhosis when the appearance is gross or when ascites is present (Fig. 4-36, C).[75] The nodularity corresponds to the presence of regenerating nodules and fibrosis.

- **Regenerating nodules** (RN)—Regenerating nodules represent regenerating hepatocytes surrounded by a fibrotic septa. Because they have a similar architecture to the normal liver, ultrasound and CT have limited ability in their detection. RN tend to be isoechoic or hypoechoic with a thin echogenic border which corresponds to fibrofatty connective tissue.[75] MRI has a greater sensitivity than both CT and ultrasound in their detection. Because some RN contain iron, gradient echo sequences demonstrate these nodules as hypointense.[76]

- **Dysplastic nodules**—Dysplastic nodules or adenomatous hyperplastic nodules are larger than RN (diameter ≥ 10mm) and are considered premalignant.[77] They contain well-differentiated hepatocytes, a portal venous blood supply and also atypical or frankly malignant cells. The portal venous blood supply can be detected with the use of color Doppler flow imaging and distinguished from the hepatic artery-supplied hepatocellular carcinoma.[78] In a patient with cirrhosis and a liver mass, percutaneous biopsy is often performed to exclude or diagnose hepatocellular carcinoma.

Doppler Characteristics of Cirrhosis. The normal Doppler waveform of the hepatic veins reflects the hemodynamics of the right atrium. The waveform is triphasic: two large antegrade diastolic and systolic waves and a small retrograde wave corresponding to the atrial "kick." Because the walls of the hepatic veins are thin, disease of the hepatic parenchyma may alter their compliance. In many patients with compensated cirrhosis (no portal hypertension), the Doppler waveform is abnormal. Two abnormal pat-

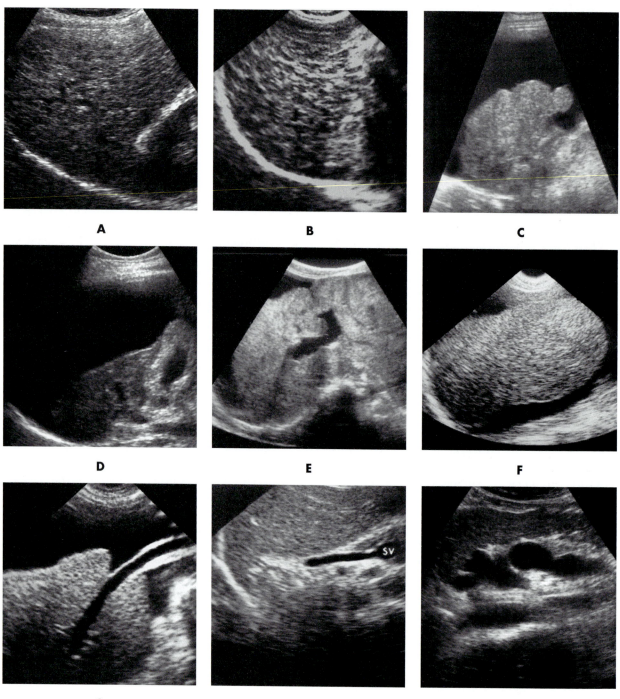

FIG. 4-36. **Cirrhosis.** **A, B,** and **C,** Parenchymal alteration. **A,** The liver is normal in size but diffusely nodular, suggesting myriads of tiny hypoechoic masses. **B,** The liver is small with diffuse coarse parenchyma. **C,** Regenerative nodules. Surface nodularity is best appreciated with ascites. **D, E,** and **F,** Size alteration. **D,** Small end-stage cirrhotic liver. **E,** Lobar redistribution. Transverse sonogram shows the right lobe is small and there is enlargement of the left lateral segment. **F,** Generous bulbous cirrhotic liver, classic for primary biliary cirrhosis, as in this case. **G, H,** and **I,** Portal hypertension. **G,** Recanalized paraumbilical vein and ascites. **H,** Enlarged coronary vein, on sagittal sonogram, running cephalad from splenic vein (SV). **I,** Varices on sagittal epigastric sonogram related to the coronary vein.

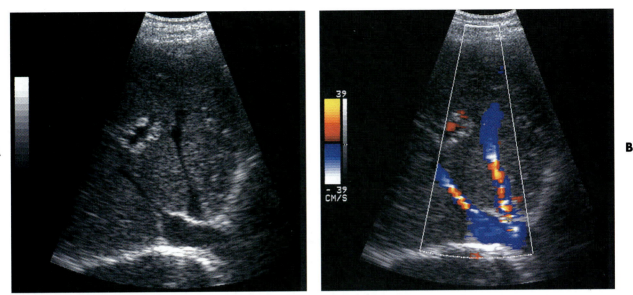

FIG. 4-37. Hepatic vein strictures-cirrhosis. A, Gray scale image of hepatic veins shows a tapered luminal narrowing. **B,** Color Doppler image shows appropriately directed flow toward the inferior vena cava in blue. There is color aliasing from the rapid velocity flow through the points of narrowing.

SONOGRAPHIC PATTERNS OF CIRRHOSIS

Volume redistribution
Coarse echotexture
Nodular surface
Nodules—regenerative and dysplastic
Portal hypertension—ascites, splenomegaly, and
   varices

---

terns have been described: decreased amplitude of phasic oscillations with loss of reversed flow; and a flattened waveform.[79,80] These abnormal patterns have also been found in patients with fatty infiltration of their livers.[80]

As cirrhosis progresses, luminal narrowing of the hepatic veins may be associated with flow alterations visible on color and spectral Doppler. High-velocity signals through an area of narrowing produce color aliasing and turbulence (Fig. 4-37).

The hepatic artery waveform also shows altered flow dynamics in cirrhosis and chronic liver disease. Lafortune et al.[81] found an increase in the resistive index of the hepatic artery following a meal in patients who had normal livers. The vasoconstriction of the hepatic artery occurs as a normal response to the increased portal venous flow stimulated by eating ($\geq$ 20% change). In patients with cirrhosis and chronic liver disease, the normal increase in postprandial resistive index is blunted.[82]

VASCULAR ABNORMALITIES

Portal Hypertension

Normal portal vein pressure is 5 to 10 mm Hg (14 cm H_2O). Portal hypertension is defined by a wedged hepatic vein pressure or direct portal vein pressure of more than 5 mm Hg greater than inferior vena cava pressure, splenic vein pressure of greater than 15 mm Hg, or portal vein pressure (measured surgically) of greater than 30 cm H_2O. **Pathophysiologically,** portal hypertension can be divided into presinusoidal and intrahepatic groups, depending on whether the hepatic vein wedged pressure is normal (presinusoidal) or elevated (intrahepatic).

Presinusoidal portal hypertension can be subdivided into extrahepatic and intrahepatic forms. The **causes of extrahepatic presinusoidal portal hypertension** include thrombosis of the portal or splenic veins. This should be suspected in any patient who presents with clinical signs of portal hypertension—ascites, splenomegaly, and varices—and a normal liver biopsy. Thrombosis of the portal venous system occurs in children secondary to umbilical vein catheterization, omphalitis, and neonatal sepsis. In adults, the causes of portal vein thrombosis include trauma, sepsis, hepatocellular carcinoma, pancreatic carcinoma, pancreatitis, portacaval shunts, splenectomy, and hypercoagulable states. The **intrahepatic presinusoidal causes of portal hypertension** are results of diseases affecting the portal zones of the liver, notably schistosomiasis, primary biliary cirrhosis,

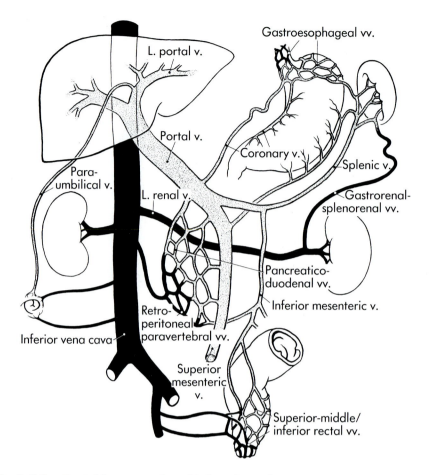

FIG. 4-38. Portal hypertension. Major sites of portosystemic venous collaterals. (Modified from Subramanyam BR, Balthazar EJ, Madamba MR, et al: Sonography of portosystemic venous collaterals in portal hypertension. *Radiology* 1983;146:161-166.)

congenital hepatic fibrosis, and toxic substances such as polyvinyl chloride and methotrexate.[83]

Cirrhosis is the most common cause of **intrahepatic portal hypertension** and accounts for greater than 90% of all cases of portal hypertension in the West. In cirrhosis, most of the normal liver architecture is replaced by distorted vascular channels that provide increased resistance to portal venous blood flow and obstruction to hepatic venous outflow. Diffuse metastatic liver disease also produces portal hypertension by the same mechanism. Thrombotic diseases of the inferior vena cava and hepatic veins, as well as constrictive pericarditis and other causes of severe right-sided heart failure, over time will lead to centrilobular fibrosis, hepatic regeneration, cirrhosis, and finally portal hypertension.

Sonographic findings of portal hypertension include the secondary signs of splenomegaly, ascites, and portosystemic venous collaterals. When the resistance to blood flow in the portal vessels exceeds the resistance to flow in the small communicating channels between the portal and systemic circulations, portosystemic collaterals form. Thus, although the caliber of the portal vein initially may be increased (≥ 1.3 cm) in portal hypertension,[84] with the development of portosystemic shunts, the portal vein caliber will decrease.[85] Five major sites of **portosystemic venous collaterals** are visualized by ultrasound (Fig. 4-38).[86,87,88]

- **Gastroesophageal junction**—Between the coronary and short gastric veins and the systemic esophageal veins. These varices are of particular importance as they may lead to life-threatening or fatal hemorrhage. Dilation of the coronary vein (> 0.7 cm) is associated with severe portal hypertension (portohepatic gradient > 10 mm Hg) (Fig. 4-36, *H*).[85]
- **Paraumbilical vein**—Runs in the falciform ligament and connects the left portal vein to the systemic epigastric veins near the umbilicus (Cruveilhier-Baumgarten syndrome).[89] Several authors have suggested that, if the hepatofugal flow in the patent paraumbilical vein exceeds the hepatopetal flow in the portal vein, patients may be

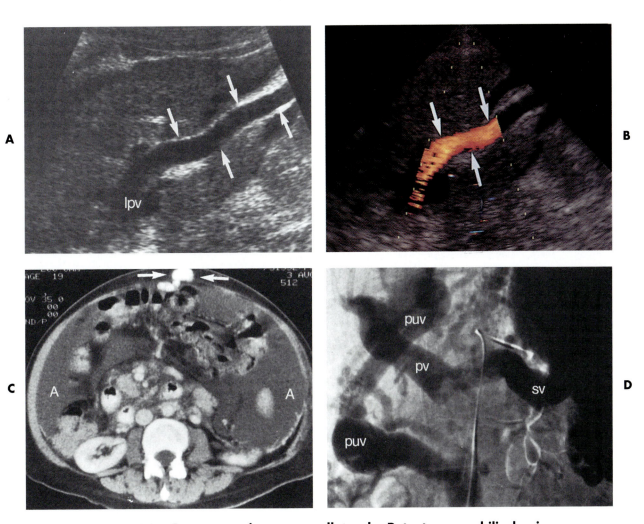

FIG. 4-39. Portosystemic venous collaterals. Patent paraumbilical vein.
A, Sagittal gray scale and B, color-flow Doppler sonograms show recanalized paraumbilical vein (*arrows*). Flow is hepatofugal. LPV—left portal vein. C, Postcontrast computed tomography scan. Communication of paraumbilical vein with systemic epigastric vein (*arrows*) is evident. A—ascites. D, Venous phase of selective splenic arterial injection shows the large paraumbilical vein (puv), equal in size to main portal vein (pv). Sv—splenic vein.

protected from developing esophageal varices (Fig. 4-36, *G* and Fig. 4-39).[90,91]

- **Splenorenal and gastrorenal**—Tortuous veins may be seen in the region of the splenic and left renal hilus (Fig. 4-40), which represent collaterals between the splenic, coronary, and short gastric veins and the left adrenal or renal veins (Fig. 4-36, *I*).
- **Intestinal**—Regions in which the gastrointestinal tract becomes retroperitoneal so that the veins of the ascending and descending colon, duodenum, pancreas, and liver may anastomose with the renal, phrenic, and lumbar veins (systemic tributaries).
- **Hemorrhoidal**—The perianal region where the superior rectal veins, which extend from the inferior mesenteric vein, anastomose with the systemic middle and inferior rectal veins.

SONOGRAPHIC IDENTIFICATION OF PORTOSYSTEMIC VENOUS COLLATERALS

Gastroesophageal junction
Paraumbilical vein, in the falciform ligament
Splenorenal and gastrorenal veins
Intestinal-retroperitoneal anastamoses
Hemorrhoidal veins

Duplex **Doppler sonography** provides additional information regarding direction of portal flow. False results may occur, however, when sampling is obtained from periportal collaterals in patients with portal vein thrombosis or hepatofugal portal flow.[92]

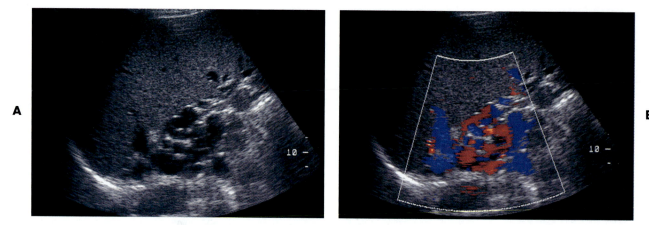

FIG. 4-40. Varices. A, Coronal view of spleen shows a plexus of tubular cystic structures in the splenic hilum. **B,** Color Doppler confirms their vascular nature.

Normal portal venous flow rates will vary in the same individual: increasing postprandially and during inspiration[82,93] and decreasing following exercise or when the patient is in the upright position.[94] An increase of less than 20% in the diameter of the portal vein with deep inspiration indicates portal hypertension with 81% sensitivity and 100% specificity.[95]

The normal portal vein demonstrates an undulating hepatopedal (toward the liver) flow. Mean portal venous flow velocity is approximately 15 to 18 cm/sec and varies with respiration and cardiac pulsation. As portal hypertension develops, the flow in the portal vein loses its undulatory pattern and becomes monophasic. As the severity of portal hypertension increases, flow becomes biphasic and finally hepatofugal (away from the liver). Intrahepatic arterial-portal venous shunting may also be seen.

Chronic liver disease is also associated with increased splanchnic blood flow. Recent evidence suggests that portal hypertension is in part caused by the hyperdynamic flow state of cirrhosis. In a study by Zwiebel et al.,[96] blood flow was increased in the superior mesenteric arteries and splenic arteries of patients with cirrhosis and splenomegaly, compared with normal controls. Of interest, in patients with cirrhosis and normal-sized livers, splanchnic blood flow was not increased. Patients with isolated splenomegaly and normal livers were not included in this study.

The limitations of Doppler sonography in the evaluation of portal hypertension include the inability to accurately determine vascular pressures and flow rates. Patients with portal hypertension are often ill, with contracted livers, abundant ascites and floating bowel, all of which create a technical challenge. In a recent article comparing duplex Doppler with MR angiography, MR imaging was superior in the assessment of patency of the portal vein and surgical shunts as well as in detection of varices.[97] However, when the

Doppler study was technically adequate, it was accurate in the assessment of normal portal anatomy and flow direction. Duplex Doppler sonography has the added advantages of decreased cost and portability of the equipment and therefore should be used as the initial screening method for portal hypertension.[97]

Portal Vein Thrombosis

Portal vein thrombosis has been associated with malignancy, including hepatocellular carcinoma, metastatic liver disease, carcinoma of the pancreas, and primary leiomyosarcoma of the portal vein;[98] as well as chronic pancreatitis; hepatitis; septicemia; trauma; splenectomy; portacaval shunts; hypercoagulable states such as pregnancy; and in neonates, omphalitis; umbilical vein catheterization; and acute dehydration.[99]

Sonographic findings of portal vein thrombosis include echogenic thrombus within the lumen of the vein, portal vein collaterals, expansion of the caliber of the vein and cavernous transformations (Figs. 4-41 and 4-42).[99] Cavernous transformation of the portal vein refers to numerous wormlike vessels at the porta hepatis, which represent periportal collateral circulation.[100] This pattern is observed in long-standing thrombosis, requiring up to 12 months to occur, and thus is more likely to develop with benign disease.[101] Acute thrombus may appear relatively anechoic and therefore overlooked unless Doppler interrogation is performed.

Doppler sonography is useful in distinguishing between benign and malignant portal vein thrombi in patients with cirrhosis. Both bland and malignant thrombi may demonstrate continuous blood flow. Pulsatile flow, however, has been found to be 95% specific for the diagnosis of malignant portal vein thrombosis (Fig. 4-43). The sensitivity was only 62%, as many malignant thrombi are hypovascular.[102]

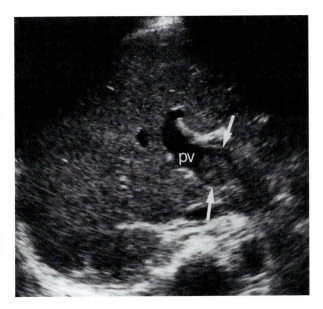

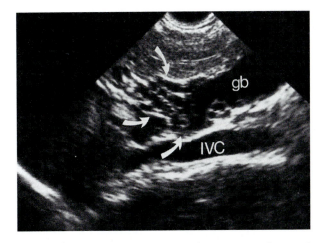

FIG. 4-42. Cavernous transformation of portal vein. Numerous periportal collateral vessels (*arrows*) are present. gb—gallbladder; IVC—inferior vena cava.

FIG. 4-41. Portal vein thrombosis. Echogenic thrombus (*arrows*) expands lumen of portal vein (pv).

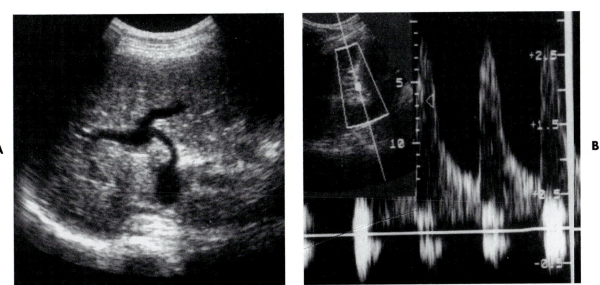

FIG. 4-43. Tumor thrombosis in portal vein with neovascularity. A, Gray scale sonogram of right portal vein shows an echogenic intraluminal filling defect. **B,** Duplex Doppler waveform of the thrombus shows arterial flow confirming neovascularity.

Budd-Chiari Syndrome

The Budd-Chiari syndrome is a relatively rare disorder characterized by occlusion of the lumina of the hepatic veins with or without occlusion of the lumen of the inferior vena cava. The degree of occlusion and the presence of collateral circulation predicts the clinical course. Some patients die in the acute phase of acute liver failure. Causes of Budd-Chiari syndrome include coagulation abnormalities such as polycythemia rubra vera, chronic leukemia and paroxysmal nocturnal hemoglobinuria; trauma; tumor extension from primary hepatocellular carcinoma, renal carcinoma, and adrenal cortical carcinoma; pregnancy; congenital abnormalities and obstructing membranes. The classic patient in North America is a young adult woman taking birth control pills who presents with an acute onset of ascites, right upper quadrant pain, hepatomegaly, and to a lesser extent, splenomegaly. In some cases, no etiologic factor is found. The syndrome is more common in other geographic areas including India, South Africa, and the Orient.

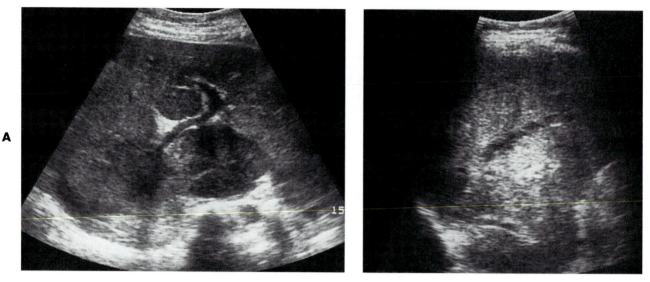

FIG. 4-44. Acute Budd-Chiari. A, Transverse view of liver shows a large, bulbous caudate lobe. **B,** Sagittal view of right hepatic vein shows echoes within the vein lumen consistent with thrombosis, with absence of the vessel toward the inferior vena cava. Doppler showed no flow in this vessel.

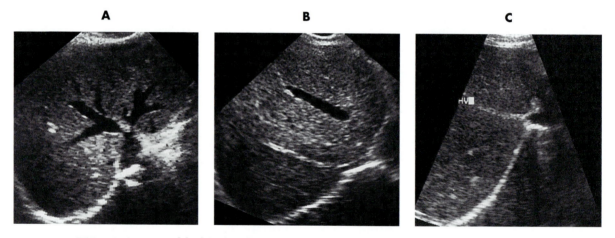

FIG. 4-45. Budd-Chiari—abnormal hepatic vein appearance in three different patients on transverse images of intrahepatic inferior vena cava (IVC). **A,** The right hepatic vein is not seen at all. The middle hepatic vein and left hepatic vein both show tight strictures just proximal to the inferior vena cava. **B,** The right hepatic vein is seen as a thrombosed cord. The middle hepatic vein does not reach the inferior vena cava. The left hepatic vein is not seen. **C,** Only a single hepatic vein, the middle hepatic vein (HV), can be seen as a thrombosed cord.

Sonographic evaluation of the patient with Budd-Chiari syndrome includes gray scale and Doppler features.[103-114] Ascites is an invariable observation. The liver is typically large and bulbous in the acute phase (Fig. 4-44, *A*). Hemorrhagic infarction may produce significant altered regional echogenicity. As infarcted areas become more fibrotic, echogenicity increases.[112] The caudate lobe is often spared in Budd-Chiari syndrome because the emissary veins drain directly into the inferior vena cava at a lower level than the involved main hepatic veins. Increased blood flow through the caudate lobe leads to relative caudate enlargement.

Real-time scanning allows the radiologist to evaluate the inferior vena cava and hepatic veins noninvasively. Sonographic features of hepatic venous involvement in Budd-Chiari syndrome include partial or complete inability to see the hepatic veins, stenosis with proximal dilatation, intraluminal echogenicity, thickened walls, thrombosis (Fig. 4-45), and intrahepatic collaterals (Fig. 4-46).[105,106] Membranous webs may be identified as echogenic or focal obliterations of the

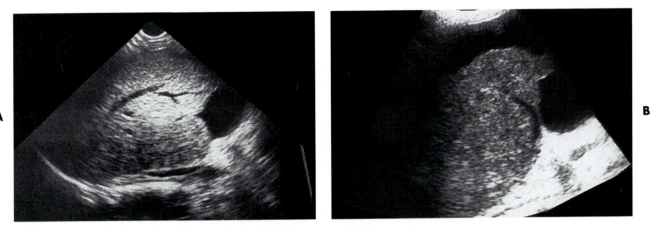

FIG. 4-46. **Budd-Chiari—abnormal intrahepatic collaterals on gray scale** in two different patients with ascites. **A,** Sagittal image of right lobe shows a normal right hepatic vein. A collateral runs from the vein to the surface of the liver, an abnormal locale for a vessel of this size. **B,** Sagittal image of right lobe shows a vessel in an abnormal locale parallel to the liver surface.

lumen.[106] Real-time ultrasonography, however, underestimates the presence of thrombosis and webs and may be inconclusive in a cirrhotic patient in whom the hepatic veins are difficult to image.[105] Intrahepatic collaterals, on gray scale images, show as tubular vascular structures in an abnormal locale and are most commonly seen extending from a hepatic vein to the liver surface where they anastomose with systemic capsular vessels (Fig. 4-46).

Duplex and color-flow Doppler imaging have considerable potential in the evaluation of patients with suspected Budd-Chiari syndrome to determine both the presence and direction of hepatic venous flow. The middle and left hepatic veins are best scanned in the transverse plane at the level of the xiphoid process. From this angle, the veins are almost parallel to the Doppler beam, allowing optimal reception of their Doppler signals. The right hepatic vein is best evaluated from a right intercostal approach.[108] The intricate pathways of blood flow out of the liver in the patient with Budd-Chiari syndrome can be mapped with documentation of hepatic venous occlusions (Fig. 4-47), hepatic-systemic collaterals (Fig. 4-48), hepatic venous-portal venous collaterals, and increased calibre of anomalous or accessory hepatic veins.

The normal blood flow in the inferior vena cava and hepatic veins is phasic in response to both the cardiac and respiratory cycles.[115] In Budd-Chiari syndrome, flow in the inferior vena cava, hepatic veins, or both, changes from phasic to absent, reversed, turbulent, or continuous.[110,114] Continuous flow has been called the pseudoportal Doppler signal and appears to reflect either partial inferior vena cava obstruction or extrinsic inferior vena cava compression.[109] The portal blood flow also may be affected and is characteristically either slowed or reversed.[110]

The addition of Doppler to gray scale sonography in the patient with suspect Budd-Chiari syndrome lends strong supportive evidence to the gray scale impression of either missing, compressed, or otherwise abnormal hepatic veins and inferior vena cava.[113,114] Associated reversal of flow in the portal vein and epigastric collaterals is also optimally assessed with this technique.[114]

Hepatic venoocclusive disease causes progressive occlusion of the small hepatic venules. The disease is endemic in Jamaica, secondary to alkaloid toxicity from bush tea. In North America, most cases are iatrogenic secondary to hepatic irradiation and chemotherapy used in bone marrow transplantation.[111] Patients with hepatic venoocclusive disease are clinically indistinguishable from those with Budd-Chiari syndrome. Duplex Doppler sonography demonstrates normal caliber, patency, and phasic forward (toward the heart) flow of the main hepatic veins and inferior vena cava.[111] Flow in the portal vein, however, may be abnormal showing either reversed or "to and fro" flow.[111,116] In addition, the diagnosis of hepatic venoocclusive disease can be suggested in a patient with decreased portal blood flow (as compared with a baseline measurement performed before ablative therapy).[111]

Portal Vein Aneurysm

Aneurysms of the portal vein are rare. Their origin is believed to be either congenital or acquired secondary to portal hypertension.[117] Portal vein aneurysms have been described proximally at the junction of the supe-

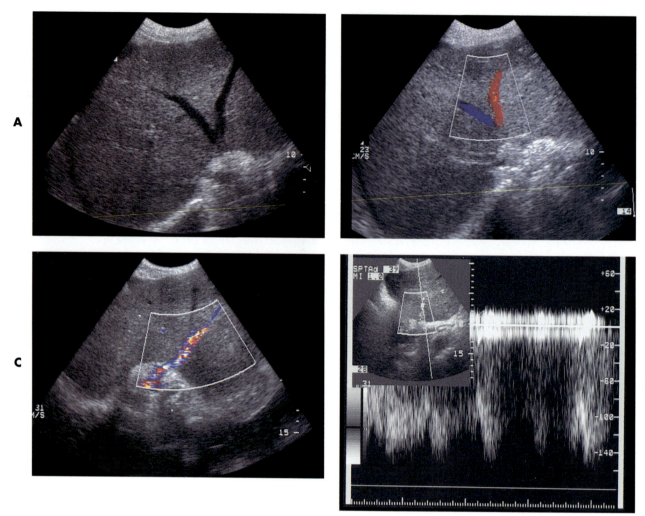

FIG. 4-47. Budd-Chiari. A, Gray scale transverse image of hepatic venous confluence shows complete absence of the right hepatic vein with obliteration of the lumen of a common trunk for the middle and left hepatic vein. **B,** Color Doppler shows the flow in the middle hepatic vein (*blue*) is normally directed towards the inferior vena cava (IVC). As the trunk is obliterated, all of the blood is flowing out of the left hepatic vein (*red*) which is abnormal. Other images showed anastomoses of the left hepatic vein with surface collaterals. **C,** Color Doppler image shows an anomalous left hepatic vein with flow to the inferior vena cava (*normal direction*) with aliasing due to a long stricture. **D,** Spectral Doppler waveform of the anomalous left hepatic vein shows a very high abnormal velocity of approximately 140 cm/sec confirming the tight stricture.

rior mesenteric and splenic veins and distally involving the portal venous radicles. The **sonographic appearance** is that of an anechoic cystic mass, which connects with the portal venous system. Pulsed Doppler sonographic examination demonstrates turbulent venous flow.[117]

Intrahepatic Portosystemic Venous Shunts

Intrahepatic **arterial-portal fistulas** are well-recognized complications of large-gauge percutaneous liver biopsy and trauma. Conversely, intrahepatic **portohepatic venous shunts** are rare. Their cause is controversial and believed to be either congenital or related to

portal hypertension.[118,119] Patients typically are middle aged and present with hepatic encephalopathy. Anatomically, portohepatic venous shunts are more common in the right lobe. **Sonography** demonstrates a tortuous tubular vessel or complex vascular channels, which connect a branch of the portal vein to an hepatic vein or the inferior vena cava.[118-120] The diagnosis is confirmed angiographically.

Hepatic Artery Aneurysm and Pseudoaneurysm

The hepatic artery is the fourth most common site of an intra-abdominal aneurysm, following the infrarenal aorta, iliac, and splenic arteries. Eighty per-

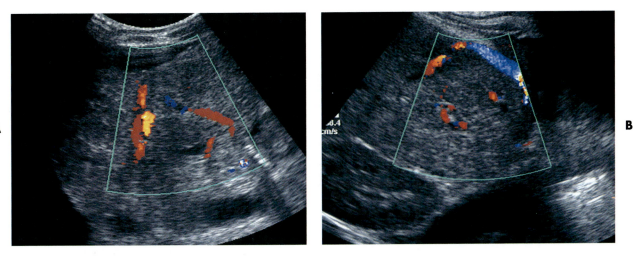

FIG. 4-48. **Budd-Chiari—intrahepatic collaterals.** **A,** Sagittal midline view shows abnormal vessels for the locale in the liver which conform with neither portal nor hepatic venous anatomy. Flow is directed toward the liver surface. **B,** Transverse scan of the right lobe shows abnormal intrahepatic vessels with flow toward the liver capsule where they anastomose with a capsular vessel shown in blue.

cent of patients with an hepatic artery aneurysm experience catastrophic rupture into the peritoneum, biliary tree, gastrointestinal tract, or portal vein.[121] Hepatic artery pseudoaneurysm secondary to chronic pancreatitis has been described. The **duplex Doppler sonographic examination** revealed turbulent arterial flow within a sonolucent mass.[121] Primary dissection of the hepatic artery is rare and in most cases leads to death prior to diagnosis.[122] Sonography may show the intimal flap with the true and false channels.

Hereditary Hemorrhagic Telangiectasia

Hereditary hemorrhagic telangiectasia, or Osler-Weber-Rendu disease, is an autosomal dominant disorder that causes arteriovenous malformations in the liver, hepatic fibrosis, and cirrhosis. Patients present with multiple telangiectasias and recurrent episodes of bleeding. **Sonographic findings** in hereditary hemorrhagic telangiectasia include: a large feeding common hepatic artery measuring up to 10 mm, multiple dilated tubular structures representing arteriovenous malformations, and large draining hepatic veins secondary to arteriovenous shunting.[123]

Peliosis Hepatis

Peliosis hepatis is a rare liver disorder characterized by blood filled cavities which range in size from less than a millimeter to many centimeters in diameter. It can be distinguished from hemangioma by the presence of portal tracts within the fibrous stroma of the blood spaces. The pathogenesis of peliosis hepatis involves rupture of the reticulin fibers that support the sinusoidal walls secondary to cell injury or nonspecific hepatocellular necrosis.[124] The diagnosis of peliosis can be made with certainty only by histologic exami-

nation. Most cases of peliosis affect the liver, although other solid internal organs and lymph nodes may be involved in the process as well.

Although early reports described incidental detection of peliosis hepatis at autopsy in patients with chronic wasting disorders, it has now been seen following renal and liver transplantation, in association with a multitude of drugs especially anabolic steroids, and with an increased incidence in patients with HIV.[125] The latter association may occur alone or as part of bacillary angiomatosis in the spectrum of opportunistic infections of AIDS.[126] Peliosis hepatis has the potential to be aggressive and lethal.

The **imaging features** of peliosis hepatis have been described in single case reports[127-129] although often without adequate histologic confirmation. Angiographically, the peliotic lesions have been described as accumulations of contrast detected late in the arterial phase and becoming more distinct in the parenchymal phase.[130] On **sonography,** described lesions are nonspecific and have shown single or multiple masses of heterogeneous echogenicity.[127,128,131] Calcifications have been reported (Fig. 4-49).[131] CT scans show low attenuation nodular lesions that may or may not enhance with contrast injection.[127,130] Peliosis hepatis is difficult to diagnose both clinically and radiologically and must be suspected in a susceptible individual with a liver mass.

BENIGN HEPATIC NEOPLASMS

Cavernous Hemangioma

Cavernous hemangiomas are the most common benign tumors of the liver, occurring in approximately

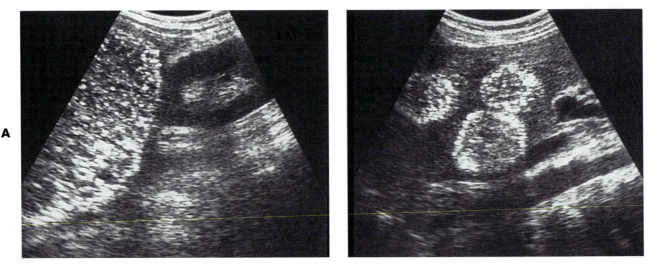

FIG. 4-49. **Peliosis hepatis** in a 34-year-old woman with deteriorating liver function necessitating transplantation. **A,** Sagittal right lobe and **B,** sagittal left lobe scans show multiple large liver masses with innumerable tiny punctate calcifications. (From Muradali D, Wilson SR, Wanless IR, et al: Peliosis hepatis with intrahepatic calcifications. *J Ultrasound Med* 1996;16:257-260.)

4% of the population. They occur in all age groups but are more common in adults, particularly women. The woman to man ratio is approximately 5:1.[132] The vast majority of hemangiomas are small, asymptomatic, and discovered incidentally. Large lesions may **rarely** produce symptoms of acute abdominal pain caused by hemorrhage or thrombosis within the tumor. Thrombocytopenia, caused by sequestration and destruction of platelets within a large cavernous hemangioma (Kasabach-Merritt syndrome), occasionally occurs in infants and is rare in adults. Once hemangiomas are identified in the adult, they usually have reached a stable size and change in appearance or size is uncommon.[133,134] Hemangiomas may enlarge, however, during pregnancy or with the administration of estrogens, suggesting the tumor is hormone-dependent. **Histologically,** hemangiomas consist of multiple vascular channels that are lined by a single layer of endothelium and separated and supported by fibrous septae. The vascular spaces may contain thrombi.

The **sonographic appearance** of cavernous hemangioma varies (Fig. 4-50). Typically the lesion is small, less than 3 cm in diameter, well-defined, homogeneous and hyperechoic (Fig. 4-50, *A*).[135] The increased echogenicity has been related to the numerous interfaces between the walls of the cavernous sinuses and the blood within them.[136] Inconsistently seen and nonspecific, posterior acoustic enhancement has been correlated with hypervascularity on angiography (Fig. 4-50, *C*).[137] It is estimated that approximately 67% to 79% of hemangiomas are hyperechoic,[138,139] and of these 58% to 73% are homogeneous.[134,137] **Atypical features** are also now fa-

miliar and include: a nonhomogeneous central area containing hypoechoic portions which may appear uniformly granular (Fig. 4-50, *H*) or lacelike in character (Fig. 4-50, *G*); an echogenic border, either a thin rim or a thick rind (Fig. 4-50, *H–I*); and a tendency to scalloping of the margin (Fig. 4-50, *D*).[140] Larger lesions tend to be heterogeneous with central hypoechoic foci corresponding to fibrous collagen scars (Fig. 4-50, *E*), large vascular spaces, or both. A hemangioma may appear hypoechoic within the background of a fatty infiltrated liver.[141] Calcification is rare (Fig. 4-50, *F*).

Hemangiomas are characterized by very slow blood flow that will not routinely be detected by either color or duplex Doppler. Occasional lesions may show a low to midrange kHz shift from both peripheral and central blood vessels. The ability of power Doppler, which is more sensitive to slow flow, to detect signals within a hemangioma is still controversial.[142,143]

Cavernous hemangiomas are commonly observed on abdominal sonograms performed for any reason and confirmation of all visualized lesions has proven to be costly and unnecessary. Therefore, it is considered acceptable practice to manage some patients conservatively without confirmation of the diagnosis. When a hyperechoic lesion typical of a cavernous hemangioma is incidentally discovered, no further examination is usually necessary, or at most, a repeat ultrasound is performed in 3 to 6 months to document lack of change.

Conversely, there are significant lesions which may mimic the morphology of a hemangioma on ultrasound and produce a single or multiple masses of uniform in-

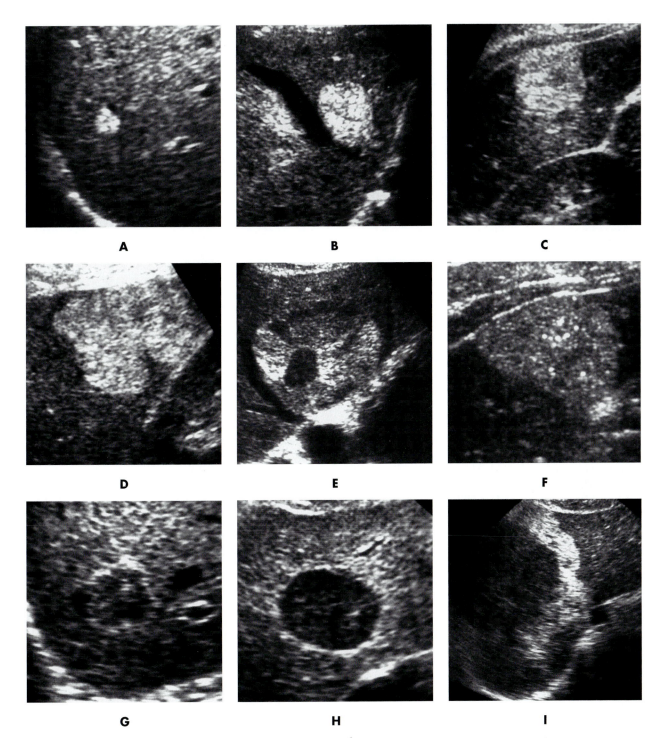

FIG. 4-50. Hemangioma—spectrum of appearances. A, B, and C, Typical appearances. A, Single, small echogenic mass. B, Larger echogenic mass. C, Echogenic mass with faint increased through transmission, a nonspecific sign. D and E, Common findings. D, Scalloped borders. E, Focal hypoechoic central area corresponding to fibrous collagen scars. F, G, H, and I, Atypical appearances. F, Rarely seen, multiple punctate calcifications. G, A hypoechoic lacelike center with a thin echogenic rim. H, A hypoechoic granular center with a thin echogenic rim. I, A hypoechoic central area with a thick echogenic rind.

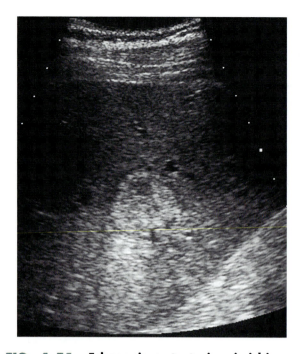

FIG. 4-51. Echogenic metastasis mimicking a hemangioma. Sonogram shows a solid, focal liver mass with increased through transmission, a nonspecific feature. There is a thin, hypoechoic halo appropriately raising the suspicion of cancer. Biopsy showed metastatic lung cancer.

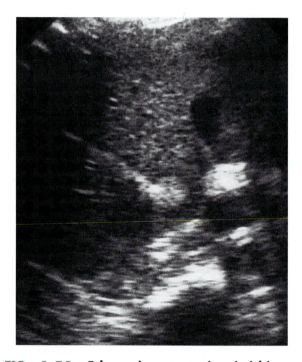

FIG. 4-52. Echogenic metastasis mimicking a hemangioma. A solitary small echogenic mass suggestive of a hemangioma is seen in the right lobe. This patient had a primary colon cancer. Hemangioma was not confirmed by either Tc-99m-labelled red blood cell SPECT or computed tomography. A biopsy needle is shown in the mass. Cytology confirmed a metastasis.

creased echogenicity (Figs. 4-51 and 4-52). Metastases from a colon primary or a vascular primary such as a neuroendocrine tumor, and small hepatocellular carcinomas, in particular, may show this morphology. Therefore, in a patient with a known malignancy, an increased risk for hepatoma, abnormal results of liver function tests, clinical symptoms referable to the liver, or an atypical sonographic pattern, one of the following additional imaging techniques is recommended **to confirm the suspicion of hemangioma:**

- **Computed tomography**—Using the strict CT criteria of: (1) hypodense lesion on precontrast scan; (2) peripheral nodular contrast enhancement during the dynamic bolus phase; and (3) complete isodense fill in of the lesion on delayed scans, up to 60 minutes after contrast material administration, between 55% to 79% of hepatic hemangiomas are specifically diagnosed.[144,145] Many of these lesions are discovered incidentally during the course of imaging for other reasons. The finding of globular peripheral enhancement during routine dynamic bolus CT is a strong indicator that the lesion is a cavernous hemangioma.[146]
- **Red blood cell scintigraphy**—Technetium-99m labelled red blood cell scintigraphy using single-photon emission CT (SPECT) has achieved a posi-

tive predictive value and specificity of almost 100% in evaluating hemangiomas.[144,147,148] The classic appearance is decreased activity on early dynamic images with increased activity on delayed blood pool scanning.

- **Magnetic resonance imaging**— MRI is more accurate than SPECT in diagnosing hemangiomas less than 2 cm and those less than 2.5 cm that are adjacent to the heart and major intrahepatic vessels.[149] Hemangiomas demonstrate marked hyperintensity on T_2-weighted images, regardless of field strength.[150] Hypervascular metastases may also appear hyperintense on T_2-weighted sequences. Heavily T_2-weighted (TE 160 msec) and gadolinium-enhanced gradient-echo imaging can better differentiate hemangiomas from malignant lesions.[151,152] The characteristic pattern of enhancement is similar to that of dynamic CT: (1) peripheral hyperintense nodules; (2) progressive centripetal enhancement; and (3) persistent homogeneous enhancement.[152]

In a minority of patients, imaging will not allow a definitive diagnosis of hemangioma to be made. **Percutaneous biopsy** of hepatic hemangiomas has been safely performed (Fig. 4-52).[153,154] Cronan et al.[154] performed biopsies on 15 patients (12 of whom

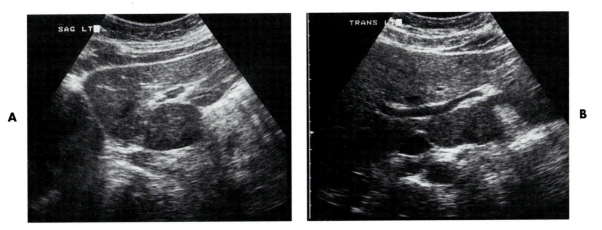

FIG. 4-53. Focal nodular hyperplasia. A, Sagittal and **B,** transverse sonograms show an isoechoic, subtle caudate lobe mass. The contour variation is the key to appreciating the presence of this mass.

were outpatients) using a 20-gauge Franseen needle. In all cases, the histologic sample was diagnostic and was characterized by large spaces with an endothelial lining. It is recommended that normal liver be interposed between the abdominal wall and the hemangioma to allow hepatic tamponade of any potential bleeding.

The best approach to the **diagnosis** of hemangiomas will depend on the clinical situation, the size and location of the lesion, the availability of imaging modalities such as MRI and SPECT, and the experience of the imager. In general, the combination of two confirmatory studies is diagnostic of hemangioma.[155] If the lesion is greater than 2.5 cm in diameter, a Tc-99m red blood cell study with SPECT is recommended. If the lesion is less than 2.5 cm in diameter, MRI with heavily T_2-weighted $\pm$ gadolinium-enhanced imaging is recommended.[151,152] MRI has the added advantage of being more specific than SPECT in diagnosis of other hepatic lesions. Dynamic contrast-enhanced CT scans, although less specific than both Tc-99m erythrocyte scintigraphy and MRI, are useful if these two modalities are unavailable. If the imaging investigation provides indeterminate results, either percutaneous biopsy or follow-up at 3 to 6 months is recommended.

Focal Nodular Hyperplasia

Focal nodular hyperplasia (FNH) is the second most common benign liver mass after hemangioma.[156] These masses are believed to be developmental hyperplastic lesions related to an area of congenital vascular malformation, likely a pre-existing arterial spiderlike malformation.[157] Hormonal influences may be factors, as focal nodular hyperplasia is more common in women than in men, particularly in the child bearing years.[158-160] Like hemangioma, FNH is invariably an incidentally detected liver mass in an asymptomatic patient.[158]

FNH is typically a well-circumscribed and most often solitary mass that has a central scar.[158] The majority of lesions are less than 5 cm in diameter. Although usually single, cases have been reported with multiple FNH. **Microscopically,** lesions include normal hepatocytes, Kupffer cells, biliary ducts, and the components of portal triads, although no normal portal venous structures are found. As a hyperplastic lesion, there is proliferation of normal, non-neoplastic hepatocytes that are abnormally arranged. Bile ducts and thick-walled arterial vessels are prominent particularly in the central fibrous scar. The excellent blood supply makes hemorrhage, necrosis, and calcification rare.[158] These lesions often produce a contour abnormality to the surface of the liver or may displace the normal blood vessels within the parenchyma.

On sonography, FNH is often a subtle liver mass which is difficult to differentiate in echogenicity from the adjacent liver parenchyma. Considering the similarities in histology of FNH to normal liver, this is not a surprising fact and has led to descriptions of FNH on all imaging as a "stealth lesion" which may be extremely subtle or hide altogether.[161] Subtle contour abnormalities (Fig. 4-53) and displacement of vascular structures should immediately raise the possibility of FNH. The central scar is seen on gray scale sonograms as a hypoechoic linear or stellate area within the central portion of the mass (Fig. 4-54).[162] On occasion, the scar may appear hyperechoic.

Doppler features of FNH are highly suggestive in that well-developed peripheral and central blood vessels are seen. Pathologic studies describe an anomalous arterial blood vessel in FNH larger than expected

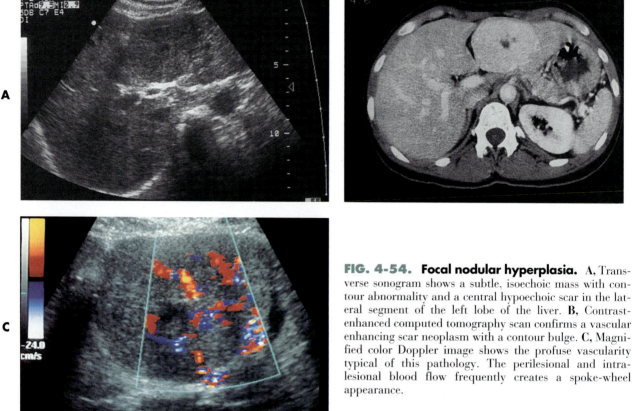

FIG. 4-54. Focal nodular hyperplasia. A, Transverse sonogram shows a subtle, isoechoic mass with contour abnormality and a central hypoechoic scar in the lateral segment of the left lobe of the liver. **B,** Contrast-enhanced computed tomography scan confirms a vascular enhancing scar neoplasm with a contour bulge. **C,** Magnified color Doppler image shows the profuse vascularity typical of this pathology. The perilesional and intralesional blood flow frequently creates a spoke-wheel appearance.

for the locale in the liver.[157] Our experience suggests that this feeding vessel is usually quite obvious on color Doppler imaging although other vascular masses may appear to have unusually large feeding vessels as well.[163] The blood vessels can be seen to course within the central scar with either a linear or stellate configuration. Doppler interrogation usually shows predominantly arterial signals centrally with a mid-range (2 to 4 kHz) shift (Fig. 4-55).

Sulfur colloid scanning is invaluable in patients with suspect FNH as 50% of lesions will take up sulfur colloid similar to the adjacent normal liver and a further 10% of lesions will be hot. Therefore, only 40% of patients with FNH will lack confirmation of their diagnosis after performing a sulfur colloid scan.[164,165]

On unenhanced **CT,** FNH is typically hypodense or isodense to surrounding normal liver parenchyma. If enhanced CT scanning is performed during the arterial phase, the lesion becomes markedly hyperdense reflecting its rich arterial blood supply. The central scar may appear hypoattenuating or hyperattenuating during the arterial phase (Fig. 4-54, *B*). There is rapid washout of contrast and during the portal venous phase, FNH may appear isointense relative to normal liver. The central scar, however, may now appear hyperdense because of delayed washout of contrast within the myxomatous stroma.[161]

Magnetic resonance imaging findings include lesion homogeneity, and isointensity or hypointensity on unenhanced T_1-weighted sequences. T_2-weighted images demonstrate the lesion to be slightly hyperintense to isointense. The central scar is hyperintense on T_2-weighted images. These "typical" findings, however, occur together in approximately 40% of cases. Following the administration of gadolinium, the enhancement pattern follows that of contrast-enhanced CT.[166,167]

Biopsy may be required in up to 40% of patients with FNH who do not have a hot or a warm lesion on sulfur colloid scanning especially if CT or MRI features are not specific. Cytologic biopsy is not confirmatory as normal hepatocytes may be found in normal liver, adenoma, and FNH. Core liver biopsy is required to show the disorganized pattern characteristic of this pathology. Because FNH rarely leads to clinical problems and does not undergo malignant transformation, conservative management is recommended.[168]

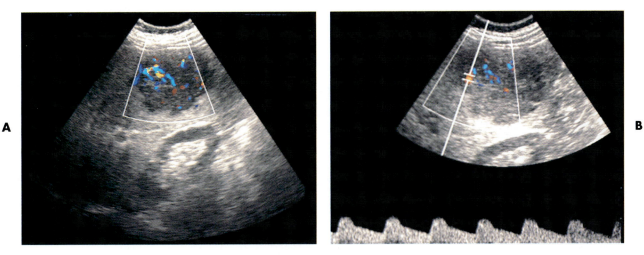

FIG. 4-55. **Focal nodular hyperplasia.** **A,** Color Doppler image shows a focal hypoechoic solid mass expanding the tip of the right lobe of the liver. The mass is vascular with prominent internal flow. **B,** Spectral waveform shows an arterial signal of 4 kHz.

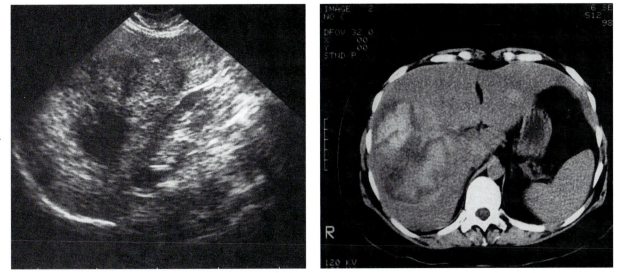

FIG. 4-56. **Hemorrhagic adenoma** in a young woman taking birth control pills presenting with severe right upper-quadrant pain. **A,** Sagittal sonogram shows a complex, inhomogeneous, large right lobe liver mass. The hypoechoic center suggests a partial fluid content. **B,** Unenhanced computed tomography scan confirms the large mass and also the presence of high density blood within the mass.

Hepatic Adenoma

Hepatic adenomas are less common than FNH. Since the 1970s, however, there has been a dramatic rise in their incidence and a link clearly established to the usage of oral contraceptive agents. The tumor may be asymptomatic, but often the patient or the physician feels a mass in the right upper quadrant. Pain may occur as a result of bleeding or infarction within the lesion. The most alarming manifestation is shock caused by tumor rupture and hemoperitoneum. Hepatic adenomas have also been reported in association with glycogen storage disease. In particular, the frequency of adenoma for type 1 GSD (von Gierke's disease) is 40%.[169] Because of its propensity to hemorrhage (Fig. 4-56) and risk of malignant degeneration,[168] surgical resection is recommended.

Pathologically, the hepatic adenoma is usually solitary and well encapsulated, and ranges in size from 8 to 15 cm. Microscopically, the tumor consists of normal or slightly atypical hepatocytes. Bile ducts and Kupffer cells are either few in number or absent.[170]

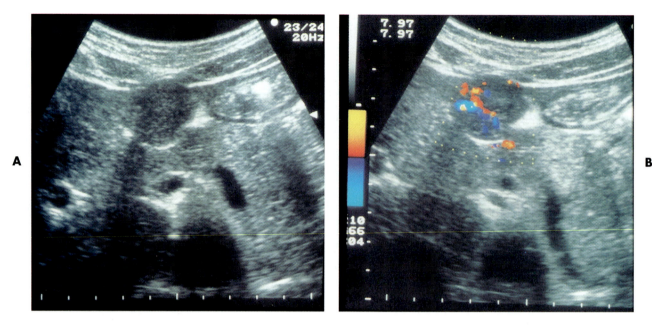

FIG. 4-57. Adenoma. Follow-up sonogram in a young woman approximately 1 year following discontinuation of birth control pills. The mass is smaller by approximately 50%. **A,** Transverse sonogram shows a solid, slightly hypoechoic, well-defined nonspecific liver mass. **B,** Color Doppler image confirms its vascular nature.

The **sonographic appearance** of hepatic adenoma is nonspecific (Fig. 4-57). The echogenicity may be hyperechoic, hypoechoic, isoechoic, or mixed.[165] With hemorrhage, a fluid component may be evident within or around the mass (Fig. 4-56) and free intraperitoneal blood may be seen. The sonographic changes with bleeding are variable, dependent on the duration and amount of hemorrhage.

It is often not possible to distinguish hepatic adenomas from FNH by their gray scale or Doppler characteristics. Both demonstrate perilesional and intralesional well-defined blood vessels with kHz shifts in the mid-range (2 to 4 kHz). Golli et al.[163] described increased venous structures within the center of the masses and a paucity of arterial vessels. In our experience, this has not been a constant finding, and we continue to identify central arterial signals in some adenomas. The majority of adenomas are cold on ^{99}Tc-sulfur colloid imaging as a result of absent or markedly decreased numbers of Kupffer cells. Isolated cases of radiocolloid uptake by the adenoma have been reported.[171] Hepatobiliary scans may be helpful in the diagnosis of hepatic adenomas. Because these lesions do not contain bile ducts, the tracer is not excreted and the mass persists as a photon-active region.

In a patient with right upper-quadrant pain and possible hemorrhage, it is important to perform an unenhanced CT scan of the liver, prior to contrast injection. The hemorrhage will appear as high density regions within the mass (Fig. 4-56, *B*). The lesion often demonstrates a rapid transient enhancement during the arterial phase.[172]

Hepatic adenomas have a variable appearance on MRI. On T_1-weighted images, the mass may be hypo- or hyperintense to the surrounding liver. The increased signal intensity on T_1-weighted images may be caused by fatty content or blood products from hemorrhage.[173,174] In the series by Arrive et al.,[174] a peripheral rim corresponding pathologically to a pseudocapsule was found in approximately one third of cases. The lesions were of variable signal intensity on T_2-weighted images with approximately half being hyperintense. Because these features can all be present in hepatocellular carcinoma, it is often not possible to distinguish between the two.

Hepatic Lipomas

Hepatic lipomas are extremely rare, and only isolated cases have been reported in the radiologic literature.[175,176,177] There is an association between hepatic lipomas and renal angiomyolipomas and tuberous sclerosis. The lesions are asymptomatic. **Ultrasound** demonstrates a well-defined echogenic mass (Fig. 4-58, *A*), indistinguishable from a hemangioma, echogenic metastasis, or focal fat unless the mass is large and near the diaphragm, in which case differential sound transmission through the fatty mass will produce a discontinuous or broken diaphragm echo.[177] The diagnosis is confirmed using CT scanning, which reveals the fatty nature of

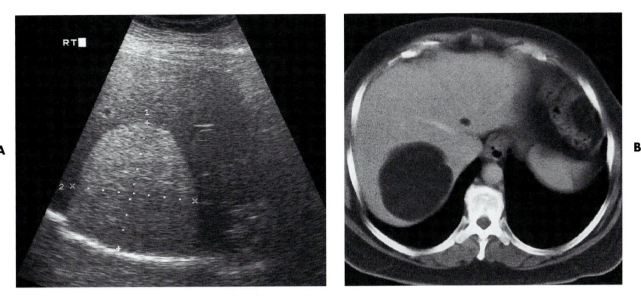

FIG. 4-58. **Hepatic lipoma mimicking a hemangioma.** **A,** Sonogram shows a focal, highly echogenic, solid liver mass. The discontinuity of the diaphragm echo due to the altered rate of sound transmission is a clue to the correct diagnosis. **B,** Confirmatory computed tomography scan shows the fat density of the mass. (From Garant M, Reinhold C: Hepatic lipoma. *C Asso Radiol J* 1996;47:140-142.)

the mass by the negative Hounsfield units (−30 HU) (Fig. 4-58, *B*).[175]

MALIGNANT HEPATIC NEOPLASMS

Hepatocellular Carcinoma

Hepatocellular carcinoma (HCC) is one of the most common malignant tumors, particularly in Southeast Asia, sub-Saharan Africa, Japan, Greece, and Italy. It occurs predominantly in men, with a sex ratio of approximately 5:1.[170] **Etiologic factors** contributing to the development of hepatocellular carcinoma depend on the geographic distribution. In the West, **alcoholic cirrhosis** is the most common condition predisposing to hepatoma. **Chronic hepatitis B and C infection** account for the high incidence of hepatocellular carcinoma in sub-Saharan Africa, Southeast Asia, China, Japan, and the Mediterranean. Aflatoxins, which are toxic metabolites produced by fungi in certain foods, have also been implicated in the pathogenesis of hepatomas in developing countries.[170] The clinical presentation is often delayed until the tumor reaches an advanced stage. Symptoms include right upper-quadrant pain, weight loss, and abdominal swelling when ascites is present.

Pathologically, hepatocellular carcinoma occurs in three forms:
• Solitary tumor
• Multiple nodules
• Diffuse infiltration

There is a propensity towards venous invasion. The portal vein is involved more commonly than the hepatic venous system, occurring in 30% to 60% of cases.[178-180]

The **sonographic appearance** of hepatocellular carcinoma is variable (Fig. 4-59). The masses may be hypoechoic, complex, or echogenic. Most small (< 5 cm) hepatocellular carcinomas are hypoechoic, corresponding histologically to a solid tumor without necrosis.[181,182] A thin, peripheral hypoechoic halo which corresponds to a fibrous capsule is seen most often in small hepatocellular carcinomas.[183] With time and increasing size, the masses tend to become more complex and inhomogeneous as a result of necrosis and fibrosis. Calcification is uncommon but has been reported.[184] Small tumors may appear diffusely hyperechoic secondary to fatty metamorphosis or sinusoidal dilation, making them indistinguishable from focal fatty infiltration, cavernous hemangiomas, and lipomas (Fig. 4-59, *A*).[181,182,185] Intratumoral fat also occurs in larger masses. However, because it tends to be focal, it is unlikely to cause confusion in diagnosis.

Preliminary studies in evaluating focal liver lesions with **duplex and color flow Doppler ultrasound** suggest hepatocellular carcinoma has characteristic high-velocity signals (Fig. 4-60).[186-188] In a study by Reinhold et al.[188] which used a frequency of 3 mHz for both imaging and Doppler examinations, 32 of 46 hepatomas and 4 of 86 metastatic lesions had Doppler shifts of ≥ 4.5 kHz. None of the 66 benign lesions were in this category. The specificity for distinguishing

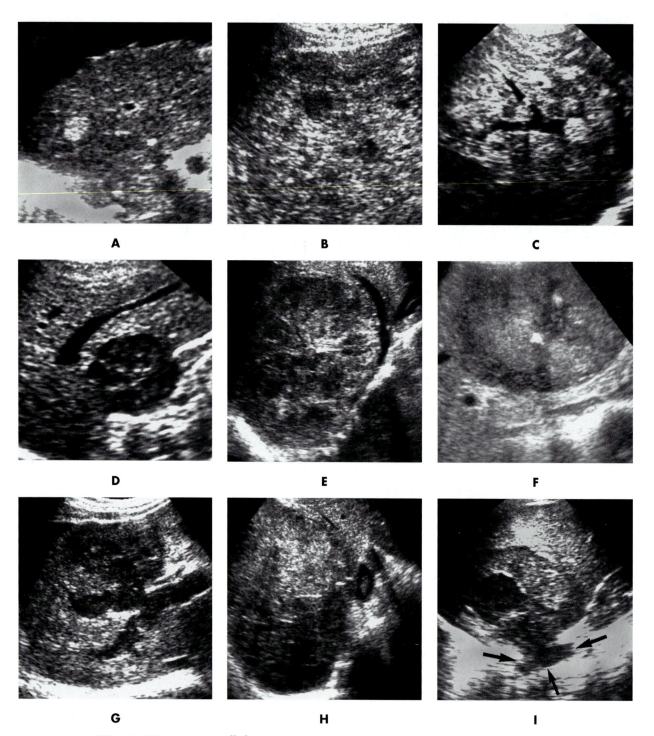

FIG. 4-59. **Hepatocellular carcinoma, pathology proven.** Early tumors may be **A,** echogenic or **B,** hypoechoic. **C,** Diffuse tumor may show as multiple tiny echogenic nodules, two of which directly involve the portal vein. Tumor features may include **D,** capsular bulging, **E,** a stellate central scar, and **F,** focal calcification. Evidence of tumor extension includes **G,** portal vein thrombus, **H,** Inferior vena cava thrombus, and **I,** direct unresectable extension through the posterior capsule *(arrows)* into the diaphragm.

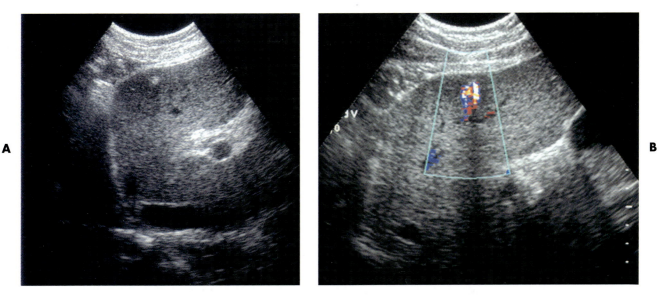

FIG. 4-60. **Proven hepatocellular carcinoma—contribution of color Doppler detection.** **A,** Sonogram shows a tiny echogenic focus in the superficial aspect of the liver, a nonspecific and often insignificant sonographic observation. **B,** A more magnified color Doppler image shows abnormal vascularity for this locale with high-velocity arterial signals suggesting arteriovenous shunting. This excludes hemangioma from consideration.

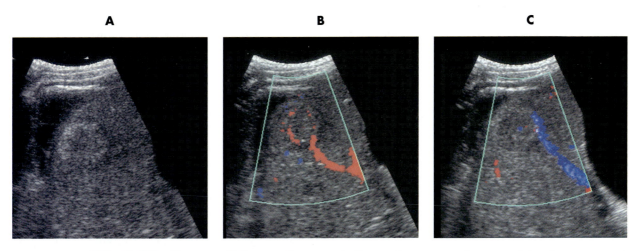

FIG. 4-61. **Hepatocellular carcinoma.** **A,** Gray scale sonogram shows a peripheral nonhomogeneous, slightly echogenic solid nodule. **B,** Color Doppler image shows an afferent artery in red and tumor vascularity. **C,** An efferent vein is seen in blue.

HCC from metastatic disease was high (95%) but the sensitivity low (70%).[188] Color Doppler can aid in the sampling for frequency shifts. It is important not to erroneously sample from displaced normal hepatic artery branches surrounding the tumor.[188] Tanaka et al.[187] have described a fine bloodflow network (branching pattern) as being characteristic of HCC (Fig. 4-61).[187] To date, although power Doppler sonography is more sensitive to blood flow in liver tumors, the patterns of signal are variable and cannot be used to reliably distinguish HCC from metastases.[142]

If **CT scanning** is being performed to screen for HCC, the study is best performed helically during both the arterial and portal venous phases. In a recent study by Baron et al.[189] 11% of patients had tumor visible only during the arterial phase of contrast enhancement. Neovascularity within portal venous thrombosis as well as arterioportal shunting are also better depicted with biphasic helical CT.[189] The pattern of contrast enhancement parallels the pathologic components of HCC. Well-vascularized neoplasms are hyperattenuating during the arterial phase, becoming hypodense during the portal venous phase. Fibrous septations and capsules may show the opposite pattern of enhancement. Necrotic tissue often appears cystic.[190] Diffuse infiltrating tumor may be difficult to detect in a patient with severe cirrhosis and portal hypertension because of the inhomogeneous hepatic parenchyma and patchy perfusion. Intratumoral fatty changes are recognized by the negative Hounsfield units.

MRI of hepatocellular carcinoma continues to improve. The ability to visualize the liver in multiple planes, with breath-hold technique and intravenous contrast agents allows increased lesion conspicuity and anatomic localization. On T_1-weighted images, HCC is usually either hypointense to surrounding liver parenchyma or hyperintense. The hyperintense signal is found more often in larger tumors and is probably related to fatty change or excess copper-binding proteins and glycogen.[191-193] On T_2-weighted sequences, small (< 2 cm) HCC may be isointense or hypointense.[194] Larger lesions are more typically hyperintense and heterogeneous. A hyperintense capsule may also be seen.[191] The features of gadolinium-enhancement parallel contrast-enhanced CT.[190]

Fibrolamellar carcinoma is a histologic subtype of hepatocellular carcinoma that is found in younger patients (adolescents and young adults) without coexisting liver disease. The serum alpha-fetoprotein levels are usually normal. The tumors are usually well-differentiated, often encapsulated by fibrous tissue and solitary. The size ranges from 6 to 22 cm.[195-197] The prognosis is generally better for fibrolamellar carcinoma compared with hepatocellular carcinoma with five-year survival rates approximately 25% to 30%.[198,199] Most patients, however, demonstrate advanced disease at the time of diagnosis. Aggressive surgical resection of tumor is recommended at the time of presentation as well as for recurrent disease.[197] The echogenicity of fibrolamellar carcinoma is variable. Punctate calcification and a central echogenic scar—features which are distinctly unusual in hepatomas—are more common in the fibrolamellar subtype. Typically the central scar is hypointense on T_2-weighted MRI (versus the scar of FNH which is hyperintense).

Hemangiosarcoma (Angiosarcoma)

Hepatic hemangiosarcoma is an extremely rare malignant tumor. It occurs almost exclusively in adults, reaching its peak incidence in the sixth and seventh decades of life. Hemangiosarcoma is of particular interest because of its association with specific carcinogens—thorotrast, arsenic, and polyvinyl chloride.[170] Very few cases of hepatic hemangiosarcoma have been reported in the radiologic literature. The **sonographic appearance** is that of a large mass of mixed echogenicity.[200,201]

Hepatic Epithelioid Hemangioendothelioma

Epithelioid hemangioendothelioma (EHE) is a rare malignant tumor of vascular origin that occurs in adults. Soft tissues, lung, and liver are affected. The prognosis is variable. Many patients survive longer than 5 years with or without treatment.[202] Hepatic EHE begins as multiple hypoechoic nodules. Over time, the nodules grow and coalesce, forming larger confluent hypoechoic masses, which tend to involve the periphery of the liver. Foci of calcification may be present.[202,203] The hepatic capsule overlying the lesions of EHE may be retracted inward secondary to fibrosis incited by the tumor. This is an unusual feature which is highly suggestive of this diagnosis. One should keep in mind that peripheral metastases postchemotherapy and tumors causing biliary obstruction may result in segmental atrophy and have a similar appearance.[204] The diagnosis is made by percutaneous liver biopsy, providing immunohistochemical staining is performed.

Metastatic Disease

In the United States, metastatic disease to the liver is 18 to 20 times more common than hepatocellular carcinoma. Its detection greatly alters the patient's prognosis and very often the management.

The incidence of hepatic metastases depends on the type of tumor and its stage at initial detection. Patients with short survival rates (< 1 year) after initial detection of liver metastases are those with hepatocellular carcinoma and carcinomas of the pancreas, stomach, and esophagus. Patients with a more prolonged survival are those with head and neck carcinomas and carcinoma of the colon. Most patients with melanoma have an extremely low incidence of hepatic metastases at diagnosis. Liver involvement at autopsy, however, may be as high as 70%.

Ultrasound is an excellent screening modality for metastatic liver disease because of its relative accuracy, speed, lack of ionizing radiation, and availability. In spite of these advantages, sonography is not uniformly used as the first line investigative technique to search for metastatic disease in the United States where CT has filled that role. However, worldwide, ultrasound is commonly used and in skilled hands is competitive with both CT and MRI for detection of metastatic lesions.[205] Contrary to popular belief, small lesions may be well seen on sonography and it is not size but echogenicity which determines lesion conspicuity on a sonogram. That is, a very tiny mass of only a few millimeters will be easily seen if it is either increased or decreased in echogenicity in contrast to the adjacent liver parenchyma. As most metastases are either hypo- or hyperechoic, a careful exam should allow for their detection. Further, the multiplanar capability of ultra-

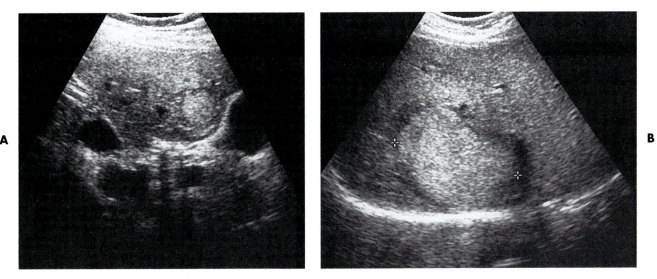

A

B

FIG. 4-62. Hepatic adenoma with a hypoechoic halo in an asymptomatic 26-year-old Chinese woman with incidentally discovered liver masses. **A,** View of left lobe of the liver and **B,** view of right lobe of the liver both show focal echogenic liver masses with definite hypoechoic halos. Neither computed tomography or magnetic resonance imaging scan was diagnostic. Liver biopsy showed adenomas with a clear zone of atrophy surrounding the mass accounting for the halo on sonography.

sound allows for excellent segmental localization of masses with the ability to detect proximity to or involvement of the vital vascular structures.

Metastatic liver disease may present as a single liver lesion although more commonly as multiple focal liver masses. All metastatic lesions in a given liver may have identical sonographic morphology; however, biopsy confirmed lesions of differing appearances may have the same underlying histology. Of importance, metastases may also be present in a liver which already has an underlying diffuse or focal abnormality, most commonly hemangioma.

Knowledge of a prior or concomitant malignancy and features of disseminated malignancy at the time of a sonogram are helpful in correct interpretation of a sonographically detected liver mass(es). Although there are no absolutely confirmatory features of metastatic disease on sonography, several are suggestive, including the presence of multiple solid lesions of varying size and the presence of a **hypoechoic halo** surrounding a liver mass. A halo around the periphery of a liver mass on sonography has been regarded as an ominous sign with a high association with malignancy, particularly metastatic disease but also hepatocellular carcinoma. In our own investigation of 214 consecutive patients with focal liver lesions, 66 patients had lesions which showed a hypoechoic halo: 13 hepatocellular carcinomas, 43 metastases, 4 focal nodular hyperplasia, and 2 adenomas (Fig. 4-62). Four lesions were unconfirmed.[206] Therefore, we conclude that al-

though a halo is not absolutely indicative of malignancy, it is seen with lesions which require further investigation and confirmation of their nature regardless of the patient's presentation or status.

Radiologic-histologic correlation has revealed that, in the majority of cases, the hypoechoic rim corresponds to normal liver parenchyma, which is compressed by the rapidly expanding tumor. Less commonly, the hypoechoic rim represents tumor fibrosis or vascularization.[207]

The following **sonographic patterns** of metastatic liver disease have been described (Fig. 4-63): echogenic, hypoechoic, target, calcified, cystic, and diffuse. Although the ultrasound appearance is not specific for determining the origin of the metastasis, certain generalities apply.

Echogenic metastases tend to arise from a gastrointestinal origin or from hepatocellular carcinoma. Also the more vascular the tumor, the more likely the lesion is to be echogenic.[187,208] Therefore metastases from renal cell carcinoma, carcinoid, choriocarcinoma and islet cell carcinoma tend to be hyperechoic (Fig. 4-63, C).

Hypoechoic metastases are generally hypovascular and are the typical pattern seen in untreated metastatic breast or lung cancer (Fig. 4-63, A). Lymphomatous involvement of the liver may also manifest as hypoechoic masses. Although at autopsy the liver is often a secondary site of involvement by Hodgkin and non-Hodgkin lymphoma, the disease

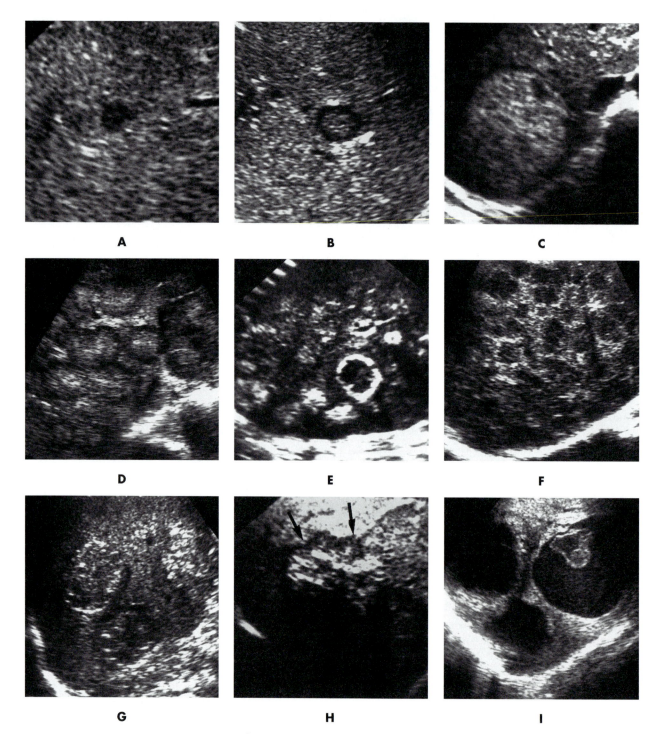

FIG. 4-63. Patterns of metastatic liver disease. A, Hypoechoic nodule—classic for breast, as in this case, lung and melanoma. **B,** Target lesion. **C,** Echogenic—classic for colon, neuroendocrine, and vascular primaries. **D, E,** and **F,** diffuse and extensive. **D,** Isoechoic masses with hypoechoic halos, classic for gastrointestinal primaries. **E,** Necrotic and echogenic, classic for gastrointestinal primaries. **F,** Hypoechoic, classic for breast, lung, and melanoma, as in this case. **G,** Calcifications seen as multiple tiny punctate rim calcifications which do not shadow. **H,** Calcified, with a large clump of shadowing echogenic material—classic for mucin-producing adenocarcinoma, chondrosarcoma, and osteosarcoma. **I,** Necrotic, classic for vascular primaries such as small bowel sarcoma.

tends to be diffusely infiltrative and undetected by sonographic examination and CT scanning.[209] The pattern of multiple hypoechoic hepatic masses is more typical of primary non-Hodgkin lymphoma of the liver or lymphoma associated with AIDS.[209,210] The lymphomatous masses may appear anechoic and septated, mimicking hepatic abscesses.

The **bull's eye** or **target pattern** is characterized by a peripheral hypoechoic zone (Fig. 4-63, *B*). The appearance is nonspecific, although it is frequently identified in metastases from bronchogenic carcinoma.[211]

Calcified metastases are distinctive by virtue of their marked echogenicity and distal acoustic shadowing (Fig. 4-63, *G* and *H*). Mucinous adenocarcinoma of the colon is most frequently associated with calcified metastases. Other primary malignancies that give rise to calcified metastases are endocrine pancreatic tumors, leiomyosarcoma, adenocarcinoma of the stomach, neuroblastoma, osteogenic sarcoma, chondrosarcoma, and ovarian cystadenocarcinoma and teratocarcinoma.[212]

Cystic metastases are fortunately uncommon and generally exhibit features that enable them to be distinguished from the ubiquitous benign hepatic cyst—for example, mural nodules, thick walls, fluid-fluid levels, and internal septations.[213,214] Primary neoplasms having a cystic component, such as cystadenocarcinoma of the ovary and pancreas and mucinous carcinoma of the colon, may produce cystic lesions, although uncommonly. More often, cystic neoplasms occur secondary to extensive necrosis, seen most commonly in metastatic sarcomas, which typically have low-level echoes and a shaggy, thickened wall (Fig. 4-63, *I*).

Diffuse disorganization of the hepatic parenchyma reflects an infiltrative form of metastatic disease and is the most difficult to appreciate. In our experience, breast and lung carcinoma as well as malignant melanoma are the most common primary tumors to give this pattern. The diagnosis can be even more difficult if the patient has a fatty liver from chemotherapy. In these patients, CT scanning or MRI may be helpful.

Cholangiocarcinoma extending to involve the liver parenchyma may also be very difficult to appreciate on sonograms. Both subtle parenchymal infiltration and invasion of the portal triads is recognized (Fig. 4-64).

Hepatic involvement by **Kaposi sarcoma,** although frequent in patients with AIDS at autopsy, is rarely diagnosed by imaging studies.[215] Sonography has demonstrated periportal infiltration and multiple, small, peripheral hyperechoic nodules (Fig. 4-65).[216,217]

Because of the nonspecific appearance of metastatic liver disease, ultrasound-guided biopsy is widely used to establish a primary tissue diagnosis. In addition, ultrasound is an excellent means to monitor the response to chemotherapy in oncology patients.

COMMON PATTERNS FOR METASTATIC LIVER DISEASE

Echogenic metastases
Gastrointestinal tract
Hepatocellular carcinoma
Vascular primaries
  Islet cell carcinoma
  Carcinoid
  Choriocarcinoma
  Renal cell carcinoma

Hypoechoic metastases
Breast cancer
Lung cancer
Lymphoma

Bull's eye or target pattern
Lung cancer

Calcified metastases
Frequently—Mucinous adenocarcinoma
Less frequently—
  Osteogenic sarcoma
  Chondrosarcoma
  Teratocarcinoma
  Neuroblastoma

Cystic metastases
Necrosis—Sarcomas
Cystic growth patterns—
  Cystadenocarcinoma of ovary and pancreas
  Mucinous carcinoma of colon

Infiltrative patterns
Breast cancer
Lung cancer
Malignant melanoma

HEPATIC TRAUMA

The approach to the management of blunt hepatic injury is becoming increasingly more conservative. Operative exploration is indicated for patients in shock or for those who are hemodynamically unstable.[218] In the hemodynamically stable patient, many institutions initially perform abdominal CT scans to assess the extent of liver trauma. Ultrasound may be used to serially monitor the pattern of healing.

The predominant site of hepatic injury in blunt trauma is the right lobe—in particular, the posterior segment.[219] In the study series by Foley et al.,[220] the most common type of injury was a perivascular laceration paralleling branches of the right and middle hepatic veins and the anterior and posterior branches of the right portal vein. Other findings were subcap-

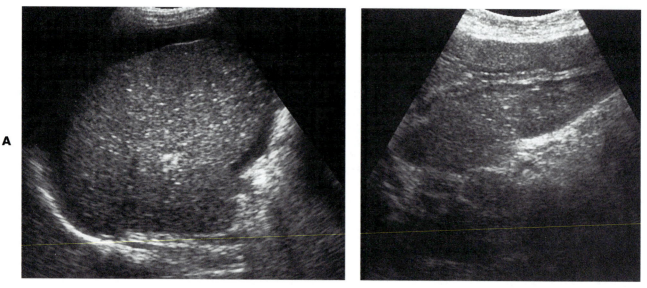

FIG. 4-64. **Cholangiocarcinoma of the liver** in two different patients. **A,** Diffuse infiltration of the liver parenchyma may be subtle as in this case. The liver however is bulbous and there are innumerable tiny echogenic parenchymal foci. Diagnosis was confirmed with an unguided tranjugular liver biopsy. **B,** Invasion of the portal triads shows as thickening and nonhomogeneity of the tissue surrounding the portal vein branches, a form of periportal cuffing.

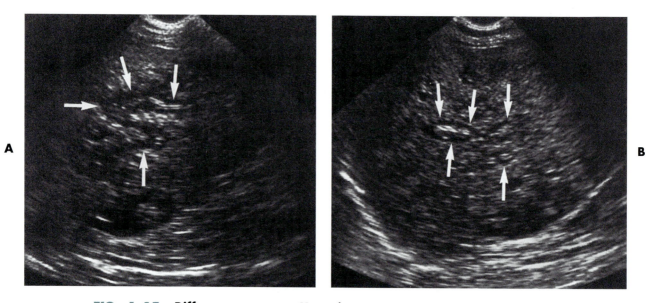

FIG. 4-65. **Diffuse metastases—Kaposi sarcoma.** **A,** Sagittal and **B,** transverse sonograms show hypoechoic periportal tumor infiltration (*arrows*). (From Towers MJ, Withers CE, Rachlis AR, et al: Ultrasound diagnosis of hepatic Kaposi sarcoma. *J Ultrasound Med* 1991;10:701.)

sular, pericapsular, or isolated hematomas, liver fracture (which was defined as a laceration extending between two visceral surfaces), lacerations involving the left lobe, and hemoperitoneum (Fig. 4-66).[220] Hepatic infarcts are rarely identified following blunt abdominal trauma because of the liver's dual blood supply.

van Sonnenberg et al.[221] evaluated the **sonographic findings** of acute trauma to the liver (< 24 hours following injury or transhepatic cholangiogram) and determined that fresh hemorrhage was echogenic (Fig. 4-67).[221] Within the first week, the hepatic laceration becomes more hypoechoic and distinct as a result of resorption of devitalized tissue and ingress of interstitial fluid. At 2 to 3 weeks later, the laceration becomes increasingly indistinct as a result of resorption of the fluid and filling of the spaces with granulation tissue.[220]

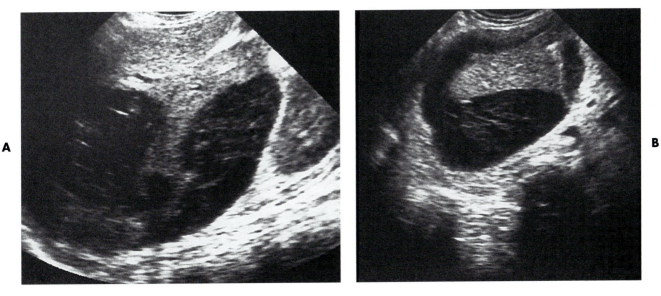

FIG. 4-66. **Post-traumatic subcapsular hematoma.** **A,** Sagittal and **B,** transverse images of the right lobe of the liver show a hypoechoic, contained, strandy fluid collection surrounding and indenting the liver parenchyma.

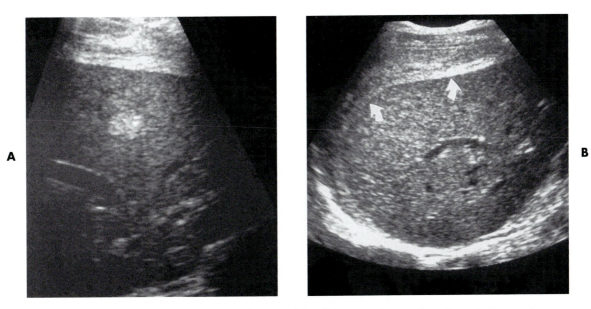

FIG. 4-67. **Acute post-core biopsy bleed into peritoneal cavity.** **A,** Image of biopsy site shows a small echogenic area in the parenchyma consistent with an acute intraparenchymal hematoma. **B,** Sagittal view of right lobe shows a thick rim of fresh perihepatic hematoma (*arrows*) between liver surface and overlying abdominal wall. This can be easily overlooked on sonography if the potential for echogenic fluid from acute bleeding is not recognized.

HEPATIC SURGERY

Liver Transplantation

Orthotopic liver transplantation is performed to eliminate irreversible disease when more conservative medical and surgical treatments have failed.[222] The procedure has the potential to restore the patient's normal lifestyle. The common indications for transplantation in adults are cirrhosis, especially secondary to chronic active hepatitis; fulminant acute hepatitis; inborn errors of metabolism; sclerosing cholangitis; Budd-Chiari syndrome; and unresectable but local hepatoma.[222,223] As a treatment for metastatic disease, transplantation is controversial and usually not performed.

The **surgical procedure** in the recipient includes hepatectomy, revascularization of the new liver, hemostasis, and biliary reconstruction.[223] Although details of the surgery are beyond the scope of this textbook, it is relevant to sonography that both venous and arterial grafts, harvested from the donor, may be used to obtain vascular anastomoses in complicated situations. Following transplantation, immunosuppression is necessary to prevent rejection of the liver. Optimal immunosuppression minimizes rejection without potentiating infection.

Complications of liver transplantation include rejection, vascular thrombosis or leak, biliary stricture or leak, infection, and neoplasia. The clinical manifestations of each are not always distinct. Biliary stricture and rejection, in particular, may cause similar manifestations including abnormal liver function. **Rejection** is the most common cause of hepatic dysfunction following transplantation and affects over one half of transplant recipients. Rejection is a clinical diagnosis confirmed by liver biopsy. Sonographic examinations and Doppler evaluations have not proved to be sensitive or specific in suggesting this diagnosis, and their role in patients with hepatic dysfunction is to eliminate causes other than rejection.[224,225]

Vascular complications include thrombosis, stricture, and arterial anastomotic pseudoaneurysms. **Vascular thrombosis** may affect the hepatic artery, the portal vein, or less commonly, the inferior vena cava and aorta. **Hepatic arterial thrombosis** affects approximately 3% to 10% of transplant recipients and may cause parenchymal ischemia and infarction or biliary stricture and necrosis.[226] Early occlusion of the hepatic artery before the development of collateral circulation is a life-threatening occurrence with a high mortality, necessitating immediate retransplantation. **IVC thrombosis** occurs most commonly in patients with an initial diagnosis of Budd-Chiari syndrome.

Biliary complications, including stricture and leak, affect approximately 15% of transplant recipients.[227] Because the hepatic artery is the sole supply of blood to the bile ducts in transplant patients, identification of a stricture of the bile duct is an indication for assessment of hepatic arterial patency. Hepatic arterial occlusion, pretransplant primary sclerosing cholangitis, choledochojejunostomy, cholangitis at liver biopsy and young age are significantly associated with biliary strictures.[228,229]

Infection is potentiated in liver transplant patients by immunosuppression and a long operative procedure. An altered immune response minimizes the overt clinical manifestations of sepsis. Therefore, all sonographically identified fluid collections should be viewed with suspicion and percutaneous aspiration performed as indicated.

Neoplasia may affect liver transplant patients either as a recurrent tumor, especially hepatocellular carcinoma, or a new neoplasia potentiated by immunosuppression, especially non-Hodgkin lymphoma (Fig. 4-68).[230] Neoplastic development should be considered in all transplant patients if new masses are identified in the abdomen or in the liver. Frequently, these tumors have a fulminant, rapidly progressive course.

Sonographic examination and **Doppler evaluation** are critical to both preoperative and postoperative noninvasive evaluation of liver transplant recipients. The **preoperative sonographic** assessment is aimed at appropriate patient selection and transplant timing and includes a general assessment of the abdomen to detect any findings that might alter patient selection, such as a large abdominal aortic aneurysm or extrahepatic malignant disease. Liver size and morphologic features are evaluated to determine the nature and extent of the liver disease. Vascular evaluation is critical, including assessment of portal vein patency; portal vein caliber; the direction of portal vein flow; the presence of venous collaterals, cavernous transformation of the portal vein, or both; hepatic arterial anatomy; and inferior vena caval size and patency. Of the preceding, identification of portal vein thrombosis or a very tiny portal vein calibre, for example, would not prevent transplantation. However, the surgeon would harvest donor veins to allow for adequate anastomosis. If the portal vein is not assessed adequately by sonography, an arteriographic or MRI examination is recommended.

Postoperative assessment includes a baseline sonogram, which is usually performed shortly after surgery. Further sonograms are performed for specific indications—most commonly, abdominal pain, fever, and abnormal liver function test results. Knowledge of the surgical procedure is essential, including the specifics of vascular anastomoses and the use of grafts, any reduction of donor liver caused by size incompatibility, details of the biliary-enteric anastomosis, and intraoperative complications such as bleeding.

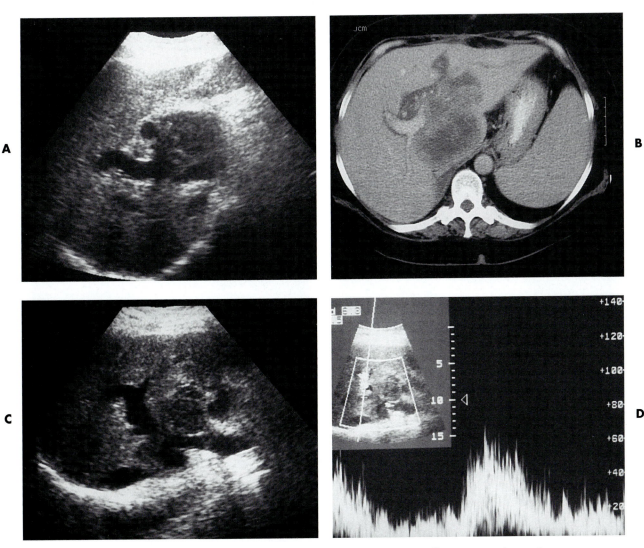

FIG. 4-68. **Lymphoproliferative disease complicating liver transplantation**
in a 46-year-old patient approximately 6 months following surgery. Biopsy showed large cell
lymphoma. **A,** Transverse sonogram shows a hypoechoic solid mass in the porta hepatis compressing the portal vein. **B,** Enhanced computed tomography scan confirms the low-density
mass and the portal venous involvement. **C,** The mass is producing a tight narrowing of the
portal vein. **D,** Portal vein spectral waveform obtained by moving cursor through the area of
narrowing confirms a focal stricture with a threefold velocity increase, from 20 to 60 cm/sec.

Sonography should include:[231]

- **Evaluation of the liver parenchyma** with assessment of any diffuse or focal abnormalities, the appearance of the periportal areas, and liver volume. Vascular occlusion, complicated by liver ischemia or gangrene, may produce a variable picture, although typically hypoechoic regions, which progress to large areas of liquefactive necrosis, are seen (Fig. 4-69). Large pockets of gas within the hepatic parenchyma necessitate angiography (Fig. 4-70). Liver infection, abscesses, and tumors have an identical appearance in the transplanted and normal liver. Transplant related non-Hodgkin lymphoma frequently appears as a large hypoechoic mass in the porta hepatis region (Fig. 4-68). These masses may be mistaken for inflammatory masses and biopsy is recommended if neoplasia is suspect.[232] Liver shrinkage may occur with chronic rejection, vascular occlusion, or chronic inflammation.

- **Bile duct evaluation,** for the presence of dilated intrahepatic or extrahepatic bile ducts, evidence of a bile duct stricture, or both (Fig. 4-71).

- **Assessment of intra-abdominal fluid collections** for size, morphologic features, and location. These may be hematomas, abscesses, bilomas, seromas, or pseudoaneurysms. In questionable cases, ultrasound-guided aspiration is most helpful to determine the nature of an identified fluid collection.

- **Evaluation of vascular patency** with both direct inspection of the vessels (portal vein, hepatic artery, and inferior vena cava) for thrombus and Doppler interrogation. The hepatic artery and main portal vein, as well as their major right and left branches, should be studied to avoid missing segmental occlusions. The hepatic artery, portal vein, hepatic veins, and inferior vena cava are all susceptible to strictures as well as thrombosis.

On color Doppler, **strictures** will show aliasing at the site of the stricture due to the high velocity flow through the narrowed segment (Fig. 4-72). **Hepatic artery stenosis** is suspected if a focal accelerated ve-

locity of greater than 200 to 300 cm per second is documented with turbulence at or distal to the stenosis (Fig. 4-73).[233] Further, a tardus parvus pattern of the intrahepatic arterial signal may also be seen (Figs. 4-73 and 4-74). Dodd et al.[234] describe parameters of the spectral hepatic arterial waveform for detection of unvisualized downstream strictures of the hepatic artery and total occlusion with collateralization to the liver. Using a threshold resistance index of less than 0.5 and a slow systolic acceleration time of greater than 0.08 seconds, they achieved a 73% sensitivity and specificity for the detection of marked hepatic arterial disease (either stenosis or thrombosis).

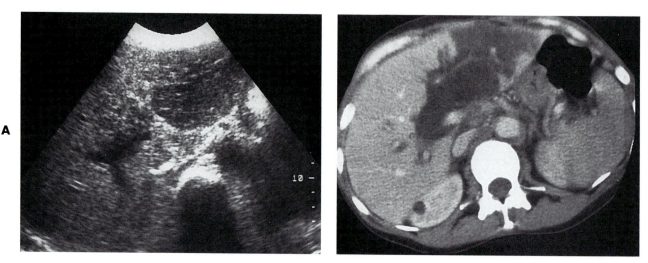

FIG. 4-69. Liver transplant, left lobe infarction. A, Transverse sonogram shows a typical hypoechoic geographic region in the left lateral segment with vague extension along the portal vein. **B,** Confirmatory computed tomography scan.

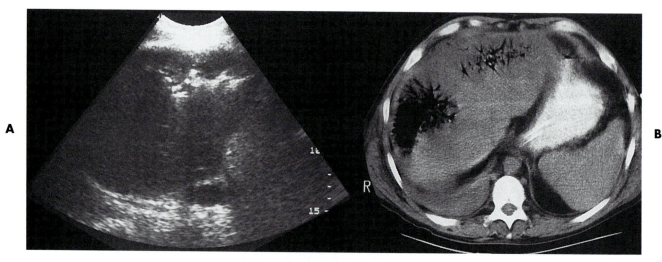

FIG. 4-70. Liver transplant, extensive portal venous gas associated with liver infarction. A, Sagittal left lobe sonogram shows bright echogenic linear streaks in the periphery of the liver. **B,** Computed tomography scan shows the branching configuration within the left lobe with a large confluent pocket in the right lobe associated with massive infarction.

Pseudoaneurysms at the anastomotic site of the hepatic artery are well-documented complications of liver transplantation. Their detection on gray scale may be obvious and straightforward with demonstration of a cystic area in continuity with the hepatic artery. More often, they appear as a nonspecific fluid collection between the porta hepatis and the region of the celiac axis (Fig. 4-75). If their vascular nature is not suspected, they may be easily overlooked; there-fore, we recommend color Doppler evaluation of all sonographically detected fluid collections post–liver transplantation.

On **color Doppler,** the waveform patterns of hepatic arterial pseudoaneurysms are variable and

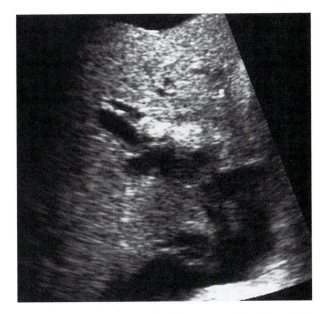

FIG. 4-71. Liver transplant complication—biliary anastomotic stricture with intrahepatic bile duct calculi. Transverse sonogram of porta hepatis shows the portal vein and a dilated right hepatic duct anteriorly. Multiple clumps of echogenic material fill the duct.

POSTOPERATIVE ASSESSMENT OF LIVER TRANSPLANT RECIPIENTS

Evaluation of the liver parenchyma
Diffuse or focal abnormality
Volume
Specific attention to:
    Infarction—hypoechoic segment(s) or lobe(s)
          —parenchymal gas
    Neoplasia—mass
    Opportunistic infection—mass or abscess

Evaluation of bile ducts
Dilated intrahepatic or extrahepatic ducts
Evidence of stricture

Assessment of fluid collections
Hematomas
Abscesses
Bilomas
Seromas
Pseudoaneurysms

Evaluation of vascular status
Thrombus
Stenosis—hepatic artery, portal and hepatic veins, IVC
Pseudoaneurysms

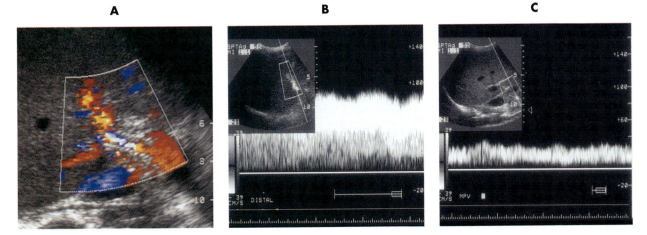

FIG. 4-72. Liver transplant recipient with a portal vein stricture. A, Color Doppler image of the portal vein shows normally directed flow toward the liver. There is aliasing in the anastomotic region consistent with a stricture. There is poststenotic turbulence. **B,** Portal vein duplex signal at the stricture shows over a fivefold velocity increase to 110 cm/sec. **C,** Portal vein duplex signal proximal to the stricture is normal, velocity approximately 20 cm/sec.

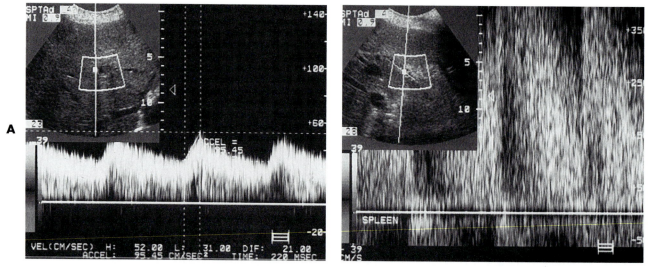

FIG. 4-73. Hepatic artery stenosis. A, Spectral waveform from intrahepatic hepatic artery shows a tardus parvus waveform with a prolonged acceleration time of 220 msec and a low RI of 0.4. **B,** Insonation of the vessel more proximally showed a focal high-velocity segment with aliasing. The tardus parvus component alone constitutes a positive test.

depend on the size of the aperture feeding the aneurysm. Internal flow may be slow and monophasic as the blood slowly circulates through the aneurysm (Fig. 4-75, *D*). However, there is usually a high velocity pulsatile jet at the entry point (Fig. 4-75, *C*). Optimal evaluation may require alteration of color scale to detect the varieties of flow within the lesion.

Portosystemic Shunts

Surgical portosystemic shunts are performed to decompress the portal system in patients with portal hypertension. The most commonly created surgical shunts include mesocaval, distal splenorenal (Warren), mesoatrial, and portacaval. **Duplex Doppler sonography** and **color Doppler imaging** appear to be reliable noninvasive methods of assessing shunt patency or thrombosis.[235-238] Both modalities are effective in assessing portacaval, mesoatrial, and mesocaval shunts.[237] Shunt patency is confirmed by demonstrating flow at the anastomotic site. If the anastomosis cannot be visualized, hepatofugal portal flow is an indirect sign of patency.[235,236]

Distal splenorenal communications are particularly difficult to examine with duplex Doppler sonography because overlying bowel gas and fat hinder accurate placement of the Doppler cursor.[237,239] Color Doppler imaging more readily locates the splenic and renal limbs of Warren shunts. The splenic limb is best imaged from a left subcostal approach, whereas the left renal vein is optimally scanned through the left flank. In the study by Grant et al.,[237] color Doppler sonog-raphy correctly inferred patency or thrombosis in all 14 splenorenal communications by evaluating the flow in both limbs of the shunt.

TRANSJUGULAR INTRAHEPATIC PORTOSYSTEMIC SHUNTS

Transjugular intrahepatic portosystemic shunts (TIPS) are the most recently developed and now most popular technique for relief of symptomatic portal hypertension, specifically varices with gastrointestinal bleeding, and less often refractory ascites. Performed percutaneously with insertion of an expandable metal stent, TIPS has less morbidity and mortality than surgical shunt procedures.[240]

The **technique** of performing TIPS requires transjugular access to the infrahepatic inferior vena cava with selection of the optimal hepatic vein on the basis of its angle and diameter is most often the right hepatic vein. After targeting the portal vein with either fluoroscopy or Doppler sonography, a transjugular puncture needle is passed from the hepatic vein to the intrahepatic portal vein and a shunt created. The tract is dilated to an approximate diameter of 10 mm with monitoring of the portal pressure gradient and filling of varices on portal venography. A bridging stent is left in place.[241]

In addition to acute problems directly attributed to the procedure itself, TIPS may be complicated by stenosis or occlusions of the stent caused by hyper-

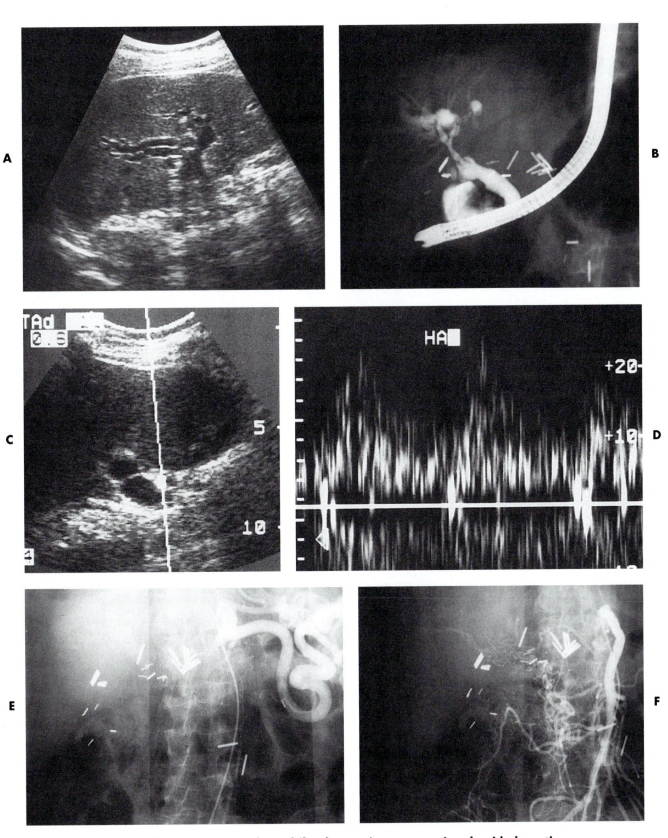

FIG. 4-74. Liver transplant, bile duct stricture associated with hepatic artery occlusion. A, Sonogram shows dilated intrahepatic bile ducts adjacent to the portal vein in the portal triads. B, Confirmatory ERCP shows stricture and proximal dilatation. C, Hepatic artery Doppler cursor shows D, a tardus parvus signal with a slow rise time and a low RI. E, Arteriogram shows an occluded hepatic artery. F, Delayed film shows collateral arterial circulation to the liver accounting for the abnormal waveform on Doppler.

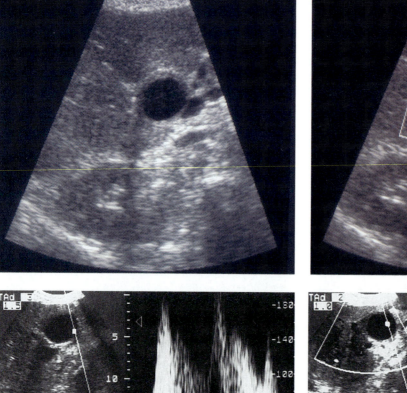

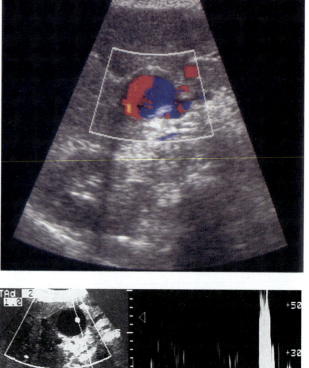

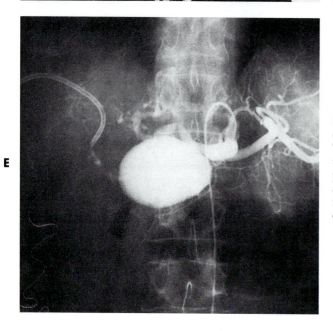

FIG. 4-75. **Liver transplant hepatic artery pseudoaneurysm.** **A,** Transverse sonogram shows the liver. There is a subhepatic cystic mass. **B,** Color Doppler shows the vascular nature of this cyst. **C,** Spectral wave form shows a pulsatile high-velocity arterial jet at the entry point to the aneurysm. **D,** Flow within the mass is low-velocity and monophasic. **E,** Confirmatory arteriogram show the false mycotic aneurysm.

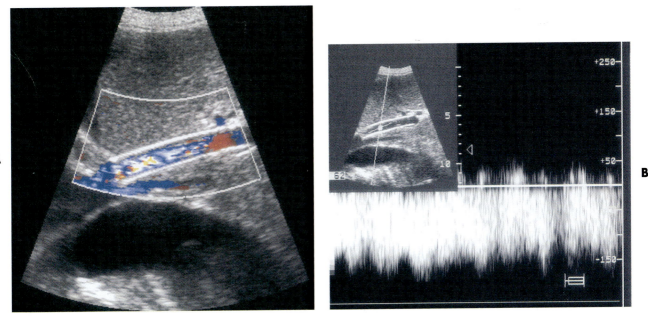

FIG. 4-76. TIPS. A, Color Doppler image of TIPS shunt shows flow throughout the shunt appropriately directed toward the heart with a turbulent pattern. **B,** Angle corrected midshunt velocity is normal at 150 cm/sec.

plasia of the pseudointimal lining. At one year, primary patency rates vary from 25% to 66% with a primary assisted patency of approximately 83%.[242,243] Sonography with Doppler provides a noninvasive method for monitoring of TIPS patients following their procedure as malfunction of the graft may be silent in its early phase. Scans should be performed immediately postprocedure, at three monthly intervals, and/or as indicated clinically.

Normal postprocedure Doppler findings include: high-velocity, turbulent blood flow (mean peak systolic velocity, 135 to 200 cm/sec)[244] throughout the stent and hepatofugal flow in the intrahepatic portal venous branches as the liver parenchyma drains through the shunt into the systemic circulation (Fig. 4-76). Increased hepatic artery peak systolic velocity is also a normal observation.

The technique of sonographic evaluation should include measurement of stent velocities at three points along the stent, as well as evaluation of the direction of flow in the intrahepatic portal vein and in the involved hepatic vein.

Sonographic detected **complications** include:
- stent occlusion;
- stent stenosis; and
- hepatic venous stenosis.

Malfunction is suggested by:
- no flow, consistent with shunt thrombosis or occlusion;
- low-velocity flow (especially at the portal venous end of the shunt) less than 50 to 60 cm per second

suggesting stenosis of the shunt beyond that point;[244,245] or
- a change in the peak shunt velocity, with either an increase or a decrease from baseline of 50 cm per second;[246]
- reversal of flow in the hepatic vein away from the inferior vena cava suggesting hepatic vein stenosis[247]
- hepatopedal intrahepatic portal venous flow;
- secondary signs including reaccumulation of ascites, reappearance of varices, and reappearance of a recanalized paraumbilical vein.

PERCUTANEOUS LIVER BIOPSY

Percutaneous biopsy of malignant disease involving the liver has a sensitivity greater than 90% in most study series.[248,249] Relative contraindications to percutaneous biopsy are an uncorrectable bleeding diathesis, an unsafe access route, and a patient who cannot adequately cooperate. Ultrasound guidance allows real-time observation of the needle tip as it is advanced into the lesion. Several biopsy attachments have been developed that allow continuous observation of the needle as it follows a predetermined path. Alternatively, many experienced radiologists prefer a "free-hand" technique. Even small masses (2.5 cm) can undergo successful biopsy using sonographic guidance.[249] Ultrasound guidance may also be used in percutaneous aspiration and drainage of complicated fluid collections in the liver. Ultrasound-guided

> **MALFUNCTION OF TIPS: SONOGRAPHIC SIGNS**
>
> **Direct signs**
> No flow
>   Consistent with shunt thrombosis or occlusion
> Low velocity flow
>   Especially at portal venous end of shunt
> Change in peak shunt velocity
>   Increase or decrease from baseline of 50 cm/sec
> Reversal of flow in hepatic vein
> Hepatopedal intrahepatic portal venous flow
>
> **Secondary signs**
> Reaccumulation of ascites
> Reappearance of varices
> Reappearance of recanalized paraumbilical vein

percutaneous ethanol injection has been used in the treatment of hepatocellular carcinoma and hepatic metastases.[250,251]

INTRAOPERATIVE ULTRASOUND

Intraoperative ultrasound is now an established application of ultrasound technology. The exposed liver is scanned with a sterile 7.5 MHz transducer, or one covered by a sterile sheath. Intraoperative ultrasound has been found to change the operative strategy in 31% to 49% of patients undergoing hepatic resection, either by allowing more precise resection or by indicating inoperability because of unsuspected masses or venous invasion.[252,253]

ACKNOWLEDGEMENT

The authors would like to thank Rose Baldwin for her assistance in the preparation of this chapter.

REFERENCES

Normal Anatomy
1. Marks WM, Filly RA, Callen PW: Ultrasonic anatomy of the liver: a review with new applications, *J Clin Ultrasound* 1979; 7:137-146.
2. Couinaud C: Le foie. In *Etudes Anatomiques et Chirurgicales*, Paris, 1957, Masson et Cie.
3. Sugarbaker PH: Toward a standard of nomenclature for surgical anatomy of the liver, *Neth J Surg* 1988;PO:100.
4. Nelson RC, Chezmar JL, Sugarbaker PH, et al.: Preoperative localization of focal liver lesions to specific liver segments: utility of CT during arterial portography, *Radiology* 1990; 176:89-94.
5. Soyer P, Bluemke DA, Bliss DF, et al.: Surgical segmental anatomy of the liver: demonstration with spiral CT during arterial portography and multiplanar reconstruction, *AJR* 1994; 163:99-103.
6. Lafortune M, Madore F, Patriquin HB, Breton G: Segmental anatomy of the liver: a sonographic approach to Couinaud nomenclature, *Radiology* 1991;181:443-448.

Normal Liver Size and Echogenicity
7. Gosink BB, Leymaster CE: Ultrasonic determination of hepatomegaly, *J Clin Ultrasound* 1981;9:37-41.
8. Niederau C, Sonnenberg A, Muller JE, et al.: Sonographic measurements of the normal liver, spleen, pancreas, and portal vein, *Radiology* 1983;149:537-540.

Developmental Anomalies
9. Belton R, Van Zandt TF: Congenital absence of the left lobe of the liver: a radiologic diagnosis, *Radiology* 1983;147:184.
10. Radin DR, Colletti PM, Ralls PW, et al.: Agenesis of the right lobe of the liver, *Radiology* 1987;164:639-642.
11. Lim JH, Ko YT, Han MC, et al.: The inferior accessory hepatic fissure: sonographic appearance, *AJR* 1987;149:495-497.
12. Fraser-Hill MA, Atri M, Bret PM, et al.: Intrahepatic portal venous system: variations demonstrated with duplex and color Doppler US, *Radiology* 1990;177:523-526.
13. Cosgrove DO, Arger PH, Coleman BG: Ultrasonic anatomy of hepatic veins, *J Clin Ultrasound* 1987;15:231-235.
14. Makuuchi M, Hasegawa H, Yamazaki S, et al.: The inferior right hepatic vein: ultrasonic demonstration, *Radiology* 1983; 148213-217.

Congenital Abnormalities
15. Gaines PA, Sampson MA: The prevalence and characterization of simple hepatic cysts by ultrasound examination, *Br J Radiol* 1989;62:335-337.
16. Bean WJ, Rodan BA: Hepatic cysts: treatment with alcohol, *AJR* 1985;144:237-241.
17. Baron RL, Campbell WL, Dodd III GD: Peribiliary cysts associated with severe liver disease: imaging-pathologic correlation, *AJR* 1994;162:631-636.
18. Levine E, Cook LT, Granthem JJ: Liver cysts in autosomal-dominant polycystic kidney disease: clinical and computed tomographic study, *AJR* 1985;145:229-233.
19. von Meyenburg H: Uber die Cystenliber, *Beitr Pathol Anat* 1918;64:477-532.
20. Chung ED: Multiple bile duct hamartomas, *Cancer* 1970; 26:287.
21. Redston MS, Wanless IR: The hepatic von Meyenburg complex: Prevalence and association with hepatic and renal cysts among 2843 autopsies, *Mod Pathol* 1996 (in press)
22. Lev-Toaff AS, Bach AM, Wechsler RJ, et al.: The radiologic and pathologic spectrum of biliary hamartomas, *AJR* 1995;165:309-313.
23. Salo J, Bru C, Vilella A, et al.: Bile-duct hamartomas presenting as multiple focal lesions on hepatic ultrasonography, *Am J Gastroenterol* 1992;87:221-223.
24. Tan A, Shen J, Hecht A: Sonogram of multiple bile duct hamartomas, *Clin Ultrasound* 1989;17:667-669.
25. Fogel EL, Heathcote EJ, Wilson SR, et al.: Cryptogenic recurrent bacterial cholangitis: possible etiologic role of multiple bile duct hamartomas, Submitted for publication *Gastroenterology*, January, 1997.
26. Burns CD, Huhns JG, Wieman TJ: Cholangiocarcinoma in association with multiple biliary microhamartomas, *Arch Pathol Lab Med* 1990;114:1287-1289.

Infectious Diseases

27. Seeft LB: Acute Viral Hepatitis. In Kaplowitz N, editor: *Liver and Biliary Disease*, ed 2, Baltimore; Williams & Wilkins; 1996;289-316.

28. Douglas DD Rakela J: Fulminant Hepatitis. In Kaplowitz N, editor: *Liver and Biliary Disease*, ed 2, Baltimore; Williams & Wilkins; 1996;317-326.

29. Davis GL: Chronic Hepatitis. In Kaplowitz N, editor: *Liver and Biliary Disease*, ed 2, Baltimore; Williams & Wilkins; 1996;327-337.

30. Zweibel WJ: Sonographic diagnosis of diffuse liver disease, *Semin US, CT, MRI* 1995;16:8-15.

31. Wilson SR, Arenson AM: Sonographic evaluation of hepatic abscesses, *J Can Assoc Radiol* 1984;35:174-177.

32. Sabbaj J, Sutter VL, Finegold SM: Anaerobic pyogenic liver abscess, *Ann Intern Med* 1972;77:629-638.

33. Lawrence PH, Holt SC, Levi CS, Gough JC: Ultrasound case of the day, *RadioGraphics* 1994;14:1147-1149.

34. Pastakia B, Shawker TH, Thaler M, et al.: Hepatosplenic candidiasis: wheels within wheels, *Radiology* 1988;166:417-421.

35. Ralls PW, Colletti PM, Quinn MF, et al.: Sonographic findings in hepatic amebic abscess, *Radiology* 1982;145:123-126.

36. Berry M, Bazaz R, Bhargava S: Amebic liver abscess: Sonographic diagnosis and management, *J Clin Ultrasound* 1986;14:239-242.

37. Ralls PW, Barnes PF, Radin DR: Sonographic features of amebic and pyogenic liver abscesses: a blinded comparison, *AJR* 1987;149:499-501.

38. Ralls PW, Barnes PF, Johnson MB, et al.: Medical treatment of hepatic amebic abscess: rare need for percutaneous drainage, *Radiology* 1987;165:805-807.

39. Ralls PW, Quinn MF, Boswell WD, et al.: Patterns of resolution in successfully treated hepatic amebic abscess: sonographic evaluation, *Radiology* 1983;149:541-543.

40. Gharbi HA, Hassine W, Brauner MW, et al.: Ultrasound examination of the hydatic liver, *Radiology* 1981;139:459-463.

41. Lewall DB, McCorkell SJ: Hepatic echinococcal cysts: sonographic appearance and classification, *Radiology* 1985;155:773-775.

42. Beggs I: Radiology of hydatid disease, *AJR* 1985;145:639-648.

43. Mueller PR, Dawson SL, Ferrucci JT Jr, et al.: Hepatic echinococcal cyst: successful percutaneous drainage, *Radiology* 1985;155:627-628.

44. Bret PM, Fond A, Bretagnolle M, et al.: Percutaneous aspiration and drainage of hydatid disease of the liver, *Radiology* 1988;168:617-620.

45. Akhan O, Ozmen MN, Dincer A, et al.: Liver hydatid disease: long-term results of percutaneous treatment, *Radiology* 1996;198:259-264.

46. Bezzi M, Teggi A, De Rosa F, et al.: Abdominal hydatid disease: ultrasound findings during medical treatment, *Radiology* 1987;162:91-95.

47. Jha R, Lyons EA, Levi CS: Ultrasound case of the day, *RadioGraphics* 1994;14:455-458.

48. Didier D, Weiler S, Rohmer P, et al.: Hepatic alveolar echinococcus: correlative ultrasound and computed tomography study, *Radiology* 1985;154:179-186.

49. McCully RM, Barron CM, Cheever AW: Schistosomiasis. In Binford CH, Connor DH, editors: *Pathology of Tropical and Extraordinary Disease*, Washington; Armed Forces Institute of Pathology; 1976;482-508.

50. Symmers W St C: Note on a new form of liver cirrhosis due to the presence of the ova of Bilharzia hematobilia, *J Pathol* 1904;9:237-239.

51. Cerri GG, Alves VAF, Magalhaes A: Hepatosplenic schistosomiasis mansoni: ultrasound manifestations, *Radiology* 1984;153:777-780.

52. Fataar S, Bassiony H, Satyanath S, et al.: Characteristic sonographic features of schistosomal periportal fibrosis, *AJR* 1984;143:69-71.

53. Kuhman JE: Pneumocystic infections: The radiologist's perspective, *Radiology* 1996;198:623-635.

54. Radin DR, Baker EL, Klatt EC, et al.: Visceral and nodal calcification in patients with AIDS-related Pneumocystis carinii infection, *AJR* 1990;154:27-31.

55. Spouge AR, Wilson SR, Gopinath N, et al.: Extrapulmonary Pneumocystis carinii in a patient with AIDS: sonographic findings, *AJR* 1990;155:76-78.

56. Telzak EE, Cote RJ, Gold JWM, et al.: Extrapulmonary Pneumocystis carinii infections, *Rev Infect Dis* 1990;12:380-386.

57. Lubat E, Megibow AJ, Balthazar EJ, et al.: Extrapulmonary Pneumocystis carinii infection in AIDS: computed tomography findings, *Radiology* 1990;174:157-160.

58. Towers MJ, Withers CE, Hamilton PA, et al.: Visceral calcification in AIDS may not be always due to Pneumocystis carinii, *AJR* 1991;156:745-747.

Disorders of Metabolism

59. Zakim D: Metabolism of glucose and fatty acids by the liver. In Zakim D, Boyer TD, editors: *Hepatology: A Textbook of Liver Disease*, Philadelphia; WB Saunders; 1982;76-109.

60. Wilson SR, Rosen IE, Chin-Sang HB, et al.: Fatty infiltration of the liver: An imaging challenge, *J Can Assoc Radiol* 1982;227-232.

61. Yates CK, Streight RA: Focal fatty infiltration of the liver simulating metastatic disease, *Radiology* 1986;159:83-84.

62. Sauerbrei EE, Lopez M: Pseudotumor of the quadrate lobe in hepatic sonography: a sign of generalized fatty infiltration, *AJR* 1986;147:923-927.

63. White EM, Simeone JF, Mueller PR, et al.: Focal periportal sparing in hepatic fatty infiltration: A cause of hepatic pseudomass on ultrasound, *Radiology* 1987;162:57-59.

64. Wanless IR, Bargman JM, Oreopoulos DG, Vas SI: Subcapsular steatonecrosis in response to peritoneal insulin delivery: a clue to the pathogenesis of steatonecrosis in obesity, *Mod Pathol* 1989;2:6974.

65. Apicella PL, Mirowitz SA, Weinreb JC: Extension of vessels through hepatic neoplasms: MR and CT findings, *Radiology* 1994;191:135-136.

66. Quinn SF, Gosink BB: Characteristic sonographic signs of hepatic fatty infiltration, *AJR* 1985;145:753-755.

67. Arai K, Matsui O, Takashima T, et al.: Focal spared areas in fatty liver caused by regional decreased blood flow, *AJR* 1988;151:300-302.

68. Ishak KG, Sharp HL: Metabolic errors and liver disease. In MacSween RNM, Anthony PP, Scheuer PJ, editors: *Pathology of the Liver*, ed 2, New York; Churchill Livingstone; 1987;99-180.

69. Grossman H, Ram PC, Coleman RA, et al.: Hepatic ultrasonography in type 1 glycogen storage disease (von Gierke disease), *Radiology* 1981;141:753-756.

70. Anthony PP: The morphology of cirrhosis: Definition, nomenclature, and classification, *Bull WHO* 1977;55:521.

71. Millward-Sadler GH: Cirrhosis. In MacSween RNM, Anthony PP, Scheuer PJ, editors: *Pathology of the Liver*, ed 2. New York; Churchill Livingstone; 1987;342-363.

72. Giorgio A, Amoroso P, Lettiri G, et al.: Cirrhosis: value of caudate to right lobe ratio in diagnosis with ultrasound, *Radiology* 1986;161:443-445.

73. Taylor KJW, Riely CA, Hammers L, et al.: Quantitative ultrasound attenuation in normal liver and in patients with diffuse liver disease: importance of fat, *Radiology* 1986;160:65-71.

74. Sandford N, Walsh P, Matis C, et al.: Is ultrasonography useful in the assessment of diffuse parenchymal liver disease? *Gastroenterology* 1985;89:186-191.

75. Freeman MP, Vick CW, Taylor KJW, et al.: Regenerating nodules in cirrhosis: sonographic appearance with anatomic correlation, *AJR* 1986;146:533-536.

76. Murakami T, Nakamura H, Hori S, et al.: Regenerating nodules in hepatic cirrhosis. MR findings with pathologic correlation, *AJR* 1990;155:1227-1231.

77. Theise ND: Macroregenerative (dysplastic) nodules and hepatocarcinomagenesis: theoretical and clinical considerations, *Semin Liver Dis* 1995;15:360-371.

78. Tanaka S, Kitamra T, Fujita M, et al.: Small hepatocellular carcinoma: differentiation from adenomatous hyperplastic nodule with color Doppler flow imaging, *Radiology* 1997;182:161-165.

79. Bolondi L, Bassi S, Gaiani S, et al.: Liver cirrhosis: changes of Doppler waveform of hepatic veins, *Radiology* 1991;178:513-516.

80. Colli A, Cocciolo M, Riva C, et al.: Abnormalities of Doppler waveform of the hepatic veins in patients with chronic liver disease: correlation with histologic findings, *AJR* 1994;162:833-837.

81. Lafortune M, Dauzat M, Pomier-Layrargues E, et al.: Hepatic artery: effect of a meal in healthy persons and transplant recipients, *Radiology* 1993;187:391-394.

82. Joynt LK, Platt JF, Rubin JM, et al.: Hepatic artery resistance before and after standard meal in subjects with diseased and healthy livers, *Radiology* 1995;196:489-492.

Vascular Abnormalities

83. Boyer TD: Portal hypertension and its complications. In Zakim D, Boyer TD, editors: *Hepatology: A Textbook of Liver Disease*, Philadelphia; WB Saunders; 1982;464-499.

84. Bolondi L, Gandolfi L, Arienti V, et al.: Ultrasonography in the diagnosis of portal hypertension: diminished response of portal vessels to respiration, *Radiology* 1982;142:167-172.

85. Lafortune M, Marleau D, Breton G, et al.: Portal venous system measurements in portal hypertension, *Radiology* 1984;151:27-30.

86. Juttner H-U, Jenney JM, Ralls PW, et al.: Ultrasound demonstration of portosystemic collaterals in cirrhosis and portal hypertension, *Radiology* 1982;142:459-463.

87. Subramanyam BR, Balthazar EJ, Madamba MR, et al.: Sonography of portosystemic venous collaterals in portal hypertension, *Radiology* 1983;146:161-166.

88. Patriquin H, Lafortune M, Burns PN, et al.: Duplex Doppler examination in portal hypertension, *AJR* 1987;149:71-76.

89. Lafortune M, Constantin A, Breton G, et al.: The recanalized umbilical vein in portal hypertension: a myth, *AJR* 1985;144:549-553.

90. DiCandio G, Campatelli A, Mosca F, et al.: Ultrasound detection of unusual spontaneous portosystemic shunts associated with uncomplicated portal hypertension, *J Ultrasound Med* 1985;4:297-305.

91. Mostbeck GH, Wittich GR, Herold C, et al.: Hemodynamic significance of the paraumbilical vein in portal hypertension: assessment with duplex ultrasound, *Radiology* 1989;170:339-342.

92. Nelson RC, Lovett KE, Chezmar JL, et al.: Comparison of pulsed Doppler sonography and angiography in patients with portal hypertension, *AJR* 1987;149:77-81.

93. Bellamy EA, Bossi MC, Cosgrove DO: Ultrasound demonstration of changes in the normal portal venous system following a meal, *Br J Radiol* 1984;57:147-149.

94. Ohnishi K, Saito M, Nakayama T, et al.: Portal venous hemodynamics in chronic liver disease: effects of posture change and exercise, *Radiology* 1985;155:757-761.

95. Bolandi L, Maziotti A, Arienti V, et al.: Ultrasonography in the diagnosis of portal hypertension and after portosystemic shunt operations, *Surgery* 1984;95:261-269.

96. Zweibel WJ, Mountford RA, Halliwell MJ, Wells PNT: Splanchnic blood flow in patients with cirrhosis and portal hypertension: investigation with duplex Doppler US, *Radiology* 1995;194:807-812.

97. Finn JP, Kane RA, Edelman RR, et al.: Imaging of the portal venous system in patients with cirrhosis: MR angiography vs. duplex Doppler sonography, *AJR* 1993;161:989-994.

98. Wilson SR, Hine AL: Leiomyosarcoma of the portal vein, *AJR* 1987;149:183-184.

99. Van Gansbeke D, Avni EF, Delcour C, et al.: Sonographic features of portal vein thrombosis, *AJR* 1985;144:749-752.

100. Kauzlaric D, Petrovic M, Barmeir E: Sonography of cavernous transformation of the portal vein, *AJR* 1984;142:383-384.

101. Aldrete JS, Slaughter RL, Han SY: Portal vein thrombosis resulting in portal hypertension in adults, *Am J Gastroenterol* 1976;65:3-11.

102. Dodd GD, Memel OS, Baron RL, et al.: Portal vein thrombosis in patients with cirrhosis. does sonographic detection of intrathrombus flow allow differentiation of benign and malignant thrombus? *AJR* 1995;165:573-577.

103. Stanley P: Budd-Chiari syndrome, *Radiology* 1989;170:625-627.

104. Makuuchi M, Hasegawa H, Yamazaki S, et al.: Primary Budd-Chiari syndrome: ultrasonic demonstration, *Radiology* 1984;152:775-779.

105. Menu Y, Alison D, Lorphelin J-M, et al.: Budd-Chiari syndrome: ultrasound evaluation, *Radiology* 1985;157:761-764.

106. Park JH, Lee JB, Han MC, et al.: Sonographic evaluation of inferior vena caval obstruction: correlative study with vena cavography, *AJR* 1985;145:757-762.

107. Murphy FB, Steinberg HV, Shires GT, et al.: The Budd-Chiari syndrome: a review, *AJR* 1986;147:9-15.

108. Grant EG, Perrella R, Tessler FN, et al.: Budd-Chiari syndrome: the results of duplex and color Doppler imaging, *AJR* 1989;152:377-381.

109. Keller MS, Taylor KJW, Riely CA: Pseudoportal Doppler signal in the partially obstructed inferior vena cava, *Radiology* 1989;170:475-477.

110. Hosoki T, Kuroda C, Tokunaga K, et al.: Hepatic venous outflow obstruction: evaluation with pulsed Duplex sonography, *Radiology* 1989;170:733-737.

111. Brown BP, Abu-Youssef M, Farner R, et al.: Doppler sonography: a non-invasive method for evaluation of hepatic venocclusive disease, *AJR* 1990;154:721-724.

112. Becker CD, Scheidegger J, Marincek B: Hepatic vein occlusion: morphologic features on computed tomography and ultrasonography, *Gastrointest Radiol* 1986;11:305-311.

113. Ralls PW, Johnson MB, Radin RD, et al.: Budd-Chiari Syndrome: detection with color Doppler sonography, *AJR* 1992;159:113-116.

114. Millener P, Grant EG, Rose S, et al.: Color Doppler imaging findings in patients with Budd-Chiari Syndrome: correlation with venographic findings, *AJR* 1993;161:307-312.

115. Taylor KJW, Burns PN, Woodcock JP, et al.: Blood flow in deep abdominal and pelvic vessels: ultrasonic pulsed Doppler analysis, *Radiology* 1985;154:487-493.

116. Kriegshauser SJ, Charboneau JW, Letendre L: Hepatic venocclusive disease after bone marrow transplantation: diagnosis with duplex sonography, *AJR* 1988;150:289-290.

117. Vine HS, Sequira JC, Widrich WC, Sacks BA: Portal vein aneurysm, *AJR* 1979;132:557-560.

118. Chagnon SF, Vallee CA, Barge J, et al.: Aneurysmal portahepatic venous fistula: report of two cases, *Radiology* 1986;159:693-695.

119. Mori H, Hayashi K, Fukuda T, et al.: Intrahepatic portosystemic venous shunt: occurrence in patients with and without liver cirrhosis, *AJR* 1987;149:711-714.

120. Park JH, Cha SH, Han JK, Han MC: Intrahepatic portosystemic venous shunt, *AJR* 1990;155:527-528.

121. Falkoff GE, Taylor KJW, Morse S: Hepatic artery pseudoaneurysm: diagnosis with real-time and pulsed Doppler ultrasound, *Radiology* 1986;158:55-56.

122. Garcia P, Garcia-Giannoli H, Meyron S, et al.: Primary dissecting aneurysm of the hepatic artery: sonographic, CT and angiographic findings, *AJR* 1996;166:1316-1318.

123. Cloogman HM, DiCapo RD: Hereditary hemorrhagic telangiectasia: Sonographic findings in the liver, *Radiology* 1984;150:521-522.

124. Wanless IR: Vascular disorders. In MacSween RNM, Anthony PP, Scheuer PJ, Burt AD, Portmann BC, editors: *Pathology of the Liver*, ed 3, Edinburgh; Churchill Livingstone; 1994;535.

125. Czapar CA, Weldon-Linne CM, Moore DM, Rhone DP: Peliosis hepatis in the acquired immunodeficiency syndrome, *Arch Pathol Lab Med* 1986;110:611.

126. Leong SS, Cazen RA, Yu GSM, et al.: Abdominal visceral peliosis associated with bacillary angiomatosis. Ultrasound evidence of endothelial destruction by bacilli, *Arch Pathol Lab Med* 1992;116:866.

127. Jamadar DA, D'Souza SP, Thomas EA, Giles TE: Radiological appearances in peliosis hepatis, *Br J Radiol* 1994;67:102.

128. Toyoda S, Takeda K, Nakagawa T, Matsuda A: Magnetic resonance imaging of peliosis hepatis: a case report, *Eur J Radiol* 1993;16:207.

129. Lloyd RL, Lyons EA, Levi CS, et al.: The sonographic appearance of peliosis hepatis, *J Ultrasound Med* 1982;1:293.

130. Tsukamoto Y, Nakata H, Kimoto T, et al.: CT and angiography of peliosis hepatis, *AJR* 1984;142:539.

131. Muradali D, Wilson SR, Wanless IR, et al.: Peliosis hepatis with intrahepatic calcifications, *J Ultrasound Med* 1996;16:257-260.

Benign Hepatic Neoplasms

132. Edmondson HA: Tumors of the liver and intrahepatic bile ducts. In *Atlas of Tumor Pathology*, Washington; Armed Forces Institute of Pathology; 1958;113.

133. Gibney RG, Hendin AP, Cooperberg PL: Sonographically detected hemangiomas: absence of change over time, *AJR* 1987;149:953-957.

134. Mungovan JA, Cranon JJ, Vacarro J: Hepatic cavernous hemangiomas: lack of enlargement over time, *Radiology* 1994;191:111-113.

135. Bree RL, Schwab RE, Neiman HL: Solitary echogenic spot in the liver: is it diagnostic of a hemangioma? *AJR* 1983;140:41-45.

136. McCardle CR.: Ultrasonic appearances of a hepatic hemangioma, *J Clin Ultrasound* 1978;6:122-123.

137. Taboury J, Porcel A, Tubiana J-M, Monnier J-P: Cavernous hemangiomas of the liver studied by ultrasound, *Radiology* 1983;149:781-785.

138. Itai Y, Ohnishi S, Ohtomo K, et al.: Hepatic cavernous hemangioma in patients at high risk for liver cancer, *Acta Radiol* 1987;28:697-701.

139. Itai Y, Ohtomo K, Araki T, et al.: Computed tomography and sonography of cavernous hemangioma of the liver, *AJR* 1983;141:315-320.

140. Moody AR, Wilson SR: Atypical hemangioma: a suggestive sonographic morphology. *Radiology* 1993;188:413-417.

141. Marsh JI, Gibney RG, Li DKB: Hepatic hemangioma in the presence of fatty infiltration: an atypical sonographic appearance, *Gastrointest Radiol* 1989;14:262-264.

142. Choi BI, Kim TK, Han JK, et al.: Power versus conventional color Doppler sonography: comparison in depiction of vasculature in liver tumors, *Radiology* 1996;200:55-58.

143. Porzio ME, Pellerito JS, D'Agostino CA, et al.: Improved characterization of hepatic hemangioma with color power angiography, In *RSNA Scientific Program 1995, Supplement to Radiology* 1995;197(P):401-402.

144. Freeny PC, Marks WM: Hepatic hemangioma: dynamic bolus computed tomography, *AJR* 1986;147:711-719.

145. Scatarige JC, Kenny JM, Fishman EK, et al.: Computed tomography of hepatic cavernous hemangioma, *J Comput Assist Tomogr* 1987;11:455-460.

146. Quinn SF, Benjamin GG: Hepatic cavernous hemangiomas: simple diagnostic sign with dynamic bolus CT, *Radiology* 1992;182:545-548.

147. Brunetti JC, Van Heertum RL, Yudd AP: SPECT in the diagnosis of hepatic hemangioma (Abstract), *J Nucl Med* 1985;26:8.

148. Birnbaum BA, Weinreb JC, Megibow AJ, et al.: Blinded retrospective comparison of MR imaging and Tc-99m-labeled red blood cell SPECT for definitive diagnosis of hepatic hemangiomas (abstract), *Radiology* 1989;173:270.

149. Birnbaum BA, Weinreb JC, Megibow AJ, et al.: Definitive diagnosis of hepatic hemangiomas: Magnetic resonance imaging versus Tc-99m-labeled red blood cell SPECT, *Radiology* 1990;176:95-101.

150. Ohmoto K, Itai Y, Yoshikawa K, et al.: Hepatocellular carcinoma and cavernous hemangioma: differentiation with MR imaging—efficacy of T2 values at 0.35 and 1.5 T, *Radiology* 1988;168:621-623.

151. McFarland EG, Mayo-Smith WW, Saini S, et al.: Hepatic hemangiomas and malignant tumors: improved differentiation with heavily T2-weighted conventional spin-echo MT images, *Radiology* 1994;193:43-47.

152. Semelka RC, Brown ED, Ascher SM, et al.: Hepatic hemangiomas: a multi-institutional study appearance on T2-weighted and serial gadolinium enhanced gradient echo MR images, *Radiology* 1994;192:401-406.

153. Solbiati L, Livraghi T, DePra L, et al.: Fine-needle biopsy of hepatic hemangioma with sonographic guidance, *AJR* 1985;144:471-474.

154. Cronan JJ, Esparza AR, Dorfman GS, et al.: Cavernous hemangioma of the liver: role of percutaneous biopsy, *Radiology* 1988;166:135-138.

155. Nelson RC, Chezmar JL: Diagnostic approach to hepatic hemangiomas, *Radiology* 1990;176:11-13.

156. Craig JR, Peters RL, Edmondson HA: Tumors of the liver and intrahepatic bile ducts. Fasc 26, 2nd ser, Washington, 1989, Armed Forces Institute of Pathology.

157. Wanless IR, Mawdsley C, Adams R: On the pathogenesis of focal nodular hyperplasia of the liver, *Hepatology* 1985;5:1194-1200.

158. Saul SH: Masses of the liver. In Sternberg SS, editor: *Diagnostic Surgical Pathology*, ed 2, New York; Raven; 1994;1517-1580.

159. Knowles DM, Casarella WJ, Johnson PM, et al.: The clinical, radiologic and pathologic characterization of benign hepatic neoplasms: alleged association with oral contraceptives, *Medicine* 1978;57:223-237.

160. Ross D, Pina J, Mirza M, et al.: Regression of focal nodular hyperplasia after discontinuation of oral contraceptives, *Ann Intern Med* 1976;85:203-204.

161. Buetow PC, Pantongrag-Brown L, Buck JL, et al.: Focal nodular hyperplasia of the liver: radiologic-pathologic correlation, *RadioGraphics* 1996;16:369-388.

162. Scatarige JC, Fishman EK, Sanders RC: The sonographic "scar sign" in focal nodular hyperplasia of the liver, *J Ultrasound Med* 1982;1:275-278.

163. Golli M, Van Nhieu JT, Mathieu D, et al.: Hepatocellular adenoma: Color Doppler US and pathologic correlations, *Radiology* 1994;190:741-744.

164. Drane WE, Krasicky GA, Johnson DA: Radionuclide imaging of primary liver tumors and tumor-like conditions of the liver, *Clin Nucl Med* 1987;12:569.

165. Welch TJ, Sheedy PF, Johnson CM, et al.: Focal nodular hyperplasia and hepatic adenoma: comparison of angiography, CT, US and scintigraphy, *Radiology* 1985;156:593.

166. Mahfouz A, Hamm B, Taupitz M, Wolf K-J: Hypervascular liver lesions: differentiation of focal nodular hyperplasia from malignant tumors with dynamic gadolinium-enhanced MR imaging, *Radiology* 1993;186:133-138.

167. Vilgrain V, Flejou J, Arrive L, et al.: Focal nodular hyperplasia of the liver. MR imaging and pathologic correlation in 37 patients, *Radiology* 1992;184:699-703.

168. Kerlin P, Davis GL, McGill DB, et al.: Hepatic adenoma and focal nodular hyperplasia: clinical, pathologic and radiologic features, *Gastroenterology* 1983;84:994-1002.

169. Brunelle R, Tammam S, Odievre M, Chaumont P: Liver adenomas in glycogen storage disease in children: ultrasound and angiographic study, *Pediatr Radiol* 1984;14:94-101.

170. Kew MC: Tumors of the liver. In Zakim D, Boyer TD, editors: *Hepatology: A Textbook of Liver Disease*, Philadelphia; WB Saunders; 1982;1048-1084.

171. Lubbers PR, Ros PR, Goodman ZD, et al.: Accumulation of Technetium-99m sulfur colloid by hepatocellular adenoma: scintigraphic-pathologic correlation, *AJR* 1987;148:1105-1108.

172. Katsuyoshi I, Kazumitsu H, Fujita T, et al.: Liver neoplasms: diagnostic pitfalls in cross sectional imaging, *RadioGraphics* 1996;16:273-293.

173. Pawson EK, McClellan JS, Washington K, et al.: Hepatic adenoma: MR characteristics and correlation with pathologic findings, *AJR* 1994;163:113-116.

174. Arrive L, Flejou JF, Vilgrain V, et al.: Hepatic adenoma: MR findings in 51 pathologically proved lesions, *Radiology* 1994;193:507-512.

175. Roberts JL, Fishman E, Hartman DS, et al.: Lipomatous tumors of the liver: evaluation with computed tomography and ultrasound, *Radiology* 1986;158:613-617.

176. Marti-Bonmati L, Menor F, Vizcaino I, et al.: Lipoma of the liver: ultrasound, computed tomography and magnetic resonance imaging appearance, *Gastrointest Radiol* 1989;14:155-157.

177. Reinhold C, Garant M: Hepatic lipoma. *C Assoc Radiol J* 1996;47:140-142.

Malignant Hepatic Neoplasms

178. Jackson VP, Martin-Simmerman P, Becker GJ, et al.: Real-time ultrasonographic demonstration of vascular invasion by hepatocellular carcinoma, *J Ultrasound Med* 1983;2:277-280.

179. Subramanyam BR, Balthazar EJ, Hilton S, et al.: Hepatocellular carcinoma with venous invasion: sonographic-angiographic correlation, *Radiology* 1984;150:793-796.

180. LaBerge JM, Laing FC, Federle MP, et al.: Hepatocellular carcinoma: assessment of resectability by computed tomography and ultrasound, *Radiology* 1984;152:485-490.

181. Sheu J-C, Chen D-S, Sung J-L, et al.: Hepatocellular carcinoma: ultrasound evaluation in the early stage, *Radiology* 1985;155:463-467.

182. Tanaka S, Kitamura T, Imaoka S, et al.: Hepatocellular carcinoma: sonographic and histologic correlation, *AJR* 1983;140:701-707.

183. Choi BI, Takayasu K, Han MC: Small hepatocellular carcinomas associated nodular lesions of the liver: pathology, pathogenesis and imaging findings, *AJR* 1993;160:1177-1188.

184. Teefey SA, Stephens DH, Weiland LH: Calcification in hepatocellular carcinoma: not always an indicator of fibrolamellar histology, *AJR* 1987;149:1173-1174.

185. Yoshikawa J, Matsui O, Takashima T, et al.: Fatty metamorphosis in hepatocellular carcinoma: radiologic features in 10 cases, *AJR* 1988;151:717-720.

186. Taylor KJW, Ramos I, Morse SS, et al.: Focal liver masses: differential diagnosis with pulsed Doppler ultrasound, *Radiology* 1987;164:643-647.

187. Tanaka S, Kitamura T, Fujita M, et al.: Color Doppler flow imaging of liver tumors, *AJR* 1990;154:509-514.

188. Reinhold C, Hammers L, Taylor CR, et al.: Characterization of focal hepatic lesions with Duplex sonography: findings in 198 patients, *AJR* 1995;164:1131-1135.

189. Baron RL, Oliver III JH, Dodd III, et al.: Hepatocellular carcinoma: evaluation with biphasic, contrast-enhanced, helical CT, *Radiology* 1996;199:505-511.

190. Johnson CD: Imaging of hepatocellular carcinoma. In Freeny PC, editor: *Radiology of the Liver, Biliary Tract and Pancreas*, San Diego; ARRS Categorical Course Syllabus 1996 96th Annual Meeting; 41-46.

191. Kadoya M, Matsui O, Takashima T, Nonomura A: Hepatocellular carcinoma: correlation of MR imaging and histopathologic findings, *Radiology* 1992;183:819-825.

192. Ebara M, Watanabe S, Kita K, et al.: MR imaging of small hepatocellular carcinoma: effect of intratumoral copper content on signal intensity, *Radiology* 1991;180:617-621.

193. Kitagawa K, Matsui O, Kadoya M, et al.: Hepatocellular carcinomas with excessive copper accumulation: CT and MR findings, *Radiology* 1991;180:623-628.

194. Winter III TC, Takayasu K, Muramatsu Y, et al.: Early advanced hepatocellular carcinoma: evaluation of CT and MR appearance with pathologic correlation, *Radiology* 1994;192:379-387.

195. Friedman AC, Lichtenstein JE, Goodman Z, et al.: Fibrolamellar hepatocellular carcinoma, *Radiology* 1985;157:583-587.

196. Brandt DJ, Johnson CD, Stephens DH, et al.: Imaging of fibrolamellar hepatocellular carcinoma, *AJR* 1988;151:295-299.

197. Stevens WR, Johnson CD, Stephens DH, Nagorney DM: Fibrolamellar hepatocellular carcinoma: stage at presentation and results of aggressive surgical management, *AJR* 1995;164:1153-1158.

198. Kanai T, Hirohashi S, Upton MP, et al.: Pathology of small hepatocellular carcinoma: a proposal for new gross classification, *Cancer* 1987;60:810-819.

199. Okuda K, Musha H, Nakajuma Y, et al.: Clinicopathologic features of encapsulated hepatocellular carcinoma: a study of 26 cases, *Cancer* 1977;40:1240-1245.

200. Mahony B, Jeffrey RB, Federle MP: Spontaneous rupture of hepatic and splenic angiosarcoma demonstrated by computed tomography, *AJR* 1982;138:965-966.

201. Fitzgerald EJ, Griffiths TM: Computed tomography of vinyl-chloride-induced angiosarcoma of liver, *Br J Radiol* 1987;60:593-595.

202. Furui S, Itai Y, Ohtomo D, et al.: Hepatic epithelioid hemangioendothelioma: report of five cases, *Radiology* 1989;171:63-68.

203. Radin R, Craig JR, Colletti PM, et al.: Hepatic epithelioid hemangioendothelioma, *Radiology* 1988;169:145-148.

204. Oliver III JH: Malignant hepatic neoplasms, excluding hepatocellular carcinoma and cholangiocarcinoma. In Freeny PC, editor: *Radiology of the Liver, Biliary Tract and Pancreas*, San Diego; ARRS Categorical Course Syllabus; 1996;27-32.

205. Kane RA, Longmaid HE, Costello P, Finn JP, Roizental M: Noninvasive imaging in patients with hepatic masses: A prospective comparison of ultrasound, CT and MR Imaging (abstract). RSNA Scientific Program 1993.

206. Misquitta A, Wanless IR, Wilson SR: The liver lesion with a hypoechoic halo on ultrasound. Submitted to JUIM.

207. Marchal GJ, Pylyser K, Tshibwabwa-Tumba EA: Anechoic halo in solid liver tumors: sonographic, microangiographic, and histologic correlation, *Radiology* 1985;156:479-483.

208. Rubaltelli L, Del Mashio A, Candiani F, et al.: The role of vascularization in the formation of echographic patterns of hepatic metastases: microangiographic and echographic study, *Br J Radiol* 1980;53:1166-1168.

209. Sanders LM, Botet JF, Straus DJ, et al.: Computed tomography of primary lymphoma of the liver, *AJR* 1989;152:973-976.

210. Townsend RR, Laing FC, Jeffrey RB, et al.: Abdominal lymphoma in AIDS: evaluation with ultrasound, *Radiology* 1989;171:719-724.

211. Yoshida T, Matsue H, Okazaki N, et al.: Ultrasonographic differentiation of hepatocellular carcinoma from metastatic liver cancer, *J Clin Ultrasound* 1987;15:431-437.

212. Bruneton JN, Ladree D, Caramella E, et al.: Ultrasonographic study of calcified hepatic metastases: a report of 13 cases, *Gastrointest Radiol* 1982;7:61-63.

213. Wooten WB, Green B, Goldstein HM: Ultrasonography of necrotic hepatic metastases, *Radiology* 1978;128:447-450.

214. Federle MP, Filly RA, Moss AA: Cystic hepatic neoplasms: complementary roles of computed tomography and sonography, *AJR* 1981;345-348.

215. Nyberg DA, Federle MP.: AIDS-related Kaposi sarcoma and lymphomas, *Sem Roentgenol* 1987;22(1):54-65.

216. Luburich P, Bru C, Ayuso MC, et al.: Hepatic Kaposi sarcoma in AIDS: ultrasound and computed tomography findings, *Radiology* 1990;175:172-174.

217. Towers MJ, Withers CE, Rachlis AR, et al.: Ultrasound diagnosis of hepatic Kaposi sarcoma, *J Ultrasound Med* 1991;10:701.

Hepatic Trauma

218. Anderson CB, Ballinger WF: Abdominal injuries. In Zuidema GD, Rutherford RB, Ballinger WF, editor. *The Management of Trauma*, ed 4, Philadelphia; WB Saunders;1985;449-504.

219. Moon KL, Federle MP: Computed tomography in hepatic trauma, *AJR* 1983;141:309-314.

220. Foley WD, Cates JD, Kellman GM, et al.: Treatment of blunt hepatic injuries: role of computed tomography, *Radiology* 1987;164:635-638.

221. vanSonnenberg E, Simeone JF, Mueller PR, et al.: Sonographic appearance of hematoma in the liver, spleen, and kidney: a clinical, pathologic, and animal study, *Radiology* 1983;147:507-510.

Hepatic Surgery

222. Tzakis AG, Gordon RD, Makowka L, et al.: Clinical considerations in orthotopic liver transplantation, *Radiol Clin North Am* 1987;25(2):289-297.

223. Starzl TE, Iwatsuki S, Shaw BW Jr: Transplantation of the human liver. In Swarts SI, editor: *Maingot's Abdominal Operations*, ed 8, Connecticut; Appleton-Century-Crofts; 1985;1687-1722.

224. Longley DG, Skolnick ML, Sheahan DG: Acute allograft rejection in liver transplant recipients: lack of correlation with loss of hepatic artery diastolic flow, *Radiology* 1988;169:417-420.

225. Marder DM, DeMarino GB, Sumkin JH, Sheahan DG: Liver transplant rejection: value of the resistive index in Doppler US of hepatic arteries, *Radiology* 1989;173:127-129.

226. Tzakis AG, Gordon RD, Shaw BW Jr, et al.: Clinical presentation of hepatic artery thrombosis after liver transplantation in the cyclosporine era, *Transplantation* 1986;40:667-671.

227. Lerut J, Gordon RD, Iwatsuki S, et al.: Biliary tract complications in human orthotopic liver transplantation, *Transplantation* 1987;43:47-51.

228. Campbell WL, Sheng R, Zajko AB, et al.: Intrahepatic biliary strictures after liver transplantation, *Radiology* 1994;191:735-740.

229. Sheng R, Zajko AB, Campbell WL, Abu-Elmagd K: Biliary strictures in hapatic transplants: prevalence and types in patients with primary sclerosing cholangitis vs. those with other liver diseases, *AJR* 1993;161:297-300.

230. Honda H, Franken Jr EA, Barloon TJ, et al.: Hepatic lymphoma in cyclosporine-treated transplant recipients: sonographic and computed tomography findings, *AJR* 1989;152:501-503.

231. Letourneau JG, Day DL, Ascher NL, et al.: Abdominal sonography after hepatic transplantation, *AJR* 1987;149:229-303.

232. Moody AR, Wilson SR, Greig PD: Non-Hodgkin lymphoma in the porta hepatis after orthotopic liver transplantation: sonographic findings, *Radiology* 1992;182:867-870.

233. Nghiem HV, Tran K, Winter III TC, et al.: Imaging of complications in liver transplantation, *RadioGraphics* 1996;16:825-840.

234. Dodd III GD, Memel DS, Zajko AB, et al.: Hepatic artery stenosis and thrombosis in transplant recipients: Doppler diagnosis with resistive index and systolic acceleration time, *Radiology* 1994;192:657-661.

235. Lafortune M, Patriquin H, Pomier G, et al.: Hemodynamic changes in portal circulation after portosystemic shunts: use of duplex sonography in 43 patients, *AJR* 1987;149:701-706.

236. Chezmar JL, Bernardino ME: Mesoatrial shunt for the treatment of Budd-Chiari syndrome: radiologic evaluation in eight patients, *AJR* 1987;149:707-710.

237. Grant EG, Tessler FN, Gomes AS et al.: Color Doppler imaging of portosystemic shunts, *AJR* 1990;154:393-397.

238. Ralls PW, Lee KP, Mayekawa DS, et al.: Color Doppler sonography of portocaval shunts, *J Clin Ultrasound* 1990;18:379-381.

239. Foley WD, Gleysteen JJ, Lawson TL, et al.: Dynamic computed tomography and pulsed Doppler sonography in the evaluation of splenorenal shunt patency, *J Comput Assist Tomogr* 1983;7:106-112.

240. Freedman AM, Sanyal AJ, Tisnado J, et al.: Complications of transjugular intrahepatic portosystemic shunt: a comprehensive review, *RadioGraphics* 1993;13:1185-1210.

241. Kerlan RK Jr, LaBerge JM, Gordon RL, Ring EJ: Transjugular intrahepatic portosystemic shunts: current status, *AJR* 1995;164:1059-1066.

242. LaBerge JM, Ring EJ, Gordon RL, et al.: Creation of transjugular intrahepatic portosystemic shunts with the Wallstent endoprosthesis: results in 100 patients, *Radiology* 1993;187:413-420.

243. Haskal ZJ, Pentecost MJ, Soulen MC, et al: Transjugular intrahepatic portosystemic shunt stenosis and revision, *AJR* 1994;163:439-444.

244. Foshager MC, Ferral H, Nazarian GK, et al.: Duplex sonography after transjugular intrahepatic portosystemic shunts (TIPS): normal hemodynamic findings and efficacy in predicting shunt patency and stenosis, *AJR* 1995;165:1-7.

245. Chong WK, Malisch TA, Mazar MJ, et al.: Transjugular intrahepatic portosystemic shunts: US assessment with maximum flow velocity, *Radiology* 1993;189:789-793.

246. Dodd GD III, Zajko AB, Orons PD, et al.: Detection of transjugular intrahepatic portosystemic shunt dysfunction: value of duplex Doppler sonography, *AJR* 1995;164:1119-1124.

247. Feldstein VA, LaBerge JM: Hepatic vein flow reversal at duplex sonography: a sign of transjugular intrahepatic portosystemic shunt dysfunction, *AJR* 1994;162:839-841.

Percutaneous Liver Biopsy

248. Charboneau JW, Reading CC, Welch TJ: CT and sonographically guided needle biopsy: current techniques and new innovations, *AJR* 1990;154:1-10.

249. Downey DB, Wilson SR: Ultrasonographically guided biopsy of small intra-abdominal masses, *Can Assoc Radiol J* 1993;44:350-353.

250. Livragi T, Festi D, Monti F, et al.: US-guided percutaneous alcohol injection of small hepatic and abdominal tumors, *Radiology* 1986;161:309-312.

251. Shiina S, Yasuda H, Muto H, et al.: Percutaneous ethanol injection in the treatment of liver neoplasms, *AJR* 1987;149:949-952.

Intraoperative Ultrasound

252. Rifkin MD, Rosato FE, Mitchell Branch H, et al.: Intraoperative ultrasound of the liver: an important adjunctive tool for decision making in the operating room, *Ann Surg* 1987;205:466-471.

253. Parker GA, Lawrence Jr J, Horsley JS, et al.: Intraoperative ultrasound of the liver affects operative decision making, *Ann Surg* 1989;209:569-577.

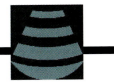

CHAPTER 5

The Spleen
•
John R. Mathieson, M.D., F.R.C.P.C.
Peter L. Cooperberg, M.D., F.R.C.P.C.

In patients with palpable splenomegaly or left upper quadrant trauma, sectional imaging techniques are indispensable to diagnose or rule out splenic abnormalities. Although in many centers computed tomography is the technique of choice for evaluation of the spleen and surrounding structures, ultrasound can be particularly useful in the first stage of the investigation and also in the follow-up of suspected or confirmed abnormalities. Particularly through the use of the real-time sector format, the spleen and other structures in the left upper quadrant can easily be ex-

amined without the patient's having to be moved. If necessary, examination can even be carried out using a portable ultrasound machine.

Because the normal spleen is uniform in echogenicity, abnormalities stand out clearly. Similarly, perisplenic fluid collections and other abnormalities are usually identified easily. Inadequate sonographic assessment of the spleen and surrounding structures is rare. Occasionally, because the spleen is located high in the left upper quadrant, difficulties can be encountered. Shadowing from ribs, overlying bowel gas, and overlying lung in the costophrenic angle can obscure visualization of the deeper structures. Expertise and persistence may be required to overcome these obstacles.

EMBRYOLOGY AND ANATOMY

Embryologically, the spleen arises from a mass of mesenchymal cells located between the layers of the dorsal mesentery, which connects the stomach to the posterior peritoneal surface over the aorta (Fig. 5-1, *A*). These mesenchymal cells differentiate to form the splenic pulp, the supporting connective tissue structures, and the capsule of the spleen. The splenic artery penetrates the primitive spleen and arterioles branch through the connective tissue into the splenic sinusoids.

As the embryonic stomach rotates 90° on its longitudinal axis, the spleen and dorsal mesentery are carried to the left along with the greater curvature of the stomach (Fig. 5-1, *B*). The base of the dorsal mesentery fuses with the posterior peritoneum over the left kidney, giving rise to the splenorenal ligament. This explains why, although the spleen is intraperitoneal, the splenic artery enters from the retroperitoneum via the splenorenal ligament (Fig. 5-1, *C*). In most adults, a portion of the splenic capsule is firmly adherent to the fused dorsal mesentery anterior to the upper left kidney, giving rise to the so-called bare area of the spleen. The size of the splenic bare area is variable, but it usually involves less than half of the posterior splenic surface (Fig. 5-2). This anatomic feature is analogous to the bare area of the liver and, similarly, can be helpful in distinguishing intraperitoneal from pleural fluid collections.[1]

The normal adult spleen is convex superolaterally, concave inferomedially, and has a very homogeneous echo pattern. The spleen lies between the fundus of the stomach and the diaphragm, with its long axis in the line of the left tenth rib. The diaphragmatic surface is convex and is usually situated between the ninth and eleventh ribs. The visceral or inferomedial surface has gentle indentations where it comes into contact with the stomach, left kidney, pancreas, and splenic flexure. The spleen is suspended by the splenorenal ligament, which is in contact with the posterior peritoneal wall and left phrenicocolic ligament, and by the gastrosplenic ligament. The gastrosplenic ligament is composed of the two layers of the dorsal mesentery, which separate the lesser sac posteriorly from the greater sac anteriorly.

The average adult spleen measures 12 cm in length, 7 cm in breadth, and 3 to 4 cm in thickness and has an average weight of 150 g, varying between 80 and 300 g. A normal spleen decreases in size and weight with advancing age. It also increases slightly during digestion and can vary in size in accordance with the nutritional status of the body.

Splenic functions include phagocytosis, fetal hematopoiesis, adult lymphopoiesis, immune response, and erythrocyte storage. Under a variety of conditions, including surgical misadventure, the spleen may be removed. It is common for a person to live successfully without a spleen. However, particularly in childhood, the immune response may be impaired, particularly to encapsulated bacteria. Recently, the surgical trend is toward splenic preservation wherever possible.

EXAMINATION TECHNIQUE

All routine abdominal sonographic examinations, regardless of the indications, should include at least one coronal view of the spleen and the upper pole of the left kidney. This view is easy to obtain with real-time scanning, particularly by using the sector format. The most common approach to visualizing the spleen is to maintain the patient in the supine position and place the transducer in the coronal plane of section posteriorly in one of the lower left intercostal spaces. The patient can then be examined in various degrees of inspiration to maximize the window to the spleen. Excessive inspiration introduces air into the lung in the lateral costophrenic angle and may obscure visualization. A modest inspiration depresses the central portion of the left hemidiaphragm and spleen inferiorly so that they can be visualized (Fig. 5-3). The plane of section should then be swept posteriorly and anteriorly to view the entire volume of the spleen. We generally find that a thorough examination in the coronal plane of section is highly accurate for ruling out any lesion within or around the spleen and for documenting approximate splenic size. If an abnormality is discovered within or around the spleen, other planes of section can be used. An oblique plane of section along the intercostal space can avoid rib shadowing (Fig. 5-4). Because the long axis of the spleen lies obliquely, this oblique plane of section is also convenient with the upper pole located posterior to the lower pole. A transverse plane from a lateral, usually intercostal approach may help to localize a lesion within the spleen anteriorly and posteriorly. In this regard, especially for beginners, it must be emphasized that the apex of the sector image is always placed at the top of the screen. However, on a left lateral intercostal transverse image, the top of the screen (the apex of the sector) is actually to the patient's left, the right side of the sector image is posterior, and the left side of the image is anterior. To look at the image appropriately, one would have to rotate it 90° in a clockwise direction or turn one's head in a 90° counterclockwise direction.

If the spleen is not enlarged and is not surrounded by a large mass, scanning from an anterior position (as one would for imaging the liver) is not helpful because of the interposition of gas within the stomach and the splenic flexure of the colon.[2] However, if the patient has a relatively large liver, one may be able to see the spleen through the left lobe of the liver and the collapsed stomach, analogous to the image seen on the transverse CT scan of the upper abdomen. Also, if the spleen is enlarged or if there is a mass in the left upper quadrant, the spleen may be visualized from an anterior approach (Fig. 5-5 on page 161). If there is free intraperitoneal fluid around the spleen or if there is a left pleural effusion, the spleen may be even better visualized from an anterolateral approach.

Often, it is beneficial to have the patient roll onto his or her right side as much as 45° or even 90° so that

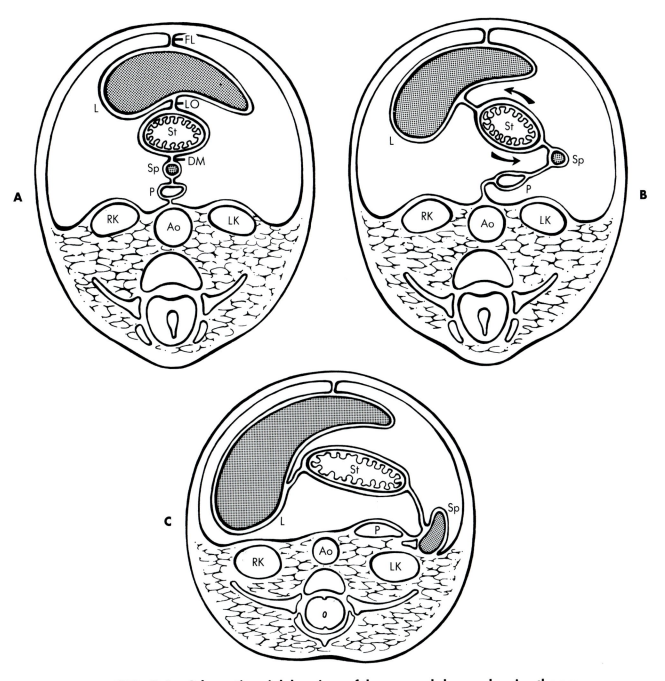

FIG. 5-1. Schematic axial drawings of the upper abdomen showing the embryologic development of splenic anatomy. **A,** Embryo of 4 to 5 weeks. The mesentery anterior to the stomach (ST) is the ventral mesentery. Posterior to the stomach is the dorsal mesentery (DM). Note the spleen and pancreas developing within the dorsal mesentery. The dorsal mesentery is divided into two portions by the spleen: the splenogastric ligament anteriorly and the splenorenal ligament posteriorly. The pancreas (P) has not yet become retroperitoneal and remains within the dorsal mesentery. The ventral mesentery is divided into the falciform ligament (FL) anteriorly and the gastrohepatic ligament, or lesser omentum (LO), posteriorly by the liver (L). **B,** 8-week embryo. The stomach rotates counterclockwise, displacing the liver to the right and the spleen to the left. The portion of the dorsal mesentery containing the pancreas, the splenic vessels, and the spleen begins to fuse to the anterior retroperitoneal surface, giving rise to the splenogastric ligament and the "bare area" of the spleen. If fusion is incomplete, the spleen will be attached to the retroperitoneum only by a long mesentery, giving rise to a mobile or "wandering" spleen. **C,** Newborn baby. Fusion of the dorsal mesentery is now complete. The pancreas is now completely retroperitoneal, and a portion of the spleen has fused with the retroperitoneum. Note the close relation of the tail of the pancreas to the splenic hilum. L, liver. ST, stomach. SP, spleen. P, pancreas. FL, falciform ligament. LO, lesser omentum, or gastrohepatic ligament. LK, left kidney. RK, right kidney. Ao, aorta.

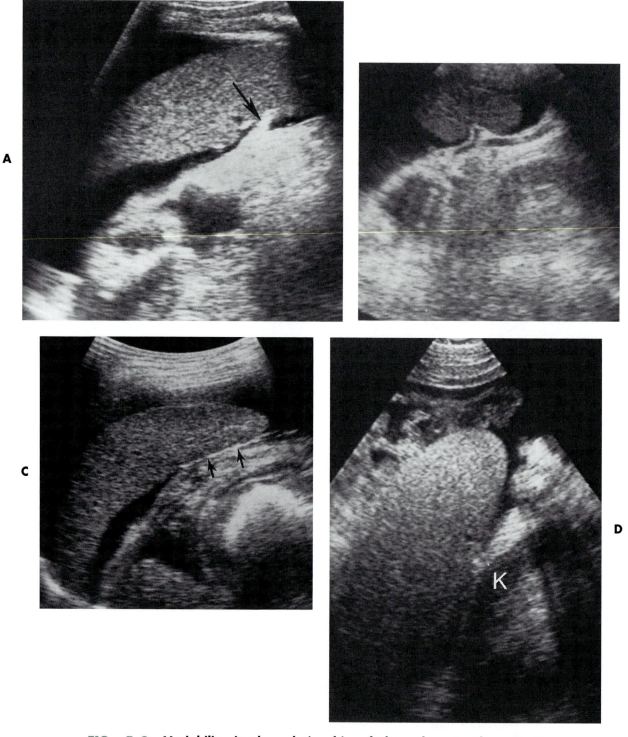

FIG. 5-2. Variability in the relationship of the spleen to the anterior retroperitoneal surface. All of these patients have gross ascites, which clearly demonstrates the extent of the splenic "bare area." **A,** This patient has no bare area. The splenorenal ligament is outlined on both sides by ascitic fluid. **B,** Part of the lower pole of the spleen is fused posteriorly. **C,** The lower pole of the spleen is fused to the retroperitoneum. **D,** A large proportion of this patient's spleen is fused posteriorly. Note the close relationship of the spleen to the left kidney.

a more posterior approach can be used to visualize the spleen. We no longer use the prone position.

Generally, the same technical settings for gain, time-gain compensation, and power are used for examination of the spleen as for examination of the other organs in the upper abdomen. Because the spleen is a superficial structure and there is generally

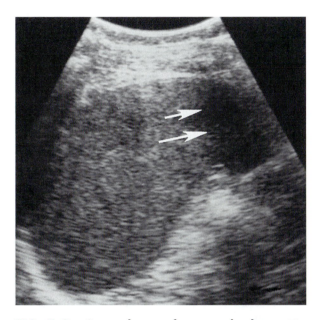

FIG. 5-3. **Coronal scan of a normal spleen.** The lower pole is partially obscured by a rib shadow *(arrows)*. Note the homogeneous echo texture.

little absorption of sound within it, a 5-MHz internally focused transducer of medium length is recommended. Although mechanical sector scanners, with or without annular array focusing, or phased array sector scanners can be used, we usually use curvilinear transducers now. There is a slight disadvantage in intercostal scanning with the larger transducer face, but the image quality is significantly improved with these transducers. It is important to appreciate that the ribs can often be broader and flatter than expected and may encroach on the intercostal spaces, making them particularly narrow. This can severely impair the quality of the image seen from an intercostal space.

SONOGRAPHY OF THE SPLEEN

The shape of the normal spleen is variable. The spleen consists of two components joined at the hilum: a superomedial component and an inferolateral component. More superiorly, on transverse scanning, the spleen has a typical fat "inverted comma" shape with a thin component extending anteriorly and another component extending medially, either superior to or adjacent to the upper pole of the kidney. This is the component that can be seen to indent the gastric fundus on plain films of the abdomen or in barium studies. As one moves the scan plane inferiorly, only the inferior component of the spleen is seen. This is the component that can be seen to be outlined by a thin

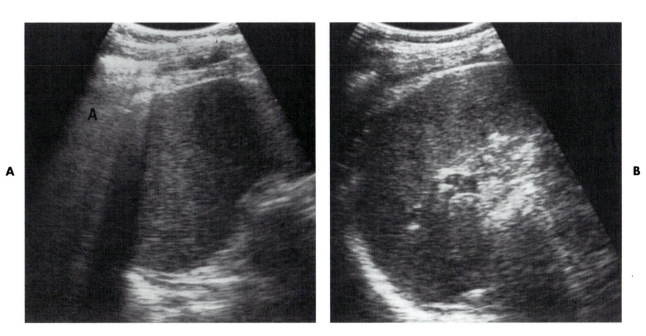

FIG. 5-4. **Importance of scan plane.** **A,** Coronal scan showing partial obscuration of the spleen by air in the lung (A) and by a rib shadow. **B,** Oblique coronal scan, aligned with the 10th interspace, shows improved visualization of the spleen.

rim of fat above the splenic flexure on a plain film of the abdomen. It may extend inferiorly to the costal margin and present clinically as a palpable spleen. However, either component can enlarge independently without the enlargement of the other component.

It is important to recognize the normal structures that are anatomically related to the spleen. The diaphragm cradles the spleen posteriorly, superiorly, and laterally. The normal liver usually does not touch the spleen. If the left lobe is enlarged, it may extend into the left upper quadrant anterior to the spleen. The fundus of the stomach and lesser sac are medial and anterior to the splenic hilum. It is important to appreciate that the fundus may contain gas or fluid. The tail of the pancreas lies posterior to the stomach and lesser sac and also approaches the hilum of the spleen, in close relation to the splenic artery and vein. The left kidney generally lies inferior and medial to the spleen. A useful landmark in identifying the spleen and splenic hilum is the splenic vein, which generally can be demonstrated, especially in splenic enlargement.

The splenic parenchyma is extremely homogeneous and therefore the spleen has a uniform mid- to low-level echogenicity. It is generally considered that the liver is more echogenic than the spleen but, in fact, the echogenicity of the parenchyma is higher in the spleen than in the liver. It is difficult to compare directly the echogenicity of these two organs. The impression that the liver has greater echogenicity occurs because of its large number of reflective vessels. When the spleen enlarges, it can become more echogenic. Unfortunately, one cannot differentiate between the different types of enlargement on the basis of the degree of echogenicity.

PATHOLOGIC CONDITIONS OF THE SPLEEN

Splenomegaly

Frequently, sonography is performed to determine the presence or absence of splenomegaly. If there is gross enlargement of the spleen, confirmation of splenomegaly is easy. However, if there is only mild enlargement, it can be difficult to make the decision based on a sonographic study. Techniques have been developed to measure serial sections of the spleen by planimetry and then compute the volume of the spleen by adding the values for each section.[3] However, these techniques are cumbersome and not popular. The most commonly used method is the "eyeball" technique: if it looks big, it is (Figs. 5-5 and 5-6). Unfortunately, this method of assessment requires considerably more experience than is necessary for other imaging techniques. Furthermore, it is relatively inaccurate. As in measuring all other structures in the

body, it is helpful to have measurements that establish the upper limits of normal. The wide range of what is considered to be a normal-sized adult spleen, combined with its complex three-dimensional shape, makes it particularly difficult to establish a normal range of sonographic measurements. Nonetheless, a study of almost 800 normal adults found that in 95% of patients, the length of the spleen was less than 12 cm, the breadth less than 7 cm, and the thickness less than 5 cm.[4] These measurements may be useful for borderline cases.

The spleen is capable of growing to an enormous size. It may extend inferiorly into the left iliac fossa. It can cross the midline and present as a mass inferior to the left lobe of the liver on longitudinal section.

The differential diagnosis of splenomegaly is exceedingly long. It includes infection, neoplasia, infiltration, trauma, blood dyscrasias, storage disorders, and portal hypertension. Sonography is not usually helpful in the specific diagnosis of splenomegaly. However, the degree of splenomegaly can help to narrow the differential diagnosis. Mild to moderate splenomegaly is usually caused by **infection, portal hypertension**, or **AIDS**. More marked splenomegaly is usually the result of hematologic disorders, including **leukemia** and **lymphoma** as well as **infectious mononucleosis**. Massive splenomegaly can be seen in **myelofibrosis**. In addition, focal lesions within the spleen may suggest **lymphomatous involvement, metastatic disease, cysts**, or **hematomas**. Nonsplenic abnormalities such as lymph node enlargement or liver involvement may suggest lymphoma, whereas recanalization of the umbilical vein or other evidence of portal systemic collaterals, such as lienorenal shunts, splenic vein varices, or ascites, can establish **portal hypertension** as the cause of splenomegaly (Fig. 5-7). However, in most cases, splenomegaly may be the sole finding or only one of several nonspecific sonographic findings.

Several investigators have attempted to quantify the degree of diffuse splenic fibrosis or tumor infiltration by analyzing various parameters of the reflected ultrasound signal. Speed and attenuation measurements have been studied, but to date, such parameters are not regarded as clinically useful.[5-7]

CAUSES OF MILD TO MODERATE SPLENOMEGAL

Portal Hypertension
Infection
AIDS

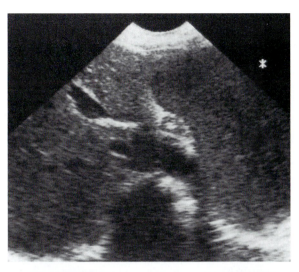

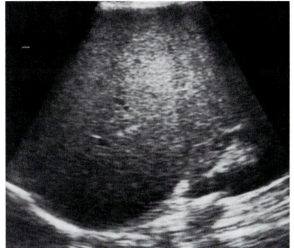

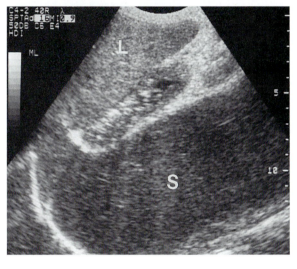

FIG. 5-5. Splenomegaly. A, Transverse scan in the upper abdomen showing the liver apparently continuous with the large spleen across the inferior aspect of the abdomen. **B,** Coronal scan showing only the midportion of the spleen, with the superior and inferior aspects beyond the sector format. **C,** Sagittal scan through the left lobe of the liver (L), with the markedly enlarged spleen (S) posterior to the stomach and liver. This is another way that the enlarged spleen may appear sonographically.

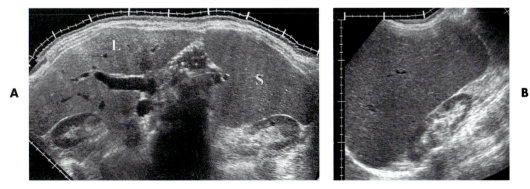

FIG. 5-6. Splenomegaly. A, Transverse and **B,** longitudinal Siescape® images show marked splenic (S) enlargement. L, liver.

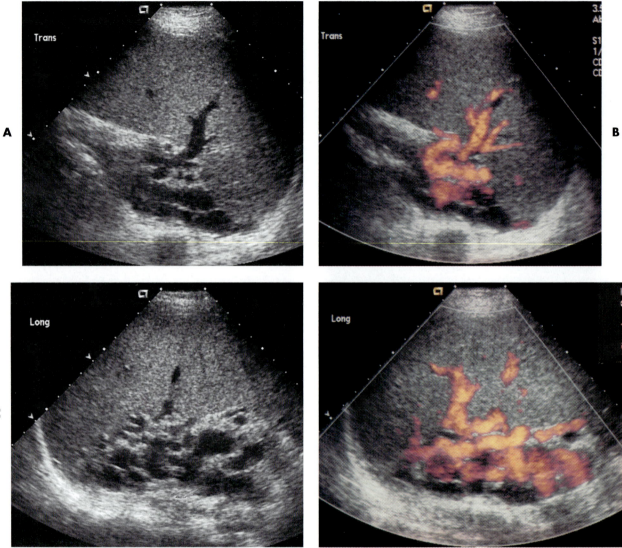

FIG. 5-7. Varices. **A** and **B**, transverse, and **C** and **D**, longitudinal power Doppler images show splenomegaly and tortuous varices medial to the spleen.

CAUSES OF MARKED SPLENOMEGALY

Leukemia
Lymphoma
Myelofibrosis

Focal Abnormalities

Cysts. Like cysts located elsewhere in the body, splenic cysts characteristically appear as echo-free areas with smooth, sharp borders and enhancement of the echoes deep into the lesions. When small, they may be located within the splenic parenchyma.

Occasionally, these cysts can grow very large and become mainly exophytic. It may then be difficult to appreciate their intrasplenic origin (Fig. 5-8).

Infectious cysts are usually caused by **echinococcus**. However, the spleen is one of the least common sites for the development of hydatid cysts. Calcification may be identified in the wall of the cyst (Fig. 5-9). The diagnosis is made with a combination of appropriate history, geographic background, serologic testing, and ultrasound appearance.[8,9] Percutaneous fine-needle aspiration can be diagnostic, provided the pathologist has been alerted to search for the scolices.

Posttraumatic cysts have no cellular lining and are also called **pseudocysts**.[10] The walls of these

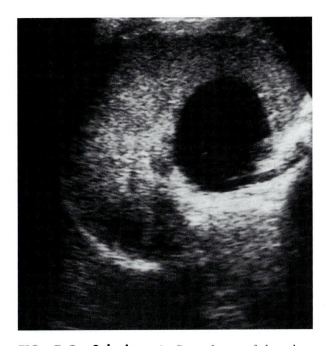

FIG. 5-8. **Splenic cyst.** Coronal scan of the spleen showing a 5-cm-diameter cyst in the hilar region of the spleen adjacent to the splenic vein. This patient had suffered trauma to the left upper quadrant several years earlier.

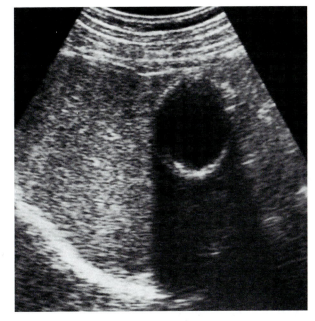

FIG. 5-9. **Calcified splenic cyst.** Note the shadowing from the near side of the splenic cyst. The calcification is incomplete in the near wall, so echoes from the deep wall can be seen through the shadow. Both "burned out" hydatid cysts and posttraumatic cysts can look like this.

CATEGORIES OF CYSTIC LESIONS OF THE SPLEEN

Infectious cysts
Posttraumatic cysts
Primary congenital cysts
Intrasplenic pancreatic pseudocysts

---

cysts, like echinococcal cysts, may become calcified. These cysts may contain low-level echoes that can be cholesterol crystals or debris.[11] Hemorrhage into any cyst also can give rise to echogenic fluid (Fig. 5-10).[12]

Primary congenital cysts, also called **epidermoid cysts,** can be differentiated from posttraumatic cysts by the presence within them of an epithelial or endothelial lining. Congenital cysts are thought to arise from embryonal rests of primitive mesothelial cells within the spleen. Endothelial-lined cysts are rare; they include lymphangiomas and, very rarely, cystic hemangiomas.[13]

Pancreatic pseudocysts extending into the spleen can be diagnosed by the associated features of pancreatitis. **Splenic abscesses** may have an appearance similar to that of simple cysts, but the diagnosis can easily be made in conjunction with the clinical findings. Frequently, there may be gas within an abscess cavity in the spleen, which should point to an infectious cause. Gas can cause a confusing picture if only a small area of increased echogenicity is seen in the spleen (Fig. 5-11). However, there may be acoustic shadowing and/or a ring-down artifact. In questionable cases, aspiration can be useful for diagnosis.[14] Furthermore, catheter drainage guided by sonography can be safely and successfully performed.[15]

Solid Masses. Solid focal lesions in the spleen are uncommon, but they can be caused by a large number of diseases. The most common focal lesions result from previous granulomatous infections, typically seen as focal, bright, echogenic lesions with or without shadowing. **Histoplasmosis** and **tuberculosis** are the most common causes, although granulomas may rarely occur in the spleen in patients with **sarcoidosis** (Fig. 5-12).[16,17] Calcification in the splenic artery is common and should not be confused with calcification in a lesion (Fig. 5-13).

Primary malignancies of the spleen are extremely rare, but primary lymphoma and angiosarcoma have been reported.[18] Metastatic involvement of the spleen generally occurs as a late phenomenon rather than as a presenting feature. Splenic **metastases** occur most commonly in **malignant melanoma, lymphoma,** and **leukemia,** but they can also occur in **carcinoma of the ovary, breast, lung,** and **stomach** (Fig. 5-14).[16,19]

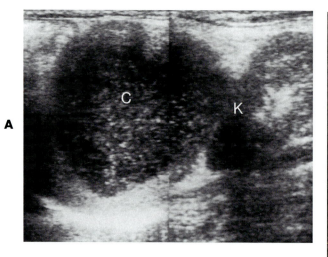

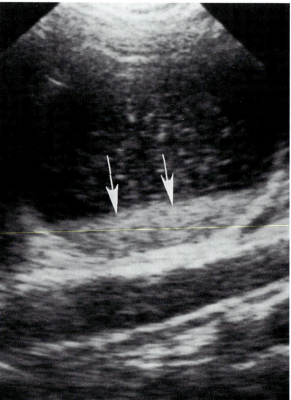

FIG. 5-10. **Splenic cyst.** **A,** Composite linear array images. Note the 8-cm-diameter splenic cyst (C). There is only a small rim of spleen noted superiorly and medially. The left kidney is displaced inferiorly toward the right of the image. The echoes from the cholesterol crystals and debris within the cyst mimic a solid lesion. **B,** The sector image shows a more echogenic, dependent layer *(arrows)*.

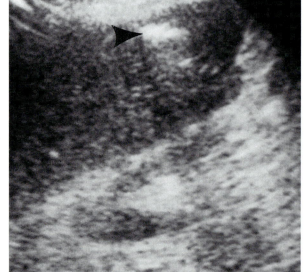

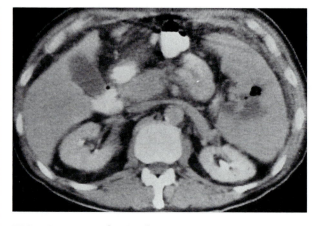

FIG. 5-11. **Splenic abscess.** **A,** Coronal scan shows a gas collection with "dirty shadowing" *(arrowhead)*. **B,** CT scan confirms the presence of gas and fluid within the spleen.

Metastases are usually hypoechoic but may be echogenic or of mixed echogenicity.

Hemangiomas of the spleen have been reported in up to 14% of patients undergoing autopsy,[20,21] but the typical appearance of hemangioma is seen far less frequently in the spleen than in the liver. Hemangiomas are usually isolated phenomena but they may occur in association with other stigmata of the Klippel-Trenaunay-Weber syndrome.[22] The sonographic appearance of hemangiomas is variable. The lesions may have a well-defined echogenic appearance, similar to the typical appearance of hemangiomas in the liver (Figs. 5-15 and 5-16). However, lesions of mixed echogenicity with cystic spaces of variable sizes have

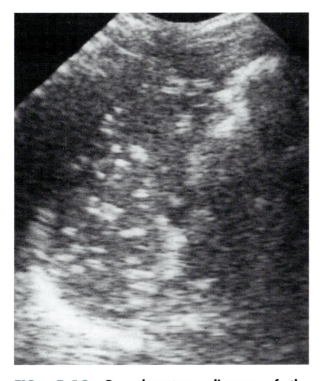

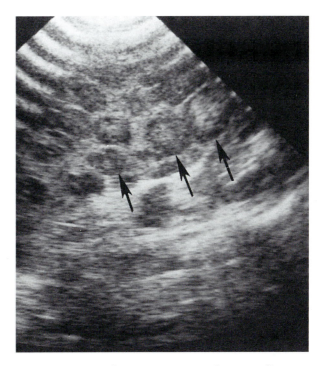

FIG. 5-12. **Granulomatous disease of the spleen.** Coronal scan showing tiny bright echoes measuring 2 to 3 mm throughout the spleen. This is a typical appearance of histoplasmosis.

FIG. 5-14. **Splenic metastases from malignant melanoma.** Note the multiple large lesions *(arrows)* in the spleen. The primary lesion is a malignant melanoma, one of the most common sources of splenic metastases.

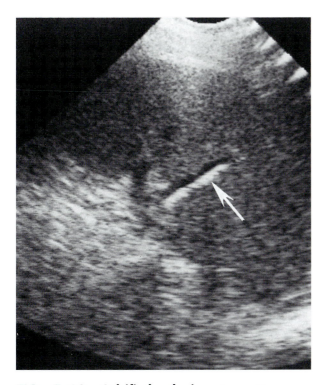

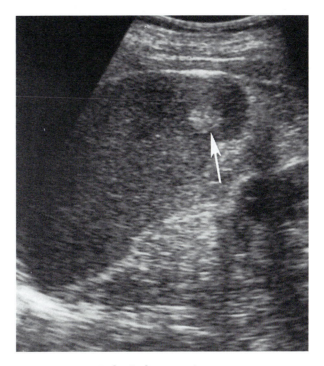

FIG. 5-13. **Calcified splenic artery.** Transverse scan of the spleen showing calcification of the splenic artery coursing parallel to the splenic vein.

FIG. 5-15. **Splenic hemangioma.** Note the small, well-defined, rounded, echogenic lesion *(arrow)* in the spleen measuring 1.4 cm in diameter. This is similar to the typical appearance of hemangiomas in the liver.

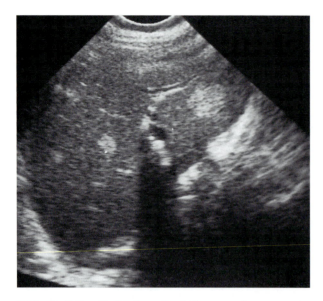

FIG. 5-16. Multiple splenic hemangiomas. The coronal scan shows multiple echogenic lesions of different sizes in the spleen. Note the calcified splenic artery adjacent to the vein in the splenic hilum.

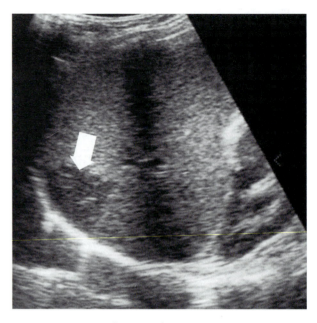

FIG. 5-17. Splenic infarct. The triangular echo-poor area *(arrow)* in the superior aspect of the spleen represents a splenic infarct. Note how the wedge-shaped area extends to the splenic capsule, analogous to the pleural wedge-shaped density seen in pulmonary infarction.

been reported. Occasionally, foci of calcification have been found.[23-25] Lymphangiomas may also occur in the spleen and may have an appearance similar to that of hemangiomas.[26] It remains to be shown whether MRI will be as helpful for confirming the diagnosis of hemangioma in the spleen as it is in the liver.

Splenic infarction is one of the more common causes of focal splenic lesions. If a typical peripheral, wedge-shaped, hypoechoic lesion is noted, splenic infarction should be the first diagnostic consideration (Figs. 5-17 and 5-18). However, splenic infarctions do not always have this typical appearance but may have a nodular appearance or, as fibrosis progresses, a hyperechoic appearance. The temporal evolution of the ultrasonic appearance of splenic infarctions has been studied and has shown that the echogenicity of the lesion is related to the age of the infarction. Infarctions are hypoechoic, or echo-free, in early stages, while they progress to hyperechoic lesions over time.[27,28]

Several relatively rare diseases have a high frequency of associated splenic abnormalities. For example, in **Gaucher's disease**, splenomegaly occurs almost universally, and approximately one third of patients have multiple splenic nodules. These nodules are frequently well-defined hypoechoic lesions, but they may also be irregular, hyperechoic, or of mixed echogenicity.[29,30] Pathologically, these nodules represent focal areas of Gaucher's cells associated with fibrosis and infarction. Rarely, the entire spleen may be involved, with ultrasound showing diffuse inhomogeneity.[29] In patients with **schistosomiasis**, splenomegaly is found universally, and focal hyperechoic nodules are seen in 5% to 10% of patients.[31]

Multiple nodules may also be found in patients with splenic infections, particularly in immunocompromised patients. The so-called wheels-within-wheels appearance has been described in patients with hepatosplenic **candidiasis**. The outer "wheel" is thought to represent a ring of fibrosis surrounding the inner echogenic "wheel" of inflammatory cells and a central hypoechoic, necrotic area. However, this appearance is not universally seen in splenic candidiasis; some patients' nodules may have a bulls-eye appearance or may be hypoechoic or hyperechoic[32] (Fig. 5-19).

Miliary tuberculosis can occur with both typical and **atypical mycobacterial infection** and is more commonly seen in immunocompromised patients. Innumerable tiny, echogenic foci can be seen diffusely throughout the spleen (Fig. 5-20). In active tuberculosis, echo-poor or cystic lesions representing tuberculous abscesses may be seen (Fig. 5-21).

In summary, although ultrasound is very helpful in finding focal splenic lesions, there is so much overlap in the appearance of the different pathologies that it is rarely possible to make a specific diagnosis. If a typical

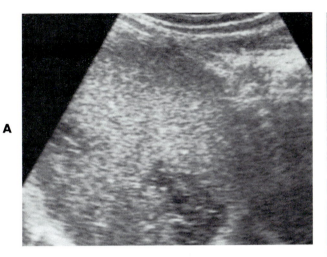

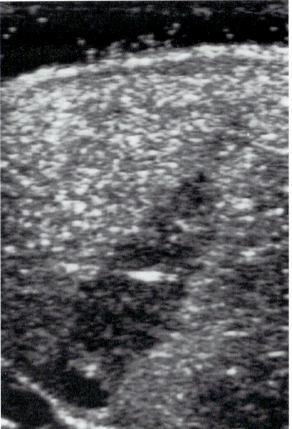

FIG. 5-18. Splenic infarct in acute myelogenous leukemia. A, *In vivo,* and **B,** *in vitro* postsplenectomy x scans showing echo-poor, wedge-shaped areas with their bases on the splenic capsule.

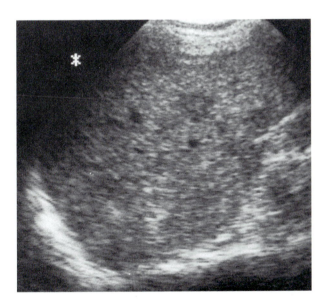

FIG. 5-19. Candida abscesses of the spleen in an AIDS patient. Note the lesion in the middle has an echogenic center characteristic of Candida.

appearance of splenic infarction is found, serial observations may be used to confirm the diagnosis and avoid a biopsy. If a very well-defined echogenic lesion is found in an asymptomatic patient, the lack of change on serial ultrasound examinations may be used to confirm the diagnosis of hemangioma. Calcified lesions in the spleen may be safely followed with serial ultrasound scanning, as they are unlikely to represent any condition requiring treatment. Otherwise, most other focal splenic lesions will require a biopsy for diagnosis.

Splenic Trauma

Ultrasound can be very useful and highly accurate in the diagnosis of subcapsular and pericapsular hematomas of the spleen. Nonetheless, this is one area in which CT has proven particularly useful because more upper-abdominal pathology can be identified in one examination.[33,34] However, splenic trauma from blunt, nonpenetrating injuries to the left upper quadrant is not always an emergency, and ultrasound can be useful.[35] In addition, if the patient is in extreme distress, the CT scanner often cannot be made available quickly enough, so ultrasound can play an important role in that circumstance, too. Furthermore, now that nonoperative management is

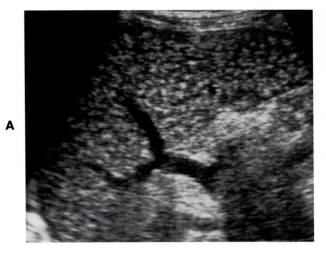

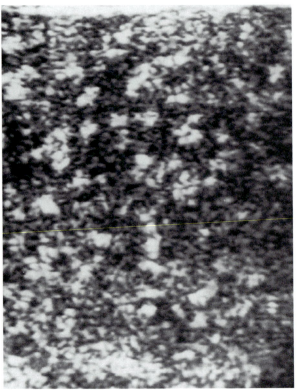

FIG. 5-20. Miliary tuberculosis of the spleen. A, Coronal and B, high-resolution linear array images showing multiple tiny echogenic foci of tuberculous granulomata. This was active tuberculosis.

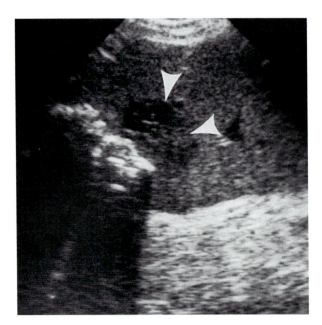

FIG. 5-21. Old and active tuberculosis in the spleen. The coronal image shows old calcified granulomas with shadowing in the superior aspect of the spleen, and echo-poor lesions *(arrows)* in the midportion resulting from reactivated tuberculosis.

preferred, ultrasound is preferable for numerous follow-up examinations.

If the spleen is involved in blunt abdominal trauma, two outcomes are possible. If the capsule remains intact, the outcome may be an intraparenchymal or subcapsular hematoma (Figs. 5-22 and 5-23). If the capsule ruptures, a focal or free intraperitoneal hematoma may result. With capsular rupture, it might be possible to demonstrate fluid surrounding the spleen in the left upper quadrant. Although blood may spread within the peritoneal cavity and be found in the flanks or in Morison's pouch, on most occasions it becomes walled off in the left upper quadrant (Figs. 5-24 and 5-25). It is important to consider the timing of the sonographic examination relative to the trauma. Immediately after the traumatic incident, the hematoma is liquid and can easily be differentiated from splenic parenchyma. However, after the blood clots, and for the subsequent 24 to 48 hours, the echogenicity of the perisplenic clot may closely resemble the echogenicity of normal splenic parenchyma. The appearance may mimic that of an enlarged spleen. Subsequently, the blood reliquefies and the diagnosis becomes easy again. Usually, by the time the patient has been admitted and has settled down, one sees only an irregularly marginated, echogenic mass that is larger than one would expect for a normal spleen. Furthermore, there are often focal areas of inhomogeneity within the spleen to indicate that there is an abnormality. Because current therapy for stable pa-

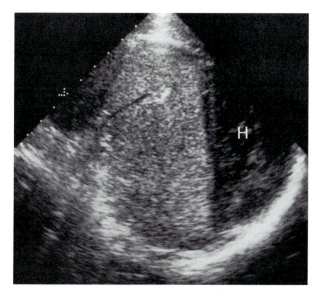

FIG. 5-22. Subcapsular hematoma of the spleen. Transverse scan showing a fluid- and debris-filled crescentic hematoma (H) in the lateral aspect of the spleen.

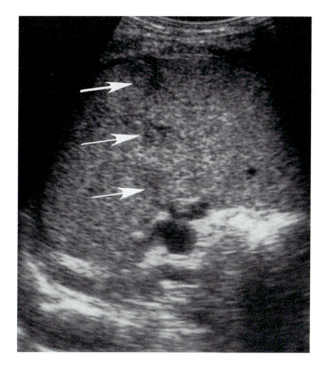

FIG. 5-24. Splenic laceration. Coronal scan showing irregular echo-poor area *(arrow)* laterally corresponding to small splenic laceration. There is a small amount of blood around the spleen. This improved and was not visible on a subsequent scan 2 weeks later.

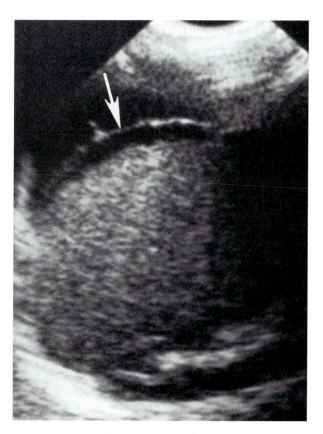

FIG. 5-23. Subcapsular and perisplenic hematomas. The thin, brightly echogenic crescentic line *(arrow)* represents the splenic capsule.

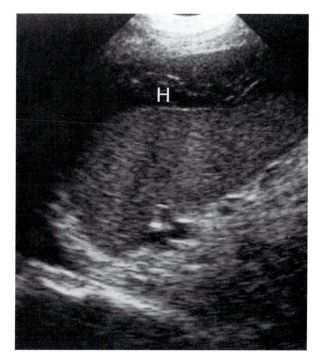

FIG. 5-25. Posttraumatic perisplenic hematoma. Coronal scan showing hematoma (H) around the lateral aspect of the spleen. There is also a left pleural effusion.

tients with suspected splenic trauma consists of nonintervention and temporization, a follow-up sonogram is suggested in 2 or 3 days to demonstrate reliquefaction of the hematoma. With time, one may clearly see the subcapsular hematoma differentiated from the pericapsular, walled-off hematoma by the capsule itself.[35] However, the splenic capsule is very thin and is frequently not visualized separately from adjacent fluid. In these cases, the shape of the fluid collection can provide an important clue to the location of the hematoma. If the collection is crescentic and conforms to the contour of the spleen, the hematoma should be assumed to be subcapsular. More irregularly shaped collections are seen with perisplenic hematomas.

Perisplenic fluid may persist for weeks or even months following the trauma. Although there may actually be a condition of delayed rupture of the spleen, it is possible that all ruptures of the spleen occurred at the time of injury and were walled off initially. Delayed rupture may only be the extension of a perisplenic hematoma into the peritoneal cavity.

Aside from splenic capsule rupture, there may be internal damage to the spleen with an intact splenic capsule. This can result in intraparenchymal or subcapsular hematoma of the spleen, which initially appears only as an inhomogeneous area in the otherwise uniform splenic parenchyma. Subsequently, the hematoma may resolve, and repeat scans can show the cyst at the site of the original injury.

Sonographically, a perisplenic hematoma can closely mimic a perisplenic abscess. The hematoma can easily become infected and transform into a left subphrenic abscess.[36] Generally, the distinction can be made clinically. If it is not clinically obvious, fineneedle aspiration can differentiate quickly between hematoma and abscess. Catheter drainage for definitive therapy can then be performed under ultrasound or CT guidance.

Acquired Immune Deficiency Syndrome (AIDS)

The most common splenic ultrasound finding in patients with AIDS is moderate splenomegaly, reported in 50% to 70% of patients referred for abdominal ultrasound.[37,38] Splenomegaly has been noted more frequently in patients with sexually transmitted HIV infection than in patients who acquired the disease through intravenous drug use. Focal lesions can occur in patients with AIDS. They may be caused by opportunistic infections such as *Candida* (Fig. 5-19), pneumocystis, or mycobacterium. There have been reports of disseminated pneumocystis appearing as tiny focal echoes throughout the liver, spleen, and kidneys.[39] We have seen an identical case caused by atypical mycobacteria (Fig. 5-26). The spleen may also be involved in Kaposi's sarcoma or lymphoma.

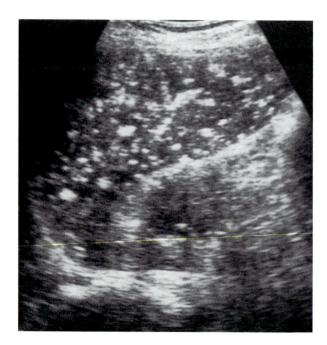

FIG. 5-26. Atypical tuberculosis of the spleen in an AIDS patient. Tiny calcifications throughout the spleen were also present throughout the liver, and isolated x foci were identified in the kidney. Several core biopsies through the liver confirmed these to be *Mycobacterium avium* intracellular granulomas. Disseminated *Pneumocystis carinii* can also look like this.

CONGENITAL ANOMALIES

Supernumerary spleens are common normal variants found in up to 30% of autopsies. They are also referred to as **splenunculi.** They may be confused with enlarged lymph nodes around the spleen or with masses in the tail of the pancreas (Fig. 5-27). When the spleen enlarges, the accessory spleens may also enlarge. Ectopic accessory spleens may be confused with abnormal masses or may undergo torsion and cause acute abdominal pain.[40-43] The vast majority of accessory spleens, however, are easy to recognize sonographically as small rounded masses, less than 5 cm in diameter (Fig. 5-28). They are located near the splenic hilum and have echogenicity identical to that of the adjacent spleen. A CT scan or nuclear scan with heat-damaged red cells can confirm the diagnosis, if necessary.

The spleen may have a long, mobile mesentery if the dorsal mesentery fails to fuse with the posterior peritoneum. The "wandering" spleen can be found in unusual locations and may be mistaken for a mass. It may undergo torsion and result in acute or chronic abdominal pain.[44-46] If the diagnosis of a wandering spleen is made in a patient with acute abdominal pain, the diagnosis of torsion may be supported by a color flow Doppler examination showing absence of blood flow.

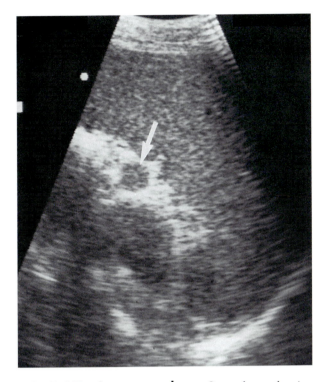

FIG. 5-27. Accessory spleen. Coronal scan showing an accessory spleen (splenunculus) in the splenic hilum, with homogeneous echogenicity identical to that of the remainder of the spleen. These are commonly seen.

The other two major congenital splenic anomalies are the **asplenia** and **polysplenia syndromes.** These conditions are best understood if viewed as part of the spectrum of anomalies known as visceral heterotaxy. A normal arrangement of asymmetric body parts is known as situs solitus. The mirror image condition is called situs inversus. In between these two extremes is a wide spectrum of abnormalities called situs ambiguous. Splenic abnormalities in patients with visceral heterotaxy consist of polysplenia and asplenia. Interestingly, patients with **polysplenia** have bilateral left-sidedness, or a dominance of left-sided over right-sided body structures. They may have two morphologically left lungs, left-sided azygous continuation of an interrupted inferior vena cava, biliary atresia, absence of the gallbladder, gastrointestinal malrotation, and, frequently, cardiovascular abnormalities. Conversely, patients with **asplenia** may have bilateral right-sidedness. They may have two morphologically right lungs, midline location of the liver, reversed position of the abdominal aorta and inferior vena cava, anomalous pulmonary venous return, and horseshoe kidneys. The wide variety of possible anomalies obviously accounts for the wide variety of presenting symptoms, but absence of the spleen per se causes impairment of the immune response, and

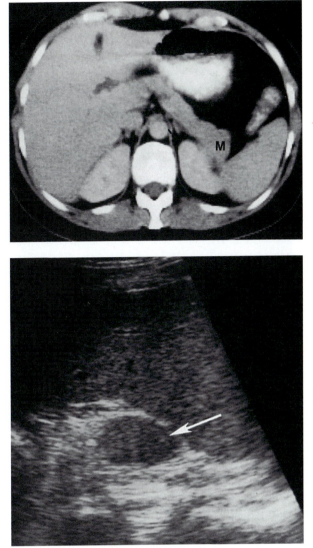

FIG. 5-28. Accessory spleen presenting as possible mass in the tail of the pancreas. A, The CT scan was done first and the patient was referred for an ultrasound-guided biopsy of the pancreatic tail. **B,** The coronal sonogram shows that the apparently enlarged pancreatic tail is actually an accessory spleen lying adjacent to the tail of the pancreas.

such patients can present with serious infections such as bacterial meningitis.

Polysplenia must be differentiated from posttraumatic splenosis. Following splenic rupture, splenic cells may implant throughout the peritoneal cavity and increase in size, resulting in multiple ectopic splenic rests.[48-50] Nuclear studies with technetium-labeled, heat-damaged red blood cells are the most sensitive studies for both posttraumatic splenosis and congenital polysplenia. Accessory spleens as small as 1 cm can be demonstrated by this method.[50]

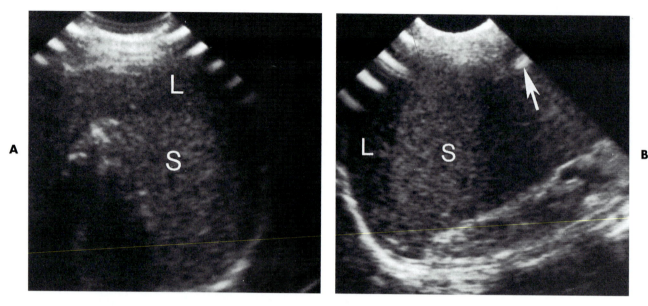

FIG. 5-29. **Pseudofluid around the spleen.** **A,** Transverse, and **B,** sagittal scans showing the crescentic, echo-poor, enlarged left lobe of the liver (L) anterior to the spleen. This should not be mistaken for a fluid collection. Note the presence of gas *(arrow)* within the stomach.

INTERVENTIONAL PROCEDURES

Despite the fact that ultrasound-guided fine-needle aspiration biopsy and catheter drainage have been established as safe and successful techniques for most areas of the abdomen, many interventional radiologists have been reluctant to apply these techniques to the spleen. The main concern has been fear of bleeding caused by the highly vascular nature of the organ. Reluctance also exists because of the frequent necessity to transgress the pleural space or colon to reach the spleen. However, in recent years a number of reports have appeared that describe ultrasound-guided interventional procedures in the spleen and demonstrate safety and success records similar to those obtained elsewhere in the abdomen.[14,51-55] Fine- and core-cutting-needle biopsies have been performed for the diagnosis of focal lesions, including abscesses, sarcoidosis, primary splenic malignancies, metastases, and lymphoma. Successful catheter drainage of abscesses, cysts, hematomas, and infected necrotic tumors has been reported. However, only very small numbers of cases have been reported, and further experience will be needed to verify the safety and efficacy of these procedures.

PITFALLS

Several sonographic pitfalls exist, and one must be wary of them when scanning the left upper quadrant and spleen. The first pitfall is the crescentic, echo-poor area superior to the spleen, which can be caused by the **left lobe of the liver** in thin individuals (Fig. 5-29).[56-59] It can mimic the appearance of a subcapsular hematoma or a subphrenic abscess. The correct interpretation can be made by noting the hypoechoic liver sliding over the more echogenic spleen during quiet respiration. It would be desirable to follow the liver from the anterior axillary line in the midline over to the posterior axillary line in the coronal plane, but this is usually not possible because of the presence of gas in the stomach. Hepatic and/or portal veins may help to identify this structure as the liver.

The **tail of the pancreas** may look large and may simulate a mass adjacent to the hilum of the spleen. This is particularly true if the plane of section is aimed along the long axis of the tail of the pancreas. Identifying the splenic artery and vein may be helpful in confirming it as the normal tail of the pancreas.

Similarly, the **fundus of the stomach** may nestle in the hilum of the spleen. A particular oblique plane of section may pass through the spleen and include the hilum, with an echogenic portion of the stomach simulating an intrasplenic lesion. Sometimes this is just the fat around the stomach. Occasionally, fluid in the fundus of the stomach can simulate an intrasplenic fluid collection or an abscess in the hilum of the spleen. This can usually be resolved by scanning transversely and, if necessary, giving the patient water to drink.

An occasional anatomic variant can occur if the inferior portion of the spleen lies posterolateral to the upper pole of the left kidney. This variant has been called the **retrorenal spleen.** Awareness of its existence can prevent the misdiagnosis of an abnormal mass. Furthermore, if visualized sonographically, it should be avoided in any interventional procedure performed on the left kidney.[60]

Finally, it can be very difficult to determine the site of origin of **large, left upper quadrant masses** arising from the spleen, left adrenal gland, left kidney, tail of the pancreas, stomach, or retroperitoneum. Differential motion observed during shallow respiration can sometimes be helpful. Additionally, the identification of the splenic vein entering the splenic hilum can be definitive. CT or MRI can usually solve difficult cases.

REFERENCES

Embryology and Anatomy

1. Vibhakar SD, Bellon EM. The bare area of the spleen: a constant computed tomography feature of the ascitic abdomen. *AJR* 1984;141(5):953-955.

Examination Technique

2. Hicken P, Sauerbrei EE, Cooperberg PL. Ultrasonic coronal scanning of left upper quadrant. *J Can Assoc Radiol* 1981;32:107-110.

Pathologic Conditions of the Spleen

3. Briarman RS, Beck JW, Corobkin M et al. *AJR* 1982;138:329-333.
4. Frank K, Linhart P, Kortsik C et al. Sonographic determination of spleen size: normal dimensions in adults with a healthy spleen. *Ultraschall Med* 1986;7(3):134-137.
5. Manoharan A, Chen CF, Wilson LS et al. Ultrasonic characterization of splenic tissue in myelofibrosis: further evidence for reversal of fibrosis with chemotherapy. *Eur J Haematol* 1988;40(2):149-154.
6. Wilson LS, Robinson DE, Griffiths KA et al. Evaluation of ultrasonic attenuation in diffuse diseases of spleen and liver. *Ultrasound Imaging* 1987;9(4):236-247.
7. Rubinson DE, Gill RW, Kossoff G. Quantitative sonography. *Ultrasound Med Biol* 1986;12(7):555-565.
8. Franquet T, Montes M, Lecumberri FJ et al. Hydatid disease of the spleen: imaging findings in nine patients. *AJR* 1990;154(3):525-528.
9. Al-Moyaya S, Al-Awami M, Vaidya MP et al. Hydatid cyst of the spleen. *Am J Trop Med Hyg* 1986;35(5):995-999.
10. Bhimji SD, Cooperberg PL, Nainan S. Ultrasound diagnosis of splenic cysts. *Radiology* 1977;122:787-789.
11. Thurber LA, Cooperberg PL, Clemente JG et al. Echogenic fluid: a pitfall in the ultrasonographic diagnosis of cystic lesions. *JCU* 1979;7:273-278.
12. Propper RA, Weinstein BJ, Skolnick ML et al. Ultrasonography of hemorrhagic splenic cysts. *JCU* 1979;7:18-20.
13. Duddy MJ, Calder CJ. Cystic hemangioma of the spleen: findings on ultrasound and computed tomography. *Br J Radiol* 1989;62(734):180-182.
14. Quinn SF, van Sonnenberg E, Casola G et al. Interventional radiology in the spleen. *Radiology* 1986;161:299-291.
15. Learner RM, Spataro RF. Splenic abscess: percutaneous drainage. *Radiology* 1994;153:643-645.
16. Kessler A, Mitchell DG, Israel L, Goldberg BB. Hepatic and splenic sarcoidosis: ultrasound and MR imaging. *Abdom Imag* 1993;18:159-83.
17. Schaeffer A, Vasile N. Computed tomography of sarcoidosis (case report). *J Comput Assist Tomogr* 1986;10(4):679-680.

18. Iwasaki M, Hiyama Y, Myojo S et al. Primary malignant lymphoma of the spleen: report of a case. *Rinsho Hoshasen* 1988;33(3):405-408.
19. Costello P, Kane RA, Oster J et al. Focal splenic disease demonstrated by ultrasound and computed tomography. *J Can Assoc Radiol* 1985;36:22-28.
20. Sammis AF Jr, Weitzman S, Arcomano JP. Hemangiolymphangioma of spleen and bone. *NY State J Med* 1971;71:1762-1764.
21. Manor A, Starinsky R, Gorfinkel D et al. Ultrasound features of a symptomatic splenic hemangioma. *J Clin Ultrasound* 1984;12:95-97.
22. Pakter RL, Fishman EK, Nussbaum A et al. Computed tomography findings in splenic hemangiomas in the Klippel-Trenaunay-Weber syndrome. *J Comput Assist Tomogr* 1987;11(1):88-91.
23. Ross PR, Moser RP, Dackman AH et al. Hemangioma of the spleen: radiologic-pathologic correlation in ten cases. *AJR* 1987;162:73-77.
24. Moss CN, Van Dyke JA, Koehler RE et al. Multiple cavernous hemangiomas of the spleen: computed tomography findings. *J Comput Assist Tomogr* 1986;10(2):338-340.
25. Kagalwala TY, Vaidya VU, Bharucha BA et al. Cavernous hemangiomas of the liver and spleen. *Indian Pediatr* 1987;24(5):427-430.
26. Pistoia F, Markowitz SK. Splenic lymphangiomatosis: computed tomography diagnosis. *AJR* 1988;150:121-122.
27. Maresca G, Mirk P, DeGaetano AM et al. Sonographic patterns in splenic infarction. *J Clin Ultrasound* 1986;14:23-28.
28. Balcar I, Seltzer SE, Davis S, Geller S. Computed tomography patterns of splenic infarction: a clinical and experimental study. *Radiology* 1984;151:723-729.
29. Hill SC, Reinig JW, Barranger JA et al. Gaucher's disease: sonographic appearance of spleen. *Radiology* 1986;160:631-634.
30. Stevens PG, Kumari-Subaiya SS, Kahn LB. Splenic involvement in Gaucher's disease: sonographic findings. *J Clin Ultrasound* 1987;15:397-400.
31. Cerri GG, Alvis VAF, Magalhaes A. Hepatosplenic schistosomiasis mansoni: ultrasound manifestations. *Radiology* 1984;153:777-780.
32. Pastakia B, Shawker TH, Thalar M et al. Hepatosplenic candidiasis: wheels within wheels. *Radiology* 1988;166:417-421.
33. Jeffrey RB, Laing FC, Federle MP et al. Computed tomography of splenic trauma. *Radiology* 1981;141:729-732.
34. Lawson DE, Jacobson JA, Spizarny DL et al. Splenic trauma: value of follow-up CT. *Radiology* 1995;194:97-100.
35. Siniuoto TM, Palvansalo MJ, Lanning FP et al. Ultrasonography in traumatic splenic. *Clin Radiol* 1992;48:39.
36. Epstein NB, Omar GM. Infective complications of splenic trauma. *Clin Radiol* 1983;34:91-94.
37. Langer R, Langer M, Schutze B, et al. Ultrasound findings in patients with AIDS. *Digitale Bilddiang* 1988;8(2):93-96.
38. Yee JM, Raghavendra BN, Horii SC, et al. Abdominal sonography in AIDS: a review. *J Ultrasound Med* 1989;8(12):705-714.
39. Spouge AR, Wilson SR, Gopinath N, et al. Extrapulmonary pneumocystis carinii in a patient with AIDS: sonographic findings. *AJR* 1990;155(1):76-78.
40. Hansen S, Jarhult J. Accessory spleen imaging: radionuclide, ultrasound and computed tomography investigations in a patient with thrombocytopenia 25 years after splenectomy for ITP. *Scand J Haematol* 1986;37(1):74-77.
41. Mostbeck G, Sommer G, Haller J et al. Accessory spleen: presentation as a large abdominal mass in an asymptomatic young woman. *Gastrointest Radiol* 1987;12:337-339.
42. Muller H, Schneider H, Ruchauer K et al. Accessory spleen torsion: clinical picture, sonographic diagnosis and differential diagnosis. *Klin Pediatr* 1988;200(5):419-421.

43. Nino-Murcia M, Friedland GW, Gross DL. Imaging the effects of an ectopic spleen on the urinary tract. *Urol Radiol* 1988;10(4):195-197.

44. Plaja Ramon P, Aso Puertolas C, Sanchis Solera L. Wandering spleen: discussion apropos of a case. *An Esp Pediatr* 1987;26(1):69-70.

45. Scicolone G, Contin I, Bano A et al. Wandering spleen: preoperative diagnosis by echotomography of the abdomen. *Chir Ital* 1986;38(1):72-79.

46. Azoulay D, Gossot D, Sarfati E et al. Volvulus of a mobile spleen: apropos of a case diagnosed in the preoperative period by ultrasonography. *J CLIR* 1987;124(10):520-522.

47. Maillard JC, Menu Y, Scherrer A et al. Intraperitoneal splenosis: diagnosis by ultrasound and computed tomography. *Gastrointest Radiol* 1989;(2):179-180.

48. Delamarre J, Capron JP, Drouard F et al. Splenosis: ultrasound and computed tomography findings in a case complicated by an intraperitoneal implant traumatic hematoma. *Gastrointest Radiol* 1988;13(3):275-278.

49. Turk CO, Lipson SB, Brandt TD. Splenosis mimicking a renal mass. *Urology* 1988;31(3):248-250.

50. Nishitani H, Hayashi T, Onitsuka H et al. Computed tomography of accessory spleens. *Radiat Med* 1984;2(4):222.

51. Vyborny CJ, Merrill TN, Reda J et al. Subacute subcapsular hematoma of the spleen complicating pancreatitis: successful percutaneous drainage. *Radiology* 1989;169:161-162.

Interventional Procedures

52. Suzuki T, Shibuya H, Yoshimatsu S et al. Ultrasonically guided staging splenic tissue core biopsy in patients with non-Hodgkin's lymphoma. *Cancer* 1987;60:879-882.

53. Taavitsainen M, Koivuniemi A, Helminen J et al. Aspiration biopsy of the spleen in patients with sarcoidosis. *Acta Radiol* 1987;28:723-725.

54. Suzuki T, Shibuya H, Yoshimatsu S et al. Ultrasonically guided staging splenic tissue core biopsy in patients with non-Hodgkin's lymphoma. *Cancer* 1987;60(4):879-882.

55. Suzuki T. Ultrasonically guided splenic biopsy in patients with malignant lymphoma. *Nippon Igaku Hoshasen Gakkai Zasshi* 1988;48(8):982-987.

Pitfalls

56. Rao MG. Enlarged left lobe of the liver mistaken for a mass in the splenic region. *Clin Nucl Med* 1989;14(2):134.

57. Li DK, Cooperberg PL, Graham MF et al. Psuedo peri-splenic "fluid collections": a clue to normal liver and spleen echogenic texture. *J Ultrasound Med* 1986;5(7):397-400.

58. Crivello MS, Peterson IM, Austin RM. Left lobe of the liver mimicking perisplenic collections. *JCU* 14(9):697-701.

59. Arenson AM, McKee JD. Left upper quadrant pseudolesion secondary to normal variants in liver and spleen. *JCU* 1986;14(7):558-561.

60. Dodds WJ, Darweesh RMA, Lawson TL et al. The retroperitoneal spaces revisited. *AJR* 1986;174:1155-1161.

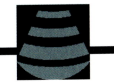

CHAPTER 6

The Gallbladder and Bile Ducts

•

Faye C. Laing, M.D.

CHAPTER OUTLINE

GALLBLADDER
  Normal Anatomy
    Congenital Variations
  Scanning Techniques
  Pathology
    Cholelithiasis
    Wall Changes
    Sludge
    Pericholecystic Fluid
    Acute Cholecystitis
  Treatment Options and the Role of Ultrasound
  Pitfalls
INTRAHEPATIC BILE DUCTS
  Normal Anatomy
  Dilated Intrahepatic Bile Ducts
  Pathology
    Intrahepatic Biliary Neoplasms
    Sclerosing and AIDS Cholangitis
    Intrahepatic Biliary Calculi

  Caroli's Disease
  Miscellaneous Rare Conditions
Pitfalls
EXTRAHEPATIC BILE DUCTS
  Normal Anatomy
  Scanning Techniques
  Pathology
    Diagnosing Obstruction
    Level and Cause of Obstruction
    Intrapancreatic Obstruction
    Suprapancreatic Obstruction
    Porta Hepatis Obstruction
    Unusual Causes for Bile Duct Dilatation
  Pitfalls
    Anatomic Problems
    Atypical Cases
    Detecting Choledocholithiasis
ENDOSCOPIC ULTRASOUND

As the number of available imaging modalities continues to expand and as their applications become more diverse and sophisticated, clinical and imaging guidelines are becoming increasingly important. Despite recent improvements in other noninvasive imaging modalities, particularly with regard to magnetic resonance imaging (MRI) and the introduction of magnetic resonance cholangiopancreatography (MRCP), sonography remains the initial screening modality of choice for evaluating the appearance of the gallbladder and bile ducts. The advantages of sonography include:
- High sensitivity and accuracy for detecting gallstones as well as intrahepatic and extrahepatic bile duct dilatation;
- Lack of ionizing radiation; no need for contrast material;
- Speed, safety, flexibility, and portability;

- Independence of gastrointestinal, hepatic, and biliary function; and
- Multiple organ examination.

Common indications for performing sonography of the gallbladder and biliary tree include signs and symptoms of acute or chronic cholecystitis, jaundice, abnormal liver function tests, and pancreatitis. New and developing uses for gallbladder and biliary ultrasound relate to laparoscopic cholecystectomy and endoluminal biliary applications.

GALLBLADDER

Normal Anatomy

A normal gallbladder should be visible in virtually all adult patients if it is physiologically distended following an 8- to 12-hour fast. Rarely, massive obesity or overlying distended bowel loops preclude a satisfactory examination. The anatomic position of the gallbladder fundus can vary dramatically from one patient to another. It may even vary markedly in a single patient depending on the patient's position. The neck of the gallbladder, however, bears a fixed anatomic relationship to the main lobar fissure and the undivided right portal vein.[1] In approximately 70% of patients a linear echo, thought to represent a portion of the main lobar fissure, can be identified connecting the gallbladder to the right or main portal vein (Fig. 6-1).[2] This anatomic consideration becomes important for conclusively identifying the gallbladder in patients with pathologic conditions such as small contracted gallbladders or gallbladders filled with calculi.

Because the **size** and **shape** of the normal gallbladder vary widely in individual patients, it is difficult to formulate precise size criteria. In general, if its transverse diameter exceeds 5 cm and if it is no longer ovoid but rounded in shape, the gallbladder is likely to be hydropic.[3] Conversely, if its diameter is less than 2 cm despite adequate fasting, the gallbladder is likely to be abnormally contracted. Gallbladder volume measurements may be useful for physiologic evaluation of gallbladder contractility.[4,5] Calculation of gallbladder volume can be obtained most easily by assuming the gallbladder has an ellipsoid shape and using the formula

$$V = 0.52 \ (L \times W \times H)$$

or by using a sonic digitizer and a digital computer.[6,7]

Although the shape of a typical gallbladder is oval or gourdlike, it frequently varies from this configuration because of apparent folding or kinking.[8] In approximately 4% of patients a **phrygian cap deformity** is present in which the gallbladder fundus appears to be folded on the body (Figs. 6-2 and 6-3).[9,10] A more frequent variation is the presence of a fold between the

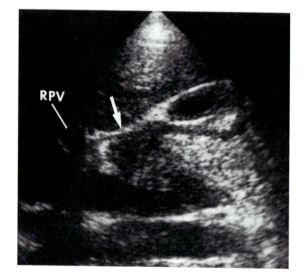

FIG. 6-1. **The interlobar hepatic fissure,** a useful anatomic landmark for identifying the gallbladder fossa, is seen on longitudinal scan through the right hepatic lobe as a linear echo *(arrow)* extending between the right portal vein *(RPV)* and the gallbladder neck. Thickening of the gallbladder wall has resulted from physiological contraction. (From Laing FC, Filly RA, Gooding GAW. Ultrasonography of the liver and biliary tract. In: Margulis AR, Burhenne HJ, eds. *Alimentary Tract Radiology.* 4th ed. St Louis: Mosby-Year Book; 1989.)

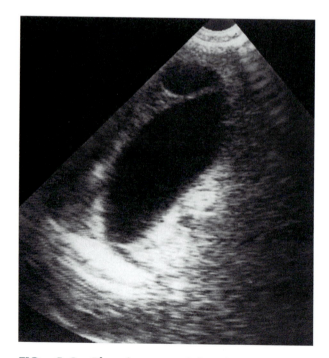

FIG. 6-2. Phrygian cap deformity. Longitudinal scan with the gallbladder fundus appearing to be folded on the body. (From Laing FC. Ultrasonography of the gallbladder and biliary tree. In: Sarti DA, ed. *Diagnostic Ultrasound: Text and Cases.* 2nd ed. St Louis: Mosby-Year Book; 1987.)

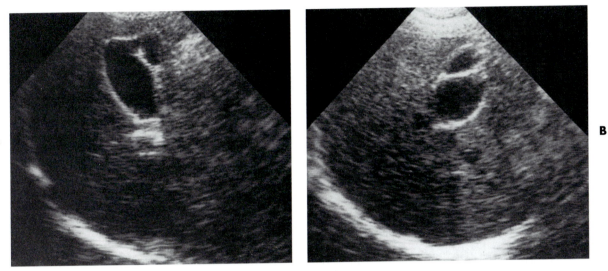

FIG. 6-3. Phrygian cap. A, Longitudinal scan shows a typical appearance. **B,** On transverse image, a confusing picture is present, suggesting that the sonolucency anterior to the gallbladder could be caused by an abscess, hematoma, or liver cyst. (From Laing FC. Ultrasonography of the gallbladder and biliary tree. In: Sarti DA, ed. *Diagnostic Ultrasound: Text and Cases.* 2nd ed. St Louis: Mosby-Year Book; 1987.)

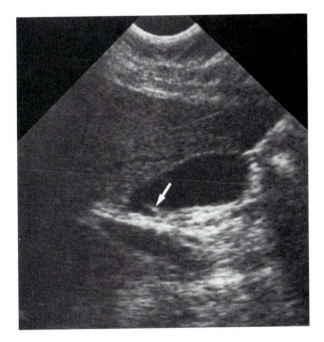

FIG. 6-4. Junctional fold *(arrow)* seen on longitudinal scan as a small linear echo in the proximal portion of the gallbladder. This appearance could be confused with a small calculus, especially if shadowing is present. A repeat scan following a deep inspiratory effort often eliminates the junctional fold. (From Laing FC. Ultrasonography of the gallbladder and biliary tree. In: Sarti DA, ed. *Diagnostic Ultrasound: Text and Cases.* 2nd ed. St Louis: Mosby-Year Book; 1987.)

body and infundibulum of the gallbladder, known as a **junctional fold** (Fig. 6-4).[10] Any fold in the gallbladder can produce high-amplitude echoes that occasionally may be associated with posterior acoustic shadowing caused by refractive effects. This appearance can cause folds to be mistaken for polyps and/or calculi. An awareness of these variations as well as meticulous scanning technique should minimize diagnostic errors.

The normal **gallbladder wall** is visible as a pencil-thin echogenic line that is less than 3 mm thick. Although the gallbladder may be normally indented by adjacent bowel loops, focal impressions on it from the liver suggest the presence of hepatic mass. Because bile does not contain particulate material, the gallbladder lumen is normally echo free.

Congenital Variations. True **gallbladder septations,**[11] **bilobed,** and **duplication anomalies** are rare,[12-14] but have each been described by ultrasound (Fig. 6-5). Gallbladder duplication is typically associated with one functioning and one nonfunctioning component. This can be documented by either cholescintigraphy or by repeating the ultrasound examination after administering a fatty meal.[13,14] **Anomalous gallbladder location** is also distinctly unusual. If it is due to an elongated cystic duct, the normal supporting mesentery may be absent, and torsion[15] or herniation through the foramen of Winslow[16] may occur. In other patients with gallbladder torsion, there may be an acquired elongation of the mesentery, about which torsion can occur. In these rare cases, ultrasound has been able

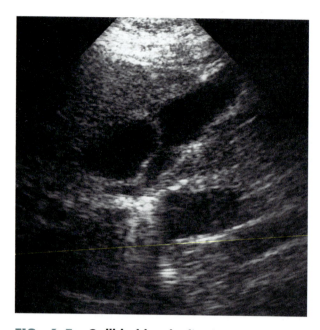

FIG. 6-5. Gallbladder duplication. Sagittal scan reveals two noncommunicating sonolucent areas that were subsequently proven to be due to a duplicated gallbladder.

to suggest the correct diagnosis by demonstrating the elongated mesentery.[17]

Scanning Techniques

To ensure adequate gallbladder distention, the examination should be performed after an overnight fast of 8 to 12 hours. Fasting is necessary to avoid diagnostic errors. Physiologic gallbladder contraction causes the gallbladder to appear small and thick-walled; this could be misinterpreted as a pathologic condition. For most patients a sector transducer is better than a linear array, because the smaller sector transducer can be more optimally positioned subcostally or within rib interspaces. The highest-frequency transducer that can satisfactorily image the gallbladder should be used. For most patients a 3.5-MHz transducer is necessary. In thin patients or in those with an anteriorly positioned gallbladder, a 5-MHz transducer should be used to provide superior resolution. Optimal images usually require the patient to suspend respiration following a deep inspiratory effort.

A thorough examination of the gallbladder can usually be accomplished in 5 to 10 minutes. The scans are performed from a lower intercostal or preferably a subcostal approach with the patient supine or in a left posterior oblique position. Occasionally, however, scans should be performed with the patient in an erect or prone position in order to convincingly demonstrate calculi mobility.[18] Cholecystosonography requires meticulous scanning technique to avoid overlooking small calculi. Special attention should be directed to the most dependent region of the gallbladder, where most calculi are found. In most patients this is the region of the gallbladder neck and the cystic duct.

Pathology

Cholelithiasis. In western countries, cholesterol stones predominate (as opposed to pigment stones, which are composed of calcium bilirubinate). The incidence of cholesterol gallstones is almost three times higher in women than in men and increases with age and possibly multiparity. Detection of cholelithiasis is the primary role of gallbladder sonography, with reported sensitivities and accuracies of greater than 95%.[19-22] Because gallstones both absorb and reflect the ultrasound beam, the net sonographic effect is a **highly reflective echo** originating from the anterior surface of the calculus with a prominent **posterior acoustic shadow.** The demonstration of a posterior acoustic shadow is important because shadowing echo densities that originate within the gallbladder correlate with cholelithiasis virtually 100% of the time, whereas nonshadowing echo densities correlate with calculi in only 50% of cases.[20] To visualize a posterior acoustic shadow optimally, it is important to use a transducer with the highest possible frequency that is focused maximally at the depth of the stone (Fig. 6-6). The combination of a narrow sound beam with the stone centrally positioned in the beam is optimal for creating an acoustic shadow. In vitro studies have shown that all gallstones whose diameters exceed 1 mm should cast an acoustic shadow, regardless of composition, surface characteristics, or shape of the calculus.[23,24] Because very small calculi may fail to demonstrate acoustic shadowing in vivo, it is sometimes advantageous to reposition the patient in an attempt to **pile small stones upon one another** (Fig. 6-7). The effect of this maneuver is to form an aggregate of small stones that acoustically behaves like a larger stone in that it casts a posterior acoustic shadow. In addition, the time-gain compensation curve should be adjusted so that acoustic enhancement behind the gallbladder does not obliterate a faint acoustic shadow.

Another sonographic feature that allows the confident diagnosis of calculus disease is to demonstrate gravity-dependent **movement** of a stone. Unless it is impacted in the gallbladder neck or is adherent to the gallbladder wall, calculi should be mobile. On rare occasions, **sludge balls**[25] or **tumefactive biliary sludge**[26] can appear as mobile masses within the gallbladder lumen (Fig. 6-8). The nature of this material varies from case to case and includes parasites, blood clots, aggregated pus, sludge, and contrast material. In contradistinction to calculi, this material is evanescent and is not associated with posterior acoustic shadowing.

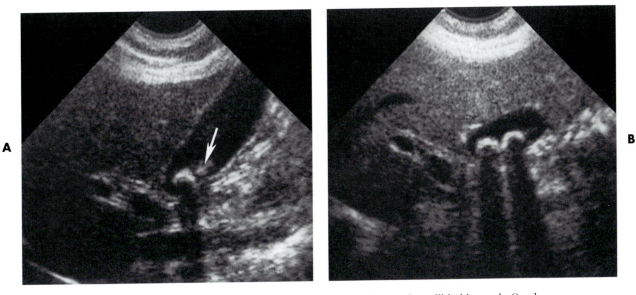

FIG. 6-6. **Cholelithiasis.** **A,** Two stones are located near the gallbladder neck. One has acoustic shadowing. Lack of shadowing from the second stone *(arrow)* is because of its position, which is slightly off center with respect to the transducer beam. **B,** A repeat scan performed with both stones in the central portion of the beam shows two acoustic shadows. (From Laing FC. Ultrasonography of the gallbladder and biliary tree. In: Sarti DA, ed. *Diagnostic Ultrasound: Text and Cases.* St Louis: Mosby–Year Book; 1987.)

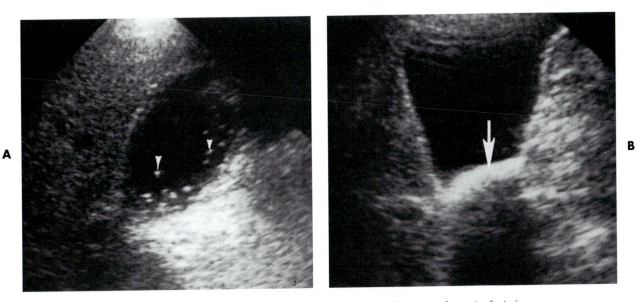

FIG. 6-7. **Cholelithiasis.** **A,** Multiple small, nonshadowing, echogenic foci *(arrowheads)* are seen in the gallbladder lumen immediately after turning the patient in an attempt to demonstrate mobility of calculi. **B,** Subsequent settling of the stones to the dependent region of the gallbladder *(arrow)* shows a prominent acoustic shadow below the stones that is caused by the additive effect of multiple small stones lying upon one another.

As the gallbladder becomes **filled with stones,** its ultrasound appearance changes dramatically. Instead of visualizing the outline of the gallbladder, a high-amplitude reflection with a prominent acoustic shadow emanates from the gallbladder fossa (Fig. 6-9). The echo-shadow complex originates from the most superficial layer of stones. The deeper calculi as well as the intraluminal bile and outline of the gallbladder are rendered invisible.[27] Close scrutiny of these images usually reveals characteristic findings that have been described as the **wall-echo-shadow (WES triad),**[28] or the **double arc shadow sign.**[29] These signs consist of two parallel, curved, echogenic lines separated by a thin anechoic space with distal acoustic shadowing. The proximal echogenic line is the result of the near wall of the gallbladder whereas the deeper echogenic line is the result of the anterior surface of the gallstone that causes the acoustic shadow. A similar appearance can also occur with calcification in the gallbladder wall (**porcelain gallbladder**)[30] or **air in the gallbladder wall.**[31,32] In patients with emphysematous cholecystitis, reverberation echoes from the air suggest the correct diagnosis.

Wall Changes. The most frequent gallbladder wall abnormality detected by sonography is **diffuse thickening,** which is diagnosed when the wall is greater than 3 mm thick. Wall thickening typically appears as a relatively hypoechoic region between two echogenic lines. Occasionally the thickened wall may have a striated or layered appearance, which was initially considered indicative of acute cholecystitis (Fig. 6-10).[33] Subsequent studies, however, have confirmed that diffuse wall thickening with or without striations is nonspecific, and that this appearance is neither sensitive nor specific for an inflammatory process. Approximately 50% to 75% of patients with acute cholecystitis have diffusely thickened gallbladder walls whereas fewer than 25% of patients with chronic cholecystitis have this finding.[3,34-36] In vitro histologic-sonographic correlation of gallbladder walls removed for suspected cholecystitis reveals that the sonographic layers associated with inflammation are determined by a variety of pathologic changes, but that because of overlap of these changes, it is not possible to predict a specific type of gallbladder pathology based on the sonographic appearance of the gallbladder wall.[37]

In addition to **inflammation,** other conditions associated with diffuse gallbladder wall thickening include **hepatic dysfunction** (associated with alco-

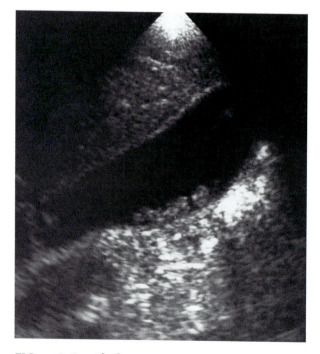

FIG. 6-8. Sludge. Three well-defined echogenic, nonshadowing, dependent sludge balls are present in the gallbladder. These were noted to be mobile on real-time examination. Nonshadowing gallstones, aggregated pus, blood clots, and a variety of other unusual entities could have a similar appearance.

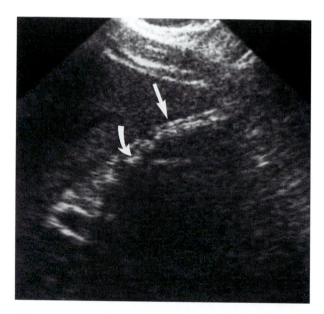

FIG. 6-9. Wall-echo shadow (WES) triad. The gallbladder is filled with multiple stones and may not be visible. Instead, the anterior gallbladder wall *(straight arrows)* may be seen with an adjacent superficial layer of calculi *(curved arrow).* (From Laing FC, Filly RA, Gooding GAW. Ultrasonography of the liver and biliary tract. In: Margulis AR, Burhenne HJ, eds. *Alimentary Tract Radiology.* 4th ed. St Louis: Mosby-Year Book; 1989.)

holism. hypoalbuminemia. ascites. and hepatitis). **congestive heart failure, renal disease, AIDS,** and **sepsis.**[38-42] Although a unifying pathophysiologic mechanism may not explain these diverse disease processes. many of these patients have decreased in-

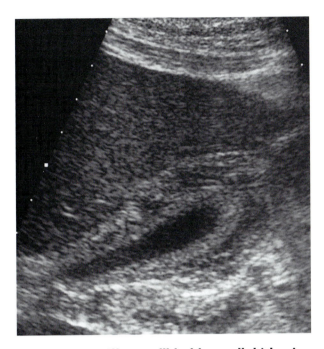

FIG. 6-10. **Diffuse gallbladder wall thickening** circumferentially surrounds the gallbladder in this patient with hepatitis. Note increased echogenicity along the inner wall of the gallbladder *(at the level of the mucosa)*, and striations within the thickened wall.

travascular osmotic pressure and elevated portal venous pressure. In addition. because of the underlying disease processes. many patients with diffuse gallbladder wall thickening also have ascites. Several investigations have suggested that ultrasound may be useful for distinguishing benign from malignant ascites by measuring the thickness of the gallbladder wall.[43-45] Malignant ascites is usually associated with normal gallbladder wall thickness whereas many benign causes are associated with an abnormally thickened gallbladder wall (Fig. 6-11). In the study by Huang et al.[43] a normal gallbladder wall thickness could predict malignant ascites with a sensitivity of 81% and a specificity of 94%.

Unusual causes of gallbladder wall thickening include **leukemic infiltration** of the gallbladder wall.[46] **interleukin-2 chemotherapy,**[47] and **gallbladder wall varices.** In the latter group of patients. serpentine sonolucencies transgress the gallbladder wall. and extrahepatic portal vein thrombosis is present in approximately one third of cases.[48] In suspicious cases, color and duplex Doppler can readily confirm abnormal vascularity within the gallbladder wall.

Although **hepatitis** frequently causes diffuse wall thickening. in exceptional cases there may be profound wall thickening with obliteration of the gallbladder lumen. In some of these unusual cases, paradoxical dilatation of the gallbladder with reduction in wall thickness may occur following administration of fat (Fig. 6-12).[49] The etiology for this unusual response is unclear. but at least in part, it may relate to increased bile flow following a fatty meal.

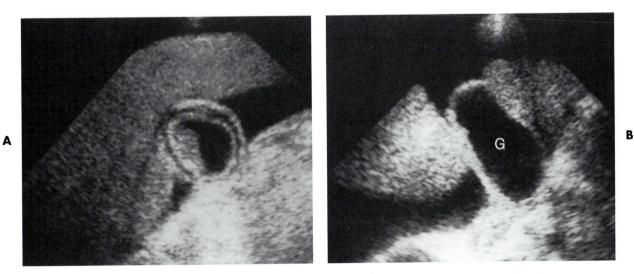

A   B

FIG. 6-11. **Ascites and gallbladder wall thickening.** **A.** Gallbladder wall is abnormally thickened: the patient had chronic liver disease and benign ascites. **B.** The gallbladder *(G)* wall is of normal thickness in this patient with malignant ascites.

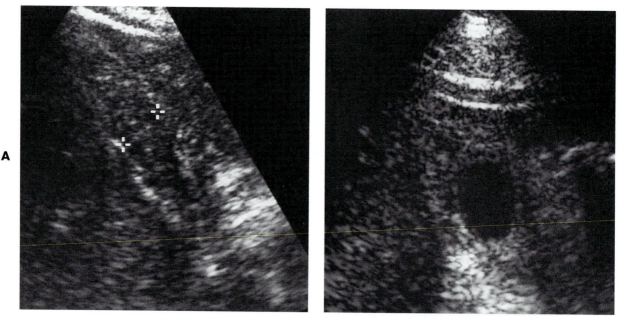

FIG. 6-12. Obliteration of gallbladder lumen associated with hepatitis.
A, Transverse scan, done while the patient was fasting, demonstrates a completely obliterated gallbladder lumen (between gradicules). **B,** A repeat scan done 1 hour after administering a fatty meal reveals paradoxical dilatation of the gallbladder. Note diffuse circumferential thickening of the gallbladder wall.

Generalized gallbladder wall thickening also occurs in the **postprandial state** (see Fig. 6-1). If the maximum diameter of the gallbladder is less than 2 cm and if diffuse wall thickening is present, the sonographer should inquire as to whether the patient fasted appropriately before the ultrasound examination.

In contrast to diffuse gallbladder wall thickening, **focal gallbladder wall thickening** strongly suggests primary gallbladder disease. **Gallbladder carcinoma** has a variety of sonographic appearances. It can present with grossly abnormal findings that include an obvious intraluminal mass (10% to 28%) (Fig. 6-13), asymmetric wall thickening (19% to 47%) (Fig. 6-14), or a mass replacing the gallbladder (28% to 39%) (Fig. 6-15).[50-52] Additional findings include gallbladder wall calcification (4% to 28%), liver metastases, evidence for direct invasion of the liver or adjacent structures (28% to 67%), adenopathy, bile duct dilatation (33% to 38%), and cholelithiasis (19% to 64%)[50-52] (see Figs. 6-13 and 6-14; Fig. 6-16). Because gallbladder carcinoma can mimic other conditions, both clinically and by imaging, particularly complicated cholecystitis (see Fig. 6-14; Fig. 6-17), polyps (Fig. 6-18), and other biliary diseases, the correct diagnosis is initially suggested by ultrasound in only 50% to 61% cases.[50,51] Preliminary work suggests that color and duplex Doppler of gallbladder masses may

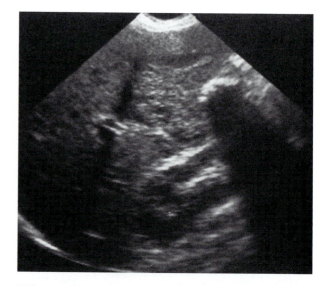

FIG. 6-13. Carcinoma of the gallbladder.
Sagittal sonogram shows a large gallstone that is trapped by a solid mass that completely fills the gallbladder. (Courtesy of Stephanie R. Wilson, M.D., Toronto Hospital, Toronto, Canada.)

be able to differentiate benign or metastatic disease from primary malignant disease by observing an abnormally high arterial velocity originating from either the gallbladder wall or the mass in patients with primary malignancy (Fig. 6-19).[53] For definitive diagnosis, ultrasound-guided fine-needle aspiration

GALLBLADDER CARCINOMA SONOGRAPHIC APPEARANCES

Intraluminal mass
Asymmetric wall thickening
Mass replacing the gallbladder
Gallbladder wall calcification
Cholelithiasis
Liver metastases
Adenopathy
Bile duct dilatation

biopsy of gallbladder masses can be done in a safe and effective manner.[54]

Metastatic nodules are most often due to melanoma (Fig. 6-20),[55,56] gastrointestinal cancer, and breast cancer; less common malignancies include carcinoid tumor[57] and lymphoma.[58] Focal gallbladder wall irregularities may also be seen in patients with complicated or **gangrenous cholecystitis.** These irregularities correspond to areas of mucosal ulceration, hemorrhage, necrosis, and/or microabscess formation.[59] Other causes for focal gallbladder wall thickening include **polyps** (adenomatous, cholesterol) (Fig. 6-21),

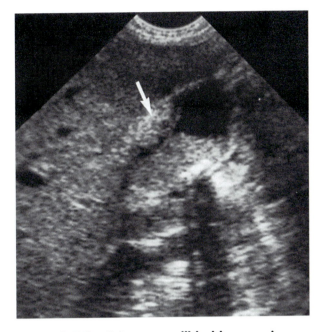

FIG. 6-14. Primary gallbladder carcinoma *(arrow)* seen as localized thickening of the anterior gallbladder wall. The dependent portion of the gallbladder is filled with sludge and numerous small stones. (From Laing FC. Ultrasonography of the gallbladder and biliary tree. In: Sarti DA, ed. *Diagnostic Ultrasound: Text and Cases.* 2nd ed. St Louis: Mosby-Year Book; 1987.)

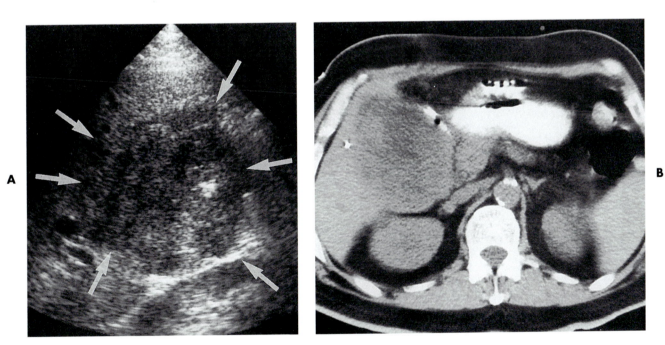

A   B

FIG. 6-15. Gallbladder carcinoma. A. Sagittal sonogram in the expected region of the gallbladder reveals a large, poorly defined heterogeneous mass *(arrows)*. Despite careful scanning, the gallbladder was not visible. **B.** CT examination reveals a large, space-occupying mass in the region of the gallbladder and nonvisualization of the gallbladder.

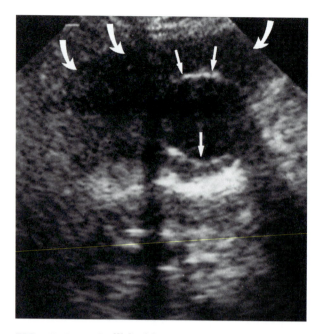

FIG. 6-16. Gallbladder carcinoma. A thin echogenic line appears to outline the gallbladder wall *(arrows)* and is caused by calcification within the wall. In addition, a poorly defined hypoechoic mass surrounds the gallbladder anteriorly and is caused by direct invitation of tumor into the liver *(curved arrows)*.

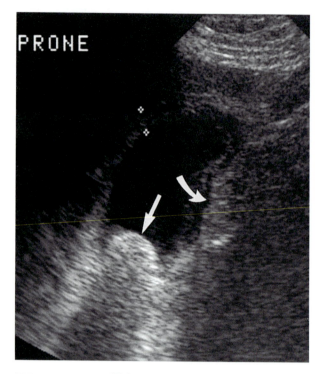

FIG. 6-17. Gallbladder cancer and acute cholecystitis. Prone sagittal scan reveals an impacted stone in the region of the neck of the gallbladder *(arrows)*. There is generalized wall thickening with a slightly more irregular area along one wall *(curved arrow)*. Pathologic examination confirmed this to be invasive gallbladder carcinoma.

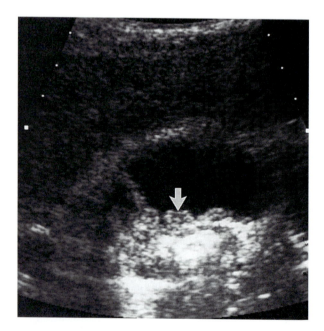

FIG. 6-18. Gallbladder cancer mimicking polyps. Prone sagittal scan reveals three well-defined, nonmobile polypoid masses on the posterior gallbladder wall *(arrow)*. Although the sonographic appearance is not particularly worrisome, pathologic examination revealed polyps with small foci of adenocarcinoma.

papillary adenomas, **adenomyomatosis** (Fig. 6-22), and occasionally, **tumefactive sludge** (Fig. 6-23). Rare conditions include villous hyperplasia[60] and cholecystitis from tuberculosis.[61]

Large (> 10 mm) cholesterol polyps can be successfully differentiated from malignancy by means of endoscopic ultrasound. In a series of 14 patients with large cholesterol polyps, a characteristic endoscopic finding associated with cholesterol was aggregation of echogenic spots; this was absent in all cases of polypoid gallbladder carcinoma (5 cases) or other benign polypoid conditions (4 cases).[62] In patients with adenomyomatosis, anechoic or echogenic foci may sometimes be visible within the thickened gallbladder wall. **Intraluminal diverticula (Rokitansky-Aschoff sinuses or RAS)** that contain bile are most likely to be responsible for the anechoic areas whereas biliary sludge or gallstones within the diverticula are most likely to be responsible for echogenic foci.[63] Not infrequently, a V-shaped reverberation artifact is seen to emanate from small cholesterol stones that are lodged within the sinuses (Fig. 6-24).[64] This artifact occurs as a result of sound reverberating within or between cholesterol crystals and may be similar in appearance to comet-

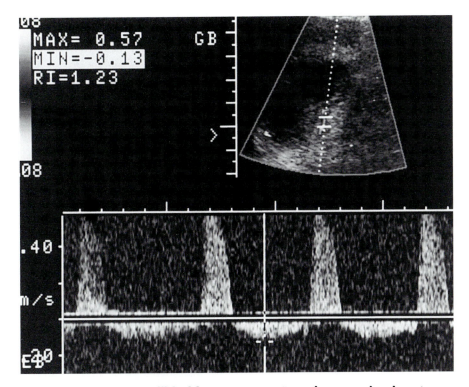

FIG. 6-19. Primary gallbladder cancer on Doppler examination (same patient as in Fig. 6-17). Note the high resistance flow pattern obtained from an area of irregular wall thickening. At surgery, there was acute and chronic cholecystitis, as well as a focal area of invasive adenocarcinoma at the site of gallbladder wall thickening.

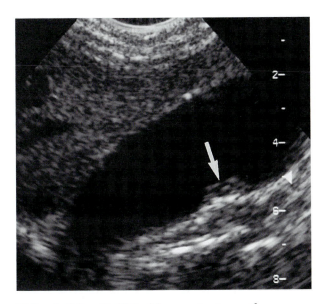

FIG. 6-20. Gallbladder metastases from malignant melanoma. A small area of wall irregularity is evident in this gallbladder *(arrow)* with a wide base of the mass.

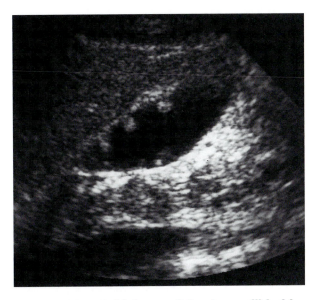

FIG. 6-21. Multiple small benign gallbladder polyps. Well-defined focal masses are visible along the luminal wall of the gallbladder. In comparison with Fig. 6-20, the base of these masses is relatively narrow.

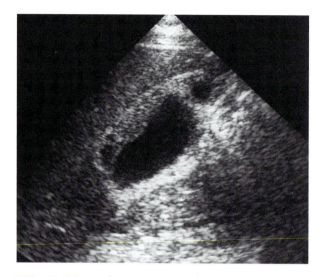

FIG. 6-22. Adenomyomatosis. Note smooth thickening along the anterior wall of the gallbladder and a small round hypoechoic area at the gallbladder fundus. This is one of the characteristic appearances for adenomyomatosis, although other conditions including a neoplasm cannot be completely excluded. (Rokitansky-Aschoff sinuses were not present.)

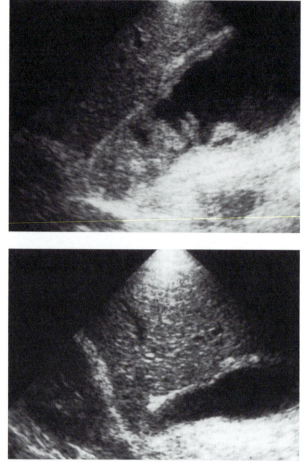

A

B

FIG. 6-23. Tumefactive sludge simulating neoplasm. A, Nonshadowing echogenic material is visible in the gallbladder, and the gallbladder wall appears to be mildly thickened. **B,** Scan obtained 10 days later shows disappearance of this echogenic material.

tail artifacts that occur when there is air in the gallbladder wall. With air, however, the reverberation artifact is usually longer (more comet-tail in appearance as opposed to V-shaped) and the patient is acutely ill.

Sludge. Echogenic bile or sludge is a term used to describe the presence of particulate material (specifically calcium bilirubinate and/or cholesterol crystals) in bile.[65] Unlike gallstones, which generate strong echoes, sludge characteristically displays low- to mid-level echoes (Fig. 6-25). It is never accompanied by posterior acoustic shadowing unless stones are also present (see Fig. 6-14). Because of its viscous nature, sludge moves sluggishly after the patient has been repositioned.

The most frequent predisposing factor associated with sludge is **bile stasis.** This can occur in patients who undergo prolonged fasting or hyperalimentation, as well as in patients with biliary obstruction at the level of the gallbladder, cystic duct, or common bile duct. In a series of fasting patients, ultrasound detected gallbladder sludge in 4% of patients within 5 days after surgery and in 31% of patients within 10 days after surgery.[66] In patients receiving total parenteral nutrition, sludge was uniformly present after 6 weeks of treatment.[67] Under certain circumstances such as following bone marrow transplantation, and for unknown reason(s), sludge has also been shown to develop without impaired gallbladder contractility.[68]

Although gallbladder sludge suggests an underlying abnormality, its presence does not necessarily imply primary gallbladder pathology. The clinical significance of sludge remains uncertain. In rare instances sludge or sludge balls have been observed to develop into gallstones.[68,69] Follow-up ultrasound studies performed on 12 postoperative patients with gallbladder sludge revealed the presence of gallstones in 3 patients who were examined 6 months after their initial surgery.[66] These studies involve limited numbers of patients; further investigation is required to determine whether sludge can irritate the gallbladder mucosa and act as a precursor to stone formation.

Pericholecystic Fluid. Localized pericholecystic fluid is most often attributable to acute cholecystitis complicated by gallbladder perforation and

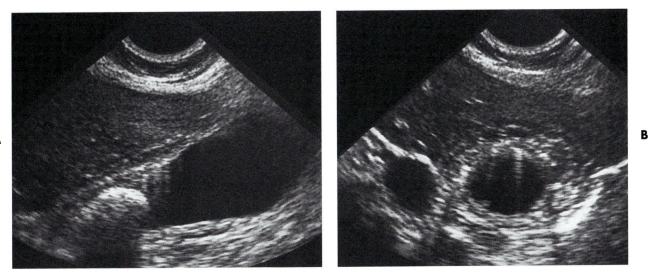

A B

FIG. 6-24. Adenomyomatosis. In this gallbladder, V-shaped reverberation artifacts emanate from anterior wall. This is due to adenomyomatosis with small cholesterol crystals lodged within Rokitansky-Aschoff sinuses. A gallstone is also visible in the neck of the gallbladder. (Courtesy of Stephanie R. Wilson, M.D., Toronto Hospital, Toronto, Canada.)

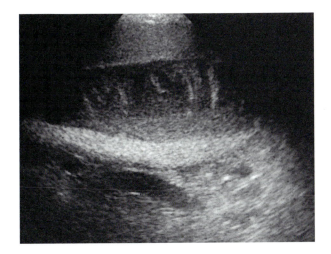

FIG. 6-25. Layering sludge. Echogenic bile or sludge creates two well-defined fluid levels in this gallbladder. The most dependent layer of sludge has the highest echogenicity due to a high concentration of crystalline material; the second layer, which is centrally located, is moderately echogenic. In addition, small amounts of echogenic sludgelike material are also visible in the anterior aspect of the gallbladder where there are vertical linear bandlike echoes probably due to unusual coalescence of sludge.

abscess formation. Ultrasound can diagnose this condition by visualizing an anechoic or complex fluid collection adjacent to or surrounding the gallbladder (Fig. 6-26).[70]

Rarely, an isolated pericholecystic fluid collection can be seen in patients with pancreatitis, peptic ulcer disease, or both (Fig. 6-27).[71] This fluid presumably results from extension of the primary inflammatory process along the hepatoduodenal ligament into the main lobar fissure, where it comes to rest adjacent to the gallbladder neck.

Acute Cholecystitis. Acute cholecystitis occurs in approximately one third of patients who have gallstones and is caused by persistent calculous obstruction of the gallbladder neck or cystic duct. This results in inflammation of the gallbladder wall with variable degrees of necrosis and infection. The physical findings in these patients range from mild to dramatic. Typically, there is some degree of right upper quadrant tenderness and guarding, although with advanced gallbladder inflammation or in elderly patients the findings may suggest diffuse peritonitis, or there may be deceptively few signs and symptoms. The differential diagnosis for acute cholecystitis is extensive and includes pancreatitis, appendicitis, peptic disease, hepatitis, perihepatitis (Fitz-Hugh–Curtis syndrome), liver abscess, or liver neoplasm, as well as renal and even intrathoracic conditions (pneumonia and cardiac disease).

Acute cholecystitis is associated with cholelithiasis in approximately 90% to 95% of patients. In the remaining 5% to 10% of patients in whom acalculous cholecystitis occurs, morbidity and mortality are much greater because this disease frequently complicates a prolonged critical illness. Although many patients with acute right upper quadrant pain are suspected of having acute cholecystitis, only one third are subsequently

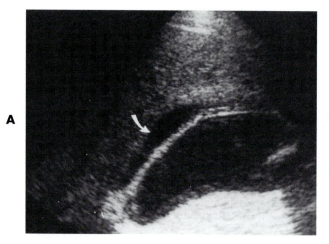

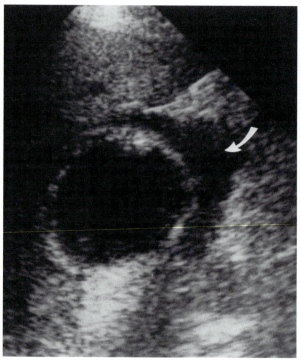

FIG. 6-26. Gangrenous cholecystitis and fundic gallbladder perforation caused localized pericholecystic fluid *(curved arrow)* on longitudinal, **A,** and transverse, **B,** scans. A gallstone is seen in the fundus of the gallbladder. (From Laing FC, Jeffrey RB, Federle MP. Gallbladder and bile ducts. In: Jeffrey RD, ed. *Computed Tomography and Sonography of the Acute Abdomen.* New York: Raven Press; 1989.)

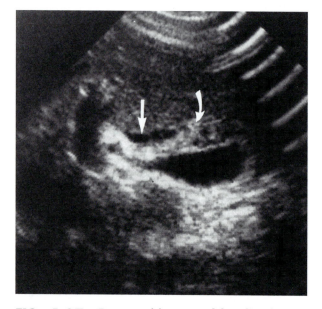

FIG. 6-27. Pancreatitis caused localized pericholecystic fluid anterior to the gallbladder neck *(arrow)* seen on longitudinal sonogram. The gallbladder wall *(curved arrow)* is thickened and irregularly sonolucent. (From Nyberg DA, Laing FC. Ultrasonographic findings in peptic ulcer disease and pancreatitis that simulate primary gallbladder disease. *J Ultrasound Med* 1983;2:303-307.)

SIGNS OF ACUTE CHOLECYSTITIS

Primary signs
Gallstones
Focally tender gallbladder (i.e., sonographic Murphy's sign)
Impacted gallstone (i.e., does not move with position change)

Secondary signs
Gallbladder dilatation
Sludge
Diffuse wall thickening

---

proved to have this disease.[35] Sonography can be used to confirm the diagnosis of acute cholecystitis;[3,35,72] it can distinguish acute from chronic cholecystitis with an accuracy of 95% to 99%,[19-21] and it can frequently suggest nonbiliary causes for the patient's symptoms. Tests using technetium-tagged IDA and IDA-like compounds are also sensitive and accurate for determining whether acute cholecystitis is present,[73] by demonstrating if there is patency of the cystic duct. The presence of a "rim sign," which consists of nonvisualization of the gallbladder with increased pericholecystic hepatic activity, is a useful secondary radionuclide sign that often accompanies severe or complicated cholecystitis.[74,75]

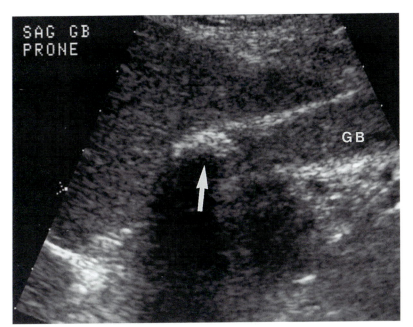

FIG. 6-28. Acute cholecystitis. Prone sagittal scan of the gallbladder shows a large stone in the gallbladder neck *(arrow)* and low-level intraluminal echoes consistent with sludge.

Because the majority of symptomatic patients do not have acute cholecystitis and because nuclear imaging is not as sensitive as ultrasound for making a nonbiliary diagnosis, many authors suggest that nuclear imaging be reserved for patients with equivocal ultrasonograms for the diagnosis of acute cholecystitis.[3,35,72] On the basis of ultrasound, most authorities diagnose **acute cholecystitis** if there are **gallstones** and the gallbladder is **focally tender** (see box on p. 188). A **sonographic Murphy's sign** is present when maximal tenderness is elicited over the sonographically localized gallbladder.[76] In the investigation reported by Ralls et al.[77] a positive sonographic Murphy's sign in conjunction with cholelithiasis had a positive predictive value of 92% for diagnosing acute cholecystitis. In Bree's more recent analysis of the sonographic Murphy's sign to diagnose acute cholecystitis, the positive predictive value and specificity were only 43% and 35%, respectively.[78] Although the reason for the discrepancy between these two reports is not absolutely clear, it is interesting to note that in Bree's investigation, physicians were involved only in questionable cases, and to elicit the sonographic Murphy's sign, the patient was asked to identify the point of maximal tenderness. This is in contrast to Ralls' technique, which relies on sonography to identify the gallbladder and to determine if it is the site of maximal tenderness. Because the sonographic Murphy's sign is a subjective and operator-dependent determination, it is important to rely on the interpretation of an experienced examiner and to use the additional maneuver of transducer palpation to detect the site of maximal tenderness.[35]

As part of the sonographic examination for acute cholecystitis, an effort should also be made to determine if a **stone is impacted** in the gallbladder neck or cystic duct (Fig. 6-28). This frequently necessitates positioning the patient in the prone, decubitus, or other positions to determine whether a calculus moves with gravitational maneuvers. Cystic duct stones are particularly difficult to detect because they are not surrounded by bile, can mimic the appearance of duodenal gas, and may be located several centimeters away from the bile-filled gallbladder.[79] Other **secondary sonographic criteria** that are sensitive but less specific for diagnosing acute cholecystitis include gallbladder dilatation, sludge, and diffuse wall thickening.

Recent interest has centered on color and duplex **Doppler of the cystic artery** in an effort to determine if this can be used to specifically diagnose acute cholecystitis. The rationale for this approach is based on in vitro arteriographic injection of acute calculous cholecystitis specimens that demonstrated arterial dilatation and extensive venous filling.[80] Unfortunately, in vivo Doppler studies of the cystic artery have reported disparate findings. In the investigation of Paulson et al. there was no significant difference in arterial flow when comparing patients with cholecystitis (both acute and chronic) to patients without cholecystitis.[81] This is in contrast to the findings of McGrath and coworkers, who noted diminished blood flow in patients with acute cholecystitis. In the latter investigation, flow was detected in only 10% of patients with acute cholecystitis, as compared with 80% of the control patients.[82] Interestingly, studies done on a canine model with induced acute cholecystitis confirm an initial loss of the vascular signal when compared with the control animals.[83] In contrast to these studies, Jeffrey et al. found that in 26% of patients with acute cholecystitis, there was increased visibility of the cystic artery such that its length exceeded 50% of the length of the anterior gallbladder wall.[84] Furthermore, visualization of the cystic artery at the level of the gallbladder fundus was significant for inflammation, as the artery was not visible at this location in the control population (Fig. 6-29). The practical usefulness of this information is limited, however, by the relatively poor sensitivity for this observation, and the fact that a false positive diagnosis can occur with diseases that increase cystic artery blood flow, such as neoplasm and severe cirrhosis.[53,84] Despite these initially disappointing results, the development of more sensitive Doppler ultrasound equipment and the potential usefulness of ultrasound contrast agents may eventually provide more clinically useful information.

As previously mentioned, acute cholecystitis occurs in only one third of patients with gallstones. The remaining patients are either asymptomatic or develop chronic cholecystitis. On pathologic examination, however, every gallbladder that contains stones will show changes of chronic inflammation (unless it is acutely inflamed). The term **chronic cholecystitis** when used clinically refers to symptomatic but nonacute cholecystolithiasis. These patients complain of

recurrent biliary colic that usually lasts for several hours and is caused by transient obstruction of the gallbladder neck or cystic duct by a stone. The diagnosis is based on the clinical findings; however, if the ultrasound examination shows gallbladder wall thickening that cannot be attributed to nonbiliary causes, the diagnosis can be confirmed on the basis of the sonogram.

Complications of acute cholecystitis include emphysematous and gangrenous cholecystitis as well as perforation. Each of these sequelae is associated with significantly increased morbidity and mortality. Large research series are not available to determine the overall sensitivity and specificity of ultrasound to detect these complications; however, ultrasound can frequently suggest the correct diagnosis.

Emphysematous cholecystitis is a relatively rare form of acute cholecystitis associated with the presence of gas-forming bacteria in the gallbladder. It differs from the usual type of acute cholecystitis in that cholelithiasis is often absent, 38% of patients are diabetic, the male to female ratio is 7:3, and gangrene with associated perforation is five times more common.[85] Gas-forming organisms invade and devitalize the gallbladder wall and release gas into the gallbladder lumen and wall. Emphysematous cholecystitis is a surgical emergency, and the diagnosis can be suggested by its characteristic ultrasound appear-

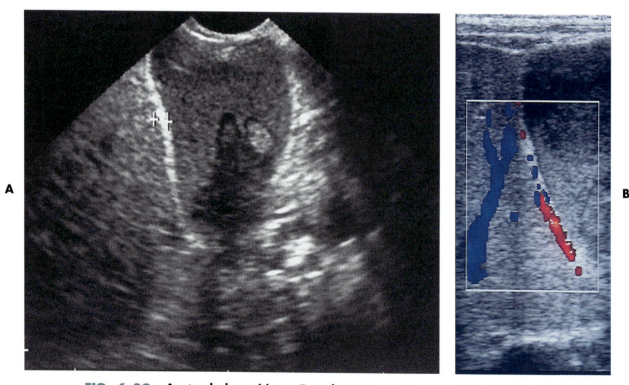

FIG. 6-29. Acute cholecystitis on Doppler. A, Thick gallbladder wall marked by cursors. B, Increased color flow Doppler vascularity in the gallbladder wall. (Courtesy of Stephanie R. Wilson, M.D., Toronto Hospital, Toronto, Canada.)

ance. If the gas is intraluminal, the sonographic image may consist of a prominent nondependent hyperechoic focus with an associated ring down or comet-tail artifact (Fig. 6-30). Intramural gas usually has a semicircular or arc-like configuration.[86,87] If a large amount of gas is present, the appearance may simulate calcification in the gallbladder wall or a gallbladder filled with stones (Fig. 6-31). Strong re-

verberative echoes should not be visible in these conditions, however. Nonetheless, suspected gas collections detected by sonography should be confirmed by either plain film radiography or computed tomography (CT).

The incidence of **gangrenous cholecystitis** ranges from 2% to 38% in patients with acute cholecystitis and is associated with gallbladder perforation in up to 10% of cases.[59] Because of the increased morbidity and mortality with perforation, specific sonographic findings that suggest gangrenous cholecystitis should be sought. In a symptomatic patient, marked irregularity or asymmetric thickening of the gallbladder wall should be viewed with suspicion (Fig. 6-32). According to Jeffrey et al.,[59] this finding was present in approximately 50% of patients and was due to ulceration, hemorrhage, necrosis, and/or microabscesses in the gallbladder wall. Despite the fact that multiple striations within a thickened gallbladder wall in and of itself is not specific for acute cholecystitis, Teefey et al. reported this appearance in 40% of patients with gangrenous cholecystitis, and suggests that when striations are present in a symptomatic patient, the diagnosis of gangrenous cholecystitis should be strongly considered.[88] Intraluminal membranes may also be present and are due to either fibrinous strands or exudate, or necrosis and sloughing of the gallbladder mucosa (Fig. 6-33). As the gallbladder

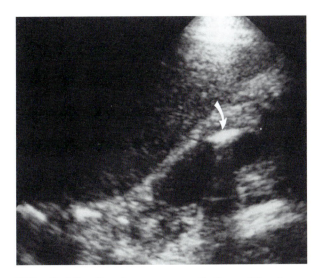

FIG. 6-30. Emphysematous cholecystitis. Intraluminal gas creates a prominent hyperechoic focus with a ring-down artifact *(curved arrow)* in a nondependent position. (From Laing FC, Jeffrey RB, Federle MP. Gallbladder and bile ducts. In: Jeffrey RD, ed. *Computed Tomography and Sonography of the Acute Abdomen.* New York: Raven Press; 1989.)

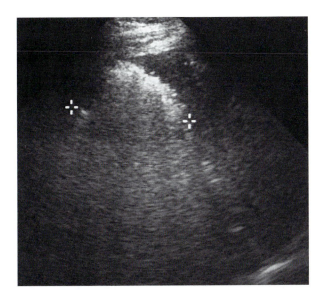

FIG. 6-31. Emphysematous cholecystitis. A prominent area of abnormal echogenicity with gradual acoustic shadowing is present in the right lobe of the liver (between gradicules) because of intraluminal air in the gallbladder.

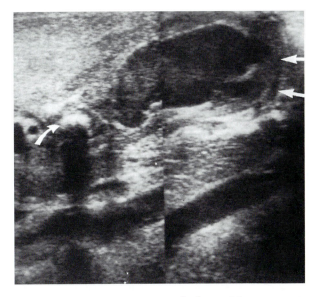

FIG. 6-32. Gangrenous cholecystitis. The gallbladder wall is markedly thickened and irregular in contour in the fundus *(arrows).* A large amount of sludge is also present. The gallbladder neck contains a high-amplitude echo with acoustic shadowing caused by an impacted cystic duct stone *(curved arrow).* (From Laing FC. Ultrasonography of the gallbladder and biliary tree. In: Sarti DA, ed. *Diagnostic Ultrasound: Text and Cases.* 2nd ed. St Louis: Mosby-Year Book; 1987.)

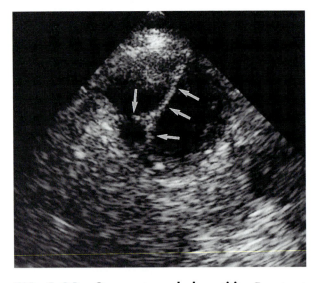

FIG. 6-33. Gangrenous cholecystitis. Prominent intraluminal membranes *(arrows)* due to sloughed mucosa are present in the gallbladder.

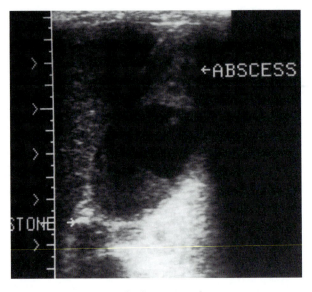

FIG. 6-34. Pericholecystic abscess. A longitudinal scan shows very subtle cystic duct stone and gallbladder sludge. An echogenic collection adjacent to the fundus of the gallbladder is surgically proven abscess.

becomes devitalized by the ravages of gangrenous cholecystitis, the patient's clinical findings paradoxically may shift away from the gallbladder. In a review by Simeone et al.[89] of 18 patients with pathologically proven gangrenous cholecystitis, the sonographic Murphy's sign was positive in only 6 patients (33%), possibly because of denervation of the gallbladder by gangrenous changes. Diffuse abdominal pain was more common (50% of patients), possibly because of generalized peritonitis with inflammation of the parietal peritoneum.

Gallbladder perforation complicates acute cholecystitis in 5% to 10% of cases and is associated with a mortality of 19% to 24%.[90] Niemeier has classified gallbladder perforation into three categories[91]:
- Acute, resulting in generalized peritonitis
- Subacute, resulting in a pericholecystic abscess
- Chronic, resulting in an internal biliary fistula

Most perforations are subacute and result in a pericholecystic abscess adjacent to the fundus (the region with the sparsest blood supply) (Fig. 6-34). In this condition, sonography may demonstrate a complex echogenic pericholecystic fluid collection with septations, or it may totally encompass the gallbladder, resulting in a nonvisible gallbladder.[88,92] Other common but nonspecific findings include a thick, hypoechoic wall and cholelithiasis.[92] Color Doppler may be useful in these cases to detect acute pericholecystic inflammation by demonstrating an echogenic pericholecystic mass that contains internal vascularity.[93] Although this is a relatively uncommon occurrence, noted in only 12 of 40 patients with right upper quadrant inflammatory

lesions (30%), approximately half of the patients with this finding had gangrenous and/or perforated gallbladders; other causes for this finding include perforated ulcers or diverticula.[93] Occasionally, ultrasound may be able to provide a definitive diagnosis by visualizing the actual site of perforation (Fig. 6-35),[94] or it may demonstrate an internal fistula between the gallbladder and adjacent bowel loop.[95] In most cases, however, CT is considered superior to ultrasound for demonstrating the actual site of perforation.[96]

Acalculous cholecystitis is a difficult diagnosis to establish both clinically and by imaging modalities. The accuracy of ultrasound and radionuclide imaging for making the correct diagnosis is significantly less for acalculous than calculous disease. Two major limitations of ultrasound are that gallstones are absent, and many patients have severe intercurrent illnesses that limit the evaluation of the sonographic Murphy's sign. The **sonographic diagnosis,** therefore, depends on gallbladder wall thickening (in the absence of hypoalbuminemia, ascites, congestive heart failure, and so on), pericholecystic fluid or subserosal edema, intraluminal or intramural gas, or sloughed mucosal membranes (Fig. 6-36). Although one investigator has suggested that a complete lack of response to cholecystokinin (CCK) should suggest the diagnosis,[97] this finding is of limited usefulness in postoperative patients because their gallbladders (proven to be normal at surgery) not infrequently also fail to contract following CCK administration.[98] In these challenging cases, if Doppler analysis reveals that the cystic artery length exceeds 50% of the anterior gallbladder wall,

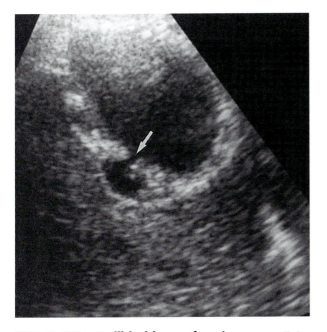

FIG. 6-35. Gallbladder perforation. A small defect is visible in the gallbladder wall at the site of this intrahepatic perforation *(arrow)*. It is unusual for ultrasound to so clearly demonstrate the actual site of perforation.

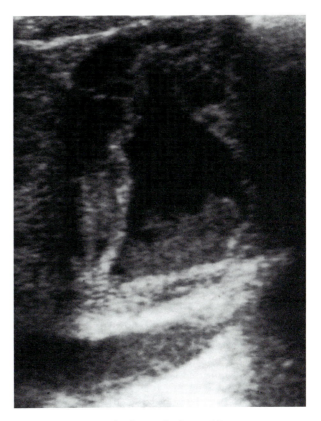

FIG. 6-36. Acalculous cholecystitis. Irregular gallbladder wall thickening and tumefactive sludge are seen.

the diagnosis of acute acalculous cholecystitis should be seriously considered (see Fig. 6-29).[84] Follow-up sonographic examination 24 hours after an initially inconclusive study may also prove useful, especially if the initial examination revealed a normal gallbladder wall thickness. Evaluation of eight such patients demonstrated progressive gallbladder wall thickening in four cases, each of whom had acute acalculous cholecystitis.[99] Before making this diagnosis, however, it is important to exclude other conditions that could result in rapidly progressive gallbladder wall edema (e.g., new onset of congestive heart failure, fluid overload).

Computed tomography is also a useful adjunct to ultrasound for diagnosing acute acalculous cholecystitis. This is primarily because of CT's superior ability to assess pericholecystic inflammation and perforation.[96,100] Although cholescintigraphy has a reported sensitivity of 90% to 95% for diagnosing acalculous cholecystitis on the basis of functional cystic duct obstruction,[97,101] the reported specificity of only 38% limits the usefulness of this study.[97] Despite using morphine augmentation, the false-positive rate (nonvisualization of a noninflamed gallbladder) remains unacceptably high, at approximately 60%.[102] False-positive examinations occur with prolonged hyperalimentation, severe intercurrent illness, and hepatocellular

dysfunction, conditions that are frequently concurrent in patients who are at risk for developing acalculous cholecystitis. Although a negative cholescintigraphic examination (gallbladder visualization) strongly suggests that acalculous cholecystitis is absent, a positive study should be interpreted with caution.

Treatment Options and the Role of Ultrasound

When **extracorporeal shock wave lithotripsy (ESWL)** was first used in 1985 to fragment gallstones, it was hoped that this form of noninvasive therapy would revolutionize the treatment of symptomatic gallstones. Unfortunately, this is not a miracle cure for several reasons. The first is that based on eligibility criteria (a functioning gallbladder and fewer than three noncalcified stones, each less than 30 mm in diameter), only 15% of patients qualify for this therapy.[103] Second, the equipment is relatively expensive and not universally available. In addition, follow-up gallbladder sonography reveals that the majority of patients undergoing this treatment have retained stone fragments at 6 and 12 months following initial therapy.[104] There is also a risk for stone recurrence, and many patients are required to be on adjunctive bile salt therapy.[105] Finally, the overwhelming acceptance of laparoscopic cholecystectomy has greatly reduced the patient population desiring ESWL. Nonetheless, despite being relegated to a secondary role, in selected cases this procedure remains attractive because it can be done on an outpatient basis and without general anesthesia. Ultrasound remains a central imaging modality for ESWL to diagnose and measure the stone burden, to monitor the appearance of the gallbladder at the time of treatment, and for long-term follow-up evaluation.

Ultrasound plays several roles in treatment of patients who are candidates for **laparoscopic cholecystectomy.** Preoperative screening of the gallbladder and bile ducts is useful because: (1) if small gallstones are present, preoperative endoscopic retrograde cholangiopancreatography (ERCP) or intraoperative cholangiography should be considered because of the propensity of these patients to have choledocholithiasis; (2) if the bile duct is dilated or if choledocholithiasis is identified, preoperative ERCP or operative bile duct exploration is probably warranted; (3) if a large gallstone is identified, to facilitate its removal, the conventional 1 cm umbilical incision may require enlargement; (4) if sonography detects gangrenous changes in the gallbladder, open cholecystectomy should be considered; and (5) other unsuspected upper abdominal pathology may be discovered that may influence the operative approach.[93,106-109]

Laparoscopic ultrasound probes have recently become available, and they may prove useful as an alternative to operative cholangiography.[110,111] In addition to detecting choledocholithiasis, unsuspected anatomic variations may be discovered. For example, by determining the length and precise insertion site of the cystic duct, or by evaluating an aberrant or accessory artery, iatrogenic complications such as transection of the common bile duct will hopefully decrease. Significant **postoperative complications** that can be evaluated by ultrasound relate to either the laparoscopic procedure (hematomas), and/or to the cholecystectomy (bilomas, abscesses, and biliary dilatation due to bile duct ligation, transection, or choledocholithiasis).[112,113] Transient and insignificant postoperative findings include borderline to mild common duct dilatation and small fluid collections in approximately 25% and 50% of patients, respectively.[114,115]

Because critically ill patients with suspected acute cholecystitis (both calculous and acalculous) may not be suitable candidates for surgery, and because percutaneous bile aspiration is falsely negative in more than half of the patients for both Gram stain and bile culture results,[116] emergency **percutaneous cholecystostomy** should be considered on these patients.[117-121] Most authorities prefer to use ultrasound guidance for this procedure and recommend a transhepatic approach to minimize bile leakage.[118-122] In

McGahan's experience, ultrasound was able to successfully guide transhepatic placement of a drainage catheter into the gallbladder 97.5% of the time (39 of 40 attempted procedures).[122] This approach may be life saving and should be considered as an alternative in patients who are unable to tolerate emergency cholecystectomy. In addition to being successful, this is a low-risk procedure with only 1 reported death directly due to catheter placement, in more than 200 reported cases.[122]

Pitfalls

Despite using high-resolution equipment and small footprint transducers to examine the gallbladder, occasional problems still arise.[123] One source of confusion involves the definitive diagnosis of cholelithiasis. **Shadows** that appear to arise from the gallbladder neck are a common source of diagnostic confusion. Because refraction from the edge of the gallbladder is associated with shadowing, it is mandatory to visualize the stone (not merely the shadow) before diagnosing cholelithiasis. Similarly, shadowing posterior to the gallbladder that originates from within the bowel should not be misinterpreted as being suggestive of primary gallbladder pathology (Fig. 6-37). Scanning after repositioning the patient in the prone or right lateral decubitus position often makes it technically easier to prove the presence of a stone. This is because repositioning causes the stone to move away from the adjacent bowel gas.

Anatomic variations in the appearance and shape of the gallbladder can also create diagnostic difficulties. Rarely, if an **enteric duplication cyst** is strategically located next to the gallbladder, it can resemble a bilobed gallbladder (see Fig. 6-5; Fig. 6-38). **Folds** that are present normally in the gallbladder can cause confusing echoes that may be associated with posterior acoustic shadowing. The junctional fold, located between the body and infundibulum of the gallbladder, and folds from the valves of Heister located in the region of the gallbladder neck are two common anatomic sites that can cause echoes that mimic stones (see Fig. 6-4; Fig. 6-39). Scanning following deep inspiration will often make these folds less apparent, especially those in the region of the junctional zone. In addition, if the patient is not acutely symptomatic and if the gallbladder is not distended, echoes that arise from the neck and the region of the valves of Heister should be viewed with suspicion because they are not likely to represent impacted gallstones.

A false-positive diagnosis of gallbladder pathology can also be made if the gallbladder is **physiologically contracted** and the gastric antrum/duodenum contains material that causes an appearance that mimics an abnormal gallbladder. In particular, it can resemble a gallbladder containing milk of calcium, or

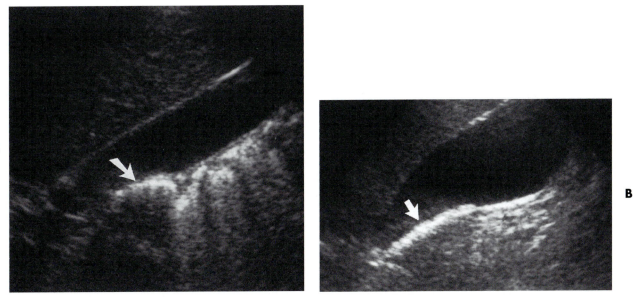

FIG. 6-37. Pitfall—bowel gas. A, Longitudinal scan shows echogenic shadowing in the region of the gallbladder neck *(arrow)*. This appearance, caused by bowel gas, may resemble subtle stones. **B,** In a different patient, an echogenic region *(arrow)* is seen on a longitudinal scan near the neck of the gallbladder. This was due to small gallstones.

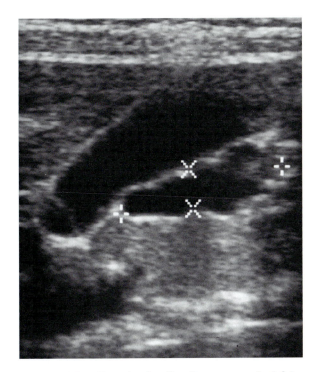

FIG. 6-38. Enteric duplication cyst mimicking gallbladder duplication. This is an unusual example because in this strategic location it mimics a bilobed gallbladder (see Fig. 6-5).

one that is filled with stones (Fig. 6-40). The latter appearance can mimic the WES triad or double arc shadow sign. Careful observation using real-time equipment and the administration of water is often required to evaluate these questionable cases. Other disorders that can mimic this appearance include a **porcelain gallbladder, emphysematous cholecystitis, milk of calcium bile,** and **gallbladder wall microabscesses.**[123] Clinical correlation, plain film radiology, and even CT may be necessary to determine the cause(s) for these sonographic findings. Rarely, particulate material may enter the gallbladder through a spontaneous or surgically created gastrointestinal fistula and may be responsible for a false-positive diagnosis of cholelithiasis.[124,125]

Although the great majority of gallstones have a classic sonographic appearance, sometimes **atypical calculi** are encountered. In almost all cases the anterior surface of gallstones is round or slightly faceted, but in unusual cases they may be pyramidal in shape, thereby imparting an unusual contour to the anterior surface of the stone (Fig. 6-41).[126] Stones either adherent to or within the gallbladder wall can be confusing because they may mimic focal air or calcification within the gallbladder wall or cholesterol polyps (cholesterolosis). These entities can sometimes be distinguished from one another by plain film radiographs, although in special circumstances CT may be required. If cholelithiasis is encountered in a patient receiving the third generation antibiotic ceftriaxone, it may represent **"pseudolithiasis"** because this drug complexes with calcium bile salts to form a precipitate that can mimic gallstones on sonographic examination.[127] Most of these patients do not develop symptoms that are referable to their gallbladder, and follow-up sonography reveals complete resolution of these precipitates with cessation of therapy.[128]

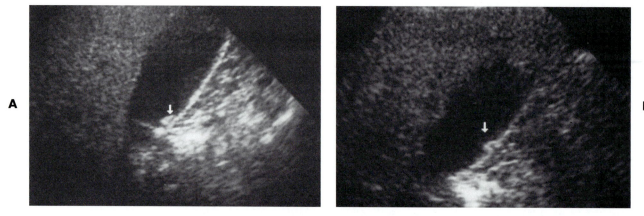

FIG. 6-39. Nonshadowing stone mimicking a junctional fold. A. Supine longitudinal scan reveals an echogenic focus near the gallbladder neck *(arrow)* without acoustic shadowing. **B.** After repositioning the patient into an erect position, the echogenic focus demonstrated mobility *(arrow)* confirming the presence of a small nonshadowing gallstone.

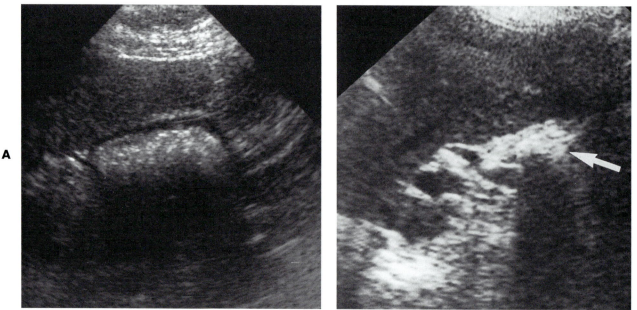

FIG. 6-40. Stomach mimics milk of calcium bile or cholelithiasis. A. Echogenic, gradually shadowing material simulates intracholecystic milk of calcium (see Fig. 6-47, *A*). The gallbladder was physiologically contracted and could not be identified. In each case, a repeat scan with the patient fasting revealed a normal gallbladder. **B.** Emergency longitudinal scan in another nonfasting patient with acute right upper quadrant pain reveals a region of acoustic shadowing *(arrow)* suggestive of a gallbladder filled with stones.

Normally, calculi are located in a dependent position within the gallbladder because their specific gravity exceeds that of bile. Rarely, however, the specific gravity of bile exceeds that of calculi, causing **gallstones to float in bile** (Fig. 6-42). The nondependent position for calculi was initially attributed to the presence of oral cholecystographic contrast material within bile.[129] It is now known that **cholesterol stones** and those **containing gas fissures** can also be observed to float.[130-132]

Echoes produced by gallstones are usually high in amplitude. Occasionally, however, they are less echogenic than expected (Fig. 6-43). This appearance occurs most often in patients with soft pigment stones that have a mudlike consistency. These calculi are unusual in the gallbladder, but are common in the intrahepatic and extrahepatic biliary tree. In addition, they are seen in patients with recurrent pyogenic cholangiohepatitis.[133] These stones may have an appearance that is identical to tumefactive sludge (see Fig. 6-8)[26] or

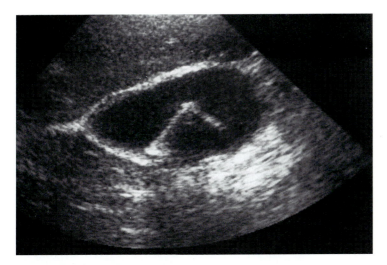

FIG. 6-41. Atypical gallstone. Instead of a round anterior surface, this unusual gallstone has a pyramidal shape. Chemical analysis revealed that it contained a variety of chemical components, including cholesterol and bilirubin.

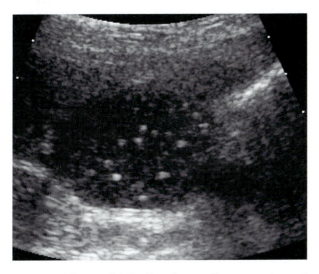

FIG. 6-42. Multiple floating gallstones. Sagittal sonogram.

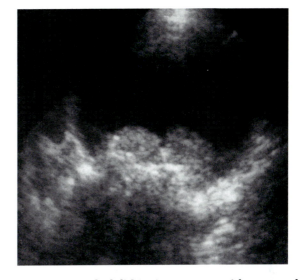

FIG. 6-43. Cholelithiasis—stones with unusual morphology. These gallstones cast acoustic shadows but are less echogenic than usual. Although this appearance may occur with soft, calcium bilirubinate pigment stones, in this patient CT suggested the stones were composed primarily of cholesterol. (From Laing FC, Filly RA, Gooding GAW. Ultrasonography of the liver and biliary tract. In: Margulis AR, Burhenne HJ, eds. *Alimentary Tract Radiology*. 4th ed. St Louis: Mosby-Year Book; 1989.)

even to a focal mass that protrudes into the gallbladder lumen (see Figs. 6-18 and 6-20). The degree to which pigment stones cast acoustic shadows also ranges widely from none to dramatic.

In a small percentage of patients, despite the use of optimal equipment and scanning techniques, neither the gallbladder nor shadowing from its fossa is seen (see box). In most of these cases the gallbladders are abnormal with an obliterated lumen (Fig. 6-44). Rarely, the gallbladder may be difficult to detect because it is filled with sludge that is isoechoic with liver parenchyma (Fig. 6-45).[134] Other causes for **gallbladder nonvisualization** include physiologic contraction, contractions associated with acute and severe hepatitis, congenital absence of the gallbladder, an unusually positioned gallbladder, or technical error.[49,135,136] In these situations, oral cholecystography or technetium-IDA imaging should be done as a confirmatory examination because the gallbladder will sometimes prove normal despite nonvisualization

SONOGRAPHIC NONVISUALIZATION OF THE GALLBLADDER:

CONSIDER

Obliterated gallbladder lumen
Sludge, isoechoic to liver, obscuring margins of gallbladder
Physiologic contraction
Contractions from acute, severe hepatitis
Congenital absence of gallbladder
Unusual position of gallbladder
Technical error

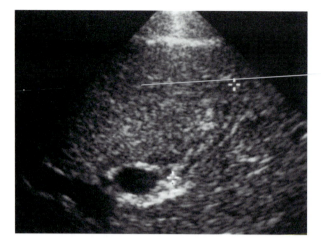

FIG. 6-44. Abnormally contracted gallbladder with an obliterated lumen *(between cursors)*. The anatomic position and shape and the fact that it did not appear to communicate with the bowel following the administration of water suggest that the cause of this unusual echogenic region is an abnormally contracted gallbladder.

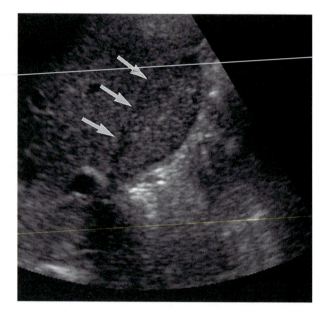

FIG. 6-45. Sludge-filled gallbladder. Sludge, isoechoic with hepatic parenchymal tissue, makes the gallbladder difficult to detect *(arrows)*. This appearance has been termed hepatization of the gallbladder.

by sonography. As previously discussed, a fatty meal can be administered in cases of severe acute hepatitis to determine if paradoxical distention of the gallbladder will occur.[49]

Sludgelike intraluminal echoes can also be a source of confusion. Both pus and blood within the gallbladder lumen can appear identical to biliary sludge. As more interventional biliary procedures and liver biopsies are performed, the incidence of hemobilia may be increasing. This can result in intracholecystic blood that in most cases resembles tumefactive as opposed to bland sludge (Fig. 6-46).[137] Patient history may be critical for evaluating the source of these echoes. Tumefactive sludge also may cause diagnostic difficulty because it can resemble either soft pigment stones or an intraluminal mass. Unlike true stones, it does not shadow and moves slowly when the patient is repositioned. Gravity dependence should be a distinguishing feature between sludge and neoplasm, but it is not always possible to demonstrate motion reliably in cases of tumefactive sludge (see Fig. 6-23).[26] A repeat examination performed several days later can usually differentiate between these two entities because tumefactive sludge will either disappear or change in appearance whereas a neoplasm will remain unchanged.

Milk of calcium or **limy bile** results in a variety of sonographic appearances.[138,139] Both an echogenic flat fluid-fluid level and a convex shadowing meniscus pattern have been reported. Occasionally the echogenicity of milk of calcium resembles sludge, although it can be distinguished from sludge by the presence of gradual acoustic shadowing (Fig. 6-47).

An unusual but potentially confusing cause of intracholecystic echoes is **parasitic infestation.** In the case

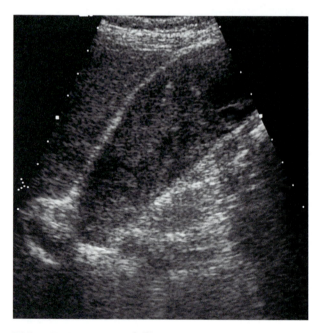

FIG. 6-46. Hemobilia. Heterogeneously echogenic material almost completely fills the gallbladder lumen. This patient had a coagulopathy due to chronic liver disease and had recently undergone a liver biopsy.

of the **trematode, *Fasciola,*** humans who live in Central or Eastern Europe and ingest water or watercress that contains the encysted larva may become an intermediate host. In the acute stage the liver is involved, and CT scanning may demonstrate peripheral tortuous lesions due to migratory tracts left by the flukes. In the chronic stage the parasite may invade the

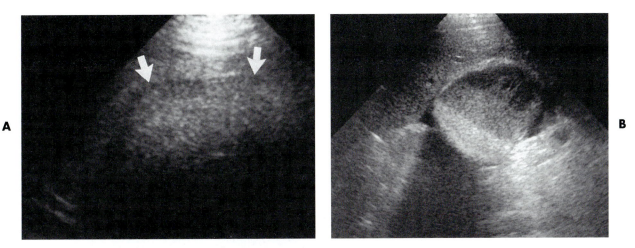

FIG. 6-47. Milk of calcium bile. A, The gallbladder is filled with isoechoic material *(arrows)*, and posterior acoustic shadowing is present. B, In another patient, there is prominent posterior acoustic shadowing behind what appears to be layering sludge. Although very small gallstones could have a similar appearance, sludge should never cause acoustic shadowing.

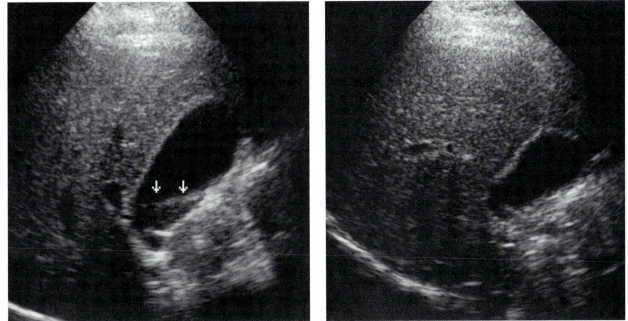

FIG. 6-48. Side-lobe artifacts. A, Sagittal scan of the gallbladder shows what appears to be a fluid level *(arrows)*, mimicking biliary sludge. B, The artifactual echoes disappear when the output setting is decreased. Alternative methods to eliminate this side-lobe artifact include changing the angle of the transducer and repositioning the patient such that the gallbladder falls away from adjacent gas-filled structures.

biliary tree and migrate into the gallbladder where it may be visible as an oval or leaf-shaped structure whose length ranges from 15 to 40 mm.[140,141] The roundworm, *Ascaris lumbricoides,* has a worldwide distribution and is the most frequent helminthic infection in humans. This worm typically lives in the intestine, but may migrate through the ampulla of Vater into the biliary tree. Owing to the length, tortuosity, and narrow diameter of the cystic duct, migration into the gallbladder

occurs but is rare.[142,143] Clinical symptoms can mimic acute cholecystitis. Sonography will reveal a nonshadowing intracystic wormlike structure that may be mobile; its shape varies depending on its position so that it may be either linear (40 to 70 mm in length) or coiled.

Occasionally, **artifacts** may be responsible for intraluminal, dependent, low-level echoes. Most often, these are due to either **slice-thickness or side-lobe artifacts** (Fig. 6-48).[144,145] Slice-thickness artifacts result from a partial volume effect and occur when a portion of the ultrasound beam interacts with the fluid-filled gallbladder lumen, while an adjacent portion of the beam interacts with a true-echo reflector. These artifactual echoes can be minimized by using a narrow sound beam focused at the level of the gallbladder and by scanning through the gallbladder's central portion.[144]

Side-lobe artifacts are caused by transducer side lobes interacting with highly reflective acoustic surfaces, such as duodenal gas located adjacent to the gallbladder. These echoes, which appear to originate within the main ultrasound beam, can be minimized by repositioning the patient so the gallbladder falls away from the adjacent gas-filled structures, by changing the angulation of the transducer, or by decreasing machine intensity.[145] Because slice-thickness and side-lobe artifacts are independent of gravity, "pseudo-sludge" will not layer with changes in patient position, unlike true sludge.

Gallbladder wall thickening is usually categorized as diffuse or focal. As previously discussed, diffuse thickening may be associated with primary gallbladder disease whereas focal wall changes are usually caused by underlying gallbladder pathology. Occasionally, however, focal gallbladder wall changes occur in patients who do not have gallbladder disease. Dilatation of the cystic veins in association with portal hypertension or extrahepatic portal vein obstruction can make the gallbladder wall look unusual because of varices located in its outer layers.[48,146] Real-time images reveal dilated tortuous vessels in the adventitial layers surrounding the gallbladder. These vessels are visible on both the peritoneal surface of the gallbladder as well as in the gallbladder bed adjacent to the liver and may protrude into the gallbladder lumen. The vascular nature of the abnormality is usually evident, and color Doppler can readily confirm the presence of varices.[147]

Edema localized to the gallbladder fossa (Fig. 6-49) may be erroneously diagnosed as gallbladder wall thickening. Careful scanning reveals that the only portion of the gallbladder wall that appears thickened is in contact with the undersurface of the liver. This appearance is nonspecific, and in our experience is usually caused by pancreatitis with inflammation that ascends the hepatoduodenal ligament. As a result, edematous changes occur in the region of the porta hepatis[71] or in the gallbladder fossa.

INTRAHEPATIC BILE DUCTS

Normal Anatomy

Because sonography can be used to identify and trace tubular fluid-filled structures, it is an ideal modality

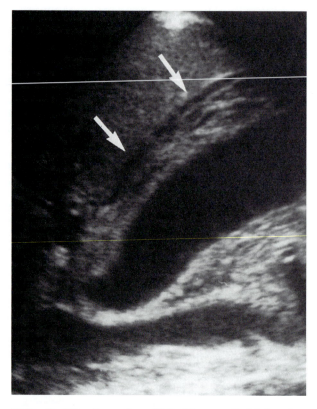

FIG. 6-49. Pseudogallbladder wall thickening caused by edema in the gallbladder fossa from acute pancreatitis. The apparent gallbladder thickening is localized to that portion of the gallbladder wall that is in contact with the undersurface of the liver (arrows).

for evaluating dilated intrahepatic bile ducts. With the advent of newer electronically focused equipment, it is now possible to see intrahepatic structures that represent normal bile ducts and/or hepatic arteries.[148] These tubular structures are considered normal if they are 2 mm or less in diameter, or not more than 40% of the diameter of the accompanying portal vein.[148] It is also routinely possible to visualize the normal right and left hepatic ducts, which are extrahepatic and do not lie within hepatic parenchyma. They course in the porta hepatis with the undivided portion of the right portal vein or initial segment of the left portal vein, respectively.

Dilated Intrahepatic Bile Ducts

Based on gray-scale imaging, four criteria enable intrahepatic bile ducts to be easily differentiated from portal veins.[149] The most reliable differentiating feature is detection of an **alteration in the normal appearance of the portal triads** (Fig. 6-50). This alteration of anatomy, which occurs in virtually all patients with generalized intrahepatic bile duct dilatation, is best seen on transverse scans of the right

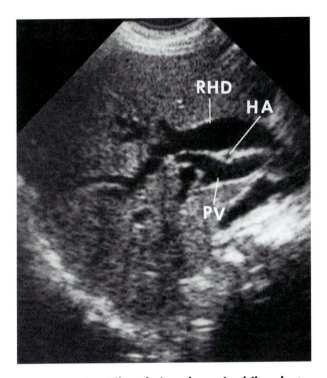

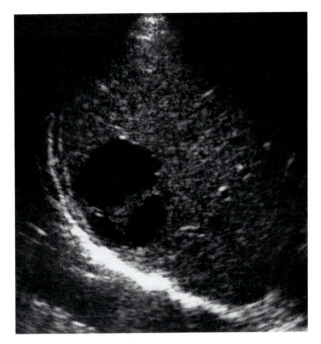

FIG. 6-51. Biliary cystadenoma. Several thick septations, which are characteristic for a cystadenoma, were evident in this incidentally discovered neoplasm.

FIG. 6-50. Dilated intrahepatic bile ducts. Oblique scan parallel to the long axis of the right portal vein shows the convergence of dilated intrahepatic bile ducts entering the dilated right hepatic duct, *RHD*. The portal vein, *PV*, is posterior and seen as a separate structure. Between the right hepatic duct and portal vein is a small circular lucency, the right hepatic artery, *HA*. (From Laing FC, Ultrasonography of the gallbladder and biliary tree. In: Sarti DA, ed. *Diagnostic Ultrasound: Text and Cases.* 2nd ed. St Louis: Mosby-Year Book; 1987.)

hepatic lobe, where the dilated intrahepatic bile ducts accompany the anterior and posterior divisions of the right portal vein. Despite the fact that the bile ducts may be anterior, posterior, or tortuous relative to the corresponding portal vein branches, the intrahepatic anatomic changes that occur with bile duct dilatation remain readily recognizable.[150,151]

The other sonographic features that characterize intrahepatic bile duct dilatation are **irregularity of the walls of dilated bile ducts, a central stellate confluence of tubular structures,** and **acoustic enhancement posterior to dilated ducts.**[149] These secondary findings are visible in approximately one half to two thirds of patients with diffuse intrahepatic biliary dilatation, and are usually most apparent with moderate to severe dilatation. If the gray-scale findings are subtle or questionable, color Doppler should be used to confirm bile duct dilatation.[152] Because the structures within the portal triads are often perpendicular to the Doppler signal with the patient supine, it may be advantageous to turn the patient into an oblique position, or to angle the Doppler signal to optimize the Doppler angle. Since it is less angle depen-

dent, power Doppler may also be advantageous in difficult cases.[153]

Pathology

In the great majority of cases, changes in the intrahepatic bile ducts occur secondary to extrahepatic bile duct obstruction. Occasionally, however, intrahepatic pathology is responsible for the biliary changes.

Intrahepatic Biliary Neoplasms. These are relatively rare and almost without exception are limited to **cystadenoma** and its malignant counterpart, **cystadenocarcinoma.** These tumors usually occur in middle-aged women who present with abdominal pain, mass, and/or jaundice. Their typical appearance is similar to ovarian cystadenoma (cystadenocarcinoma) in that the tumors are cystic masses with multiple septae and, frequently, papillary excrescences (Fig. 6-51).[154] Variations can occur with occasional tumors described as unilocular, calcified, or multiple. The **differential diagnosis** includes cysts complicated by hemorrhage or infection, echinococcal cyst, abscess, hematoma, or cystic metastasis. Cyst aspiration should be considered to differentiate a primary biliary neoplasm from other causes, but surgical resection is necessary to distinguish a benign cystadenoma from a cystadenocarcinoma. Primary bile duct carcinoma (**cholangiocarcinoma**) is rarely confined to the intrahepatic ducts unless the patient is predisposed by infection with the liver fluke *Opisthorchis viverrini*.[155] Affected individuals who frequently live in northeastern Thailand develop tumors whose appearance mimics hepatocellular carcinoma. In a report of 107 patients with peripheral cholangiocarcinoma, the most typical sonographic finding, found in 78% of patients, was a solitary mass that was of either mixed or increased echogenicity. The remaining patients had multiple masses, or infiltrating tumors. The right hepatic lobe was involved in 80% of cases, and peripheral bile duct dilatation was detected 31% of the time.[155]

Sclerosing and AIDS Cholangitis.
These two entities can have intrahepatic bile duct changes that are virtually identical on sonography. Clinically, more than 50% of patients with sclerosing cholangitis have ulcerative colitis. Liver function tests typically reveal markedly obstructive liver chemistries (increased alkaline phosphatase and bilirubin), while imaging demonstrates relatively minimal luminal bile duct dilatation. In both of these conditions, sonography may reveal smooth or irregular wall thickening of the intrahepatic bile ducts.[156-158] In some cases the wall thickening may be marked, such that it compromises the lumen of the bile duct (Fig. 6-52). In approximately 25% of patients with primary sclerosing cholangitis, the intrahepatic ducts appear falsely normal by ultrasound. Cholangiographic comparison reveals multiple strictures and pruning, but no dilatation.[159] Although in theory, primary or metastatic tumors may have a similar appearance, cholangitis usually involves the bile ducts in a more generalized fashion.

Intrahepatic Biliary Calculi.
Intrahepatic biliary calculi are uncommon in patients with gallstones, but characteristically occur in patients with **recurrent pyogenic cholangitis (RPC)**.[133] This condition has a variety of names, including **Oriental cholangiohepatitis, intrahepatic pigment stone disease,** and **biliary obstruction syndrome of the Chinese.** Although extremely common in Asia, RPC can occur in any patient with prolonged bile stasis. In many cases of RPC, bile stasis develops because of biliary parasites *(Clonorchis sinensis* or *Ascaris lumbricoides).*[160] This contributes to infection (especially with coliform organisms), which in turn causes bile to deconjugate and results in precipitates of calcium bilirubinate pigment crystals that form soft, mudlike stones. In contrast to extrahepatic cholesterol stones seen in the western hemisphere, in Asia intrahepatic pigment stones tend to form in younger patients, with no sexual preference. The stones are usually multiple and develop in the intrahepatic and extrahepatic ductal system (Figs. 6-53 and 6-54).[161] Not infrequently, they form a cast of the biliary tree. The lateral segment of the left lobe is the most common site of involvement, and intrahepatic ductal dilatation typically involves the first and second order branches. This distribution may be due to relatively more profound bile stasis in this anatomic distribution.[133,162] Because these ducts may be completely obstructed, cholangiographic visualization (retrograde and/or antegrade) may be unsuccessful; in these difficult cases sonography is often successful to precisely

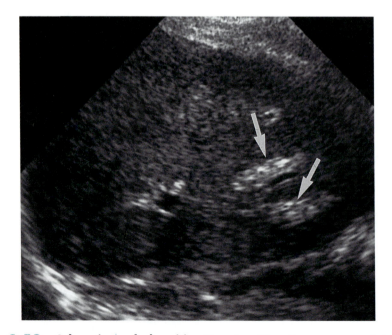

FIG. 6-52. Sclerosing cholangitis. Two bandlike linear areas of increased echogenicity *(arrows)* are visible in the hepatic parenchyma. Most likely this represents thickened bile duct walls that compromise the lumen of the ducts.

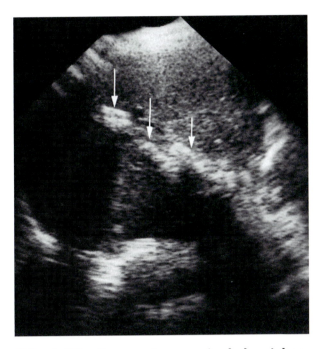

FIG. 6-53. Recurrent pyogenic cholangiohepatitis (RPC). Longitudinal scan shows multiple high-amplitude echoes *(arrows)* with acoustic shadowing caused by intrahepatic biliary calculi. (From Laing FC. Ultrasound diagnosis of choledocholithiasis. *Sem Ultrasound CT MR* 1987;8:103-113.)

delineate the site and degree of pathology.[163] Sonography reveals these stones to have a dramatic range of appearances. They can be of moderate echogenicity and lack acoustic shadowing, in which case they can mimic sludge, pus, blood, or even a biliary neoplasm. With very large stones, acoustic shadowing frequently predominates and results in a dramatic appearance that obliterates visualization of the bile ducts in a manner similar to a gallbladder filled with small stones.[161] Because ultrasound is often used as the initial examination, it is important for sonographers to recognize the varied appearances of this disease process. In contrast to patients with choledocholithiasis caused by gallstone disease, surgical treatment differs considerably in these patients. If RPC is suggested by sonography, CT should usually be obtained preoperatively because the results may complement the sonographic findings and allow more precise delineation of the ductal system.

Sonography is limited in patients with RPC who have undergone biliary-enteric anastomoses. This is because reflux of gas into the biliary tree can obscure and/or mimic intrahepatic calculi (Fig. 6-55). In addition, gas-containing abscesses, a rather common complication in patients with this condition, may also be obscured.

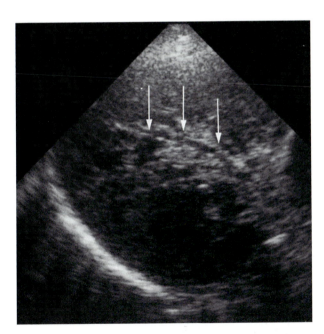

FIG. 6-54. Recurrent pyogenic cholangiohepatitis. Nonshadowing intraductal echogenic material *(arrows)* is due to soft pigment stones. Biliary sludge could have an identical appearance. (From Laing FC. Ultrasound diagnosis of choledocholithiasis. *Sem Ultrasound CT MR* 1987;8:103-113.)

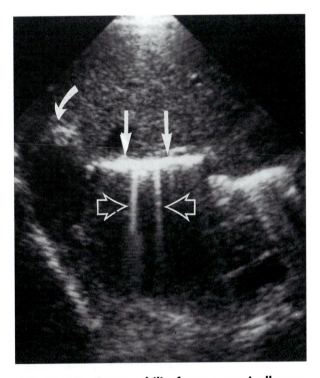

FIG. 6-55. Pneumobilia from a surgically created biliary enteric anastomosis. Intensely echogenic linear foci due to air in the biliary tree *(arrows)*. Comet-tail artifacts *(open arrows)* are also present. This patient (with recurrent pyogenic cholangitis) also has intrahepatic biliary calculi *(curved arrow)*. Pneumobilia may mask the presence of intrahepatic stones.

Caroli's Disease. Caroli's disease is a congenital abnormality that is most likely inherited in an autosomal recessive fashion. A recent review defines two distinct forms of this disease.[164] The originally described "pure" form can occur in a focal or diffuse manner and is characterized by saccular, communicating intrahepatic bile duct ectasia. Complications include pyogenic cholangitis, hepatic abscess, intrahepatic biliary obstruction and calculi, and in 7% of cases the development of cholangiocarcinoma. In the pure form of this disease a variety of imaging modalities, including ultrasound, have been used to demonstrate and prove the existence of diverticulum-like sacculi of the intrahepatic biliary tree (Fig. 6-56). Communication between the sacs and bile ducts is important to distinguish this condition from polycystic liver disease. Because the sacs often have either a characteristic bulge on one wall, a central dot, or a linear bridging structure that contains a portal vein and hepatic artery radical, Doppler can be used to show the relationship of these vascular structures to the sac itself.[164,165]

The second form of Caroli's disease presents in childhood, has relatively less bile duct dilatation, and is associated with hepatic fibrosis that results in portal hypertension and terminal liver failure. Associated conditions include choledochal cyst and infantile polycystic kidney disease. When Caroli's disease is associated with hepatic fibrosis, sonography reveals that the biliary changes are less pronounced, with portal hypertension and cystic disease of the kidneys predominating.

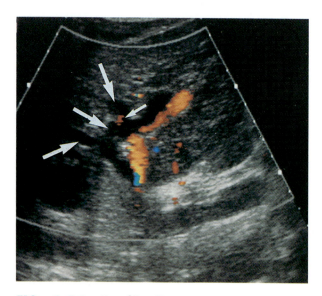

FIG. 6-56. Caroli's disease. Color Doppler scan demonstrates dilated intrahepatic bile ducts. Several small saccules appear to communicate with the bile ducts *(arrows)*, and in the periphery of one of these saccules, a vascular structure is also visible *(small arrow)*.

Miscellaneous Rare Conditions. Even though multiple **bile duct hamartomas** are discovered at autopsy in 0.6% to 2.8% of individuals, because of their small size and the fact that they typically occupy only a small part of the liver, they are rarely visible by cross-sectional imaging. These hamartomas are considered a developmental bile duct malformation that is characterized by bile duct duplication with surrounding dense, hyalinized fibrous stroma. These hamartomatous lesions contain a lumen, but do not usually communicate with bile ducts. In unusual cases with multiple, large hamartomas, sonography may reveal focal masses that can range in echogenicity from hypoechoic to hyperechoic.[166] These lesions can simulate malignancy not only on sonographic evaluation, but also on CT and MRI evaluation. This appears to be a nonprogressive and asymptomatic condition that requires liver biopsy for definitive diagnosis.

Peribiliary cysts represent another rare condition, which are found in patients with severe liver disease.[167] These simple-appearing cysts, which are located in the peribiliary tissue near the porta hepatis, vary in size from several millimeters to several centimeters. Histopathologically, they are serous cysts that most likely represent obstructed periductal glands. In most cases they are incidentally discovered and are of no clinical significance. Rarely, they may be sufficiently large to cause biliary obstruction. Because a linear collection of these cysts can mimic an enlarged bile duct, careful sonographic examination is necessary to detect the thin walls that separate adjacent cysts. If the cysts are clustered, they can simulate a cystic neoplasm or abscess.

Pitfalls

Although dilated intrahepatic bile ducts are specific for active biliary obstruction, this finding is not highly sensitive because up to 23% of patients with biliary obstruction lack intrahepatic bile duct dilatation.[168] In most cases **false-negative results** are due to **lack of intrahepatic dilatation despite distal obstruction.** In these cases neither the level of hyperbilirubinemia nor the duration of jaundice appears to bear any relation to the presence or absence of intrahepatic biliary dilatation.[168]

Segmental biliary obstruction can also cause a false-negative ultrasound examination. This may be due to intrahepatic calculi (especially in patients with RPC), strictures, or neoplasm. Although detecting dilated intrahepatic ducts usually and reliably can be made by scanning the region of the right portal vein, it is important to observe the entire portal venous system when the liver is being scanned.

Because blood clot can be isoechoic with hepatic parenchymal tissue, it may be difficult to detect dilated bile ducts in the presence of **hemobilia.**[169,170] Hemobilia occurs in at least 4% to 13% of patients who undergo percutaneous biliary drainage procedures.[170a] The sonographic appearance for acute intraductal clot consists of diffuse, homogeneous echoes that may be isoechoic with the ductal system and/or surrounding liver parenchyma. As the clot evolves, a soft-tissue mass may be visible within a portion of the duct. After 48 hours, clot retraction occurs and appears as a discrete, tubular, soft-tissue mass. Occasionally the sonolucent portion of the duct immediately adjacent to the retracted clot can be misconstrued as the entire duct; this can cause a false-negative result with regard to ductal dilatation.[169] The varying appearances of intraductal clot may be identical to intraductal sludge, pus, or pigment stones.

Shadowing from either the biliary tree or adjacent structures can also limit sonographic ability to evaluate the ductal system. **Pneumobilia** can be due to a surgically created biliary-enteric anastomosis, incompetence of the sphincter of Oddi, or wall erosion by a gallstone or ulcer into the common bile duct (see Fig. 6-55). On ultrasound, pneumobilia is characterized by variable length echogenic foci in the distribution of the biliary tree. Intermittent acoustic shadowing, especially of the comet-tail variety, is typically seen.[171] Because of the geometry of the bile ducts, when a patient is supine, the gas usually rises to the most anterior structure, which is the left ductal system. Occasionally intrahepatic arterial calcification has been reported to mimic pneumobilia.[172] In difficult cases plain film radiography should be performed so that a definitive diagnosis can be made.

Intrahepatic parenchymal calcifications may be difficult to differentiate from intrahepatic biliary stones.[173] This is especially true in patients with peripherally impacted intrahepatic ductal stones that do not appear to be continuous with the biliary tree. Criteria that may be useful for suggesting intrahepatic calculi as opposed to parenchymal calcification include the presence of bile duct dilatation, multiple lesions, left lobe involvement, and elevated alkaline phosphatase.[173]

Although false-negative diagnoses for intrahepatic bile duct dilatation are common, **false-positive diagnoses** are unusual. They can be made, however, in patients with abnormally **large hepatic arteries,** in which case the dilated intrahepatic arteries mimic dilated intrahepatic bile ducts (Fig. 6-57).[174] This situation occurs most often in patients with severe cirrhosis and portal hypertension. Pseudodilated intrahepatic bile ducts can usually be distinguished from truly dilated bile ducts; in the former the extrahepatic artery is large whereas the common bile duct is normal in size. The changes are manifest primarily in the left hepatic lobe, and there is evidence of portal

hypertension (recanalized umbilical vein, varices, splenomegaly, ascites). In suspicious cases color Doppler should be used because of its ability to rapidly and effectively differentiate between dilated intrahepatic bile ducts and vascular structures.[152]

As mentioned previously, patients with severe liver disease may have **peribiliary cysts** in the region of the porta hepatis.[167] Occasionally these cysts may be arranged in a linear fashion, in which case they can mimic bile duct dilatation. In most cases careful sonographic examination will reveal the thin walls that separate adjacent cysts.

Patients may occasionally have a hypoechoic rim of periportal tissue (**periportal cuffing**) that can resemble biliary dilatation. In some cases this may occur following liver transplantation, or it may be evident in patients with malignant periportal adenopathy.[175,176] Based on the fact that an identical appearance has been created in animals following interruption of the

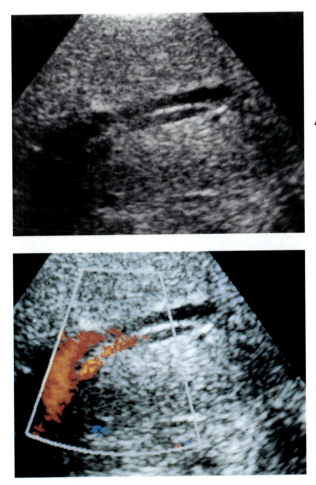

FIG. 6-57. Pitfall—large hepatic artery mimicking dilated intrahepatic bile ducts. A, Transverse scan over the left lobe of the liver demonstrates two parallel tubular structures. **B,** Color Doppler shows blood flowing within both tubular structures.

hepatic lymphatics, it has been suggested that periportal cuffing is due to lymphedema.[175] Additionally, these changes regress following chemotherapy with resolution of portal adenopathy.[175,176] Occasionally, however, a similar appearance is visible with AIDS cholangitis (Fig. 6-58).[158] The etiology for this finding and its association with HIV are as yet unexplained.

EXTRAHEPATIC BILE DUCTS

Normal Anatomy

The most easily visualized portion of the extrahepatic ductal system is the **common hepatic duct,** which results from the union of the **right and left intrahepatic bile ducts.** The anatomic position of the common hepatic duct is constant, and it can be readily detected in the porta hepatis as it crosses anterior to the undivided right portal vein. At this level the right hepatic artery is usually visible in cross section between the posteriorly positioned portal vein and the anteriorly positioned bile ducts. As the common hepatic duct leaves the porta hepatis, it joins the cystic duct and forms the **common bile duct** (CBD) (Fig. 6-59).[2] The **normal cystic duct** lies posterior to the CBD, has an average diameter of slightly less than 2 mm, and is visible in approximately 50% of patients.[177]

After its union with the cystic duct, the CBD descends within the hepatoduodenal ligament in a fixed but somewhat confusing anatomic relationship with two other tubular structures, the main portal vein and the proper hepatic artery. Recognition of these three tubular structures requires an understanding of their fixed and reproducible anatomic relationship. Proximally within the hepatoduodenal ligament the portal vein is posterior; the bile duct is anterior and somewhat laterally positioned (on the same side as the gallbladder). The proper hepatic artery is anterior and medially positioned (on the same side as the aorta) relative to the portal vein. As these three structures descend within the hepatoduodenal ligament, their anatomic relationship changes in accordance with their sites of termination. Because the CBD terminates in the retroperitoneally located second part of the duodenum, it courses posteriorly as it descends. The portal vein descends in a relatively anterior direction to form the splenic and superior mesenteric veins. The third component of this tubular triad, the proper hepatic artery, remains anterior as it gives off the gastroduodenal artery, which enters the anterior aspect of the pancreatic head. Proper identification of these similar-appearing but very differently functioning anatomic structures is crucial to analyze the extrahepatic biliary tree correctly. Although their positional relationship usually allows confident identification of these anatomic structures, in confusing or difficult cases, duplex and color Doppler should be used to confirm the anatomy.

The **size** of the extrahepatic bile duct is the most sensitive means of distinguishing medical from surgical jaundice. There are discrepant reports in the literature regarding the maximal normal diameter of the CBD; measurements as small as 4 mm or as large as 8 mm have been reported.[178,179] The literature is simi-

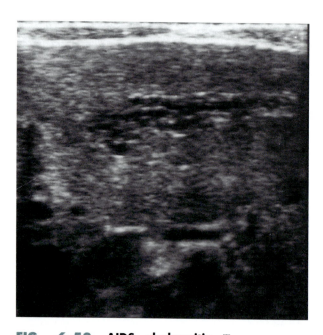

FIG. 6-58. AIDS cholangitis. Transverse scan through the left lobe of the liver shows irregular thickening of the walls of the intrahepatic bile ducts. (From Dolmatch BL, Laing FC, Federle MP et al. AIDS-related cholangitis: radiographic findings in nine patients. *Radiology* 1987;163:313-316.)

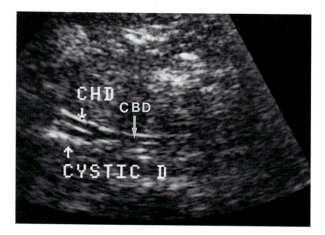

FIG. 6-59. Normal porta hepatis. Parasagittal scan shows posteriorly a normal-appearing cystic duct joining the anteriorly positioned common hepatic duct, *CHD,* to form the common bile duct, *CBD.* In this scan, neither the portal vein nor the hepatic artery is visible.

larly unclear as to whether the CBD dilates postcholecystectomy. Articles can be found that both support[178,180] and refute[181-183] the claim that CBD dilatation occurs after cholecystectomy.

Studies also suggest that the diameter of the CBD may increase slightly with aging and that 10 mm should be considered the upper normal value in elderly patients.[184] A simple **rule of thumb** is to consider as normal a 4-mm mean duct diameter at age 40, a 5-mm mean duct diameter at age 50, a 6-mm mean duct diameter at age 60, and so on.

It is generally accepted that the diameter of the CBD is normally slightly greater in its distal than its proximal portion. In most patients this discrepancy in size is barely perceptible, but occasionally the duct becomes funneled and the distal diameter is several millimeters wider than the proximal diameter (Fig. 6-60). In this situation, if the duct is measured solely in the porta hepatis, it may be of normal caliber. When measured more distally, it may be borderline or even frankly enlarged. The significance of the funneled appearance is that it may indicate early extrahepatic bile duct obstruction. This finding is nonspecific, however, because a similar appearance may be seen in patients whose obstruction has been relieved.

Sonographic measurements are smaller than corresponding measurements made during radiographic procedures such as transhepatic cholangiography, intravenous cholangiography, or ERCP. The usual explanation for this discrepancy is that the ul-

trasonograms do not include the effects of radiographic magnification or the choleretic effect of contrast agents. A recent comparative study between sonographic and cholangiographic diameters of the extrahepatic duct, however, revealed a surprising twofold discrepancy, with the sonographic diameter less than one half the cholangiographic diameter.[185] The explanation for this difference was determined following careful retrospective analysis and revealed that the sonographic measurement was most often obtained at the level of the right hepatic duct, as opposed to the extrahepatic duct (where the cholangiographic measurement was obtained).

The size of the common hepatic or common bile duct may be somewhat larger in patients who have undergone previous biliary surgery or following liver transplantation.[186] Postoperatively the common hepatic duct may measure up to 10 mm in diameter.[181] Unless baseline postoperative scans are obtained, however, a single measurement of 10 mm should be followed with sequential scans and liver function tests (especially alkaline phosphatase) to evaluate the possibility of early obstruction. If a symptomatic postoperative patient has a large or equivocal duct measurement (by nonoperated size criteria), further evaluation should be undertaken.

Scanning Techniques

To minimize obscuration by overlying bowel gas, the **distal CBD** should be examined initially. This is most satisfactorily accomplished by performing scans with the patient in an **erect RPO or right lateral decubitus position** and by relying on **transverse scans** as opposed to the parasagittal approach (Fig. 6-61).[187] These positions **minimize gas in the antrum and duodenum** while the transverse scan plane maximizes the ability to trace the course of the intrapancreatic distal duct. Using a curvilinear transducer with compression over the pancreatic head may also be useful because the large transducer footprint can help to eliminate intervening gastric and colonic gas.[188] If overlying bowel gas continues to obscure this region, the patient should be given 16 ounces of water to drink, then placed in a right lateral decubitus position for 2 to 3 minutes, and rescanned.

Although the **proximal CBD** can also be evaluated in this position, it is usually seen to better advantage in the **parasagittal plane** after the patient has been repositioned into a supine LPO position.[187] In most patients examination of the proximal and distal bile ducts can be completed in 5 to 10 minutes. In difficult cases the study may take as long as 15 to 30 minutes.

Pathology

As a screening modality, the primary function of ultrasound is to determine whether biliary obstruction is

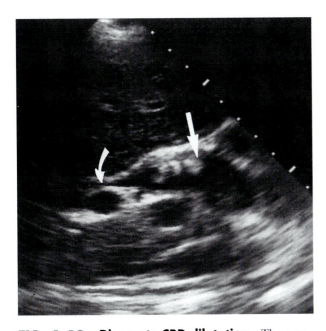

FIG. 6-60. Disparate CBD dilatation. The extrahepatic duct *(arrow)* is much larger than the common hepatic duct *(curved arrow)*. This funneled appearance was caused by an acute obstruction from choledocholithiasis. Many nonobstructing stones are also visible.

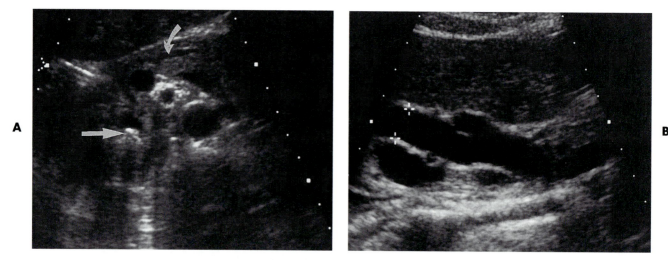

FIG. 6-61. Dilated common bile duct. A, A transverse scan obtained with the patient in an erect position reveals a stone *(arrow)* in the dilated distal common bile duct. The pancreatic duct *(arrowheads)* is also dilated. **B,** A parasagittal scan with the patient in an LPO position shows a markedly dilated proximal duct *(between gradicules)*. The distal duct, which contained the calculus, is not visible on this view.

present. A secondary function is to determine the level and cause of the obstruction.

Diagnosing Obstruction. Because bile ducts expand centrifugally from the point of obstruction, extrahepatic dilatation occurs before intrahepatic dilatation.[189] It is not unusual, therefore, to see isolated or disparate dilatation of the extrahepatic duct in patients with obstructive jaundice (see Fig. 6-60). Furthermore, in patients with fibrosed or infiltrated livers, intrahepatic dilatation cannot readily occur because of lack of compliance of the hepatic parenchyma. Because intrahepatic bile ducts may not always dilate in patients with surgical jaundice, most authorities consider the diameter of the common hepatic duct as the most sensitive indicator for diagnosing biliary obstruction.

In many ultrasound laboratories, biliary obstruction is suggested if the common hepatic duct diameter is 8 mm or greater.[168] A diameter of 6 to 7 mm is equivocal, and smaller diameters are not suggestive of this diagnosis. Dilated intrahepatic ducts also suggest obstruction.

Level and Cause of Obstruction. Localizing the anatomic site and cause for biliary obstruction is important for determining what other examinations, if any, should be performed for further diagnostic evaluation. This information may also be useful for determining whether additional procedures such as surgery, endoscopy, or percutaneous drainage are necessary. In cases of biliary obstruction, the ultrasonographer should attempt to place the level of obstruction at one of three sites: the intrapancreatic common duct, the suprapancreatic common duct, or the porta hepatis.

With refinements in real-time equipment and improved scanning techniques, ultrasound has been reported to define the level of dilatation in up to 92% of cases and to suggest the correct cause in up to 71% of cases.[190]

Intrapancreatic Obstruction. The three most common conditions that cause 90% of biliary obstructions occur at the level of the distal duct and cause the extrahepatic duct to be dilated throughout its entire course. These conditions include (1) pancreatic carcinoma (Fig. 6-62); (2) choledocholithiasis; and (3) chronic pancreatitis with stricture formation. In the United States, choledocholithiasis is the single most common cause for biliary obstruction, occurring in approximately 15% of patients with cholelithiasis. If ultrasound indicates a distal site of obstruction but fails to determine the cause, ERCP should be performed for precise diagnosis.

In a technically adequate examination, solid **pancreatic masses** larger than 2.5 cm in diameter should be readily visible. Masses smaller than 2.5 cm in diameter may not be visible, but their presence may be inferred because their strategic anatomic location within the head and/or uncinate process frequently results in a double duct sign. Pancreatic neoplasm

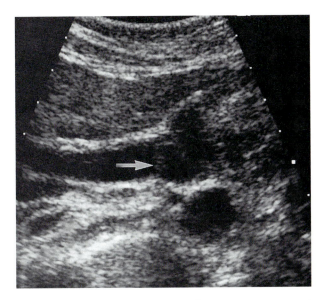

FIG. 6-62. Pancreatic carcinoma. Longitudinal scan shows common bile duct dilatation and a mass invading the distal common duct *(arrows)*. This was due to a carcinoma in the head of the pancreas.

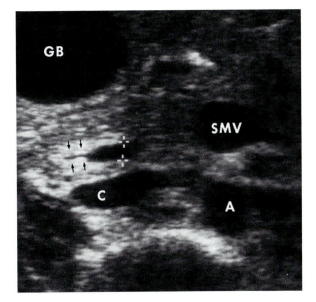

FIG. 6-63. **AIDS cholangitis—stricture of CBD.** Transverse scan through the head of the pancreas shows abrupt distal tapering of the duct as well as echogenic thickening of the distal duct wall *(arrows)*. *A,* Aorta; *C,* inferior vena cava; *SMV,* superior mesenteric vein; *GB,* gallbladder. (From Dolmatch BL, Laing FC, Federle MP et al. AIDS-related cholangitis: radiographic findings in nine patients. *Radiology* 1987;163:313-316.)

and focal pancreatitis may be indistinguishable causes of distal biliary obstruction unless secondary findings such as adenopathy or distant metastases are visible. If a focal polypoid, intraluminal mass is visible in the distal common duct, an ampullary neoplasm should be considered.[191,192] The histologic origin of these tumors, which are named on the basis of their location, includes distal CBD (cholangiocarcinoma), mucous membrane of the duodenum, ampulla, and, occasionally, Brunner glands.

With optimal scanning technique, distal **CBD calculi** can be visualized in up to 70% of patients.[187] As with gallstones, acoustic shadowing is almost always present (see Fig. 6-61, *A*). Choledocholithiasis may be detected in a normal size bile duct, but calculi are more readily identified in a dilated system. Not surprisingly, ultrasound's sensitivity for diagnosing choledocholithiasis diminishes dramatically if the region over the head of the pancreas is obscured because of overlying bowel gas or obesity.

Strictures, the third most common cause for distal obstruction, are a problem for sonography. Apart from abrupt termination of the dilated distal CBD, the stricture per se is not usually visible, and the precise cause of obstruction is not usually apparent. If a patient is known to have AIDS, careful scanning will sometimes reveal echogenic thickening of the distal duct wall, indicative of a stricture due to AIDS cholangitis (Fig. 6-63).[158,193]

Suprapancreatic Obstruction. Suprapancreatic obstruction is defined as obstruction that originates between the pancreas and the porta hepatis. Sonographically, the head of the pancreas is normal, as are the diameters of the intrapancreatic bile duct and pancreatic duct. **Malignancy** (both primary and secondary) is the most common cause for these obstructions. Ultrasound may reveal a mass or adenopathy at this level. Rarely, a mass may be visible within the intraluminal portion of the duct.[194] In approximately one fourth of patients with primary extrahepatic bile duct tumors, the sonographic appearance can mimic a dilated duct filled with echogenic material. In reality the tumor is causing diffuse and extensive wall thickening with obliteration of the lumen.[194,195] Careful inspection may sometimes reveal a thin, centrally reflecting line that is caused by the compressed and obliterated lumen (Fig. 6-64). Calculi and inflammatory strictures are uncommon causes of suprapancreatic obstruction.

Porta Hepatis Obstruction. Obstruction at the level of the porta hepatis is also usually due to **neoplasm,** either primary or secondary. In a prospective study that included 40 patients with hilar lesions, 31 (78%) had lesions caused by neoplasms.[196] In patients with obstruction at the level of the porta, sonography discloses intrahepatic ductal dilatation and a normal size CBD. The gallbladder may be obstructed, depending on the level of the lesion relative to the

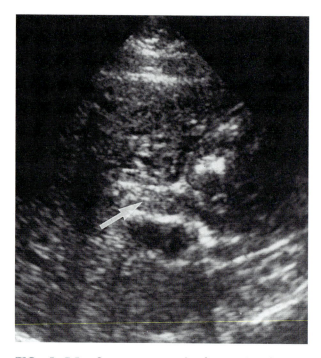

FIG. 6-64. **Suprapancreatic obstruction from a primary bile duct tumor.** An abnormal area of echogenicity is present within the dilated bile duct. Careful inspection reveals a thin centrally reflecting line *(arrow)* due to apposition of the thickened bile duct walls.

position of the cystic duct. Several recently reported studies have evaluated ultrasound's ability to stage primary hilar tumors.[197-200] Criteria used to establish unresectability include hepatic and/or nodal metastases, portal vein occlusion involving either the main or both major branches, or extensive bile duct obstruction with atrophy of the contralateral hepatic lobe. Unfortunately, the sonographic findings reported in these studies lacked uniformity, making it difficult to draw definitive conclusions. For example, two studies suggested that Doppler ultrasound can successfully predict vascular patency or involvement of the portal vein in 83% to 100% of patients,[97,198] while a third study detected main portal vein involvement only 50% of the time.[199] The literature also varies between 21%[201] and 96%[194] with respect to ultrasound's ability to visualize the actual tumor. Nonetheless, most authors agree that sonography is useful because it can detect biliary obstruction, and it is often complementary to other imaging modalities, including CT and cholangiography.

Unusual Causes for Bile Duct Dilatation.

Bile duct carcinoma (cholangiocarcinoma) is a relatively rare malignancy, accounting for fewer than 1% of all cancers.[202,203] Predisposing conditions include ulcerative colitis, sclerosing cholangitis, Caroli's disease, choledochal cyst, parasitic infestation *(Clonorchis sinensis, Opisthorchis viverrini*[155]*)*, and

exposure to a variety of chemicals.[202] This tumor originates within the larger bile ducts and in more than two thirds of cases is located in either the CBD or CHD.[202] A Klatskin tumor is a specific type of cholangiocarcinoma that occurs in 10% to 25% of cases and is named after the physician who described its anatomic location at the hepatic hilum.[204] In 95% of cases this tumor is an adenocarcinoma that can be morphologically subdivided into sclerosing, nodular, or papillary forms.[194,202] Because this neoplasm clinically presents with biliary obstruction while it is relatively small, sonography is often the initial imaging examination. The most suggestive sonographic feature to indicate cholangiocarcinoma is isolated intrahepatic bile duct dilatation. Although the obstructing tumor mass may not be visible, nonunion of the right and left ducts is characteristic for a hilar (Klatskin) tumor (Fig. 6-65). In a recently reported series that evaluated the sonographic features in 49 patients with cholangiocarcinoma, infiltrating tumors occurred in 84% of patients and caused mural thickening that, on sonography, appeared as a small mass. This is because sonography cannot usually discern that the mass is actually caused by apposition of the walls of a focally thickened bile duct. Additional characteristics of this tumor include local invasion of the liver and porta hepatis (including the portal vein), a normal size extrahepatic duct, absent intraductal calculi, normal pancreas, and absence of a primary tumor. The differential diagnosis includes sclerosing or suppurative cholangitis, benign stricture, benign bile duct tumor, metastasis, and proximal spread of distal bile duct carcinoma.[195-205]

Mirizzi syndrome is an uncommon cause for extrahepatic biliary obstruction due to an impacted stone in the cystic duct creating extrinsic mechanical compression of the common hepatic duct.[206] Not uncommonly, the stone penetrates into the common hepatic duct or the gut, resulting in a cholecystobiliary or cholecystenteric fistula. In most cases the cystic duct inserts unusually low into the common hepatic duct. This results in the two ducts having parallel alignment, which geometrically allows for the development of the syndrome. The sonographic findings include intrahepatic bile duct dilatation, a normal size CBD, and a large stone in the neck of the gallbladder or cystic duct (Fig. 6-66).[206] Failure to recognize these changes can lead to surgical complications that include ligation and transection of the CBD. Unfortunately, ultrasound findings are not always classic, and in suspicious cases CT and especially cholangiography should be performed for confirmation and for detection of the extrinsic compression of the CBD or a cholecystobiliary fistula.[207]

Choledochal cyst is a third uncommon lesion that may cause bile duct dilatation. This congenital

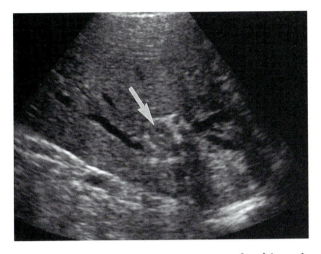

FIG. 6-65. Cholangiocarcinoma (Klatskin primary bile duct tumor). Transverse scan at the level of the porta hepatis reveals intrahepatic dilatation of the right and left bile ducts. A poorly defined isoechoic mass *(arrow)* is causing the obstruction. The anatomic site is characteristic for a Klatskin tumor.

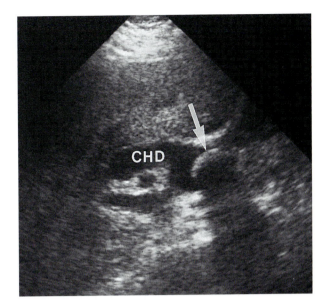

FIG. 6-66. Mirizzi syndrome. A large calculus *(arrow)* is located in the cystic duct and is causing proximal dilatation of the common hepatic duct, *CHD*. Although the appearance of this scan suggests that the stone may be in the common hepatic duct, careful scanning and surgery confirmed that the calculus was in the cystic duct.

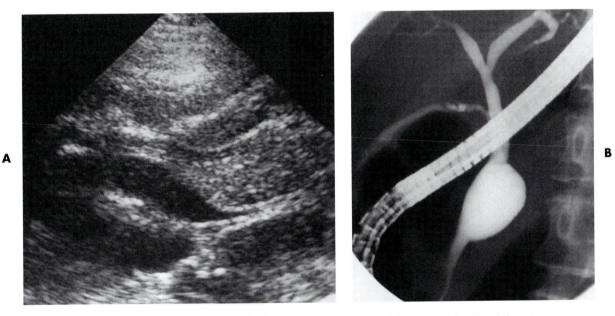

FIG. 6-67. Type I choledochal cyst. A, The common bile duct is dilated and there is gradual distal tapering. **B,** Cholangiogram of the same patient confirms fusiform dilatation of the common bile duct.

anomaly has been subdivided into various types, including:
- Type I—Cystic fusiform dilatation of the CBD, often with an anomalous junction of the pancreaticobiliary ductal system (the most common form) (Fig. 6-67);
- Type II—A diverticulum protruding from the wall of the CBD (rare); and

- Type III—A choledochocele or herniation of the CBD into the duodenum (rare).[208]

This entity usually occurs in Asian women whose symptoms vary from none to the classic triad of pain, jaundice, and an abdominal mass.[208] The sonographic findings will reflect the specific type of choledochal cyst present, although typically a cystic extrahepatic mass will be present. Not infrequently, a portion of the proximal bile duct can be seen extending into the choledochal cyst. Complications associated with the presence of a choledochal cyst may result in additional sonographic findings that include choledocholithiasis, changes due to pancreatitis and/or biliary cirrhosis, portal vein thrombosis, hepatic abscess, and malignant neoplasm within the cyst wall or gallbladder.[208] Despite reports to the contrary, intrahepatic bile duct dilatation is also commonly present.[209] In most cases the ultrasound findings are sufficient to suggest the correct diagnosis. If the cyst is large and round and if the intrahepatic ducts are normal, the diagnosis may not be evident. In these challenging cases the differential diagnosis includes other fluid-filled masses such as a hepatic cyst, pancreatic pseudocyst, or enteric duplication cyst. Hepatobiliary scintigraphy may be diagnostic in these cases to demonstrate excretion of radiopharmaceutical into the abnormal cystic structure.[209,210]

Biliary parasites. Because the clinical presentation of patients with biliary parasites includes symptoms of biliary colic, cholangitis, and acute cholecystitis, ultrasound is often performed as the initial imaging study. The most common parasite, estimated to infect up to 75% of the population in endemic areas, is the roundworm *Ascaris lumbricoides.*[211] Because the adult worm is greater than 10 cm in length, 3 to 6 mm thick, and has a propensity to enter the biliary tree, it may be visible by sonography where it may cause biliary obstruction (Fig. 6-68). Characteristic sonographic findings include visualizing the worm(s) in the extrahepatic bile duct as one or more nonshadowing tubelike structures that may either be straight or coiled.[212] Aggregates of multiple worms have been described as having an appearance like spaghetti.[213] Rarely, a worm may be visible in the gallbladder;[142,143] when impacted in an intrahepatic bile duct, it may appear as a curvilinear nonshadowing tubular structure with a central sonolucent center.[212] Occasionally a macerated roundworm in the extrahepatic bile duct can mimic a mass and be misdiagnosed as cholangiocarcinoma.[212] In addition to ultrasound's ability to diagnose ascariasis, it can also be used to document disappearance of the worm(s) following treatment.

Clonorchis sinensis, a liver fluke that is endemic to populations living in the Far East, frequently infests medium or small intrahepatic bile ducts. In some patients the extrahepatic bile ducts and/or gallbladder may be affected.[214] Although the diagnosis of clonorchiasis depends on detecting eggs or adult worms in the feces or bile, ultrasound can suggest the diagnosis. Characteristic sonographic findings include diffuse dilatation of small intrahepatic ducts with minimal or absent dilatation of the extrahepatic ductal system. Increased echogenicity and

thickening of the involved bile duct walls are also present. Because these parasites are 8 to 15 mm long and 1.5 to 5 mm thick, they are not usually visible as they obstruct the intrahepatic bile ducts. Aggregates of adult worms or individual worms may occasionally be seen in the extrahepatic bile duct and gallbladder, respectively.[214] Their appearance can be distinguished from gallstones on the basis of their fusiform outline and the fact that they may show spontaneous movement. In addition, they are less echogenic than typical gallstones and do not cause acoustic shadowing. A consequence of chronic biliary infestation by this liver fluke is an increased incidence of cholangiocarcinoma and possibly recurrent pyogenic cholangitis.[215]

Fasciola hepatica is a trematode that usually infests cattle and sheep. Humans are uncommonly infected by drinking or eating contaminated water or plants.[141,216] Sonography may reveal these relatively small (15 to 40 mm) flukes as echogenic foci in the gallbladder and dilated extrahepatic ducts.[140,141,216] Their appearance can mimic sludge, small nonshadowing stones, or even an irregularly thickened bile duct.[141,216] When present, active motility is extremely useful for restricting the differential diagnosis.

Pitfalls

To maximize the use of ultrasound in evaluating the extrahepatic duct, sonographers must have a clear understanding of the problems and pitfalls pertaining to examining the CBD.

Anatomic Problems. In approximately 8% of patients, redundancy, elongation, or folding of the gallbladder neck on itself can each cause a pattern that

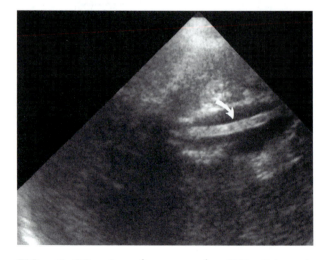

FIG. 6-68. *Ascaris* worm in CBD. Echogenic tubular structure *(curved arrow)* is visible in a markedly dilated CBD. (From Laing FC. Ultrasonography of the gallbladder and biliary tree. In: Sarti DA, ed. *Diagnostic Ultrasound: Text and Cases.* 2nd ed. St Louis: Mosby-Year Book; 1987.)

mimics dilatation of either the common hepatic or proximal CBD.[2,217] To avoid misinterpreting a redundant or elongated gallbladder neck for a dilated CBD, scans should be done in deep inspiration and in expiration. A redundant gallbladder neck will elongate on the inspiratory scan whereas there will be little if any change in the appearance of a dilated extrahepatic duct. In addition, careful real-time scanning should allow the CHD or CBD to be identified in its normal position medial to the gallbladder neck (Fig. 6-69).

Variations in the course of the extrahepatic bile duct can occasionally occur. In approximately 20% of patients with CBD dilatation, the duct assumes a relatively transverse course, in which case it may be confused for the portal and splenic veins.[218] The course of the duct may also vary in the presence of a pancreatic mass, particularly within the uncinate process. This may result in anterior elevation of the distal duct, such that it mimics the course of the gastroduodenal artery. In addition, patients who have undergone biliary surgery may have anatomic deviations in the position of the extrahepatic bile ducts.

Variations in the anatomic position of the hepatic artery, which occur in approximately 30% of patients, can also cause diagnostic problems.[219] Because the diameters of both the aberrant artery and duct are usually small, in most circumstances it is not necessary to determine which structure is the duct and which the artery. A problem may develop, however, if the hepatic artery (aberrant or normally positioned) dilates and becomes larger in diameter than the CBD. Color Doppler is essential to correctly analyze any case in which there is a question regarding the anatomic relationship(s) of vascular and/or biliary structures in the porta hepatis or hepatoduodenal ligament.

Atypical Cases. Although ultrasound can distinguish medical from surgical jaundice in more than 90% of cases, atypical cases will be encountered. Infrequently, **dilatation** of the biliary tree can occur **without jaundice.**[220,221] In these patients partial or incomplete biliary obstruction is usually present, or only one hepatic duct is dilated. In general the ultrasound findings and the serum alkaline phosphatase level are more sensitive than the serum bilirubin for suggesting obstruction. Occasionally, anicteric dilatation of the extrahepatic bile duct may be seen in postcholecystectomy patients or in patients with prior obstruction who exhibit dilatation without obstruction. Intestinal hypomotility may also be responsible for some cases of nonobstructed bile duct dilatation as it relates to factors that inhibit the relaxation of the sphincter of Oddi or prolongs its contraction.[222]

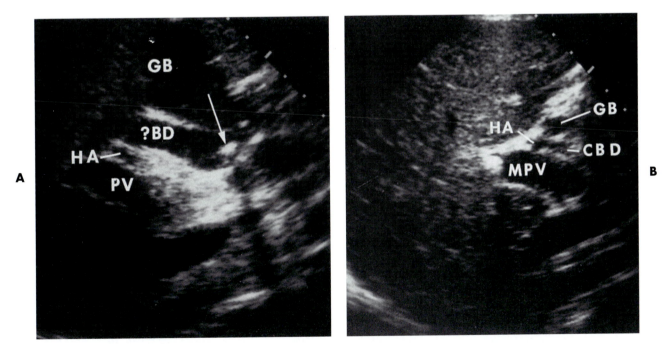

FIG. 6-69. **Pitfall—stone in a redundant gallbladder neck mimicking choledocholithiasis.** **A,** Calculus with acoustic shadowing *(arrow)* is visible in what might be mistaken for a dilated bile duct. The gallbladder, *GB,* is anterior, the portal vein, *PV,* and hepatic artery, *HA,* are posterior to this structure. **B,** Longitudinal scan obtained in a slightly more medial direction confirms a normal size bile duct, *CBD,* posterior to the gallbladder neck, *GB.* *MPV,* Main portal vein; *HA,* hepatic artery. (From Laing FC, Filly RA, Gooding GAW. Ultrasonography of the liver and biliary tract. In: Margulis AR, Burenne HJ, eds. *Alimentary Tract Radiology.* 4th ed. St Louis: Mosby-Year Book; 1989.)

The converse can also occur if a patient with **obstructive jaundice lacks dilatation** of the intrahepatic and extrahepatic bile ducts.[168,223] Cholangitis, partial obstruction, or intermittent obstruction from choledocholithiasis is usually responsible for these cases (Fig. 6-70). Rarely, a patient may have an extrahepatic duct that changes rapidly in size (over a period of several minutes to several days).[224,225] These prominent fluctuations most probably relate to the elasticity and associated distensibility of the duct.

In questionable cases biliary dynamics can be assessed by repeating the scan after administering a fatty meal (Fig. 6-71). **Indications for administering a fatty meal include:**

- Equivocal extrahepatic duct diameter;
- Mildly abnormal caliber duct with normal laboratory values;
- Normal caliber duct with abnormal laboratory values;
- A persistent question of choledocholithiasis;
- Asymptomatic bile duct dilatation[226]; and
- An attempt to detect choledocholithiasis.[227]

In true-negative cases a normal size duct remains unchanged or decreases in size following a fatty meal whereas an initially enlarged duct decreases in caliber. In true-positive cases an initially normal or slightly dilated duct increases in size.[226,228,229] The literature is discrepant with regard to interpreting an initially dilated duct that fails to change in size following a fatty meal. According to Simeone et al., this is an abnormal finding suggestive of obstruction.[226] Willson et al.[228]

claim that a dilated CBD that does not decrease in size following a fatty meal is not a specific indicator of obstruction because in their experience 84% of such cases fail to show obstruction. In general this test has been most useful for detecting patients with partial CBD obstruction; in the experience of Darweesh et al.[229] it had a sensitivity of 74% and a specificity of 100% for detecting partial common duct obstruction. When performing this test it is important to measure the duct at precisely the same location before and after the fatty meal. Simeone et al.[226] consider a 1 mm size change significant; other investigators conclude that differences in duct diameters of 1 mm are within the range of measurement error; therefore they consider changes of 2 mm or greater as significant.[229] When critically ill patients are examined, they often fail to show any biliary response following the administration of either oral fat (Lipomul) or intravenous cholecystokinin (sincalide). If gallbladder contraction fails to occur, the test loses its validity in these patients.

Another approach to a patient with a questionably obstructed duct is to measure the effect of the Valsalva maneuver on the diameter of the common hepatic duct.[230] With true extrahepatic biliary obstruction, the duct should not change in caliber as a result of the Valsalva maneuver whereas it should decrease by 1 mm if obstruction is absent. Quinn and co-investigators reported on 25 consecutive patients (12 with and 13 without obstruction) and noted that this maneuver was able to correctly predict the status of the duct with a sensitivity of 100% and a specificity of 92%.[230] The authors speculate that in the absence of biliary obstruction the Valsalva maneuver compresses the liver and common hepatic duct; with obstruction, increased pressure in the duct prevents this change.[230]

Detecting Choledocholithiasis. Modern ultrasound equipment and careful scanning techniques currently allow approximately 75% of CBD stones to be visualized.[187,227] Nonetheless recent reports continue to acknowledge that the sensitivity of ultrasound may be significantly less than these figures, with the range between 20% to 36%.[231,232] Although experienced sonographers can usually diagnose choledocholithiasis with confidence, there are several possible sources of confusion. Distally, gas or particulate material in the adjacent duodenum can mimic a CBD stone. Transverse scanning with fluid in the duodenum can minimize this problem. Pancreatic calcification can also be confused for a distal calculus. Careful transverse scanning over the distal duct can usually differentiate between these two entities, but CT or a radiographic contrast examination of the bile duct may be required for definitive diagnosis.

Occasionally soft pigment stones will be difficult if not impossible to distinguish from intrabiliary sludge, pus, blood, or even neoplasm (Figs. 6-72 and 6-73).

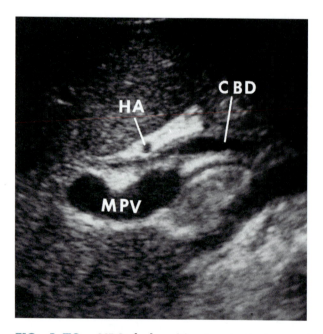

FIG. 6-70. AIDS cholangitis. Longitudinal scan of the CBD reveals diffuse wall thickening without dilatation. Note the aberrant location of the hepatic artery, *HA*. *CBD*, Common bile duct; *MPV*, main portal vein.

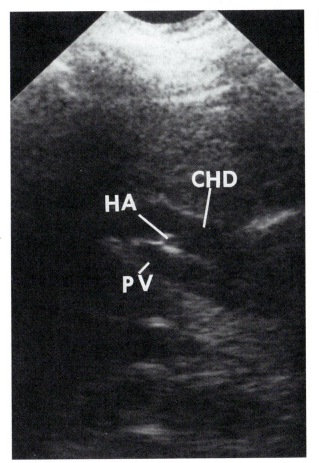

A

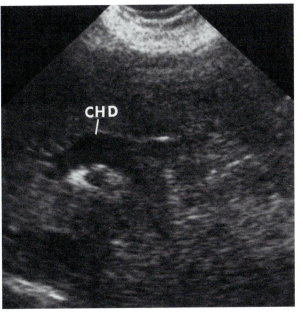

B

FIG. 6-71. Fatty meal. A, Longitudinal scan over the porta hepatitis shows mild dilatation of the common hepatic duct (diameter of 9 mm). **B,** A repeat scan performed 45 minutes after a fatty meal shows progressive dilatation of the common hepatic duct, *CHD* (diameter of 11 mm), indicating active obstruction. The cause was a distal bile duct stricture in a patient with AIDS cholangitis. *CHD,* Common hepatic duct; *PV,* portal vein; *HA,* hepatic artery.

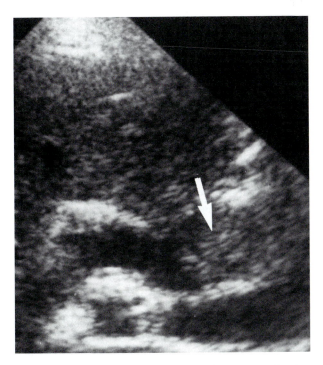

FIG. 6-72. Biliary obstruction due to a soft pigment stone in the distal CBD *(arrow).*

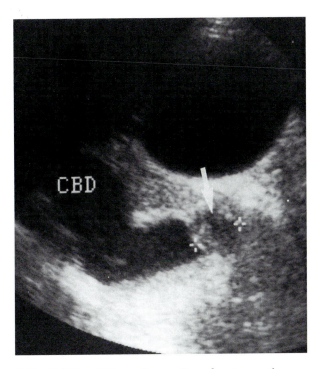

FIG. 6-73. Biliary obstruction due to a primary bile duct tumor *(arrow). CBD,* Common bile duct.

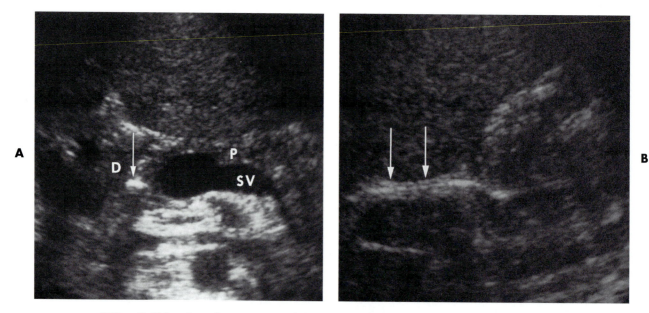

FIG. 6-74. **Gas in common bile duct mimicking choledocholithiasis.** **A,** Transverse scan over the body and head of the pancreas obtained with the patient in an erect position reveals an echogenic shadowing focus that suggests distal choledocholithiasis *(arrow).* **B,** Longitudinal scan of the same patient reveals a linear area of echogenicity *(arrows)* in the expected position of the common bile duct, *CBD,* suggesting air. Choledocholithiasis was not present. *SV,* Splenic vein; *P,* pancreas; *D,* duodenum.

As sonographic resolution has improved, it is now possible to visualize the normal papilla of Vater.[233] To the unwary, this 3 to 6 mm cylindrical or oval structure projecting into the duodenal lumen could be misconstrued as a nonshadowing stone, small mass, sludge, or blood. Gas anywhere in the biliary tree can sometimes mimic choledocholithiasis and will also limit ultrasound's ability to detect and diagnose biliary calculi confidently (Figs. 6-74 and 6-75). Patients known to have biliary gas as a result of prior surgery or biliary-enteric fistula should probably undergo CT or cholangiography for bile duct evaluation.

Ultrasound will also be limited in its ability to detect choledocholithiasis in the absence of bile duct dilatation. Because patients with impacted distal calculi frequently seek medical help soon after the onset of their symptoms, it is not surprising that one third of CBD calculi are found in nondilated bile ducts (Fig. 6-76).[79,234] In our limited experience for detecting choledocholithiasis in normal size ducts, our sensitivity was 60% (3 of 5 patients).[187] In Cronan's series of 78 patients with choledocholithiasis, 26 patients (33%) had normal size ducts and the detection rate for calculi in this group was only 12% (3 of 26 patients).[235]

The sensitivity of ultrasound for detecting calculi in the proximal CBD approximates 90%.[187] Despite this high sensitivity, there are several pitfalls that can cause problems for the unwary. Sources of this confusion include the right hepatic artery, postcholecystec-tomy surgical clips, the cystic duct, tortuosity of the duct, and reverberation echoes within the bile duct. It must be emphasized that appropriate equipment and scanning technique, as well as familiarity with these causes of echogenic foci within the common duct, should minimize false-positive diagnoses of choledocholithiasis.

ENDOSCOPIC ULTRASOUND

The relatively recent development of high-resolution and miniaturized ultrasound transducers, flexible endoscopes, and increasingly sophisticated catheters and interventional techniques allow ultrasound to explore the gallbladder and hepatobiliary tree using a variety of new approaches.

Endoscopic ultrasound typically uses transducers that range in frequency from 7.5 MHz to 12 MHz.[62,236] In a comparative study of 62 consecutive patients, choledocholithiasis was detected in 25% versus 97% of patients using a transabdominal versus endoscopic ultrasound approach, respectively.[237] Other indications are to evaluate the appearance of large gallbladder polyps[62] and to determine the extent of gallbladder carcinoma.[238] With respect to the gallbladder, a significant limitation is the presence of multiple and/or large stones that can obscure evaluation of the wall. Endoscopic ultrasound has also been used to evaluate

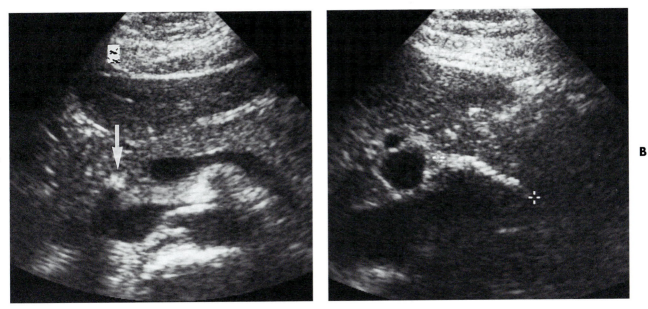

FIG. 6-75. **Choledocholithiasis.** **A,** Transverse pancreatic scan reveals an echogenic focus in the distal common duct *(arrow)* consistent with choledocholithiasis. **B,** Parasagittal scan reveals a linear area of echogenicity with acoustic shadowing between the gradicules. Although the appearance of these images is virtually identical to Fig. 6-74, in this case multiple small stones were present within a normal size common duct.

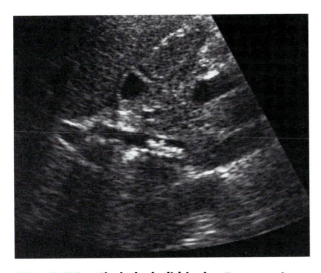

FIG. 6-76. **Choledocholithiasis.** Parasagittal scan shows multiple small echogenic foci in a normal size common bile duct.

the precise anatomic configuration and anatomy of a choledochal cyst,[236] and it can be useful in patients with carcinoma of the papilla of Vater with respect to precisely determining tumor size, depth of invasion, and lymph node metastasis.[239] This technique cannot, however, detect microscopic invasion; nor can it evaluate lymph nodes that are out of the field of view.

Intraluminal or intraductal approaches into the gallbladder or bile ducts, respectively, can be accomplished

by introducing the transducer through a previously established percutaneous tract.[240-242] Alternatively, an endoscopic approach can be used to place a miniaturized transducer through the papilla into the CBD.[243] These transducers, which range in frequency from 20 MHz to 30 MHz, have been shown to be more accurate than either CT or angiography for determining the depth of invasion of bile duct tumors and to evaluate whether the portal vein is involved.[242] In patients with biliary tumors, it may also be useful to guide intraluminal brachytherapy,[244] and it may help define response to therapy.[241] This technique can also be used in benign conditions as an adjunct to remove retained biliary stones,[240] to differentiate blood clot or debris from stones, and to image biliary strictures.[241]

As these techniques are still in their infancy, it will be interesting to observe future technical developments and applications.

REFERENCES

The Gallbladder

1. Callen PW, Filly RA. Ultrasonographic localization of the gallbladder. *Radiology* 1979;133:687-691.
2. Laing FC, Filly RA, Gooding GAW. Ultrasonography of the liver and biliary tract. In: Margulis AR, Burhenne HJ, eds. *Alimentary Tract Radiology.* 4th ed. St Louis: Mosby-Year Book; 1989.
3. Worthen NJ, Uszler JM, Funamura JL. Cholecystitis: prospective evaluation of sonography and 99 mTc-HIDA cholescintigraphy. *AJR* 1981;137:973-978.

4. Donald JJ, Fache JS, Buckley AR et al. Gallbladder contractility: variation in normal subjects. *AJR* 1991;157:753-756.

5. Bucceri AM, Brogna A, Ferrara R. Sonographic study of postprandial gallbladder emptying and common bile duct changes in patients with diabetes or cholelithiasis. *Abdom Imag* 1994;19:427-429.

6. Dodds WJ, Groh WJ, Darweesh RMA et al. Sonographic measurement of gallbladder volume. *AJR* 1985;145:1009-1011.

7. Hopman WPM, Brouwer WFM, Rosenbusch G et al. A computerized method for rapid quantification of gallbladder volume from real-time sonograms. *Radiology* 1985;154:236-237.

8. Meilstrup JW, Hopper KD, Thieme GA. Imaging of gallbladder variants. *AJR* 1991;157:1205-1208.

9. Laing FC. Ultrasonography of the gallbladder and biliary tree. In: Sarti DA, ed. *Diagnostic Ultrasound: Text and Cases.* 2nd ed. St Louis: Mosby-Year Book; 1987.

10. Sukov RJ, Sample WF, Sarti DA et al. Cholecystosonography: the junctional fold. *Radiology* 1979;133:435-436.

11. Strauss S, Starinsky R, Alon Z. Partial multiseptate gallbladder: sonographic appearance. *J Ultrasound Med* 1993;4:201-203.

12. Martinoli C, Derchi LE, Pastorino C, et al. Case report: imaging of a bilobed gallbladder. *Br J Radiol* 1993;66:734-736.

13. Diaz MJ, Fowler W, Hnatow BJ. Congenital gallbladder duplication: preoperative diagnosis by ultrasonography. *Gastrointest Radiol* 1991;16:198-200.

14. Gupta S, Kumar A, Gautam A. Preoperative sonographic diagnosis of gallbladder duplication: importance of challenge with fatty meal. *J Clin Ultrasound* 1993;21:399-401.

15. Cameron EW, Beale TJ, Pearson RH. Case report: torsion of the gallbladder on ultrasound-differentiation from acalculous cholecystitis. *Clin Radiol* 1993;47:285-286.

16. Bach DB, Satin R, Palayew M et al. Herniation and strangulation of GB through foramen of Winslow. *AJR* 1884;142:541.

17. Safadi RR, Abu-Yousef MM, Farah AS et al. Preoperative sonographic diagnosis of gallbladder torsion: report of two cases. *J Ultrasound Med* 1993;5:296-298.

18. Parulekar SG. Evaluation of the prone view for cholecystosonography. *J Ultrasound Med* 1986;5:617-624.

19. Cooperberg PL, Burhenne HJ. Real-time ultrasonography. Diagnostic technique of choice in calculus gallbladder disease. *N Engl J Med* 1980;302:1277-1279.

20. Crade M, Taylor KJW, Rosenfield AT et al. Surgical and pathologic correlation of cholecystosonography and cholecystography. *AJR* 1978;131:227-229.

21. McIntosh DMF, Penney HF. Gray scale ultrasonography as a screening procedure in the detection of gallbladder disease. *Radiology* 1980;136:725-727.

22. Marzio L, Innocenti P, Genovesi N et al. Role of oral cholecystography, real-time ultrasound, and CT in evaluation of gallstones and gallbladder function. *Gastrointest Radiol* 1992;17:257-261.

23. Carroll BA. Gallstones: in vitro comparison of physical, radiographic, and ultrasonic characteristics. *AJR* 1978;131:223-226.

24. Filly RA, Moss AA, Way LW. In vitro investigation of gallstone shadowing with ultrasound tomography. *J Clin Ultrasound* 1979;7:255-262.

25. Jeanty P, Ammann W, Cooperberg P et al. Mobile intraluminal masses of the gallbladder. *J Ultrasound Med* 1983;2:65-71.

26. Fakhry J. Sonography of tumefactive biliary sludge. *AJR* 1982;139:717-719.

27. Laing FC, Gooding GAW, Herzog KA. Gallstones preventing ultrasonographic visualization of the gallbladder. *Gastrointest Radiol* 1977;1:301-303.

28. MacDonald FR, Cooperberg PL, Cohen MM. The WES triad: a specific sonographic sign of gallstones in the contracted gallbladder. *Gastrointest Radiol* 1981;6:39-41.

29. Raptopoulos V, D'Orsi C, Smith E et al. Dynamic cholecystosonography of the contracted gallbladder: the double arc shadow sign. *AJR* 1982;138:275-278.

30. Kane RA, Jacobs R, Katz J, et al. Porcelain gallbladder: ultrasound and computed tomography appearance. *Radiology* 1984;152:137-141.

31. Hunter ND, Macintosh PK. Acute emphysematous cholecystitis: an ultrasonic diagnosis. *AJR* 1980;134:592-593.

32. Parulekar SG. Sonographic findings in acute emphysematous cholecystitis. *Radiology* 1982;145:117-119.

33. Cohan RH, Mahony BS, Bowie JD et al. Striated intramural gallbladder lucencies on ultrasound studies: predictors of acute cholecystitis. *Radiology* 1987;164:31-35.

34. Teefey SH, Baron RL, Bigler SA. Sonography of the gallbladder: the significance of striated (layered) thickening of the gallbladder wall. *AJR* 1991;156:945-947.

35. Laing FC, Federle MP, Jeffrey RB et al. Ultrasonic evaluation of patients with acute right upper quadrant pain. *Radiology* 1981;140:449-455.

36. Sanders RC. The significance of sonographic gallbladder wall thickening. *J Clin Ultrasound* 1980;8:143-146.

37. Teefey SA, Kimmey MB, Bigler SA et al. Gallbladder wall thickening: an in vitro sonographic study with histologic correlation. *Acad Radiol* 1994;1:121-127.

38. Shlaer WJ, Leopold GR, Scheible FW. Sonography of the thickened gallbladder wall: a nonspecific finding. *AJR* 1981;136:337-339.

39. Ralls PW, Quinn MF, Juttner HU. Gallbladder wall thickening: patients without intrinsic gallbladder disease. *AJR* 1981;137:65-68.

40. Wegener M, Borsch G, Schneider J et al. Gallbladder wall thickening: a frequent finding in various nonbiliary disorders—a prospective ultrasonographic study. *J Clin Ultrasound* 1987;15:307-312.

41. Romano AJ, VanSonnenberg E, Casola G et al. Gallbladder and bile duct abnormalities in AIDS: sonographic findings in eight patients. *AJR* 1988;150:123-127.

42. Maresca G, De Gaetano AM, Mirk P et al. Sonographic patterns of the gallbladder in acute viral hepatitis. *J Clin Ultrasound* 1984;12:141-146.

43. Huang Y-S, Lee S-D, Wu J-C et al. Utility of sonographic gallbladder wall patterns in differentiating malignant from cirrhotic ascites. *J Clin Ultrasound* 1989;17:187-192.

44. Tsujimoto F, Miyamoto Y, Tada S. Differentiation of benign from malignant ascites by sonographic evaluation of gallbladder wall. *Radiology* 1985;157:503-504.

45. Marti-Bonmati L, Andres JC, Aguado C. Sonographic relationship between gallbladder wall thickness and the etiology of ascites. *J Clin Ultrasound* 1989;17:497-501.

46. Finlay DE, Mitchell SL, Letourneau JG et al. Leukemic infiltration of the gallbladder wall mimicking acute cholecystitis. *AJR* 1993;160:63-64.

47. Dickey KW, Barth RA, Stewart JA. Recurrent transient gallbladder wall thickening associated with interleukin-2 chemotherapy. *J Clin Ultrasound* 1993;21:58-61.

48. Chawla Y, Dilawari JB, Katariya S. Gallbladder varices in portal vein thrombosis. *AJR* 1994;162:643-645.

49. David V, Laing FC. Paradoxical dilatation of the gallbladder after fat ingestion in patients with acute hepatitis. *J Ultrasound Med* 1996;15:179-182.

50. Daly BD, Cheung H, Arnold M et al. Ultrasound in the diagnosis of gall-bladder carcinoma in Chinese patients. *Clin Radiol* 1993;48:41-44.

51. Franquet T, Montes M, Ruiz de Azua Y et al. Primary gallbladder carcinoma: imaging findings in 50 patients with pathologic correlation. *Gastrointest Radiol* 1991;16:143-148.

52. Rooholamini SA, Tehrani NS, Razavi MK et al. Imaging of gallbladder carcinoma. *RadioGraphics* 1994;14:291-306.

53. Li D, Dong B, Wu Y et al. Image-directed and color Doppler studies of gallbladder tumors. *J Clin Ultrasound* 1994;22:551-555.

54. Zargar SA, Khuroo MS, Mahajan R et al. US-guided fine-needle aspiration biopsy of gallbladder masses. *Radiology* 1991;179:275-278.

55. Avila NA, Shawker TH, Fraker D. Color-flow Doppler ultrasonography in metastatic melanoma of the gallbladder. *J Clin Ultrasound* 1994;22:342-347.

56. Hahn ST, Park SH, Choi HS et al. Ultrasonographic features of metastatic melanoma of the gallbladder. *J Clin Ultrasound* 1993;21:542-546.

57. Salimi Z, Sharafuddin M. Ultrasound appearance of primary carcinoid tumor of the gallbladder associated with carcinoid syndrome. *J Clin Ultrasound* 1995;23:435-437.

58. O'Boyle MK. Gallbladder wall mass on sonography representing large-cell non-Hodgkin's lymphoma in an AIDS patient. *J Ultrasound Med* 1994;13:67-68.

59. Jeffrey RB, Laing FC, Wong W et al. Gangrenous cholecystitis: diagnosis by ultrasound. *Radiology* 1983;148:219-221.

60. Dixon JT, Foster SC, Gauvin GP et al. Villous hyperplasia of the gallbladder: an unusual sonographic appearance. *J Ultrasound Med* 1993;12:619-620.

61. Jain R, Sawhney S, Bhargava D et al. Gallbladder tuberculosis: sonographic appearance. *J Clin Ultrasound* 1995;23:327-329.

62. Sugiyama M, Atomi Y, Kuroda A et al. Large cholesterol polyps of the gallbladder: diagnosis by means of US and endoscopic US. *Radiology* 1995;196:493-497.

63. Raghavendra BN, Subramanyam BR, Balthazer EJ et al. Sonography of adenomyomatosis of the gallbladder: radiologic-pathologic correlation. *Radiology* 1983;146:747-752.

64. Lafortune M, Gariepy G, Dumont A et al. The V-shaped artifact of the gallbladder. *AJR* 1986;147:505-508.

65. Filly RA, Allen B, Minton MJ et al. In vitro investigation of the origin of echoes within biliary sludge. *J Clin Ultrasound* 1980;8:193-200.

66. Bolondi L, Gaiani S, Testa S et al. Gallbladder sludge formation during prolonged fasting after gastrointestinal tract. *Gut* 1985;26:734-738.

67. Messing B, Bories C, Kustlinger F et al. Does total parenteral nutrition induce gallbladder sludge formation and lithiasis? *Gastroenterology* 1983;84:1012-1019.

68. Teefey SA, Hollister MS, Lee SP et al. Gallbladder sludge formation after bone marrow transplant: sonographic observations. *Abdom Imag* 1994;19:57-60.

69. Britten JS, Golding RH, Cooperberg PL. Sludge balls to gallstones. *J Ultrasound Med* 1984;3:81-84.

70. Laing FC, Jeffrey RB, Federle MP. Gallbladder and bile ducts. In: Jeffrey RB, ed. *Computed Tomography and Sonography of the Acute Abdomen.* New York: Raven Press; 1989:59-62.

71. Nyberg DA, Laing FC. Ultrasonographic findings in peptic ulcer disease and pancreatitis that simulate primary gallbladder disease. *J Ultrasound Med* 1983;2:303-307.

72. Shuman WP, Mack LA, Rudd TG et al. Evaluation of acute right upper quadrant pain: sonography and 99mTc-PIPIDA cholescintigraphy. *AJR* 1982;139:61-64.

73. Weissman HS, Frank MS, Bernstein LH et al. Rapid and accurate diagnosis of acute cholecystitis with 99mTc-HIDA cholescintigraphy. *AJR* 1979;132:523-528.

74. Brachman MB, Goodman MD, Waxman AD. The rim sign in acute cholecystitis: comparison of radionuclide, surgical, and pathologic findings. *Clin Nucl Med* 1993;18:863-866.

75. Bohdiewicz PJ. The diagnostic value of grading hyperfusion and the rim sign of cholescintigraphy. *Clin Nucl Med* 1993;18:867-871.

76. Sherman M, Ralls PW, Quinn M et al. Intravenous cholangiography and sonography in acute cholecystitis: prospective evaluation. *AJR* 1980;135:311-313.

77. Ralls PW, Colletti PM, Lapin SA et al. Real-time sonography in suspected acute cholecystitis. *Radiology* 1985;155:767-771.

78. Bree RL. Further observations on the usefulness of the sonographic Murphy sign in the evaluation of suspected acute cholecystitis. *J Clin Ultrasound* 1995;23:169-172.

79. Laing FC, Jeffrey RB Jr. Choledocholithiasis and cystic duct obstruction: difficult ultrasonographic diagnosis. *Radiology* 1983;146:475-479.

80. Warren BL. Small vessel occlusion in acute acalculous cholecystitis. *Surgery* 1992;111:163-168.

81. Paulson EK, Kliewer MA, Hertzberg BS et al. Diagnosis of acute cholecystitis with color Doppler sonography: significance of arterial flow in thickened gallbladder wall. *AJR* 1994;162:1105-1108.

82. McGrath FP, Lee SH, Gibney RG. Color Doppler imaging of the cystic artery. *J Clin Ultrasound* 1992;20:433-438.

83. Lee FT, DeLone DR, Bean DW et al. Acute cholecystitis in an animal model: findings on color Doppler sonography. *AJR* 1995;165:85-90.

84. Jeffrey RB, Nino-Murcia M, Ralls PW et al. Color Doppler sonography of the cystic artery: comparison of normal controls and patients with acute cholecystitis. *J Ultrasound Med* 1995;14:33-36.

85. Mentzer RM, Golden CT, Chandler JC et al. A comparative appraisal of emphysematous cholecystitis. *Am J Surg* 1975;129:10-15.

86. Bloom RA, Libson E, Lebensart PD et al. The ultrasound spectrum of emphysematous cholecystitis. *J Clin Ultrasound* 1989;17:251-256.

87. Parulekar SG. Sonographic findings in acute emphysematous cholecystitis. *Radiology* 1982;145:117-119.

88. Teefey SA, Baron RL, Radke HM et al. Gangrenous cholecystitis: new observation on sonography. *J Ultrasound Med* 1991;10:603-606.

89. Simeone JF, Brink JA, Mueller PR et al. The sonographic diagnosis of acute gangrenous cholecystitis: importance of the Murphy sign. *AJR* 1989;152:289-290.

90. Strohl EL, Diffenbaugh WG, Baker JH et al. Collective reviews: gangrene and perforation of the gallbladder. *Int Obstet Surg* 1962;114:1-7.

91. Niemeier OW. Acute free perforation of the gallbladder. *Ann Surg* 1934;99:922-924.

92. Smith R, Rosen JM, Alderson PO. Gallbladder perforation: diagnostic utility of cholescintigraphy in suggested subacute or chronic cases. *Radiology* 1986;158:63-66.

93. McDonnell CH, Jeffrey RB, Vierra MA. Inflamed pericholecystic fat: color Doppler flow imaging and clinical features. *Radiology* 1994;193:547-550.

94. Chau WK, Na AT, Feng TT et al. Ultrasound diagnosis of perforation of the gallbladder: real-time application and the demonstration of a new sonographic sign. *J Clin Ultrasound* 1988;16:358-360.

95. Chau WK, Wong KB, Chan SC et al. Ultrasonic "hole sign": a reliable sign of perforation of the gallbladder? *J Clin Ultrasound* 1992;20:294-299.

96. Kim PN, Lee KS, Kim IY et al. Gallbladder perforation: comparison of US findings with CT. *Abdom Imag* 1994;19:239-242.

97. Mirvis SE, Vainright JR, Nelson AW et al. The diagnosis of acute acalculous cholecystitis: a comparison of sonography, scintigraphy, and computed tomography. *AJR* 1986;147:1171-1175.

98. Raduns K, McGahan JP, Beal S. Cholecystokinin sonography: lack of utility in diagnosis of acute acalculous cholecystitis. *Radiology* 1990;175:463-466.

99. Jeffrey RB, Sommer FG. Follow-up sonography in suspected acalculous cholecystitis: preliminary clinical experience. *J Ultrasound Med* 1993;412:183-187.

100. Blankenberg F, Wirth R, Jeffrey RB et al. Computed tomography as an adjunct to ultrasound in the diagnosis of acute acalculous cholecystitis. *Gastrointest Radiol* 1991;16:149-153.

101. Swayne LC. Acute acalculous cholecystitis: sensitivity in detection using technetium-99m iminodiacetic acid cholescintigraphy. *Radiology* 1986;160:33-38.

102. Fig LM, Wahl RL, Stewart RE et al. Morphine-augmented hepatobiliary scintigraphy in the severely ill: caution is in order. *Radiology* 1990;175:467-474.

103. Ferrucci JT. Biliary lithotripsy. *AJR* 1989;153:15-22.

104. Torres WE, Baumgartner BR, Nelson RC et al. Shock wave lithotripsy of gallstones: results and 12-month follow-up in 174 patients. *Radiology* 1991;179:699-701.

105. Zeman RK, Al-Kawas F, Benjamin SB. Gallstone lithotripsy: is there still cause for optimism? *Radiology* 1991;178:33-35.

106. Cox MR, Wilson TG, Luck, AJ et al. Laparoscopic cholecystectomy for acute inflammation of the gallbladder. *Ann Surg* 1993;218:630-634.

107. Chen RC, Liu MH, Tu HY et al. The value of ultrasound measurement of gallbladder wall thickness in predicting laparoscopic operability prior to cholecystectomy. *Clin Radiol* 1995;50:570-572.

108. Metcalf AM, Ephgrave KS, Dean TR et al. Preoperative screening with ultrasonography for laparoscopic cholecystectomy: an alternative to routine intraoperative cholangiography. *Surgery* 1992;112:813-817.

109. Wachsberg RH. Sonographic evaluation of patients before laparoscopic cholecystectomy: imaging findings. *AJR* 1995;164:1419-1423.

110. Ascher SM, Evans SRT, Zeman RK. Laparoscopic cholecystectomy: intraoperative ultrasound of the extrahepatic biliary tree and the natural history of postoperative transabdominal ultrasound findings. *Sem Ultrasound CT MR* 1993;14:331-337.

111. Ascher SM, Evans SRT, Goldberg JA et al. Intraoperative bile duct sonography during laparoscopic cholecystectomy: experience with a 12.5 MHz catheter-based US probe. *Radiology* 1992;185:493-496.

112. Ray CE, Hibbeln JF, Wilbur AC. Complications after laparoscopic cholecystectomy: imaging findings. *AJR* 1993;160:1029-1032.

113. vanSonnenberg E, D'Agostino HB, Easter DW et al. Complications of laparoscopic cholecystectomy: coordinated radiologic and surgical management in 21 patients. *Radiology* 1993;188:399-404.

114. Kang EH, Middleton WD, Balfe DM et al. Laparoscopic cholecystectomy: evaluation with sonography. *Radiology* 1991;181:439-442.

115. Farrell TA, Geraghty JG, Keeling F. Abdominal ultrasonography following laparoscopic cholecystectomy: a prospective study. *Clin Radiol* 1993;47:111-113.

116. McGahan JP, Lindfors KK. Acute cholecystitis: diagnostic accuracy of percutaneous aspiration of the gallbladder. *Radiology* 1988;167:669-671.

117. Takada T, Yasuda H, Uchiyama K et al. Pericholecystic abscess: classification of ultrasound findings to determine the proper therapy. *Radiology* 1989;172:693-697.

118. Boland GW, Lee MJ, Mueller PR et al. Gallstones in critically ill patients with acute calculous cholecystitis treated by percutaneous cholecystostomy: nonsurgical therapeutic options. *AJR* 1994;162:1101-1103.

119. Browning PD, McGahan JP, Gerscovich EO. Percutaneous cholecystostomy for suspected acute cholecystitis in the hospitalized patient. *JVIR* 1993;4:531-538.

120. Lee MJ, Saini S, Brink JA et al. Treatment of critically ill patients with sepsis of unknown cause: value of percutaneous cholecystostomy. *AJR* 1991;156:1163-1166.

121. Lo LD, Vogelzang RL, Braun MA et al. Percutaneous cholecystostomy for the diagnosis and treatment of acute calculous and acalculous cholecystitis. *JVIR* 1995;6:629-634.

122. McGahan JP, Lindfors KK. Acute cholecystitis: diagnostic accuracy of percutaneous aspiration of the gallbladder. *Radiology* 1988;167:669-671.

123. Fitzgerald EJ, Toi A. Pitfalls in the ultrasonographic diagnosis of gallbladder diseases. *Postgrad Med J* 1987;63:525-532.

124. White M, Simeone JF, Mueller PR. Imaging of cholecystocolic fistulas. *J Ultrasound Med* 1983;2:181-185.

125. Gooding GAW. Food particles in the gallbladder mimic cholelithiasis in a patient with a cholecystojejunostomy. *J Clin Ultrasound* 1981;9:346-347.

126. Wall DT, Cooperberg PL, Mathieson JR. An unusual sonographic appearance: the pyramidal gallstone. *J Ultrasound Med* 1992;11:521-525.

127. Kirejczyk WM, Crowe HM, Mackay IM et al. Disappearing "gallstones": biliary pseudolithiasis complicating ceftriaxone therapy. *AJR* 1992;159:329-330.

128. Schaad UB, Wedgwood-Krucko J, Tschaeppeler H. Reversible ceftriaxone-associated biliary pseudolithiasis in children. *Lancet* 1988;2:1411-1413.

129. Scheske GA, Cooperberg PL, Cohen MM. Floating gallstones: the role of contrast material. *J Clin Ultrasound* 1980;8:227-231.

130. Rubaltelli L, Talenti E, Rizzatto G et al. Gas-containing gallstones: their influence on ultrasound images. *J Clin Ultrasound* 1984;12:279-282.

131. Mitchell DG, Needleman L, Frauenhoffer S et al. Gas-containing gallstones: the sonographic "double echo sign." *J Ultrasound Med* 1988;7:39-43.

132. Yeh HC, Goodman J, Rabinowitz JG. Floating gallstones in bile without added contrast material. *AJR* 1986;146:49-50.

133. Federle MP, Cello JP, Laing FC et al. Recurrent pyogenic cholangitis in Asian immigrants. *Radiology* 1982;143:151-156.

134. Reinig JW, Stanley JH. Sonographic hepatization of the gallbladder: a cause of nonvisualization of the gallbladder by cholecystosonography. *J Clin Ultrasound* 1984;12:234-236.

135. Hammond DI. Unusual causes of sonographic nonvisualization or nonrecognition of the gallbladder: a review. *J Clin Ultrasound* 1988;16:77-85.

136. Ferin P, Lemer RM. Contracted gallbladder: a finding in hepatic dysfunction. *Radiology* 1985;154:769-770.

137. Laing FC, Frates MC, Feldstein VA et al. Hemobilia: sonographic appearances in the gallbladder and biliary tree with emphasis on intracholecystic blood. *J Ultrasound Med*, in press.

138. Childress MH. Sonographic features of milk calcium cholecystitis. *J Clin Ultrasound* 1986;14:312-314.

139. Chun GH, Deutsch AL, Scheible W. Sonographic findings in milk of calcium bile. *Gastrointest Radiol* 1982;7:371-373.

140. Pandolfo I, Zimbaro G, Bartiromi G et al. Ultrasonographic and cholecystographic findings in a case of fascioliasis of the gallbladder. *J Clin Ultrasound* 1991;19:505-507.

141. Van Beers B, Pringot J, Geubel A et al. Hepatobiliary fascioliasis: noninvasive imaging findings. *Radiology* 1990;174:809-810.

142. Filice C, Marchi L, Meloni C et al. Ultrasound in the diagnosis of gallbladder ascariasis. *Abdom Imag* 1995;20:320-322.

143. Khuroo MS, Zargar SA, Yattoo GN et al. Sonographic findings in gallbladder ascariasis. *J Clin Ultrasound* 1992;20:587-591.

144. Fiske CE, Filly RA. Pseudo-sludge: a spurious ultrasound appearance within the gallbladder. *Radiology* 1982;144:631-632.

145. Laing FC, Kurtz AB. The importance of ultrasonic side-lobe artifacts. *Radiology* 1982;145:763-768.

146. Marchal GJ, Holsbeeck MV, Tshibwabwa-Ntumba E. Dilatation of the cystic veins in portal hypertension: sonographic demonstration. *Radiology* 1985;154:187-189.

147. Ralls PW, Mayekawa DS, Lee KP et al. Gallbladder wall varices: diagnosis with color flow doppler sonography. *J Clin Ultrasound* 1988;16:595-598.

Intrahepatic Bile Ducts

148. Bressler EL, Rubin JM, McCracken S et al. Sonographic parallel channel sign: a reappraisal. *Radiology* 1987;164:343-346.

149. Laing FC, London LA, Filly RA. Ultrasonographic identification of dilated intrahepatic bile ducts and their differentiation from portal venous structures. *J Clin Ultrasound* 1978;6:90-94.

150. Bret PM, de Stempel JV, Atri M et al. Intrahepatic bile duct and portal vein anatomy revisited. *Radiology* 1988;169:405-407.

151. Lim JH, Ryu KN, Ko YT et al. Anatomic relationship of intrahepatic bile ducts to portal veins. *J Ultrasound Med* 1990;9:137-143.

152. Ralls PW, Mayekawa, Lee KP et al. The use of color Doppler sonography to distinguish dilated intrahepatic ducts from vascular structures. *AJR* 1988;152:291-292.

153. Rubin JM, Bude RO, Carson PL et al. Power Doppler US: a potentially useful alternative to mean frequency-based color Doppler US. *Radiology* 1994;190:853-856.

154. Byung IC, Lim JH, Han MC et al. Biliary cystadenoma and cystadenocarcinoma: computed tomography and sonographic findings. *Radiology* 1989;171:57-61.

155. Wibulpolprasert B, Dhiensiri T. Peripheral cholangiocarcinoma: sonographic evaluation. *J Clin Ultrasound* 1992;20:303-314.

156. Carroll BA, Oppenheimer DA. Sclerosing cholangitis: sonographic demonstration of bile duct wall thickening. *AJR* 1982;139:1016-1018.

157. Singcharoen T, Baddeley H, Benson M et al. Primary sclerosing cholangitis: sonographic findings. *Aust Radiol* 1986;30:99-102.

158. Dolmatch BL, Laing FC, Federle MP et al. AIDS-related cholangitis: radiographic findings in nine patients. *Radiology* 1987;163:313-316.

159. Majoie CBLM, Smits NJ, Phoa SSKS et al. Primary sclerosing cholangitis: sonographic findings. *Abdom Imag* 1995;20:109-112.

160. Schulman A. Intrahepatic biliary stones: imaging features and a possible relationship with ascaris lumbricoides. *Clin Radiol* 1993;47:325-332.

161. Laing FC. Ultrasound diagnosis of choledocholithiasis. *Sem Ultrasound CT MR* 1987;8:103-113.

162. Chan FL, Man SW, Leong LLY et al. Evaluation of recurrent pyogenic cholangitis with CT: analysis of 50 patients. *Radiology* 1989;170:165-169.

163. Changchien CS, Chen JJ, Tai DI et al. Sonographic detection of stones in poorly opacified left intrahepatic ducts. *J Clin Ultrasound* 1992;20:121-125.

164. Miller WJ, Sechtin AG, Campbell WL et al. Imaging findings in Caroli's disease. *AJR* 1995;165:333-337.

165. Lee MG, Cho KS, Auh YH et al. Hepatic arterial color Doppler signals in Caroli's disease. *Clin Imag* 1992;16:234-238.

166. Bravo SM, Laing FC. Multiple bile duct hamartomas: Von Meyenburg complexes detected on sonography and CT scanning. *J Ultrasound Med* 1994;13:649-651.

167. Baron RL, Campbell WL, Dodd GD. Peribiliary cysts associated with severe liver disease: imaging-pathologic correlation. *AJR* 1994;162:631-636.

168. Sample WF, Sarti DA, Goldstein Ll et al. Gray-scale ultrasonography of the jaundiced patient. *Radiology* 1978;128:719-725.

169. Laffey PA, Teplick SK, Haskin PH. Hemobilia: a cause of false-negative ductal dilatation. *J Clin Ultrasound* 1986;14:636-638.

170. Laffey PA, Brandon JC, Teplick SK et al. Ultrasound of hemobilia: a clinical and experimental study. *J Clin Ultrasound* 1988;16:167-170.

170a. Monden M, Okamura J, Kobayashi N et al. Hemobilia after percutaneous transhepatic biliary drainage. *Arch Surg* 1980;115:161-164.

171. Lewandowski BJ, Withers C, Winsberg F. The air-filled left hepatic duct: the saber sign as an aid to the radiographic diagnosis of pneumobilia. *Radiology* 1984;153:329-332.

172. Desai RK, Paushter DM, Armistead J. Intrahepatic arterial calcification mimicking pneumobilia. *J Ultrasound Med* 1989;8:333-335.

173. Lin HH, Changchien CS, Lin DY. Hepatic parenchymal calcifications: differentiation from intrahepatic stones. *J Clin Ultrasound* 1989;17:411-415.

174. Wing VW, Laing FC, Jeffrey RB. Sonographic differentiation of enlarged hepatic arteries from dilated intrahepatic bile ducts. *AJR* 1985;145:57-61.

175. Marincek B, Barbier PA, Becker CD et al. CT appearance of impaired lymphatic drainage in liver transplants. *AJR* 1986;147:519-523.

176. Kedar RP, Cosgrove DO. Echo-poor periportal cuffing: ultrasonographic appearance and significance. *J Clin Ultrasound* 1993;21:464-467.

Extrahepatic Bile Ducts

177. Parulekar SG. Sonography of the distal cystic duct. *J Ultrasound Med* 1989;8:367-373.

178. Niederau C, Muller J, Sonnenberg A et al. Extrahepatic bile ducts in healthy subjects, in patients with cholelithiasis, and in postcholecystectomy patients: a prospective ultrasonic study. *J Clin Ultrasound* 1983;11:23-27.

179. Behan M, Kazam E. Sonography of the common bile duct: value of the right anterior oblique view. *AJR* 1978;130:701-709.

180. Paruleker SG. Ultrasound evaluation of common bile duct size. *Radiology* 1979;133:703-707.

181. Graham MF, Cooperberg PL, Cohen MM et al. The size of the normal common hepatic duct following cholecystectomy: an ultrasonographic study. *Radiology* 1980;135:137-139.

182. Mueller PR, Ferrucci JT, Simeone JF et al. Postcholecystectomy bile duct dilatation: myth or reality? *AJR* 1981;136:355-358.

183. Bucceri AM, Brogna A, Ferrara R. Common bile duct caliber following cholecystectomy: a two-year sonographic survey. *Abdom Imag* 1994;19:251-252.

184. Wu CC, Ho YH, Chen CY. Effect of aging on common bile duct diameter: a real-time ultrasonographic study. *J Clin Ultrasound* 1984;12:473-478.

185. Davies RP, Downey PR, Moore WR et al. Contrast cholangiography versus ultrasonographic measurement of the "extrahepatic" bile duct: a two-fold discrepancy revisited. *J Ultrasound Med* 1991;10:653-657.

186. Campbell WL, Foster RG, Miller WJ et al. Changes in extrahepatic bile duct caliber in liver transplant recipients without evidence of biliary obstruction. *AJR* 1992;158:997-1000.

187. Laing FC, Jeffrey RB, Wing VW. Improved visualization of choledocholithiasis by sonography. *AJR* 1984;143:949-952.

188. Ralls PW. The gallbladder and bile ducts. In: Jeffrey RB, Ralls PW, eds. *CT and Sonography of the Acute Abdomen.* 2nd ed. Philadelphia, Pa: Lippincott-Raven; 1996:101.

189. Shawker TH, Jones BL, Girton ME. Distal common bile duct obstruction: an experimental study in monkeys. *J Clin Ultrasound* 1981;9:77-82.

190. Laing FC, Jeffrey RB Jr, Wing VW. Biliary dilatation: defining the level and cause by real-time ultrasound. *Radiology* 1986;160:39-42.

191. Buck JL, Elsayed AM. Ampullary tumors: radiologic-pathologic correlation. *RadioGraphics* 1993;13:193-212.

192. Robledo R, Prieto ML, Perez M et al. Carcinoma of the hepaticopancreatic ampullar region: role of US. *Radiology* 1988;166:409-412.

193. Da Silva F, Boudghene F, Lecomte I et al. Sonography in AIDS-related cholangitis: prevalence and cause of an echogenic nodule in the distal end of the common bile duct. *AJR* 1993;160:1205-1207.

194. Robledo R, Muro A, Prieto ML. Extrahepatic bile duct carcinoma: US characteristics and accuracy in demonstration of tumors. *Radiology* 1996;198:869-873.

195. Middleton WD, Surratt RS. Thickened bile duct wall simulating ductal dilatation on sonography. *AJR* 1992;159:331-332.

196. Gibson RN, Yeung E, Thompson J et al. Bile duct obstruction: radiologic evaluation of level, cause, and tumor resectability. *Radiology* 1986;160:43-47.

197. Looser C, Stain SC, Baer HU et al. Staging of hilar cholangiocarcinoma by ultrasound and duplex sonography: a comparison with angiography and operative findings. *Br J Radiol* 1992;65:871-877.

198. Neumaier CE, Bertolotto M, Perrone R et al. Staging of hilar cholangiocarcinoma with ultrasound. *J Clin Ultrasound* 1995;23:173-178.

199. Hann LE, Fong Y, Shriver CD et al. Malignant hepatic hilar tumors: can ultrasonography be used as an alternative to angiography with CT arterial portography for determination of resectability? *J Ultrasound Med* 1996;15:37-45.

200. Garber SJ, Donald JJ, Lees WR. Cholangiocarcinoma: ultrasound features and correlation of tumor position with survival. *Abdom Imag* 1993;18:66-69.

201. Choi BI, Lee JH, Han MC et al. Hilar cholangiocarcinoma: comparative study with sonography and CT. *Radiology* 1989;172:689-692.

202. Perret RS, Thorsen MK, Lawson TL. Neoplastic diseases of the gallbladder and biliary tract. In: Freeny PC, Stevenson GW, eds. *Alimentary Tract Radiology.* 5th ed. St Louis: Mosby-Year Book 1994:1333-1342.

203. Nesbit GM, Johnson CD, James EM et al. Cholangiocarcinoma: diagnosis and evaluation of resectability by computed tomography and sonography as procedures complementary to cholangiography. *AJR* 1988;151:933-938.

204. Klatskin G. Adenocarcinoma of the hepatic duct at its bifurcation within the porta hepatis: an unusual tumor with distinctive clinical and pathologic features. *Am J Med* 1965;38:241-256.

205. Wang JH, Wang LY, Lin ZY et al. Doppler sonography of common hepatic duct tumor invasion in hepatocellular carcinoma: report of two cases. *J Ultrasound Med* 1995;14:471-474.

206. Jackson VP, Lappas JC. Sonography of the Mirizzi syndrome. *J Ultrasound Med* 1984;3:281-283.

207. Becker CD, Hassler H, Terrier F. Preoperative diagnosis of the Mirizzi syndrome: limitations of sonography and computed tomography. *AJR* 1984;143:591-596.

208. Kim OH, Chung HJ, Choi BG. Imaging of the choledochal cyst. *RadioGraphics* 1995;15:69-88.

209. Han BK, Babcock DS, Gelfand MH. Choledochal cyst with bile duct dilatation: sonography and 99mTc-IDA cholescintigraphy. *AJR* 1981;136:1075-1079.

210. Miller TT, Palestro CJ, Groisman GM et al. Choledochal cyst: preoperative sonographic and scintigraphic assessment. *Clin Nucl Med* 1993;18:1001-1002.

211. World Health Organization. Intestinal Protozoan and Helminthic Infections. Geneva: World Health Organization; 1981:27. Technical report series 666.

212. Ali M, Khan AN. Sonography of hepatobiliary ascariasis. *J Clin Ultrasound* 1996;24:235-241.

213. Schulman A, Loxton AJ, Heydenrych JJ et al. Sonographic diagnosis of biliary ascariasis. *AJR* 1982;139:485-489.

214. Lim JH, Ko YT, Lee DH. Clonorchiasis: sonographic findings in 59 proved cases. *AJR* 1989;152:761-764.

215. Lim JH. Radiologic findings of clonorchiasis. *AJR* 1990; 155:1001-1008.

216. Ooms HWA, Puylaert JBCM, van der Werf SDJ. Biliary fascioliasis: US and endoscopic retrograde cholangiopancreatography findings. *Eur Radiol* 1995;5:196-199.

217. Laing FC, Jeffrey RB. The pseudo-dilated common bile duct: ultrasonographic appearance created by the gallbladder neck. *Radiology* 1980;135:405-407.

218. Jacobson JB, Brody PA. The transverse common duct. *AJR* 1981;136:91-95.

219. Berland LL, Lawson TL, Foley WD. Porta hepatis: sonographic discrimination of bile ducts from arteries with pulsed Doppler with new anatomic criteria. *AJR* 1982;138:833-840.

220. Weinstein BJ, Weinstein DP. Biliary tract dilatation in the nonjaundiced patient. *AJR* 1980;134:899-906.

221. Zemen R, Taylor KJW, Burrell MI et al. Ultrasound demonstration of anicteric dilatation of the biliary tree. *Radiology* 1980;134:689-692.

222. Raptopoulos V, Smith EH, Cummings T et al. Bile-duct dilatation after laparotomy: a potential effect of intestinal hypomotility. *AJR* 1986;147:729-731.

223. Muhletaler CA, Gerlock AJ Jr, Fleischer AC et al. Diagnosis of obstructive jaundice with nondilated bile ducts. *AJR* 1980;134:1149-1152.

224. Glazer GM, Filly RA, Laing FC. Rapid change in caliber of the nonobstructed common duct. *Radiology* 1981;140:161-162.

225. Mueller PR, Ferrucci JT Jr, Simeone JF et al. Observations on the distensibility of the common bile duct. *Radiology* 1982;142:467-472.

226. Simeone JF, Butch RJ, Mueller PR et al. The bile ducts after a fatty meal: further sonographic observations. *Radiology* 1986;160:29-31.

227. Dong B, Chen M. Improved sonographic visualization of choledocholithiasis. *J Clin Ultrasound* 1987;15:185-190.

228. Willson SA, Gosink BB, vanSonnenberg E. Unchanged size of a dilated common bile duct after fatty meal: results and significance. *Radiology* 1986;160:29-31.

229. Darweesh RM, Dodds WJ, Hogan WJ. Fatty meal sonography for evaluating patients with suspected partial common duct obstruction. *AJR* 1988;151:63-68.

230. Quinn RJ, Meredith C, Slade L. The effect of the Valsalva maneuver on the diameter of the common hepatic duct in extrahepatic biliary obstruction. *J Ultrasound Med* 1992;11:143-145.

231. Pasanen P, Partanen K, Pikkarainen P et al. Ultrasonography, CT, and ERCP in the diagnosis of choledochal stones. *Acta Radiol* 1992;33:53-56.

232. Stott MA, Farrands PA, Guyer PB et al. Ultrasound of the common bile duct in patients undergoing cholecystectomy. *J Clin Ultrasound* 1991;19:73-76.

233. Lim JH. Papilla of Vater: normal sonographic appearance. *J Ultrasound Med* 1996;15:33-35.

234. Cronan JJ, Mueller PR, Simeone JF et al. Prospective diagnosis of choledocholithiasis. *Radiology* 1983;146:467-469.

235. Cronan J. Ultrasound diagnosis of choledocholithiasis: a reappraisal. *Radiology* 1986;161:133-134.

Endoscopic Ultrasound

236. Pham CAN, Valette PJ, Barkun A. Endoscopic ultrasound exploration of a choledochal cyst. *Abdom Imag* 1993;18:29-31.

237. Amouyal P, Amouyal G, Levy P et al. Diagnosis of choledocholithiasis by endoscopic ultrasonography. *Gastroenterology* 1994;106:1062-1067.

238. Mitake M, Nakazawa S, Naitoh Y et al. Endoscopic US in diagnosis of the extent of gallbladder carcinoma. *Gastrointest Endosc* 1990;36:562-566.

239. Mitake M, Nakazawa S, Tsukamoto Y et al. Endoscopic ultrasonography in the diagnosis of depth invasion and lymph node metastasis of carcinoma of the papilla of Vater. *J Ultrasound Med* 1990;9:645-650.

240. Lossef SV, Garra BS, Barth KH et al. Percutaneous extraction of biliary stones: value of endoluminal sonography. *AJR* 1992;159:411-412.

241. vanSonnenberg E, D'Agostino HB, Sanchez RL et al. Percutaneous intraluminal US in the gallbladder and bile ducts. *Radiology* 1992;182:693-696.

242. Kuroiwa M, Tsukamoto Y, Naitoh Y et al. New technique using intraductal ultrasonography for the diagnosis of bile duct cancer. *J Ultrasound Med* 1994;13:189-195.

243. Furukawa T, Naitoh Y, Tsukamoto Y et al. New technique using intraductal ultrasonography for the diagnosis of diseases of the pancreatobiliary system. *J Ultrasound Med* 1992;11:607-612.

244. Minsky B, Botet J, Gerdes H et al. Ultrasound directed extrahepatic bile duct intraluminal brachytherapy. *Int J Radiat Oncol Biol Phys* 1992;23:165-167.

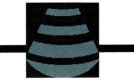

CHAPTER 7

The Pancreas

•

Mostafa Atri, M.D., F.R.C.P.(C)
Paul W. Finnegan, M.D., C.M., F.R.C.P.(C)

CHAPTER OUTLINE

EMBRYOLOGY
ANATOMY
  Surrounding Structures
    Gastrointestinal Tract, Ligaments, and
      Peritoneal Spaces
    Vessels
    Common Bile Duct
PANCREATIC SONOGRAPHY
  Head
    Transverse Plane
    Sagittal Plane
  Neck, Body, and Tail
    Transverse Plane
    Sagittal Plane
  Pancreatic Duct
  Pancreatic Echotexture
  Dimensions
  Pitfalls and Normal Variants
    Pancreas
    Pancreatic Duct
    Intrapancreatic Common Bile Duct
  Technical Aspects
    Patient Preparation
    Considerations of Technique
    Sonographic Examination of the Pancreas
CONGENITAL ANOMALIES
  Agenesis
  Congenital Cysts

Cystic Fibrosis
Pancreas Divisum
von Hippel-Lindau Syndrome
INFLAMMATORY PROCESSES
  Acute Pancreatitis
    Sonography
    Complications
  Chronic Pancreatitis
NEOPLASMS
  Adenocarcinoma
    Sonography
    Comparative Imaging
    Differential Diagnosis
  Cystic Neoplasms
    Sonography
    Comparative Imaging
  Islet-Cell Tumors
    Functioning Tumors
    Sonography
    Comparative Imaging
  Nonislet-Cell Tumors
ULTRASOUND-GUIDED PANCREATIC
  INTERVENTION
  Biopsy
  Percutaneous Pancreatography
PANCREATIC TRANSPLANTATION
ENDOSCOPIC ULTRASONOGRAPHY

Before 1970, imaging of the pancreas was limited to the assessment of its surrounding structures or its vascular tree by angiography. With the advent of ultrasonography, visualization of the pancreas itself became a reality. Since then, other imaging modalities such as computerized tomography (CT) and magnetic resonance imaging (MRI) have become available to examine the pancreatic parenchyma. The development of fiber optic technology has allowed physicians to examine the pancreatic duct with endoscopic retrograde cholangiopancreatography (ERCP) and, more recently, has allowed the examiner to apply high-resolution sonography with the use of endoscopic ultrasonography (EUS). Although CT has played a major role, ultrasound remains the most widely available and least expensive means of visualizing the pancreas.

Although a spectrum of pathological processes affects the pancreas, the major tasks of the imager are to distinguish a normal from an abnormal pancreas and to differentiate pancreatitis from malignancies. With the development of ultrasound-guided percutaneous fine-needle aspiration (PFNA) biopsy, accuracy in differentiating pancreatitis from carcinoma has significantly improved. Ultrasound guidance has also helped to promote the percutaneous interventional procedure as an alternative to surgical treatment for a number of pathologies related to the pancreas.

EMBRYOLOGY

The primitive pancreas consists of a dorsal and a ventral bud.[1] The dorsal bud arises as a diverticulum of the dorsal aspect of the duodenum, whereas the ventral bud originates as a common diverticulum with the primitive common bile duct (Fig. 7-1, *A*). At 6 weeks' gestation, the ventral bud rotates 270° to lie posteroinferior to the dorsal bud (Fig. 7-1, *B*). Fusion of these two buds forms the final pancreas. The dorsal bud develops into the cephalad aspect of the head, neck, body, and the tail, whereas the caudad aspect of the head and the uncinate process originate from the ventral bud (Fig. 7-1, *C*). Initially, each pancreatic bud has its own duct, which drains separately into the duodenum at two different openings, the major and minor papillas. Following fusion of the two buds, the ventral duct in the head anastomoses with the proximal part of the dorsal duct in the body and tail to form the final *main pancreatic duct* (**duct of Wirsung**), which drains most of the pancreas (Fig. 7-1, *C*). This main duct empties into the duodenum through the major papilla together with the common bile duct. The remaining portion of the dorsal pancreatic duct, called the *accessory pancreatic duct* (**duct of Santorini**), opens into the duodenum at the minor papilla. Various degrees of regression affecting the terminal part of the

dorsal pancreatic duct result in multiple anatomic variants of the pancreatic duct (Fig. 7-2).[2]

ANATOMY

The pancreas can be localized with ultrasound by identifying its parenchymal architecture and the surrounding anatomical landmarks. The level of the pancreas is known to change slightly, depending on the phase of respiration. With maximal inspiration and expiration, the organ has been shown to shift 2 to 8 cm in the craniocaudad axis.[3] These respiratory migrations should be taken into consideration when imaging the pancreas and especially during ultrasound-guided biopsy.

The pancreas is a nonencapsulated, retroperitoneal structure that lies in the anterior pararenal space between the duodenal loop and the splenic hilum over a length of 12.5 to 15 cm.[1] The head, uncinate process, neck, body, and tail constitute the different parts of the pancreas (Fig. 7-3). The superior mesenteric vessels course posterior to the neck of the pancreas, separating the head from the body. The uncinate process represents the medial extension of the head and lies behind the superior mesenteric vessels. No anatomic landmark separates the body from the tail.

The pancreas comprises of exocrine and endocrine tissues. The exocrine pancreas constitutes 80% of the pancreatic tissue and is made up of ductal and acinar cells. The endocrine islet cells of Langerhans form only 2% of the pancreatic substance. The remaining 18% consists of fibrous stroma that contains blood vessels, nerves, and lymphatics.[4]

Surrounding Structures
Gastrointestinal Tract, Ligaments, and Peritoneal Spaces. The antrum of the **stomach** lies transversely across the midline, usually anterior to the pancreas, with the gastric body located anterior to the pancreatic tail. However, depending on the patient's body habitus, which alters the shape and orientation of the stomach, the pancreas may occupy a position cephalad or caudad to the stomach. The **duodenal loop**, except for the first segment, is retroperitoneal and encircles the pancreatic head.

The **transverse mesocolon** attaches posteriorly to the anterior aspect of the head, body, and proximal tail of the pancreas and anteriorly to the greater omentum. At the level of the head of the pancreas, the mesocolon joins midway between the superior and the inferior borders; at the level of the body, it suspends from the inferior border of the pancreas, dividing the organ into supra- and inframesocolic portions. The stomach, omentum, and lesser sac lie anterior to the pancreas in the **supramesocolic portion**.[1]

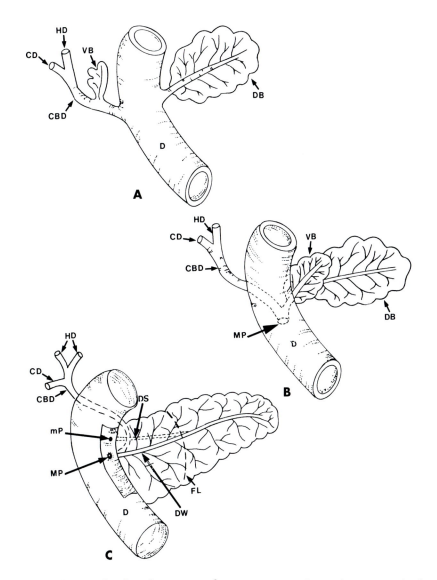

FIG. 7-1. **Stages in development of pancreas.** **A,** Original pancreatic buds ventral and dorsal. **B,** 270-degree rotation of ventral bud. **C,** Fusion of two buds and formation of final pancreatic duct. CBD—Common bile duct; CD—cystic duct; D—duodenum; DB—dorsal bud; DS—duct of Santorini; DW—duct of Wirsung; FL—fusion line; HD—hepatic duct; MP—major papilla; mP—minor papilla; VB—ventral bud.

The **lesser omentum**, which is a double layer of peritoneum, bridges the abdominal part of the esophagus, lesser curvature of the stomach, and first portion of the duodenum to the fissure for the ligamentum venosum of the liver. The **greater omentum,** which is also double-layered, hangs down from the greater curvature of the stomach and attaches to the transverse colon after looping back on itself. The lesser sac is a potential space situated between the lesser omentum, greater omentum, and the stomach anteriorly and the parietal peritoneum posteriorly. Depending on the position of the stomach, different parts of the lesser and greater omentum, stomach, and lesser sac are related to the pancreas anteriorly.[1] The **lesser sac** is often partially or completely obliterated by adhesions, and therefore, the stomach and greater and lesser omentum come in close contact with the anterior surface of the pancreas. The jejunal loops, duodenojejunal junction, and splenic flexure of the colon lie anterior to the pancreas in the **inframesocolic space.**[1] The tip of the tail of the pancreas is intraperitoneal because it is ensheathed in the lienorenal ligament.[1]

Vessels

Arteries. The **abdominal aorta** runs posterior to the body of the pancreas. The **celiac axis** arises from the abdominal aorta at the superior border of the pancreas and divides into the left gastric, common hepatic, and splenic arteries. The common hepatic artery proceeds anteriorly to the right, cephalad to the head of the pancreas. At the inferior border of the epiploic

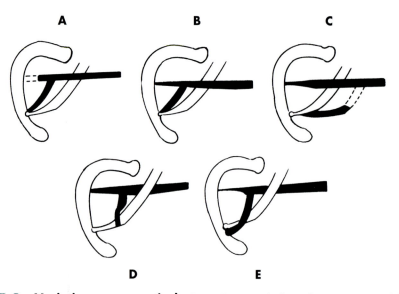

FIG. 7-2. **Variations, pancreatic duct anatomy.** **A,** Complete regression of duct of Santorini (40% to 50%). **B,** Persistence of the duct of Santorini (35%). **C,** Persistence of both Santorini and Wirsung ducts without communication (5% to 10%). **D,** Communication of Santorini and Wirsung ducts, with duct of Wirsung entering common bile duct proximal to ampulla (5% to 10%). **E,** Separate entrance of duct of Wirsung and common bile duct with variable persistence of duct of Santorini (5%). (From Berman LG, Prior JT, Abramow SM, et al.: A study of the pancreatic duct system in man by the use of vinyl acetate casts of postmortem preparations, *Surg Gynecol Obstet* 1960;110:391-403.)

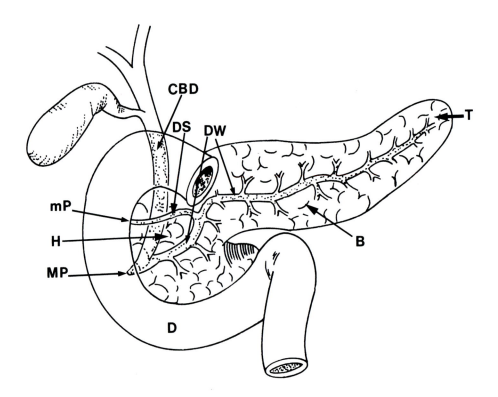

FIG. 7-3. **Schematic drawing, pancreas, duodenum, and bile duct.** B—Body of pancreas; CBD—common bile duct; DS—duct of Santorini; DW—duct of Wirsung; H—head of pancreas; mP—minor papilla; MP—major papilla; T—tail of pancreas.

foramen, the common hepatic artery divides into its two terminal branches: the hepatic proper and the gastroduodenal arteries. The hepatic artery proper travels superiorly toward the liver along the free edge of the lesser omentum anterior to the portal vein and to the left of the bile duct. A common normal variant, present in 25% of the population, consists of a completely or incompletely replaced hepatic artery, which arises from the right lateral aspect of the superior mesenteric artery. This accessory (or replaced hepatic artery) usually courses between the portal vein and the inferior vena cava as opposed to the normal hepatic artery that runs anterior to the portal vein. The gastroduodenal artery travels a short distance posterior to the junction of the pylorus and the first portion of the duodenum within a groove on the superior border of the pancreas lateral to the neck. Then, passing anterior to the head of the pancreas, it divides into its terminal branches, the right gastroepiploic and the superior pancreaticoduodenal arteries.[1] The splenic artery follows a tortuous course along the superior border of the body and the tail of the pancreas. The **superior mesenteric artery** arises from the abdominal aorta just caudad to the inferior border of the pancreas, descending anterior to the uncinate process of the pancreas and the third portion of the duodenum to enter the mesentery.

Veins. The **inferior vena cava** lies posterior to the head of the pancreas. Depending on the level at which the renal veins drain into the inferior vena cava, the left renal vein may travel posterior to the head of the pancreas, although it is usually more caudal.

The **splenic vein** runs from its origin in the splenic hilum along the posteroinferior aspect of the pancreas to join the superior mesenteric vein. The **superior mesenteric vein** travels to the right of the superior mesenteric artery and ascends anterior to the third portion of the duodenum and the uncinate process of the pancreas. The superior mesenteric vein and the splenic vein join posterior to the neck of the pancreas to form the portal vein. The **portal vein** ascends toward the porta hepatis cephalad to the head of the pancreas.[1]

Common Bile Duct. The common bile duct passes inferiorly in the free edge of the lesser omentum to the level of the duodenum. It then travels posterior to the first portion of the duodenum and the head of the pancreas to lie to the right of the main pancreatic duct. The common bile duct then opens into the duodenum at the hepaticopancreatic ampulla on the summit of the major papilla after forming a common trunk with the pancreatic duct (80%). In 20% of people, the common bile duct has its own separate ampulla but still enters the duodenum at the major papilla.[5] In its course behind the head of the pancreas, it lies in a groove on the posterior aspect of the pancreas or is embedded in its substance.

PANCREATIC SONOGRAPHY

Head

Transverse Plane. The pancreatic head may be quite long, extending over several centimeters. The sonographic appearance varies from the most cephalad to the most caudal image. **Cephalad to the pancreatic head,** the hepatic artery and bile duct are seen anterior to the portal vein. The air- or fluid-filled pylorus and the first portion of the duodenum may also be seen at this level. In the **superior aspect of the head,** two circular structures can be identified on the right lateral aspect of the head that represent a cross-sectional view of the **gastroduodenal artery** anteriorly and the **common bile duct** posteriorly. The latter structures demarcate the lateral aspect of the pancreatic head, allowing for separation of the head of the pancreas from the more laterally placed duodenum (Fig. 7-4, A). However, in some individuals, the lateral extent of the head may extend beyond a line drawn between the gastroduodenal artery and common bile duct (Fig. 7-4, B).[6] At this level, the medial extent of the head merges with the neck of the pancreas. The inferior vena cava lies posterior to the head. However, the relation of the pancreas to the inferior vena cava and aorta is variable and can occasionally be off-center to the left of the major vessels, especially in thin patients and in patients lying in the left decubitus position (Fig. 7-4, C). The main pancreatic duct and its branches may be seen extending obliquely between the neck of the pancreas more superiorly, and to the second portion of the duodenum more inferiorly, where it may or may not join the common bile duct before entering the duodenum. In its most **inferior aspect,** the medial portion of the pancreatic head tapers to form the **uncinate process.** At this level in cross-section, the superior mesenteric vein is seen to the right and the superior mesenteric artery to the left between the uncinate process and the neck of the pancreas (Fig. 7-4, D). A replaced hepatic artery is commonly shown by sonographic examination,[7] arising from the right lateral aspect of the superior mesenteric artery and running toward the liver between the portal vein and inferior vena cava (Fig. 7-5). **Caudally to the head,** the third portion of the duodenum may be seen running transversely from right to left.

Sagittal Plane. On the right and lateral to the head, the second portion of the duodenum projects in a cephalocaudal direction. In the lateral aspect of the head in some patients, the gastroduodenal artery may be seen coursing in a cephalocaudal direction anterior to the pancreas with the common bile duct running parallel but more posteriorly (Fig. 7-6, A). The latter may lie posterior to the pancreas or be embedded in its posterior aspect. The third portion of the duodenum is seen in cross-sectional views caudally to the pancreas.

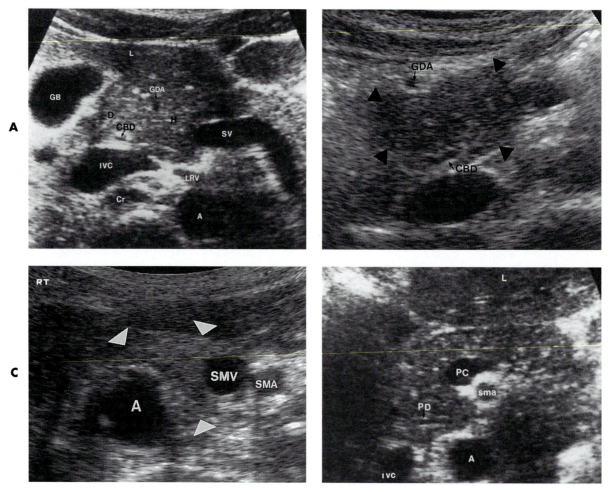

FIG. 7-4. Head of pancreas, transverse scans. A, Superior aspect of head. Duodenum is as echogenic as pancreas and can only be distinguished from head because of visualization of gastroduodenal artery (GDA) and common bile duct (CBD). **B,** Normal variant of the head. Head of pancreas (*arrowheads*) extends lateral to a line drawn between the GDA and CBD. **C,** Head of pancreas (*arrowheads*) lies anterior and to the left of abdominal aorta (A). **D,** Inferior aspect of head. Arrow points to branch of pancreatic duct (PD). A—aorta; CBD—common bile duct; Cr—crus of diaphragm; D—duodenum; GB—gallbladder; GDA—gastroduodenal artery; H—head of pancreas; IVC—inferior vena cava; L—liver; LRV—left renal vein; PC—portal confluence; PV—portal vein; sma—superior mesenteric artery; smv—superior mesenteric vein; sv—splenic vein.

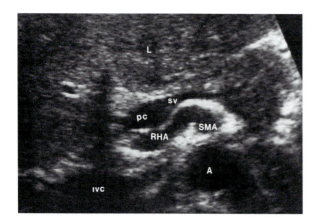

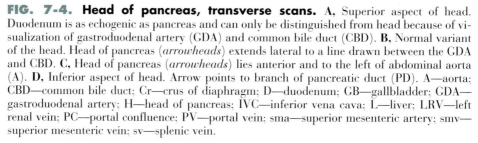

FIG. 7-5. Replaced hepatic artery (RHA) running between portal confluence (PC) and inferior vena cava (IVC). Transverse scan. A—aorta; L—liver; SMA—superior mesenteric artery; SV—splenic vein.

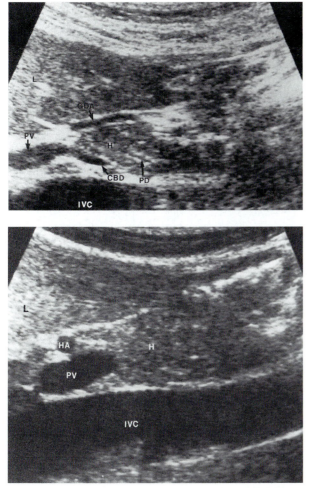

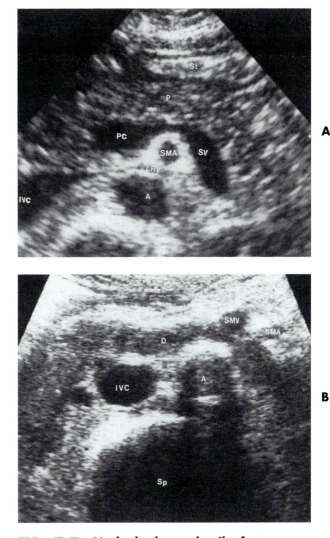

FIG. 7-6. Head of pancreas, sagittal view. A, Lateral aspect of head. B, Medial aspect of head. CBD—Common bile duct; GDA—gastroduodenal artery; H—head of pancreas; HA—hepatic artery; IVC—inferior vena cava; L—liver; PD—pancreatic duct; PV—portal vein.

FIG. 7-7. Neck, body, and tail of pancreas, transverse view. A, Through pancreas. B, Caudad to pancreas. A—aorta; D—duodenum; IVC—inferior vena cava; L—liver; LRV—left renal vein; P—pancreas; PC—portal confluence; SMA—superior mesenteric artery; Sp—spine; St—stomach; SV—splenic vein.

More medially, the longest cephalocaudal dimension of the head is displayed. A longitudinal view of the main portal vein projects superior to the head of the pancreas at this level (Fig. 7-6, B).

Neck, Body, and Tail

The pancreatic neck lies between the head and body anterior to the portal venous confluence. There is no anatomic landmark separating the body and the tail of the pancreas, but the left lateral border of the vertebral column is considered the arbitrary plane demarcating these two segments. The level of the tail in relation to the body of the pancreas on the horizontal plane varies depending on the body habitus. It may be located cephaladly, at the same level, or (rarely) lower than the body.

Transverse Plane. The celiac axis is seen **cephalad** to the body of the pancreas at this level,

dividing similar to a "Y" into the hepatic and splenic arteries. At the **level of the neck**, the confluence of the splenic and superior mesenteric veins is seen posterior to the pancreas. More laterally, the splenic vein runs posterior to the body and the tail. The abdominal aorta lies posterior to the proximal body of the pancreas. The left renal vein courses between the superior mesenteric artery and the aorta and posterior to the pancreas to drain into the inferior vena cava. The upper pole of the left kidney and the left renal vessels may also be seen posterior to the tail of the pancreas. Depending on the location of the stomach, its posterior wall may be visualized anterior to the pancreas (Fig. 7-7, A). **Caudad** to the pancreas lie the third and fourth portions of the duodenum (Fig. 7-7, B).

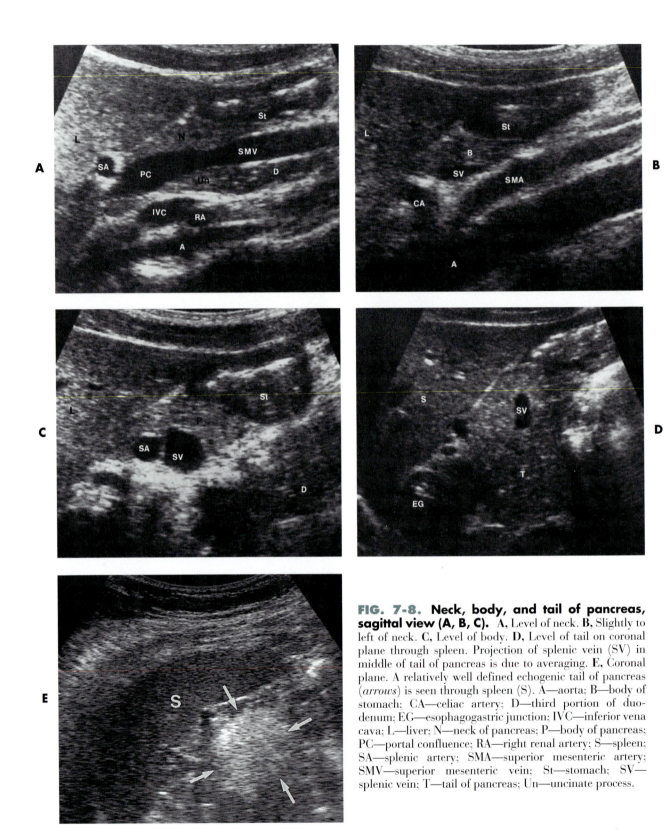

FIG. 7-8. **Neck, body, and tail of pancreas, sagittal view (A, B, C).** A, Level of neck. B, Slightly to left of neck. C, Level of body. D, Level of tail on coronal plane through spleen. Projection of splenic vein (SV) in middle of tail of pancreas is due to averaging. E, Coronal plane. A relatively well defined echogenic tail of pancreas (*arrows*) is seen through spleen (S). A—aorta; B—body of stomach; CA—celiac artery; D—third portion of duodenum; EG—esophagogastric junction; IVC—inferior vena cava; L—liver; N—neck of pancreas; P—body of pancreas; PC—portal confluence; RA—right renal artery; S—spleen; SA—splenic artery; SMA—superior mesenteric artery; SMV—superior mesenteric vein; St—stomach; SV—splenic vein; T—tail of pancreas; Un—uncinate process.

Caution should be exercised not to mistake a jejunal branch draining into the superior mesenteric vein as a splenic vein. In the presence of splenic vein thrombosis, this jejunal branch may be mistaken for a patent splenic vein.

Sagittal Plane. At the level of the neck, the superior mesenteric vein is seen posterior to the pancreas (Fig. 7-8, *A*). The uncinate process of the head is seen posterior to the superior mesenteric vein. A longitudinal view of the aorta is identified with the **body** of

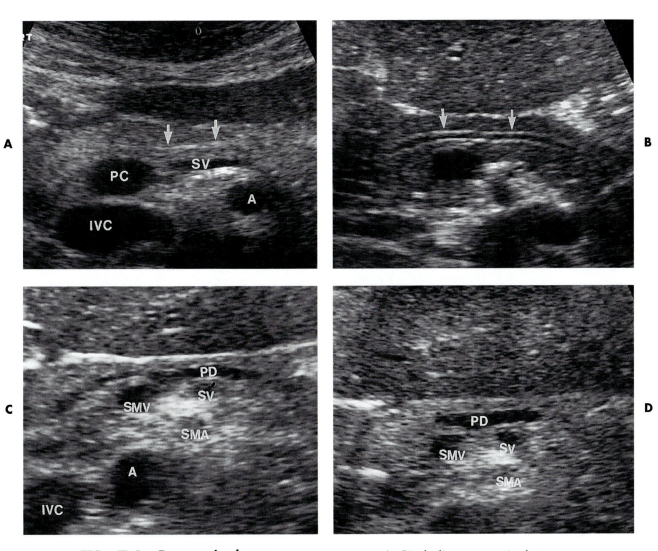

FIG. 7-9. Pancreatic duct, transverse scan. A, Single line pancreatic duct (*arrows*). **B,** Double-line pancreatic duct (*arrows*). **C,** Small caliber pancreatic duct (PD), **D,** changing to a larger caliber during the same examination. A—aorta; IVC—inferior vena cava; L—liver; PC—portal confluence; SMA—superior mesenteric artery; SMV—superior mesenteric vein; SV—splenic vein.

the pancreas situated between the celiac axis and the superior mesenteric artery (Fig. 7-8, *B*). At the levels of the body and the tail, the stomach lies anteriorly (Fig. 7-8, *C*). A cross-section of the splenic vein is seen posteriorly, whereas a cross-section of the splenic artery appears cephaladly. The third portion of the duodenum projects inferiorly. Using the spleen as an acoustic window, the **tail** of the pancreas is occasionally seen medial to that organ on both transverse and coronal planes (Fig. 7-8, *D*). When the pancreas is echogenic, a distinct echogenic structure representing the tail may be seen through the spleen (Fig. 7-8, *E*).

Pancreatic Duct

The normal pancreatic duct is seen at least partially in 86% of patients.[8] On the transverse plane, it is opti-

mally visualized in the central portion of the body where the duct is perpendicular to the ultrasound beam. Based on the resolution of the ultrasound system, the patient's body habitus, and the angle of insonation, the pancreatic duct is seen as a single linear structure (Fig. 7-9, *A*) or as double-parallel lines (Fig. 7-9, *B*). The mean internal diameter on sonographic examination has been reported to measure 3 mm in the head, 2.1 mm in the body, and 1.6 mm in the tail.[9] The dimensions of the pancreatic duct obtained sonographically are smaller than the corresponding ERCP measurements as a result primarily of x-ray magnification and overdistention of the duct.[10] Its diameter increases with age, probably because of parenchymal atrophy. Although 2- to 2.5-mm[8,10] diameter has been reported as the upper limit of normal, for practical purposes the

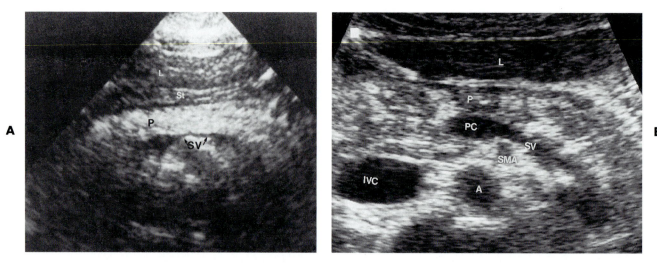

FIG. 7-10. Pancreas echotexture. A, Echogenic pancreas. Transverse scan. **B,** Mottled appearance of pancreas (P). A—aorta; IVC—inferior vena cava; L—liver; P—pancreas; PC—portal confluence; SMA—superior mesenteric artery; St—stomach; SV—splenic vein.

pancreatic duct is probably normal as long as the walls maintain their parallel course and the duct can be followed along its whole length to the duodenum. When the pancreatic duct becomes dilated, its side branches may also be seen and may be mistaken for pancreatic cysts. Occasionally, the accessory duct of Santorini and some normal branches of the main pancreatic duct can be identified in the pancreatic head. The normal pancreatic duct can change caliber during the examination (Fig. 7-9, C and D).

Pancreatic Echotexture

The normal pancreas is usually homogeneous. The echogenicity, when compared with the normal liver, is either isoechoic (Fig. 7-4, B) or hyperechoic (Fig. 7-8, E and Fig. 7-10, A). Sometimes a mottled appearance may be seen (Fig. 7-7, A and Fig. 7-10, B). The contour of the pancreas is distinct when its echogenicity is less than the surrounding retroperitoneal fat. The gland usually appears smoothly contoured, although a lobulated contour is occasionally discerned. With aging and obesity, the pancreas becomes more echogenic as a result of the presence of **fatty infiltration**, and in up to 35% of cases may be as echogenic as the adjacent retroperitoneal fat (Figs. 7-8, E and 7-10, A).[11] The increased echogenicity resulting from excessive body fat is reversible.[12] Hyperechogenicity may account for difficulty in visualizing the pancreas as it blends with the adjacent retroperitoneal fat, making its contour and true size impossible to identify. In such patients, the gland can be assessed only by describing the pancreatic fossa using the vascular anatomy as landmarks. Because the size of the pancreas cannot be evaluated in these patients, pancreatic atrophy resulting in

pancreatic insufficiency should not be excluded.[11] Also, retroperitoneal fat in the bed of a congenitally absent or atrophic body and tail of the pancreas may mimic pancreatic tissue on ultrasound (Fig. 7-11). CT scans are indicated in these patients. **Causes of fatty infiltration of the pancreas** include: aging, obesity, chronic pancreatitis, dietary deficiency, viral infection, steroid therapy, cystic fibrosis, diabetes mellitus, hereditary pancreatitis, and obstruction caused by a stone or pancreatic carcinoma.[12] In lipomatous pseudohypertrophy, the pancreas is massively enlarged as a result of fatty replacement.[13]

Dimensions

The normal head of the pancreas generally has the largest dimensions with the neck having the smallest.[14] The body and most of the tail are slightly smaller than the head. In one study,[15] the anteroposterior dimension of the normal head measured 2.2 to 0.3 cm, with the body measuring 1.8 to 0.3 cm. The cephalocaudal dimension of the head has been reported as 2.01 to 0.39 cm and that of the body as 1.18 to 0.36 cm.[14] The pancreas may appear larger in obese patients, because it blends with the excessive retroperitoneal fat. The size of the pancreas diminishes with age.[16]

Pitfalls and Normal Variants

Pancreas. Structures that may be mistaken for the pancreas or pancreas pathology include the **posterior part (segment 2) of the lateral segment of the left lobe of the liver,** when it is less echogenic than the anterior part (segment 3) because of sound attenuation by perivascular fat. **Papillary process of the caudate lobe,** when it is completely separated

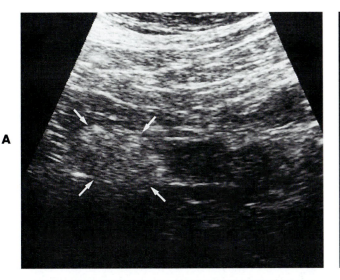

A

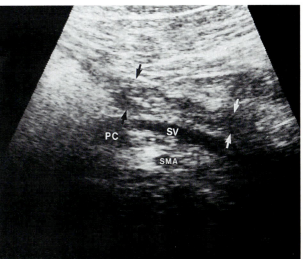

B

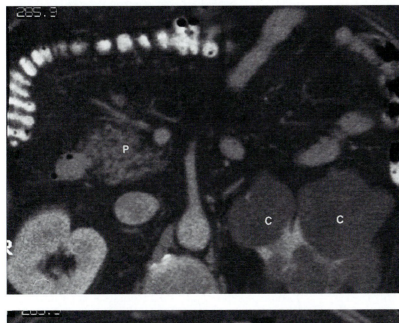

C

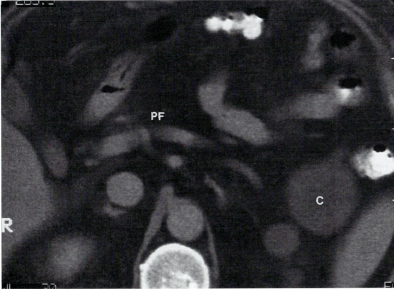

D

FIG. 7-11. Congenital absence of body and tail of pancreas confirmed on CT scan. **A,** Transverse view of region of head shows a well-defined echogenic structure (*arrows*). **B,** Transverse view of the region of body and tail. An inhomogeneous area of increased echogenicity (*arrows*) representing retroperitoneal fat mimicks body and tail of pancreas. **C,** Normal head of pancreas (P). **D,** Absent body and tail of pancreas in the pancreatic fossa (PF). C—renal cysts.

STRUCTURES THAT MAY BE MISTAKEN FOR THE PANCREAS OR PANCREAS PATHOLOGY

Posterior part of the lateral segment of the left lobe of the liver because of sound attenuation by perivascular fat

Papillary process of the caudate lobe when it is completely separated from the liver

Third part of the duodenum
  Collapsed or filled with echogenic fluid

Retroperitoneal fibrosis
  When seen as a midline band inferior to the pancreas between the aorta and the mesenteric vessels

Horseshoe kidney
  Usually inferior and posterior to the mesenteric vessels

Lymph nodes simulate a bandlike pancreas

Intrapancreatic collateral veins secondary to portal vein thrombosis may mimic intrapancreatic cystic lesions (Fig. 7-12, *A* and *B*).

Ventral aspect of the head and uncinate process may be hypoechoic relative to the rest of the pancreas (Fig. 7-12, *C* and *D*)

STRUCTURES THAT ARE CONFUSED WITH THE PANCREATIC DUCT

Layers of the posterior wall of the stomach and the splenic vein (Fig. 7-13, *A*)

Jejunal branch of the superior mesenteric vein
  May be surrounded by retroperitoneal fat that can simulate pancreatic tissue

Averaging of a tortuous splenic artery within the pancreas

Significant pancreatic atrophy
  Erroneous interpretation of a vascular structure

Venous branches draining into the portal vein

Intrapancreatic collateral veins

Air in the pancreatic duct
  Mistaken for ductal calculi

---

from the liver. **Third part of the duodenum,** when it is collapsed or filled with echogenic fluid (bowel wall layers and peristalsis differentiate). **Retroperitoneal fibrosis,** when seen as a midline band (it usually occurs inferior to the pancreas between the aorta and the mesenteric vessels). **Horseshoe kidney,** which is usually inferior and posterior to the mesenteric vessels, continuous with kidneys, and reniform in shape. **Lymph nodes,** which can simulate a bandlike pancreas (associated aortocaval, retrocaval, or retroaortic lymphadenopathy help to differentiate them from the pancreas). **Intrapancreatic collateral veins** secondary to portal vein thrombosis which may mimic intrapancreatic cystic lesions (Fig. 7-12, *A* and *B*). The embryologic **ventral aspect of the head and uncinate process of the pancreas** may be hypoechoic relative to the rest of the pancreas in some individuals (Fig. 7-12, *C* and *D*).[17-19] The distribution of the hypoechogenicity and geographic appearance, sharp demarcation from the rest of the pancreas, and the identification of the normal pancreatic duct and common bile duct (Fig. 7-12, *C*) within this zone help to distinguish it from pathological process.

We have shown on correlation of ultrasound and pathology *in vitro* that this area of hypoechogenicity corresponds to less fatty infiltration of the embryologic ventral pancreas.[19] The corresponding finding on CT scan is higher attenuation of the ventral pancreas. In our series, the prevalence of this finding was 54% on the pancreas autopsy specimens and 22% on the CT scan. *In vivo* prevalence of this finding on ultrasound was 28.1% in Donald et al. series.[17] CT may or may not show an area of high density corresponding to the hypoechogenicity on ultrasound, presumably depending on the discrepancy in fat content.

Pancreatic Duct. Structures that are confused with the pancreatic duct and errors of interpretation include the layers of the posterior wall of the stomach and the outline of the splenic vein (Fig. 7-13, *A*). No pancreatic parenchyma surrounds them, they are not located in the middle of an apparent pancreas, and their course is not toward the second portion of the duodenum. A jejunal branch of the superior mesenteric vein may have an appearance and orientation similar to the pancreatic duct because it may be surrounded by retroperitoneal fat that can simulate pancreatic tissue on ultrasonograms. Following the vessel to its junction with the superior mesenteric vein and Doppler interrogation help to differentiate a vascular structure from the pancreatic duct. Artifacts inherent to the ultrasound technology, such as beam width, can cause averaging of a tortuous splenic artery within the pancreas and may simulate a dilated pancreatic duct. With significant pancreatic atrophy caused by obstruction, no pancreatic tissue is seen around the dilated duct, creating the potential for an erroneous interpretation of a vascular structure. This is more likely to happen when the pancreas is very anterior as a result of significant emaciation caused by pancreatic carcinoma. On rare occasions, venous branches draining into the portal vein are seen in the head of the pancreas,

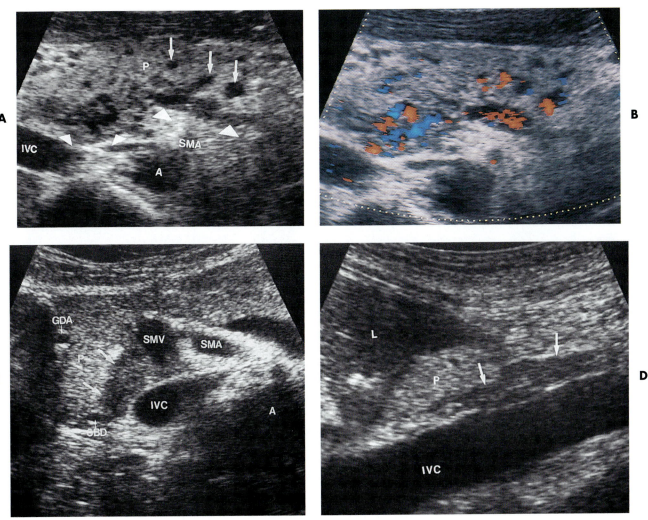

FIG. 7-12. Pitfalls and normal variants of pancreas. Thrombosis of the splenoportal circulation in a patient with pancreatic carcinoma. Transverse views. **A,** Splenoportal vein thrombosis (*arrowheads*). Collateral veins (*arrows*) in pancreas (P). **B,** Color Doppler examination of the same patient demonstrating color flow in the vascular spaces of the pancreas. **Hypoechoic ventral aspect of head of pancreas. C,** Transverse and **D,** Sagittal views show well-defined hypoechogenicity of embryologic ventral aspect of head of pancreas (*arrows*). Notice the undisturbed common bile duct (CBD). A—aorta; GDA—gastroduodenal artery; IVC—inferior vena cava; L—liver; P—pancreas; SMA—superior mesenteric artery; SMV—superior mesenteric vein.

which can be mistaken for the pancreatic duct (Fig. 7-13, *B* and *C*). Intrapancreatic collaterals in the presence of portal vein thrombosis may be mistaken for a pancreatic duct. The course of these structures and documentation of flow on Doppler help differentiation (Fig. 7-13, *D, E,* and *F*). Air in the pancreatic duct, usually secondary to pancreaticoenterostomy, may be mistaken for ductal calculi.

Intrapancreatic Common Bile Duct. A normal posterior-superior pancreaticoduodenal vein is occasionally seen running in the cephalocaudal di-

mension in the head of the pancreas to insert on the caudal aspect of the portal vein (Fig. 7-14, *A, B,* and *C*). This vein is reported to parallel the common bile duct posteriorly in 98% and anteriorly in 2% in one series.[20] It can potentially be mistaken for the common bile duct.

Technical Aspects

Patient Preparation. Evaluation of the pancreas is usually performed as part of the ultrasound examination of the upper abdomen and especially in con-

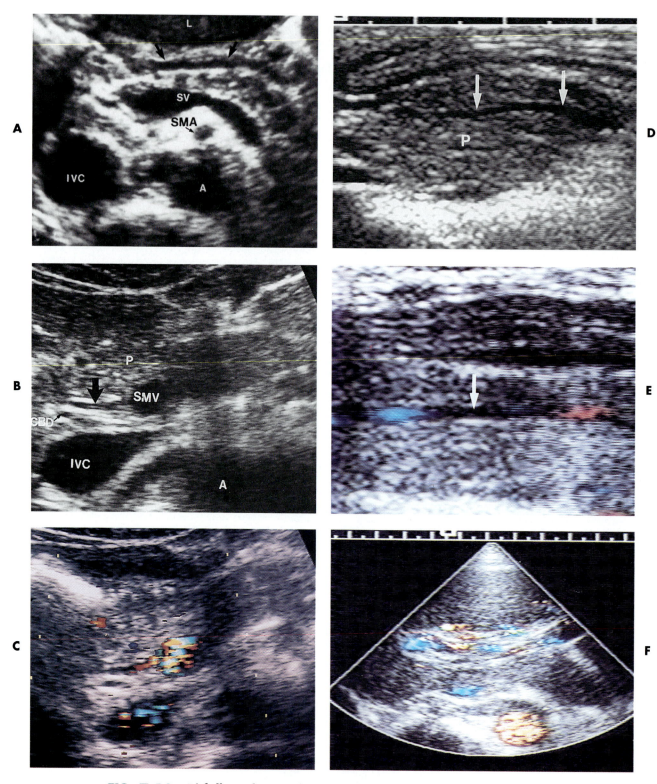

FIG. 7-13. Pitfalls and normal variants of pancreatic duct. Muscular layer of posterior wall of stomach *(arrows)* mimicking pancreatic duct. **A,** Transverse view. Branch of portal vein *(arrow)* lying transversely in the head of pancreas. **B,** Gray scale and, **C,** color Doppler transverse views. **Cavernous transformation of portal vein with collateral veins in the pancreas in a patient with history of pancreatitis. D,** Transverse view of head of pancreas (P) demonstrates a tubular structure *(arrows)*. **E,** Color Doppler shows the tubular structure *(arrow)* is a vessel. **F,** Cavernous transformation of portal system. Transverse view of porta hepatis. Pulsed Doppler interrogation proved these were veins. A—aorta; IVC—inferior vena cava; L—liver; P—pancreas; SMA—superior mesenteric artery; SMV—superior mesenteric vein; SV—splenic vein.

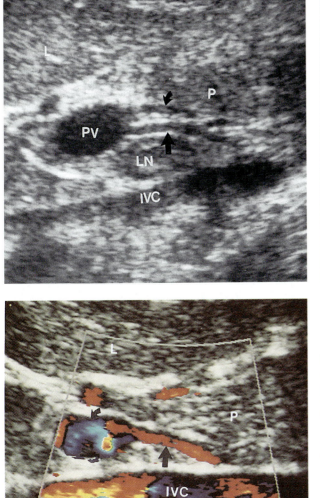

A

B

C

FIG. 7-14. Normal posterior superior pancreaticoduodenal vein (PSPDV). A, Sagittal view of head of pancreas (P) shows parallel course of PSPDV (*straight arrow*) posterior to common bile duct (*curved arrow*). **B,** Transverse plane of head of pancreas demonstrates PSPDV (*straight arrow*) posterior to common bile duct (*curved arrow*). **C,** Color Doppler view showing PSPDV (*straight arrow*) entering caudal aspect of portal vein (*curved arrow*). A—aorta; IVC—inferior vena cava; L—liver; LN—lymph node; P—pancreas; PC—portal confluence. (Courtesy of R. H. Wachsberg, MD, New Jersey Medical Center, Newark, New Jersey)

junction with assessment of the biliary system. Because optimal gallbladder distention requires fasting, ultrasound examination of the pancreas has been traditionally performed following a minimum fast of 6 hours. Theoretically, fasting also diminishes gaseous distension of the upper gastrointestinal tract, which can interfere with the visualization of the pancreas. However, in some patients, evaluating the pancreas alone appears to be feasible in postfasting state.[21]

Considerations of Technique. There are two major factors preventing optimal visualization of the pancreas: fat and interfering gastrointestinal gas. As the pancreas is retroperitoneal, it is a deep structure in larger patients and a particular technical challenge because it is covered by the gas-filled gastrointestinal tract. Scanning principles used for the examination of the pancreas include the following:

- Place the area of interest within the focal zone of the transducer.
- Alter the patient's position to include erect, supine, both obliques, both decubituses, and even prone positions, to displace the gas-containing structures or transfer the gas into another part of the gastrointestinal tract. The erect position displaces the gas-filled stomach or colon away from the pancreas and causes the liver to move down over the pancreas, becoming an acoustic window. The erect position appears to be most effective if used in the beginning of the examination because aerophagia caused by deep inspirations during the examination may fill the stomach with gas.
- Further, breathing mechanisms, including suspended inspiration or expiration, and a Valsalva maneuver may be helpful. Differentiation of a pan-

creatic mass from a lesion arising from surrounding structures may be helped by evaluating the mobility of the mass relative to these structures during respiration. The mobility of the pancreas is not as great as the intraperitoneal structures.[3]

- Lastly, increasing stomach distention with fluid when there is a large amount of interfering gas and when the upright position has failed to demonstrate the pancreas may allow pancreatic visualization. Ultrasonic oral contrast agents are also being developed to reduce artifacts from a gas-filled gastrointestinal tract, which may help visualization of the pancreas.[22] The fluid-filled stomach provides an acoustic window, causes movement of the intragastric gas, and acts as a balloon, displacing the gas-filled colon and small bowel loops inferiorly. Ingestion of deionized water through a straw minimizes air swallowing. Some investigators have advocated the use of tubeless hypotonic duodenography with glucagon to facilitate visualization of the head of the pancreas.[23] Alternatively, some authors have shown that using agents such as metoclopramide, which increases gastric and duodenal contractility, can improve visualization of the pancreas.[24] However, in practice, ingestion of water alone is adequate for most patients and no additional medication is required. In patients who have had barium studies of the upper gastrointestinal tract, ultrasound evaluation of the pancreas with a water-filled stomach one hour after the upper gastrointestinal study has been shown to provide better results than an ultrasound examination performed immediately after or 1 hr after the barium examination without a fluid-filled stomach.[25]

Sonographic Examination of the Pancreas.
Sonographic examination of the pancreas should begin with the patient in the erect position. Transverse scans in the midline below the xiphoid are made using the related vascular landmarks to identify the region of the pancreas. The probe may need to be oblique to visualize the gland in its entirety. Angling the transducer cephalad and caudal from the level of the longitudinal view of the splenic vein appears to be adequate in most patients to scan through the entire gland.

Sagittal scanning of the pancreas is initiated with the transducer in the midline below the xiphoid. The level of the pancreas is easily localized by identification of the portal splenic confluence. There should be minimal movement of the transducer to the left or right of the midline, and in practice, side-tilting of the probe has proved more effective than a lateral-sliding displacement.

Using the left kidney as an acoustic window, the tail of the pancreas may be visualized anterior to its upper pole with a left coronal view. In some thin patients, the tail of the pancreas can also be seen through the spleen from the left lateral intercostal approach using a coronal plane. The head can occasionally be seen through the right lateral approach on a coronal plane.

CONGENITAL ANOMALIES

Agenesis

Congenital absence of the body and tail of pancreas has been reported (Fig. 7-11).[26] The remaining head may show compensatory hypertrophy. This condition should be differentiated from acquired atrophy by CT scan.

Congenital Cysts

Epithelium-lined true cysts of the pancreas are believed to be congenital in origin, representing anomalous development of the pancreatic ducts.[27] Multiple congenital cysts, ranging in size from microscopic to 3 to 5 cm,[27] are associated with cystic disease of the pancreas, liver, spleen, and kidneys as part of the broad spectrum of adult type polycystic kidney disease. Von Hippel-Lindau syndrome is another entity associated with multiple true pancreatic cysts.[27] Solitary congenital pancreatic cysts are rare and usually seen in infancy and childhood.[28]

Cystic Fibrosis

Cystic fibrosis is characterized by viscous secretions and dysfunction of multiple glands including the pancreas. It can lead to pancreatic insufficiency with the majority of patients showing evidence of exocrine pancreas dysfunction. When severely affected, the pancreas is shrunken with marked fibrosis, fatty replacement, and cysts secondary to the obstruction of small ducts.[29]

The most common **sonographic manifestation** is increased echogenicity caused by fibrosis or fatty replacement resulting from glandular atrophy.[30,31] In one study series, all patients demonstrated abnormal pancreatic echopatterns when compared with an age- and gender-matched normal population.[30] The pancreas may be small,[32] but this can only be appreciated in cases in which the pancreas is less echogenic than the adjacent retroperitoneal fat. If the pancreas is enlarged, it indicates the presence of complicating pancreatitis, and it is usually associated with a hypoechoic parenchyma.[32] The pancreatic duct is less often visualized in patients with cystic fibrosis than in the normal population.[33] Small cysts of 1 to 3 mm are seen on pathologic examination of the pancreas but are uncommonly seen on sonography.[32] Individual larger cysts, less than 5 cm in diameter, have been reported on ultrasound examinations.[31] Rarely, pancreatic cytosis or multiple cysts can completely replace the pancreatic parenchyma. A high amylase content has been shown on aspiration biopsy of these cysts.[34]

Pancreas Divisum

Pancreas divisum, caused by the lack of fusion of the dorsal and ventral pancreatic buds, occurs in 10% of the population on anatomic studies.[35,36] Drainage of the entire dorsal pancreas is through the minor papilla, with only the ventral part draining through the major papilla. There is controversy regarding the predisposition of patients with pancreas divisum to pancreatitis, which may be related to the drainage of most of the pancreatic secretions through the relatively small orifice of the minor papilla. In a group of patients with recurrent idiopathic pancreatitis, Cotton[35] reported an incidence of 25.6% with associated pancreas divisum.[36] Involvement of the pancreas with acute pancreatitis is usually limited to the dorsal part of the gland.[36] However, isolated ventral pancreatitis has also been documented.[37] A persistent dorsal pancreatic duct in the head may be identified on ultrasound but the presence or absence of communication with the ventral duct is difficult to ascertain. Increased prominence of the ventral pancreas, suggesting preservation of this part of pancreas from chronic pancreatitis, has been reported as an indication of pancreas divisum.[16]

Von Hippel-Lindau Syndrome

Pancreatic cysts are common in von Hippel-Lindau syndrome and are described in 72% of autopsy results[38] and 25% of patients on sonographic examination.[38] Other associated lesions include apudomas, microcystic adenomas, ductal cell adenocarcinomas, ampullary cell carcinomas, and hemangioblastomas.[39]

INFLAMMATORY PROCESSES

Acute Pancreatitis

The diagnosis of acute pancreatitis is usually based on clinical and laboratory findings, with clinical severity best determined by Ranson's criteria[40] or APACHE II criteria.[41] Radiologic examinations are helpful for patients with a confusing history or clinical findings. The role of ultrasound lies in the detection of gallstones or common bile duct calculi, survey of possible complications such as peripancreatic fluid, follow-up of complications arising from acute pancreatitis, and guidance of interventional procedures. Ultrasound is limited in its usefulness as part of the early investigation of acute pancreatitis or traumatic pancreatic injury,[42] whereas CT has been shown to be useful in helping to predict the outcome of acute pancreatic inflammation and to detect necrosis and fracture of the pancreas.[43,44]

Pathologic changes in acute pancreatitis depend on the severity of the disease. Mild forms consist of interstitial edema limited to the gland with no or slight peripancreatic inflammation. Although parenchymal necrosis is not visible grossly, small foci of acinar cell necrosis occasionally may be found. Necrosis of intra- and peripancreatic adipose tissue is commonly seen. Inflammation is associated with extravasation of enzymes into the surrounding tissues. More severe cases show fat necrosis, parenchymal necrosis, and necrosis of blood vessels with subsequent hemorrhage and more severe peripancreatic inflammatory changes appearing in 1 to 2 days.[45] If the patient survives, the necrotic tissue is replaced by diffuse or focal parenchymal or stromal fibrosis, calcifications, and irregular ductal dilations. Pseudocysts may form by the accumulation of enzyme-rich fluid and necrotic debris confined by a nonepithelialized capsule of connective tissue.[27]

Acute pancreatitis has numerous causes; however, the precise pathophysiologic factors are yet to be elucidated. Congenital causes include hereditary pancreatitis and compression from a congenital choledochal cyst. The role of pancreas divisum as a predisposing factor to pancreatitis is controversial with some studies showing increased[36] and others showing similar[46] incidence of acute pancreatitis in these patients. Acquired conditions such as alcohol abuse and biliary

---

CAUSES OF ACUTE PANCREATITIS

Biliary tract disease
Ethyl alcohol abuse
Peptic ulcer
Trauma, surgery (cardiopulmonary bypass surgery), hypotensive shock
Pregnancy
Hyperlipoproteinemias (types I, IV, and V)
Hypercalcemia (primary and secondary, hyperparathyroidism, multiple myeloma)
Drugs (azathioprine, estrogens, corticosteroids, and thiazides)
Hereditary pancreatitis, idiopathic fibrosing pancreatitis
Infectious agents (mumps, ascaris, *Campylobacter* and *Mycoplasma* spp infections, and hydatid)
Methyl alcohol, L-asparaginase
Scorpion bites
Carcinoma of pancreas (primary and metastatic); ductal obstruction by tumor
Endoscopic retrograde cholangiopancreatography, upper-gastrointestinal endoscopy, percutaneous transhepatic biliary tract drainage
Posttransplantation
Legionnaires' disease

Modified from Geokas MC, moderator: Acute pancreatitis, *Ann Intern Med* 1985;103:87.

calculi account for the majority of the cases of acute pancreatitis. Trauma and other less common entities (see box on p. 241) can induce acute pancreatitis.[47]

Because the natural history of acute pancreatitis is variable, serial examination by ultrasound plays an important role in monitoring the inflammatory process of the pancreas after an initial attack. The process can take several directions: resolution, pseudocyst formation, or chronic pancreatitis. Cases of mild pancreatitis, or self-limiting disease, often revert to normal organ echotexture and size. More severe disease may result in increased echogenicity of the pancreas. This increase may be homogeneous and accompanied by scattered, random, bright reflections representing minute calcifications (often without acoustic shadowing) or inhomogeneous and mottled in appearance. These changes reflect the healing of the pancreas by fibrosis accompanied by calcifications deposited along the main pancreatic duct or in the branches within the parenchyma.

Pseudocyst formation is an attempt by the body to wall off the pancreatic secretions to prevent further autodigestion of the peripancreatic tissue or other structures. In many instances patients feel better at the time of pseudocyst formation because it acts as a cordon, enclosing the active inflammation.

Chronic pancreatitis usually results from repeated bouts of acute pancreatitis. This condition is progressive, with indolent destruction and fibrosis of the organ leading to functional exocrine and endocrine glandular failure.

Sonography. **Sonographic findings of acute pancreatitis** can be classified by distribution (focal or diffuse) and by severity (mild, moderate, and severe).[48] Ultrasound findings may be negative in the milder forms of acute pancreatitis. The examination may, however, find the cause of pancreatitis, such as choledocholithiasis, or an alternative diagnosis in questionable cases. Mild pancreatitis is a self-limiting disease responding to conservative treatment. In more severe cases, CT is the primary modality of choice to identify necrotic parenchyma and extraparenchymal involvement because the associated ileus limits ultrasonographic visualization.[49] The technical success of the ultrasound examination improves 48 hours after the acute episode, as the paralytic ileus resolves.[48] Complications may be found, such as **inflammatory mass, hemorrhage, intrapancreatic** and **extrapancreatic fluid collections,** and **pseudocyst formation.** Sonograms may differentiate between inflammatory masses and fluid collections and can also be used to guide needle aspiration that would help to differentiate between infected and noninfected inflammatory masses and pseudocysts.

Focal pancreatitis, presenting as focal isoechoic or hypoechoic enlargement of the pancreas without extrapancreatic manifestations, poses a dilemma to the imager. This presentation generally occurs in the pancreatic head (Fig. 7-15).[50] These patients usually are alcohol abusers and have a previous history of pancreatitis or pain. This suggests that focal pancreatitis tends to occur in the background of chronic pancreatitis.[50] Differentiation from neoplasm may be difficult because both conditions create a focal hypoechoic mass on sonograms. If the serum amylase level is normal and the patient is asymptomatic, the mass is likely to represent a neoplasm. If the patient's symptoms and signs are severe, the focal hypoechogenicity is more likely to be caused by pancreatitis than by a tumor. The presence of calcification within the mass and abnormal ductal changes outside the focal enlargement on ERCP (suggestive of chronic pancreatitis) also favor an inflammatory mass.[50] In addition, serial sonographic examination while the patient is undergoing treatment may differentiate focal pancreatitis from tumor. Endoscopic ultrasound (EUS) may provide better resolution of the pancreas and reveal parenchymal features suggestive of chronic pancreatitis other than a mass.[51-52] CT scans can be helpful by showing peripancreatic soft tissue inflammation (Fig. 7-15, *C*). Percutaneous biopsy should be performed on patients whose diagnoses remain questionable, keeping in mind that a negative biopsy finding does not exclude malignancy. Focal pancreatitis may also be caused by an adjacent inflammatory process, such as a penetrating peptic ulcer (Fig. 7-16).

In **diffuse pancreatitis,** the pancreas becomes increasingly hypoechogenic relative to the normal liver and increases in size (Fig. 7-17). The assessment of relative pancreatic echogenicity may be difficult because of the alcohol-induced fatty liver present in a large number of these patients. Therefore, comparison of the echogenicity of the pancreas with the liver may be of little practical value. In mild acute pancreatitis, sonograms show a normal pancreas with abnormal clinical and laboratory findings. As the condition worsens, decreased echogenicity and increased size are more evident as a result of the increased fluid content in the interstitium secondary to inflammation. The pancreas may also appear inhomogeneous (Fig. 7-18). The pancreatic duct may be compressed or dilated. Ductal dilation is usually caused by a focal pancreatic inflammation located upstream from the dilated pancreatic duct. Rarely, another cause of duct obstruction such as a calculus, tumor, or ascaris can be detected by transcutaneous or endoscopic sonography.[53]

Differentiation cannot be made between necrotic and non-necrotic pancreatitis by ultrasound but is evident on CT (Fig. 7-19). Focal hemorrhage is detected as a focal echogenic mass. When acute inflammation of the pancreas becomes masslike and is accompanied by severe symptoms and clinical findings, the term *in-*

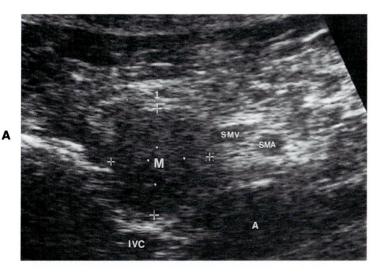

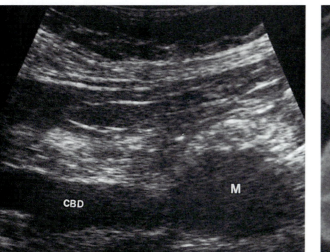

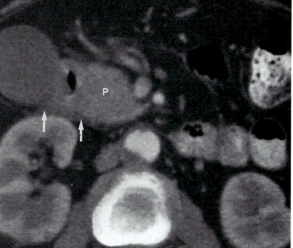

FIG. 7-15. Focal pancreatitis proven by surgery. A, Transverse and, B, sagittal scans of head of pancreas in a patient with a large hypoechoic mass (M) in the region of head of pancreas. Dilated common bile duct (CBD) is seen extending to this mass. C, Enhanced computed tomography scan shows slightly inhomogeneous head of pancreas (P) with a small amount of peripancreatic fluid (*arrows*). Multiple percutaneous and surgical biopsies did not yield any malignancy. A—aorta; CBD—common bile duct; IVC—inferior vena cava; M—mass; P—pancreas; SMA—superior mesenteric artery; SMV—superior mesenteric vein.

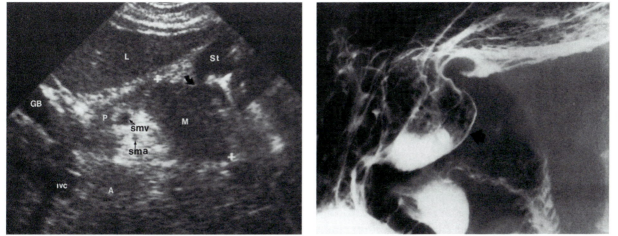

FIG. 7-16. Focal pancreatitis caused by penetrating benign gastric ulcer. A, Transverse scan of pancreas shows hypoechoic masslike enlargement (M) of body and tail. No fat plane is present between this mass and adjacent stomach (St). A—aorta; GB—gall bladder; IVC—inferior vena cava; L—liver; P—pancreas; sma—superior mesenteric artery; smv—superior mesenteric vein. B, Large ulcer of posterior wall of body of stomach (*arrow*).

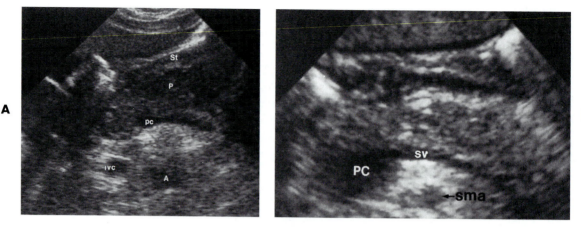

FIG. 7-17. Acute pancreatitis with resolution. A, Transverse scan of enlarged hypoechoic pancreas (P). B, Same patient following resolution. Pancreas has returned to normal size and echogenicity. A—aorta; IVC—inferior vena cava; PC—portal confluence; sma—superior mesenteric artery; St—stomach; sv—splenic vein.

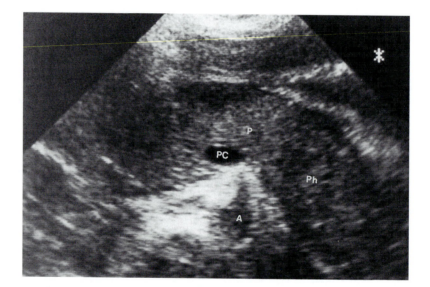

FIG. 7-18. Severe acute pancreatitis. Transverse scan shows large pancreas (P) with inhomogeneous, hypoechoic area in tail, which represents phlegmon (Ph) or an inflammatory mass. A—aorta; PC—portal confluence.

flammatory mass can be employed (Fig. 7-18). Conservative management with serial ultrasonographic imaging is advised because most inflammatory masses resolve without intervention.[54]

Extrapancreatic manifestations in patients with acute pancreatitis are important and should be sought because intrapancreatic changes tend to be subjective.[49] They consist of **fluid collections** and **edema** along the different soft tissue planes and are generally seen in severe cases. The common spaces for the extrapancreatic fluid to collect include the lesser sac, anterior pararenal spaces, mesocolon, perirenal spaces, and peripancreatic soft tissues.[49]

Lesser sac fluid located between the pancreas and the stomach is the easiest to visualize with ultrasonography (Fig. 7-20, A). If the fluid is located in the superior recess of the lesser sac, it tends to surround the caudate lobe (Fig. 7-20, B).[49] The free edge of the gastrohepatic ligament may be visualized with a combination of lesser sac and greater sac fluid (Fig. 7-20, C). Perirenal fluid is also readily demonstrated. However, edema or fluid in the anterior pararenal space is more difficult to see and may require coronal scanning; a hypoechoic band separated from the kidney by the echogenic perirenal fat would represent fluid in the pararenal space.[49] Fluid collections in the

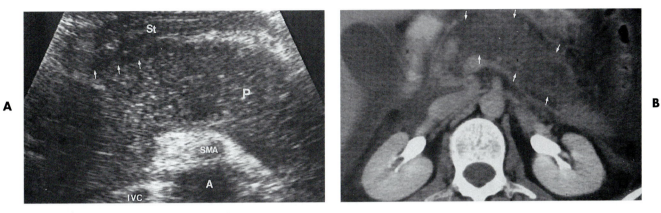

FIG. 7-19. **Acute pancreatitis with pancreatic necrosis.** **A.** Transverse ultrasonic view. Enlarged hypoechoic inhomogeneous pancreas (P) surrounded by a small amount of fluid anteriorly (*arrows*). **B.** Corresponding computed tomography scan shows lack of enhancement of body and most of tail of pancreas (*arrows*). A—aorta; IVC—inferior vena cava; SMA—superior mesenteric artery; St—stomach.

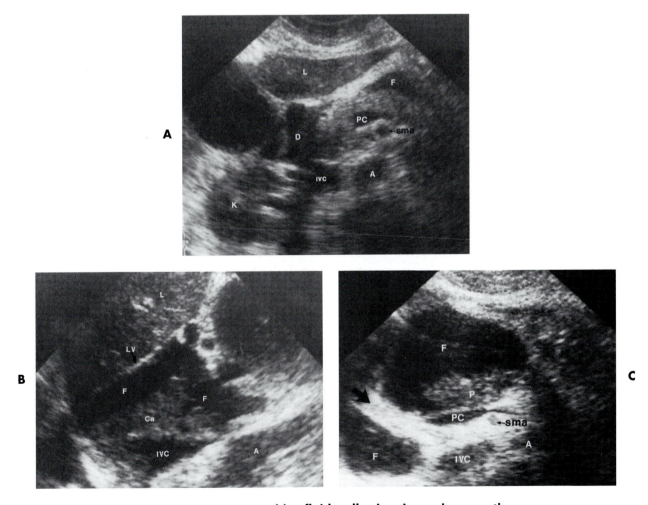

FIG. 7-20. **Acute pancreatitis, fluid collection in peripancreatic spaces.** **A.** Fluid (F) anterior to pancreas in lower lesser sac. **B.** Fluid (F) surrounding caudate lobe (Ca) in sagittal plane. **C.** Fluid (F) on both sides of gastrohepatic ligament (*arrow*) in transverse plane. A—aorta; D—duodenum; IVC—inferior vena cava; K—kidney; L—liver; P—pancreas; PC—portal confluence; sma—superior mesenteric artery.

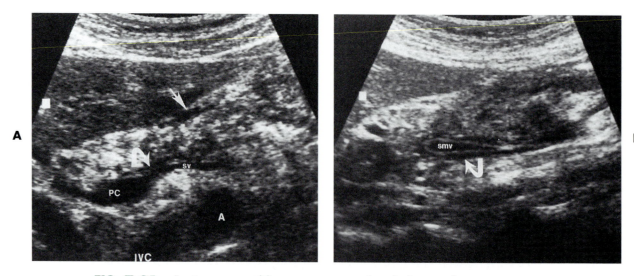

FIG. 7-21. **Acute pancreatitis, extrapancreatic soft tissue edema.** **A,** Transverse scan. **B,** Longitudinal scan. Pancreas echotexture is inhomogeneous. Peripancreatic edema (*straight arrow*) and periportal system edema (*curved arrow*) are present. A—aorta; IVC—inferior vena cava; PC—portal confluence; smv—superior mesenteric vein; SV—splenic vein.

mesocolon are the most difficult to identify by ultrasonographic examination. They present in the midline just caudal to the pancreas. Peripancreatic soft tissue changes are seen as hypoechoic bands adjacent to the pancreas or surrounding the portal venous system (Fig. 7-21).[49] In less severe cases, the only finding may be a small amount of fluid (Fig. 7-22, *A*) or hypoechoic linear edema (Fig. 7-22, *B* and *C*) in the retroperitoneal fat immediately surrounding the pancreas anteriorly or posteriorly. The presence of fluid between the pancreas and the splenic vein has been reported as the only indication of pancreatic injury on CT scan in trauma patients.[55] Fluid or edema may also be visualized around the ligamentum teres (Fig. 7-23).

Pancreatic fluid is either clear or septated as a result of associated hemorrhage or infection. Retroperitoneal or intraperitoneal fluid collections may be inhomogeneous and solid looking as a result of the inflammatory nature of the edematous retroperitoneal tissues (Fig 7-24). Extrapancreatic fluid collections occur within four weeks from the onset of an acute attack and have a high incidence of spontaneous regression; therefore, they can be treated conservatively in conjunction with serial ultrasonographic scanning.[56] The term **"pseudocyst"** is used when a pancreatic fluid collection has developed into a well-defined, walled-off fluid structure that persists on serial imaging examinations for an interval of at least four weeks from the onset of acute inflammation.[57]

Other extrapancreatic findings include **ascites, thickening of the adjacent GI tract** (stomach, duodenum, and colon), and a **thickened gallbladder wall** with or without pericholecystic fluid, which may simulate acute cholecystitis (Fig. 7-24, *D*).[58]

Complications

Pancreatic pseudocysts. A pancreatic pseudocyst is a fluid collection that has developed a well-defined nonepithelialized wall in response to extravasated enzymes.[59] It is generally spherical in shape and distinct from other structures. Approximately 4 to 6 weeks are necessary for a fluid collection to enclose itself by forming a wall composed of collagen and vascular granulation tissue.[60] Pseudocysts occur in 10% to 20% of patients who have had acute pancreatitis.[61] Most commonly, pseudocyst formation is associated with alcoholic or biliary etiology. However, it may also occur following blunt trauma or secondary to pancreatic malignancy (Fig. 7-25). Persistent pain and elevation of amylase levels suggest the diagnosis; however, it can be confirmed by imaging. Classically, a pseudocyst is seen on ultrasonographic examination as a well-defined, smooth-walled, anechoic structure with acoustic enhancement. Occasionally, they may also appear solid or complex, especially during formation.[59,62] As a pseudocyst matures, serial scanning will generally reveal gradual clearing of the internal echoes. Debris within a pseudocyst may occur with complications such as hemorrhage or infection (Fig. 7-26).[59] A pseudocyst may also remain multiloculated without complications and may develop calcifications within its walls (Fig. 7-26). A heavily calcified pseudocyst may be difficult to see on ultrasonograms because of the pres-

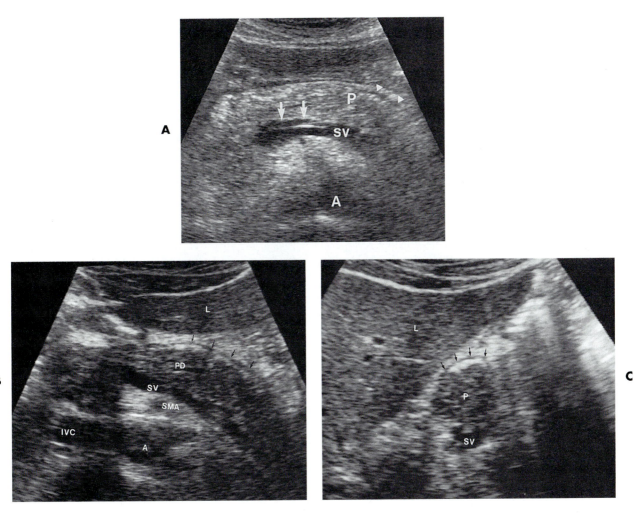

FIG. 7-22. Subtle peripancreatic changes in acute pancreatitis. A, Transverse view. Small amount of fluid is seen posterior *(arrows)* and anterior *(arrowheads)* to the pancreas (P) as the only indication of acute pancreatitis. **B,** Transverse. **C,** sagittal views of another patient with proven pancreatitis demonstrate a hypoechoic band *(arrows)* anterior to the pancreas (P) *(arrows).* A—aorta; IVC—inferior vena cava; M—mass; PD—pancreatic duct; SMA—superior mesenteric artery; SMV—superior mesenteric vein.

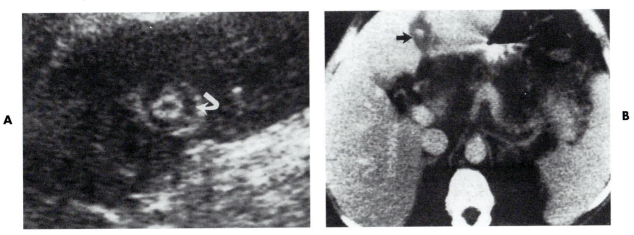

FIG. 7-23. Acute pancreatitis, edema around ligamentum teres. A, Transverse ultrasound scan shows hypoechoic edema *(curved arrow)* around ligamentum teres. **B,** Hypodense edema *(arrow)* is seen in same area on computed tomography scan.

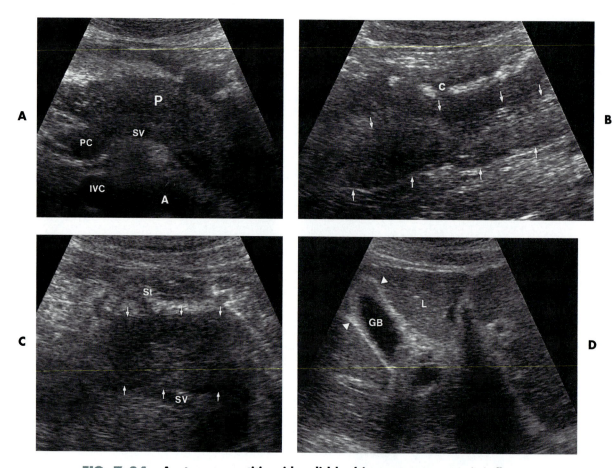

FIG. 7-24. **Acute pancreatitis with solid-looking extrapancreatic inflammation** (*arrows*). **A,** Transverse view of inflamed pancreas (P). **B,** Sagittal view of left flank and **C,** Transverse view of lesser sac. **D,** Transverse view of gallbladder (GB). With thickening of gallbladder wall (*arrowheads*). A—aorta; C—colon; GB—gallbladder; IVC—inferior vena cava; L—liver; P—pancreas; PC—portal confluence; St—stomach; SV—splenic vein.

ence of shadowing (Fig. 7-27). Pseudocysts can migrate outside the abdomen and have been reported to occur in the mediastinum and the thigh.[63,64]

Complications have been reported in 30% to 50% of the patients with a pancreatic pseudocyst.[65] These lesions may become large or may be strategically placed and cause obstruction of the stomach, small bowel (especially duodenum), colon, or the bile ducts.[66] The latter may progress from obstructive jaundice to obstructive cholangitis. Bowel obstruction occurs by extrinsic compression or by intramural extension of the pseudocyst between the serosa and muscularis or between the muscularis and mucosa (Fig. 7-28).[67] Pseudocysts can also **dissect** into the parenchyma of the adjacent organs such as the liver, spleen, and kidney (Fig. 7-29).[68]

Gastrointestinal hemorrhage may occur from direct erosion of the pseudocyst into the stomach, or from variceal bleeding secondary to local portal hyper-

COMPLICATIONS OF PANCREATITIS

Pancreatic pseudocyst
Obstruction of the stomach, small bowel, colon, or the bile ducts
Pseudocysts dissect into adjacent organs
Gastrointestinal hemorrhage
    From direct erosion
    From variceal bleeding
Acute peritonitis
Chronic pancreatitis

tension caused by portosplenic venous compression or thrombosis.[65,69] A pseudocyst or pancreatic secretion alone may erode into an adjacent visceral artery, most commonly the splenic, with resultant intracystic hemorrhage or formation of a pseudoaneurysm. Hemor-

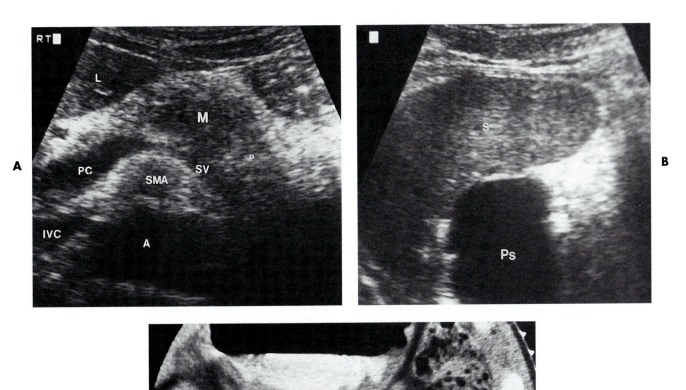

FIG. 7-25. **Pseudocyst of pancreas tail from pancreatic body carcinoma.**
A, Transverse view of pancreas (P) shows a poorly defined hypoechoic mass in the body (M).
B, Coronal view of spleen (S) demonstrates a pseudocyst (Ps) in the splenic hilum. **C,** Enhanced
computed tomography scan shows the pseudocyst (Ps) and inflammatory changes in the adjacent stomach wall (St). A—aorta; IVC—inferior vena cava; L—liver; P—pancreas; PC—portal
confluence; PS—pseudocyst; S—spleen; SMA—superior mesenteric artery; St—stomach; SV—
splenic vein.

rhage may also occur with a pancreatic abscess and severe necrotizing pancreatitis without pseudocyst formation.[70,71] Hemorrhage can be suspected by identifying areas of increased echogenicity. With the addition
of Doppler insonation, the presence of a **pseudoaneurysm** and **portosplenic thrombosis** can be revealed.[72] If thrombosis becomes chronic, cavernous
transformation of the portal venous system may follow.
   Acute peritonitis can ensue with rupture of a pseudocyst into the peritoneal cavity. This serious complica-

tion should be differentiated clinically from pancreatic
ascites, which is caused by a slow leakage of fluid into
the peritoneal cavity, unassociated with peritonitis.
   A pseudocyst that forms during acute necrotizing
pancreatitis has a high propensity toward spontaneous regression, whereas a pseudocyst that forms as
a result of chronic pancreatitis does not generally resolve on its own, especially when calcifications occur
within the walls.[73] Spontaneous decompression of the
pseudocyst may occur by rupturing into the pancre-

atic duct, the adjacent portion of the gastrointestinal tract (usually the stomach) or the common bile duct.[74] In general, pseudocysts that persist beyond 6 weeks require decompression and the risk of complications rises significantly.[59] A pseudocyst will persist as long as disruption of the pancreatic ducts exists; upon healing of this disruption, spontaneous resorption will occur.[74] The **criteria for decompression** of a pancreatic pseudocyst include: (1) persistence greater than 6 weeks; (2) size larger than 5 cm in diameter without evidence of ongoing regression on follow-up ultrasonographic or CT examination; (3) smaller pseudocysts causing symptoms; and (4) presence of

complications such as infection, internal hemorrhage, or intra-abdominal perforation.

Nonsurgical decompression is becoming more popular, with more favorable results obtained in the past few years.[72] There remains controversy over the choice of approach; some large series advocate the transgastric approach as the primary route,[75] whereas others initially prefer the direct approach and reserve the transgastric, transduodenal, or transhepatic approaches for inaccessible locations.[75] Single aspiration has been abandoned because of a high recurrence rate.[75] Percutaneous transgastric pseudocyst drainage is a combined technique of percutaneous gastrostomy with cystogastrostomy using a Mitty-Pollack needle (Cook, Bloomingdale, IN) performed under fluoroscopy and ultrasound guidance. There is a minimal chance of pseudocyst recurrence because of internal drainage to the stomach. In one study series using this technique, a success rate of 67% was observed with a recurrence rate of 12.5%.[76] This approach is consid-

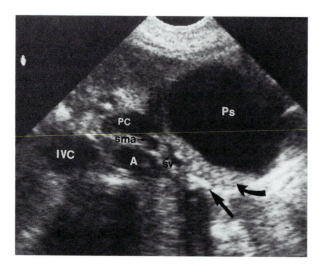

FIG. 7-26. Complicated pseudocyst. Transverse scan of partially calcified (*straight arrow*) pseudocyst (Ps) containing debris (*curved arrow*) in tail of pancreas. A—aorta; IVC—inferior vena cava; PC—portal confluence; sma—superior mesenteric artery; SV—splenic vein.

CRITERIA FOR DECOMPRESSION OF A PANCREATIC PSEUDOCYST

Persistence greater than 6 weeks
Larger than 5 cm in diameter without evidence of ongoing regression
Smaller pseudocysts causing symptoms
Complications such as infection, internal hemorrhage, or intra-abdominal perforation

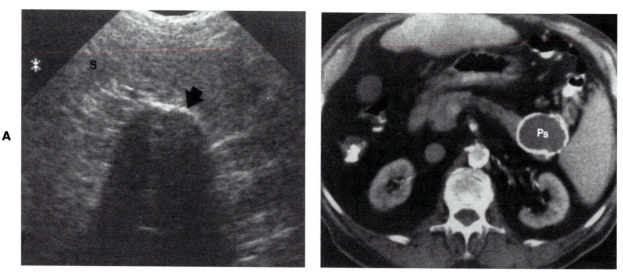

FIG. 7-27. Calcified pseudocyst. A, Heavily calcified pseudocyst (*arrow*) in splenic hilum causing shadowing. **B,** Confirmatory computed tomography scan. Ps—pseudocyst; S—spleen.

ered the route of choice in pseudocysts associated with obstruction of the pancreatic duct. The direct approach is performed using the usual percutaneous technique. The reported success rate for the combined approach (with the majority being drained directly) is 86%.[75] The catheter is left in place until drainage ceases, the pseudocyst resolves, and there is no communication with the pancreatic duct.[75] The drainage period is generally longer than an uncomplicated abscess and closer to abscesses associated with fistula to the gastrointestinal tract.[75] Recently, the systemic administration of octreotide acetate, to reduce pancre-

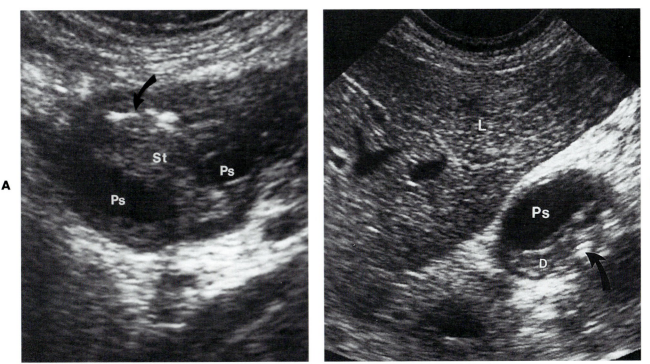

FIG. 7-28. Pseudocyst in the wall of gut. A, Intramural pseudocyst in the wall of stomach (St). Transverse view of antrum showing multiple pseudocysts (Ps) in thickened wall. B, Intramural pseudocyst (Ps) in the wall of duodenum in a different patient. D—duodenum; L—liver; Ps—pseudocyst. Notice gas (*curved arrow*) in lumen.

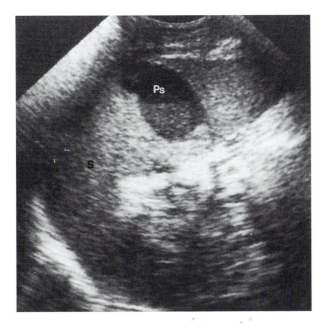

FIG. 7-29. Pseudocyst of spleen. Sagittal view of spleen (S) shows cyst (Ps) containing a fluid level.

atic exocrine function, is suggested to improve the success rate of percutaneous drainage of pseudocyst.[77]

Endoscopic cystogastrostomy or duodenostomy is an alternative approach; however, it may be more time consuming than the radiologically guided percutaneous approach.[78] If the above techniques are unavailable, the anatomy precludes their usage, or a pseudocyst is extensively multiloculated, a surgical decompression should be used.

Infected pancreatic lesions. The uncircumscribed infected pancreatic focus consists of secondarily infected entities that are not delimited by a wall, such as pancreatic necrosis, pancreatic fluid collections, and pancreatic hemorrhage. Bacterial contamination of necrotic pancreatic tissue and fluid rises to a significant rate (71.4%) after two weeks of acute necrotic pancreatitis.[79] Sonographically, a sterile, uncircumscribed focus cannot be distinguished from an infected one. Therefore, a high index of suspicion is necessary to detect these lesions, and an ultrasound-guided (or CT-guided) needle aspiration with Gram stain and culture of the aspirate should be performed to confirm the presence of infection. An uncircumscribed infected pancreatic focus is best treated by surgical debridement.[80] Percutaneous catheter drainage is reserved for cases in which the patient is in refractory shock or cannot withstand immediate surgery.[81]

Sonographically, an **infected pancreatic pseudocyst** cannot be distinguished from a sterile pseudocyst with certainty. Clinically, the patient may appear well with stable vital signs, except for an elevated temperature. Therefore, a high degree of suspicion is again necessary and a percutaneous ultrasound-guided aspiration with Gram stain and culture should be employed whenever the question of infection arises. An infected pseudocyst is best treated (94% reported success) by percutaneous image-guided catheter drainage.[75,76]

A **pancreatic abscess** is distinguished from an infected pseudocyst by its greater risk of mortality (near 100% mortality if left untreated) and its need for surgical debridement when associated with pancreatic necrosis (versus percutaneous catheter drainage).[80,82] The organisms obtained are usually gram-negative enteric bacteria, and approximately half of the cultures are polymicrobial.[83] Pancreatic abscesses occur more frequently in postoperative patients than in those with alcohol or biliary pancreatitis.[84] **Sonographically,** one sees a thick-walled, mostly anechoic mass containing debris with bright echoes from gas bubbles. However, gas collections can also arise from uninfected fistulous communications with the gastrointestinal tract.[85] Whether one sees gas bubbles, the absence of gas, a cystic, complex, or a solid structure, suspicious areas must be aspirated with a fine needle (22-gauge) under ultrasound or CT guidance in order to obtain specimens for Gram stain, culture, and sensitivity tests. Pancreatic abscesses require surgical debridement. CT scan is required to evaluate the extent of the disease before catheter placement or surgical intervention. The information obtained from the CT scan may help to predict the success of draining a pancreatic abscess with a radiologic catheter.[86] However, ultrasound and more recently MRI is superior to CT scan for determining the nature of fluid and thus its drainability by a percutaneous image-guided catheter (Fig. 7-30). An uncomplicated clear pancreatic abscess without necrotic tissue is likely to respond to percutaneous drainage.[75] Residual collections left after surgery can also have a percutaneous catheter placed radiologically to help affect a complete cure.[86]

Vascular complications. Vascular complications may be related to the pancreatitis or may occur secondary to the pseudocyst formation. They include venous or arterial thrombosis with splenic infarct as a rare complication of vascular involvement (Fig. 7-31, *A* and *B*)[87] or pseudoaneurysm formation (Fig. 7-31, *C* and *D*).[88] A high degree of suspicion is crucial to diagnose a pseudoaneurysm because of the potential to mistake them for a much more common complication of this condition (e.g., a pseudocyst). The presence of an echogenic crescent in the periphery of a cystic mass is highly suspicious for an aneurysm. Doppler should be used to confirm the existence of these vascular complications.

Pancreatic ascites and pleural effusion. Pancreatic ascites results from slow leakage of pancreatic enzymes into the peritoneal cavity from a disruption of the main pancreatic duct or a poorly walled pseudocyst.[89] Anterior enzyme leakage enters the lesser sac and the peritoneal cavity, causing ascites. Posterior enzyme leakage moves cephalad into the mediastinum and the pleural space, resulting in pancreatic pleural effusion (classically, left sided).[90] A "leaky" diaphragm or a pleural-subdiaphragmatic fistula may also allow ascites to become a pleural effusion. Pancreatic ascites is asymptomatic, causing an enlarging abdomen. ERCP can detect the location of pancreatic duct disruption.

Chronic Pancreatitis

Chronic pancreatitis is a progressive, irreversible destruction of the pancreas by repeated bouts of mild or subclinical pancreatitis resulting from high-alcohol intake or biliary tract disease. In chronic alcoholic pancreatitis, the chronic alcohol intake causes increased pancreatic protein secretion with subsequent obstruction of the ducts by the protein-rich plugs, resulting in the more common type, namely **chronic calcifying pancreatitis.**[27] The fibrous connective tissue proliferates around ducts and between parenchymal lobules causing interstitial scarring ac-

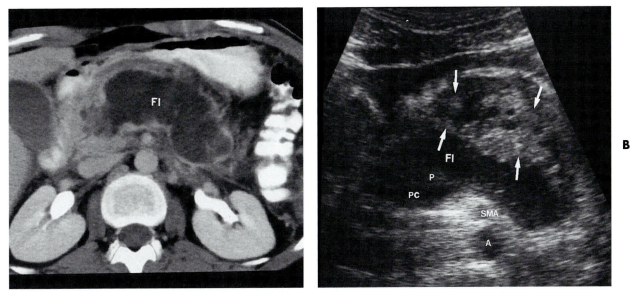

FIG. 7-30. Value of ultrasound to determine the nature of pancreatic fluid collection following pancreatic necrosis. Same patient as in Fig. 7-22, 15 days later. **A,** Enhanced computed tomography scan shows a walled-off homogeneous fluid collection (FI). **B,** Transverse ultrasound confirms fluid nature of the posterior aspect of this mass (FI) but the anterior aspect is solid (*arrows*). Residual pancreatic tissue is seen posteriorly (P). A—aorta; PC—portal confluence; SMA—superior mesenteric artery.

companied by loss of acini.[91] This process eventually leads to an irregular, nodular appearance of the surface of the pancreas and pancreatic calculi.[27,91] The less common type is **chronic obstructive pancreatitis** with a nonlobular distribution, less ductal epithelial damage, and rare calcified stones. This is usually caused by stenosis of the sphincter of Oddi by cholelithiasis or pancreatic carcinoma.[27]

Sonographic findings of chronic pancreatitis consist of changes in the size and echotexture of the pancreas, focal mass lesions, calcifications, pancreatic duct dilation, and pseudocyst formation. Bile duct dilation and portal vein thrombosis are other associated findings.[16] The echotexture of the pancreas is usually a mixture of patches of hypoechoic and hyperechoic foci. The hyperechoic foci are probably caused by a combination of fibrosis and calcification. Hypoechoic areas are likely due to the associated inflammation.[16,92] The echotexture changes are relatively sensitive but nonspecific.[16] The size of the pancreas depends on the degree of associated inflammation. In the absence of significant acute inflammation, the pancreas tends to be atrophied.

A **focal mass** or enlargement is found in approximately 40% of patients.[92,93] These changes result from progressive, mostly perilobular scarring in the interstitium accompanied by chronic edema and inflammatory infiltration. The presence of calcification helps to differentiate these focal enlargements from neoplasms (Fig. 7-32). However, in some cases differen-

tiation is not possible (Fig. 7-15). Irregular **dilation of the pancreatic duct** occurs in chronic pancreatitis. In advanced cases, the duct becomes very tortuous (Fig. 7-33). The differential diagnosis between chronic pancreatitis and pancreatic carcinoma in a patient with duct dilation can be difficult. However, as a general rule, chronic pancreatitis is more highly suspected when the duct contains calcification and no obstructing mass lesion is seen, whereas carcinoma is suggested when a parenchymal mass lesion is identified at the site of obstruction of the pancreatic duct.[94] In normal subjects, it has been shown that variable degrees of pancreatic duct dilation occur following a standard meal or secretin stimulation.[16] An absent or diminished response has been shown in patients with chronic pancreatitis.[16]

Pancreatic calcifications are mostly intraductal in location and result from deposition of calcium carbonate on intraductal protein plugs.[95] They may (Figs. 7-34 and 7-35) or may not (Fig. 7-32) be obstructive. The presence of these calcifications has been used diagnostically and as a basis for treatment of chronic pancreatitis because they were believed to be associated with clinical pancreatic insufficiency. However, contrary to previous opinion, a recent study showed a poor correlation between exocrine function and pancreatic calcification.[96] Moreover, the degree and pattern of pancreatic calcification have been shown to change with time.[97] Three phases were identified: (1) increasing calcifications; (2) stationary calcifications; and (3) decreasing calcifications. The third phase,

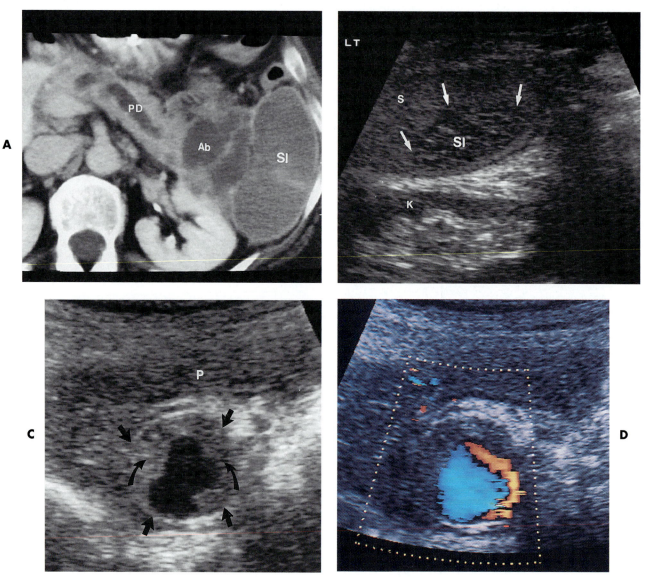

FIG. 7-31. Vascular complications of acute pancreatitis. Splenic infarct (SI) dilatation of pancreatic duct (PD), and an abscess (Ab) in the tail of pancreas **A,** Enhanced computed tomography scan and **B,** ultrasound shows a wedge-shaped area of hypoechogenicity with multiple interfaces (*arrows*) in the spleen (S) diagnostic of infarct. Pseudoaneurysm in a pancreas transplant with history of acute pancreatitis. **C,** Gray scale transverse view, and **D,** color Doppler of left lower quadrant show a rounded cystic mass (*straight arrows*) with a crescent of peripheral solid tissue (*curved arrows*) is seen posterior to pancreas transplant (P). Ab—abscess; K—kidney; S—spleen; SI—splenic infarct. **D,** Color Doppler confirms the aneurysmal nature of this mass.

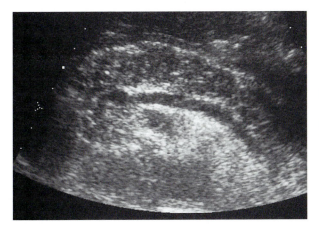

FIG. 7-32. Chronic calcific pancreatitis.
The pancreas is generous and nonhomogeneous. The parenchyma is less echogenic than normal and there are tiny foci of increased echogenicity.

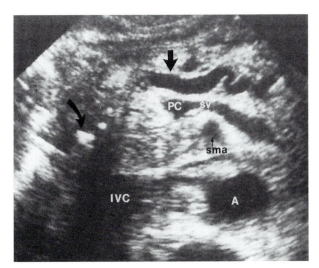

FIG. 7-33. Chronic calcific pancreatitis.
Transverse scan shows a dilated tortuous pancreatic duct (*straight arrow*) and a large head with calcification (*curved arrow*). A—aorta; IVC—inferior vena cava; PC—portal confluence; sma—superior mesenteric artery; sv—splenic vein.

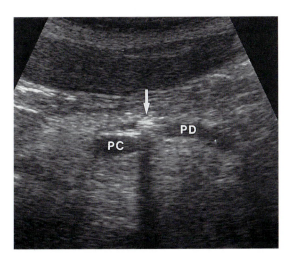

FIG. 7-34. Pancreatic duct calculus, transverse scan. A stone (*arrow*) is present obstructing the pancreatic duct (PD). PC—Portal confluence; PD—pancreatic duct.

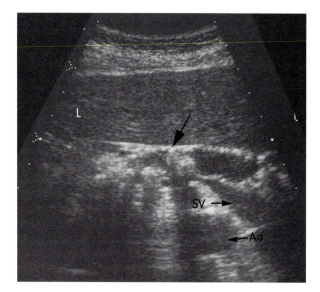

FIG. 7-35. **Chronic calcific pancreatitis with obstructive duct calculus.** Transverse sonogram shows multiple calcifications as bright echogenic foci in the dilated pancreatic duct. There is a large stone (*arrow*) in the duct with distal duct dilatation. L—left lobe of liver; SV—splenic vein; Ao—aorta. (Courtesy of J. William Charboneau, MD, Mayo Clinic, Rochester, Minnesota)

not previously recognized, occurred to a significant degree in one third of the patients studied; some of this loss resulted from drainage procedures, whereas others occurred spontaneously with continued loss of exocrine function.

Pancreatic pseudocysts are reported in 25% to 40% of patients with chronic pancreatitis.[16] They are better walled-off in chronic pancreatitis than in the acute stage and tend not to resolve spontaneously.

Dilation of the common bile duct is present in 5% to 10% of the patients with chronic pancreatitis and characteristically causes smooth gradual tapering although abrupt tapering is rarely seen.[16]

Portosplenic vein thrombosis may occur as a complication of chronic pancreatitis and was recently reported as occurring in 5.1% of patients.[98] Because of the chronic nature of the disease, cavernous transformation may be present.

There is relatively good functional and morphologic correlation in advanced pancreatic disease, but poor correlation for mild-to-moderate disease. In chronic pancreatitis, bicarbonate secretion seems to correlate best with ductal imaging (i.e. ERCP), whereas enzyme secretion correlates with gland imaging (i.e. ultrasound and CT).[99] However, recently a revised "Cambridge" classification of chronic pancreatitis was proposed and preliminary studies indicate good correlations based on findings of ERCP and ultrasound (Table 7-1). Ductal abnormalities of more than three side branches are diagnostic of the early stages of chronic pancreatitis, whereas abnormality of

the main duct indicates at least moderate disease.[100] The finding of intraductal calculi constitutes sufficient evidence for grading as advanced chronic pancreatitis.[101] Therefore, correlation of ultrasound findings with that of ERCP has recently become part of the basis of treatment of chronic pancreatitis.

NEOPLASMS

Adenocarcinoma

Pancreatic carcinoma is the fourth leading cause of death from cancer in the United States, preceded by cancer of the lung, colon, and breast. The incidence of this neoplasm has increased threefold in the past 40 years. Carcinoma of the pancreas is extremely rare before 40 years of age, and two thirds of patients present after age 60 years.[102] The prognosis is particularly poor, with a median survival time of 2 to 3 months and a 1-year survival of 8%. **Clinical symptoms** depend on the location. Tumors arising in the pancreatic head present earlier because of associated bile duct obstruction. A palpable, nontender gallbladder accompanied by jaundice (Courvoisier's sign) is present in approximately 25% of patients.[4] Tumors in the body and tail present later with less specific symptoms—most commonly weight loss, pain, jaundice, and vomiting when the gastrointestinal tract is invaded by the tumor. Diabetes and malabsorption are late findings.

Pathologically, almost all adenocarcinomas originate in the ductal epithelium, with less than 1% arising in the acini. They may be either mucinous or nonmucinous secreting.[27] Approximately 70% of the pancreatic cancers arise in the region of the head, 15% to 20% in the body, and 5% in the tail. In 20% of cases, the tumor is distributed diffusely throughout the gland.[27]

Because pancreatic head tumors present earlier, they can be fairly small and cause little or moderate expansion of the head. They may be inapparent on external examination and only create an impression of abnormal consistency or nodularity. On cut cross-section, they are poorly defined and present an irregular margin with few, if any, foci of hemorrhage.[27] Carcinoma of the body and tail of the pancreas are, on the average, larger than those of the head and tend to invade adjacent organs including the stomach, transverse colon, spleen, and adrenal gland. Carcinomas in the region of the body and tail are more likely to present with metastases, probably as a result of late presentation.[102] Massive hepatic metastases are characteristic. Metastases occur most frequently in the regional lymph nodes, liver, lungs, peritoneum, and adrenal glands. Peripancreatic, gastric, mesenteric, omental, and portohepatic nodes are frequent sites of spread.

TABLE 7-1
REVISED "CAMBRIDGE" CLASSIFICATION OF CHRONIC PANCREATITIS

Class*	Ultrasound
1. Normal	Visualisation of entire gland and demonstration and measurement of main pancreatic duct
2. Equivocal	Less than two abnormal signs
	Main duct enlarged (less than 4 mm)
	Gland enlarged (up to twice normal)
	Cavities (less than 10 mm)
	Irregular ducts
3. Mild	Focal reduction in parenchymal echogenicity
4. Moderate	Two or more abnormal signs
	Echogenic foci in parenchyma
	Increased or irregular echogenicity of wall of main duct
	Irregular contour to gland, particularly focal enlargement
5. Marked	Large cavities (greater than 10 mm)
	Calculi
	Duct obstruction (greater than 4 mm)
	Major duct irregularity
	Gross enlargement (greater than 4 mm)
	Contiguous organ invasion

*If pathologic changes are limited to one third of the gland or less, they are classified as focal.
Modified from Jones SN, Lees WR, Frost RA: Diagnosis and grading of chronic pancreatitis by morphological criteria derived by ultrasound and pancreatography. *Clin Radiol* 1988;39:43-48.

Sonography

Direct signs. The most common ultrasonographic finding in pancreatic carcinoma is a **poorly defined, homogeneous or inhomogeneous hypoechoic mass** in the pancreas or pancreatic fossa.[103] This may or may not be associated with expansion of the pancreas or compression of the adjacent structures. In patients whose pancreas shows increased echogenicity, the tumor will be better visualized as the contrast between the neoplasm and the normal pancreatic echotexture is accentuated. When an isoechoic mass is identified, attention should be given to the size of the pancreas and nodularity of its contour. In the uncinate process, the presence of a mass changes its pointed contour to a rounded appearance (Figs. 7-36 and 7-37). Necrosis, seen as a cystic area within the mass, is a rare manifestation of pancreatic carcinoma.[104] However, pseudocysts caused by associated pancreatitis may be seen adjacent to the carcinoma (Fig. 7-25). The less common diffuse tumors can be mistaken for acute pancreatitis. The lobulated appearance of the pancreatic mass and clinical presentation help in differentiation. At the time of diagnosis by ultrasonography, pancreatic carcinomas usually measure more than 2 cm. The tumor size is usually larger at surgery or autopsy than on the ultrasonograms. This may be caused by the presence of microscopic infiltration of the tissues surrounding the tumor itself, which is undetected by ultrasound.

Indirect signs. Dilation of the pancreatic duct proximal to a pancreatic mass is a common finding. A normal pancreatic duct usually measures less than 2 to 3 mm and has parallel walls and a straight course. When obstructed, it loses its parallel nature, becomes tortuous, and ends or tapers abruptly. The pancreatic duct distends with aging, but it maintains its parallel straight course and can be followed to its entrance into the duodenum. Recognition of a dilated pancreatic duct is an important observation, because it can lead to detection of small pancreatic carcinoma (Fig. 7-38). However, in the absence of a mass, the appearances of the pancreatic duct in both pancreatic carcinoma and pancreatitis may overlap.

Bile duct dilation is commonly seen with lesions in the head of the pancreas. The gallbladder and cystic duct may or may not be dilated. The level of obstruction may be in the head, above the head, or in the porta hepatis, depending on the extent of the lesion or associated lymphadenopathy. Abrupt termination of the dilated bile duct is strongly suggestive of malignancy. Thick, echogenic sludge in the common bile duct proximal to a tumor should not be mistaken for the tumor itself. These patients also often have thick sludge in the gallbladder. Uncommonly, the mass itself extends inside the bile duct. Dilation of the common bile duct (Fig. 7-38), pancreatic duct, or both may occasionally be the only ultrasonographic finding. Although the **double-duct sign** (combined dilation

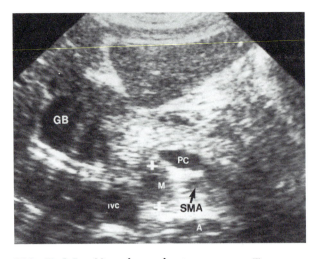

FIG. 7-36. Mass in uncinate process. Transverse view shows hypoechoic mass (M) bulging contour of uncinate process. A—aorta; GB—gallbladder; IVC—inferior vena cava; PC—portal confluence; SMA—superior mesenteric artery.

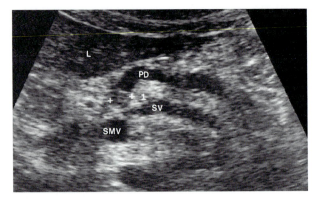

FIG. 7-38. Small pancreatic carcinoma. Transverse ultrasound. Detection of this small slightly hypoechoic mass (between calipers) was facilitated by following the dilated pancreatic duct (PD). This mass was not evident on computed tomography scan. L—liver; PD—pancreatic duct; SMV—superior mesenteric vein; SV—splenic vein.

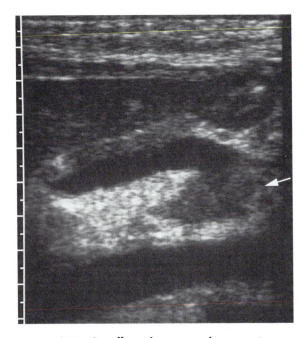

FIG. 7-37. Small uncinate carcinoma. Longitudinal scan shows a small hypoechoic mass *(arrow)* posterior to the superior mesenteric vein. (Courtesy of J. William Charboneau, MD, Mayo Clinic, Rochester, Minnesota)

of the pancreatic and common bile duct) is also seen with chronic pancreatitis, it usually indicates the presence of pancreatic adenocarcinoma (Fig. 7-39).

Displacement and involvement of adjacent vascular structures may occur (Fig. 7-40). Compression of the inferior vena cava by the head of the pancreas has been reported as an indication of a mass lesion.[105]

Associated pancreatitis proximal to the mass may obscure the underlying primary tumor because of

the similar echogenicity. This is especially true when pseudocyst formation from pancreatitis distorts the gland and the underlying tumor. In these cases, sonographic differentiation may be difficult (Fig. 7-25).

Atrophy of the gland proximal to an obstructing mass in the head may occur and may appear hypo- or hyperechoic. In the presence of a hypoechoic body and tail, disproportionate size of the head may be the only clue to the presence of a mass (Fig. 7-41).

Some patients presenting with carcinoma of the pancreas are very cachectic. In these circumstances, because the pancreas is situated anteriorly and close to the abdominal wall, a 7.5-MHz transducer or a transducer with a good near field should be used. Occasionally, when there is occlusion of the pancreatic duct, the dilated duct may be the only structure left in the atrophied pancreas and the entire pathologic state can be overlooked if the duct is mistaken for a blood vessel. When dilation of the pancreatic duct or common bile duct or both are present, meticulous scanning should be performed in the region where one or both dilated ducts terminate, in order to identify the mass.

Doppler findings. Pancreatic carcinoma appears to have Doppler features similar to other malignant lesions (increased velocity and diminished flow impedance).[106] Taylor et al.[106] have reported a velocity greater than 3 KHz and a systolic/diastolic ratio of less than 3 in pancreatic carcinomas. These results are similar to those reported for primary liver, kidney, and adrenal neoplasms. The increased velocity is attributed to arteriovenous shunting and the diminished impedance to vascular spaces that lack muscular walls.[106] However, Doppler has not proven effective in differentiating benign from malignant pancreatic masses.

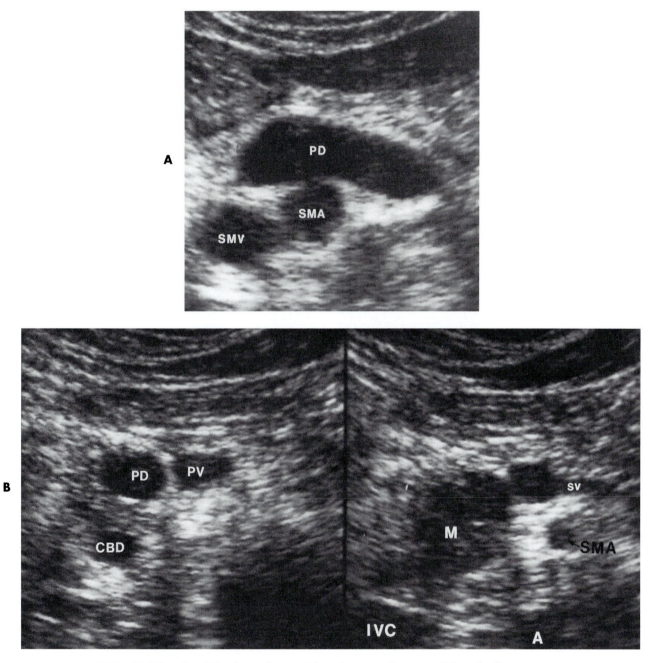

FIG. 7-39. Double-duct sign, with adenocarcinoma of head of pancreas.
A, Transverse view of body shows dilated pancreatic duct (PD). B, Two adjacent cuts of head of pancreas show dilated common bile duct (CBD) and PD, leading to mass (M). A—aorta; IVC—inferior vena cava; PV—portal vein; SMA—superior mesenteric artery; SMV—superior mesenteric vein.

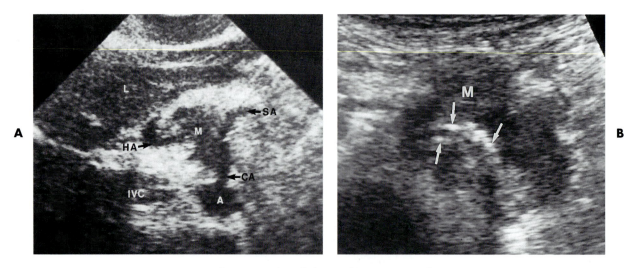

FIG. 7-40. Pancreatic cancer involving adjacent vascular structures in two patients. A. Encasement of celiac artery (CA). Transverse view. **B.** Encasement of calcified splenic artery (*arrows*). M—mass lesion; A—aorta; HA—hepatic artery; IVC—inferior vena cava; L—liver; SA—splenic artery.

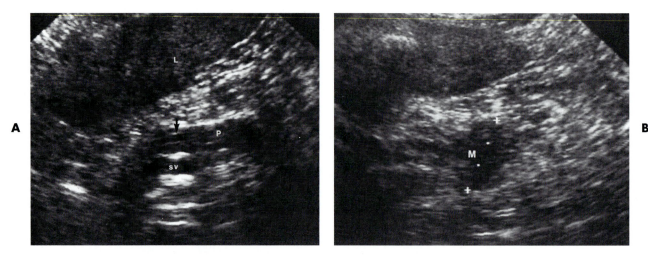

FIG. 7-41. Atrophy of pancreas proximal to obstructing mass. A. Transverse view shows small atrophied pancreas (P) slightly dilated pancreatic duct (*arrow*). **B.** Head (caliper) is disproportionate in size, indicating presence of mass (M). L—liver; P—pancreas; sv—splenic vein.

Color and pulsed Doppler can be used to evaluate venous and arterial structures for the presence or absence of encasement, occlusion, or thrombosis. Increased focal arterial or venous flow velocity indicates the presence of compression or encasement of a vessel.

Staging of pancreatic carcinomas. The role of ultrasound is important not only in diagnosing pancreatic carcinomas but also in assessing the tumor's resectability. Surgery is still the treatment of choice in carcinomas that are considered resectable. However, surgery still carries a high rate of mortality and morbidity, and provides poor results. Therefore, every at-

tempt should be made to preoperatively confirm the diagnosis and properly stage the disease to prevent unnecessary surgery.

Extension of pancreatic carcinomas beyond the pancreatic parenchyma—including venous invasion, involvement of the retroperitoneal fat and adjacent organs, lymphadenopathy, and liver metastasis—precludes the feasibility of surgery. Some surgeons also consider arterial involvement a contraindication to surgery. It is generally difficult to differentiate between **compression** and **invasion** of the **venous structures**. Occlusion or thrombosis of the splenic vein is suggested

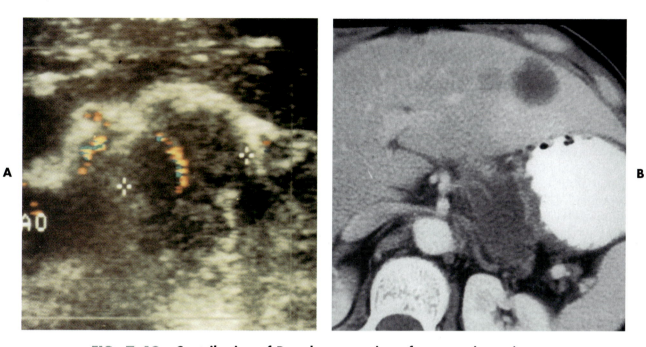

FIG. 7-42. **Contribution of Doppler to staging of pancreatic carcinoma.**
A, Color Doppler image shows a hyopechoic mass in the pancreatic tail and the splenic artery encased by the tumor. **B,** Contrast-enhanced computed tomography scan confirms encasement of the splenic artery. (Courtesy of J. William Charboneau, MD, Mayo Clinic, Rochester, Minnesota)

with interruption of the vein, splenomegaly, and collateral formation in the peripancreatic and periportal region and along the stomach wall. Intrapancreatic collaterals are rarely seen (Fig. 7-12, *A* and *B* and Fig. 7-13, *D* and *E*). Enlargement of the gastrocolic vein draining into the superior mesenteric vein providing a collateral pathway via the gastroepiploic vein may be seen when there is involvement of the splenic vein or superior mesenteric portal vein confluence above the gastrocolic trunk. A gastrocolic vein greater than 5 mm is reported to be suggestive of occlusion of the splenic vein or superior mesenteric portal vein confluence above gastrocolic trunk on CT examination.[107] Also, lack of visualization of the splenic vein should be regarded as suspicious for its invasion. The superior mesenteric and portal veins' involvement may also result in collateral formation in the mesentery. Although cavernous transformation is rare because of the short duration of portal thrombosis in these patients, it can occur. **Encasement** of the celiac axis or superior mesenteric artery as a result of lymphatic involvement is more easily recognizable and may be the only indication of the presence of the disease (Fig. 7-40). Vascular structures should be evaluated with the help of the Doppler examination (Fig. 7-42). Ascites is seen in more advanced cases.

Comparative Imaging. There is controversy concerning the role of ultrasound and CT in the detection of pancreatic carcinoma.[108-110] The superiority of ultrasound over CT for tissue characterization is generally accepted. Because sonography relies more on tissue characterization, which is a more objective sign than pancreatic enlargement for the diagnosis of pancreatic carcinoma, ultrasonography should be more accurate than CT when the pancreas is optimally seen. Because CT relies more on indirect signs, such as enlargement of the pancreas, it has a lower specificity than ultrasound.[108] In one study, 59% of the CT results falsely suggested a pancreatic mass solely on the basis of apparent localized enlargement of the pancreas without any other findings. All proved to be normal on the ultrasonographic examination.[108] In another series comparing CT and ultrasound for the detection of pancreatic carcinoma, ultrasound showed the tumor itself in 86% as compared with 69% with CT. Ultrasound identified secondary signs but not the tumor in 11% of patients compared with 25% for CT, and the findings were normal in 3% as compared with 6% for CT.[109] However, with the advent of helical CT and the possibility of visualizing the normal pancreas at its peak enhancement, which occurs early, the increased contrast between the very vascular normal parenchyma and the hypovascular adenocarcinoma of the pancreas has improved the sensitivity and specificity of CT scan for diagnosing pancreatic carcinoma.[111] The sensitivity of ultrasound for the detection of pancreatic carcinoma is more operator-dependent and is related to the time spent in visualizing the entire pancreas. Generally speaking, if the pancreas is optimally seen in its entirety and is normal, pancreatic carcinoma can be excluded with a high degree of certainty, considering the reported 98% sensitivity of ultrasound for detection of pancreatic carcinoma.[108] However, if the whole length of the pancreas is not seen, pancreatic carcinoma cannot be excluded.

CT should be performed following the ultrasonographic diagnosis of pancreatic carcinoma to assess resectability. CT appears to be more sensitive when assessing local extension with regards to involvement of the adjacent retroperitoneal fat. However, if ultrasound confirms unresectability, no additional information is gained by performing CT.[108] Angiography is useful for the assessment of vascular invasion. ERCP should only be used in conjunction with ultrasound or CT, when there is a question of differentiation of malignant from inflammatory masses.[112] ERCP has no role if the malignant nature of a pancreatic mass is confirmed on ultrasound or CT.

Differential Diagnosis. The main differential diagnosis of pancreatic carcinoma is **focal pancreatitis,** or a focal mass associated with chronic pancreatitis. If the findings are localized to the pancreas and limited to a hypoechoic area with or without mass effect, pancreatic carcinoma cannot be differentiated from focal pancreatitis unless the area has foci of calcification. With pancreatitis, CT scan may show more diffuse involvement of the pancreas or soft tissue changes in the adjacent fat. ERCP may show smooth tapering of the ducts at the site of the mass and associated changes of pancreatitis, especially upstream to the mass.[112]

Peripancreatic lymphadenopathy can usually be differentiated from pancreatic cancer by the identification of echogenic septa between individual nodes. The absence of jaundice when a large pancreatic head mass is present close to the distal common bile duct favors lymphadenopathy.

Ampullary adenocarcinomas should be differentiated from pancreatic adenocarcinomas because the former has a better prognosis. For the three gross patterns of ampullary adenocarcinoma—intra-ampullary, periampullary, and mixed—the prognosis diminishes respectively. Masses larger than 2 cm have a similar prognosis to that of pancreatic carcinoma.[113] Most patients present with dilation of both the common bile duct and the pancreatic duct. However, the bile duct may be the only involved duct. Occasionally, an intraluminal mass is seen at the distal end of a dilated bile duct.[114] EUS has improved the accuracy of ultrasound for diagnosing ampullary carcinoma, allowing its differentiation from pancreatic carcinoma and the staging of ampullary carcinoma (see the section on EUS).

Cystic Neoplasms

Cystic neoplasms of the pancreas represent 10% to 15% of all pancreatic cysts and 1% of all pancreatic cancers. There are two main categories of cystic neoplasms: microcystic or serous type and macrocystic or mucinous type. Both types of cystic neoplasms have a woman to man preponderance that is 3:2 for the microcystic and 6:1 for the macrocystic group.[115,116] Microcystic neoplasms are usually seen in patients over 60 years of age, whereas macrocystic tumors occur in both middle and old age.[116] Patients present with nonspecific abdominal symptoms, weight loss, abdominal mass, or jaundice. Tumors may be found incidentally at surgery or autopsy.[117] Microcystic neoplasms constitute a high percentage of cysts seen in patients with von Hippel-Lindau syndrome.[115]

Microcystic or serous cystadenoma is a moderately well-circumscribed, multilocular mass, without a true capsule, often containing a central stellate scar with occasional calcification within this scar. Microcystic neoplasms are always benign and therefore do not require surgery, especially because they usually present in older patients. The cysts vary in size from less than 1 mm to 2 cm and are more numerous peripherally (Fig. 7-43). The cysts are lined with glycogen-containing cells.[115] In one study series, almost 30% of these cysts were located in the pancreatic head, with the rest distributed between the body and the tail.[115]

Macrocystic or mucinous cystadenoma and cystadenocarcinoma are unilocular or multilocular smooth-surfaced cystic masses with occasional papillary projections or calcification. The cysts usually measure more than 2 cm and are lined with cells containing mucinous material.[116] These tumors are malignant or potentially malignant. Differentiation of benign and malignant forms is difficult (except when there are ob-

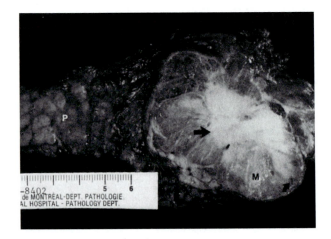

FIG. 7-43. Microcystic neoplasm of pancreas. Pancreatectomy specimen. Mass (M) in pancreas (P) with multiple tiny cysts (*curved arrow*) peripherally and a central radiating scar (*straight arrow*).

vious papillary projections) even at surgery, and tumors presumed to be benign can present a few years later with metastasis. However, even the malignant macrocystic tumors have a better prognosis than adenocarcinomas. Therefore, these tumors should be surgically removed if possible.

Sonography. **Microcystic adenomas** are relatively well-defined tumors with external lobulation. Depending on the size of the individual cysts, the ultrasound appearance may vary from a well-defined, slightly echogenic, solid-appearing mass (because the smaller cysts are only depicted as interfaces) to a partly solid-looking mass with cystic areas, more commonly peripherally (Fig. 7-44) and to a multicystic mass (Fig. 7-45). Individual cysts range in size from 1 to 20 mm. The scar that is present in some of these lesions is depicted at the ultrasonographic examination as a central, stellate-shaped echogenic area. Calcifications may be present within this scar (Fig. 7-44).[117] The scar is present in up to 20% of cases.[117,118] The pseudocapsule and septa of these tumors tend to be very vascular. This increased vascularity may be detected on Doppler. Although pancreatic and common bile duct dilatation is uncommonly seen, these tumors tend not to obstruct these ducts, presumably because of their soft nature.

Macrocystic neoplasms commonly manifest sonographically as well-circumscribed, smooth-surfaced, thin- or thick-walled, unilocular or multilocular cystic lesions of variable sizes, usually more than 2 cm in diameter and less than six in number.[117-119] The appearances of these cysts have been classified into four types[120]:

- Clear cysts
- Echogenic cysts containing debris
- Cysts with solid mural vegetations
- Completely filled or solid-looking cysts

The presence of a solid component in a predominantly cystic mass is diagnostic of this condition (Fig. 7-46). Cysts with multiple thick septa (Fig. 7-47) as well as multicystic masses with dominant cysts larger than 2 cm are also very suggestive of a macrocystic tumor. In fact, these tumors have gross features similar to those of an ovarian surface epithelial tumor. The first two types must be differentiated from a pseudocyst. The cysts may show peripheral or mural calcifications.[119] Although it is not possible to definitely differentiate between benign and malignant types, the lesions demonstrating more solid components or papillary projections are usually malignant.[117,119]

A **ductectatic mucinous cystic neoplasm** is a form of mucinous cystic neoplasm that has been recently reported.[121] It is seen in older age groups and is preponderant in men. These tumors are usually located in the uncinate process and result from cystic dilation of a branch of the pancreatic duct. They present as a multilocular cyst without nodularity, measuring less than 3 cm in diameter. ERCP shows a single or grapelike cluster of filling defects within the dilated ducts. Mucinous material may be seen exuding from the ampulla if the cysts are communicating with the pancreatic duct. Dilation of the pancreatic duct and intraluminal filling defects may be seen as a result of mucinous secretion.[121]

Comparative Imaging. Small cysts and mural nodules are better recognized on sonographic examinations than CT scans, whereas calcification is more evident on CT scan. Also, CT may show septal or mural enhancement.[117] Angiography shows significant vascularity of the microcystic tumors (Fig. 7-45, *C*).

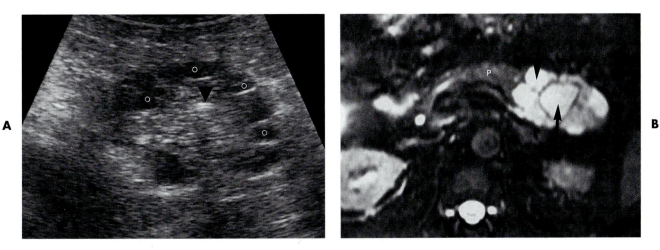

FIG. 7-44. Partially solid, partially cystic-looking microcystic neoplasm.
A, Predominantly solid-looking mass with a central cyst, calcification (*arrowhead*), and smaller peripheral cysts (*circles*). **B,** T₂-weighted axial MRI sequence with fat saturation shows cystic nature of the entire mass *(arrows)*. P—pancreas.

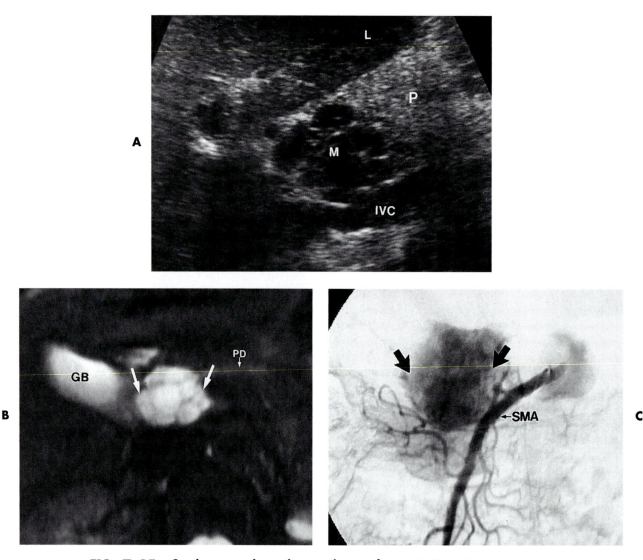

FIG. 7-45. Cystic-appearing microcystic neoplasm. A, Sagittal ultrasound scan shows multicystic mass (M) in head of pancreas (P) containing multiple small cysts. B, Confirmatory heavily T₂-weighted axial MRI with fat saturation confirms the multicystic mass (*arrows*) and no solid component. C, Superior mesenteric angiogram demonstrates an intensely vascular mass (*arrows*). GB—gallbladder; IVC—inferior vena cava; L—liver; M—mass; P—pancreas; PD—pancreatic duct; SMA—superior mesenteric artery.

MRI, particularly heavily T₂-weighted sequences, helps resolve these cysts irrespective of their size (Figs. 7-44, *B* and 7-45, *B*).[122] The combination of an apparent, solid, echogenic mass on ultrasound that appears cystic on MRI is very suggestive of a microcystic tumor (Fig. 7-44). ERCP rarely shows communication with the pancreatic duct in macrocystic neoplasms.[123]

Differential diagnosis. The microcystic type can be differentiated from an **adenocarcinoma** by its well-circumscribed nature and if tiny cysts are visualized on ultrasound or the multicystic nature of an apparently solid mass on ultrasound is confirmed on MRI. Multilocularity with solid components and multiple septa are more in keeping with a mucinous cystic

tumor than a serous type. Communication with the pancreatic duct and parenchymal changes of pancreatitis on ERCP and lack of multilocularity or septa on ultrasound favor the diagnosis of a pseudocyst. Uncommonly, necrotic or cystic islet cell and solid and papillary neoplasms can mimic mucinous tumors.[122] **Choledochal cysts** may present as a cystic mass in the region of the head of the pancreas, but their communication with the common bile duct on cholangiography or direct opacification helps to differentiate them from the cystic neoplasms.[124]

Percutaneous fine-needle aspiration (PFNA) has been used to differentiate between pancreatic cystic masses. Despite the findings of recent reports,[125-128]

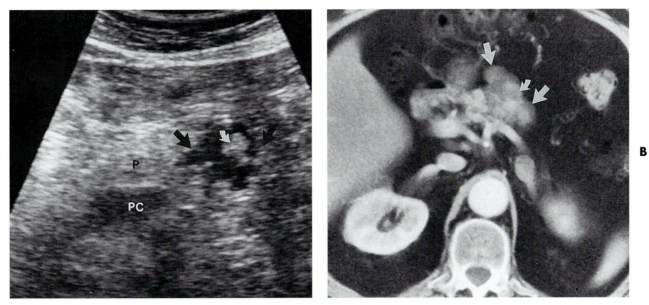

FIG. 7-46. Macrocystic neoplasm. A, Transverse ultrasound. Multicystic mass (*arrows*) with a solid nodule (*curved arrow*). **B,** Computed tomography scan shows a lobular mass (*arrows*) with enhancing nodule (*curved arrow*) corresponding to the solid nodule seen on ultrasound. P—pancreas; PC—portal confluence.

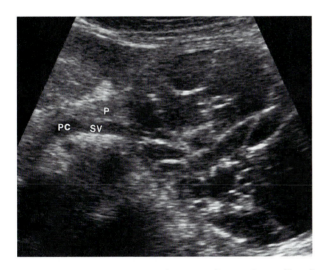

FIG. 7-47. Macrocystic neoplasm in tail of pancreas. Large cyst with multiple thick septa. P—pancreas; PC—portal confluence; SV—splenic vein.

experience with cyst fluid analysis is still limited. Some authors have shown a high accuracy for aspiration cytology by identifying inflammatory cells in pseudocysts, hypocellular material with rare strips of cuboidal cells and positive stain for glycogen in microcystic tumors, and moderately cellular material with columnar cells containing mucin in macrocystic tumors.[127,128] Other experts question the diagnosis of pseudocyst made on the basis of the presence of an inflammatory smear.[125] Also, some smears from cystic tumors lack epithelial cells.[125] The amylase content of

pseudocysts is almost always high, whereas the level in neoplastic cysts is generally low.[126] However, cystic tumors of all types may exhibit elevated amylase levels.[125] Some tumor markers, especially carcinoembryonic antigen (CEA), are high in mucinous tumors and low in pseudocysts and microcystic tumors.[125] High viscosity of the cyst content has been shown to be highly specific for mucinous tumors.[125]

Islet-Cell Tumors

Islet-cell tumors of the pancreas appear to arise from multipotential stem cells in ductal epithelium, referred to as the *amine precursor uptake* and *decarboxylation (APUD) system.* Islet-cell tumors can be part of the multiple endocrine neoplasia (MEN) syndrome, in which multiple tumors can secrete different polypeptides.[129] Although each specific tumor secretes multiple peptides, the clinical picture depends on the dominant hormone. Each of the syndromes may be caused by diffuse hyperplasia, benign adenoma, and malignant neoplasm.

Islet-cell tumors are equally distributed throughout the gland.[27] Electron microscopy and immunoassay techniques are required for specific marking of the tumor.[27] Necrosis, hemorrhage, and calcification are more prominent in larger, malignant types, but malignancy cannot be differentiated microscopically and only dissemination provides indisputable evidence of malignancy. Even malignant tumors are slow growing, and spread beyond regional lymph nodes and liver is rare. Islet-cell tumors are classified as functioning or nonfunctioning (silent). Silent tumors secrete a biologically inactive polypeptide hormone, or target cells are unresponsive or have blocked receptors.[130]

Functioning Tumors

B-cell tumors (insulinomas). Insulinomas are the most common type of islet-cell tumors. They are usually benign, presenting in the fourth through six decades of life with hypoglycemic symptoms. B-cell tumors are most commonly found in the body or tail of the pancreas.[27] They are usually well encapsulated and do not differ from normal islet cells on microscopic examination. Of these lesions, 70% are solitary adenomas, 10% are multiple adenomas, and 10% are malignant. The remaining 10% are diffuse hyperplasia or extrapancreatic. Tumors range in size from minute lesions, difficult to locate on the dissecting table, to huge masses over 1500 g (90% < 2 cm in diameter).[131] Ten percent to 27% of patients with biochemical and clinical indication of insulinomas have no tumor discovered at the time of the initial operation, in which case a blind distal pancreatectomy may be performed.[132]

G-cell tumors (gastrinomas). Gastrinomas, which produce the Zollinger-Ellison syndrome, are the second most common islet-cell tumors after insulinomas. The presenting symptoms include diarrhea and peptic ulcer disease with a patient mean age of 50 at presentation.[133] Most gastrinomas are in the pancreas, with 10% to 15% arising in the duodenum.[27] Of those located in the pancreas, only 25% are solitary. Earlier reported malignancy rates were as high as 60% at presentation,[134] but recent studies confirm a decline in malignant cases, probably as a result of earlier detection because of radioimmunoassay tests for plasma gastrin levels.[135] However, it should be noted that all lesions are potentially malignant. Current management consists of medical treatment of the symptoms. Surgical intervention is limited to patients whose lesions are accurately localized.[135]

Rare islet-cell tumors. Glucagonoma, vipoma, somatostatinoma, and carcinoid and multihormonal tumors constitute rare functioning islet-cell tumors. There is a high incidence of malignancy in glucagonomas and vipomas.[136] Vipomas are also associated with dilation of the gallbladder (caused by its paralysis as it fills with diluted bile), fluid-filled distended bowel loops (caused by inhibition of bowel motility), and excessive secretion of fluid and electrolytes. The gastric wall may also be thickened.[137]

Nonfunctioning islet-cell tumors constitute one third of all islet-cell neoplasms and have a tendency to present as large tumors with a high incidence of malignancy (Fig. 7-48). They are usually located in the head of the pancreas.[133]

Sonography. Preoperative ultrasonographic examination for the detection of islet-cell tumors is generally difficult, with identification varying from 25% to 60%.[136,137] This difficulty is the small size of these tumors in patients who are generally obese because of overeating for fear of hypoglycemic episodes. Gastrinomas are even smaller, with an average detection rate of 20%.[138] However, recent experience with endoscopic ultrasonography has allowed more reliable detection of these intrapancreatic endocrine neoplasms, increasing the detection rate to a level of 80%.[139] The usual small islet-cell tumors are hypoechoic and well-defined without calcifications or necrosis. However, these lesions can be isoechoic and only detectable by contour changes.[140] The larger tumors can be echogenic and irregular and may contain calcifications or areas of necrosis (Fig. 7-48). The latter findings are usually associated with malignancy.[141] The metastatic lesions tend to be echogenic.[141]

One of the most important contributions of **intraoperative ultrasound** (IOUS) is in the detection of the islet cell tumors (Fig. 7-49).[138,139] IOUS has improved the sensitivity of ultrasonographic detection from 61% to 84%,[138] and combined with palpation, it has a reported sensitivity of 100%.[132] In another study series, 86% of insulinomas and 83% of gastrinomas were detected by IOUS, and intrapancreatic lesions were identified in 100% of cases.[142] IOUS can also outline the relation of the neoplasm to the pancreatic or common bile duct.[138] Although more sensitive than both CT and preoperative ultrasonography, IOUS is less accurate for the detection of multiple adenomas, with a sensitivity of 36% because of the small size of the tumors.[136]

Comparative Imaging. Preoperative localization of islet-cell tumors remains extremely difficult because of the small size and rare occurrence, which limits the experience of individual institutions.[142-145] Preoperative ultrasonographic, CT, and angiographic examinations appear to be comparable in the detection of islet-cell tumors that are larger than 2 cm. For smaller tumors, the accuracy of various modalities for the investigation of islet-cell tumors depends on the specific expertise available in different institutions.

The reported sensitivity of CT for the detection of insulinomas is 40% to 66%,[143] whereas angiographic sensitivity varies from 29% to 90%.[142,143] Success rates of as high as 97% have been reported with venous sampling.[144] The advent of helical CT appears to have improved the detectability of islet cell tumors by CT. Considering that these tumors are generally vascular, the addition of early arterial (parenchymal) phase helical CT with thin slices enhances the detection of these tumors. Van Hoe et al.[145] detected 9 of 11 islet-cell tumors including a 4-mm gastrinoma using both arterial and venous phase helical CT. Also, combinations of fat-suppressed T_1-weighted spin-echo, T_2-weighted spin-echo, dynamic gadolinium DTPA gradient recalled echo, and gadolinium-enhanced fat-

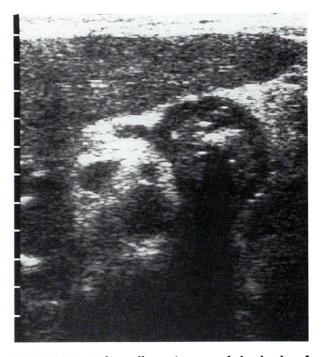

FIG. 7-48. Islet cell carcinoma of the body of the pancreas. Transverse sonogram shows a sharply marginated focal hypoechoic mass with internal calcifications which casts an acoustic shadow. (Courtesy of J. William Charboneau, MD, Mayo Clinic, Rochester, Minnesota.)

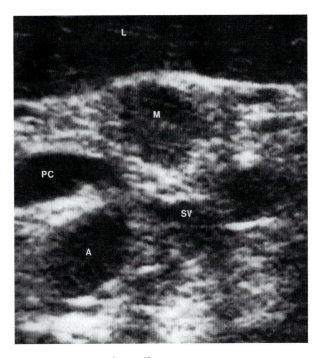

FIG. 7-49. Islet-cell tumor. Intraoperative scan shows hypoechoic mass (M) in body. A—aorta; L—liver; PC—portal confluence; SV—splenic vein.

suppressed T_1 images appear to be superior to conventional CT and ultrasound.[146-148] Further studies are required to compare the performance of helical CT and MRI.

Nonislet-Cell Tumors

The rare nonislet-cell tumors of the pancreas include giant cell tumors, adenosquamous carcinomas, mucinous adenocarcinomas, anaplastic carcinomas, solid and papillary epithelial neoplasms, acinar cell carcinomas, pancreaticoblastomas, connective tissue tumors, metastases, lymphomas, and plasmacytomas.[149] There is no reported sonographic description for most of these tumors.

Solid and papillary tumors are usually seen in young women as large, well-defined, encapsulated tumors that may contain thick-walled cystic areas as a result of hemorrhage and necrosis. They have a predilection for the pancreatic tail and have a better prognosis and a tendency for long patient survival because of their local invasion and lack of metastases.[150]

Metastasis to the pancreas is not common and usually occurs as direct extensions from adjacent structures, such as the stomach, or contiguous lymphadenopathy. On autopsy, only 3% of all patients with a proven malignancy had metastasis to the pancreas.[151] Metastases to the pancreas occur in 8.4% of patients with lung cancer,[152] 19% of those with breast cancer,[153] and 37.5% of those with malignant melanomas.[154] Pancreatic metastasis[155] is usually hypoechoic and small, so the contour of the pancreas is not always affected. Larger lesions, especially from the ovary and melanoma, may show cystic changes. Single lesions may be mistaken for primary adenocarcinomas and multiple ones for acute pancreatitis, diffuse adenocarcinoma, or lymphoma.[155]

Non-Hodgkin's lymphomas, especially the histiocytic type, tend to involve the extra lymph node organs. The extranodal involvement is usually associated with concomitant intra-abdominal lymphadenopathy. Involvement of the pancreas may be either solitary or diffuse,[156] with multiple discrete nodules (Fig. 7-50) or diffuse involvement. In some cases, the pancreas is embedded in massive peripancreatic lymphadenopathy, in which case it is not possible to know if the pancreas is involved or merely compressed.

ULTRASOUND-GUIDED PANCREATIC INTERVENTION

Biopsy

A percutaneous biopsy of pancreatic masses is in general performed to differentiate an inflammatory process from a pancreatic carcinoma. Although the sensitivity of PFNA biopsy for the diagnosis of pancreatic malignancy (50% to 86%)[157,158] is not as high as for

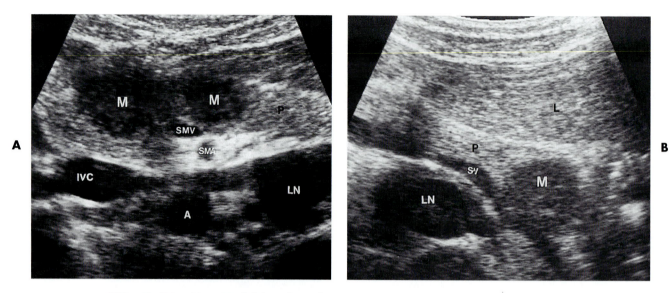

FIG. 7-50. Non-Hodgkin's lymphoma. A, Transverse ultrasound of head, body, and **B,** tail of pancreas demonstrate multiple well-defined hypoechoic masses (M) throughout pancreas (P). A—aorta; IVC—inferior vena cava; L—liver; LN—lymph node; P—pancreas; SMA—superior mesenteric artery; SMV—superior mesenteric vein; SV—splenic vein.

the diagnosis of liver malignancy, its reported specificity is as high as 100%.[157-159] Lower sensitivity results, both percutaneous and at surgery, are the result of several factors:

- Presence of necrosis that is not visible on ultrasonograms
- Tendency for the neoplasm to produce significant desmoplastic fibrous reaction,[159] causing a negative biopsy result
- Associated pancreatitis that may complicate localization of the tumor
- Well-differentiated tumors that can be difficult to diagnose on cytologic examinations.[159]

However, more recent reports using larger cutting needles to obtain core biopsy have shown better results with sensitivities of 92% and 94% without increase in complication rate.[160,161] It is most efficacious to obtain biopsy specimens in the region where the pancreatic duct tapers. A positive biopsy result prevents unnecessary surgery when unresectability is confirmed by prior imaging.

The main complication of PFNA of the pancreas is the induction of pancreatitis, and a few deaths have been reported from fulminant pancreatitis.[162-164] This usually occurs when a normal pancreas has undergone biopsy. There have also been isolated reports of seeding of pancreatic cancer along the path of the biopsy needle.[162,165]

Percutaneous Pancreatography

Although performing percutaneous pancreatography is feasible in a nondilated system (considering the fact that the pancreatic duct is almost always seen under ultrasound guidance), the opacification of a nondilated pancreatic duct should be left to ERCP. In patients with a dilated duct, a plain radiograph is obtained to document calcifications. The pancreatic duct is then punctured under ultrasound guidance using a 22-gauge needle. A small amount of pancreatic juice is aspirated for cytologic assessment, and water-soluble contrast medium is injected at a low pressure using fluoroscopy.[166] The amount of contrast injected varies with visualization of the pancreatic duct or, in cases of occlusion, the amount of pressure needed to opacify the duct and the patient's response to the injection. Excessive injection should be avoided, and the contrast medium should be aspirated at the end of the procedure.[166] A success rate of 89% has been obtained in the largest study series reported.[166] No complications are reported, except for one case of bile leakage as a result of transgression of a dilated intrahepatic bile duct.[166]

Indications for percutaneous pancreatography include:

- Technical difficulty with ERCP, either as a result of failure of the procedure or modified anatomy from previous surgery (such as prior gastrectomy, pancreaticojejunostomy, or a Whipple procedure)[166]
- Lack of ERCP visualization of the pancreatic duct in spite of opacification of the common bile duct
- Poor or nonopacification of the proximal pancreatic duct caused by significant narrowing or occlusion of the distal pancreatic duct
- Determination of the presence of stones and creation of a surgical map before pancreatic surgery

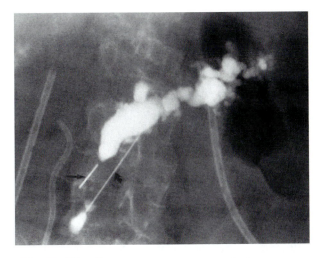

FIG. 7-51. **Percutaneous pancreatogram, performed under ultrasound guidance using 22-gauge needle** (*curved arrow*). Site of occlusion has been biopsied using 22-gauge needle (*straight arrow*) under fluoroscopic guidance.

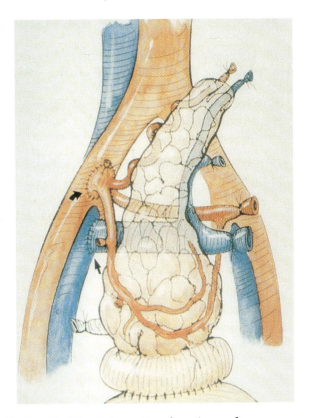

FIG. 7-52. Schematic drawing of pancreas transplant. During pancreaticoduodenal transplantation, the venous anastomosis is performed by suturing the end of the donor portal vein to the anterior side of the recipient external or common iliac vein, or occasionally to the distal inferior vena cava. The arterial anastomosis (which most commonly involves a patch of aorta of donor, including both celiac trunk and superior mesenteric artery) is anastomosed to the anterior wall of the common iliac artery or occasionally to the aorta.

- A dilated pancreatic duct but no demonstrable mass on ultrasonographic or CT examinations (a pancreatogram can precisely localize a lesion for biopsy) (Fig. 7-51).

The introduction of magnetic resonance cholangiopancreatography (MRCP) may obviate the need for percutaneous pancreatography in some cases of failed or inadequate ERCP, because it provides noninvasive visualization of the pancreatic duct.[167]

PANCREATIC TRANSPLANTATION

A number of techniques are used for pancreatic transplantation that are beyond the scope of this book.[168] Knowledge of the initial operative procedure, however, is essential to the radiological assessment of these patients, especially with respect to the evaluation of the vascular structures. The most commonly used technique involves transplantation of the complete pancreas with a section of the duodenal loop anastomosed to the bladder for the management of the exocrine function, which is done by measuring the urine amylase (Fig. 7-52).[168]

Pancreatic transplants are complicated by ischemia, rejection, anastomotic leak, other arterial and venous anastomotic complications, and infection. Pancreatitis is the only complication unique to the pancreas.[169] There is no sensitive test for early detection of transplant rejection, and pancreatic biopsy is seldom performed because of the high risk of complications. However, when combined renal and pancreatic transplantations are performed, the two organs tend to be rejected at the same time.[169] The only established roles of ultrasound in pancreatic transplantation are to detect peripancreatic fluid collections and pancreatic enlargement[169] and to guide aspiration to characterize fluid.[170] Cystoscopic transduodenal ultrasound-guided biopsy of the transplant pancreas has been shown to be safe and produces increased diagnostic yield.[171] Transplant rejection may cause an inhomogeneous echopattern,[169] but this is not specific.[169,170] Pulsed Doppler imaging with an RI of more than 0.7 in diagnosing early signs of transplant rejection has resulted in a low sensitivity and specificity of 20% and 73%, respectively.[172] Currently, the main role of color Doppler imaging is in the evaluation of the main vasculature of pancreas transplants to look for arterial and venous thrombosis, especially in the early postoperative period.[173] Graft thrombosis is seen as a primary event or as a secondary process in association with rejection, inflammation, or infection.[168]

ENDOSCOPIC ULTRASONOGRAPHY

Endoscopic ultrasonography is a technique that combines endoscopy with high-resolution ultrasonography. High-resolution sonograms of the pancreas can be obtained because of the proximity to the pancreas provided by the intra-gastrointestinal position of the endoscopic probe. EUS can overcome factors that limit transabdominal sonography, such as overlying bowel gas, morbid obesity, or the patient's inability to cooperate with respiratory instructions.[174] As in all forms of sonography, this procedure is highly operator-dependent. In addition, it is available in only a few institutions. With increased expertise, the rate of technical failure has decreased from 25% to a level below 5% in the hands of experienced endoscopists.[175] The few remaining failures relate to the inability to pass the endoscope into the third portion of the duodenum in cases where a detailed view of the uncinate and head of pancreas is needed.

Two types of endosonographic scopes are commercially available. The radial type uses a high-frequency (7.5 and 12 MHz) radial scanner capable of producing 360° cross-sectional images. This type of scope is useful for surveying the gastrointestinal tract and the surrounding organs. The orientation within the scan plane is relatively straightforward. The commercially available unit does not have color Doppler capability and has relatively limited scanning depth. Biopsy capability is not yet commercially available. The commercially available sector-type scanner employs a lower-frequency (5 and 7.5 MHz) transducer. At this level of transducer frequency, detection of small intrapancreatic lesions is still excellent. Color Doppler and biopsy capabilities are available with the sector units, although endosonographic-guided biopsies have not currently matured as a widely employed technique. The lower transducer frequencies permit deeper tissue penetration, which is useful in identifying deep lesions, such as intrapancreatic endocrine tumors. However, the smaller field of view can make it difficult to maintain scan orientation.

Transverse and coronal oblique views of the pancreatic head can be obtained from the duodenal bulb or the second part of the duodenum. The body and tail of the pancreas can be visualized through the greater curvature of the stomach. High-resolution images of the entire pancreas, as well as the portal venous confluence, the common bile duct, the pancreatic duct, and the superior mesenteric vessels, can be obtained (Fig. 7-53).[176] Two methods of contact are employed to provide adequate interface between the gut wall and the transducer. The first is the balloon method, which is preferred when examining the pancreas and uses a water-filled balloon at the tip of the scope surrounding the transducer. The

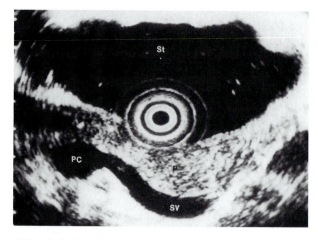

FIG. 7-53. **Transgastric endosonography, body and tail of normal pancreas** (P). PC—portal confluence; St—stomach; SV—splenic vein. (Courtesy of P.J. Valette, MD, Hopital Edouard Herriot, Lion, France.)

second is the water-filled stomach method, which consists of placing an uncovered transducer in the stomach filled with 300 to 800 ml of deaerated water.[177] The complete examination lasts approximately 15 to 30 minutes.[178]

EUS is highly accurate in identifying the presence of a pancreatic abnormality. The sensitivity of EUS in detecting **pancreatic lesions** has been reported to be 98% to 100%. In comparison, the sensitivities of TA-US (transabdominal), CT scan, and ERCP are 67% to 72%, 71% to 78%, and 88% to 94%, respectively.[175,179,180] EUS is especially useful in detecting pancreatic lesions that are less than 3 cm. In one study, the EUS detection rate was 100% versus 50% for TA-US, 55% for CT, and 90% for ERCP.[180]

Indications for EUS include detection and staging of pancreatic adenocarcinoma (especially tumors < 3 cm), evaluation for pancreatic neuroendocrine tumors, assessment of the pancreas in morbidly obese patients, and high-resolution anatomic assessment of the pancreatic head and the ampulla.[174,175] EUS is showing promise in the assessment of patients with abdominal pain who are suspected of having chronic pancreatitis.[181]

EUS appears to be the single most accurate technique in both localizing pancreatic lesions and assessing resectability of a pancreatic malignancy (Fig. 7-54). Accuracies of EUS, TA-US, CT, and MRI for detecting pancreatic cancers are reported to be 91% to 96%, 64% to 88%, 66% to 88% and 83% respectively.[182,183,184] EUS has also been shown to be accurate both in localizing and staging the ampullary tumors and differentiating them from the pancreatic cancer (Fig. 7-55).[185] The ultrasonographic appearance of pancreatic carcinoma on EUS is similar to that of con-

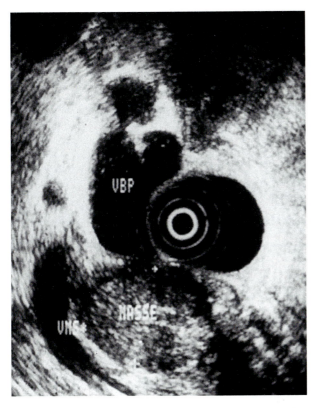

FIG. 7-54. Transduodenal endosonography of pancreatic carcinoma. MASSE—pancreatic mass; VBP—common bile duct; VMS—superior mesenteric vein. (Courtesy of P. Taourel, MD, Hopital St. Eloi, Montpellier, France.)

ventional ultrasound; however, EUS affords better characterization of the mass in regards to tumor margin, shape, echogenicity, and echotexture. Although most pancreatic carcinomas are described as being hypoechoic with irregular margins and mottled echotexture, substantial overlap exists with the features seen in chronic pancreatitis.[175,184] Moreover, examination of a pancreatic mass greater than 5 cm greatly hampers the ability of EUS because of the limited field of view and acoustic penetration (a function of the high-frequency transducer). In determining resectability of a pancreatic carcinoma, EUS has been found to be particularly useful in evaluating the presence or absence of invasion into the portal, splenic, and superior mesenteric veins, the duodenal wall, or the ampulla.[186] Clinical utility of EUS in determining the presence of lymph node metastasis as well as invasion of the celiac and superior mesenteric arteries is not convincing at this time when compared with other imaging modalities. EUS shortcomings include the difficulty in performing EUS-guided needle biopsy with currently available instrumentation and its inability to accurately detect the liver, peritoneal, and omental metastases. At present, there seems to be no substitute for laparoscopy in detecting these metastases when they are

small, which is crucial in determining the resectability status for a patient with pancreatic carcinoma.[187]

EUS is an important nonsurgical localization study in patients with insulinomas and gastrinomas. In patients with sporadic insulinomas, EUS provides a detection rate of 80% to 90%.[181] If an insulinoma is identified by EUS, no other study is required. Pancreatic angiography and arterial stimulation study are performed only if EUS is negative in a patient suspected of having sporadic insulinomas. IOUS as a stand-alone diagnostic procedure has disadvantages, such as extended intraoperative time. IOUS is therefore recommended as an image-guidance adjunct to insulinoma enucleation or as a second-line diagnostic modality when all other studies fail.

In patients with hyperinsulinoma secondary to MEN I syndrome, EUS is used to evaluate only the head and uncinate process because a distal pancreatectomy is performed regardless of other findings. In patients with clinical diagnosis of Zollinger-Ellison syndrome, EUS can detect virtually all intrapancreatic gastrinomas. Sensitivity of a negative EUS of the pancreas predicting extrapancreatic gastrinoma is 100%.[181] A negative EUS in combination with a negative CT scan in a patient with Zollinger-Ellison syndrome strongly suggests the probability that a small submucosal gastrinoma will be found in the duodenum.

The superior resolution of EUS over TA-US can help to characterize cystic neoplasms. The cystic nature of serous cystadenomas can be better appreciated on EUS by identification of small cysts in an apparent solid mass on TA-US (Fig. 7-56).

EUS is sensitive to parenchymal changes associated with chronic pancreatitis. Eight EUS features have been described: (1) inhomogeneous echogenicities; (2) accentuation of parenchymal lobulations; (3) irregular margin of the pancreas; (4) increased thickness or echogenicity of the main pancreatic ductal wall; (5) dilatation of the main pancreatic duct and side branches; (6) echogenic foci within the gland; (7) intraductal calcifications; and (8) pancreatic or peripancreatic cystic structures.[188,189] Specificity and accuracy of EUS in the diagnosis of chronic pancreatitis is reported to be in the range of 80% to 86%.[189] However, no major double-blinded or histologically confirmed study has been published to date. Therefore, the observed EUS features in patients suspected of having chronic pancreatitis with a normal ERCP result may represent either greater sensitivity of EUS to early chronic pancreatic changes or false-positive results. Nevertheless, in doubtful cases where chronic pancreatitis is clinically suspected but cannot be confirmed by TA-US or CT scan, EUS is recommended (prior to ERCP), because it has been shown to be sensitive to parenchymal changes and also does not carry the risk of procedure-related acute pancreatitis.

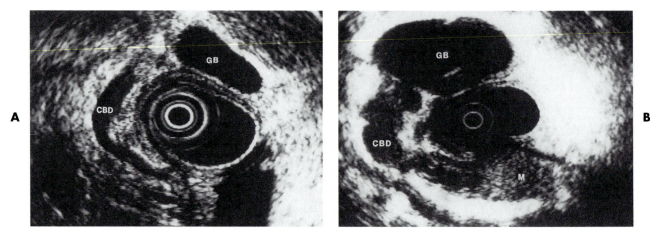

FIG. 7-55. Transduodenal endosonography, common bile duct (CBD) and gallbladder (GB). A, Normal common bile duct. **B,** Solid intraluminal mass (M) in distal dilated common bile duct is ampullary carcinoma. Gallbladder is distended. (Courtesy of P.J. Valette, MD, Hopital Edouard Herriot, Lion, France.)

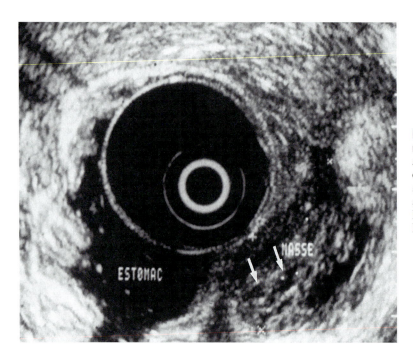

FIG. 7-56. Transgastric endosonography of solid-appearing pancreatic serous cystadenoma on TA-ultrasound exam. Endoscopic ultrasound shows multiple small cysts (*arrows*) that were not seen by transabdominal ultrasound. Estomac—stomach; Masse—mass. (Courtesy of P. Taourel, MD, Hopital St. Eloi, Montpellier, France.)

EUS is still a developing sonographic modality, although its use outside the university teaching centers is beginning to be accepted. It requires the combined expertise of an endoscopist and a sonologist. EUS–guided biopsy capability is yet to be refined to the level of consistent reliability. Development of the anticipated EUS biopsy guide and needle system would make EUS an even more powerful investigative modality. Finally, high-frequency mini-probes (daughter scopes introduced through the interventional channel of a mother scope) with 20 to 30 MHz scan heads are being developed for examination of the pancreatic duct, which may prove to be useful in the search of an intraductal papillary carcinoma.[161]

REFERENCES
Embryology
1. Clemente CD: The digestive system. In *Gray's Anatomy*, ed 30, Philadelphia, Lea & Febiger 1985;1502-1507.
2. Berman LG, Prior JT, Abramow SM, et al.: A study of the pancreatic duct system in man by the use of vinyl acetate casts of postmortem preparations, *Surg Gynecol Obstet* 1960; 110:391-403.

Anatomy
3. Suramo I, Peivensalo M, Myllyle V: Cranio-caudal movements of the liver, pancreas and kidneys in respiration, *Acta Radiol* 1984;25(2):129-131.
4. Valenzvela JE: Pancreas. In Gitnick G, Hollander D, Samloff IM, editors: *Principles and Practice of Gastroenterology and Hepatology*. New York, 1988, Elsvier Science Publishing.

5. Newman BM, Lebenthal E: In Vay Liang WG, Gardner JD, Brooks FP, et al., editors: *Congenital Anomalies of the Exocrine Pancreas*, New York, 1986, Raven Press.

6. Ross BA, Brooke Jeffrey R, Mindelzun RE. Normal variations in the lateral contour of the head and neck of the pancreas mimicking neoplasm: Evaluation with dual-phase helical CT, *Am J Roentgenol* 1996;166:799-801.

Pancreatic Sonography

7. Bret PM, Reinhold C, Herba M, et al.: Replaced or right accessory hepatic artery: Can ultrasound replace angiography, *J Clin Ultrasound* 1988;16:245-249.

8. Bryan PJ: Apperance of normal pancreatic duct: A study using real-time ultrasound, *J Clin Ultrasound* 1982;10:63-66.

9. Hadidi A: Pancreatic duct diameter: sonographic measurement in normal subjects, *J Clin Ultrasound* 1983;11:17-22.

10. Didier D, Deschamps JP, Rohmer P, et al.: Evaluation of the pancreatic duct: a reappraisal based on a retrospective correlative study by sonography and pancreatography in 117 normal and pathologic subjects, *Ultrasound Med Biol* 1983;9(5):509-518.

11. So CB, Cooperberg PL, Gibney RG, et al.: Sonographic findings in pancreatic lipomatosis, *Am J Roentgenol* 1987; 149:67-68.

12. Patel S, Bellon EM, Haaga J, et al.: Fat replacement of the exocrine pancreas, *Am J Roentgenol* 1980;135:843-845.

13. Nakamura M, Katada N, Sakakibara, et al.: Huge lipomatous pseudohypertrophy of the pancreas, *Am J Gastroenterol* 1979;72(2):171-174.

14. de Graaff CS, Taylor KJW, Simonds BD, et al.: Gray-scale echography of the pancreas: re-evaluation of normal size, *Radiology* 1978;129:157-161.

15. Niederau C, Sonnenberg A, Muller JE, et al.: Sonographic measurements of the normal liver, spleen, pancreas, and portal vein, *Radiology* 1983;149:537-540.

16. Bolondi L, Bassi, SL, Gaiani S: Sonography of chronic pancreatitis, *Radiol Clin North Am* 1989;27(4):815-833.

17. Donald JJ, Shorvon PJ, Lees WR: A hypoechoic area within the head of the pancreas: a normal variant, *Clin Radiol* 1990;41:337-338.

18. Marchal G, Verbeken E, Van Steenbergen W, et al.: Uneven lipomatosis: A pitfall in pancreatic sonography, *Gastrointest Radiol* 1989;14:233-237.

19. Atri M, Nazarnia S, Mehio A, et al.: Hypoechogenic embryologic ventral aspect of the head and uncinate process of the pancreas: *In vitro* correlation of US with histopathologic findings, *Radiology* 1994;190:441-444.

20. Wachsberg RH: Posterior superior pancreaticoduodenal vein: Mimic of distal common bile duct at sonography, *Am J Roentgenol* 1993;160:1033-1037.

21. Tszekessy D, Pochhammer KF: Diurnal sonographic imaging of the pancreas, *Ultraschall Med* 1985;6:134-136.

22. Muradali D, Wilson SR, Hope-Simpson D, Burns PN: Oral contrast agents for sonography: improved visualization of the abdomen and gut, *RSNA* 1995;197(P):611.

23. Odo Op den Orth J: Tubeless hypotonic duodenography with water: a simple aid in sonography of the pancreatic head, *Radiology* 1985;154:826.

24. duCret RP, Jackson VP, Rees C, et al.: Pancreatic sonography: enhancement by metoclopramide, *Am J Roentgenol* 1986;146:341-343.

25. Rauch RF, Bowie JD, Rosenberg ER, et al.: Can ultrasonic examination of the pancreas and gallbladder follow a barium UGI series on the same day? *Invest Radiol* 1983;18(6):523-525.

Congenital Anomalies

26. Gold RP: Agenesis and pseudo-agenesis of the dorsal pancreas, *Abd Imaging* 1993;18:141-144.

27. Cotran RC, Kumar V, Robbins SL: *The Pancreas: Robins' Pathologic Basis of Disease*, ed 4, Philadelphia, 1989, W B Saunders.

28. Mares AJ, Hirsch M: Congenital cysts of the head of the pancreas, *J Pediatr Surg* 1977;12:547-552.

29. Oppenheimer EH, Esterly JR: Pathology of cystic fibrosis review of the literature and comparison with 146 autopsied cases, *Perspect Pediatr Pathol* 1975;2:241-278.

30. Swobodnik W, Wolf A, Wechsler JG, et al.: Ultrasound characteristics of the pancreas in children with cystic fibrosis, *J Clin Ultrasound* 1985;13:469-474.

31. Dobson RL, Johnson MA, Henning RC, et al.: Sonography of the gallbladder, biliary tree, and pancreas in adults with cystic fibrosis, *Can Assoc Radiol J* 1988;39:257-259.

32. Daneman A, Gaskin K, Martin DJ, et al.: Pancreatic changes in cystic fibrosis: Computed tomography and sonographic appearances, *Am J Roentgenol* 1983;141:653-655.

33. Graham N, Manhire AR, Stead RJ, et al.: Cystic fibrosis: Ultrasonographic findings in the pancreas and hepatobiliary system correlated with clinical data and pathology, *Clin Radiol* 1985;36(2):199-203.

34. Hernanz-Schulman M, Teele RL, Perez-Atayde A, et al.: Pancreatic cytosis in cystic fibrosis, *Radiology* 1986;158:629-631.

35. Cooperman M, Ferrara JJ, Fromkes JJ, et al.: Surgical management of pancreas divisum, *Am J Surg* 1982;143:107-112.

36. Cotton PB: Congenital anomaly of pancreas divisum as cause of obstructive pain and pancreatitis, *Gut* 1980;21:105-114.

37. Brinberg DE, Carr MF Jr, Premkumar A, et al.: Isolated ventral pancreatitis in an alcoholic with pancreas divisum, *Gastrointest Radiol* 1988;13(4):323-326.

38. Jennings CM, Gaines PA: The abdominal manifestation of von Hippel-Lindau disease and a radiological screening protocol for an affected family, *Clin Radiol* 1988;39(4):363-367.

39. Levine E, Collins DL, Horton WA, et al.: Computed tomography screening of the abdomen in von Hippel-Lindau disease, *Am J Roentgenol* 1982;139:505-510.

Inflammatory Processes

40. Ranson JHC, Ratkind KM, Turner JW: Prognostic signs and non-operative peritoneal lavage in acute pancreatitis, *Surg Gynecol Obstet* 1976;143:209-219.

41. Knaus W, Draper E, Wagner D, et al.: APACHE II: A severity of disease classification system, *Crit Care Med* 1985;13:818-829.

42. Jeffrey RB, Laing FC, Wing VW: Ultrasound in acute pancreatic trauma, *Gastrointest Radiol* 1986;11:44-48.

43. Jeffrey RB Jr., Federle MP, Crass RA: Computed tomography of pancreatic trauma, *Radiology* 1983;147:491-494.

44. Balthazar EJ, Robinson DL, Megibow AJ, et al.: Acute pancreatitis: Value of CT in establishing prognosis, *Radiology* 1990;174:331-336.

45. Gyr KE, Singer MV, Sarles H: Pancreatitis: Concepts and classification, *International Congress Ser*, vol 642, February 1985.

46. Delhaye M, Engelholm L, Cremer M: Pancreas divisum: Congenital anatomic variant or anomaly?—contribution of endoscopic retrograde dorsal pancreatography, *Gastroenterology* 1985;89:951-958.

47. Goekas MC: Etiology and pathogenesis of acute pancreatic inflammation: Acute pancreatitis, *Ann Intern Med* 1985;103:86-100.

48. Freeny PC: Classification of pancreatitis, *Radiol Clin North Am* 1989;27:1-3.

49. Jeffrey RB, Laing FC, Wing VW: Extrapancreatic spread of acute pancreatitis: New observations with real-time ultrasound, *Radiology* 1986;159:707-711.

50. Neff CC, Simeone JF, Wittenberg J, et al.: Inflammatory pancreatic masses: Problems in differentiating focal pancreatitis from carcinoma, *Radiology* 1984;150:35-40.

51. Zuccaro G Jr, Sivak MV Jr: Endoscopic ultrasonography in the diagnosis of chronic pancreatitis, *Endoscopy* 1992;24:347-349.

52. Nattermann D, Goldschmidt AJ, Dancygier H: Endosonography in chronic pancreatitis—a comparison between ERCP and EUS, *Endoscopy* 1993;25:565-570.

53. Price J, Leung JWC: Ultrasound diagnosis of *Ascaris lumbricoides* in the pancreatic duct: The "four-lines" sign, *Br J Radiol* 1988;61:411-413.

54. Warshaw AL: Inflammatory masses following acute pancreatitis, *Surg Clin North Am* 1974;54:621-636.

55. Lane MJ, Mindelzun RE, Sandhu JS, et al.: CT diagnosis of blunt pancreatic trauma: Importance of detecting fluid between the pancreas and the splenic vein, *Am J Roentgenol* 1994;163:833.

56. Bradley EL III, Clements JL Jr, Gonzalez AC: The natural history of pancreatic pseudocysts: A unified concept of management, *Am J Surg* 1979;137:135-141.

57. Donovan PJ, Sanders RC, Siegelman SS: Collections of fluid after pancreatitis: Evaluation of computed tomography and ultrasonography, *Radiol Clin North Am* 1982;20:653-665.

58. Nyberg DA, Laing F: Ultrasonographic findings in peptic ulcer disease and pancreatitis that simulate primary gallbladder disease, *J Ultrasound Med* 1983;2:303-307.

59. Lee CM, Chang-Chien CS, Lim DY, et al.: Real-time ultrasonography of pancreatic pseudocyst: Comparison of infected and uninfected pseudocysts, *J Clin Ultrasound* 1988;16:393-397.

60. Bradley EL III: *Pancreatic pseudocyst.* In Bradley EL III, editor: *Complications of Pancreatitis: Medical and Surgical*, Philadelphia, 1982, WB Saunders.

61. Rattner DW, Warshaw AL: Surgical intervention in acute pancreatitis, *Crit Care Med* 1988;16:85-95.

62. Laing FC, Gooding GAW, Brown T, et al.: Atypical pseudocysts of the pancreas: An ultrasonographic evaluation, *J Clin Ultrasound* 1979;7:27-33.

63. Maier W, Roscher R, Malfertheinar P, et al.: Pancreatic pseudocyst of the mediastinum: Evaluation by computed tomography, *Eur J Radiol* 1986;6:70-72.

64. Lye DJ, Stark RH, Cullen GM, et al.: Ruptured pancreatic pseudocysts: Extension into the thigh, *Am J Roentgenol* 1987;49:937-938.

65. Grace RR, Jordan PH Jr: Unresolved problems of pancreatic pseudocysts, *Ann Surg* 1976;184:16-21.

66. Rheingold OJ, Wilbar JA, Barkin JS: Gastric outlet obstruction due to pancreatic pseudocyst: A report of two cases, *Am J Gastroenterol* 1978;69:92-96.

67. Bellon EM, George CR, Schreiber H, et al.: Pancreatic pseudocysts of the duodenum, *Am J Roentgenol* 1979;133:827-831.

68. Vick CW, Simeone JF, Ferrucci JT, et al.: Pancreatitis associated fluid collection involving the spleen: Sonographic and computed tomographic appearance, *Gastrointest Radiol* 1981;6:247-250.

69. Stanley JL, Frey CF, Miller TA, et al.: Major arterial hemorrhage: A complication of pancreatic pseudocyst and chronic pancreatitis, *Arch Surg* 1976;111:435-440.

70. Frey CF, Lindenaver SM, Miller TA: Pancreatic abscess, *Surg Gynecol Obstet* 1979;149:722-726.

71. White AF, Barum S, Buranasiri S: Aneurysms secondary to pancreatitis, *Am J Roentgenol* 1976;127:393-396.

72. Falkoff GE, Taylor KJW, Morse SS: Hepatic artery pseudoaneurysm: Diagnosis with real-time and pulsed doppler ultrasound, *Radiology* 1986;58:55-56.

73. Crass RA, Way LW: Acute and chronic pancreatic pseudocysts are different, *Am J Surg* 1981;142:660-663.

74. Sarti DA: Rapid development and spontaneous regression of pancreatic pseudocysts documented by ultrasound, *Radiology* 1977;125:789-793.

75. vanSonnenberg E, Wittich GR, Casola G, et al.: Percutaneous drainage of infected and noninfected pancreatic pseudocysts: experience in 101 cases, *Radiology* 1989;170:757-761.

76. Matzinger FRK, Ho CS, Yee AC, et al.: Pancreatic pseudocysts drained through a percutaneous transgastric approach: Further experience, *Radiology* 1988;167:431-434.

77. D'Agostino HB, vanSonnenberg E, Sanchez RB, et al.: Treatment of pancreatic pseudocyst with percutaneous drainage and octreotide: Work in progress, *Radiology* 1993;187:685-688.

78. Cremer M: Endoscopic cystoduodenostomy, *Endoscopy* 1981;2:29-30.

79. Beger HG, Bittner R, Block S, et al.: Bacterial contamination of pancreatic necrosis: A prospective clinical study, *Gastroenterology* 1986;91:433-438.

80. Doglietto GB, Gui D, Pacelli F, et al.: Open vs closed treatment of secondary pancreatic infection: Review of 42 cases, *Arch of Surg* 1994;129:689-693.

81. van Sonnenberg E, Wittich GR, Casola G, et al.: Complicated pancreatic inflammatory disease: Diagnostic and therapeutic role of interventional radiology, *Radiology* 1985;155:340-355.

82. Banks PA: Clinical manifestations and treatment of pancreatitis, *Ann Intern Med* 1985;103:91-95.

83. Seiler JG, Polk HC: Factors contributing to fatal outcome after treatment of pancreatic abscess, *Ann Surg* 1986;203:605-612.

84. Ranson JHC, Spencer FC: Prevention, diagnosis and treatment of pancreatic abscess, *Surgery* 1977;82:99-105.

85. Federle MP, Jeffrey RB, Crass RA, et al.: Computed tomography of pancreatic abscess, *Am J Roentgenol* 1981;136:879-882.

86. Vernacchia FS, Jeffrey RB Jr, Federle MP, et al.: Pancreatic abscess: Predictive value of early abdominal computed tomography, *Radiology* 1987;162:435-438.

87. Fishman EK, Soyer P, Bliss DF, et al.: Splenic involvement in pancreatitis: Spectrum of CT findings, *Am J Roentgenol* 1995;164:631-635.

88. Kahn LA, Kamen C, McNamara MP Jr: Variable color Doppler appearance of pseudoaneurysm in pancreatitis, *Am J Roentgenol* 1994;162:187-188.

89. Sankaran S, Walt A: Pancreatic ascites: Recognition and management, *Arch Surg* 1976;(3):430-434.

90. Belfar HL, Radecki PD, Friedman AC, et al.: Pancreatitis presenting as pleural effusions: Computed tomography demonstration of pleural extension of pancreatic exudate, *Comput Tomogr* 1987;11:184-186.

91. Howard JM, Nedurich A: Correlation of the histologic observations and operative findings in patients with chronic pancreatitis, *Surg Gynecol Obstet* 1971;132:387-395.

92. Alpern MB, Sandler MA, Kellman GM, et al.: Chronic pancreatitis: Ultrasonic features, *Radiology* 1985;155:215-219.

93. Ferrucci J Jr, Wittenberg J, Black EB, et al.: Computed body tomography in chronic pancreatitis, *Radiology* 1979;130:175-182.

94. Fishman EK, Siegelman SS: Pancreatitis and its complications. In Tavares JM, Ferrucci JT, editors: *Radiology: Diagnosis, Imaging, Intervention*, Philadelphia 1986, JB Lippincott.

95. Weinstein BJ, Weinstein DP, Brodmeckel GJ Jr: Ultrasonography of pancreatic lithiasis, *Radiology* 1980;134:185-189.

96. Lankish PG, Otto J, Erkelenz I, et al.: Pancreatic calcifications: No indicator of severe exocrine pancreatic insufficiency, *Gastroenterology* 1986;90:617-621.

97. Ammann RW, Meunch R, Otto R, et al.: Evolution and regression of pancreatic calcification in chronic pancreatitis, *Gastroenterology* 1988;95:1018-1028.

98. Rosch N, Lux G, Rieman JF, et al.: Chronic pancreatitis and the neighboring organs, *Fortschr Med* 1981;99:1118-1125.

99. Malfertheiner P, Buchler M: Correlation of imaging and function in chronic pancreatitis, *Radiol Clin North Am* 1989;27: 51-64.

100. Ason ATA: Endoscopic retrograde cholangiopancreatography in chronic pancreatitis: Cambridge classification, *Radiol Clin North Am* 1989;27:39-50.

101. Jones SN, Lees WR, Frost RA: Diagnosis and grading of chronic pancreatitis by morphological criteria derived by ultrasound and pancreatography, *Clin Radiol* 1988;39:43-48.

Neoplasms

102. Kissane JM: *Anderson's Pathology*, ed 9, St Louis 1990, Mosby-Year Book.

103. Weinstein DP, Weinstein BJ: Pancreas. In Goldberg BB, editor: *Clinics in Diagnostic Ultrasound: Ultrasound in Cancer*, New York 1981, Churchill Livingston.

104. Kaplan JO, Isikoff MB, Barkin J, et al.: Necrotic carcinoma of the pancreas: "The pseudo-pseudocyst," *J Comput Assist Tomogr* 1980;4(2):166-167.

105. Walls WJ, Templeton AW: The ultrasonic demonstration of inferior vena caval compression: A guide to pancreatic head enlargement with emphasis on neoplasm, *Radiology* 1977; 123:165-167.

106. Taylor KJW, Ramos I, Carter D: Correlation of doppler US tumor signals with neovascular morphologic features, *Radiology* 1988;166:57-62.

107. Mori H, McGrath FP, Malone DE, et al.: *Radiology* 1992; 182:871-877.

108. Campbell JP, Wilson S: Pancreatic neoplasms: How useful is evaluation with ultrasound? *Radiology* 1988;167:341-344.

109. Peivensalo M, Lehde S: Ultrasonography and computed tomography in pancreatic malignancy, *Acta Radiologica* 1988;29(3):343-344.

110. Kamin PD, Bernardino ME, Wallace S, et al.: Comparison of ultrasound and computed tomography in the detection of pancreatic malignancy, *Cancer* 1980;46:2410-2412.

111. Bluemke DA, Cameron JL, Hruban RH, et al.: Potentially resectable pancreatic adenocarcinoma: Spiral CT assessment with surgical and pathologic correlation, *Radiology* 1995; 197:381-385.

112. Hildell J, Aspelin P, Wehlin L: Gray scale ultrasound and endoscopic ductography in the diagnosis of pancreatic disease, *Acta Chir Scand* 1979;145:239-245.

113. Cubilla AL, Fitzgerald PJ: Surgical pathology aspects of cancer of the ampulla-head-of-pancreas region, *Monogr Pathol* 1980;21:67-81.

114. Robledo R, Prieto ML, Perez M, et al.: Carcinoma of the hepaticopancreatic ampullar region: Role of ultrasound, *Radiology* 1988;166:409-412.

115. Compagno J, Oertel JE: Microcystic adenomas of the pancreas (glycogen-rich cystadenomas): A clinicopathologic study of 34 cases, *Am J Clin Pathol* 1978;69(3):289-298.

116. Compagno J, Oertel JE: Mucinous cystic neoplasms of the pancreas with overt and latent malignancy (cystadenocarcinoma and cystadenoma): A clinicopathologic study of 41 cases, *Am J Clin Pathol* 1978;69(6):573-580.

117. Friedman AC, Lichtenstein JE, Dachman AH: Cystic neoplasms of the pancreas: radiological-pathological correlation, *Radiology* 1983;149:45-50.

118. Johnson CD, Stephens DH, Charboneau JW, et al.: Cystic pancreatic tumors: Computed tomography and sonographic assessment, *Am J Roentgenol* 1988;151:1133-1138.

119. Bastid C, Sahel J, Sastre B, et al.: Mucinous cystadenocarcinoma of the pancreas: Ultrasonographic findings in 5 cases, *Acta Radiologica* 1989;30(1):45-47.

120. Busilacchi P, Rizzatto G, Bazzocchi M, et al.: Pancreatic cystadenocarcinoma: Diagnostic problems, *Br J Radiol* 1982; 55:558-561.

121. Itai Y, Ohhashi K, Nagai H, et al.: "Ductectatic" mucinous cystadenoma and cystadenocarcinoma of the pancreas, *Radiology* 1986;161:697-700.

122. Ros PR, Hamrick-Turner JE, Chiechi MV, et al.: Cystic masses of pancreas, *Radiographics* 1992;12:673-686.

123. Herrera L, Glassman CI, Komins JI: Mucinous cystic neoplasm of the pancreas demonstrated by ultrasound and endoscopic retrograde pancreatography, *Am J Gastroenterol* 1980;73(6):512-515.

124. Markle BM, Friedman AC, Sachs L: Anomalies and congenital disorders, In Friedman AC, editor: *Radiology of the Liver, Biliary Tree, Pancreas, and Spleen*, Baltimore 1987, Williams & Wilkins.

125. Lewandrowski K, Lee J, Southern J, et al.: Cyst fluid analysis in the differential diagnosis of pancreatic cysts: A new approach to the preoperative assessment of pancreatic cystic lesions, *Am J Roentgenol* 1995;164:815-819.

126. Hammel P, Levy P, Voitot H, et al.: Preoperative cyst fluid analysis is useful for the differential diagnosis of cystic lesions of the pancreas, *Gastroenterology* 1995;108:1230-1235.

127. Laucirica R, Schwartz MR, Ramzy I: Fine needle aspiration of pancreatic cystic epithelial neoplasms, *Acta Cytol* 1992; 36:881-886.

128. Jorda M, Essenfeld H, Garcia E, et al.: The value of fine-needle aspiration cytology in the diagnosis of inflammatory pancreatic masses, *Diagn Cytopathol* 1992;8:65-67.

129. Friesen SR: Tumors of the endocrine pancreas, *N Engl J Med* 1982;306:580-590.

130. Toledo-Pereyra LH: *The Pancreas: Principles of Medical and Surgical Practice*, New York 1985, Wiley Medical Publication.

131. van Heerden JA, Edis AJ, Service FJ: The surgical aspects of insulinomas, *Ann Surg* 1979;189:677-682.

132. Grant CS, van Heerden J, Charboneau JW, et al.: Insulinoma: The value of intraoperative ultrasonography, *Arch Surg* 1988;123:843-848.

133. Rossi P, Allison DJ, Bezzi M, et al.: Endocrine tumors of the pancreas, *Radiol Clin North Am* 1989;27(1):129-161.

134. Jensen RT, Gardner JD, Raufman JP, et al.: Zollinger-Ellison syndrome: Current concepts and management, *Ann Intern Med* 1983;98:59-75.

135. Stadil F: Gastrinomas: Clinical syndromes, *Acta Oncologica* 1989;28(3):379-381.

136. Galiber AK, Reading CC, Charboneau JW, et al.: Localization of pancreatic insulinoma: Comparison of pre- and intraoperative ultrasound with computed tomography and angiography, *Radiology* 1988;166(2):405-408.

137. Gorman B, Charboneau JW, James EM, et al.: Benign pancreatic insulinoma: Preoperative and intraoperative sonographic localization, *Am J Roentgenol* 1986;147:929-934.

138. Kuhn FP, Gunther R, Ruckert K, et al.: Ultrasonic demonstration of small pancreatic islet cell tumors, *J Clin Ultrasound* 1982;10:173-175.

139. Norton JA, Cromack DT, Shawker TH: Intraoperative ultrasonographic localization of islet cell tumors, *Ann Surg* 1988;207:160-168.

140. Katz LB, Aufses AH, Rayfield E, et al.: Preoperative localization and intraoperative glucose monitoring in the manage-

ment of patients with pancreatic insulinoma, *Surg Gynecol Obstet* 1986;163:509-512.

141. Rossi P, Baert A, Passariello R. et al.: Computed tomography of functioning tumors of the pancreas, *Am J Roentgenol* 1985;144:57-60.

142. Montenegro-Rodas F, Samaan NA: Glucagonoma tumors and syndrome, *Curr Prob Cancer* 1981;6:1-54.

143. Roche A, Raisonnier A, Gillon-Savouret MC: Pancreatic venous sampling and arteriography in localizing insulinomas and gastrinomas: Procedure and results in 55 cases, *Radiology* 1982;145:621-627.

144. Tjon A Tham RT, Jansen JB, et al.: Magnetic resonance, computed tomography, and ultrasound findings of metastatic vipoma in pancreas, *J Comput Assist Tomogr* 1989;13:142-144.

145. Van Hoe L, Gryspeerdt S, Marchal G, et al.: Helical CT for the preoperative localization of islet cell tumors of the pancreas: Value of arterial and parenchymal phase images, *AJR* 1995; 165:1437-1439.

146. Moore NR, Rogers CE, Britton BJ: Magnetic resonance imaging of endocrine tumours of the pancreas, *Br J Radiol* 1995;68:341-347.

147. Aspestrand F, Kolmannskog F, Jacobsen M: CT, MR imaging and angiography in pancreatic apudomas, *Acta Radiologica* 1993;34:468-473.

148. Semelka RC, Cumming MJ, Shoenut JP, Magro CM: Islet cell tumors: Comparison of dynamic contrast-enhanced CT and MR imaging with dynamic gadolinium enhancement and fat suppression, *Radiology* 1993;186:799-802.

149. Rice NT, Woodring JH, Mostowycz L, et al.: Pancreatic plasmacytoma: Sonographic and computerized tomographic findings, *J Clin Ultrasound* 1981;9:46-48.

150. Lin JT, Wang TH, Wei TC, et al.: Sonographic features of solid papillary neoplasm of the pancreas, *J Clin Ultrasound* 1985;13:339-342.

151. Willis RA: *The Spread of Tumors in the Human Body*, New York, 1975, Butterworths.

152. Budinger JM: Untreated bronchogenic carcinoma: A clinicopathological study of 250 autopsied cases, *Cancer* 1958; 11:106-116.

153. de la Monte SM, Hutchins GM, Moore GW: Endocrine organ metastases from breast carcinoma, *Am J Pathol* 1984;114: 131-136.

154. Patel JK, Didolkar MS, Pickren JW, et al.: Metastatic pattern of malignant melanoma: A study of 216 autopsy cases, *Am J Surg* 1978;135:807-810.

155. Wernecke K, Peters PE, Galanski M: Pancreatic metastases: Ultrasound evaluation, *Radiology* 1986;160:339-402.

156. Glazer HS, Lee JKT, Balfe DM, et al.: Non-Hodgkin lymphoma: Computed tomographic demonstration of unusual extranodal involvement, *Radiology* 1983;149:211-217.

Ultrasound-Guided Pancreatic Intervention

157. Pilotti S, Rilke F, Claren R, et al.: Conclusive diagnosis of hepatic and pancreatic malignancies by fine needle aspiration, *Acta Cytol* 1988;32(1):27-38.

158. Ekberg O, Bergenfeldt M, Aspelin P, et al.: Reliability of ultrasound-guided fine-needle biopsy of pancreatic masses, *Acta Radiologica* 1988;29(5):535-539.

159. Yamamoto R, Tatsuta M, Noguchi S, et al.: Histocytologic diagnosis of pancreatic cancer by percutaneous aspiration biopsy under ultrasonic guidance, *Am J Clin Pathol* 1985; 83(4):409-414.

160. Brandt KR, Charboneau JW, Stephens DH, et al.: CT- and US-guided biopsy of the pancreas, *Radiology* 1993;187:99-104.

161. Elvin A, Andersson T, Scheibenpflug L, et al.: Biopsy of the pancreas with a biopsy gun, *Radiology* 1990;176:677-679.

162. Hancke S, Holm HH, Koch F: Ultrasonically guided puncture of solid pancreatic mass lesions, *Ultrasound Med Biol* 1984;10(5):613-615.

163. Evans WK, Ho CS, McLoughlin MJ, et al.: Fatal necrotizing pancreatitis following fine-needle aspiration biopsy of the pancreas, *Radiology* 1981;141:61-62.

164. Levin DP, Bret PM: Percutaneous fine-needle aspiration biopsy of the pancreas resulting in death, *Gastrointest Radiol* 1991;16:67-69.

165. Caturelli E, Rapacci GL, Anti M, et al.: Malignant seeding after fine-needle aspiration biopsy of the pancreas, *Diagn Imaging Clin Med* 1985;54(2):88-91.

166. Matter D, Bret PM, Bretagnolle M, et al.: Pancreatic duct: Ultrasound guided percutaneous opacification, *Radiology* 1987;163:635-636.

167. Soto JA, Barish MA, Yucel EK, et al.: MR cholangiopancreatography with a three-dimensional fast spin-echo technique, *Radiology* 1995;196:459-464.

Pancreatic Transplantation

168. Dunn DL, Sutherland DER: Pancreas transplantation. In Letourneau JL, Day DL, Ascher NL, editors: *Radiology of Pancreas Transplantation*, St. Louis, 1991, Mosby-Year Book.

169. Patel B, Markivee C, Mahanta B, et al.: Pancreatic transplantation: Scintigraphy, ultrasound and computed tomography, *Radiology* 1988;167:685-687.

170. Letourneau JG, Maile CW, Sutherland DER, et al.: Ultrasound and computed tomography in the evaluation of pancreatic transplantation, *Radiol Clin North Am* 1987; 25:345-355.

171. Nelson NL, Lowell JA, Taylor RJ, et al.: Pancreas transplants: Efficacy of US-guided cystoscopic biopsy, *Radiology* 1994;191:283-284.

172. Wong JJ, Krebs TL, Klassen DK, et al.: Sonographic evaluation of acute pancreatic transplant rejection: Morphology-Doppler analysis versus guided percutaneous biopsy, *AJR* 1996;166:803-807.

173. Nghiem DD, Ludrosky L, Young JC: Evaluation of pancreatic circulation by duplex color Doppler flow sonography, *Trans Proc* 1994;26:466.

Endoscopic Ultrasonography

174. Kaplan DS, Heisig DG, Roy AK, et al.: Endoscopic ultrasound in the morbidly obese patient: A new indication, *Am J Gastroenterol* 1993;88:593-594.

175. Kelsey PJ, Warshaw AL: EUS: An added test or a replacement for several? *Endoscopy* 1993;25:179-181.

176. Zerbey AL, Lee MJ, Brugge WR, et al.: Endoscopic sonography of the upper gastrointestinal tract and pancreas, *Am J Roentgenol* 1996;166:45-50.

177. Boyce GA, Sivak MV Jr: Endoscopic ultrasonography in the diagnosis of pancreatic tumors, *Gastrointest Endosc* 1990; 36:S28-S32.

178. Kaufman AR, Sivak MV Jr: Endoscopic ultrasonography in the differential diagnosis of pancreatic disease, *Gastrointest Endosc* 1989;35:214-219.

179. Rosch T, Lorenz R, Braig C, et al.: Endoscopic ultrasound in pancreatic tumor diagnosis, *Gastrointest Endosc* 1991;37: 347-352.

180. Snady H, Cooperman A, Siegel J: Endoscopic ultrasonography compared with computed tomography and ERCP in patients with obstructive jaundice or small peripancreatic mass, *Gastrointest Endosc* 1992;38:27-34.

181. Thompson NW, Czako PF, Fritts LL, et al.: Role of endoscopic ultrasonography in the localization of insulinomas and gastrinomas, *Surgery* 1994;116:1131-1138.

182. Palazzo L, Roseau G, Gayet B, et al.: Endoscopic ultrasonography in the diagnosis and staging of pancreatic adenocarcinoma. Results of a prospective study with comparison to ultrasonography and CT scan, *Endoscopy* 1993;25:143-150.

183. Nakaizumi A, Uehara H, Iishi H, et al.: Endoscopic ultrasonography in diagnosis and staging of pancreatic cancer, *Digest Dis Sci* 1995;40:696-700.

184. Yasuda K, Mukai H, Fujimoto S, et al.: The diagnosis of pancreatic cancer by endoscopic ultrasonography, *Gastrointest Endosc* 1988;34:1-8.

185. Tio TL, Tytgat GN, Cikot RJ, et al.: Ampullopancreatic carcinoma: Preoperative TNM classification with endosonography, *Radiology* 1990;175:455-461.

186. Snady H, Bruckner H, Siegel J, et al.: Endoscopic ultrasonographic criteria of vascular invasion by potentially resectable pancreatic tumors, *Gastrointest Endosc* 1994;40:326-333.

187. Cuesta MA, Meijer S, Borgstein PJ, et al.: Laparoscopic ultrasonography for hepatobiliary and pancreatic malignancy, *Br J Surg* 1993;12(80):1571-1574.

188. Wiersema MJ, Hawes RH, Lehman GA, et al.: Prospective evaluation of endoscopic ultrasonography and endoscopic retrograde cholangiopancreatography in patients with chronic abdominal pain of suspected pancreatic origin, *Endoscopy* 1993;25:555-564.

189. Rosch T: Endoscopic ultrasonography—more questions than answers? *Endoscopy* 1993;25:600-602.

CHAPTER 8

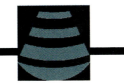

The Gastrointestinal Tract

•

Stephanie R. Wilson, M.D., F.R.C.P.C.

BASIC PRINCIPLES

Gastrointestinal tract sonography is frequently frustrating and always challenging. Gas content within the gut lumen can make visibility difficult and even impossible, intraluminal fluid may mimic cystic masses, and fecal material may create a variety of artifacts and pseudotumors. Nevertheless, normal gut has a reproducible pattern or **"gut signature,"** and a variety of gut pathologies create recognizable sonographic abnormalities. In addition, in a few conditions—such as acute appendicitis and acute diverticulitis—sonography may play a major primary investigative role. Further, endosonography, performed with high-frequency transducers in the lumen of the gut, is an increasingly popular technique for assessing the esophagus, stomach, and rectum.

The Gut Signature

The gut is a continuous hollow tube with **four concentric layers** (Fig. 8-1). From the lumen outward, they are: (1) mucosa, which consists of an epithelial lining, loose connective tissue or lamina propria, and muscularis mucosa; (2) submucosa; (3) muscularis propria, with inner circular and outer longitudinal fibers; and (4) serosa or adventitia.

These layers create a characteristic appearance or **gut signature** on sonography, where up to **five layers** may be visualized (Fig. 8-2). The correlation of the histologic layer with the sonographic appearance is depicted in Fig. 8-3.[1-3] The sonographic layers are alternately echogenic and hypoechoic: the first, third, and fifth layers are echogenic; and the second and fourth layers are hypoechoic. On routine sonograms, the gut signature (Fig. 8-4) may vary from a bull's eye in cross-section, with an echogenic central area and a hypoechoic rim, to full depiction of the five sonographic layers. The quality of the scan and the resolu-

---

FOUR HISTOLOGIC LAYERS OF THE GUT

Mucosa
Consists of an epithelial lining, loose connective tissue or lamina propria, and muscularis mucosa

Submucosa

Muscularis propria
With inner circular and outer longitudinal fibers

Serosa or adventitia

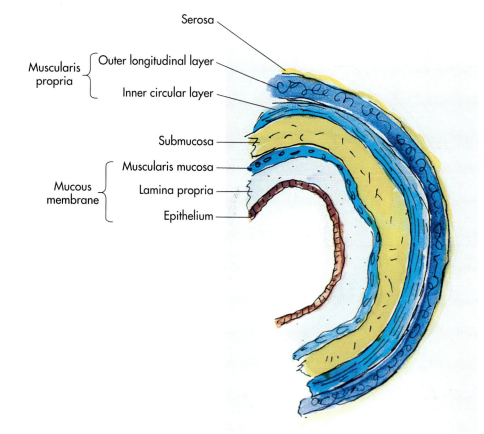

FIG. 8-1. **Schematic depiction of the histologic layers of the gut wall.**

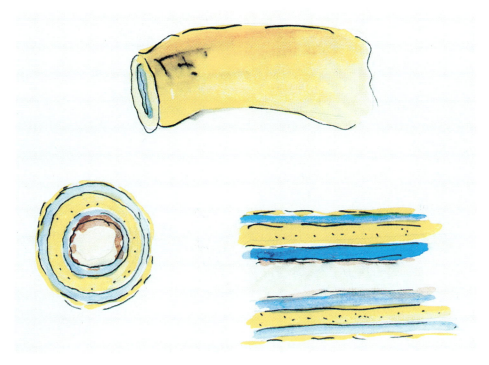

FIG. 8-2. **Gut signature, schematic.** Top figure is a loop of gut. Bottom left is a cross-sectional and bottom right a longitudinal representation of the five layers seen on a sonographic image. Blue layers—hypoechoic. Yellow and pink layers—hyperechoic.

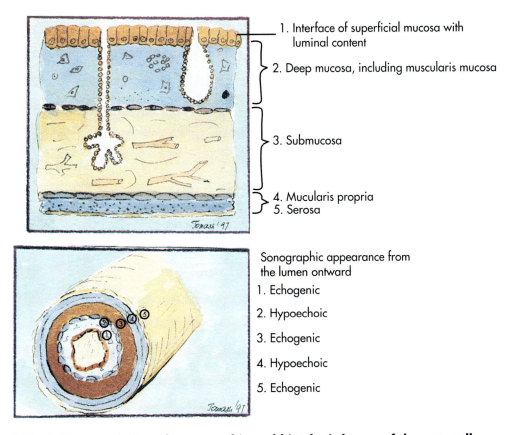

1. Interface of superficial mucosa with luminal content

2. Deep mucosa, including muscularis mucosa

3. Submucosa

4. Mucularis propria
5. Serosa

Sonographic appearance from the lumen ontward

1. Echogenic

2. Hypoechoic

3. Echogenic

4. Hypoechoic

5. Echogenic

FIG. 8-3. **Correlation of sonographic and histologic layers of the gut wall.**
Top schematic shows histologic layers of the gut wall which correspond with the sonographic layering. **Bottom** schematic shows gut in cross section with documented layer echogenicity as it relates to the histologic image shown above.

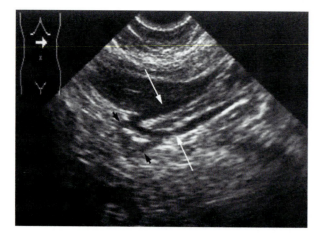

FIG. 8-4. Normal gut signature. Transverse sonogram in epigastrium shows normal gastric antrum (*white arrows*), pylorus, and duodenal bulb (*black arrows*) with depiction of a normal gut signature with five sonographic layers. The submucosa is the thickest echogenic layer surrounded by the hypoechoic muscularis propria.

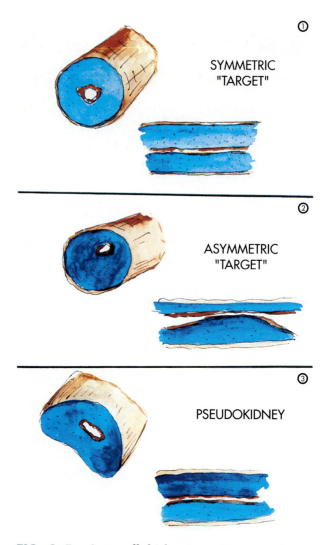

FIG. 8-5. Gut wall thickening. Schematic of sonographic appearances. 1 and 2—"target sign" with 1, symmetric, and 2, asymmetric wall involvement. 3—"Pseudokidney sign."

tion of the transducer determine the degree of layer differentiation. The normal gut wall is uniform and compliant, with an average thickness of 3 mm if distended and 5 mm if not.

The **content** and **diameter** of the gastrointestinal lumen and the **motor activity** of the gut are also assessed. Hypersecretion, mechanical obstruction, and ileus are implicated when gut fluid is excessive. Peristalsis is normally seen in the small bowel and stomach. Activity may be increased with mechanical obstruction and with some inflammatory enteritides. Decreased activity is seen with paralytic ileus.

Gut Wall Pathology

Gut wall pathology creates characteristic sonographic patterns. The most familiar, the **"target" pattern** (Fig. 8-5), was first described by Lutz and Petzoldt[4] in 1976 and later by Bluth et al.[5] who referred to the pattern as a **"pseudokidney"** (Fig. 8-5), noting that a pathologically significant lesion was found in more than 90% of patients with this pattern. In both descriptions, the hypoechoic external rim corresponds to **thickened gut wall**, whereas the echogenic center relates to residual gut lumen or mucosal ulceration (Fig. 8-6). The target and pseudokidney are the abnormal equivalents of the gut signature created by normal gut.

Gut wall masses, as distinct from thickened gut wall, may be intraluminal, mural, or exophytic, all with or without ulceration (Fig. 8-7). Intraluminal gut masses and mucosal masses may have a variable appearance on sonography (Fig. 8-8) but are frequently hidden by gas or luminal content. In contrast, gut pathology creating an **exophytic mass** without (Fig. 8-9) or with (Fig. 8-10) mucosal involvement or ul-

ceration may form masses that are more readily visualized. They may be difficult to assign to a gastrointestinal tract origin if typical gut signatures, targets, or pseudokidneys are not seen on sonography. Consequently, intraperitoneal masses of varying morphology, which do not clearly arise from the solid abdominal viscera or the lymph nodes, should be considered to have a potential gut origin (Fig. 8-11).

Technique

Routine sonograms are best performed when the patient has fasted. A real-time survey of the entire abdomen is performed with a 3.5- and/or a 5-MHz transducer in which any obvious masses or gut signatures are observed. The pelvis is scanned before and after the bladder is emptied because the full bladder

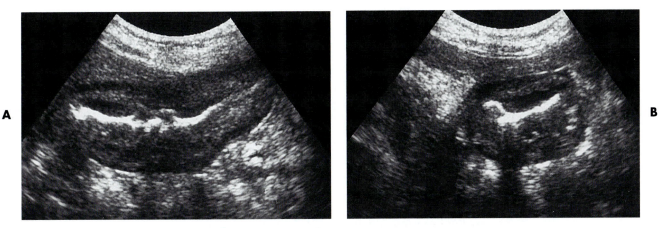

FIG. 8-6. Pseudokidney morphology of gut thickening in a patient with linitis plastica of the stomach. A, Long axis and B, transverse images of the stomach show a hypoechoic rim, representing the tumor, surrounding an echogenic center, representing the residual mucosa and luminal content.

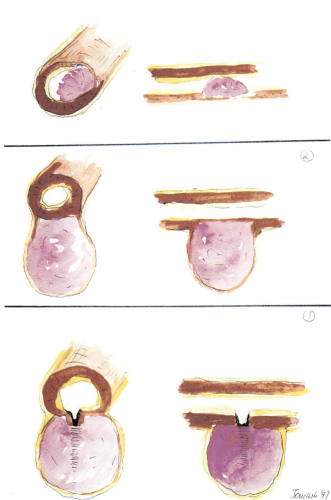

FIG. 8-7. Focal gut wall masses. Schematic depiction shows: 1. Intraluminal mass, 2. Exophytic mass, 3. Exophytic and ulcerated mass. Type 1 may be hidden on sonography by luminal content and gas. This growth pattern may reflect a mucosal or mural origin. Type 2 and 3 are usually mural or serosal in origin. Gas within an ulcer crater will produce characteristic bright echogenicity with ringdown on sonographic images.

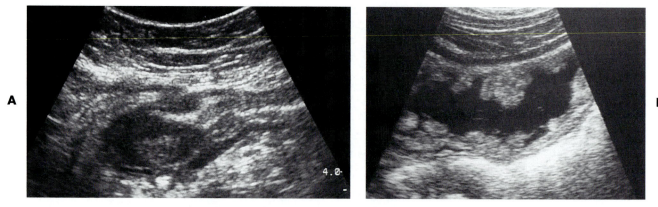

FIG. 8-8. **Intraluminal masses in two different patients**—analogous to #1 in Fig. 8-7. **A,** Polypoid intraluminal carcinoma of cecum. Transverse sonogram of right lower quadrant shows the normal terminal ileum at the ileocecal valve. The cecum shows a solid hypoechoic intraluminal mass. (From Wilson SR: Gastrointestinal tract sonography. *Abdom Imaging* 1996;21:1-8) **B,** Jejunal postinflammatory polyps, Crohn disease. Long axis sonogram in the left upper-quadrant shows segmental dilatation of the gut. The lumen is fluid filled potentiating visualization of multiple polypoid projections arising from both walls of the gut. (From Sarrazin J, Wilson, SR: Manifestations of Crohn disease at US. *RadioGraphics* 1996;16:499-520.)

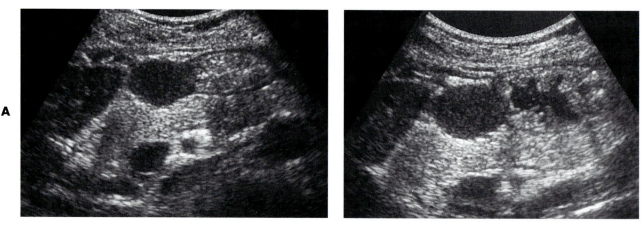

FIG. 8-9. **Exophytic gut mass**—analogous to #2 from Fig. 8-7. A gastric leiomyoma. **A,** Transverse sonogram of epigastrium shows the normal gastric gut signature and the focal exophytic mass. **B,** Following water ingestion, the lumen contains fluid which appears black. The solid mass is now clearly seen to be related to the outer hypoechoic layer of the gastric wall, the muscularis propria.

facilitates visualization of pathologic conditions in some patients and displaces abdominal bowel loops in others. Areas of interest then receive detailed analysis, including **compression sonography.**[6,7] Although this technique was initially described using high-frequency linear probes, 5-MHz convex linear and some sector probes work extremely well. The critical factor is a transducer with a short focal zone allowing optimal resolution of structures close to the skin. Slow graded pressure is applied. Normal gut will be compressed, and gas pockets displaced away from the region of interest. In contrast, thickened abnormal loops of bowel and/or obstructed noncom-

pressible loops will remain unchanged (Fig. 8-12). Patients with peritoneal irritation or local tenderness will usually tolerate the slow gentle increase in pressure of compression sonography, whereas they show a marked painful response if rapid uneven scanning is performed.

On occasion, oral fluid or a fluid enema may be helpful aids to sonography, particularly when one is attempting to determine the origin of a documented fluid collection or to confidently establish the gastric origin of intraluminal or intramural gastric masses.

Doppler evaluation of the gut wall. Doppler used as a tool to differentiate inflammatory from is-

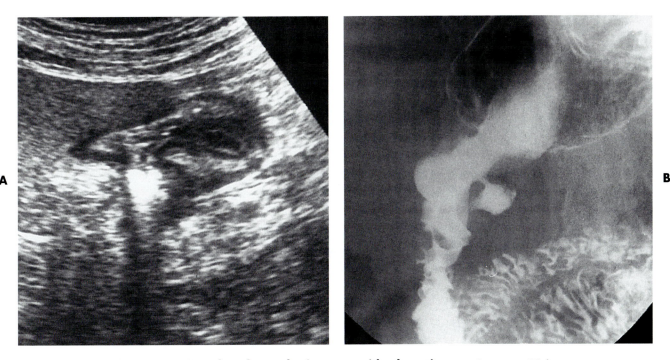

FIG. 8-10. **Mural and exophytic mass with ulceration**—analogous to #3 from Figure 8-7. Peptic ulcer, gastric antrum. **A,** sonogram shows the normal gastric gut signature. A bright echogenic focus with dirty shadowing represents gas in the ulcer crater. A hypoechoic soft tissue mass surrounding the gas is the ulcer mound. **B,** Confirmatory barium swallow. The presence of gas on a sonogram may be helpful in localizating a mass to a gut origin or, as here, the artifact from the gas may hide all or part of the associated mass.

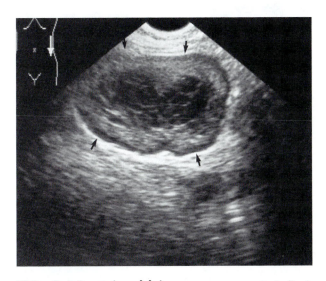

FIG. 8-11. **Jejunal leiomyosarcoma.** Left flank sagittal sonogram shows a well-defined mass (*arrows*) with solid rim and nonuniform cystic center consistent with necrosis. The gut origin of this mass was not definite on the sonogram.

chemic gut wall thickening is a relatively recent advancement which requires sophisticated high-quality Doppler capability.[8] Teefey et al.[8] examined 35 patients and found absence or barely visible blood flow on color Doppler and absence of arterial signal to be

suggestive of ischemia. In contrast, readily detected color Doppler flow and a resistance index less than 0.6 were consistent with inflammation. In our own experience, we have found color Doppler to be of particular additional value in differentiating thick inflamed gut from gut adjacent to an inflammatory focus with sympathetic wall thickening and in confirming our suspicion of an inflammatory gut process (Fig. 8-13).

GASTROINTESTINAL TRACT NEOPLASMS

The role of sonography in the evaluation of gastrointestinal tract neoplasms is similar to that of computed tomography (CT) scan. Visualization is rarely obtained in early mucosal lesions or with small intramural nodules, whereas tumors growing to produce an exophytic mass, a thickened segment of gut with or without ulceration, or a sizable intraluminal mass may all be seen. Sonograms are frequently performed early in the diagnostic work-up of patients with gastrointestinal tract tumors, often before their initial identification. Vague abdominal symptomatology, abdominal pain, a palpable abdominal mass, and anemia are common indications for these scans. Appreciation of the typical morphologies associated with gastrointestinal tract neoplasia may lead to accurate recognition, localization, and even staging of

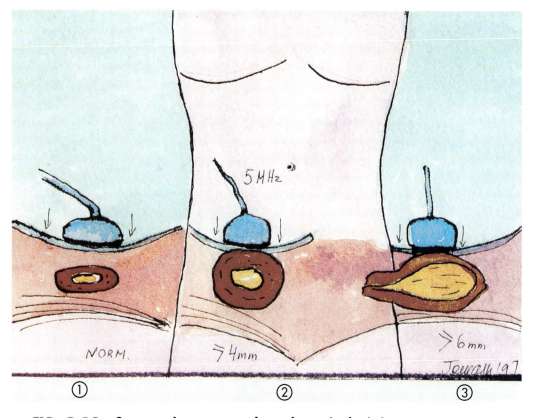

FIG. 8-12. Compression sonography, schematic depiction. 1, Normal gut is compressed. **2,** Abnormally thickened gut or, **3,** an obstructed loop such as that seen in acute appendicitis will be noncompressible. (Modified from Puylaert JBCM: Acute appendicitis: Ultrasound evaluation using graded compression. *Radiology* 1986;158:355-360.)

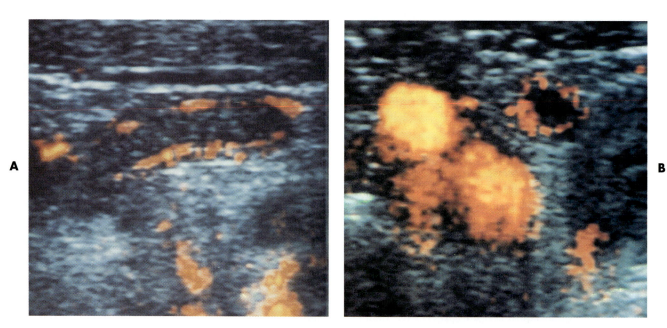

FIG. 8-13. Contribution of Doppler to gut assessment. A, Long axis and **B,** transverse power Doppler images of an inflamed appendix show extensive mural blood flow not seen in noninflamed or normal gut.

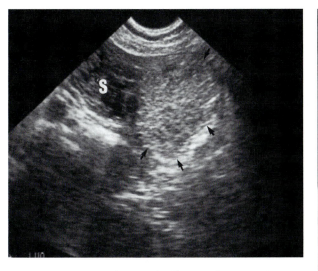

FIG. 8-14. Intraluminal villous adenocarcinoma of the stomach. A, Transverse sonogram following oral fluid ingestion shows a relatively well-defined, nonhomogeneous, echogenic mass (*arrows*) within the body of the stomach. Fluid is in the stomach lumen (S). **B,** Confirmatory barium swallow shows the villous tumor (*arrows*).

disease with the opportunity for directing appropriate further investigation, including sonography-guided aspiration biopsy.

Adenocarcinoma

Pathology. Adenocarcinoma is the most common malignant tumor of the gastrointestinal tract. It accounts for 80% of all malignant gastric neoplasms. These tumors arise most commonly in the prepyloric region, the antrum and the lesser curve, which are the most optimally assessed portions of the stomach on sonography. Grossly their growth patterns are polypoid, fungating, ulcerated, and infiltrative. Infiltration may be superficial or transmural, the latter creating a linitis plastica or a "leather bottle" stomach.

Adenocarcinoma is much less frequent in the small bowel than in either the stomach or the large bowel. It accounts for approximately 50% of the tumors found in this region, 90% of them arising in either the proximal jejunum or the duodenum.[9] Crohn disease is associated with a significantly increased incidence of adenocarcinoma that usually develops in the ileum. Small bowel adenocarcinomas are generally annular in gross morphology, frequently with ulceration.

Colon carcinoma is very common, its incidence surpassed only by lung and breast cancer. Colon carcinoma accounts for virtually all malignant colorectal neoplasms. Colorectal adenocarcinoma grows with two major gross morphologic patterns: polypoid intraluminal tumors, which are most prevalent in the cecum and ascending colon, and annular constricting lesions, which are most common in the descending and sigmoid colon.

Sonography of Adenocarcinoma. Most GI tract mucosal cancers are not visualized on sonography; however, large masses, either intraluminal (Figs. 8-14 and 8-8) or exophytic, and annular tumors (Fig. 8-15) create sonographic abnormalities.[10,11] Tumors of variable length may thicken the gut wall in either a concentric symmetric or an asymmetric pattern. A target (Fig. 8-16) or pseudokidney (Fig. 8-6) morphology may be created. Air in mucosal ulcerations typically produces linear echogenic foci, often with ring-down artifact, within the bulk of the mass. Tumors are usually, but not invariably, hypoechoic. Annular lesions may produce gut obstruction with dilatation, hyperperistalsis, and increased luminal fluid of the gut proximal to the tumor site.[11] Evidence of direct invasion, regional lymph node enlargement, and liver metastases should be specifically sought in all cases.

Mesenchymal Tumors

Pathology. Of the mesenchymal tumors affecting the gut, those of smooth muscle origin are the most common and account for about 1% of all gastrointestinal tract neoplasms. Although they may be found as an incidental observation at surgery, sonography, or autopsy, these vascular tumors frequently become very large and may undergo ulceration, degeneration, necrosis, and hemorrhage.[12]

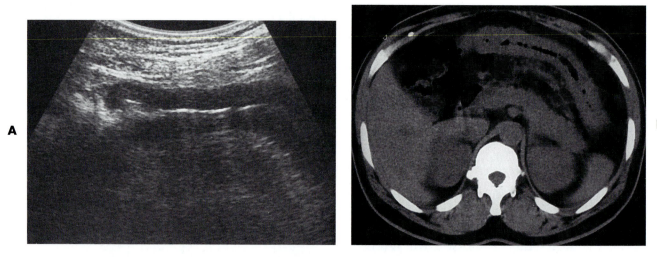

FIG. 8-15. **Infiltrative carcinoma of the transverse colon in a 42-year-old black man who presented to the emergency room with acute abdominal pain. A,** Transverse view of the epigastrium shows a featureless segment of thick gut with total loss of wall layering in the location of the transverse colon. Deep to the gut is a diffuse echogenic "mass effect" suggesting infiltrated or inflamed fat. **B,** Confirmatory computed tomography scan. Neoplasia was not suspected on the basis of either imaging test or at surgery.

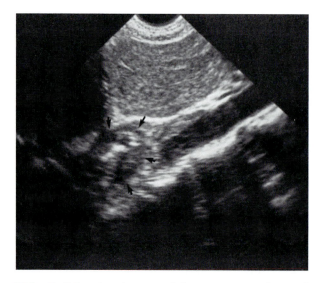

FIG. 8-16. **Carcinoma of the gastroesophageal junction.** Sagittal sonogram in the left paramedian area shows target pattern (*arrows*).

Sonography of Smooth Muscle Tumors.

Smooth muscle tumors typically produce round mass lesions of varying size and echogenicity often with central cystic areas (Fig. 8-17).[13] Their gut origin is not always easily determined but if ulceration is present, pockets of gas in an ulcer crater may suggest the presence of tumors. Smooth muscle tumors of gut origin should be considered in the differential diagnosis of incidentally noted, indeterminate abdominal masses in asymptomatic patients. These tumors are very amenable to sonographic-guided aspiration biopsy.

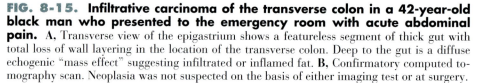

GROWTH PATTERNS OF LYMPHOMA

Nodular or polypoid
Carcinoma-like ulcerative lesions
Infiltrating tumor masses
    Invade the adjacent mesentery and lymph nodes

Lymphoma

Pathology. The gut may be involved with lymphoma in two basic forms: as widespread dissemination in stage III or IV lymphoma of any cell type or, more commonly, as primary lymphoma of the GI tract, which is virtually always a non-Hodgkin lymphoma. Primary tumors constitute only 2% to 4% of all GI tract malignant tumors[14] but account for 20% of those found in the small bowel. Three predominant **growth patterns** are observed: nodular or polypoid, carcinoma-like ulcerative lesions, infiltrating tumor masses that frequently invade the adjacent mesentery and lymph nodes.[9]

Sonography of Lymphoma. Although small submucosal nodules may be easily overlooked, many affected patients have large, very hypoechoic, ulcerated masses in the stomach or small bowel (Fig. 8-18).[15,16] Long, linear, high-amplitude echoes with ring-down artifacts, indicating gas in the residual lumen or ulcerations, are frequently seen. This particular pathology has been recognized as one of the more frequent presentations of patients with AIDS–related lymphoma as compared with other lymphoma popu-

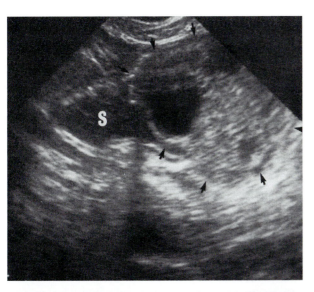

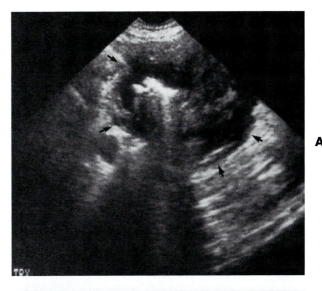

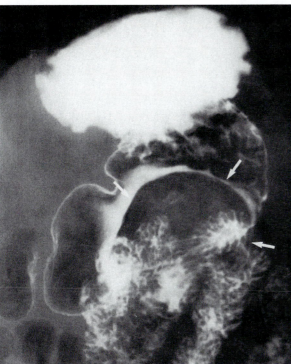

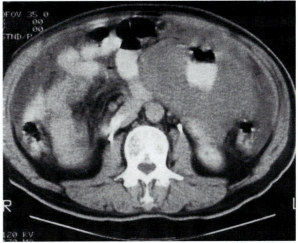

FIG. 8-18. Small bowel lymphoma. A, Transverse left paramedian sonogram shows hypoechoic round mass lesion (*arrows*). Central echogenicity with ring-down gas artifact suggests gut origin. **B,** Confirmatory computed tomography scan shows large soft tissue mass with corresponding residual gut lumen.

FIG. 8-17. Gastric leiomyosarcoma. A, Transverse sonogram following oral ingestion of fluid shows a complex intramural mass (*arrows*) projecting into the fluid-filled stomach lumen (S). **B,** Confirmatory barium swallow shows the intramural tumor (*arrows*).

lations (Fig. 8-19). Regional lymph node enlargement may be visualized, although generalized lymph node abnormality is uncommon.

Metastatic Tumors

Malignant melanoma and primary tumors of the lung and breast are the tumors most likely to have secondary involvement of the GI tract.[17] In order of fre-

quency, the stomach, small bowel, and colon are involved. Small submucosal nodules, with a tendency to ulcerate, are rarely seen on sonography. However, large diffusely infiltrative tumors with large ulcerations are common, particularly in the small bowel (Fig. 8-20), where they create hypoechoic well-defined masses that often have bright, specular echoes with ring-down artifacts in areas of ulceration.

Secondary neoplasm affecting the omentum and peritoneum may cause ascites, tiny or confluent superficial secondary nodules on the gut surface (Fig. 8-21), or extensive omental cakes that virtually engulf the involved gut loops.[18,19] Metastases to the peritoneum most commonly arise from primary tumors in the ovary or the gut.

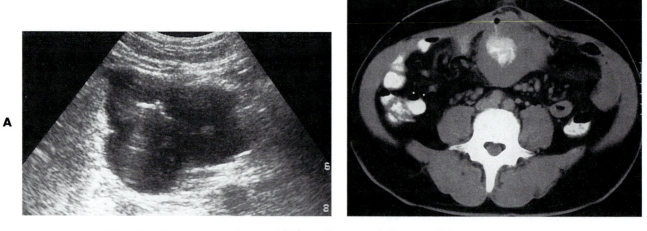

FIG. 8-19. AIDS patient with lymphoma of the small bowel. A, Sonogram shows a focal mid-abdominal very hypoechoic (*black*) mass with no wall layer definition, classic for gut lymphoma. The luminal gas appears as central bright echogenicity with dirty shadowing. **B,** Confirmatory computed tomography scan.

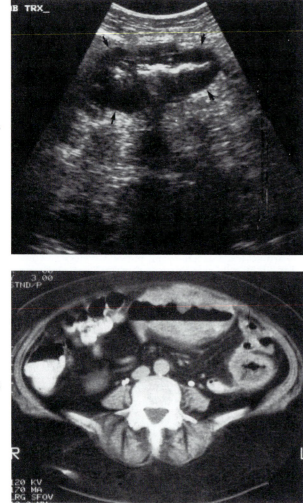

FIG. 8-20. Metastatic malignant melanoma to small bowel. A, Transverse paraumbilical sonogram shows well-defined, hypoechoic mass (*arrows*) with central irregular echogenicity with gas artifact suggesting gut origin. **B,** Confirmatory computed tomography scan.

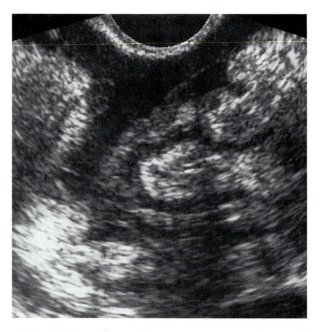

FIG. 8-21. Visceral gut metastases in peritoneal carcinomatosis from ovarian carcinoma. Transvaginal sonogram shows ascites. There is a hypoechoic nodular rim of tissue encasing adjacent loops of gut.

INFLAMMATORY BOWEL DISEASE

Inflammatory bowel disease includes Crohn disease and ulcerative colitis. Although barium study and endoscopy remain the major tools to evaluate mucosal and luminal abnormality, sonography, like CT, may offer valuable additional information about the gut wall, the lymph nodes, the mesentery, and the regional soft tissues.[20] The chronic nature of inflammatory bowel disease, characterized by multiple remissions and exacerbations, is well assessed by a noninvasive,

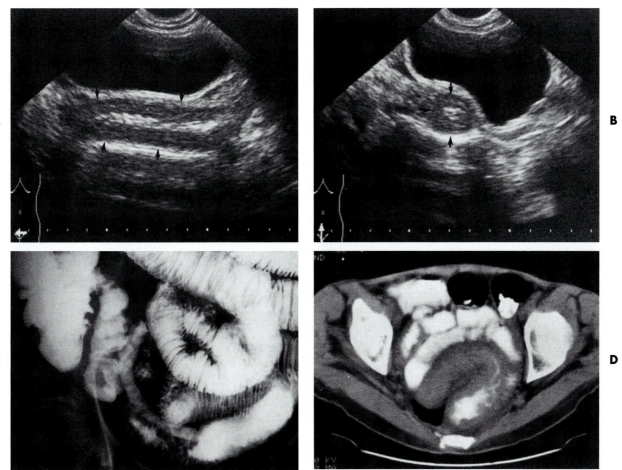

FIG. 8-22. **Crohn disease of ileum.** **A,** Long axis, and **B,** short axis sonograms of a diffusely thickened loop of gut (*arrows*) with narrowing of the central echogenic lumen. **C,** Confirmatory small bowel enema. **D,** Confirmatory computed tomography scan.

sensitive modality such as sonography. The degree of thickening of the gut wall and the frequent association of extraluminal disease make Crohn disease the most optimally studied disorder. Baseline examination with follow-up predicts complications such as abscess, fistula, or obstruction; detects postoperative recurrence; and identifies patients who require more invasive imaging techniques.[21]

Crohn Disease

Pathology. Crohn disease, a chronic inflammatory disorder of the GI tract of unknown pathogenesis and etiology, most commonly affects the terminal ileum and the colon although any portion of the gut may be involved. It is a transmural granulomatous inflammatory process affecting all layers of the gut wall. Grossly, the gut wall is typically very thick and rigid with secondary luminal narrowing. Discrete or continuous ulcers and deep fissures are characteristic, frequently leading to fistula formation. Mesenteric lymph node enlargement and matting of involved loops are common. The mesentery may be markedly

thickened and fatty, creeping over the edges of the gut to the antimesenteric border. Recurrence after surgery, skip lesions, and perianal disease are classic features.

Sonography of Crohn Disease. Sonography may be used in patients with Crohn disease to document the **classic features** including gut wall thickening, strictures, creeping fat, hyperemia, mesenteric lymphadenopathy, and uncommonly mucosal abnormalities or **complications** including inflammatory masses (phlegmon or abscess), fistula, obstruction, perforation or appendicitis.[21]

Detect thickened loops of gut (Fig. 8-22). This may be appropriate for initial detection, for detection of recurrence,[22] for determining the extent of disease, and in follow-up in the assessment of improvement. Gut wall thickening is most frequently concentric and may be quite marked.[23,24] Wall echogenicity varies depending on the degree of inflammatory infiltration and fibrosis. Stratification with retention of the gut layers may occur, or a target or pseudokidney appearance is possible. Involved gut appears rigid and fixed with no visible peristalsis.

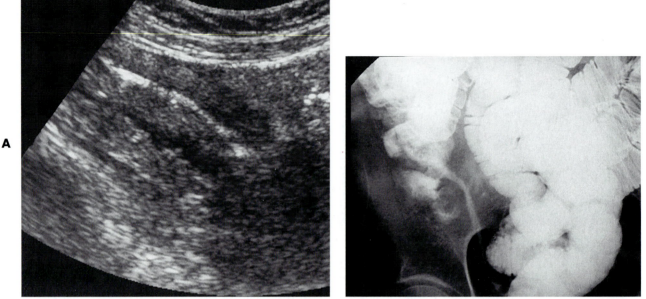

FIG. 8-23. Acute Crohn disease of ileum. A, Sagittal sonogram shows a loop of very thick gut. The wall layers are not defined. The luminal surfaces, seen as a central echogenic line, are in apposition. **B,** Small bowel enema confirms a long tight stricture in left lower quadrant.

SONOGRAPHIC FEATURES OF CROHN DISEASE

Classic features
Gut wall thickening
Strictures
Creeping fat
Hyperemia
Mesenteric lymphadenopathy
Mucosal abnormalities

Complications
Inflammatory masses
Fistula
Obstruction
Perforation
Appendicitis

Skip areas are frequent. Involved segments vary in length from a few millimeters to several centimeters.

Assess strictures. The caliber of the lumen and the length of involved segments are readily assessed; the lumen appears as a linear echogenic central area within a thickened gut loop (Fig. 8-23). Peristaltic waves from the obstructed gut, proximal to a narrowed segment, may produce visible movement through the strictured segment. Incomplete mechanical obstruction is inferred if dilated hyperperistaltic segments are seen proximal to a stricture. Involved segments of gut may show luminal dilatation with sacculation as well as narrowing (Fig. 8-24).

Detect creeping fat. Edema and fibrosis of the adjacent mesentery produce a mass in the mesentery adjacent to the diseased gut which may "creep" over the border of the abnormal gut or completely engulf it. The sonographic appearance is that of a hyperechoic "mass effect" which is most prominent medial and cephalad to the ileocecal valve in the expected location of the small bowel mesentery. Mesenteric fat creeping onto the margins of the involved gut creates a uniform echogenic halo around the mesenteric border of the gut with a "thyroidlike" appearance in cross-section (Fig. 8-25). It may become more heterogeneous and even hypoechoic in long-standing disease. Creeping fat is the most common cause found to explain gut loop separation as seen on contrast GI studies.[21] It is also the most striking and easy to detect abnormality on sonography of patients with perienteric inflammatory processes. Its detection should provoke the examiner to perform a detailed evaluation of the regional gut.

Assess hyperemia. Although subjective, the addition of color Doppler to gray-scale sonography is valuable supportive evidence of inflammatory change in the gut (Fig. 8-26) and adjacent inflamed fat (Fig. 8-27).[21]

Characterize conglomerate masses. These may have clumps of matted bowel, inflamed edematous mesentery, increased fat deposition in the mesentery, and uncommonly mesenteric lymphadenopathy (Fig. 8-28). Involved loops may demonstrate angulation and

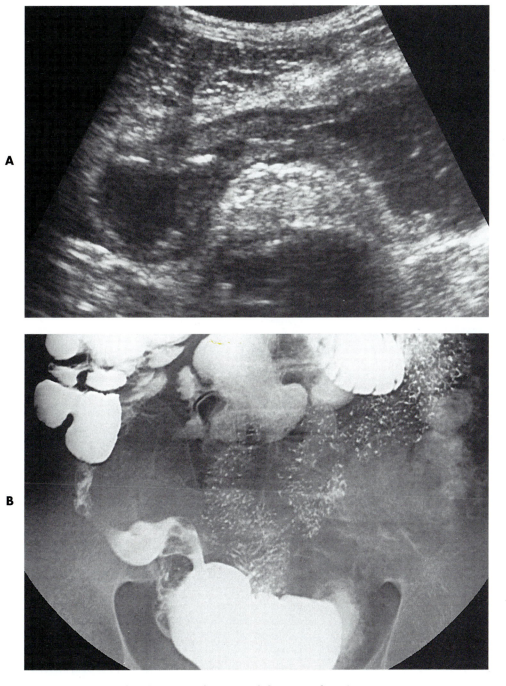

FIG. 8-24. **Crohn disease of terminal ileum with stricture.** A, Transverse sonogram shows two dilated fluid filled segments of gut, on the right and left of the image, separated by a segment of thick walled gut with a narrowed lumen. **B,** Small bowel follow through confirms stricture with sacculations.

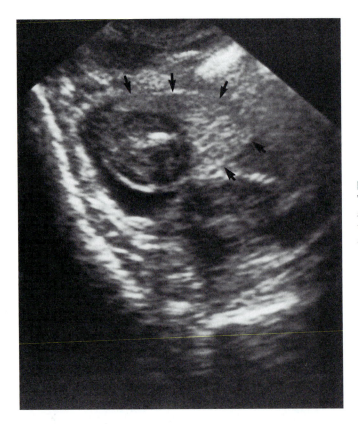

FIG. 8-25. Crohn disease—creeping fat. Transverse sonogram of thickened ascending colon shows fat (*arrows*) creeping onto the gut from the mesenteric margin. It produces a "thyroidlike" echogenic halo along the anteromedial aspect of the loop of gut.

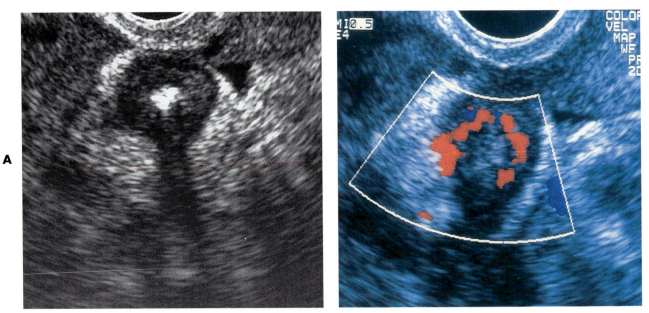

FIG. 8-26. Crohn disease—hyperemia of actively inflamed gut. A. Cross-sectional sonogram shows thickening of the wall of the terminal ileum with abundant vascularity. **B.** Corresponding color Doppler image shows thickening of the wall of the terminal ileum with abundant vascularity. (From Sarrazin J, Wilson SR: Manifestations of Crohn disease at US. *RadioGraphics* 1996;16:499-520.)

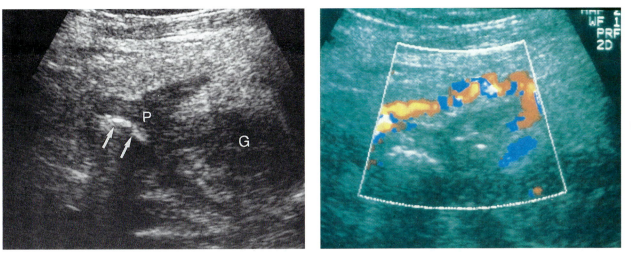

FIG. 8-27. Crohn disease—hyperemic extraintestinal inflammatory mass.
A, Long axis sonogram of the right lower quadrant shows an ill-defined phlegmon (P) with an extraintestinal focus of gas which is seen as a bright echogenic area (*arrows*). The inflamed adjacent fat produces a uniformly echogenic surrounding "mass effect." Gut (G). **B,** Color Doppler shows abundant vascularity of the inflamed fatty tissues surrounding the phlegmon. (From Sarrazin J, Wilson SR: Manifestations of Crohn disease at US. *RadioGraphics* 1996;16:499-520.)

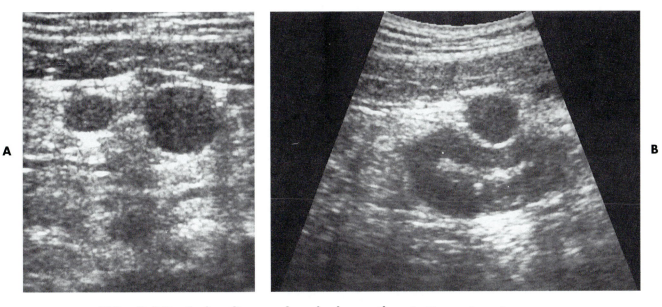

FIG. 8-28. Crohn disease—lymphadenopathy. A, Mesenteric nodes are most commonly shown as hypoechoic round or oval masses of varying size in the region of the mesentery of the involved gut. Linear array transducers are optimal. **B,** Occasionally, as in this case, large nodes may be seen closely juxtaposed to the pathological gut.

fixation resulting from retraction of the thickened fibrotic mesentery.

Identify inflammatory masses or abscesses.
Abscesses are a frequent complication of Crohn disease, producing complex or fluid-filled masses (Fig. 8-29). Gas content within an abscess is both helpful in raising suspicion of an abscess (Fig. 8-30) and also a potential source of sonographic error, particularly if

large quantities are present. Abscesses may be intraperitoneal or extraperitoneal (Fig. 8-31) or may be in remote locations such as the liver. Prior to the stage of liquefaction, phlegmonous change may be noted as ill defined hypoechoic zones without fluid content within areas of inflamed fat (Fig. 8-32).

Assess fistula formation. Although mucosal ulcerations are not well assessed on sonography, deep

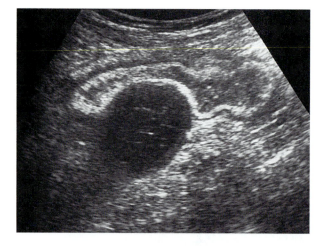

FIG. 8-29. Crohn ileitis—interloop abscess. A strandy well-defined fluid collection to a loop of mildly thickened gut.

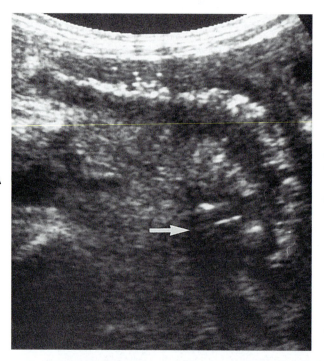

A

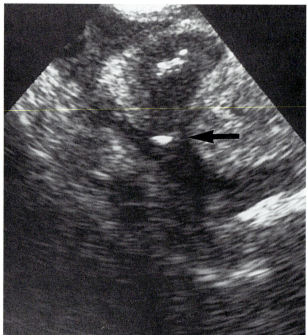

B

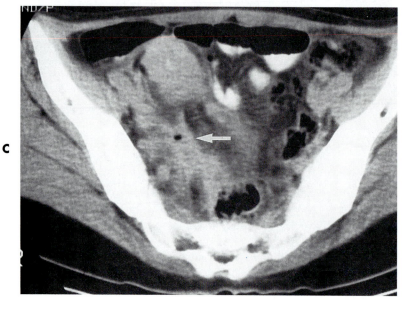

C

FIG. 8-30. Crohn disease—abscess. A, Longitudinal sonogram through the terminal ileum shows thickening of the gut, echogenic inflamed fat and a poorly defined focal hypoechoic area deep to the gut (*arrow*). Bubbles of gas outside of the gut are seen as bright echogenic foci. B, Cross-sectional sonogram through the terminal ileum shows thickening of the gut, echogenic inflamed fat and a poorly defined focal hypoechoic area deep to the gut (*arrow*). Bubbles of gas outside of the gut are seen as bright echogenic foci. C, Confirmatory computed tomography scan shows the thickened terminal ileum, inflamed fat and the abscess (*arrow*), with an extraluminal bubble of gas. (From Sarrazin J, Wilson SR: Manifestations of Crohn disease at US. *RadioGraphics* 1996; 16:499-520.)

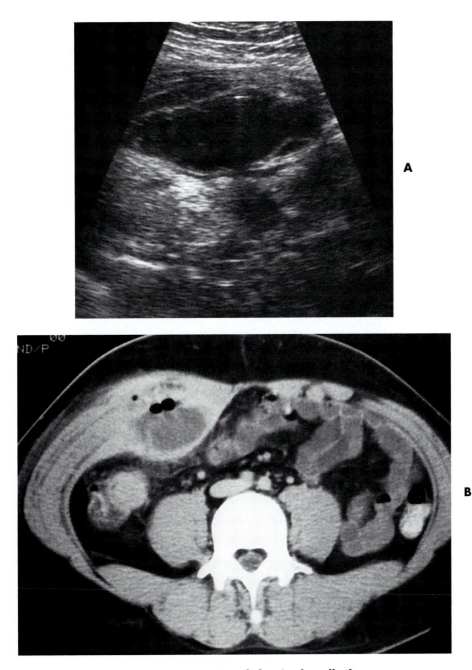

FIG. 8-31. Crohn disease—anterior abdominal wall abscess. A, Transverse sonogram shows a gas containing fluid collection superficial to the parietal peritoneum. **B,** Confirmatory computed tomography scan. (From Sarrazin J, Wilson SR: Manifestations of Crohn disease at US. *RadioGraphics* 1996;16:499-520.)

fissures in the gut wall appear as echogenic linear areas penetrating deeply into the wall beyond the margin of the gut lumen (Fig. 8-33). With fistula formation, linear bands of varying echogenicity can be seen extending from segments of abnormal gut to the skin (Fig. 8-34), bladder (Fig. 8-35), or to other abnormal loops. If there is gas or movement in the fistula during sonographic study, the fistula will usually appear bright or echogenic, with or without ring-down artifact related to the presence of air in the tract. Conversely, if the tract is empty or partially closed it may appear as a black or hypoechoic tract.

Transrectal ultrasound (TRUS) is frequently ordered in patients with rectal Crohn disease or perianal

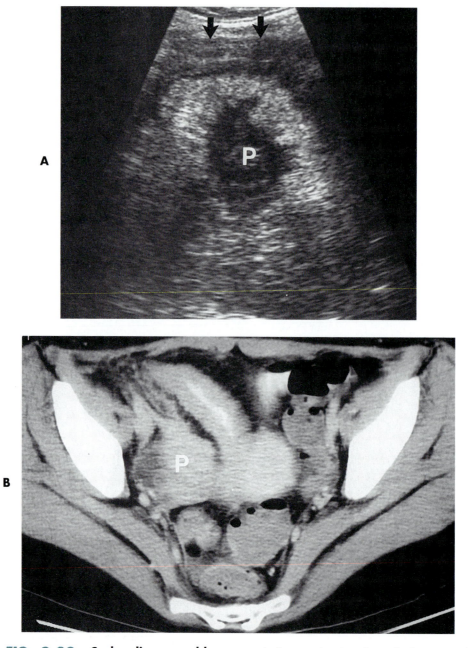

FIG. 8-32. Crohn disease—phlegmon. A, Long axis view through the terminal ileum shows a relatively superficial loop of thickened gut (*arrows*). Deep to the abnormal gut there is inflamed fat seen as a uniformly echogenic "mass effect." Within the inflamed fat there is a phlegmon (P) seen as a serpiginous bordered hypoechoic mass. **B,** Confirmatory computed tomography scan showing the thickened gut and the adjacent inflamed fat and phlegmonous mass. Within the inflamed fat there is a phlegmon (P) seen as a serpiginous bordered hypoechoic mass. (From Sarrazin J, Wilson SR: Manifestations of Crohn disease at US. *RadioGraphics* 1996;16:499-520.)

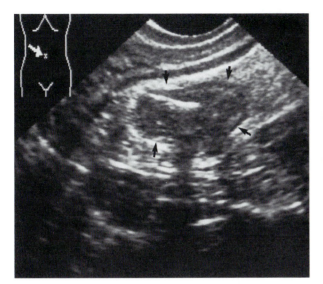

FIG. 8-33. Crohn disease—deep fissure.
Transverse sonogram of ascending colon (*arrows*) shows deep fissure, seen as an echogenic linear line, extending from the gut lumen to the serosa of the involved segment.

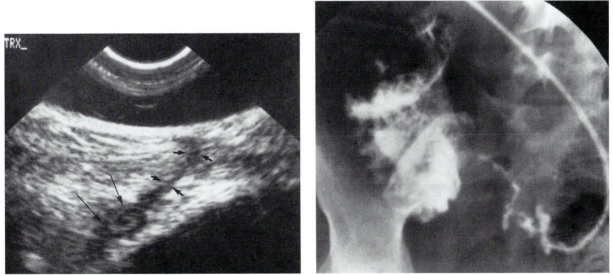

FIG. 8-34. Crohn disease—fistula to skin. A, Sonogram shows a mildly thickened loop of gut (*long arrows*) communicating with the skin by a faint linear hypoechoic fistulous tract (*short arrows*). Image has been taken with a small stand-off pad to place the fistula within the focal zone of the transducer. **B,** Confirmatory sinogram.

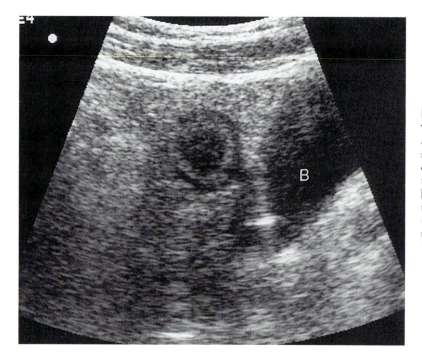

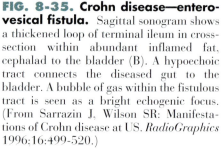

FIG. 8-35. Crohn disease—enterovesical fistula. Sagittal sonogram shows a thickened loop of terminal ileum in cross-section within abundant inflamed fat, cephalad to the bladder (B). A hypoechoic tract connects the diseased gut to the bladder. A bubble of gas within the fistulous tract is seen as a bright echogenic focus. (From Sarrazin J, Wilson SR: Manifestations of Crohn disease at US. *RadioGraphics* 1996;16:499-520.)

pathology and may successfully show regional abscesses and fistulous tracts. However, we have not had uniform success with this procedure which is often painful and noncontributory in this particular population. In contrast, in patients of either gender, we have found **transperineal** scanning to be a more comfortable and often more informative technique used alone or in combination with transrectal ultrasound (Fig. 8-36). Further, in women, we have found **transvaginal** scan to contribute greatly to our assessment of rectal (Fig. 8-37) and perirectal disease. It is also ideal for showing enterovesicle (Fig. 8-38), enterovaginal and rectovaginal fistulas.[25]

If bladder symptoms are present, we recommend transvaginal sonography be performed with a partially full bladder. Further, the probe should be fully inserted and slowly withdrawn while elevating the examining hand to allow for evaluation of the entire rectum and anal canal in both sagittal and transverse planes (Fig. 8-37).

ACUTE ABDOMEN

Sonography is a valuable imaging tool in patients who may have specific GI disease such as acute appendicitis or acute diverticulitis; however, its contribution to the assessment of patients with **possible** GI tract disease is less certain. Seibert et al.[26] emphasized its great value in assessing the patient with a distended and gasless abdomen, in detecting ascites, unsuspected masses, and abnormally dilated fluid-filled loops of small

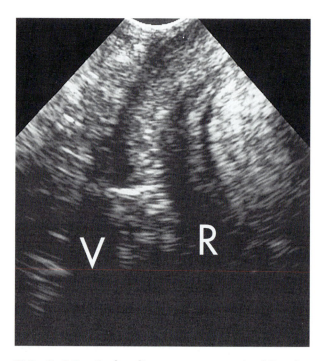

FIG. 8-36. Crohn disease—rectovaginal fistula. Transperineal sagittal scan shows a bright echogenic focus representing gas in a fistulous tract running between the rectum (R) and the vagina (V).

bowel. In my experience, sonography has been helpful not only in the gasless abdomen but also in a wide variety of other situations. Sonography may add greatly to diagnostic acumen if used in conjunction with plain film radiography, CT, and other imaging modalities.

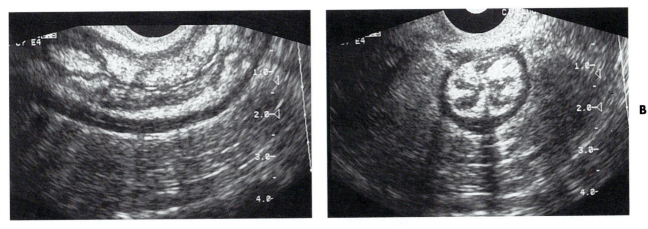

FIG. 8-37. Transvaginal assessment of rectal Crohn disease. Left, long axis and right, cross sectional views of the rectum show circumferential symmetric wall thickening. The mucosal surfaces are in apposition. Wall layering is preserved. (From Damani N, Wilson SR: Nongynocologic findings of transvaginal sonography. Submitted to *RadioGraphics* August 1997.)

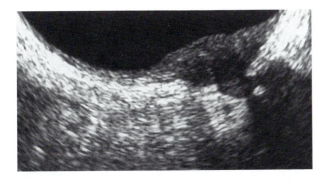

FIG. 8-38. Transvaginal demonstration of an enterovesicle fistula. There is an inflammatory mass involving the bladder wall. The fistulous tract is seen as a black hypoechoic tract with only a single echogenic gas bubble. (From Damani N, Wilson SR: Nongynocologic findings of transvaginal sonography. Submitted to *RadioGraphics* August 1997.)

SONOGRAPHIC APPROACH TO THE PATIENT WITH AN ACUTE ABDOMEN

Gas	Intraluminal	
	Extraluminal	Intraperitoneal
		Retroperitoneal
		Gut wall
		Gallbladder/biliary ducts
		Portal veins
Fluid	Intraluminal	Normal calibre gut
		Dilated gut
	Extraluminal	Free
		Loculated
Masses		Neoplastic
		Inflammatory
Perienteric soft tissues		Inflamed fat
Gut		Wall
		Calibre
		Peristalsis
Clinical interaction		Palpable mass
		Maximal tenderness
		Sonographic Murphy sign
		Sonographic McBurney sign

Similar to the radiographic approach to plain film interpretation, a **systematic approach** is invaluable in the sonographic assessment of the abdomen in a patient with an acute abdomen of uncertain etiology.

Gas within the abdomen should be assessed as to its intraluminal or extraluminal origin. Dirty shadowing or ring-down artifact help identify gas in a site where it is not normally found (Figs. 8-39 and 8-40). **Extraluminal gas** may be intraperitoneal or retroperitoneal and its presence should raise the possibility of either hollow viscus perforation or infection with gas-forming organisms.[27] Nonluminal gas may be easily overlooked, particularly if the collection is large. Gas in the **wall of the GI tract,** pneumatosis intestinalis, with or without gas in the portal veins raises the possibility of ischemic gut. Gas in the **biliary ducts or**

gallbladder may be seen with spontaneous biliary enteric anastomosis or emphysematous cholecystitis.

Free intraperitoneal gas may be difficult to detect on sonography and suspicion of its presence should prompt recommendation for further imaging. The potential for large artifacts from gas to obscure visualization of part or all of a sonographic image leads many to

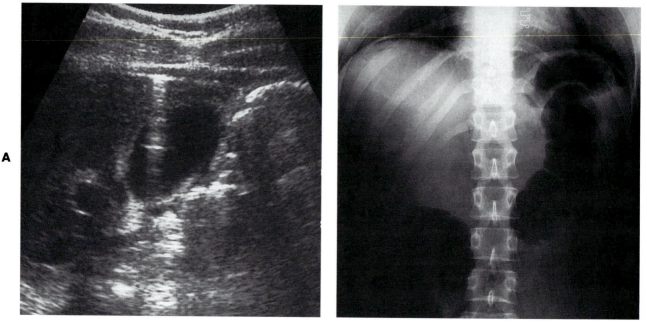

FIG. 8-39. **Pneumoperitoneum.** **A,** Sonogram shows a bright echogenic focus representing free air between the abdominal wall and liver. Also shown is enhancement of the peritoneal stripe (*arrows*). **B,** Confirmatory plain film. (From Muradali D, Burns P, Wilson SR: A specific sign for pneumoperitoneum on sonography: Enhanced peritoneal stripe, Submitted for publication April 1997.)

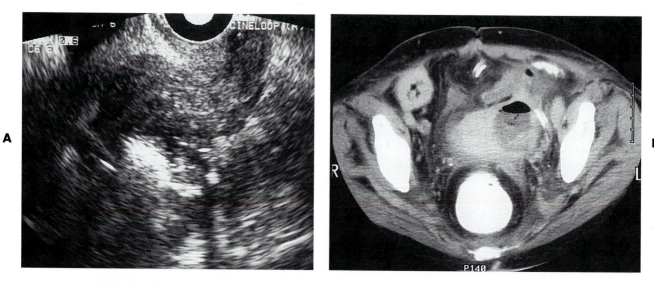

FIG. 8-40. **Unsuspected gas containing abscess secondary to acute diverticulitis in a renal transplant recipient.** **A,** Transvaginal image shows a large gas containing mass posterior to the uterus. **B,** Computed tomography scan confirms gas containing abscess. This kind of abscess may be very difficult to appreciate on suprapubic scan.

avoid the challenge of ultrasound interpretation with a preference for CT scan. However, there are useful clues to the presences of intraperitoneal gas on sonography.

The likelihood of gas artifacts between the abdominal wall and the underlying liver to be related to free intraperitoneal gas was nicely described by Lee, et al.[27] In our own work, we have found that the peritoneal stripe appears as a bright continuous echogenic line and that air adjacent to the peritoneal stripe produces enhancement of this layer as the gas has a higher acoustic impedance to sound waves than does the peritoneum itself (Fig. 8-39). Careful peritoneal

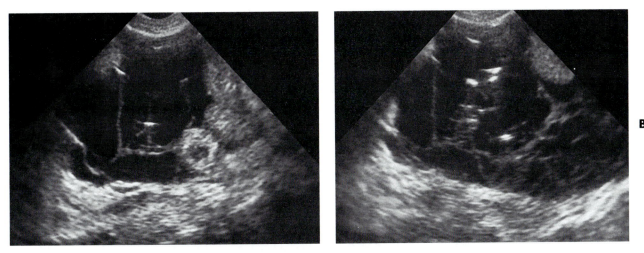

FIG. 8-41. Purulent peritonitis. A. Sagittal and **B.** transverse images of left flank show no normal landmarks. There is gross strandy ascites with acute angles at the margins of the gut. Multiple air bubbles from gas forming organisms show as bright echogenic foci with ring-down artifact.

assessment is best done with a 5- or even 7.5-mHz probe with the focal zone set at the expected level of the peritoneum. In a clinical situation, enhancement of the peritoneal stripe is a highly specific but insensitive sign to detect pneumoperitoneum.[28]

Similarly, **fluid** should be assessed to determine whether it is luminal or extraluminal. Loculated fluid collections can mimic portions of the GI tract. Left upper-quadrant and pelvic collections suggestive of the stomach and rectum may be clarified by adding fluid orally and rectally. Assessing peristaltic activity and wall morphology also help in distinguishing luminal from extraluminal collections. Interloop and flank collections are aperistaltic and tend to correspond in contour to the adjacent abdominal wall or intestinal loops, frequently forming acute angles, which are rarely seen with intraluminal fluid (Fig. 8-41).

The appearance of the **perienteric soft tissues** is frequently the first and most obvious clue to abdominal pathology on abdominal sonograms. Inflammation of the perienteric fat shows as a hyperechoic "mass effect" often with absence of the usual appearance created by normal gut with its contained small pockets of gas. Neoplastic infiltration of the perienteric fat is often indistinguishable from inflammatory infiltration on ultrasound (Fig. 8-15).

The realtime aspect of sonographic study allows for direct interaction of the sonographer/physician with the patient with confirmation of palpable masses and/or focal points of tenderness. This has led sonographers to describe the value of the sonographic equivalent to clinical examination with such descriptors as a **Sonographic Murphy or Sonographic McBurney sign.**

Mesenteric adenopathy is another manifestation of both inflammatory and neoplastic processes of the gut which should be specifically sought when performing abdominal sonography. As elsewhere, lymph nodes tend to change in size and shape when they are replaced by abnormal tissue. A normal oval or flattened lymph node with a normal linear hilar echo becomes increasingly round and hypoechoic with either inflammatory or neoplastic replacement. In contrast to the sonographic appearance of loops of gut, mesenteric lymph nodes typically appear as focal discrete hypoechoic masses of varying size (Fig. 8-42). Their identification on sonography suggests enlargement as they are not normally seen on routine examinations.

Abnormal **masses** related to or causing GI tract abnormality should also be sought. These are most commonly neoplastic or inflammatory in origin.

Acute Appendicitis

Acute appendicitis is the most common cause of the acute abdomen. Although many patients have a classic presentation, allowing prompt diagnosis and treatment, some patients have atypical and frequently confusing presentations, leading to misdiagnoses. This is especially problematic in women of child-bearing age.[29] In the clinical literature, laparotomy resulting in removal of normal, noninflamed appendices is reported in 16% to 47% of cases, mean 26%.[30-32] Equally distressing, perforation may occur in up to 35%.[33]

Current medical practice recognizes the necessity of removing some normal appendices to minimize perforation rates. In 1986, Julien Puylaert described the value of **graded compression sonography** in the

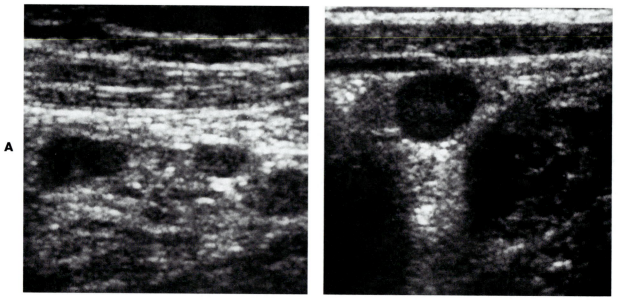

FIG. 8-42. Mesenteric adenopathy in two patients with acute terminal ileitis. A, Three hypoechoic nodes are seen. **B,** A single round hypoechoic node is seen close to a loop of abnormal gut.

evaluation of 60 consecutive patients suspected of having acute appendicitis.[7] Since then, other investigators have improved the sonographic criteria for diagnosis, firmly establishing the value of sonography in assessing patients with equivocal evidence of this disease. The accuracy afforded by sonography should keep negative laparotomy rates at approximately 10%,[34] clearly an improvement over the rate achieved by instinct alone.

Pathology and Clinical Features. The underlying factor in the development of acute appendicitis is believed to be obstruction of the appendiceal lumen, 35% of cases demonstrating a fecalith.[35] Mucosal secretions continue, increasing the intraluminal pressure and compromising venous return. The mucosa becomes hypoxic and ulcerates. Bacterial infection ensues with ultimate gangrene and perforation. Walled-off abscess is more common than free peritoneal contamination.

Acute appendicitis begins with transient, visceral, or referred crampy pain in the periumbilical area associated with nausea and vomiting. Coincident with inflammation of the serosa of the appendix, the pain shifts to the right lower quadrant and may be associated with physical signs of peritoneal irritation.

Both clinical and experimental data support the belief that some patients have repeated attacks of appendicitis.[36,37] Surgical specimens have shown chronic inflammatory infiltrate in patients with recurrent attacks of right lower-quadrant pain before appendectomy.

Sonography. Puylaert's[7] initial reports of success in **diagnosing acute appendicitis** with **compression**

SONOGRAPHIC DIAGNOSIS OF ACUTE APPENDICITIS

Patient with right lower-quadrant pain/ elevated white blood cell count

Identify appendix
Blind ended
Aperistaltic tube
Gut signature
Arising from base of cecum
Diameter greater than 6 mm

Supportive features
Inflamed perienteric fat
Pericecal collections
Appendicolith

sonography depended solely on visualization of the appendix: a blind-ended, aperistaltic tube, arising from the tip of the cecum with a gut signature (Fig. 8-43). However, other investigators have reported seeing normal appendices on a sonogram.[38,39] The normal appendix is compressible with wall thickness of less than or equal to 3 mm.[40] Jeffrey[39] and his colleagues concluded that the size of an appendix can differentiate normal from acutely inflamed. Sonographic visualization of an appendix with a total diameter greater than 6 mm (Fig. 8-44) in an adult patient with right lower-quadrant pain is highly suggestive of acute appendicitis. Sonographic visualization of an appendix with

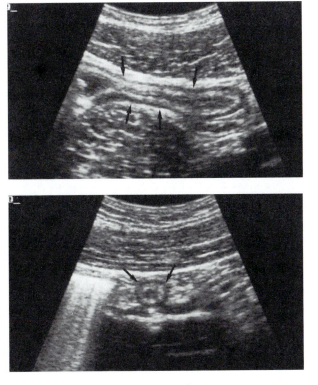

FIG. 8-43. Normal appendix. A, Long axis, and B, short axis sonograms of a normal appendix (*arrows*) show a normal gut signature and a diameter less than 6 mm.

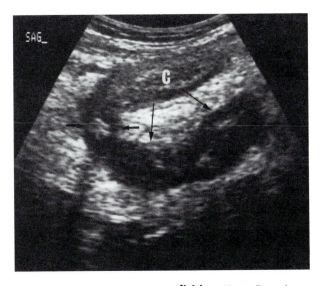

FIG. 8-44. Acute appendicitis. The inflamed appendix (*long arrows*) is seen as a blind-ended, aperistaltic, noncompressible tubular structure, arising from the cecum (C). A faintly shadowing appendicolith (*small arrows*) is seen.

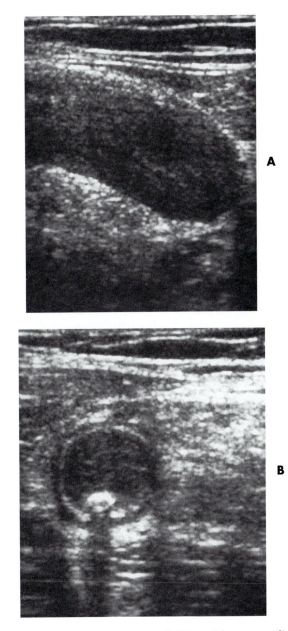

FIG. 8-45. Acute appendicitis with appendicolith. A, Linear array image of the right lower quadrant shows the blind end of a dilated appendix. B, Transverse image close to the cecum shows an echogenic luminal shadowing focus, appendicolith, and the layered wall.

an appendicolith, regardless of appendiceal diameter, should also be regarded as a positive test (Fig. 8-45).

Although the sensitivity of sonography decreases with **perforation**, features statistically associated with its occurrence include[41] loculated pericecal fluid, phlegmon (Fig. 8-46) or abscess (Fig. 8-47), promi-

SONOGRAPHY OF APPENDICEAL PERFORATION

Loculated pericecal fluid
Phlegmon
Abscess
Prominent pericecal fat
Circumferential loss of the submucosal layer

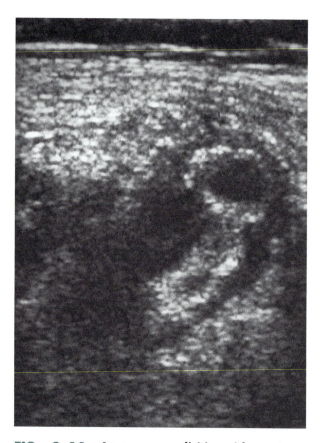

FIG. 8-46. Acute appendicitis with rupture. Sonogram of right lower quadrant shows the blind ended appendix with a pus-filled lumen surrounded by a hypoechoic mass representing a phlegmon.

nent pericecal fat (Fig. 8-48), and circumferential loss of the submucosal layer of the appendix.

Differential Diagnosis. False-positive diagnosis for acute appendicitis may occur if a normal appendix or a thickened terminal ileum is mistaken for an inflamed appendix. Awareness of the diagnostic criteria stated previously, particularly related to appendiceal diameter and morphology, should minimize these errors.

Clinical misdiagnosis occurs most frequently in young women with gynecologic conditions, especially acute pelvic inflammatory disease and rupture or torsion of ovarian cysts. Gastrointestinal illnesses clinically misdiagnosed as acute appendicitis include acute terminal ileitis with mesenteric adenitis,[42] acute typhlitis, acute diverticulitis, especially of a cecal tip diverticulum, and Crohn disease in the ileocecal area or involving the appendix itself.[43] Urologic disease, especially stone-related and right-sided segmental omental infarction, may also mimic acute appendicitis. The **value of sonography** in establishing an **alternative diagnosis** in patients with suspected acute appendicitis was addressed by Gaensler et al.[44] who found that 70% of patients with another diagnosis had abnormalities visualized on the sonogram.

Acute Diverticulitis

Pathology and Clinical Features. Diverticula of the colon are usually acquired deformities and are found most frequently in western urban civi-

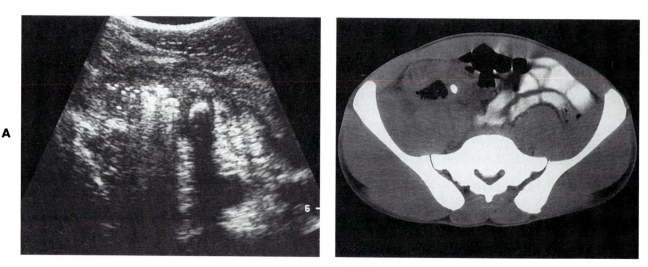

FIG. 8-47. Ruptured appendix—retrocecal gas containing abscess. **A,** Transverse sonogram shows inflamed regional fat as streaky increased echogenicity. A bright shadowing focus suggests an appendicolith. On the left side of the image, adjacent to the appendicolith, is a pocket of gas bubbles suggesting an extraluminal location. **B,** Confirmatory computed tomography scan shows the appendicolith and the gas-containing retrocecal abscess. (From Wilson SR: Gastrointestinal tract sonography. *Abdom Imaging* 1996;21:1-8.)

lizations.[45] The incidence of diverticula increases with age,[46] affecting approximately half the population by the ninth decade. Muscular dysfunction and hypertrophy are constant associated features. Diverticula are usually multiple; their most common location is the sigmoid and left colon. Acute diverticulitis and spastic diverticulosis may both be associated with a classical triad of presentation: left lower-quadrant pain, fever, and leukocytosis. Diverticula may also be found singly and in the right colon, where no association with muscular hypertrophy and dysfunction has been established. These congenital or true diverticula with muscular walls are relatively rare. Their inflammation produces a clinical picture most often identical to that of acute appendicitis.

Inspissated fecal material is believed to incite the initial inflammation in the apex of the diverticulum leading to acute diverticulitis.[47] Spread to the peridiverticular tissues and microperforation or macroperforation may follow. Localized abscess formation occurs more commonly than peritonitis. Fistula formation, with communication to the bladder, vagina, skin, or other bowel loops, is present in the minority of cases.

Surgical specimens demonstrate shortening and thickening of the involved segment of colon, associated with muscular hypertrophy. The peridiverticular inflammatory response may be minimal or very extensive.

Sonography. Sonography appears to be of value in early assessment of patients suspected of having acute diverticulitis[48,49] in which segments of thickened gut are detected and inflamed diverticula are identified. A negative scan combined with a low clinical suspicion

is usually a good indication to stop investigation. However, a negative scan in a patient with a highly suggestive clinical picture justifies a CT scan. Similarly, demonstration of pericolonic inflammatory disease on the sonogram may be appropriately followed by CT scan to define the nature and extent of the pericolonic disease before surgery or other intervention.

Since diverticula and smooth muscle hypertrophy of the colon are so prevalent, it seems likely that they would be commonly seen on routine sonography but this is not the usual experience. However, with the development of acute diverticulitis, both the inflamed diverticulum and the thickened colon become evident. Presumably the impacted fecalith, with or without microabscess formation, accentuates the diverticulum, whereas smooth muscle spasm, inflammation, and edema accentuate the gut wall thickening. **Identification of diverticula** on the sonogram strongly **indicates diverticulitis.**[48]

Diverticula are arranged in parallel rows along the margins of the teniae coli; therefore careful **technique** is required to make their identification. Following demonstration of a thickened loop of gut, the long axis of the loop should be determined. Slight tilting of the transducer to the margins of the loop will potentiate visualization of the diverticula because they may be on the lateral and medial edges of the loop rather than directly anterior or posterior. Cross-sectional views are then obtained running along the entire length of the thickened gut. Abnormalities must be confirmed on both views. Errors related to overlapping gut loops, in particular, can be virtually eliminated with this careful technique.

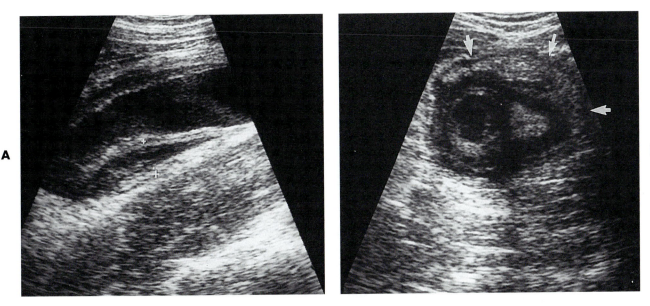

FIG. 8-48. Perforated appendix. A, Long axis view shows a distended appendix with a fluid-filled lumen and surrounding inflammatory mass. **B,** Transverse image close to the base of the appendix shows a rim of thick fat (*arrows*) anteriorly marginating the appendix, on the left, and the inflamed mesoappendix, on the right side of the image.

Failure to identify gas-containing abscesses and interloop abscesses are the major potential sources of error when using sonography. The meticulous technique of following involved thickened segments of colon in long axis and transverse section will help detect even small amounts of extraluminal gas.

Sonographic features of diverticulitis include: segmental **concentric thickening** of the gut wall that is frequently strikingly hypoechoic, reflecting the predominant thickening in the muscular layer; **inflamed diverticula**, seen as bright echogenic foci, with acoustic shadowing or ring-down artifact, within or beyond the thickened gut wall (Figs. 8-49 and 8-50);

acute **inflammatory changes** in the **pericolonic fat**, seen as poorly defined hyperechoic zones without obvious gas or fluid content; **abscess formation**, seen as loculated fluid collections in an intramural, pericolonic, or remote location (Fig. 8-51). With the development of extraluminal inflammatory masses, the diverticulum may no longer be identified on sonography, presumably being incorporated into the inflammatory process. Therefore, demonstration of a thickened segment of colon with an adjacent inflammatory mass may be consistent with diverticulitis but also with neoplastic or other inflammatory disease. Intramural **sinus tracts** appear as high-amplitude linear echoes,

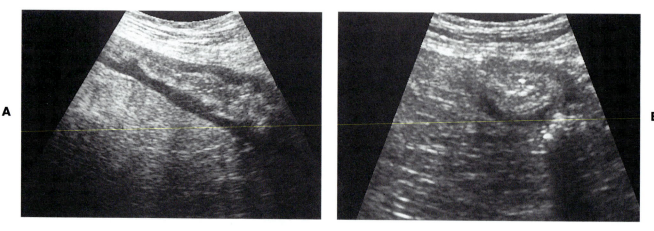

FIG. 8-49. Acute diverticulitis. A, Long axis view of descending colon shows a long segment of thickened gut with prominent muscularis propria. Edema of the perienteric fat is striking and shows as a homogeneous echogenic "mass effect" deep to the gut. **B,** Cross-sectional image shows the thick gut. The large inflamed diverticulum shows as a pocket of increased echogenicity projecting beyond the contour of the gut with distal acoustic shadowing. The diverticulum shows only on the cross-sectional image.

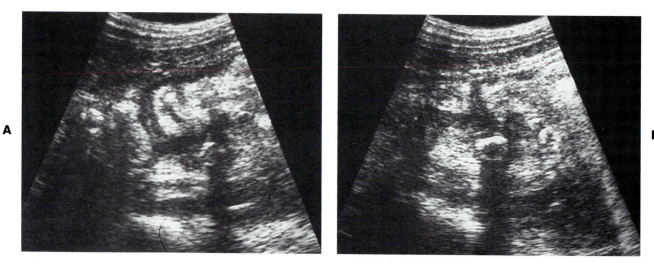

FIG. 8-50. Acute cecal diverticulitis in a man with right lower-quadrant pain and suspect appendicitis. A, Sagittal scan of right flank shows a prominent ascending colon. A bright shadowing echogenic focus projects beyond the gut. **B,** Transverse scan through the region of interest shows the cecum collapsed anteriorly, and the inflamed diverticulum on the posterior wall as a bright shadowing echogenic focus with surrounding inflamed fat.

often with ring-down artifact, within the gut wall (Fig. 8-52). Typically they are deep, between the muscularis propria and the serosa. **Fistulae** appear as linear tracts that extend from the involved segment of gut to the bladder, vagina, or adjacent loops. Their echogenicity depends on their content, usually gas or fluid. **Thickening** of the **mesentery** and inflamed mesenteric fat (Fig. 8-49) may also be seen.

The sonographic and clinical features of diverticulitis are more specific than those of acute appendicitis and the errors of diagnosis occur less often. However, **torsion** of an **appendix epiploicae** may produce a sonographic appearance so closely resembling acute diverticulitis that differentiation may be difficult.[50] The inflamed/infarcted fat of the appendix shows as a shadowing area of increased echogenicity

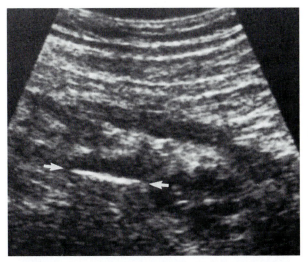

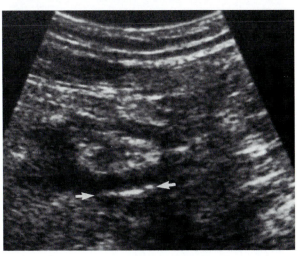

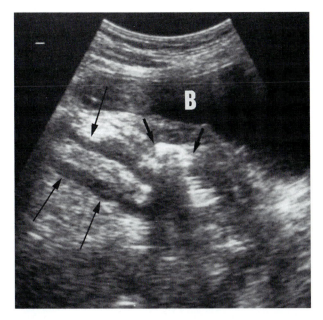

FIG. 8-51. Acute diverticulitis—gas-containing abscess. This patient had recurring pelvic pain and cystitis. Sagittal pelvic sonogram shows a diffusely thickened loop of sigmoid colon (*long arrows*), a large abscess containing a large focus of gas (*small arrows*), and the urinary bladder (B).

FIG. 8-52. Acute diverticulitis-intramural sinus tract. A, Long axis, and **B,** short axis, sonograms of thickened sigmoid colon show linear echogenic tract (*arrows*) deep to the muscularis propria (From Wilson SR, Toi A: The value of sonography in the diagnosis of acute diverticulitis of the colon. *AJR* 1990;154:1199-1202.)

related to the margin of the colon mimicking an inflamed diverticulum. Regional perienteric inflammatory change however is usually minimal and systemic symptoms are less. The noninflamed colonic appendices epiploicae are not visible except with ascites where they are seen as uniformly spaced echogenic foci along the margins of the colon.

Gastrointestinal Tract Obstruction

Occlusion of the gastrointestinal tract lumen producing obstruction may be **mechanical**, where an actual physical impediment to the progression of the luminal content exists, or may be **functional**, where paralysis of the intestinal musculature impedes progression (paralytic ileus).[51]

SONOGRAPHY IN BOWEL OBSTRUCTION	
Ideal	The gasless abdomen
Do not see	Gas filled loops
	Dilated fluid filled gut
Do see	Dilated fluid filled gut
	Altered peristalsis increased to-and-fro
Site of obstruction	Assess caliber of stomach, duodenum, small bowel, and large bowel
	Assess for caliber alteration
Obstruction site	Mass—luminal, mural, extrinsic
	Gut wall thickening
	Abnormal gut location

Mechanical Bowel Obstruction. Mechanical bowel obstruction (MBO) is characterized by dilatation of the intestinal tract proximal to the site of luminal occlusion, accumulation of large quantities of fluid and/or gas, and hyperperistalsis as the gut attempts to pass the luminal content beyond the obstruction. If the process is prolonged, exhaustion and over distention of the bowel loops may occur with secondary decrease in the peristaltic activity. There are three broad categories of mechanical obstruction: **obturation obstruction**, related to blockage of the lumen by material in the lumen; **intrinsic abnormalities** of the gut wall associated with luminal narrowing; and **extrinsic bowel lesions**, including adhesions. **Strangulation obstruction** develops when the circulation of the obstructed intestinal loop becomes impaired.

Sonography in Suspected Mechanical Obstruction. In most patients with intestinal obstruction, sonography is not helpful. This is easily appreciated if one remembers that adhesions, the most common cause of intestinal obstruction, are not visible on the sonogram. Also, the presence of abundant gas in the intestinal tract, characteristic of most patients with obstruction, frequently produces sonograms of nondiagnostic quality. However, in the minority of patients with mechanical obstruction who do not have significant gaseous distention, sonography may be very helpful. In a prospective study of 48 patients, Meiser et al.[52] found that ultrasound was positive in 25% of the patients when the plain film was considered normal. Ultrasound alone allowed complete diagnosis of the cause of obstruction in six patients. Lim et al.[11] in a retrospective study of sonography on 26 patients with known colonic obstruction correctly predicted the location of colonic obstruction in 22 cases (85%) and the etiology of the obstruction in 21 cases

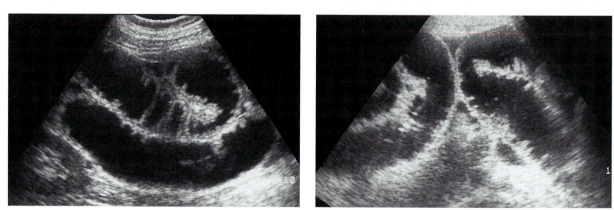

A   **B**

FIG. 8-53. Mechanical small bowel obstruction. **A,** Sagittal image of right flank shows multiple adjacent long loops of dilated fluid-filled small bowel with the classic morphology for a distal mechanical small bowel obstruction. **B,** Transverse image in the left lower quadrant confirms the multiplicity of dilated loops involved in the process. A small amount of ascites is seen between the dilated loops.

(81%). Of 13 patients ultimately proven to have adenocarcinoma, five had a mass on sonography, five had segmental thickening and 11 others showed a target sign of intussusception.

Sonographic study of **potential bowel obstruction** should include assessment of:

- **GI tract caliber** from the stomach to the rectum, noting any point at which the caliber alters (Fig. 8-53).
- **Content** of any dilated loops, with special attention to their fluid and/or gaseous nature.
- **Peristaltic activity** within the dilated loops, which is typically markedly exaggerated and abnormal, frequently producing a to-and-fro motion of the luminal content (Fig. 8-54). With strangulation, peristalsis may decrease or cease (Fig. 8-55).
- **Site** of obstruction for **luminal** (large gallstones, bezoars,[53] foreign bodies, intussusception, and oc-

casional polypoid tumors); **intrinsic** (segmental gut wall thickening and stricture formation from Crohn disease and annular carcinomas); and **extrinsic** (abscesses, endometriomas) abnormality as a cause of the obstruction.

- **Location of gut loops,** noting any abnormal position. Obstruction associated with external hernias is ideal for sonographic detection in that dilated loops of gut may be traced to a portion of the gut with normal caliber but abnormal location (Fig. 8-56). Spigelian and inguinal hernias are the disorders most commonly seen on sonograms.

Unique sonographic features are seen in the following:

Closed loop obstruction occurs if the bowel lumen is occluded at two points along its length, a serious condition that facilitates strangulation and necrosis. As the obstructed loop is closed off from the more proximal portion of the GI tract, little or no gas is present within the obstructed segments, which may become very dilated and fluid filled (Fig. 8-57). Consequently, the abdominal radiograph may be quite unremarkable (Fig. 8-57, *C*) and sonography may be most helpful by showing the dilated involved segments and often the normal calibre bowel distal to the point of obstruction. The CT features of closed loop obstruction are well described and include dilated small bowel, a C- or U-shaped bowel loop, a whirl sign, and two adjacent collapsed loops.[54,55] The latter important specific observation is very difficult to observe on ultrasound, in contrast to CT scan. However, we have correctly suspected closed loop obstruction in many patients on the basis of virtually normal plain films, small bowel dilatation and a U- or C-shaped bowel loop (Fig. 8-57, *A*) especially if there is gut wall thickening and/or pneumatosis intestinalis suggesting gut infarction.

Afferent loop obstruction is an uncommon complication of subtotal gastrectomy, with Billroth II gastrojejunostomy, that may occur by twisting at the anastomotic site, internal hernias, or with anastomotic stricture. Again, a gasless dilated loop may be readily recognized on sonography in a location consistent with the enteroenteric anastomosis running from the right upper quadrant across the midline. Its detection, location and shape should allow for correct sonographic diagnosis of this condition.[56]

Intussusception, invagination of a bowel segment (the intussusceptum) into the next distal segment (the intussuscipiens), is a relatively infrequent cause of mechanical obstruction in the adult where it is usually associated with a tumor as a lead point. A sonographic appearance of **multiple concentric rings,** related to the invaginating layers of the telescoped bowel, seen in cross-section is virtually pathognomonic (Fig. 8-58).[57]

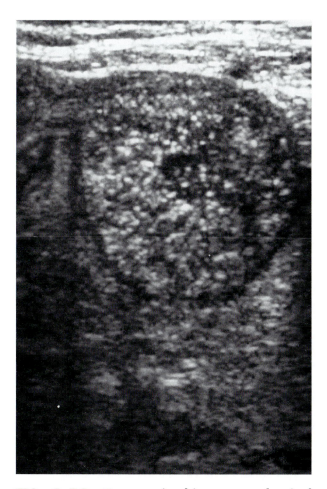

FIG. 8-54. Hyperperistaltic gut—mechanical bowel obstruction. Sonogram shows a dilated loop of small bowel in cross section. Hyperperistalsis often shows innumerable bright echogenic foci within the lumen, on a still frame, as in this case, due to the agitation of the luminal content.

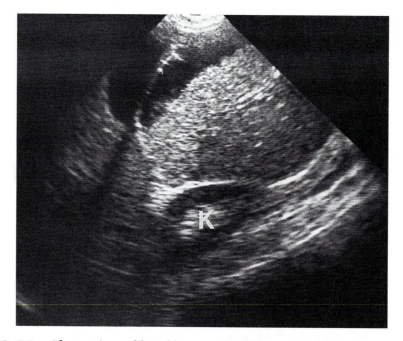

FIG. 8-55. Obstruction—dilated hypoperistaltic segments. Sagittal sonogram in the right flank shows gross dilatation of the ascending colon. There is a long fluid sediment level seen as a reflection of the hypoperistalsis of this segment of gut. Kidney (K). (From Sarrazin J, Wilson SR: Manifestations of Crohn disease at US. *RadioGraphics* 1996;16:499-520.)

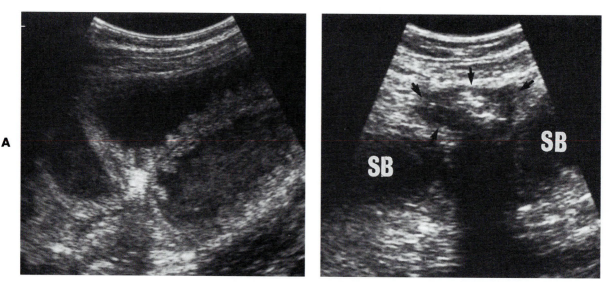

FIG. 8-56. Mechanical small bowel obstruction—ventral hernia. A, Sonogram shows dilated fluid-filled loops of small bowel with edematous valvulae conniventes. B, Transverse paraumbilical sonogram shows normal caliber gut (*arrows*) lying in abnormal superficial location. Dilated loops of small bowel (SB) could be traced to this point.

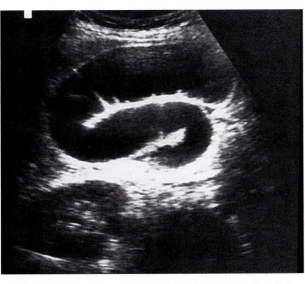

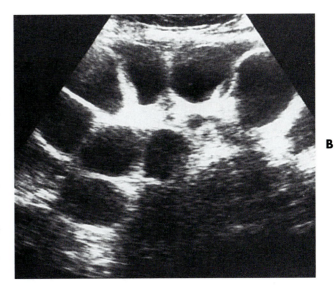

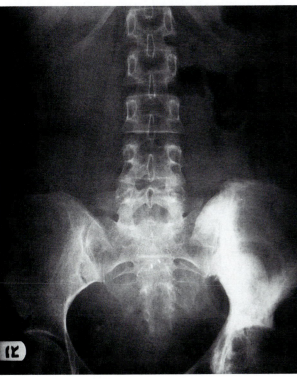

FIG. 8-57. **Closed loop obstruction.** A, and B, Sonograms show grossly dilated gasless fluid-filled small bowel loops. The loop on the left image is C- or U-shaped. C, Plain film is unremarkable.

Occasionally, only a target appearance may be seen.[58] The longitudinal appearance suggesting a "**hay fork**"[59] is not as reliably detected (Figs. 8-59 and 8-60).

Midgut malrotation predisposes to bowel obstruction and infarction. It is infrequently encountered in adults. Sonographic abnormality related to the superior mesenteric vessels is suggestive of malrotation.[60] On transverse sonograms, the **superior mesenteric vein is seen on the left ventral aspect of the superior mesenteric artery,** a reversal of the normal relationship.

Paralytic Ileus. Paralysis of the intestinal musculature, in response to general or local insult, may impede the progression of luminal content. Although the lumen remains patent, no progression occurs. Sonography is usually of little value because these patients characteristically have poor quality sonograms resulting from large quantities of gas in the intestinal tract. However, on rare occasions, the sonogram may demonstrate dilated, fluid-filled, very quiet, or aperistaltic loops of intestine. A **fluid-fluid level in a dilated loop** is characteristic of paralytic ileus, reflecting lack of movement of the intestinal contents (Fig. 8-61).

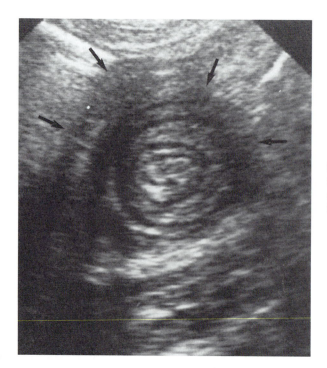

FIG. 8-58. Intussusception—submucosal metastatic nodule as lead point. Sonogram shows multiple, concentric rings (*arrows*) representative of the invaginating intussuscipiens and the intussusceptum.

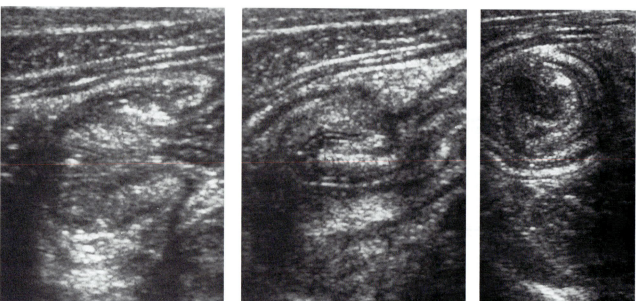

FIG. 8-59. Acute terminal ileitis with ileocolic intussusception. **A.** Region of ileocecal valve shows transient hay fork appearance of intussusception in long axis. **B.** Moments later the appearance has resolved showing a thick terminal ilium and no intussusception. **C.** At the time of intussusception, cross-sectional view shows a series of concentric rings related to the intussusceptum within the intussuscipiens.

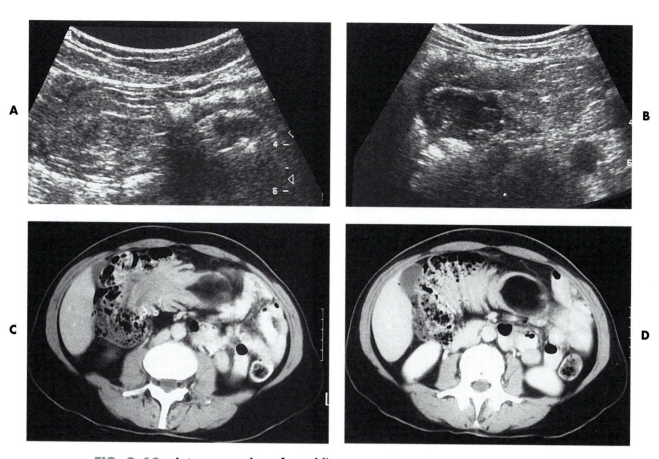

FIG. 8-60. **Intussusception of cecal lipoma.** **A,** Transverse epigastric image to the left side of the patient's abdomen shows an echogenic mass, suggesting fat, and its continuity with normal gut distally on the right side of this image. **B,** Transverse image of right epigastrium shows a hypoechoic mass with a central echo with features of "a hay fork of intussusception" in long axis. At the leading edge, on the right of the image, is the focal echogenic mass of fat density. **C** and **D,** Computed tomography images show the features of intussusception and the large leading mass of fat density, a surgically confirmed cecal lipoma.

GASTROINTESTINAL TRACT INFECTIONS

Although fluid-filled, actively peristaltic gut may be seen with infectious viral or bacterial gastroenteritis, most affected patients do not demonstrate a sonographic abnormality. However, some pathogens, notably *Yersinia enterocolitica*, *Mycobacterium tuberculosis*, and *Campylobacter jejuni*, produce highly suggestive sonographic abnormalities in the ileocecal area. Also, certain high-risk populations, such as those with AIDS and neutropenia,[61] appear to be susceptible to acute typhlitis and colitis, which also have a highly suggestive sonographic appearance.

Mesenteric Adenitis and Acute Ileitis

Mesenteric adenitis, in association with acute terminal ileitis, is the most frequent GI cause of misdiagnosis of acute appendicitis. Patients typically have right lower-quadrant pain and tenderness. During the sonographic examination, enlarged mesenteric lymph

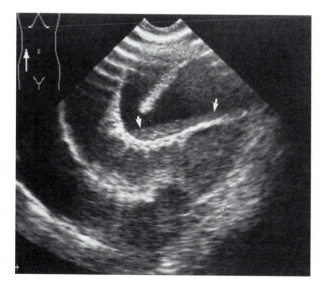

FIG. 8-61. **Paralytic ileus.** Sagittal sonogram shows extensive small bowel dilatation. Loops are fluid-filled and quiet with fluid-fluid level (*arrows*).

nodes and mural thickening of the terminal ileum are noted. *Yersinia enterocolitica* and *Campylobacter jejuni* are the most common causative agents.[62,63]

The AIDS Population

Sonography is frequently performed on AIDS patients; thus, awareness of the GI tract infections that produce sonographic abnormalities may lead to improved diagnosis and treatment. AIDS patients are at increased risk for development of both GI tract neoplasia, especially lymphoma (Fig. 8-19), and unusual opportunistic infections, most commonly candida esophagitis and cytomegalovirus (CMV) colitis.[64,65] The relative incidence of infection compared with neoplasia is about four or five to one. Acute abdominal catastrophe in patients with AIDS is usually a complication of CMV colitis and may result in hemorrhage, perforation, and peritonitis.[66]

Typhlitis and Colitis

Cytomegalovirus and *Mycobacterium tuberculosis* are the pathogens isolated most commonly in patients with typhlitis and colitis, although other organisms have been implicated. Immunocompromised patients are most often affected with AIDS accounting for the overwhelming majority of cases in the last decade. Sonographic study most commonly demonstrates **striking concentric, uniform thickening of the colon wall, usually localized to the cecum and the adjacent ascending colon** (Fig. 8-62). The colon wall may be several times normal in thickness, reflecting inflammatory infiltration throughout the gut wall. Cytomegalovirus is associated with deep ulcerations that may be complicated by perforation.

Tuberculous colitis is frequently associated with lymphadenopathy (particularly involving the mesenteric and omental nodes), splenomegaly, intrasplenic masses, ascites, and peritoneal masses, all of which may be assessed using sonography.

Pseudomembranous Colitis

Pseudomembranous colitis is a necrotizing inflammatory bowel condition that may occur as a response to a heterogeneous group of insults. Today, antibiotic therapy with effects from the toxin of *Clostridium difficile*, a normal inhabitant of the GI tract, is most commonly implicated.[67] Watery diarrhea is the most common symptom and usually occurs during antibiotic therapy but may be quite remotely associated, occurring up to 6 weeks later. Endoscopic demonstration of pseudomembranous exudative plaques on the mucosal surface of the gut and culture of the enterotoxin of *C. difficile* are diagnostic. Superficial ulceration of the mucosa is associated with inflammatory infiltration of the lamina propria and the submucosa, which may be thickened to many times normal size.[68]

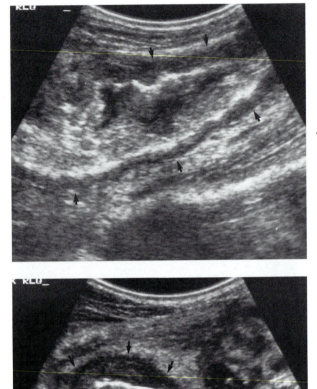

FIG. 8-62. **AIDS—acute typhlitis.** **A,** Sagittal, and **B,** transverse sonograms of the cecum show diffuse concentric thickening of the cecal wall (*arrows*). The cecal lumen is distended and partially fluid filled.

Sonography is frequently performed before pseudomembranous colitis is diagnosed, often based on a history of fever, abdominal pain, and watery diarrhea. **Sonographic features** have only rarely been described[69,70] but are suggestive of pseudomembranous colitis. Usually the entire colon is involved in a process that may produce striking **thickening of the colon wall. Exaggerated haustral markings** and a **nonhomogeneous thickened submucosa**, with **virtual apposition of the mucosal surfaces of the thickened walls**, are characteristic (Fig. 8-63). Pseudomembranous colitis should be suspected in any patient with diffuse colonic wall thickening without a previous history of inflammatory bowel disease. Because the history of concurrent or prior antibiotic therapy is not always given, direct questioning of the patient is frequently helpful.

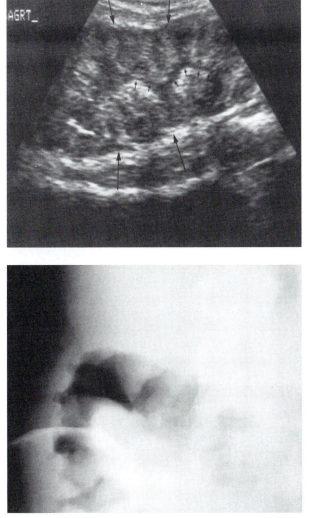

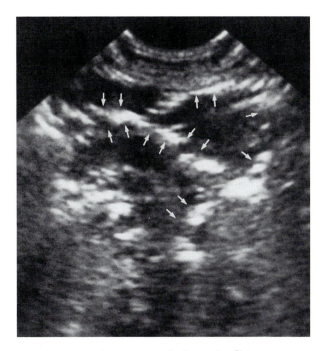

FIG. 8-64. Pneumatosis intestinalis. Sonogram shows three loops of gut with bright, high-amplitude echoes (*arrows*) originating within the gut wall.

FIG. 8-63. Pseudomembranous colitis. A, Long-axis scan of ascending colon shows grossly thickened gut (*long arrows*), exaggerated haustral pattern, and virtual apposition of the mucosal surfaces of the gut wall (*short arrows*). **B,** Plain abdominal radiograph shows thumbprinting.

MISCELLANEOUS GASTROINTESTINAL TRACT ABNORMALITIES

Congenital Abnormalities of the Gastrointestinal Tract

Duplication cysts, characterized by the presence of the normal layers of the gut wall, may occur in any portion of the GI tract. These cysts may be visualized on the sonogram, either routine or endoscopic, and should be considered as diagnostic possibilities whenever unexplained abdominal cysts are seen.

Ischemic Bowel Disease

Ischemic bowel disease most commonly affects the colon and is most prevalent in elderly persons who

have arteriosclerosis. In younger patients, it may complicate cardiac arrhythmia, vasculitis, coagulopathy, embolism, shock, or sepsis.[71] Sonographic features have been poorly described, although gut wall thickening may be encountered. Pneumatosis intestinalis may complicate gut ischemia with a characteristic sonographic appearance.

Pneumatosis Intestinalis

Pneumatosis intestinalis is a relatively rare condition in which intramural pockets of gas are found throughout the GI tract. It has been associated with a wide variety of underlying conditions including obstructive pulmonary disease, collagen vascular disease, inflammatory bowel disease, traumatic endoscopy, and postjejunoileal bypass. In many situations, affected patients are asymptomatic and the observation is incidental. However, its demonstration is of great clinical significance when necrotizing enterocolitis or ischemic bowel disease is present. Both conditions are associated with mucosal necrosis in which gas from the lumen passes to the gut wall.

Sonographic description is limited to isolated case reports. **High-amplitude echoes** may be demonstrated **in the gut wall with typical air artifact or shadowing** (Fig. 8-64).[72,73] Gut wall thickening may be noted if the pneumatosis is associated with underlying inflammatory bowel disease. If gut ischemia is suspect, careful evaluation of the liver is recommended to look for evidence of portal venous air.

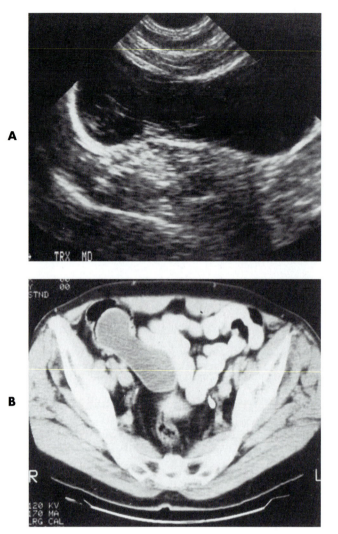

FIG. 8-65. Mucocele of the appendix. A, Sonogram of right lower quadrant shows well-defined cystic mass with some low-level echogenicity. **B,** Confirmatory computed tomography scan.

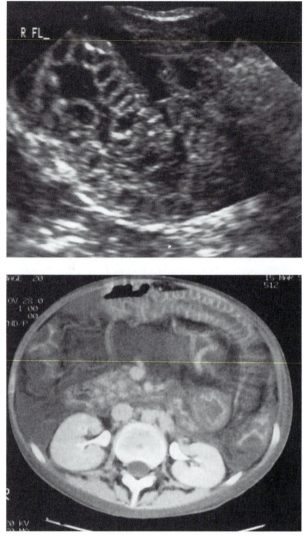

FIG. 8-66. Grossly edematous small bowel wall in a patient with septic shock. A, Sonogram shows ascites and dilated grossly edematous small bowel characterized by strikingly edematous valvulae conniventes. **B,** Confirmatory computed tomography scan.

Mucocele of the Appendix

Mucocele of the appendix is relatively uncommon, occurring in about 0.25% of 43,000 appendectomy specimens in one series.[74] Many patients with this condition are asymptomatic. A mass may be palpated in approximately 50% of cases. Both benign and malignant varieties occur in a ratio of approximately 10:1.[75] In the **benign form,** the appendiceal lumen is obstructed by either inflammatory scarring or fecaliths. The glandular mucosa in the isolated segment continues to secrete sterile mucus. The **neoplastic variety** of mucocele is associated with primary mucous cystadenoma or cystadenocarcinoma of the appendix. Although the gross morphology of the appendix may be similar in the benign and malignant varieties, the malignant form is often associated with pseudomyxoma peritonei if rupture occurs.

Mucoceles typically produce **large, hypoechoic, well-defined right lower-quadrant cystic masses** with variable internal echogenicity, wall thickness, and wall calcification (Fig. 8-65). These masses are frequently retrocecal and may be mobile. Although their sonographic appearance is not always specific, this diagnostic possibility should be considered when an elongated oval cystic mass is found in the right lower quadrant in any patient with an appendix.[76]

Gut Edema

Hypoalbuminemia, congestive heart failure, and venous thrombosis may all be associated with diffuse edema of the gut wall. **Prominent thickened hypoechoic valvulae conniventes** (Fig. 8-66) and

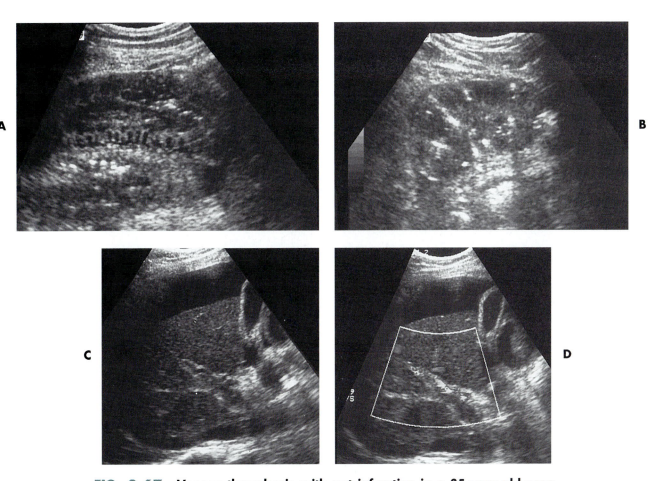

FIG. 8-67. Venous thrombosis with gut infarction in a 35-year-old pregnant woman with abdominal pain and distention. **A,** Sonogram shows a loop of small bowel with edematous valvulae conniventes. **B,** A different loop shows pneumatous intestinalis with multiple gas bubbles within the gut wall. **C,** Sagittal image of porta hepatis shows the portal vein filled with echogenic thrombus. **D,** There is no flow in the portal vein on color Doppler. (From Wilson SR: Gastrointestinal tract sonography. *Abdom Imaging* 1996;21:1-8.)

gastric rugae are relatively easy to recognize on the sonographic study, which should also include Doppler evaluation of the mesenteric and portal veins (Fig. 8-67).

Gastrointestinal Tract Hematoma

Blunt abdominal trauma, complicated by duodenal hematoma and rectal trauma, either sexual or iatrogenic following rectal biopsy, are the major causes of local hematomas seen on sonography. Hematoma is usually localized to the submucosa. Larger or more diffuse hematomas may complicate anticoagulation therapy or bleeding disorders associated with leukemia. If hematomas are large, diffuse gut wall thickening may be seen on sonograms.

Peptic Ulcer

Peptic ulcer, a defect in the epithelium to the depth of the submucosa, may be seen in either gastric or duo-

denal locations. Although rarely visualized, peptic ulcer has a fairly characteristic sonographic appearance. A gas-filled ulcer crater is seen as a **bright echogenic focus with ring-down artifact, either in a focal area of wall thickening or beyond the wall,** depending on the depth of penetration. Edema in the acute phase and fibrosis in the chronic phase may produce localized wall thickening and deformity (Fig. 8-68).

Bezoars

Bezoars are masses of foreign material or food typically found in the stomach after surgery for peptic ulcer disease (phytobezoars) or after ingestion of indigestible organic substances such as hair (trichobezoars). These masses may produce **shadowing intraluminal densities on the sonogram** and have been documented as a rare cause of small bowel obstruction.[53] They may also form in the small bowel in association with chronic stasis (Fig. 8-69).

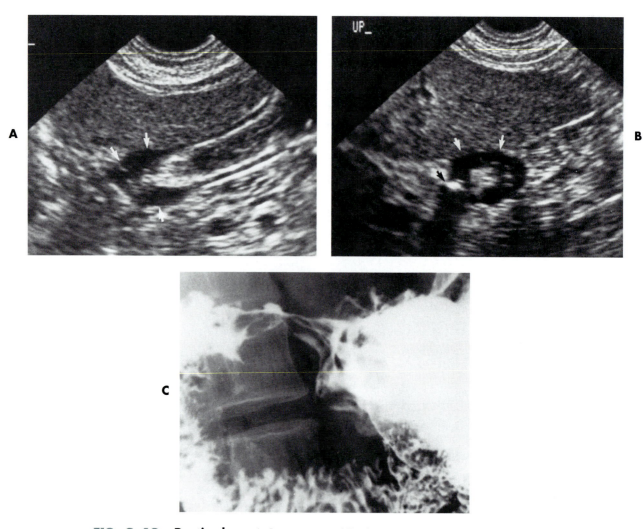

FIG. 8-68. Peptic ulcer. A, Long-axis, and B, short-axis sonograms show focal hypo-echoic thickening (*white arrows*) of the wall of the gut in the region of the pyloric channel. The ulcer crater (*black arrow*) is seen as an echogenic focus with acoustic shadowing. This focus projects beyond the lumen of the gut wall. C, Confirmatory barium swallow.

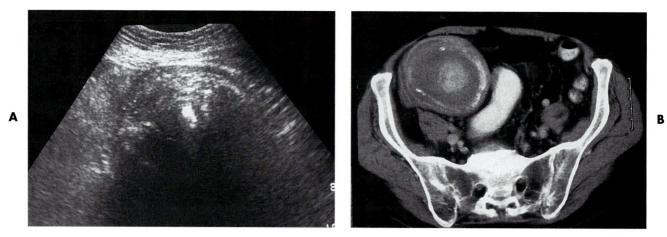

FIG. 8-69. Small bowel bezoar in a patient with Crohn disease with strictures. A, Sonogram of right lower quadrant shows a highly attenuating intraluminal mass. B, Confirmatory computed tomography scan.

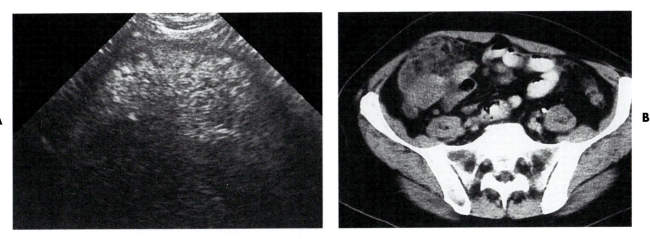

FIG. 8-70. Acute omental infarction in an elderly man with acute right lower-quadrant pain. **A,** Sonogram shows a large tender mass in the right lower quadrant. The mass is uniformly echogenic and attenuating with an ultrasound appearance suggesting inflamed fat. **B,** Confirmatory computed tomography scan.

Intraluminal Foreign Bodies

Large foreign bodies, including bottles, candles, sexual vibrators, contraband, tools, and food, may be identified, particularly in the rectum and sigmoid colon where they produce fairly sharp, distinct specular echoes with sharp acoustic shadows. Their recognition is enhanced by suspicion of their presence.

Right Sided Segmental Omental Infarction

Right-sided segmental infarction of the omentum is a rare condition which is virtually always mistaken clinically for acute appendicitis.[77] Of unknown etiology, it is postulated to occur with an anomalous and fragile blood supply to the right lower omentum, making it susceptible to painful infarction.[78] Patients present with right lower-quadrant pain and tenderness. On sonography, **a plaque or cakelike area of increased echogenicity suggesting inflamed or infiltrated fat** is seen superficially in the right flank with adherence to the peritoneum (Fig. 8-70).[77] No underlying gut abnormality is shown. As segmental infarction is a self-limited process, its correct diagnosis will prevent unnecessary surgery. If necessary, CT scan is confirmatory showing streaky fat in a masslike configuration in the right side of the omentum.

ENDOSONOGRAPHY

Endosonography, performed with high-frequency transducers in the lumen of the gut, allows for detection of mucosal abnormality, delineation of the layers of the gut wall, and definition of the surrounding soft tissues to a depth of 8 to 10 cm from the transducer crystal. Thus, tumors hidden below normal mucosa, tumor penetration into the layers of the gut wall, and tumor involvement of surrounding vital structures or lymph nodes may be well evaluated. Staging of previously identified mucosal tumors is one of the major applications of this technique.

Upper Gastrointestinal Tract Endosonography

Technique. Rotating high-frequency transducers, using 7.5-MHz crystals fitted into a fiberoptic endoscope, are most suitable for endosonography of the esophagus, stomach, and duodenum. Light sedation of the patient is usually required. The patient is placed in the left lateral decubitus position, and the endoscope is inserted to the desired location. Intraluminal gas is aspirated, and a balloon covering the transducer crystal is inflated with deaerated water. Localization is determined from the distance of insertion from the teeth and identification of anatomic landmarks, such as the spleen, liver, pancreas, and gallbladder. Rotation and deflection of the transducer tip allow scanning of visualized lesions in different planes.[79]

Benign Lesions. Identification, localization, and characterization of benign masses are possible with endoscopic sonography. **Varices** are seen as compressible hypoechoic or cystic masses deep to the submucosa or in the outer layers of the esophagus, gastroesophageal junction, or gastric fundus.[80] **Benign tumors,** such as fibromas or leiomyomas, are well-defined solid masses without mucosal involvement that can be localized to the layer of the wall from which they arise, usually the submucosa and the muscularis propria respectively. **Peptic ulcer** typically produces marked thickening of all layers of the gastric wall with a demonstrated ulcer crater. **Menetrier's disease** produces thickening of the mucosal folds.

Malignant Tumors. Staging of esophageal carcinoma involves assessment of depth of tumor invasion and evaluation of involvement of the local lymph nodes and adjacent vital structures.[81] Constricting lesions that do not allow passage of the endoscope may produce technically unsatisfactory or incomplete examinations.

Gastric lymphoma is typically very hypoechoic, its invasion is along the gastric wall or horizontal, and involvement of extramural structures and lymph nodes is less than with gastric carcinoma. Thus, localized mucosal ulceration with extensive infiltration of the deeper layers suggests lymphoma that may also grow with a polypoid pattern or as a diffuse infiltration without ulceration.[82] **Gastric carcinoma,** in contrast, arises from the gastric mucosa, is usually more echogenic, tends to invade vertically or through the gastric wall, and frequently involves the perigastric lymph nodes by the time of diagnosis.

Rectal Endosonography

Although a variety of pathologic conditions may be assessed with endorectal sonography, the **staging** of previously detected **rectal carcinoma** is its major role. Patients are scanned in the left lateral decubitus position following a cleansing enema. Both axial and sagittal images are obtained. A variety of rigid intrarectal probes are now commercially available using a range of transducer technologies with phased array, mechanical sector, and rotating crystals. A sterile condom covers an inner balloon, which is inflated with 35 to 70 cc of deaerated water. The probe is moved to allow for visualization of the tumor within the focal zone of the transducer. Axial images demonstrate the rectum as a multilayered circle (Fig. 8-71).

Tumors are staged according to the Astler-Coller modification of the Dukes classification[83] or more simply with the primary tumor (T) component of the "Union Internationale Contre le Cancer" (UICC) TNM classification[84] where T represents the primary tumor, N the nodal involvement, and M the distant metastases (Figs. 8-72 through 8-74).

Rectal carcinoma arises from the mucosal surface of the gut. Tumors appear as relatively hypoechoic masses that may distort the rectal lumen. Invasion of the deeper layers, the submucosa, the muscularis propria, and the perirectal fat produces discontinuity of these layers on the sonogram. Superficial ulceration or crevices that allow small bubbles of gas to be trapped deep to the inflated balloon may demonstrate ringdown artifact and shadowing, with loss of layer definition deep to the ulceration. Lymph nodes appear as round or oval hypoechoic masses in the perirectal fat. Sonographically, many visible nodes may be reactive

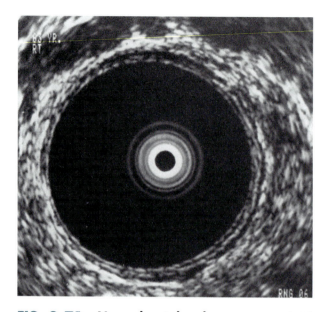

FIG. 8-71. **Normal rectal endosonogram.** Axial view shows the probe centrally within the rectal lumen. The five layers of the gut wall are most optimally seen between the three o'clock and seven o'clock positions.

T COMPONENT FOR STAGING TUMORS— TNM UICC CLASSIFICATION

T_1—Tumor confined to mucosa or submucosa
T_2—Invasion of the muscularis propria or serosa
T_3—Tumor invading the perirectal fat
T_4—Tumor involving an adjacent organ

---

rather than neoplastic, and normal-sized nodes may have microscopic invasion. Therefore, definitive staging requires pathological assessment of both the tumor and the regional nodes.

Wang et al.[85] studied 6 normal and 16 neoplastic colorectal specimens *in vitro* with an 8.5-MHz ultrasound transducer. They accurately demonstrated invasion of the submucosa in 92.5% and invasion of the muscularis propria in 77%. Invasive tumors with extension beyond the muscularis propria were accurately predicted 90% of the time. *In vivo* studies support this excellent result.[86,87] Comparing preoperative transrectal ultrasound and CT staging in 102 consecutive patients, Rifkin et al.[88] found transrectal sonography superior to CT in assessment of tumor extent and in the detection of lymph node involvement.

Limitations of sonography include:
- Inability to identify microscopic tumor invasion
- Inability to image stenotic tumors
- Inability to image tumors greater than 15 cm from the anal verge

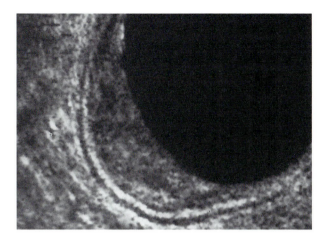

FIG. 8-72. Rectal carcinoma—T₁. A hypoechoic mass between the six o'clock and eight o'clock positions is noted. The submucosa, the echogenic line, and the muscularis propria, the external hypoechoic line, are intact.

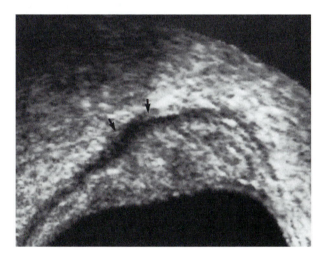

FIG. 8-73. Rectal carcinoma—T₂. A tumor is seen anteriorly. The muscularis propria (*arrows*) is the hypoechoic line that is thickened and nodular consistent with tumor involvement.

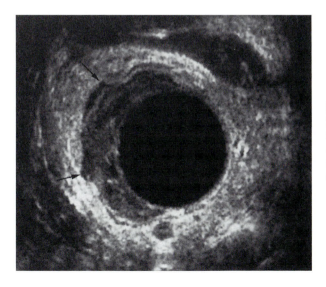

FIG. 8-74. Rectal carcinoma—T₃. A large tumor involves the entire right lateral wall of the rectum. Invasion of the perirectal fat (*arrows*) is noted in several locations. A large node is seen at the six o'clock position; smaller nodes are seen at the five o'clock and eight o'clock positions.

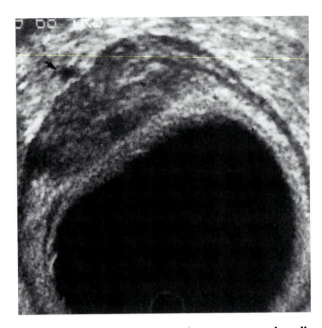

FIG. 8-75. Metastatic carcinoma to rectal wall.
A hypoechoic mass is seen between the ten o'clock and one
o'clock positions. It involves the deep layers of the rectal
wall and not the rectal mucosa. There is a small lymph node
(*arrow*).

- Inability to distinguish nodes involved with tumor
  from those with reactive change
- Inability to identify normal-sized nodes with microscopic tumor invasion.

Despite these limitations, endorectal ultrasound appears to be an excellent imaging tool for preoperative
staging of accessible rectal cancers.

Recurrent Rectal Carcinoma. Recurrent rectal cancer after local resection is usually extraluminal,
involving the resection margin secondarily. Serial
transrectal sonography may be used in conjunction
with serum chorioembryonic antigen levels to detect
these recurrences. A pericolic hypoechoic mass or
local thickening of the rectal wall, in either deep or superficial layers, is taken as evidence of recurrence.
Previous radiation treatment may produce a diffuse
thickening of the entire rectal wall, usually of moderate or high echogenicity with an appearance that is
usually easily differentiated from the focal hypoechoic
appearance of recurrent cancer. Sonographic-guided
biopsy of a detected abnormality facilitates histologic
differentiation of recurrence from postoperative, inflammatory, or postradiation change.

Metastatic Rectal Carcinoma. Prostatic carcinoma may invade the rectum directly, or more remote
tumors may involve the rectum, usually as a result of
seeding to the posterior peritoneal pouch. Because these
tumors initially involve the deeper layers of the rectal
wall with mucosal involvement occurring as the disease
progresses, their sonographic appearance is distinct
from that of primary rectal carcinoma (Fig. 8-75).

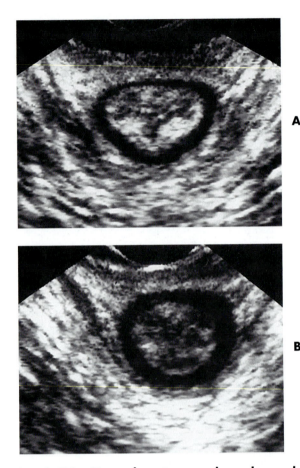

FIG. 8-76. Normal rectum and anal canal.
A, Cross sectional image of rectum taken with probe in the
vagina showing the normal convoluted rectal mucosa,
prominent submucosa (*white*) and the muscularis propria as
a black thin rim. The rectum is usually oval, as shown here.
B, The anal canal shows the thick well-defined internal anal
sphincter as a continuous black ring which is in continuity
with the muscularis propria of the rectal wall above. The external anal sphincter is less well-defined and echogenic.

Miscellaneous Rectal Abnormalities. Benign
mesenchymal tumors, especially of smooth muscle
origin, are uncommon in the rectum. When seen, their
sonographic features are the same as elsewhere. Mucous
retention cysts, caused by the obstruction of mucous
glands, produce cystic masses of varying size that are located deep in the rectal wall.

Anal Evaluation

Anal endosonography, performed with addition of a
hard cone attachment to a radial 7.5-MHz probe, allows accurate assessment of the anal canal, including
the internal and external sphincters.[89] Performed primarily for assessment of fecal incontinence, this test
shows the integrity of the sphincters with documentation of the degree and size of muscle defects.

Young women following traumatic obstetric delivery
are most often afflicted with fecal incontinence. We have

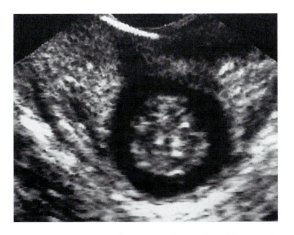

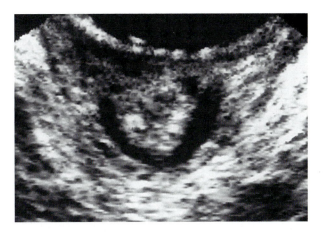

FIG. 8-77. Tear of external anal sphincter in a young woman with fecal incontinence following traumatic obstetric delivery. Transvaginal scan shows the tear as a black wedge-shaped defect (*arrow*) at approximately 11:00 o'clock.

FIG. 8-78. Tear of internal anal sphincter and external anal sphincter with loss of perineum in a young woman following traumatic obstetric delivery. Transvaginal scan shows a large disruption of the internal and external anal sphincters between the ten o'clock and one o'clock positions with loss of the soft tissue of the perineum anteriorly.

A

B

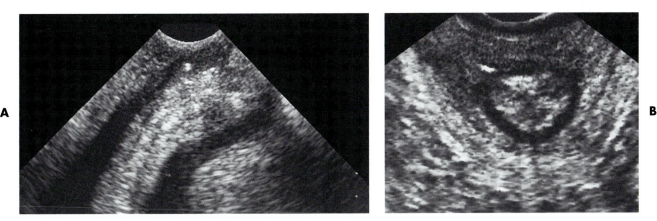

FIG. 8-79. Rectovaginal fistula in a young women with Crohn colitis. **A,** Sagittal transvaginal view of rectum shows a diffusely thick rectal wall. Close to the introitus, there are air bubbles projecting anteriorly through the rectal wall. **B,** Transvaginal scan with side-fired probe shows the cephalad portion of the anal sphincter in cross section. The fistula shows as a small echogenic gas pocket at the eleven o'clock position external to the hyperechoic ring of the internal anal sphincter.

found **transvaginal assessment** of the anal sphincter performed with a side firing transvaginal probe close to the introitus equally effective as a transanal approach.[25]

The internal anal sphincter, in continuity with the muscularis propria of the rectum above, is seen as a circular hypoechoic or black ring just deep to the convoluted mucosal echoes (Fig. 8-76). The external anal sphincter, in contrast, is less well defined and more echogenic appearing gray on the ultrasound examination. Traumatic disruption of the muscle layers will show as defects in the continuity of the normal muscle texture most commonly anterior (Fig. 8-77). Post-traumatic scarring may be associated with a change of shape of the anal canal from round to oval (Fig. 8-78). Involvement of the anal canal with fistula is also well assessed with a transvaginal approach in women (Fig. 8-79).

ACKNOWLEDGEMENTS

The author would like to acknowledge Rose Baldwin for her assistance with the preparation of this chapter and Jenny Tomashpolskaya for her artwork.

REFERENCES
Basic Principles

1. Heyder N, Kaarmann H, Giedl J. Experimental investigations into the possibility of differentiating early from invasive carcinoma of the stomach by means of ultrasound, *Endoscopy* 1987;19:228-232.
2. Bolondi L, Caletti G, Casanova P, et al.: Problems and variations in the interpretation of the ultrasound feature of the normal upper and lower gastrointestinal tract wall, *Scan J Gastroenterol* 1986;21:16-26.
3. Kimmey MB, Martin RW, Haggitt RC, et al.: Histologic correlates of gastrointestinal ultrasound images, *Gastroenterology* 1989;96:433-441.
4. Lutz H, Petzoldt R: Ultrasonic patterns of space occupying lesions of the stomach and the intestine, *Ultrasound Med Biol* 1976;2:129-131.
5. Bluth EI, Merritt CRB, Sullivan MA: Ultrasonic evaluation of the stomach, small bowel, and colon, *Radiology* 1979;133:677-680.
6. Wilson SR: Gastrointestinal sonography, *Abdom Imaging* 1996;21:1-8.
7. Puylaert JBCM: Acute appendicitis: Ultrasound evaluation using graded compression, *Radiology* 1986;158:355-360.
8. Teefey SA, Roarke MC, Brink JA, et al.: Bowel wall thickening: Differentiation of inflammation from ischemia with color Doppler and duplex US, *Radiology* 1996;198:547-551.

Gastrointestinal Tract Neoplasms

9. Winawer SJ, Sherlock P: Malignant neoplasms of the small and large intestine. In Sleisenger MH, Fordtran JS, editors: *Gastrointestinal disease: Pathophysiology Diagnosis Management*, ed 3, Philadelphia, 1983, WB Saunders.
10. Lim JH: Colorectal cancer: Sonographic findings, *AJR* 1996;167:45-47.
11. Lim JH, Ko YT, Lee DH, et al.: Determining the site and causes of colonic obstruction with sonography, *AJR* 1994;163:1113-1117.
12. Mesenchymal tumors. In Fenoglio-Preiser CM, Lantz PE, Listrom MB, et al. editors: *Gastrointestinal Pathology: An Atlas and Text*, New York, 1989, Raven Press.
13. Kaftori JK, Aharon M, Kleinhaus U: Sonographic features of gastrointestinal leiomyosarcoma, *J Clin Ultrasound* 1981;9:11-15.
14. Primary lymphomas of the gastrointestinal tract. In Fenoglio-Preiser CM, Lantz PE, Listrom MB, et al., editors: *Gastrointestinal Pathology: An Atlas and Text*, New York, 1989, Raven Press.
15. Salem S, Hiltz CW: Ultrasonographic appearance of gastric lymphosarcoma, *J Clin Ultrasound* 1978;6:429-430.
16. Derchi LE, Bandereali A, Bossi MC, et al.: Sonographic appearance of gastric lymphoma, *J Ultrasound Med* 1984;3:251-256.
17. Telerman A, Gerend B, Van der Heul B, et al.: Gastrointestinal metastases from extra-abdominal tumors, *Endoscopy* 1985;17:99.
18. Rubesin SE, Levine MS: Omental cakes: Colonic involvement by omental metastases, *Radiology* 1985;54:593-596.
19. Yeh H-C: Ultrasonography of peritoneal tumors, *Radiology* 1979;133:419-424.

Inflammatory Bowel Disease

20. Seitz K, Rettenmaier G: Inflammatory bowel disease, *Sonographic Diagnostics*, Dr. Falk Pharma, West Germany, GmbH, 1988.
21. Sarrazin J, Wilson SR: Manifestations of Crohn Disease at US, *RadioGraphics* 1996;16:499-520.
22. DiCandio G, Mosca F, Campatelli A, et al.: Sonographic detection of postsurgical recurrence of Crohn's disease. *AJR* 1986;146:523-526.

23. Worlicek H, Lutz H, Heyder N, et al.: Ultrasound findings in Crohn's disease and ulcerative colitis: A prospective study. *J Clin Ultrasound* 1987;15:153-163.
24. Dubbins PA: Ultrasound demonstration of bowel wall thickness in inflammatory bowel disease, *Clin Radiol* 1984;35:227-231.
25. Damani N, Wilson SR: Nongynocologic findings of transvaginal sonography. Submitted to *RadioGraphics* August 1997.

Acute Abdomen

26. Seibert JJ, Williamson SL, Golladay ES, et al.: The distended gasless abdomen: a fertile field for ultrasound, *J Ultrasound Med* 1986;5:301-308.
27. Lee DH, Lim JH, Ko YT, et al.: Sonographic detection of pneumoperitoneum in patients with acute abdomen. *AJR* 1990;154:107-109.
28. Muradali D, Burns P, Wilson SR: A specific sign for pneumoperitoneum on sonography: Enhanced peritoneal stripe, Submitted for publication April 1997.
29. Berry J Jr, Malt RA: Appendicitis near its centenary, *Ann Surg* 1984;200(5):567-575.
30. Kazarian KK, Roeder W, Mersheiner WL: Decreasing mortality and increasing morbidity from acute appendicitis, *Am J Surg* 1970;119:681-685.
31. Pieper R, Fonsell P, Kagen L: Perforating appendicitis: A nine year survey of treatment and results, *Acta Clin Scand* 1986;530:51-57.
32. Go PMNYH, Luyendijk R, Murting JDK: Metronidazo-protylaxe bij appendectomie, *Med Tijdschr Geneejk* 1986;130:775-778.
33. Van Way CW III, Murphy JR, Dunn EL, et al.: A feasibility study in computer-aided diagnosis in appendicitis, *Surg Gynecol Obstet* 1982;155:685-688.
34. Jeffrey RB Jr, Laing FC, Lewis FR: Acute appendicitis: High-resolution real-time ultrasound findings, *Radiology* 1987;163:11-14.
35. Shaw RE: Appendix calculi and acute appendicitis, *Br J Surg* 1965;52:452-459.
36. Savrin RA, Clauren K, Martin EW Jr, et al.: Chronic and recurrent appendicitis, *Am J Surg* 1979;137:355-357.
37. Dachman AH, Nichols JB, Patrick DH, et al.: Natural history of the obstructed rabbit appendix: Observations with radiography, sonography, and computed tomography, *AJR* 1987;148:281-284.
38. Abu-Yousef MM, Bleicher JJ, Maher JW, et al.: High-resolution sonography of acute appendicitis, *AJR* 1987;149:53-58.
39. Jeffrey RB Jr, Laing FC, Townsend RR: Acute appendicitis: Sonographic criteria based on 250 cases, *Radiology* 1988;67:327-329.
40. Rioux M: Sonographic detection of the normal and abnormal appendix, *AJR* 1992;158:887-778.
41. Borushok KF, Jeffrey RB Jr, Laing FC, et al.: Sonographic diagnosis of perforation in patients with acute appendicitis, *AJR* 1990;154:275-278.
42. Puylaert JBCM, Lalisang RI, van der Werf SDJ, et al.: Campylobacter ileocolitis mimicking acute appendicitis: Differentiation with graded-compression ultrasound, *Radiology* 1988;166:737-740.
43. Agha FP, Ghahremani GG, Panella JS, et al.: Appendicitis as the initial manifestation of Crohn's disease: Radiologic features and prognosis, *AJR* 1987;149:515-518.
44. Gaensler EHL, Jeffrey RB Jr, Laing FC, et al.: Sonography in patients with suspected acute appendicitis: Value in establishing alternative diagnoses, *AJR* 1989;152:49.
45. Painter NS, Burkitt DP: Diverticular disease of the colon, a 20th century problem, *Clin Gastroenterol* 1975;4:3.
46. Parks TG: Natural history of diverticular disease of the colon, *Clin Gastroenterol* 1975;4:53.

47. Ming SC, Fleischner FG: Diverticulitis of the sigmoid colon: Reappraisal of pathology and pathogenesis, *Surgery* 1965; 58:627.

48. Wilson SR, Toi A: The value of sonography in the diagnosis of acute diverticulitis of the colon, *AJR* 1990;154:1199-1202.

49. Parulekar SG: Sonography of colonic diverticulitis, *J Ultrasound Med* 1985;4:659-666.

50. Derchi LE, Reggiani L, Rebaudi F, Bruschetta M: Appendices epiploicae of the large bowel. Sonographic appearance and differentiation from peritoneal seeding, *J Ultrasound Med* 1988; 7:11-14.

51. Jones RS: Intestinal obstruction, pseudo-obstruction, and ileus. In Sleisenger MH, Fordtran JS, editors: *Gastrointestinal Disease: Pathophysiology Diagnosis Management*, ed 4, Philadelphia, 1988, WB Saunders.

52. Meiser G, Meissner K: Sonographic differential diagnosis of intestinal obstruction. Results of a prospective study of 48 patients, *Ultraschall Med* 1985;6:39-45.

53. Tennenhouse JE, Wilson SR: Sonographic detection of a small bowel bezoar, *J Ultrasound Med* 1990;9:603-605.

54. Siewert B, Raptopoulos V: CT of the acute abdomen: Findings and impact on diagnosis and treatment, *AJR* 1994;163:1317-1324.

55. Balthazar EJ: CT of small-bowel obstruction, *AJR* 1994;162:255-261.

56. Lee DH, Lim JH, Ko YT: Afferent loop syndrome: Sonographic findings in seven cases, *AJR* 1991;157:41-43.

57. Parienty RA, Lepreux JF, Gruson B: Sonographic and computed tomography features of ileocolic intussusception, *AJR* 1981;136:608-610.

58. Weissberg DL, Scheible W, Leopold GR: Ultrasonographic appearance of adult intussusception, *Radiology* 1977;124:791-792.

59. Alessi V, Salerno G: The "hay-fork" sign in the ultrasonographic diagnosis of intussusception, *Gastrointest Radiol* 1985;10:177-179.

60. Gaines PA, Saunders AJS, Drake D: Midgut malrotation diagnosed by ultrasound, *Clin Radiol* 1987;38:51-53.

Gastrointestinal Tract Infections

61. Teefey SA, Montana MA, Goldfogel, et al.: Sonographic diagnosis of neutropenic typhlitis, *AJR* 1987;149:731-733.

62. Puylaert JBCM: Mesenteric adenitis and acute terminal ileitis: Sonographic evaluation using graded compression, *Radiology* 1986;161:691-695.

63. Puylaert JBCM, Lalisang RI, van der Werf SDJ, et al.: Campylobacter ileocolitis mimicking acute appendicitis: Differentiation with graded-compression ultrasound, *Radiology* 1988;166:737-740.

64. Frager DH, Frager JD, Brandt LJ, et al.: Gastrointestinal complications of AIDS: radiologic features, *Radiology* 1986; 158:597-603.

65. Balthazar EJ, Megibow AJ, Fazzini E, et al.: Cytomegalovirus colitis in AIDS: Radiographic findings in 11 patients, *Radiology* 1985;155:585-589.

66. Teixidor HS, Honig CL, Norsoph E, et al.: Cytomegalovirus infection of the alimentary canal: Radiologic findings with pathologic correlation, *Radiology* 1987;163:317-323.

67. Bartlett JG: The pseudomembranous enterocolitides. In Sleisenger MH, Fordtran JS, editors: *Gastrointestinal Disease: Pathophysiology Diagnosis Management*, ed 4, Philadelphia, 1988, WB Saunders.

68. Totten MA, Gregg JA, Fremont-Smith P, et al.: Clinical and pathological spectrum of antibiotic associated colitis, *Am J of Gastroenterol* 1978;69:311.

69. Bolondi L, Ferrentino M, Trevisani F, et al.: Sonographic appearance of pseudomembranous colitis, *J Ultrasound Med* 1985;4:489-492.

70. Downey DB, Wilson SR: The role of sonography in pseudomembranous colitis, *Radiology* 1991;180:61-64.

Miscellaneous Gastrointestinal Tract Abnormalities

71. The Non-neoplastic Large Intestine. In Fenoglio-Preiser CM, Lantz PE, Listrom MB, et al. editors: *Gastrointestinal Pathology: An Atlas and Text*, New York, 1989, Raven Press.

72. Sigel B, Machi J, Ramos JR, et al.: Ultrasonic features of pneumatosis intestinalis, *JCU* 1985;13:675-678.

73. Vernacchia FS, Jeffrey RB, Laing FC, et al.: Sonographic recognition of pneumatosis intestinalis, *AJR* 1985;145:51-52.

74. Woodruff R, McDonald JR: Benign and malignant cystic tumors of the appendix, *Surg Gynecol Obstet* 1940;71:750-755.

75. The gastrointestinal tract. In Robbins SL, Cotran RS, Kumar V, editors: *Pathologic Basis of Disease*, ed 3, Philadelphia, 1984, WB Saunders.

76. Horgan JG, Chow PP, Richter JO, et al.: Computed tomography and sonography in the recognition of mucoceles of the appendix, *AJR* 1984;143:959.

77. Puylaert JBCM: Right-sided segmental infarction of the omentum: Clinical, US, and CT findings, *Radiology* 1992; 185:169-172.

78. Bender MD, Ockner RK: Diseases of the peritoneum, mesentery and diaphragm. In Sleisenger MH, Fordtran JS, editors: *Gastrointestinal Disease*, ed 3, Philadelphia, 1983, WB Saunders.

Endosonography

79. Shorvon PJ, Lees WR, Frost RA, et al.: Upper gastrointestinal endoscopic ultrasonography in gastroenterology, *Br J Radiol* 1987;60:429-438.

80. Strohm WD, Classen M: Benign lesions of the upper GI tract by means of endoscopic ultrasonography, *Scand J Gastroenterol* 1986;21(123):41-46.

81. Takemoto T, Ito T, Aibe T, et al.: Endoscopic ultrasonography in the diagnosis of esophageal carcinoma, with particular regard to staging it for operability, *Endoscopy* 1986;18(3):22-25.

82. Bolondi L, Casanova P, Caletti GC, et al.: Primary gastric lymphoma versus gastric carcinoma: Endoscopic ultrasound evaluation, *Radiology* 1987;165:821-826.

83. Astler VB, Coller FA: The prognostic significance of direct extension of carcinoma of the colon and rectum, *Ann Surg* 1954;139:816.

84. Spiessel B, Schiebe O, Wagner G: Union International Contre le cancer (UICC) TNM Atlas, New York, 1982, Springer Verlag.

85. Wang KY, Kimmey MB, Nyberg DA, et al.: Colorectal neoplasms: Accuracy of ultrasound in demonstrating the depth of invasion, *Radiology* 1987;165:827-829.

86. Yamashita Y, Machi J, Shirouzu K, et al.: Evaluation of endorectal ultrasound for the assessment of wall invasion of rectal cancer: Report of a case, *Dis Col & Rect* 1988;31(8):617-623.

87. Hildebrandt U, Feifel G: Preoperative staging of rectal cancer by intrarectal ultrasound, *Dis Col & Rect* 1985;28(1):42-46.

88. Rifkin MD, Ehrlich SM, Marks G: Staging of rectal carcinoma: Prospective comparison of endorectal ultrasound and computed tomography, *Radiology* 1989;170:319-322.

89. Law PJ, Bartman CI: Anal endosonography: Technique and normal anatomy, *Gastrointest Radiol* 1989;14:349-353.

CHAPTER 9

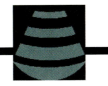

The Urinary Tract

•

Wendy Thurston, M.D., B.Sc., F.R.C.P.C.
Stephanie R. Wilson, M.D., F.R.C.P.C.

CHAPTER OUTLINE, cont'd.

The prime function of the kidney is excretion of metabolic waste product. The kidneys do this by converting more than 1700 liters of blood per day into 1 liter of highly concentrated urine.[1] The kidney is an endocrine organ secreting many hormones including erythropoietin, renin, and prostaglandins. The kidneys also function to maintain homeostasis by regulating water/salt and acid/base balance. The renal collecting system, ureters, and urethra function as conduits and the bladder as a reservoir for urinary excretion.

EMBRYOLOGY

Development of the Kidneys and Ureter

Three sets of kidneys develop in human embryos: the **pronephros, mesonephros** and **metanephros** (the permanent kidney).[2] The **pronephros** appear early in the fourth embryologic week and are rudimentary and nonfunctioning. The **mesonephros** form late in the fourth week and function as interim kidneys until the **metanephros** develop (fifth week) and begin to function (ninth week).

The **metanephros** (permanent kidneys) develop from two sources: (1) the **ureteric bud** and (2) the **metanephrogenic blastema.**[2] The ureteric bud which forms the ureter, renal pelvis, calyces, and collecting ducts interacts with and penetrates the blastema. This interaction is necessary to initiate ureteric bud branching and differentiation of nephrons within the metanephrogenic blastema (Fig. 9-1). Initially, the permanent kidneys are found in the pelvis. With fetal growth the kidneys come to lie in the upper retroperitoneum. With ascent, the kidneys rotate medially 90° so that the renal pelvis is directed anteromedially. The kidneys are in their adult location and position by the ninth gestational week. As the kidneys ascend they derive their blood supply from nearby vessels. Their adult blood supply is from the abdominal aorta.

Development of the Bladder

In the seventh gestational week the **urorectal septum** fuses with the **cloacal membrane** dividing it into a **ventral urogenital sinus** and a **dorsal rectum.** The bladder develops from the urogenital sinus. Initially, the bladder is continuous with the allantois, which eventually becomes a fibrous cord called the **urachus** (known as the *median umbilical ligament* in the adult). As the bladder enlarges, the distal portion of the mesonephric ducts are incorporated as connective tissue into the bladder trigone.[2] At the same time, the ureters come to open separately into the bladder.[2] In infants and children, the bladder is an abdominal organ and it is not until after puberty that it becomes a true pelvic structure (Fig. 9-2).[2]

Development of the Urethra

The epithelium of most of the male urethra and the entire female urethra is derived from the endoderm of the urogenital sinus.[2] The urethral connective tissue

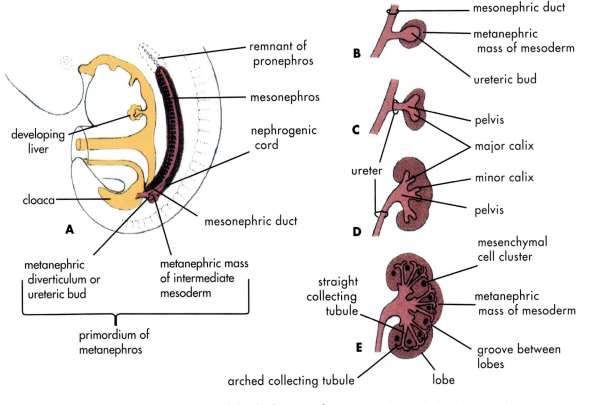

FIG. 9-1. Embryology of the kidney and ureter. A, Lateral view of a 5-week embryo showing the three embryologic kidneys that develop. **B** through **E,** Successive stages of development of the ureteric bud (fifth to eighth week) into the ureter, pelvis, calyces, and collecting tubules. (Modified from Moore KL, Persaud TVN. *The Developing Human. Clinically Oriented Embryology.* 5 ed. Philadelphia: WB Saunders; 1993.)

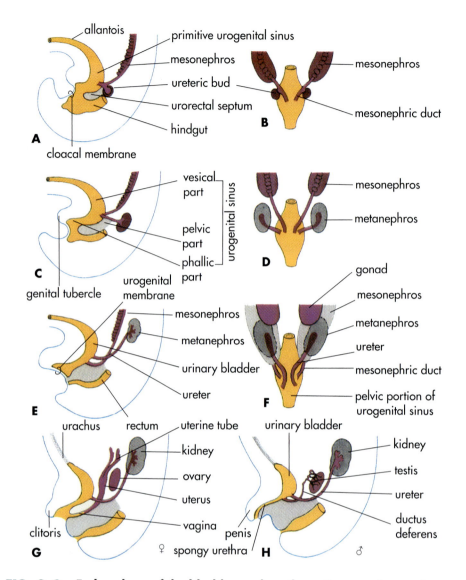

FIG. 9-2. Embryology of the bladder and urethra. Diagrams showing division of the cloaca into the urogenital sinus and rectum; absorption of the mesonephric ducts; development of the urinary bladder, urethra and urachus; and change in location of the ureters. **A** and **B**, 5-week embryo. **C** through **H**, 7- to 12-week embryo. (Modified from Moore KL, Persaud TVN. *The Developing Human. Clinically Oriented Embryology*, 5 ed. Philadelphia: WB Saunders; 1993.)

and smooth muscle form from adjacent splanchnic mesenchyme.[2]

ANATOMY

Kidney

In the adult, each kidney is about 11 cm long, 2.5 cm thick, 5 cm wide and weighs between 120 and 170 grams.[3] Emamian et al.[4] demostrated, using 665 volunteers, that parenchymal volume of the right kidney is smaller than the left. Possible explanations for this include: (1) the spleen is smaller than the liver and

there is more space for left kidney growth, and (2) the left renal artery is shorter than the right and therefore increased blood flow on the left results in increased renal volume. They also demonstrated that renal length correlates best with body height and renal size decreases with advancing age because of parenchymal reduction.

The left kidney usually lies 1 to 2 cm higher than the right.[3] The kidneys are mobile and will move depending on body position. In the supine position, the superior pole of the left kidney is at the level of the twelfth thoracic vertebrae and the inferior pole at the level of the third lumbar vertebrae.

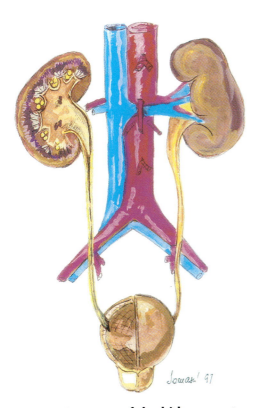

FIG. 9-3. Anatomy of the kidney, ureter, and bladder.

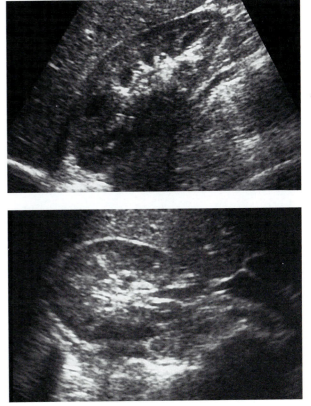

FIG. 9-4. **Normal kidney.** **A,** Sagittal and **B,** transverse sonograms demonstrating normal anatomy with corticomedullary differentiation.

The normal adult kidney is bean-shaped with a smooth convex contour anteriorly, posteriorly, and laterally. Medially, the surface is concave and known as the **renal hilum.** The renal hilum is continuous with a central cavity called the **renal sinus.** Within the renal sinus are the major branches of the renal artery, major tributaries of the renal vein, and the collecting system.[3] The remainder of the renal sinus is packed with fat. The collecting system (renal pelvis) lies posterior to the renal vessels in the renal hilum (Fig. 9-3).

The **renal parenchyma** is composed of **cortex** and **medullary pyramids.** The renal medullary pyramids are hypoechoic relative to renal cortex and can be identified in most normal adults (Fig. 9-4). The normal renal cortex has classically been described as being less echogenic than adjacent liver and spleen. Platt et al.[5] evaluated 153 patients and found that 72% of patients with renal cortical echogenicity equal to liver had normal renal function. If renal echogenicity greater than liver were used as the criterion, both specificity and positive predictive value for abnormal renal function rose to 96% and 67%, respectively. However, sensitivity is poor—only 20%.[5]

During normal development there is partial fusion of two parenchymal masses called renunculi. **Paren-**chymal junctional defects occur at the site of fusion and must not be confused with pathologic processes such as renal scars and angiomyolipoma. The junctional parenchymal defect is most typically located anteriorly and superiorly and can be traced medially and inferiorly into the renal sinus. Usually, it is oriented more horizontally than vertically, and therefore, is best appreciated on sagittal scans (Fig. 9-5).[6] It is seen more often on the right; however, when a good acoustic window is present (splenomegaly), it can also be seen on the left.

Hypertrophied column of Bertin (HCB) is a normal variant and represents unresorbed polar parenchyma from one or both of the two subkidneys that fuse to form the normal kidney.[7] **Sonographic criteria** used to allow **diagnosis** of HCB include indentation of the renal sinus laterally and bordered by a junctional parenchymal line and defect. It is usually at the junction of the upper and middle thirds of the kidney and contains renal cortex that is continuous with the adjacent renal cortex of the same subkidney. HCB contains renal pyramids. The largest dimension is less than 3 cm.[7,8]

Echogenicity of the HCB and renal cortex depends on the scan plane in relation to the tissue structures. The differences in tissue orientation produce different

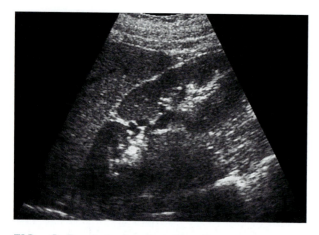

FIG. 9-5. Anterior junction line. Sagittal sonogram demonstrating the echogenic line that extends from the renal sinus to the perinephric fat.

SONOGRAPHIC CRITERIA FOR HYPERTROPHIED COLUMN OF BERTIN

Indentation of the renal sinus laterally
Bordered by a junctional parenchymal defect
Location at the junction of the upper and middle thirds
Continuous with adjacent renal cortex
Contains renal pyramids
Less than 3 cm in size

---

acoustic reflectivity.[7] The echoes of the HCB are brighter than those of adjacent renal cortex when seen en face (Fig. 9-6).[7] It may be difficult to differentiate a small avascular tumor from an HCB; however, demonstration of arcuate arteries by color Doppler indicates HCB rather than tumor. Occasionally, intravenous pyelography (IVP), computed tomography (CT) or renal scintigraphy will be required to make the differentiation.

Renal duplication artifact can occur as a result of sound beam refraction between the lower portion of the spleen or liver and adjacent fat.[9] Middleton et al.[9] analyzed duplication artifact in 20 patients and found that it mimicked duplication of the collecting system, suprarenal mass, and upper-pole renal cortical thickening. This artifact is seen most commonly on the left and in obese patients. Changing the transducer position or using deep inspiration so that the liver and spleen are interposed as an acoustic window will eliminate the false impression.

The kidney has a thin, fibrous true capsule. Outside this capsule is the perirenal fat. The fat is encased anteriorly by the **fibrous fascia of Gerota** and posteri-

orly by the **fibrous fascia of Zuckerkandl.**[10] The perirenal space is open superiorly on the right to the bare area of the liver allowing communication between the retroperitoneum and intraperitoneal space.[11] The perirenal spaces communicate with one another at the level of the third to fifth lumbar vertebrae.[11]

Ureter

The ureter is a long (30 to 34 cm)[3] mucosal-lined conduit that delivers urine from the renal pelvis to the bladder. Each ureter varies in diameter from 2 to 8 mm.[3] As the ureter enters the pelvis, it passes anterior to the common or external iliac artery. The ureter has an oblique course through the bladder wall (Fig. 9-3).

Bladder

The bladder is in the pelvis inferior and anterior to the peritoneal cavity and posterior to the pubic bones.[3] Superiorly, the peritoneum is reflected over the anterior aspect of the bladder. Within the bladder the ureteric and urethral orifices demarcate an area known as the **trigone** (Fig. 9-3). The urethral orifice marks the area known as the **bladder neck**. The bladder neck and trigone remain constant in shape and position; however, the remainder of the bladder will change shape and position depending on the volume of urine within it. Deep to the peritoneum covering the bladder lies a loose, connective tissue layer of subserosa which forms the adventitial layer of the bladder wall. Adjacent to the adventitia are three muscular layers which include: (1) outer or longitudinal muscle layer; (2) middle or circular muscle layer; and (3) internal longitudinal muscle layer. Adjacent to the muscle, the innermost layer of the bladder is composed of mucosa. The bladder wall should be smooth and of uniform thickness. The wall thickness depends on the degree of bladder distention.

GENITOURINARY TRACT SONOGRAPHY

Technical Aspects

Ability to visualize organs of the genitourinary tract sonographically is multifactorial related to (1) body habitus; (2) operator experience; and (3) type of equipment. The patient should fast a minimum of 6 hours before the examination in an attempt to limit bowel gas. High-resolution, real-time sector scanners should be used.

Scanning Technique

Kidney. The kidneys should be assessed in the transverse and coronal plane. Patient position should include the supine, oblique, lateral decubitus, and, occasionally, prone position. Usually, a combination of subcostal and intercostal approaches is necessary to

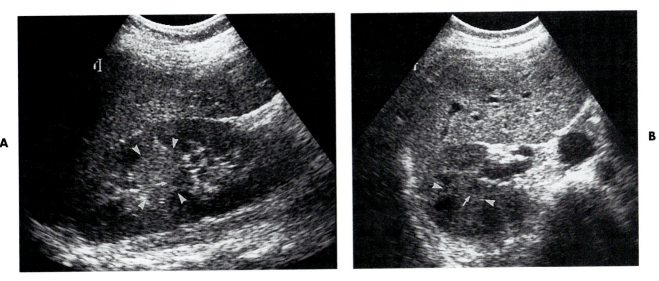

FIG. 9-6. Hypertrophied column of Bertin. A, Sagittal and B, transverse sonograms demonstrate variable echogenicity of the column (*arrowheads*) depending on the scan plane. Medullary pyramids can be seen within the hypertrophied column of Bertin (*arrow*).

fully evaluate the kidneys, particularly the upper pole of the left kidney.

Ureter. The proximal ureter is best visualized using a coronal-oblique view with the kidney as an acoustic window. An attempt is made to follow the ureter to the bladder maintaining the same approach. A nondilated ureter may be impossible to visualize because of overlying bowel gas. Transverse scanning of the retroperitoneum will often demonstrate a dilated ureter which can then be followed caudally with both transverse and sagittal imaging. In women, a dilated distal ureter can be well seen with transvaginal scanning if visualization through the abdominal wall is poor because of intervening bowel gas or if the bladder is empty.

Bladder. The bladder is best evaluated when it is moderately filled. When overfilled, patient discomfort occurs. The bladder should be scanned in the transverse and sagittal plane and occasionally in a decubitus position. To better visualize the bladder wall in women, transvaginal scanning can be helpful. If the nature of a large fluid-filled mass in the pelvis is uncertain either voiding or insertion of a Foley catheter will clarify the location and appearance of the bladder relative to the fluid-filled mass.

Urethra. The urethra in a woman can be scanned with transvaginal, transperineal or translabial sonography (Fig. 9-7).[12] The posterior or prostatic urethra in men is best visualized with endorectal probes (Fig. 9-8).

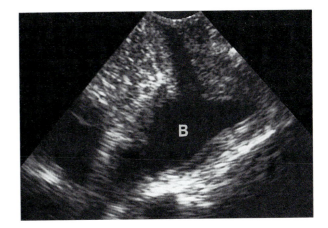

FIG. 9-7. Translabial ultrasound of the female urethra. Sagittal sonogram shows the tubular hypoechoic urethra extending from the bladder (B) to the skin surface.

CONGENITAL ANOMALIES OF THE GENITOURINARY TRACT

Anomalies Related to Renal Growth

Hypoplasia. Renal hypoplasia represents a renal parenchymal anomaly in which there are too few nephrons. Renal function is normal in proportion to the mass of the kidney. True hypoplasia is a rare anomaly. Many patients with unilateral hypoplasia are asymptomatic and the condition is found as an incidental finding. Patients with bilateral hypoplasia

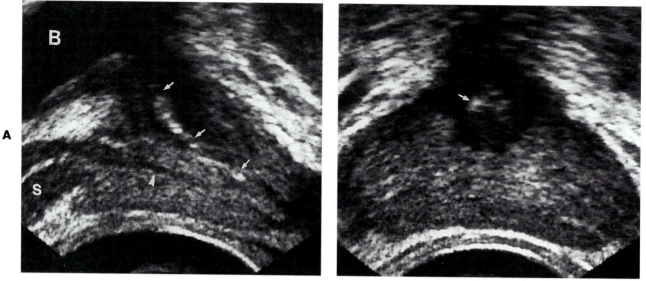

FIG. 9-8. Transrectal ultrasound of the male urethra. A. Sagittal and **B,** transverse sonograms show the urethra with calcifications in the urethral glands (*arrows*) surrounded by the echo-poor muscle of the internal urethral sphincter. Bladder, B, ejaculatory duct (*arrowhead*), seminal vesicles, S. (Courtesy of Ants Toi, MD, The Toronto Hospital.)

often have evidence of renal insufficiency. Hypoplasia is believed to result from the ureteral bud making contact with the caudal most portion of the metanephrogenic blastema. This can occur with delayed development of the ureteric bud or from delayed contact of the bud with the cranially migrating blastema. Morphologically, the diagnosis is established by the finding of fewer renal lobules which otherwise have a normal microscopic appearance.[13] **Sonographically,** the kidney is small but otherwise normal.

Fetal Lobulation. Fetal lobulation is usually present until 4 or 5 years of age; however, persistent lobulation is seen in 51% of adult kidneys.[14] There is infolding of the cortex without loss of cortical parenchyma. **On sonography,** sharp clefts are seen overlying the septa of Bertin.[15]

Compensatory Hypertrophy. Compensatory hypertrophy may be diffuse or focal and occurs when existing healthy nephrons enlarge to allow the healthy renal parenchyma to perform more work. The diffuse form is seen with **nephrectomy, renal agenesis, renal hypoplasia, renal atrophy,** or **renal dysplasia.** The focal form is seen when **residual islands of normal tissue** enlarge in an otherwise diseased kidney (**reflux nephropathy**). On sonography, **diffuse compensatory hypertrophy** reveals an enlarged but otherwise normal kidney. In **nodular compensatory hypertrophy,** large areas of nodular normal renal tissue are seen between scars and may mimic a solid renal mass (Fig. 9-9).[15]

Anomalies Related to Ascent of the Kidney

Ectopia. Failure of the kidney to ascend during embryologic development results in a **pelvic kidney** which is estimated to occur in 1 in 724 pediatric autopsies.[15] These kidneys are often small and abnormally rotated. Fifty percent of pelvic kidneys have decreased function.[15] The ureters are often short. These kidneys are prone to poor drainage and may develop dilatation of the collecting system with susceptibility to infection and stone formation. The blood supply is derived from the regional vessels, usually the common or internal iliac artery, and is often multiple. If the kidney ascends too high, it may pass through the foramen of Bochdalek and became a true **thoracic kidney.** This is usually of no clinical significance. On sonography, the kidney location can usually be ascertained if not found in its normal location (Fig. 9-10). Particularly with kidneys that have ascended too high, ultrasound is helpful to determine whether or not the diaphragm is intact.

Crossed Renal Ectopia. In crossed renal ectopia, both kidneys are found on the same side. In 85% to 90% of cases, the ectopic kidney will be fused to the other kidney. The upper pole of the ectopic kidney is usually fused to the lower pole of the other kidney, although fusion may occur anywhere. The incidence at autopsy is one in 1000 to 1500.[14] Embryologically, there is fusion of the metanephrogenic blastema, which does not allow proper rotation

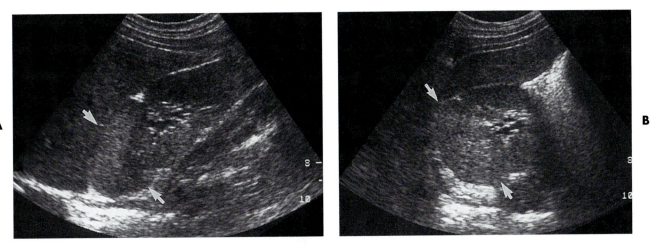

FIG. 9-9. Nodular compensatory hypertrophy. A, Sagittal and B, transverse sonograms demonstrate nodular compensatory hypertrophy predominantly in the upper pole related to reflux and chronic asymmetric pyelonephritis. This area of nodular hypertrophy mimics a solid renal mass (*arrows*).

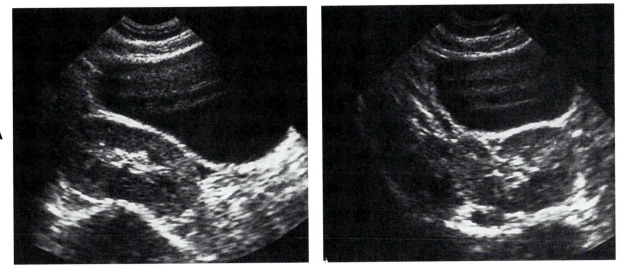

FIG. 9-10. Pelvic kidney. A, Sagittal and B, transverse sonograms demonstrate a kidney posterior to the bladder.

or ascent; therefore, both kidneys are more caudally located. The ureterovesicle junctions will be located in their normal position. **On sonography,** both kidneys will be on the same side with the majority demonstrating fusion (Fig. 9-11). In patients with renal colic, the knowledge that the ureterovesicle junctions are normally located is particularly important.

Horseshoe Kidney. Horseshoe kidney occurs with an incidence of 0.01% to 0.25%. These kidneys fail to rotate properly and often demonstrate ureteropelvic junction obstruction, which leads to an increased incidence of infection and stone formation. The horseshoe kidney sits anterior to the abdominal great vessels and derives its blood supply from the

aorta and other regional vessels such as inferior mesenteric, common iliac, internal iliac, and external iliac arteries. Fusion of the metanephrogenic blastema usually at the lower poles (95%) prior to ascent will result in a horseshoe kidney. Usually, the isthmus is composed of functioning renal tissue, although sometimes it may be a fibrous connection. Associated anomalies include ureteropelvic junction obstruction, vesicoureteral reflux, collecting system duplication, renal dysplasia, retrocaval ureter, supernumerary kidney, anorectal malformation, esophageal atresia, rectovaginal fistula, omphalocoele, and cardiovascular and skeletal abnormalities. **On sonography,** the kidneys are usually lower than normal with the lower

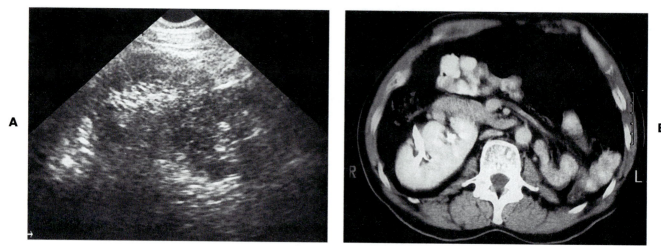

FIG. 9-11. Cross-fused ectopia. A, Sagittal sonogram demonstrates two kidneys fused to each other. B, Confirmatory computed tomography.

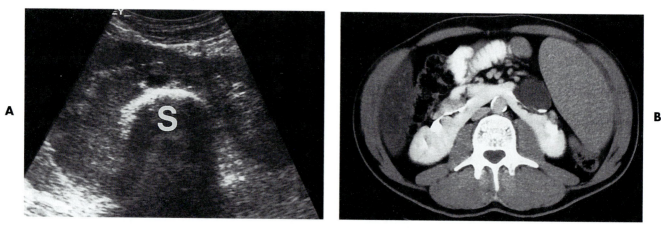

FIG. 9-12. Horseshoe kidney. A, Transverse sonogram shows the isthmus crossing anterior to the retroperitoneal great vessels with the renal parenchyma of each limb of the horseshoe draping over the spine (S). B, Confirmatory computed tomography.

poles projecting medially. Transverse imaging of the retroperitoneum will demonstrate the renal isthmus crossing the midline anterior to the abdominal great vessels (Fig. 9-12). Pelvicaliectasis and collecting system stones may be evident.

Anomalies Related to the Ureteral Bud

Renal Agenesis. Renal agenesis may be unilateral or bilateral. Bilateral renal agenesis is a rare anomaly incompatible with life and found in 0.04% of autopsies with a 3:1 male predominance.[14] Unilateral renal agenesis is usually an incidental finding with the remaining kidney demonstrating compensatory hypertrophy. Renal agenesis will occur when there is: (1) absence of the metanephrogenic blastema; (2) absence of ureteral bud development; or (3) absence of interaction and penetration of the ureteral bud with the metanephrogenic blastema. Renal agenesis is as-

sociated with genital tract anomalies which are often cystic pelvic masses in both men and women. Other associated anomalies include skeletal abnormalities, anorectal malformations, and cryptorchism. **On sonography,** the kidney is absent; however, a normal adrenal gland is usually found. The adrenal gland will be absent in 8% to 17%.[15] It may be difficult to differentiate between renal agenesis and a small hypoplastic or dysplastic kidney. The other kidney will demonstrate compensatory hypertrophy with all these conditions. Usually, the colon falls into the empty renal bed and care should be taken not to confuse a loop of gut as a normal kidney.

Supernumerary Kidney. Supernumerary kidneys are an exceedingly rare anomaly. The supernumerary kidney is usually smaller than normal and can be found above, below, in front of, or behind the normal kidney. The supernumerary kidney often has

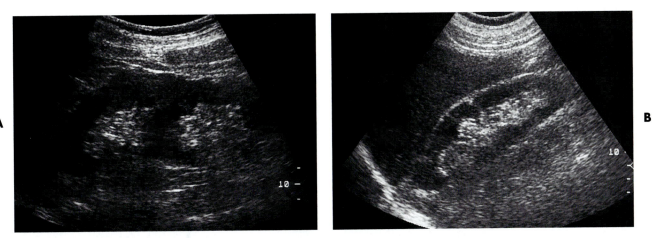

FIG. 9-13. Supernumerary kidney. Sagittal sonograms demonstrate **A,** two fused kidneys on the left and **B,** normal right kidney.

only a few calyces and a single infundibulum. The formation of a supernumerary kidney is likely caused by the same mechanism as that which gives rise to a duplex collecting system.[14] Two ureteric buds reach the metanephrogenic blastema which then divides or there are two blastema initially present. **On sonography,** an extra kidney will be found (Fig. 9-13).

Duplex Collecting System and Ureterocoele.
Duplex collecting system is the most common congenital anomaly of the urinary tract with a reported incidence of 0.5% to 10% of all live births.[14] The degree of duplication is variable. Duplication is **complete** when there are two separate collecting systems and two separate ureters, each with their own ureteral orifice. Duplication is **incomplete** when the ureters join and enter the bladder through a single ureteral orifice. Ureteropelvic duplication arises when two ureteral buds form and join with the metanephrogenic blastema or when there is division of a single ureteral bud early in embryogenesis. Normally during embryologic development, the ureteral orifice migrates superiorly and laterally to become part of the bladder trigone. With complete duplication, the ureter from the lower pole of the kidney migrates to assume its normal location, whereas the ureter draining the superior pole of the kidney doesn't migrate normally resulting in a more medial and inferior located ureteral orifice. There is an increased incidence of ureteropelvic junction obstruction and uterus didelphys.[15]

In complete duplication, the ureter draining the lower pole has a more perpendicular course through the bladder wall making it more prone to reflux. The ectopic ureter from the upper pole is prone to obstruction, reflux or both. If obstruction is present, it can result in cystic dilatation of the intramural portion of the ureter giving rise to a **ureterocoele.** Ureterocoeles may

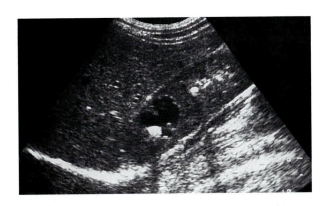

FIG. 9-14. Duplex collecting system. Sagittal sonogram shows central parenchyma separating the upper- and lower-pole moieties. There is moderate dilatation of the upper moiety. Each moiety contains an echogenic focus with distal acoustic shadowing representing small stones.

be uni- or bilateral and may occur in normal, duplicated, and ectopic ureters. Clinically, ureterocoeles may produce obstruction and give rise to recurrent or persistent urinary tract infections. If large, they may block the contralateral ureteral orifice and/or the urethral orifice at the bladder neck. Ureterocoele treatment is surgical. Ureterocoeles are a common observation at sonography on asymptomatic patients. They are often transient, incidental, and insignificant.

On sonography, a duplex collecting system is seen as two central echogenic renal sinuses with intervening bridging renal parenchyma. Unfortunately, this sign is insensitive and only seen in 17% of duplex kidneys.[16] Hydronephrosis of the upper pole moiety and visualization of two distinct collecting systems and ureters are diagnostic (Fig. 9-14). The bladder should always

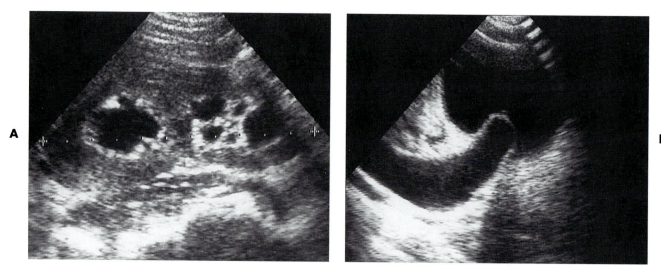

FIG. 9-15. Duplex kidney with a ureterocoele. Sagittal sonograms reveal **A,** duplex system with dilatation in both the upper and lower moiety. **B,** Ureterocoele of the upper moiety at the ureterovesicle junction.

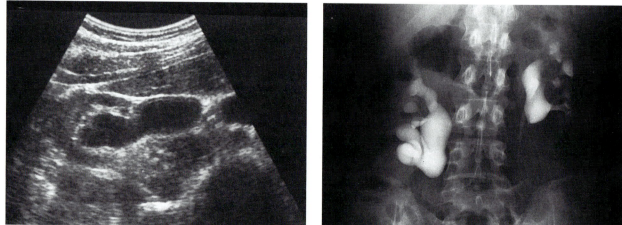

FIG. 9-16. Ureteropelvic junction obstruction. **A,** Transverse sonogram demonstrates marked ballooning of the renal pelvis with associated proximal caliectasis. **B,** Intravenous pyelogram reveals bilateral ureteropelvic junction obstruction.

be carefully evaluated for the presence of a ureterocoele. A ureterocoele will appear as a round, cystlike structure within the bladder (Fig. 9-15). Occasionally, it may be large enough to occupy the entire bladder with obstruction of the bladder neck.

Ureteropelvic Junction Obstruction. Ureteropelvic junction (UPJ) obstruction is a common anomaly and found in men with a 2:1 predominance. The left kidney is affected twice as frequently as the right. It is bilateral in 10% to 30%.[17] Most adult patients will present with chronic vague back or flank pain. Symptomatic patients or patients with complications including superimposed infection, stones, or impairment of renal function will be treated. There is an increased incidence of contralateral multicystic

dysplastic kidney and renal agenesis. It is believed that most idiopathic UPJ obstructions are functional rather than anatomic.[17] Histologic evaluation of affected resected specimens has demonstrated excessive collagen between muscle bundles, deficient or absent muscle, and excessive longitudinal muscle.[17] Occasionally, intrinsic valves, true luminal stenosis, and aberrant arteries are the cause of obstruction. **On sonography,** pelvicaliectasis is present to the level of the UPJ (Fig. 9-16). Often marked ballooning of the renal pelvis is present, and if long-standing, there will be associated renal parenchymal atrophy. The ureter is of normal caliber. Careful evaluation of the contralateral kidney should be performed to assess for the presence of associated anomalies.

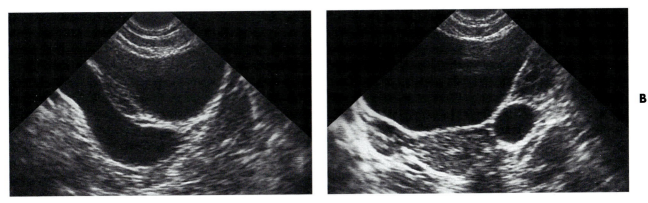

FIG. 9-17. Congenital megaureter. A, Sagittal and B, transverse sonograms show fusiform dilatation of the distal ureter. Associated pelvicaliectasis may or may not be present.

Congenital Megacalyces. Congenital megacalyces is an entity producing nonobstructive enlargement of the calyces which is usually unilateral. It is nonprogressive and patients have normal renal function and parenchyma. There is an increased incidence of infection and stone formation because of calyceal enlargement. The exact pathogenesis is speculative. The most common association is with primary megaureter.[18] **On sonography,** enlarged clubbed calyces are seen which are usually increased in number. Papillary impressions are absent. Cortical thickness is maintained.

Congenital Megaureter. Congenital megaureter results in functional ureteric obstruction. The distal most segment of ureter is aperistaltic giving rise to a wide spectrum of findings, ranging from insignificant distal ureterectasis to progressive hydroureteronephrosis. Men are more commonly affected as is the left side.[17] Eight percent to 50% of patients will demonstrate bilateral involvement. **On sonography,** fusiform dilatation of the distal third of the ureter is classic (Fig. 9-17). Depending on the severity, associated pelvicaliectasis may or may not be present. The ureter will demonstrate normal or increased peristalsis with the waves disappearing at the distal aperistaltic segment. Calculi may form just proximal to the adynamic segment.

Anomalies Related to Vascular Development

Aberrant Vessels. As the kidney ascends during embryologic development, it derives its blood supply from the aorta at successively higher levels with regression of the lower level vessels. If the lower level vessels persist, aberrant renal arteries will be present. Aberrant vessels can compress the ureter anywhere along its course, giving rise to obstruction. With color Doppler, aberrant vessels may be seen crossing the ureter at the level of ureteric obstruction.

Retrocaval Ureter. Retrocaval ureter is a rare but well-recognized congenital anomaly. There is a 3:1 predominance in men with most patients presenting with pain in the second to fourth decade of life. Normally, the infrarenal inferior vena cava (IVC) develops from the supracardinal vein. If this portion of the cava develops from the subcardinal vein, the ureter will pass posterior to the IVC. The ureter then passes medially and anteriorly between the aorta and IVC to cross the right iliac vessels. It then enters the pelvis and bladder in a normal fashion. **On sonography,** there will be pelvicaliectasis and proximal hydroureter to the level where the ureter turns medial to pass posterior to the IVC.

Anomalies Related to Bladder Development

Agenesis. Bladder agenesis is a rare anomaly. Most infants with bladder agenesis are stillborn with virtually all surviving infants being female.[19] Often, many associated anomalies are present. **Sonographically** the bladder is absent.

Duplication. Bladder duplication has been divided into three types:
- **Type 1**—A peritoneal fold, which may be complete or incomplete, separates the two bladders.
- **Type 2**—An internal septum is present dividing the bladder. The septum may be complete or incomplete and be oriented in a sagittal or coronal plane. There may be multiple septae.
- **Type 3**—There is a transverse band of muscle dividing the bladder into two unequal cavities.[15]

Exstrophy. Bladder exstrophy occurs in 1 in 30,000 live births.[15] There is a 2:1 predominance in males.[15] Failure in development of the mesoderm below the umbilicus leads to absence of the lower abdominal and anterior bladder wall. There is a high incidence of associated musculoskeletal, gastrointestinal,

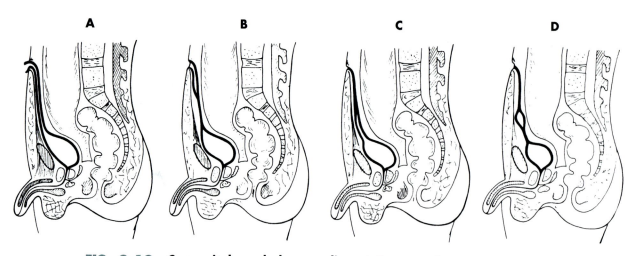

FIG. 9-18. **Congenital urachal anomalies.** **A,** Patent urachus. **B,** Urachal sinus. **C,** Urachal diverticulum. **D,** Urachal cyst. (Modified from Schnyder P, Candardjis G. Vesicourachal diverticulum: CT diagnosis in two adults. *AJR* 1981;137:1063-1065.)

and genital tract anomalies. These patients have an increased incidence of bladder carcinoma (200×) which is adenocarcinoma in 90% of cases.[15]

Urachal Anomalies. Normally, the urachus closes in the last half of fetal life.[15] There are four types of congenital urachal anomalies.[15,20,21] There is a 2:1 predominance in males.

- **patent urachus** (50%)
- **urachal cyst** (30%)
- **urachal sinus** (15%)
- **urachal diverticulum** (5%) (Fig. 9-18)

A **patent urachus** is usually associated with urethral obstruction and serves as a protective mechanism to allow normal fetal development. A **urachal cyst** forms if the urachus closes at the umbilical and bladder ends but remains patent in between. The cyst is usually situated in the lower one third of the urachus. There is an increased incidence of adenocarcinoma. On sonography, a cyst with or without internal echoes is seen superior to the bladder near the midline. A **urachal sinus** forms when the urachus closes at the bladder end but remains patent at the umbilicus. A **urachal diverticulum** forms if the urachus closes at the umbilical end but remains patent at the bladder. They are usually incidentally found. There is, however, an increased incidence of carcinoma and stone formation. Sonographically, an outpouching at the bladder fundus is noted.

Anomalies Related to Urethral Development

Diverticulum. The majority of **urethral diverticula** are acquired through injury or infection, although some are congenital developmental anomalies. Most urethral diverticula in women form as a result of infection of the periurethral glands. Some may be related to childbirth. Most are found in the midurethra and are bilateral. Often, a fluctuant anterior vaginal mass is felt. Stones may develop because of urinary stasis. **Transvaginal** or **translabial scanning** may demonstrate a simple or complex cystic structure communicating with the urethra through a thin neck.

INFECTIONS OF THE GENITOURINARY TRACT

Pyelonephritis

Acute Pyelonephritis. Acute pyelonephritis is a tubulointerstitial inflammation of the kidney. Two routes may give rise to inflammation and these are: (1) **ascending infection** (*Escherichia coli*) 85% and (2) **hematogenous seeding** (*Staphylococcus aureus*) 15%. Women 15 to 35 years of age are most commonly affected.[22] Two percent of pregnant women will develop acute pyelonephritis.[23] Most adults present with flank pain and fever and can be diagnosed clinically with the aid of laboratory studies (bacteriuria, pyuria, leukocytosis). Treatment with appropriate antibiotics results in rapid improvement in both clinical and laboratory findings. Imaging is only necessary to rule out potential complications (such as renal or perirenal abscess development) when symptoms and laboratory abnormalities persist. The Society of Uroradiology has proposed a simplified terminology describing acutely infected kidneys.[24] The term *acute pyelonephritis* should be used, thus eliminating the need for terms such as *bacterial nephritis, lobar nephronia, renal cellulitis, lobar nephritis, renal phlegmon,* and *renal carbuncle.*[24]

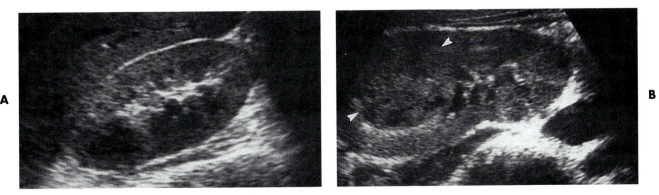

FIG. 9-19. Acute pyelonephritis. Sagittal sonograms show **A,** enlarged swollen kidney with loss of corticomedullary differentiation. **B,** Focal hypoechoic mass (*arrowheads*) with compression of the central renal sinus.

On sonography, the majority of kidneys with acute pyelonephritis appear normal. If abnormality is present, the following can be seen (Fig. 9-19):

- **renal enlargement**
- **compression of the renal sinus**
- **alteration of the echotexture which may be hypoechoic (edema) or hyperechoic (hemorrhage)**
- **loss of corticomedullary differentiation**
- **poorly marginated mass(es)**
- **gas within the renal parenchyma.**[23,24]

Sonography is less sensitive than CT or Tc-99m DMSA cortical scintigraphy for demonstrating changes of acute pyelonephritis but is more accessible and less expensive and therefore an excellent screening modality for the development and follow-up of complications. Ultrasound also is an excellent modality in the assessment of pregnant patients with acute pyelonephritis because of its lack of ionizing radiation.[23,24]

Renal and Perinephric Abscess. Untreated or inadequately treated acute pyelonephritis may lead to parenchymal necrosis with abscess formation. Patients at increased risk for abscess development include those with diabetes, urinary tract obstruction, infected renal stones, immune compromise, IV drug abuse, or chronic debilitating disease.[23,25] **Renal abscesses** tend to be solitary and may spontaneously decompress into the collecting system or perinephric space. **Perinephric abscess** may also result from a ruptured pyonephrosis, direct extension of peritoneal or retroperitoneal infection, or following intervention such as surgery, endoscopy, or percutaneous procedures.[23] Small abscesses may be treated conservatively with antibiotics, whereas larger ones will require percutaneous drainage and, if unsuccessful, surgery.

On sonography, a renal abscess will appear as a round, thick-walled hypoechoic complex mass often with some through transmission (Fig. 9-20). Internal

ACUTE PYELONEPHRITIS ON SONOGRAPHY
Renal enlargement
Compression of the renal sinus
Abnormal echotexture
Loss of corticomedullary differentiation
Poorly marginated mass(es)
Gas within the renal parenchyma

mobile debris may be seen. Occasionally, gas with dirty shadowing may be noted within the abscess. Septations may be present. The **differential diagnosis** includes: (1) hemorrhagic or infected cysts; (2) parasitic cysts; (3) multiloculated cysts; and (4) cystic neoplasm. Sonography is not as accurate as CT in determining the presence and extent of perinephric abscess extension.[23] Sonography is, however, an excellent modality for following patients with abscesses that are being treated conservatively to document resolution.

Pyonephrosis. Pyonephrosis implies purulent material in an obstructed collecting system. Depending on the level of obstruction, any portion of the collecting system including the ureter can be affected. Early diagnosis and treatment are crucial to prevent development of bacteremia and life-threatening septic shock. The mortality rate of bacteremia and septic shock is 25% and 50%, respectively.[26] Fifteen percent of patients will be asymptomatic at presentation.[27] In the young adult, ureteropelvic junction obstruction and stones are the most frequent cause of pyonephrosis development, whereas malignant ureteral obstruction is usually the cause in the elderly.[23] **On sonography,** hydronephrosis with or without hydroureter will be seen. Mobile collecting system debris

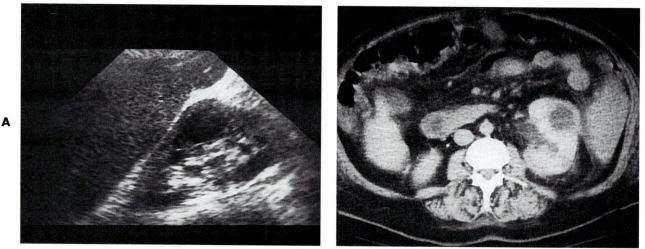

FIG. 9-20. **Renal abscess.** **A,** Sagittal sonogram shows a hypoechoic mass in the renal parenchyma. **B,** Confirmatory computed tomography reveals the abscess with inflammatory change in the perinephric fat.

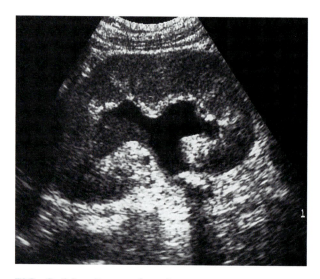

FIG. 9-21. **Pyonephrosis.** Sagittal sonogram shows an echogenic focus with shadowing at the ureteropelvic junction representing a stone. Associated hydronephrosis is present, containing debris in the upper-pole calyces.

with or without a fluid-debris level, collecting system gas, and stones can be seen (Fig. 9-21).

Emphysematous Pyelonephritis. Emphysematous pyelonephritis (EPN) is an uncommon, life-threatening infection of the renal parenchyma characterized by gas formation. Most patients are women (2:1) and diabetic (90%) with a mean age of 55. Twenty percent of diabetic patients with EPN will have urinary obstruction compared with nondiabetic patients in whom urinary tract obstruction is present in 75%. Bilateral disease occurs in 5% to 10%. *Escherichia coli* is the offending organism in 62% to 70%, Klebsiella 9%, Pseudomonas 2%, with Proteus,

Aerobacter, and Candida occasionally involved.[23,25] At presentation most patients are extremely ill with fever, flank pain, hyperglycemia, acidosis, dehydration, and electrolyte imbalance.[28] Eighteen percent of patients will present only with fever of unknown origin.[29]

Wan et al.[30] retrospectively studied 38 patients with EPN and identified two types of disease. **EPN1** was characterized by parenchymal destruction with presence of streaky or mottled gas. **EPN2** was characterized as either renal or perirenal fluid collections with bubbly or loculated gas or gas in the collecting system. They found the mortality rate for EPN1 and for EPN2 was 69% and 18%, respectively. They postulate that the difference between EPN1 and EPN2 is related to the severity of immune compromise of the patient as well as to the vascular insufficiency of the affected kidney. Emergency nephrectomy is the treatment of choice of EPN1, whereas percutaneous drainage is recommended for patients with EPN2. CT is the preferred method to image patients with EPN to determine the location and extent of renal and perirenal gas. **Sonographic evaluation** can be difficult, because gas will produce echogenic foci with distal dirty shadowing obscuring visualization of deeper structures. The gas could potentially be misinterpreted as bowel gas or renal calculi (Figs. 9-22 and 9-23).[31]

Chronic Pyelonephritis. Chronic pyelonephritis is an interstitial nephritis often associated with vesicoureteric reflux. Reflux nephropathy is believed to cause 10% to 30% of all cases of end-stage renal disease.[32] Chronic pyelonephritis usually begins in childhood and is more common in women. The renal changes may be unilateral or bilateral but usually are asymmetric. Reflux into the collecting tubules occurs when the papillary duct orifices are

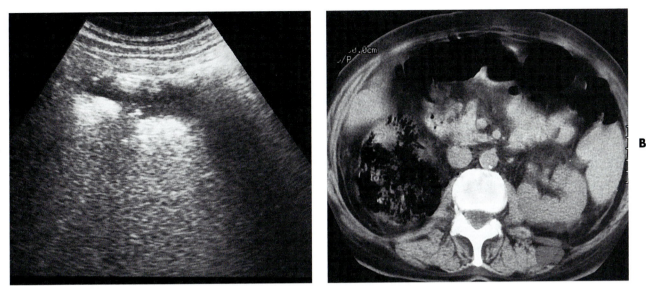

FIG. 9-22. Emphysematous pyelonephritis (type 1). A, Sagittal sonogram of right renal bed reveals extensive air obscuring visualization. The kidney cannot be visualized. B, Computed tomography demonstrates diffuse parenchymal destruction of the right kidney with extensive mottled gas. Caution must be exercised to avoid missing this diagnosis altogether on ultrasound. Failure to see a kidney in a septic patient warrants computed tomography scan.

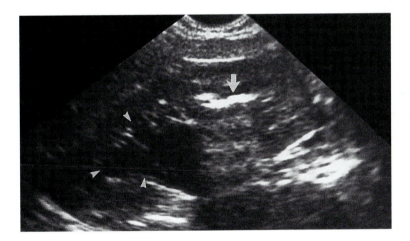

FIG. 9-23. Emphysematous pyelonephritis (type 2). Sagittal sonogram shows a dilated collecting system (*arrowheads*) containing air (*arrow*) which appears as a bright, non-dependent echogenic line with dirty shadowing.

incompetent. This occurs more often in compound papillae which are typically found at the poles of the kidneys. Cortical scarring, therefore, tends to be predominantly polar overlying the involved calyx. There is associated papillary retraction with calyceal clubbing. **On sonography,** a dilated blunt calyx is seen associated with an overlying cortical scar or cortical atrophy (Fig. 9-24).[33] These changes may be multicentric and bilateral. If the disease is unilateral, there may be compensatory hypertrophy of the contralateral kidney. If the disease is multicentric,

compensatory hypertrophy of normal intervening parenchyma may create islands of normal tissue simulating a tumor (Fig. 9-9).

Xanthogranulomatous Pyelonephritis. Xanthogranulomatous pyelonephritis (XGP) is a chronic, suppurative renal infection causing destruction of renal parenchyma and replacement of it with lipid-laden macrophages. The disease is usually unilateral and may be **diffuse, segmental,** or **focal.** XGP is usually associated with nephrolithiasis (70%) and obstructive nephropathy.[34,35,36] The disease is found

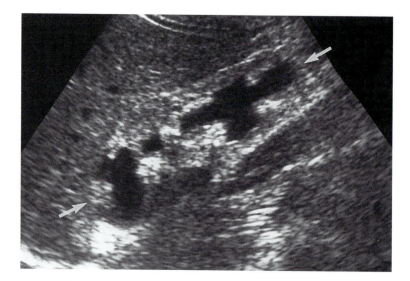

FIG. 9-24. Chronic pyelonephritis. Sagittal sonogram demonstrates echogenic parenchyma with atrophy most marked at the renal poles (*arrows*). Dilatation of the collecting system is from chronic vesicoureteric reflux.

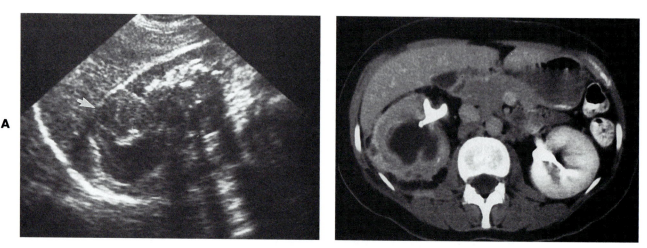

A

B

FIG. 9-25. Xanthogranulomatous pyelonephritis. **A,** Sagittal sonogram demonstrates a large central mass with calcification. Calyceal dilatation with purulent debris is noted (*arrow*). **B,** Confirmatory computed tomography shows a large staghorn calculus with proximal hydronephrosis and multiple intrarenal abscesses.

most commonly in middle-aged women and diabetics.[36] Presenting signs are nonspecific and include pain, mass, weight loss, and urinary tract infection (Proteus or *E. coli*).[34] In the diffuse variety, the kidney is usually nonfunctioning. **On sonography,** the **diffuse variety** will show renal enlargement with maintenance of the reniform shape and lack of corticomedullary differentiation. Multiple hypoechoic areas are seen corresponding to dilated calyces or inflammatory parenchymal masses.[34] Through transmission is variable depending on the degree of liquefaction of the parenchymal masses. The central renal sinus may be extremely echogenic with shadowing corresponding to a large staghorn calculus (Fig. 9-25). Perinephric extension may be present and is

often best appreciated with CT. Occasionally, in the diffuse variety, the kidney demonstrates large complex cystic masses with irregular thick walls and fluid levels mimicking pyonephrosis. **Segmental XGP** will be seen as one or more hypoechoic masses often associated with a single calyx.[34,37] An obstructing calculus may be seen near the papilla.[34] **Focal XGP** arises in the renal cortex and does not communicate with the renal pelvis. It cannot be distinguished sonographically from tumor or abscess.[34]

Papillary Necrosis

Many causative factors are implicated in the ischemia leading to the development of papillary necrosis and these include: (1) **analgesic abuse,** (2) **diabetes,** (3)

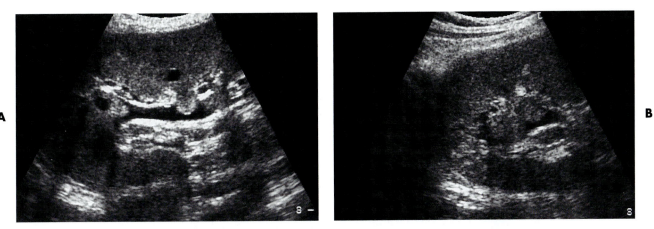

FIG. 9-26. **Papillary necrosis.** **A,** Sagittal and **B,** transverse sonograms show swollen bulbous papillae.

SONOGRAPHIC FINDINGS OF PAPILLARY NECROSIS

Swollen pyramids
Papillary cavitation
Adjacent clubbed calyx
Sloughed papilla in the collecting system that can
    calcify and simulate a stone
Sloughed papilla may cause obstruction

---

urinary tract infection; (4) **renal vein thrombosis**; (5) **prolonged hypotension**; (6) **urinary tract obstruction**; (7) **dehydration**; (8) **sickle cell anemia; and** (9) **hemophilia.**[38] Initially, the papilla swells and then a communication with the calyceal system occurs. Central papillary cavitation then occurs and the papilla may slough. Occasionally, a necrotic papilla may calcify. The **sonographic findings** parallel the pathologic changes. Swollen pyramids may be seen but are difficult to recognize sonographically (Fig. 9-26). With papillary cavitation, cystic collections within the medullary pyramids will be noted. If the papilla sloughs, the affected adjacent calyx will be clubbed. The sloughed papilla can be seen in the collecting system as an echogenic nonshadowing structure. If it calcifies distal acoustic shadowing simulating a stone will be seen.[39] If the sloughed papilla passes into the ureter, obstruction may occur with development of hydronephrosis.

Tuberculosis

Urinary tract tuberculosis (TB) occurs with hematogenous seeding of the kidney by *Mycobacterium tuberculosis* from an extraurinary source, most commonly the lung. Urinary tract TB usually will manifest itself 5 to 10 years following the initial pulmonary infection.[40] Chest x-rays can be normal (35% to 50%) or demonstrate active (10%) or inactive healed TB (40% to 55%).[40] Most patients present with lower urinary tract signs and symptoms which include frequency, dysuria, nocturia, urgency, and gross (25%) or microscopic (75%) hematuria. Approximately 10% to 20% of patients will be asymptomatic.[40] Urinalysis demonstrating sterile pyuria, microscopic hematuria, and acid pH suggests urinary tract TB. Definitive diagnosis is demonstration of acid-fast bacilli in the urine however, this usually requires 6 to 8 weeks for growth.

Even though both kidneys are seeded initially, clinical manifestations are usually unilateral. The **early or acute changes** include development of bilateral multiple small tuberculomas. Das et al.[41] reviewed the sonographic features of genitourinary TB in 20 patients. They found the most frequently encountered abnormality was focal renal lesions. Small focal lesions (5 to 15 mm) were echogenic or were hypoechoic with an echogenic rim. Larger focal lesions (> 15 mm) were of mixed echogenicity with poorly defined borders. Bilateral disease was noted in 30% of their patients. Most will heal spontaneously or following antituberculous therapy. At some later date (can be years), one or more of the tubercles may enlarge. With enlargement, cavitation and communication with the collecting system will occur with changes resembling papillary necrosis. Papillary involvement is noted when a sonolucent linear tract is seen extending from the involved calyx into the papilla. Soft tissue calyceal masses representing sloughed papilla can be seen. Following rupture into the collecting system, *M. tuberculosis* bacilluria develops and allows the spread of the renal infection to other parts of the urinary tract. Spasm or edema in the region of the ureterovesicle junction (UVJ) may occur, giving rise to pelvicaliectasis and

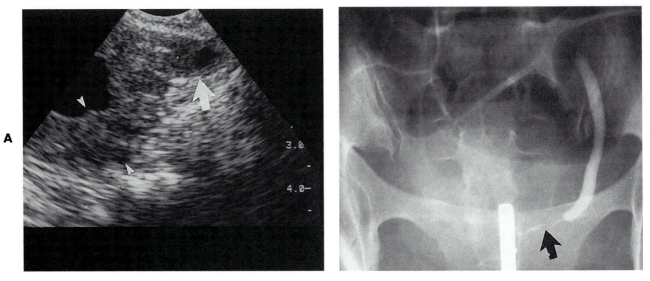

FIG. 9-27. Acute urinary bladder tuberculosis. A, Transverse transvaginal sonogram shows marked urothelial thickening of left bladder wall (*arrowheads*) and of the distal left ureter at the ureterovesicle junction (*arrow*). B, Retrograde pyelogram on left shows a ureterovesicle junction stricture (*arrow*).

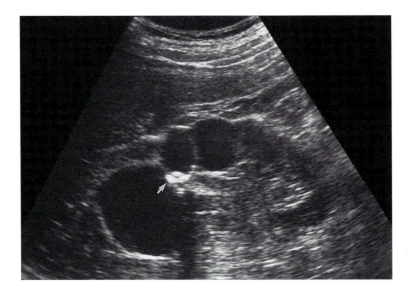

FIG. 9-28. Chronic renal tuberculosis. Sagittal sonogram shows upper- and midpole calyceal clubbing with marked overlying parenchymal atrophy. A focal area of calcification (*arrow*) in the region of the upper-pole infundibulum is noted.

hydroureter. Ureteric linear ulcers may also occur most commonly in the distal portion. Involvement of the bladder is frequent and is responsible for the initial clinical symptoms of dysuria and frequency. The early bladder manifestations include mucosal edema and ulceration. If edema occurs at the bladder trigone, ureteric obstruction may occur. Bladder involvement will be seen in 33% of patients with genitourinary tract TB.[41] Bladder wall tuberculomas may be single or multiple and can be quite large (Fig. 9-27).

The **later or more chronic changes** of genitourinary tract TB include fibrotic strictures, extensive cavitation, calcification, mass lesions, perinephric abscess, and fistula.[40] It is the chronic changes, in particular those related to fibrotic strictures that result in significant renal damage. Strictures may occur anywhere in the intrarenal collecting system and ureter. The obstruction then results in proximal collecting system dilatation and pressure atrophy of the renal parenchyma (Fig. 9-28). With time, calcification in the areas of caseation or sloughed papilla may occur. If renal infection ruptures into the perinephric space, an abscess may develop. If the perinephric abscess extends to involve adjacent viscera, fistula formation can occur. Eventually, the

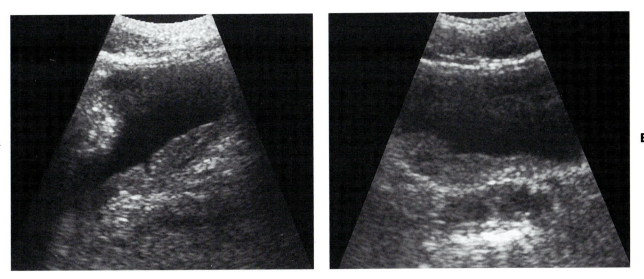

FIG. 9-29. **Bladder schistosomiasis.** **A,** Sagittal and **B,** transverse sonograms reveal asymmetric bladder wall thickening.

kidney will become nonfunctioning, small and totally calcified (**autonephrectomy or putty kidney**). In the bladder, chronic fibrotic healing results in a thick-walled, small symmetric bladder.[40] Speckled or curvilinear calcification of the bladder wall may occur but is rare.[42]

Most cases of genitourinary tract TB can be diagnosed with a combination of IVP, retrograde pyelography, ultrasound, and CT. Premkmar et al.[43] demonstrated in 14 patients with advanced urinary tract TB that detailed morphologic information and functional renal status are best assessed with CT and urography. Das et al.[44] demonstrated that ultrasound-guided, fine-needle aspiration is useful in making the diagnosis of renal TB in patients with negative urine cultures and in defining the nature of obvious sonographic lesions in patients with positive urine cultures.

Unusual Infections

Fungal. Patients with diabetes mellitus, indwelling catheters, malignancy, hematopoietic disorders, chronic antibiotic or steroid therapy, transplant, and IV drug abuse are at increased risk for developing fungal infections of the urinary tract.[45]

Candida albicans. Candida albicans is the most common fungal agent that affects the urinary tract. Renal parenchymal involvement usually occurs with diffuse systemic involvement. Multiple small focal parenchymal abscesses occur which may calcify with time.[46] Extension into the perinephric space is possible. Invasion of the collecting system may occur ultimately resulting in formation of **fungal balls.** They need to be differentiated from **blood clot, radiolucent stones, transitional cell tumors, sloughed** **papilla, fibroepithelial polyps, cholesteatomas,** and **leukoplakia.**[47,48] On sonography, the microabscesses appear similar to bacterial abscesses and are small hypoechoic parenchymal masses. **Fungus balls** appear as echogenic nonshadowing soft tissue masses within the collecting system. Fungus balls are mobile and may cause obstruction leading to development of hydronephrosis.

Parasitic. In third-world countries parasitic infections are common. For all practical purposes, there are three parasitic infections of the urinary tract that need to be considered: (1) **schistosomiasis;** (2) **echinococcus (hydatid disease);** and (3) **filariasis.**

Schistosomiasis. *Schistosoma haematobium* is the most common agent to affect the urinary tract. The worms enter the human host by penetrating the skin. They are then carried via the portal venous system to the liver where they mature into their adult form. *S. haematobium* likely enters the perivesical venous plexus from the hemorrhoidal plexus.[50] The female worm then deposits eggs into the venules of the bladder wall and ureter. Granuloma formation and obliterative endarteritis occur. Serological tests demonstrating ova allow diagnosis. Hematuria is the most frequent complaint.[50] **On sonography,** the kidneys are normal until late in the disease. Pseudotubercles develop in the ureter and bladder and the urothelium becomes thickened (Fig. 9-29). With time, the pseudotubercles will calcify. The calcification may be fine and granular, fine and linear, or thick and irregular.[51] If repeated infections occur, the bladder will become small and fibrosed. There is an increased incidence of ureteral and bladder calculi.[50] With chronic disease,

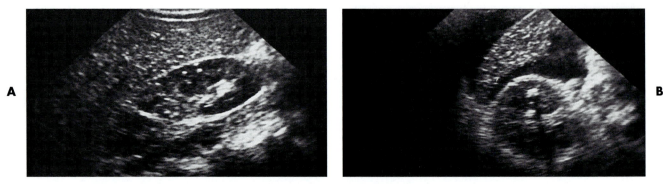

FIG. 9-30. **AIDS nephropathy.** **A,** Sagittal and **B,** transverse sonograms show multiple scattered echogenic foci within the renal parenchyma. Some foci demonstrate the distal acoustic shadowing of calcification. Similar findings are seen in the liver. Proven pneumocystis. (From Spouge AR, Wilson S, Gopinath N, et al: Extrapulmonary *Pneumocystis carinii* in a patient with AIDS. Sonographic findings. *AJR* 1990;155:76-78.)

there is also an increased incidence of squamous cell carcinoma.[50]

Echinococcus (hydatid disease). Two major types of hydatid disease exist that affect the urinary tract: (1) *Echinococcus multilocularis*; and (2) *Echinococcus granulosus*. The latter is the more common offending organism. Renal hydatid disease is found in 2% to 5% of patients with hydatid disease[50] and is usually solitary involving the renal poles.[52] Hydatid cysts may occur along the ureter or in the bladder. Each hydatid cyst consists of: (1) **the pericyst;** (2) the **ectocyst;** and (3) **the endocyst.** The disease is often silent until the cyst has grown large enough to either rupture or cause pressure on adjacent structures. **On sonography,** early in its development an anechoic cyst is seen which may have a perceptible wall. Mural nodularity suggests scolices. When daughter cysts are present, a multiloculated cystic mass will be seen. The membranes from the endocyst may detach and precipitate to the bottom of the hydatid fluid to become **"hydatid sand."**[53] Calcification is variable in its appearance ranging from eggshell to dense reticular. Ring-shaped calcifications inside a larger calcified lesion suggests calcified daughter cysts.[50,53]

Filariasis. Most people with **filariasis (*Wuchereria bancrofti*)** are infected between 10 and 12 years of age, although the signs and symptoms of elephantiasis, chyluria, and chylous ascites usually don't develop for many years (5 to 20 years).[50] Filariasis is transmitted to humans by mosquitoes and the worms migrate into the lymphatics.[50] A granulomatous inflammatory reaction occurs. Obstruction of the retroperitoneal lymphatics occurs leading to dilatation, proliferation, and subsequent rupture of these lymphatics into the pelvicalyceal system. Diagnosis is usually made by lymphangiography.[54] **Sonography** is not helpful.

AIDS. Many renal abnormalities have been described in AIDS patients including: **acute tubular necrosis, nephrocalcinosis, and interstitial nephritis.**[55] Pathologic changes in the kidney include focal and segmental glomerulosclerosis and tubular abnormalities.[55] These changes lead to increased renal parenchymal echogenicity on ultrasound.[55,56] There is also an increased incidence of **opportunistic infection** (Cytomegalovirus, *Candida albicans*, Cryptococcus, *Pneumocystis carinii, Mycobacterium avium-intracellulare* and *mucormycosis*[57]) and **tumor** (lymphoma and Kaposi's sarcoma) in these patients. Pyelonephritis, renal abscess, and cystitis may occur. Diffuse visceral calcifications, including renal, may be seen with disseminated *P. carinii*, cytomegalovirus and *M. avium-intracellulare* infections (Fig. 9-30).[58,59,60]

Cystitis

Infectious. **Cystitis** is a disease found predominantly in women and involves colonization of the urethra by rectal flora. In men, it is associated with bladder outlet obstruction or prostatitis. The most common offending pathogen is *E. coli*.[61] Mucosal edema and decreased bladder capacity are common. Findings may be more prominent at the trigone and bladder neck. Patients will present with bladder irritability and hematuria. **On sonography,** the most typical finding is that of diffuse bladder wall thickening. If cystitis is focal, pseudopolyps may form which are impossible to differentiate from tumor (Fig. 9-31).[62]

Malakoplakia. Malakoplakia is rare granulomatous infection with a predilection for the urinary bladder. The remainder of the urothelium can be affected. The disease is seen more commonly in women (4:1) with a peak incidence in the sixth decade.[63] Pathogenesis is not known; however, its increased association in patients with diabetes mellitus, alcoholic

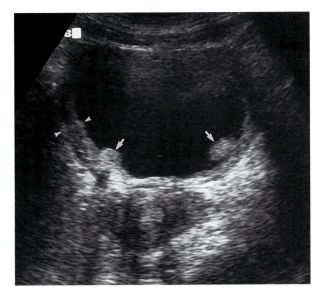

FIG. 9-31. Infectious cystitis. Transverse decubitus sonogram reveals bladder wall thickening (*arrowheads*) with pseudopolyp formation (*arrows*).

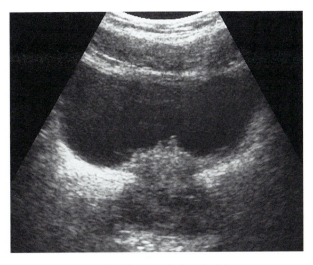

FIG. 9-32. Bladder malakoplakia. Transverse sonogram shows a mucosal-based mass with focal invasion of the prostate gland.

CAUSES OF BLADDER WALL THICKENING

FOCAL	DIFFUSE
Neoplasm	Neoplasm
Transitional cell	Transitional cell
carcinoma	carcinoma
Squamous cell	Squamous cell
carcinoma	carcinoma
Adenocarcinoma	
Lymphoma	Infectious/Inflammatory
Metastases	Cystitis
	Tuberculosis (chronic)
Infectious/Inflammatory	Schistosomiasis
Tuberculosis (acute)	(chronic)
Schistosomiasis (acute)	
Cystitis	Medical Diseases
Malakoplakia	Interstitial cystitis
Cystitis cystica	Amyloidosis
Cystitis glandularis	
Fistula	Neurogenic Bladder
	Detrusor hyper-
Medical Diseases	reflexia
Endometriosis	
Amyloidosis	Bladder Outlet Obstruc-
	tion with Muscular
Trauma	Hypertrophy
Hematoma	

liver disease, mycobacterial infections, sarcoidosis, and following transplantation suggests an altered immune response.[64] Patients may present with hematuria and symptoms of bladder irritability.[65] **On sonography,** single or multiple mucosal-based mass(es) ranging from 0.5 to 3.0 cm are seen most commonly at the bladder base. The disease may be locally invasive (Fig. 9-32).[63]

Emphysematous Cystitis. Emphysematous cystitis occurs most commonly in patients with diabetes. Patients present with symptoms of cystitis and occasionally have pneumaturia.[61] The most common offending organism is *E. coli*. Both intraluminal and intramural gas is present. Frank gangrene of the bladder rarely occurs. In these severely ill patients, the urothelium is ulcerated, necrotic, and may slough completely. The **sonographic identification** of this entity depends on the demonstration of echogenic foci with ringdown or dirty shadowing (air) within the bladder wall (Fig. 9-33).[66]

Chronic Cystitis. Chronic inflammation of the bladder causes predictable histologic change. Brunn's nests are solid nests of urothelium in the lamina propria.[67] If the central portion of a Brunn's nest degenerates, a cyst results (**cystitis cystica**). If chronic irritation persists, the Brunn's nests may develop into glandular structures (**cystitis glandularis**) and may be a precursor of adenocarcinoma.[61] **Sonographically,** these chronic inflammatory changes may be visible. Cysts or solid papillary masses may be seen (Fig. 9-34). Differentiation from malignancy is impossible with imaging, and cystoscopy with biopsy is necessary for diagnostic confirmation.

Bladder Fistula. Bladder fistula may be congenital or acquired. When acquired, etiologies in-

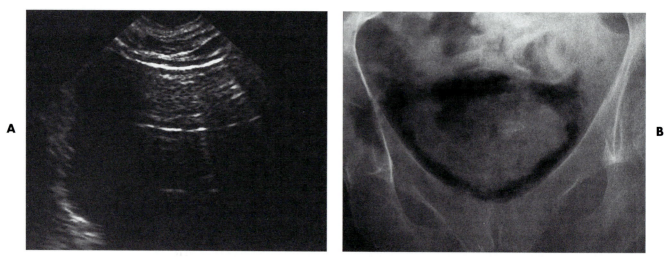

FIG. 9-33. Emphysematous cystitis. A, Transverse sonogram shows an anterior linear echogenic line with dirty shadowing and a multiple reflection artifact distally in the bladder representing air. **B,** Plain film demonstrates extensive air in the bladder wall.

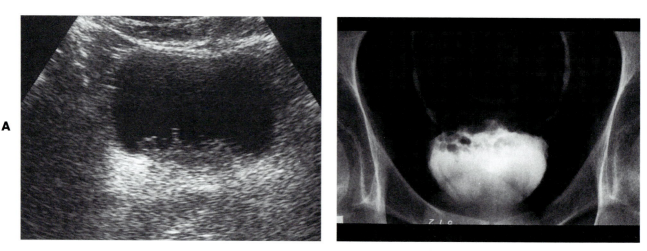

FIG. 9-34. Cystitis glandularis. A, Transverse sonogram shows a solid, papillary mass. **B,** Intravenous pyelogram demonstrates the rounded filling defects superiorly in the bladder.

clude: **trauma, inflammation, radiation, and neoplasm.** Fistula formation may occur with: (1) the vagina; (2) the gut; (3) the skin; (4) the uterus; and (5) the ureter. **Vesicovaginal fistulas** are most commonly related to gynecologic or urologic surgery, bladder carcinoma, and carcinoma of the cervix. **Vesicoenteric fistulas** are most commonly related to diverticulitis and Crohn disease. **Vesicocutaneous fistulas** occur following surgery or trauma. **Vesicouterine fistulas** occur most commonly following cesarean section. **Vesicoureteral fistulas** are rare and usually occur following hysterectomy.[68] **On sonography,** fistulas are difficult to diagnose, because they are often thin, short communications. Occasionally, linear bands of varying echogenicity[69,70] are seen extending from the bladder to the organ with which fistulous communica-

tion exists. If the bladder communicates with gut, vagina, or skin, an abnormal collection of air may be seen in the bladder lumen as a nondependent linear echogenic focus with distal dirty shadowing. Palpation of the abdomen during scanning may cause gas to percolate through the fistula enhancing its detection (Fig. 9-35).[70]

GENITOURINARY TRACT STONES AND CALCIFICATION

Stones

Renal stones are very common, affecting 12% of the population at some time in their life.[71] Stone disease increases with advancing age and white men are most

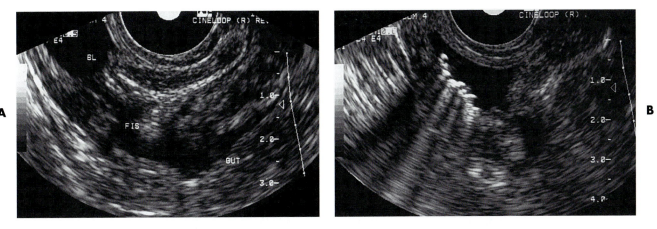

FIG. 9-35. Bladder fistula. Sagittal transvaginal sonograms showing **A,** Fistulous tract extending from the gut to the bladder. **B,** Echogenic foci with ring-down representing air within the bladder lumen. (From Damani N, Wilson S. Non-gynecologic applications of transvaginal sonography. Submitted to *RadioGraphics* August 1997.)

commonly affected. The most common type of stone is calcium oxalate (60% to 80%).[72] The etiology of stone formation is largely unknown, although it is believed to be multifactorial. Calyceal stones which are nonobstructing are usually asymptomatic, although patients may have hematuria (gross or microscopic) or pain. If a stone moves and causes infundibular or UPJ obstruction, clinical signs and symptoms of flank pain and infection often occur. If a stone passes into the ureter, there are **three areas of ureteric narrowing** where the stone may lodge: (1) just past the UPJ; (2) as the ureter crosses the iliac vessels; and (3) at the UVJ. The majority of stones will lodge at the UVJ (75% to 80%) where the ureter has its smallest diameter of 1 to 5 mm.[72] Approximately 80% of stones smaller than 5 mm will pass spontaneously.

Renal calculi can be detected using many different imaging modalities including: (1) plain films; (2) tomography; (3) ultrasound; and (4) CT. Many studies have been undertaken evaluating the sensitivity for stone detection utilizing these various imaging modalities. Middleton et al.[73] demonstrated that sonography has a 96% sensitivity for renal stone detection which was slightly inferior to a combination of plain radiography with tomography. They also found that stones greater than 5 mm in size were detected with 100% sensitivity sonographically. **On sonography, renal calculi** are seen as echogenic foci with sharp distal acoustic shadowing (Figs. 9-36 and 9-37). Smith et al.[74] have demonstrated that annular array transducers are able to demonstrate stone shadowing to better advantage than mechanical sector transducers. Certain entities may **mimic renal calculi** sonographically including: (1) intrarenal gas; (2) renal artery calcification; (3) calcified sloughed papilla; and (4) calcified transitional cell tumor.

ENTITIES THAT MIMIC RENAL CALCULI

Intrarenal gas
Renal artery calcification
Calcified sloughed papilla
Calcified transitional cell tumor

For patients presenting with **acute renal colic,** the role of imaging is to confirm the diagnosis, define stone size, stone location, stone number, and to assess for associated complications. Normally, this is accomplished by plain renal tomography followed by intravenous pyelography (IVP). The ability of urography to provide information regarding anatomy and function still makes it a widely performed test. Alternatively, a **plain film** of the abdomen combined with **renal sonography** has been advocated as a replacement.[75-78] This approach has not gained universal acceptance.[79,80] There are many sonographic pitfalls for this approach including: (1) evaluation before hydronephrosis develops leading to a false-negative result; and (2) mistaking parapelvic cysts and nonobstructive pelvicaliectasis as hydronephrosis.[80]

On sonography, the search for **ureteral calculi** can be difficult because of overlying bowel gas and the deep retroperitoneal location of the ureter. However, transvaginal or transperineal scanning may be an optimal way to detect and demonstrate distal ureteral calculi not seen with a transabdominal suprapubic approach.[70,81,82] When the ureter is dilated, the distal 3 cm will be seen as a tubular hypoechoic structure entering the bladder obliquely. A stone will be identified as an echogenic focus with distal sharp acoustic shad-

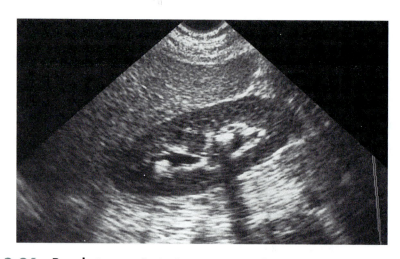

FIG. 9-36. **Renal stones.** Sagittal sonogram reveals two central echogenic foci with sharp distal acoustic shadowing. Mild caliectasis is present.

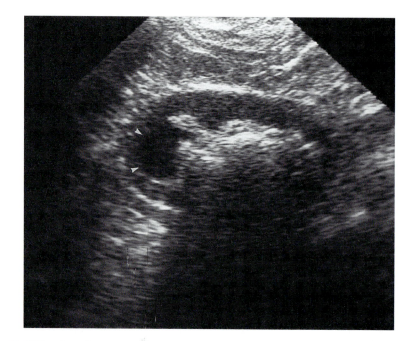

FIG. 9-37. **Staghorn renal stone.** Large central echogenic focus with sharp distal acoustic shadowing. Associated proximal caliectasis is present in the upper pole (*arrowheads*).

owing within the ureteric lumen (Fig. 9-38). There may be associated mucosal edema at the bladder trigone. Transabdominal evaluation of the ureteral orifices for **jets** is helpful to assess for obstruction.[83] On **gray scale,** a stream of low level echoes can be seen entering the bladder from the ureteral orifice. It is believed that density differences between the jet and bladder urine allow its sonographic visualization.[84] Good hydration prior to the study is important. In addition, patients should not be allowed to completely empty their bladder following hydration, prior to the study, so that concentrated urine remains in the bladder. This will then cause a density difference between the ureteric and bladder urine, allowing a jet to be seen.[85] In addition to gray-scale evaluation, **Doppler** improves detection of ureteric jets. The use of color Doppler over duplex Doppler has the advantage of being less prone to sampling error and also allowing simultaneous visualization of both ureteral orifices (Fig. 9-39).[83] Depending on the state of hydration, jet frequency may vary from less than one per minute to continuous flow; however, both sides should be symmetric in a healthy individual. Patients with high-grade ureteric obstruction will have asymmetric jets on

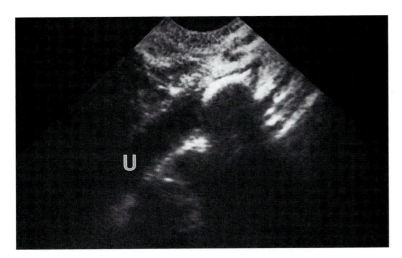

FIG. 9-38. Ureteric stone. Sagittal transvaginal scan shows the dilated tubular hypoechoic ureter (U) containing an echogenic stone with shadowing.

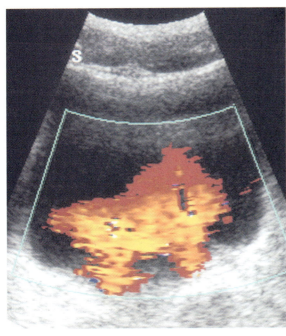

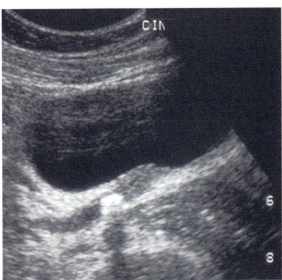

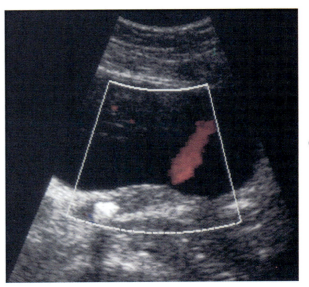

FIG. 9-39. Value of color Doppler evaluation of ureteric jets to discriminate degree of urinary tract obstruction. A, Transverse color sonogram in a normal patient shows bilateral symmetric ureteric jets. B, Sagittal sonogram in a patient with renal colic reveals a dilated ureter containing a stone distally. The urothelium at the ureterovesicle junction is thickened, representing edema. C, Sagittal color sonogram on the patient in B, shows a color jet indicative of incomplete obstruction.

color Doppler imaging which will be detected as either: (1) complete absence of the jet on the affected side; or (2) continuous, low-level flow from the symptomatic side. Patients with low-grade obstruction may or may not have asymmetry of their jets.[83] The use of color Doppler should be adjunctive in assessing for ureteric obstruction (Fig. 9-39).[83]

Recently, it has been suggested that the addition of **duplex renal Doppler** to the gray-scale examination may allow diagnosis of both **acute and chronic urinary tract obstruction.**[86] It is believed that with obstruction, the renal pelvic wall tension increases resulting in elevation of prostaglandins which initially causes vasodilatation.[87] With prolonged obstruction, many hormones including renin-angiotensin, kallikrein-kinin, and prostaglandin-thromboxane reduce vasodilatation and produce diffuse vasoconstriction. Platt et al.[86] used a threshold resistance index (RI) of greater than 0.70 to indicate obstruction. They also noted a difference in RI of 0.08 to 0.1 when comparing the patients' obstructed and nonobstructed kidney. Others have not had the same success using duplex Doppler.[80,87] Some of the potential problems include: (1) no elevation of RI with partial obstruction; (2) the use of nonsteroidal anti-inflammatory medication for pain control appears to alter the RI by interfering with vasodilatation and vasoconstriction; and (3) antecedent IVP causes vasoconstriction, altering the RI.[80,87]

At the present time, IVP is most accepted as the initial imaging test in patients with acute renal colic (with the exception of pregnant patients) when sonography should be used in an attempt to eliminate radiation exposure.[80] Recently, unenhanced helical CT has been advocated as the imaging procedure of choice in patients with acute renal colic.[88,89,90] Helical CT can be performed rapidly with no patient preparation required, no risk of contrast reaction and the associated findings of hydronephrosis, hydroureter, perinephric stranding and ureteric edema easily assessed although at a higher cost than ultrasound.[88] In addition, extraurinary tract causes of acute flank pain may also be noted with helical CT.

Bladder calculi occur most commonly as a result of either migration from the kidney or urinary stasis in the bladder. Urinary stasis is usually related to bladder outlet obstruction, cystocele, neurogenic bladder, or a foreign body in the bladder. Bladder calculi may be asymptomatic. If symptomatic, patients will complain of bladder pain or foul smelling urine with or without hematuria. **On sonography,** a mobile, echogenic focus with distal acoustic shadowing will be seen in the bladder (Fig. 9-40). If the stone is large, edema of the ureteral orifices and thickening of the bladder wall may be seen. Occasionally, stones can adhere to the bladder wall because of adjacent inflammation, and these are known as **"hanging" bladder stones.**

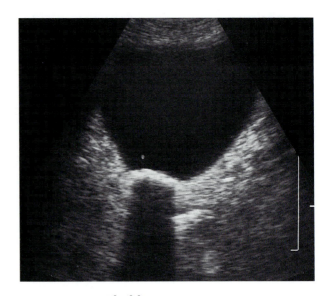

FIG. 9-40. Bladder stone. Transverse sonogram shows a dependent echogenic focus with distal sharp acoustic shadowing.

Nephrocalcinosis

Nephrocalcinosis refers to renal parenchymal calcification. The calcification may be **dystrophic** or **metastatic.** With **dystrophic calcification,** there is deposition of calcium in devitalized tissue, usually resulting from ischemia or necrosis.[91] This type occurs in tumors, abscesses, and hematomas. **Metastatic nephrocalcinosis** occurs most commonly with hypercalcemic states caused by hyperparathyroidism, renal tubular acidosis, and renal failure. **Metastatic nephrocalcinosis** can be further categorized by the location of the calcium deposits into **cortical** or **medullary nephrocalcinosis.** Causes of **cortical nephrocalcinosis** include acute cortical necrosis, chronic glomerulonephritis, chronic hypercalcemic states, ethylene glycol poisoning, sickle cell disease, and rejected renal transplants. Causes of **medullary nephrocalcinosis** include hyperparathyroidism (40%), renal tubular acidosis (20%), medullary sponge kidney, bone metastases, chronic pyelonephritis, Cushing's syndrome, hyperthyroidism, malignancy, renal papillary necrosis, sarcoidosis, sickle cell disease, vitamin D excess, and Wilson's disease.[91]

The **Anderson-Carr-Randall theory** of stone progression postulates that the concentration of calcium is high in the fluid around the renal tubules. The calcium is removed by lymphatics and if the amount exceeds lymphatic capacity, deposits of calcium in the forniceal tips and margins of the medulla will occur, producing a striking appearance on **sonography** with nonshadowing echogenic rims surrounding all medullary pyramids (Fig. 9-41). Plaques form which may perforate the calyx and form a nidus for further stone growth.[92]

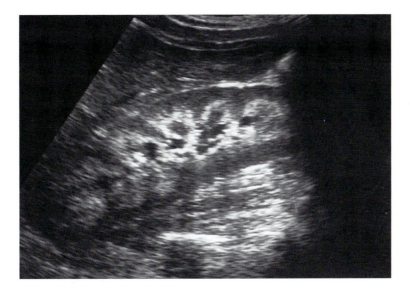

FIG. 9-41. Anderson-Carr kidney. Sagittal sonogram demonstrates increased echogenicity in a rimlike pattern around all medullary pyramids.

Sonographically, cortical nephrocalcinosis is seen as increased cortical echogenicity which may produce acoustic shadowing. **Medullary nephrocalcinosis** is apparent when the medullary pyramids become more echogenic than the adjacent cortex. With time, further calcium deposition and stone formation occur with acoustic shadowing becoming apparent (Fig. 9-42).

TUMORS OF THE GENITOURINARY TRACT

Renal Cell Carcinoma

Renal cell carcinoma (RCC) accounts for approximately 3% of all adult malignancies and 86% of all primary malignant renal parenchymal tumors.[93] There is a 2:1 predominance in men. Peak age is between 50 and 70 years. The etiology is unknown although a moderate association with smoking has been shown.[94] Although most RCCs occur sporadically, a **familial variety** does occur.[95] This variety occurs at an earlier age, is multifocal and bilateral, and affects men and women equally.[95] There is also an association with **von Hippel-Lindau disease,** in which 24% to 45% of affected patients develop RCC.[96] Seventy-five percent of the patients will have multicentric and bilateral tumors.[97] There is also an increased incidence of RCC in patients with **tuberous sclerosis.** Patients with chronic renal failure who have been on long-term hemodialysis or peritoneal dialysis develop **acquired cystic kidney disease (ACKD)** and have an increased incidence of RCC. RCC associated with ACKD is often small and hypovascular.[98,99]

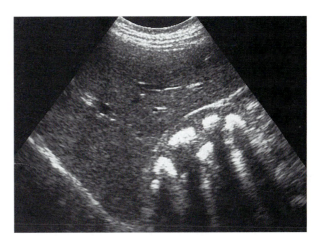

FIG. 9-42. Medullary nephrocalcinosis. Sagittal sonogram shows extensive medullary calcification.

The classic diagnostic triad of flank pain, gross hematuria, and palpable renal mass is seen in 4% to 9% of patients at presentation.[100] Systemic symptoms, such as anorexia and weight loss, are common. Many manifestations secondary to hormone production occur including erythrocytosis (erythropoietin); hypercalcemia (parathormone, vitamin D metabolites, prostaglandins); hypokalemia (ACTH); galactorrhea (prolactin); hypertension (renin); gynecomastia (gonadotropin). RCC has been described as having metastases to virtually every organ in the body. Spontaneous regression of the primary tumor may occur, although the mechanism for this is unclear.[101]

With the rapidly changing and improved superior technology of current cross-sectional imaging techniques, we are able to detect smaller renal masses. The prevalence rate of incidentally discovered occult renal cell carcinoma on CT is 0.3%.[102] Before the advent of CT, renal tumors less than 3 cm represented 5% of lesions, whereas now these small lesions represent 9% to 38% of all renal tumors.[103] Warshauer et al.[104] demonstrated the relative insensitivity of excretory urography/linear tomography for renal masses less than 3 cm in diameter and of ultrasound for masses less than 2 cm. Jamis-Dow et al.[105] found that CT was more sensitive than ultrasound for the detection of small renal masses (< 1.5 cm) and that both ultrasound and CT were equally able to characterize a mass larger than 1 cm. They also demonstrated that a combination of ultrasound and CT allowed accurate characterization of a lesion larger than 1.0 cm 95% of the time. Neither method was able to accurately characterize lesions less than 1 cm in diameter. Therefore, a combination of both ultrasound and CT is superior to either one alone. With the advent of helical CT, respiratory misregistration and partial volume averaging can be eliminated. Many authors[106-109] have demonstrated that nephrographic phase helical CT scans enable better lesion detection and characterization. With the combined use of ultrasound and helical CT, there is usually no need for other imaging in the evaluation of renal masses.

Magnetic resonance imaging (MRI) for renal mass characterization has improved significantly with the development of phased-array multicoils, fast breath-hold imaging and gadopentetate dimeglumine contrast enhancement. This method is assuming an increasingly important role in the detection and characterization of some renal masses.[110,111] This is particularly so in patients with allergy to iodinated contrast, renal failure, pregnancy, and when indeterminate renal masses or extent of vascular involvement cannot be adequately sorted out with a combination of ultrasound and CT.

With the detection of a small (< 3 cm) renal mass, the controversy now is how to manage them. The choice is either watchful waiting or surgery (radical nephrectomy, partial nephrectomy or enucleation). Bosniak et al.[112] as a result of preliminary experience, suggest watchful waiting in some elderly patients and those patients at risk for surgery, who have these small incidentally discovered lesions.

On sonography, most tumors are **solid** with no predilection for either kidney nor for the upper, mid-, or lower pole. Tumors may be hypoechoic, isoechoic, or hyperechoic (Fig. 9-43). Charboneau et al.[113] demonstrated that the majority (86%) are isoechoic, whereas the minority were hypoechoic (10%) or echogenic (4%). More recently, it has been demonstrated that small renal tumors (< 3 cm) tend to be echogenic compared with normal renal parenchyma. Forman et al.[114] found that 77% of their small RCCs

(< 3 cm) and Yamashita et al.[115,116] found 61% of their small RCCs were more **echogenic** than renal parenchyma. In comparing hyperechoic RCCs and angiomyolipomas (AMLs), Yamashita et al.[115,116] found considerable overlap in the echogenicity of these two tumors. They demonstrated a **hypoechoic rim** sonographically, which represented a pseudocapsule histologically, in 84% of the RCCs and in none of the AMLs. As well, **intratumoral cystic spaces** were noted in their hyperechoic RCCs and not in any of the AMLs (Fig. 9-43). The exact pathologic basis for the hyperechoic appearance of RCC is not understood but in their study this appearance was seen in RCCs with papillary, tubular, or microcystic architecture or in tumors with minute calcification, necrosis, cystic degeneration, or fibrosis.[116] RCC will demonstrate **calcification** in 8% to 18% of cases. This calcification may be punctate, curvilinear, diffuse (rare), central, or peripheral.[117-121] Daniels et al.[120] demonstrated that central calcification was associated with a malignant tumor 87% of the time. Rim or diffuse calcification of a renal mass may obscure adequate sonographic visualization and CT is advised to look for features of malignancy including the presence of a soft tissue mass extending beyond the calcification.[122]

Five percent to 15% of RCCs will be of a **papillary variety**.[123] This type of tumor is characterized by slower growth, lower stage at presentation, and better prognosis.[124] These tumors tend to be hypoechoic or isoechoic, although no consistent sonographic pattern exists as some may also be hyperechoic.[123] Five percent to 7% of all RCCs will be of a **cystic variety**.[125] **Four histologic growth patterns** have been described: (1) multilocular; (2) unilocular; (3) cystic necrosis; and (4) tumors originating in a simple cyst (Fig. 9-44).[126] Yamashita et al.[125] feel that recognition of subtypes may have clinical significance as the multilocular and unilocular subtypes seem to be less aggressive. On sonography, **multilocular cystic RCC** will demonstrate a cystic mass with internal septations. These septations may be thick (>2 mm), nodular, and contain calcification. **Unilocular cystic RCC** will demonstrate a debris-filled cystic mass with thick, irregular walls which may be calcified. **Necrotic RCCs** show various sonographic findings depending on the degree of necrosis. **Tumors originating in a simple cyst** are rare and a mural tumor nodule will be found at the base of a simple cyst. Spiral-enhanced CT in conjunction with ultrasound will usually allow accurate characterization of the internal nature of a cystic renal lesion. Silverman et al.[127] demonstrated that spiral CT alone can underestimate the number of septations in small (≤ 3 cm) cystic renal lesions. The majority of cystic RCCs will demonstrate features of malignancy in 88% of cases (Fig. 9-43)[128]

The use of **Doppler ultrasound** for detection of tumor vascularity has shown high sensitivity for ma-

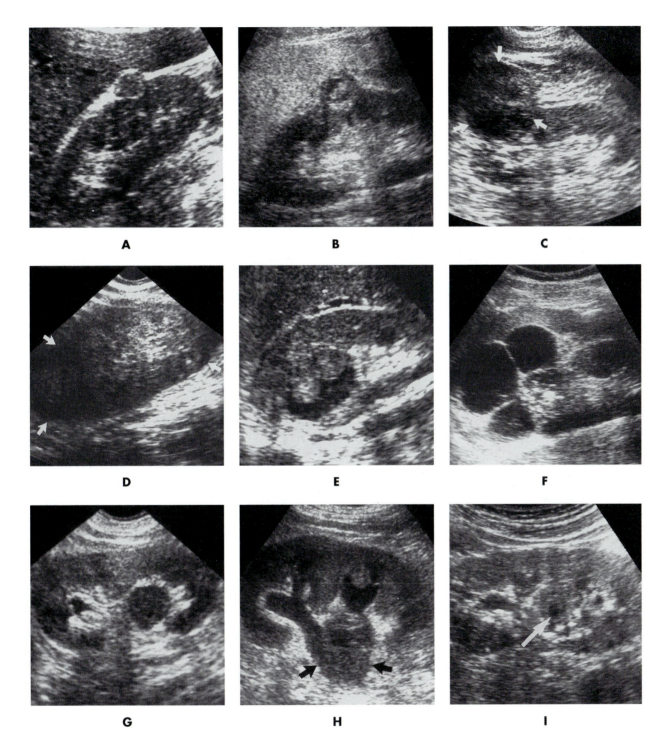

FIG. 9-43. Renal cell carcinoma. A, B, and C, Sagittal renal sonograms showing the morphologic spectrum of solid tumors. A, Tiny incidental hyperechoic tumor. B, Small echogenic tumor with central cystic spaces and a thin, hypoechoic peripheral halo. C, Isoechoic tumor (*arrows*). D, Sagittal sonogram demonstrates a diffuse, infiltrative tumor with maintenance of the reniform shape (*arrows*). E, and F, Sagittal sonograms demonstrate cystic renal cell carcinomas. E, Cystic necrotic tumor. F, Multiloculated cystic tumor with multiple punctate echogenic foci centrally representing cribriform loculation. G, H, and I, Sagittal renal sonograms demonstrate central renal masses. G, Renal cell carcinoma. H, Expansile tumor thrombus in the renal vein (*arrows*). I, Pseudotumor. Medullary pyramid is seen (*arrow*) in this column of Bertin (Fig. 9-43E, F from Vanderburgh L, Thurston W: Imaging features of cystic renal cell carcinoma. In press.)

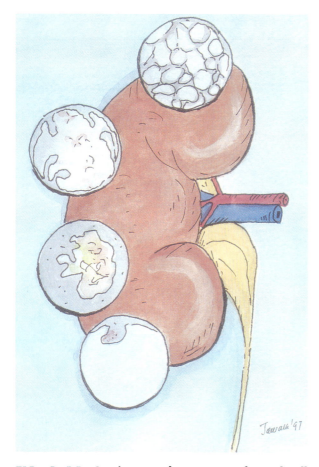

FIG. 9-44. Cystic growth patterns of renal cell carcinoma. Upper pole, multilocular; upper lateral, unilocular; lower lateral, cystic necrosis; lower pole, origin in the wall of a simple cyst. (From Vanderburgh L, Thurston W: *Imaging features of cystic renal cell carcinoma.* In press.)

lignant lesions in the liver, kidneys, adrenal glands, and pancreas. Most malignant renal tumors (70% to 83%) will have Doppler shift frequency of 2.5 KHz.[131-133] Similar changes may be noted with inflammatory masses however, patients with renal infection should be clinically apparent. Absence of high-frequency Doppler shift does not exclude malignancy.[131]

Tumor stage at diagnosis is important for patient prognosis. **Robson staging is: I—tumor confined within the renal capsule; II—tumor invasion of perinephric fat; III—tumor involvement of regional lymph nodes or venous structures; IV—invasion of adjacent organs or distant metastases.** Five-year survival rates for Robson stage I, II, III, and IV are 67%, 51%, 33.5%, and 13.5%, respectively.[134] Patients with stage I and II disease are treated surgically (partial or radical nephrectomy). Patients with stage III disease, with extensive metastatic lymphadenopathy are often treated palliatively. Patients with stage III disease and with tumor thrombus, are

treated with radical nephrectomy and thrombectomy. Patients with stage IV disease usually receive palliative treatment only.[135] Ultrasound is inferior to CT and MRI for staging RCC. Unfortunately, obese patients and overlying bowel gas make it difficult to assess for lymphadenopathy and/or vascular involvement. Sonography is, however, excellent for assessment of the intrahepatic IVC and determination of the cephalad extent of venous tumor thrombus (Fig. 9-45). Habboub et al.[136] found the accuracy of detecting renal vein and IVC involvement on sonography was 64% and 93%, respectively. They also demonstrated that addition of color Doppler improved accuracy for diagnosing both renal vein and IVC thrombus to 87% and 100%, respectively (Fig. 9-46). It is crucial to determine the location and extent of vascular tumor thrombus to plan the surgical approach. Many **staging limitations,** however, are shared by ultrasound, CT, and MRI. These include: (1) microscopic tumor invasion of the renal capsule; (2) detection of metastatic tumor deposits in normal sized lymph nodes; and (3) differentiation of inflammatory hyperplastic nodes from neoplastic ones.[137]

Transitional Cell Carcinoma

Transitional cell carcinoma (TCC) of the renal pelvis accounts for 7% of all primary renal tumors.[138] They are two to three times more common than ureteral neoplasms. Bladder TCC, because of its large surface area, is 50 times more common than renal pelvic TCC.[139] The multifocal and bilateral nature of this disease requires accurate diagnosis and staging to allow appropriate surgical planning. Yousem et al.[140] retrospectively reviewed 645 cases of TCC of the bladder, ureter, and kidney and found that 3.9% of patients with bladder cancer developed an upper tract lesion (mean = within 61 months). Thirteen percent of patients with ureteral TCC and 11% of patients with renal TCC developed metachronous tumors (mean = within 28 and 22 months respectively). Synchronous TCC was present in 2.3% of patients with bladder TCC, 39% with ureteral TCC, and 24% with renal TCC. Surveillance with IVP, retrograde pyelography, and cystoscopy is recommended. Some patients at increased risk for development of TCC may require closer surveillance and include those with: (1) Balkan nephritis; (2) vesicoureteric reflux; (3) multifocal recurrent bladder TCC; (4) high-grade bladder tumors; (5) carcinoma *in situ* of the distal ureters following cystectomy; (6) analgesic abuse; (7) heavy smoking; (8) exposure to carcinogens; and (9) treatment with cyclophosphamide.[140]

TCC may be **papillary** or **nonpapillary.** Papillary forms are exophytic polypoid lesions attached to the mucosa by a stalk. This type tends to be low grade, slow to infiltrate, late to metastasize, and follows a more benign course. Nonpapillary tumors, on the

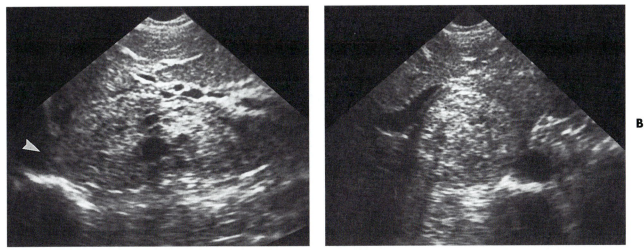

FIG. 9-45. Tumor thrombus in inferior vena cava. A, Sagittal and B, transverse sonograms demonstrate a large, expansile tumor thrombus extending cephalad to the diaphragm (*arrowhead*).

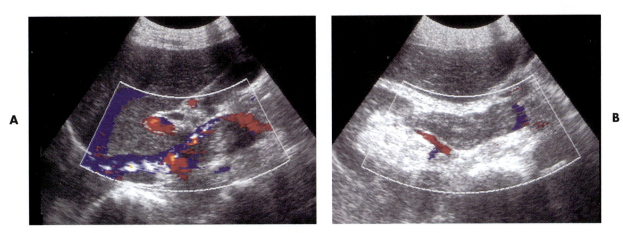

FIG. 9-46. Renal cell carcinoma with venous tumor thrombosis in the renal vein and inferior vena cava. A, Sagittal color Doppler sonogram showing thrombus in the inferior vena cava, which remains patent. B, Transverse sonogram showing occlusive renal vein thrombus extending into the inferior vena cava. The inferior vena cava (*blue*) is patent as noted by flow at the thrombus margin. The renal artery (*red*) is seen posterior to the occluded renal vein.

other hand, present as nodular or flat tumors demonstrating mucosal thickening. These tumors are usually high grade and infiltrating.[139]

Kidney. **Transitional cell tumors of the kidney** are more common in men than women (4:1) with a mean age at diagnosis of 65 years.[139] Seventy-five percent of patients with renal pelvic tumors will present with gross or microscopic hematuria. Twenty-five percent of patients will have flank pain. Incidental tumor discovery occurs in less than 5%.[139]

Sonographic assessment of the **renal sinus** poses unique problems and is a challenge to evaluate for pathologic processes because of its variable morphologic appearance. The presence of fat within the renal sinus can appear as a hypoechoic mass simulating a solid TCC (Fig. 9-47). In uncertain cases, confirmation with IVP is recommended to rule out neoplasm particularly in patients with hematuria.

The sonographic appearance of renal TCC is quite variable and depends on tumor morphology (papillary, nonpapillary, or infiltrative), location, size, and presence, or absence of hydronephrosis (Fig. 9-48). Small, nonobstructing tumors may be impossible to visualize. With growth papillary tumors will be seen as a discrete, solid, central, hypoechoic renal sinus mass with or without associated proximal caliectasis (Fig. 9-47). The **differential diagnosis** includes blood clots, sloughed papilla, and fungus ball.

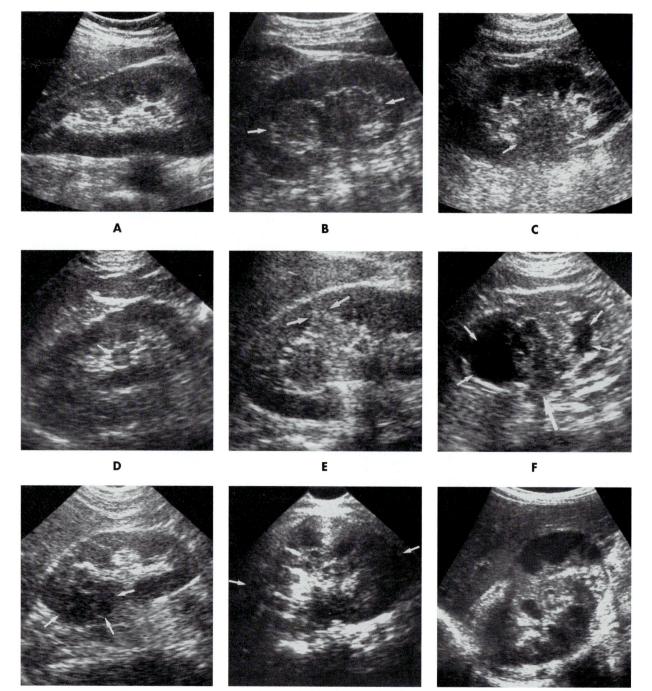

FIG. 9-47. Transitional cell carcinoma of the kidney. A, B, and C, The morphologic spectrum of normal and fat-filled renal pelves. **A,** Normal. **B,** Lobulated fat (*arrows*) mimicking solid tumor. **C,** Irregular central fat (*arrows*). **D, E,** and **F,** The morphologic spectrum of central transitional cell carcinoma. **D,** Small, central nonobstructing hypoechoic mass. **E,** Solid upper-pole expansile calyceal tumor invading the renal parenchyma (*arrows*). **F,** Central solid mass (*large arrow*) causing hydronephrosis (*small arrows*). **G, H,** and **I,** The morphologic spectrum of infiltrative transitional cell carcinoma. **G,** Large, lobulated solid parenchymal infiltrative mass (*arrows*) with no associated caliectasis. **H,** Diffusely destructive tumor with the reniform shape maintained (*arrows*). **I,** Perirenal tumor extension. (From Ramji F, Thurston W, Wilson S: Transitional cell carcinoma of the kidney: sonographic appearance. In press.)

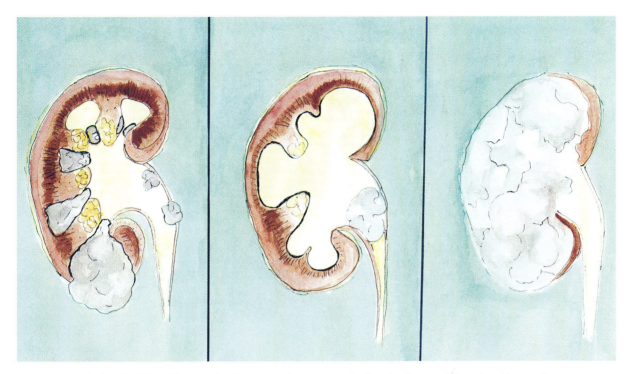

FIG. 9-48. Morphologic growth patterns of renal transitional cell carcinoma. (From Ramji F, Thurston W, Wilson S: Transitional cell carcinoma of the kidney: sonographic appearance. In press.)

The tumor may demonstrate peripelvic or parenchymal extension. Tumor growth may be in a diffusely infiltrative pattern. These destructive tumors distort and enlarge the renal architecture with maintenance of reniform shape (Fig. 9-47).[141] Flat tumors are difficult to see, although the associated pelvicaliectasis may be visualized sonographically. Both sessile and papillary TCCs may demonstrate dystrophic calcification creating difficulty in the differentiation of tumor from stones or sloughed calcified papilla.[142] TCC may invade the renal vein in 7% of cases.[143] This is usually a late finding.

Ureter. **TCC of the ureter** is rare accounting for only 1% to 6% of all upper urinary tract cancers.[139,144] Men are more commonly affected (3:1), with peak prevalence between the fifth and seventh decade.[139] The tumors are usually found in the lower third of the ureter (70% to 75%).[139,144] Sixty percent of the tumors are **papillary** and 40% **nonpapillary.**[139] The most frequent symptoms are hematuria, frequency, dysuria, and pain.[144] The imaging modalities of choice for evaluation include retrograde pyelography for direct ureteral visualization and CT for evaluation of extraureteral tumor extent. **On sonography,** hydronephrosis and hydroureter will be seen and occasionally a solid ureteral mass will be depicted.[144]

Bladder. **TCC of the bladder** is a common malignant tumor. These tumors occur more commonly in men (3:1), with a peak incidence in the sixth and seventh decades. They occur most frequently at the trigone and along the lateral and posterior walls of the bladder. Approximately 70% of bladder cancers are superficial, whereas the remaining 30% are invasive. Patients most commonly present with hematuria. Frequency, dysuria, and suprapubic pain may also be present. **Sonographic detection** of bladder tumors is excellent and is greater than or equal to 95%.[145] The appearance is that of a focal nonmobile mass or of urothelial thickening (Fig. 9-49). The appearances, however, are nonspecific and the **differential diagnosis** is extensive and includes cystitis; wall thickening due to bladder outlet obstruction; postradiation change; postoperative change; adherent blood clot; invasive prostate carcinoma; lymphoma; metastases; endometriosis; and neurofibromatosis. Cystoscopy and biopsy are necessary for diagnosis. Both transvaginal and transrectal ultrasound may be used to assess a bladder wall mass if suprapubic visualization is poor (Fig. 9-50). Transitional tumors may also arise within urinary bladder diverticula. Many diverticula have narrow necks, making them inaccessible for cystoscopic examination and imaging plays an important role in the detection of these tumors. The periureteric and posterolateral wall locations of most bladder diverticula allow for adequate sonographic visualization.[146] Diverticular tumors are seen as a

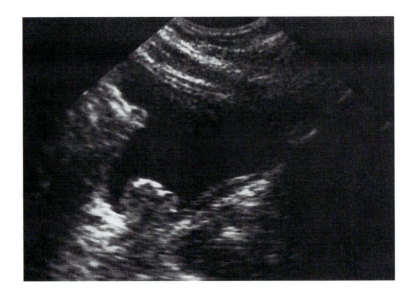

FIG. 9-49. Calcified bladder transitional cell carcinoma. Sagittal sonogram demonstrates a polypoid solid mass with superficial echogenic foci representing calcification.

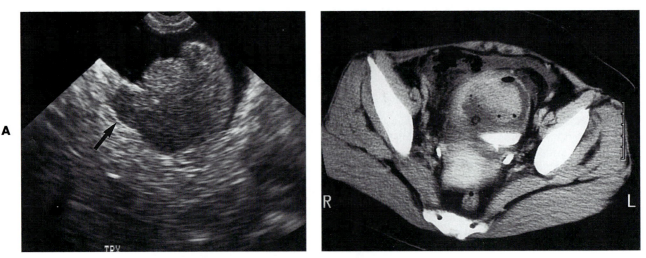
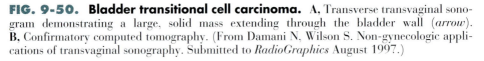

FIG. 9-50. Bladder transitional cell carcinoma. **A,** Transverse transvaginal sonogram demonstrating a large, solid mass extending through the bladder wall (*arrow*). **B,** Confirmatory computed tomography. (From Damani N, Wilson S. Non-gynecologic applications of transvaginal sonography. Submitted to *RadioGraphics* August 1997.)

moderately echogenic nonshadowing mass. Although ultrasound is good for tumor detection, staging is still best performed clinically in combination with CT or contrast-enhanced MRI.[147]

Squamous Cell Carcinoma

Squamous cell carcinoma (SCC) is rare but is the second most common malignant tumor arising from urothelium after TCC. It represents 6% to 15% of renal pelvic tumors and 5% to 8% of all bladder tumors.[148,149] Chronic infection, irritation, and stones lead to squamous metaplasia and leukoplakia of the urothelium. Leukoplakia is felt to be premalignant.

SCC tends to be solid, flat, and infiltrative with extensive ulceration and very rarely is exophytic and fungating. Distant metastases are usually present at the time of diagnosis. **On sonography, renal SCC** is seen as a diffusely enlarged kidney which has maintained its reniform shape. The normal renal echotexture is destroyed and often a stone (47% to 58%)[148] will be present. It may be impossible to differentiate this from xanthogranulomatous pyelonephritis. Often, perinephric tumor extension and metastases are present. **Ureteral SCC** is rare and hydronephroureterectasis proximal to the tumor mass will be apparent. Occasionally, the tumor mass is seen as a poorly defined, irregular, solid mass. Associated stones are often present. **Bladder SCC** tend to be large, solid, and infiltrating. Ultrasound is an effective modality for detection but less reliable in its ability to stage these tumors. Staging is best done with CT or MRI.

Adenocarcinoma

Adenocarcinoma of the kidney, ureter, and bladder is rare. Almost all patients with adenocarcinoma of the kidney will have urinary tract infection[150] and two thirds will have a stone, usually a staghorn. Most will have hematuria. One must be careful to differentiate adenocarcinoma of the bladder from adenocarcinoma of the rectum, uterus, or prostate that has invaded the bladder. The prognosis of this tumor is poor. **On sonography,** a renal pelvic, ureteric, or bladder mass will be seen occasionally with calcification. An associated stone will often be present.

Oncocytoma

Oncocytes are large epithelial cells with granular eosinophilic cytoplasm caused by extensive cytoplasmic mitochondria. **Oncocytomas** may occur in the parathyroid glands, the thyroid gland, the adrenal glands, the salivary glands, and the kidneys. They represent 3.1% to 6.6% of all renal tumors.[151,152] They occur most commonly in men (1.7:1), with a peak incidence in the sixth and seventh decade.[153] Most patients are asymptomatic.[151] Oncocytomas may be small or extremely large (mean = 3 to 8 cm). On cut surface, they have a mahogany color. Hemorrhage and calcification are uncommon. These tumors histologically may have a benign or more malignant appearance. Patients with benign appearing tumors clinically do well. Pathologically these tumors are multicentric and bilateral in 5% to 10% and 3%, respectively.[152]

On the basis of imaging, oncocytoma and renal cell adenocarcinoma cannot be differentiated. Davidson et al.[154] demonstrated that CT homogeneity, lack of homogeneity, and a central stellate "scar" are poor predictors in differentiating oncocytomas from RCCs. Oncocytomas represent about 5% of all tumors originally diagnosed as RCC on imaging.[155] **On sonography,** oncocytomas are variable in appearance and may be isoechoic, hypoechoic, or hyperechoic. These tumors may be homogeneous or heterogeneous with a well- or poorly demarcated wall depending on its size (Fig. 9-51).[156] A central scar, central necrosis, or calcification may be seen. These features may also be seen with RCC. If a solid mass is found in the kidney on sonography, CT is required for both staging and to look for the presence of fat. Most nonfat containing solid renal mass(es) are either RCC or oncocytoma.[154] With a large oncocytoma, perinephric engulfment of fat may occur.[157] In these cases, care must be taken not to mistakenly diagnose angiomyolipoma.

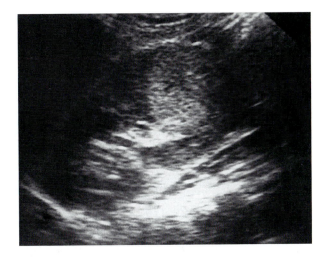

FIG. 9-51. Oncocytoma. Sagittal sonogram shows a large hyperechoic tumor at the lower pole of the kidney. It cannot be differentiated from renal cell carcinoma.

Angiomyolipoma

Angiomyolipomas (AML) are benign renal tumors composed of varying proportions of adipose tissue, smooth muscle cells, and blood vessels. Angiomyolipomas may occur sporadically or be found in patients with tuberous sclerosis. Tumors in patients, without stigmata of tuberous sclerosis, most commonly are unilateral and demonstrate a middle-aged predominance in women. Up to 50% of patients with AML will have stigmata of tuberous sclerosis (mental retardation, epilepsy, and sebaceous adenomas of the face) and up to 80% of patients with tuberous sclerosis will have one or more AML.[158] AMLs associated with tuberous sclerosis are usually small, multiple, and bilateral with no sex predilection. Sporadic tumors are histologically identical to those associated with tuberous sclerosis. It is unusual for small tumors (< 4 cm)[159] to be symptomatic; however, with growth, these tumors may hemorrhage giving rise to signs and symptoms of hematuria, flank pain, or palpable flank mass.

On sonography, the echopattern of the AML depends on the proportion of fat, smooth muscle, vascular elements, and hemorrhage. Classically, AMLs are markedly hyperechoic relative to renal parenchyma (Fig. 9-52). The tumors may be within the parenchyma or exophytic (Fig. 9-53). If muscle, vascular elements or hemorrhage predominate, the tumor may be hypoechoic (Fig. 9-54). Small (< 3 cm) renal cell carcinomas (RCC) are also hyperechoic and may stimulate AML up to 33% of the time.[114,115] Therefore, CT imaging is necessary to demonstrate that the presence of fat and helical CT is superior to conventional CT.[160] Yamashita et al.[116] demonstrated that intratumoral cystic spaces and a peripheral hypoechoic rim in an echogenic solid lesion suggest RCC rather than AML.

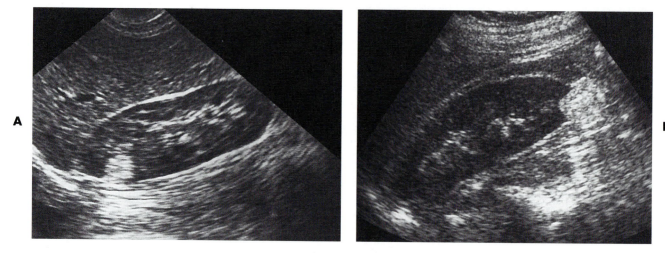

FIG. 9-52. Angiomyolipoma. Sagittal sonograms on two patients show **A,** classic small hyperechoic intraparenchymal tumor and **B,** large echogenic tumor at the lower pole of the kidney.

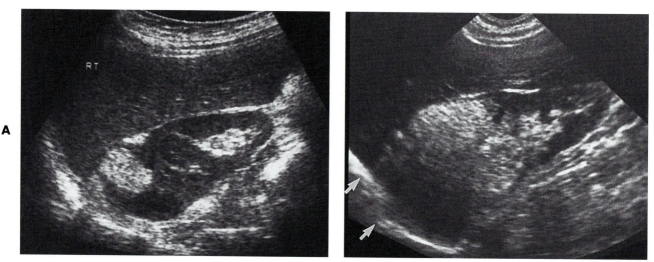

FIG. 9-53. Exophytic angiomyolipomas in two patients. A, Sagittal sonogram showing an exophytic echogenic tumor with perirenal hemorrhage. **B,** Sagittal sonogram demonstrating a large exophytic tumor with shadowing. Diaphragmatic interruption (*arrows*) indicates fatty nature of the mass.

Siegel et al.[161] have also shown that the multiple fat and nonfat interfaces in an AML along with the large acoustic impedance differences at these interfaces cause scattering and attenuation of the sound waves giving rise to an echogenic lesion with detectable shadowing (Fig. 9-53). Shadowing was seen in 33% of their AMLs and in none of their RCCs. Involvement of regional lymph nodes and extension of tumor into the inferior vena cava have been described.

Small, asymptomatic AMLs may be followed for growth. If they are large, symptomatic, or have hemorrhaged, surgery is often performed. If possible, renal sparing surgery is preferable, particularly because these tumors are benign or may be multiple. Embolization may also be used to treat actively bleeding AMLs.[163]

Lymphoma

Kidney. The kidney does not contain lymphoid tissue and lymphomatous involvement of the kidney occurs from either **hematogeneous dissemination** or **contiguous extension** of retroperitoneal disease. Renal disease is more commonly **non Hodgkin lymphoma** than Hodgkin lymphoma. By the time renal disease is evident, there is usually apparent disseminated disease. Urinary tract symptoms are uncommon. Occasionally flank pain, flank mass, or hematuria may occur. At autopsy, renal involvement will be found in one third of lymphoma patients[164] and bilateral renal disease is more common than unilateral disease. Isolated renal disease may be seen in patients undergoing treatment.

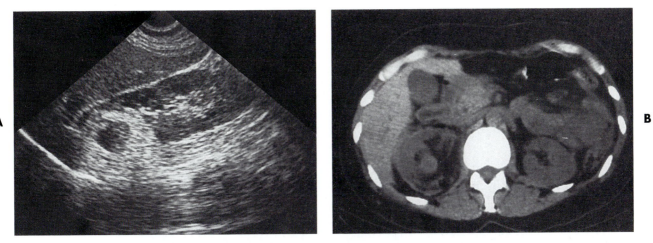

FIG. 9-54. Angiomyolipoma with central hemorrhage. A, Sagittal sonogram demonstrates an echogenic mass with a central hypoechoic component. B, Confirmatory nonenhanced computed tomography shows the fatty component of the tumor with central hemorrhage.

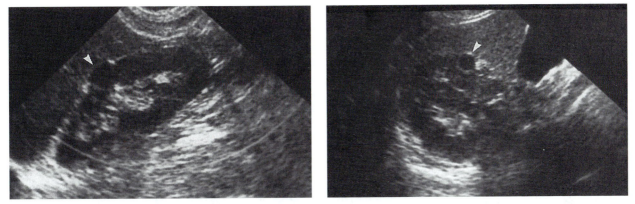

FIG. 9-55. Lymphoma. A, Sagittal and B, transverse sonograms demonstrate a small hypoechoic renal mass (*arrowhead*) simulating a cyst. Through transmission is not seen indicating a solid lesion.

The **sonographic appearance** of renal lymphoma is variable depending on the pattern of involvement. **Four patterns are recognized and include focal parenchymal involvement; diffuse infiltration; invasion from a retroperitoneal mass; perirenal involvement.**

Focal parenchymal involvement may manifest itself as solitary or multiple nodules. These masses appear homogeneous and hypoechoic or anechoic (Fig. 9-55). They may simulate cysts however, appropriate through transmission, for the size of the lesion, is not apparent.[165,166] **Diffuse infiltration** is seen as complete disruption of the normal renal architecture with maintenance of the reniform shape. The kidney may be enlarged (Fig. 9-56). The tumor may invade the renal sinus and destroy the echogenic central echo complex.[167] **Direct invasion** of the kidney by large retroperitoneal lymph node masses may occur with

> ### SONOGRAPHIC APPEARANCE OF RENAL LYMPHOMA
>
> Focal parenchymal involvement
> Diffuse infiltration
> Invasion from a retroperitoneal mass
> Perirenal involvement

associated vascular and ureteral encasement. Large retroperitoneal hypoechoic lymph node masses will be seen extending into the kidney causing hydronephrosis. Rarely, **perirenal involvement** is noted as a surrounding hypoechoic perirenal mass/rind which may be confused with hematoma or extramedullary hematopoiesis (Fig. 9-57).[168,169]

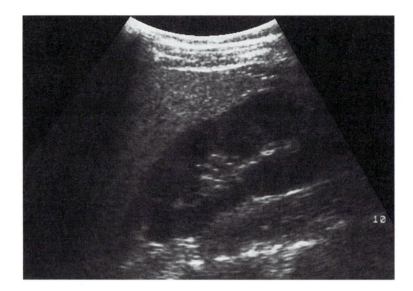

FIG. 9-56. Lymphoma. Diffuse infiltration and parenchymal destruction are seen. The kidney is diffusely hypoechoic however reniform shape is maintained.

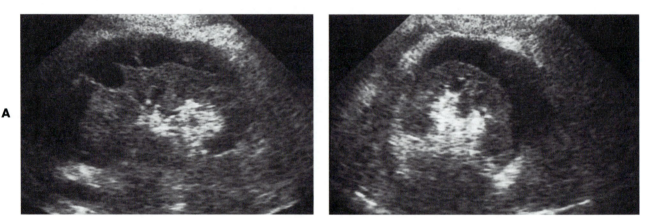

FIG. 9-57. Lymphoma. A, Sagittal and **B,** transverse sonograms demonstrate a rind of hypoechoic tissue surrounding and indenting the renal margin.

Ureter. Lymphomatous involvement of the ureter occurs with either displacement or encasement. Displacement is more common with encasement representing 1% to 16%. Of these cases, actual invasion of the ureter wall occurs in only one third.[144] The result is usually dilatation of the intrarenal collecting system and ureter to the level of the retroperitoneal mass. This is usually easily appreciated on sonography.

Bladder. Primary bladder lymphoma arises from lymph follicles in the submucosa and usually does not infiltrate the other layers of the bladder wall.[170] Most patients are between 40 to 60 years of age with women more commonly affected. **On sonography,** a bladder wall mass is seen usually covered by intact epithelium. If large, ulceration may occur (Fig. 9-58).

Leukemia

Leukemic involvement of the kidney may be **diffuse** or **focal.** Sixty-five percent of patients with leukemia will have renal infiltrates at autopsy.[171] Although seen with great frequency at autopsy, the sonographic changes may be hard to appreciate. **On sonography,** bilateral diffuse renal enlargement may occur; however, 15% of patients demonstrating enlargement will have no evidence of leukemic infiltrate.[172] The renal parenchyma may demonstrate a coarsened echopattern with distortion of the central sinus echo complex.[173] Alternatively, diffuse decreased echogenicity of the renal parenchyma may be seen. Focal mass(es) may occur which may be single or multiple.[174] Renal, subcapsular, or perinephric

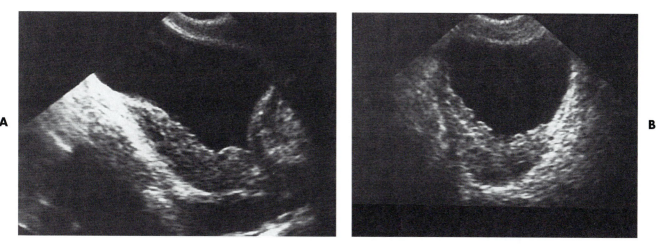

FIG. 9-58. Bladder lymphoma. A, Sagittal and **B,** transverse sonograms show extensive bladder wall thickening with intact overlying mucosa.

hemorrhage may be present as these patients are prone to bleed.

Metastases

Kidney. Metastatic disease to the kidneys is common with metastases to the lung, liver, bone, and adrenal glands only surpassing the kidney in frequency.[175] Spread to the kidneys is via a hematogenous route. The **most common primary tumors** giving rise to renal metastases are: (1) lung carcinoma; (2) breast carcinoma; and (3) renal cell carcinoma of the contralateral kidney.[93] Other tumors that may produce renal metastases include: colon, stomach, cervix, ovary, pancreas, and prostate.[93] Most remain clinically silent, although some patients may develop hematuria or flank pain. Morphologically, the pattern of renal metastases may be: (1) **a solitary mass;** (2) **multiple masses;** or (3) **diffusely infiltrative** enlarging the kidney with maintenance of reniform shape.[176] Choyke et al.[177] evaluated 27 patients with renal metastases and found that metastases are usually multifocal; however, solitary large tumors may occur which are otherwise indistinguishable from primary renal cell carcinoma. They also found that a new renal lesion in a patient with advanced cancer is more likely a metastatic tumor than a primary one. If a single renal lesion is discovered synchronously in a patient with a known primary tumor or one in remission, with no evidence of other metastases, renal biopsy is necessary to differentiate a primary renal cell carcinoma from a renal metastasis.

Contrast-enhanced CT is the best radiographic technique for detecting renal metastasis, although ultrasound is almost as sensitive.[177] **On sonography,** the appearance will depend on the pattern of involvement. **A solitary metastasis** will be seen as a solid mass indistinguishable from renal cell carcinoma (Fig.

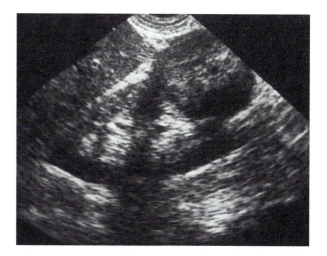

FIG. 9-59. Renal metastasis. Sagittal renal sonogram demonstrates a solitary renal metastasis. This cannot be differentiated from renal cell carcinoma.

9-59). This occurs often with colon carcinoma.[177] Central necrosis, hemorrhage, and calcification may be evident. **Multiple metastases** are usually small, poorly marginated hypoechoic masses. Involvement of the perinephric space is possible, particularly with malignant melanoma and lung cancer.[177] **Diffuse tumor infiltration** will be seen as renal enlargement with distorted architecture and loss of the normal corticomedullary differentiation (Fig. 9-60).[176]

Ureter. **Ureteric metastases** are rare and evidence of diffuse metastases elsewhere will be seen in 90% of cases.[178] Metastatic disease to the ureter occurs either by **hematogenous** or **lymphatic dissemination.** Tumors that may secondarily involve the ureter include: (1) melanoma; (2) bladder; (3) colon; (4) breast; (5) stomach; (6) lung; (7) prostate; (8) kidney; and (9) cervix. **Three types of ureteral in-**

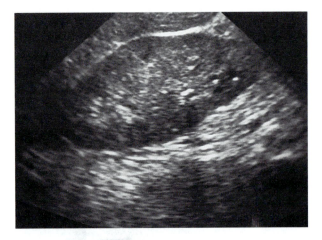

FIG. 9-60. Renal metastases. Sagittal sonogram demonstrating diffuse parenchymal tumor infiltration. Reniform shape is maintained.

volvement occur and these are: (1) infiltration of the periureteral soft tissues; (2) transmural involvement of the ureteral wall; and (3) submucosal nodules. The first two types demonstrate stricture formation with or without an associated mass, whereas the third type demonstrates an intraluminal mass(es).[144] **On sonography,** the site of tumor involvement may be seen if a mass is present. Usually, the secondary sign of hydronephroureterosis is present.

Bladder. Metastases to the bladder may occur with malignant melanoma, lung, gastric, or breast cancer. This is, however, a rare occurrence. **Sonographically,** a solid mass may be seen in the bladder wall. Often, metastatic malignant melanoma will be recognized cystoscopically by its deep brown color.

Urachal Adenocarcinoma

The urachus measures 3 to 10 cm in length and represents the obliterated remnant of the allantois. It is lined by transitional epithelium and neoplasms of the urachus are rare. They represent 0.01% of all adult cancers, 0.17% to 0.34% of all bladder cancers and 20% to 39% of all primary bladder adenocarcinomas.[179] Seventy-five percent of patients are men.[180] Most tumors arise at the bladder dome at the vesicourachal junction. The tumors have a poor prognosis and tend to invade the anterior abdominal wall. Most patients present with hematuria, although other common clinical presentations include frequency, dysuria, and mucosuria.[180] **On sonography,** a bladder dome mass is seen which is often calcified. Tumor extension into the perivesicle fat, space of Retzius and the abdominal wall is common.

Rare Neoplasms

Kidney. **Juxtaglomerular tumors** are rare benign tumors which occur most frequently in women. They produce renin that causes hypertension. On sonography, they are usually small, solid, and hyperechoic.[181] Excision will alleviate the hypertension. **Leiomyomas** are benign tumors. They are usually discovered incidentally but may grow large enough to become clinically evident. On sonography, a solid, well-defined mass is seen. They may be peripheral, arising from the renal capsule. **Carcinoid tumor** is a rare renal tumor which tends to be solid, often showing peripheral or central calcification.[182] Other benign tumors have been described including **lipoma and hemangioma.**

Renal sarcomas represent approximately 1% of all malignant renal tumors. **Leiomyosarcoma** is the most common, accounting for 58% of all renal sarcomas. Patients have a poor prognosis. **Hemangiopericytoma** represents 20% of all renal sarcomas. On sonography, these tumors cannot be distinguished from renal cell carcinoma. **Liposarcoma** accounts for 20% of all renal sarcomas. Depending on the amount of mature fat present, these tumors can be quite hyperechoic and indistinguishable from an angiomyolipoma. **Less common sarcomas** include **rhabdomyosarcoma, fibrosarcoma, and osteogenic sarcoma.**

Wilms' tumor may rarely occur in adults and cannot be differentiated radiologically from renal cell carcinoma.

Bladder. Mesenchymal bladder tumors are rare, accounting for 1% of all bladder tumors. **Leiomyoma** is the most common benign bladder tumor. Most arise from the submucosa near the bladder trigone.[183] These tumors may show intravesical (63%), intramural (7%), or extravesicle (30%) growth.[183] On sonography, a well-defined round or oval solid mass will be seen. Cystic degeneration may occur. **Neurofibromas** of the bladder may be seen as an isolated finding or occur with diffuse systemic disease. Sonographically, these tumors are similar to leiomyomas. **Cavernous hemangiomas** are most commonly found in the dome and posterolateral bladder wall.[184] Cystoscopically, they are bluish-red in color. On sonography, two types have been described: (1) a round, well-defined, solid, hyperechoic, intraluminal mass which is highly vascular on color Doppler ultrasound; and (2) diffuse wall thickening with multiple hypoechoic spaces and calcification.[184] **Bladder pheochromocytomas** are rare and represent only 1% of all pheochromocytomas.[183] Patients may have symptoms including headache, sweating, and tachycardia related to bladder distention or voiding. These tumors arise in the submucosa and may be found anywhere in the bladder, although are commonly found at the dome. Sonographically, a well-defined, solid, intramural bladder wall mass will be seen (Fig. 9-61).

Malignant mesenchymal bladder tumors are rare. The most common ones include **leiomyosar-**

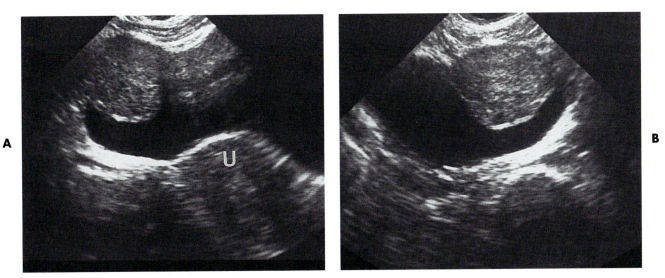

FIG. 9-61. **Bladder pheochromocytoma.** **A,** Sagittal and **B,** transverse sonograms showing a well-defined, homogeneous mural mass at the bladder dome. U—uterus.

coma and rhabdomyosarcoma. On sonography, a large, infiltrative mass is seen.

RENAL CYSTIC DISEASE

Cortical Cysts

Simple. **Simple renal cysts** are benign and fluid-filled. Their exact pathogenesis is unknown, although they are believed to be acquired lesions. Their incidence increases with advancing age and they are found in at least 50% of people over the age of 50. Most are asymptomatic, however, if large, flank pain and hematuria may occur. The **sonographic criteria** used to diagnose a simple cyst include:

- anechoic
- acoustic enhancement
- sharply defined, imperceptible, smooth far wall
- round or ovoid shape

If all these sonographic criteria are met, further evaluation or follow-up of the cyst is not required (Fig. 9-62). If the renal cyst is large and symptomatic, cyst puncture and sclerosis may be performed. Several simple cysts may be found in both kidneys and rarely, several simple cysts may involve only one kidney or a localized portion of one kidney (Fig. 9-63).

Complex. **Complex renal cysts** are those that do not meet the strict criteria of a simple renal cyst. These include cysts containing **internal echoes, septations, calcification, perceptible defined wall, and mural nodularity.** Depending on the degree of abnormality most of these cysts require further imaging with CT. A combination of ultrasound and

---

APPROACH TO A SONOGRAPHICALLY DISCOVERED COMPLEX RENAL CYST

Internal echoes
Follow-up with ultrasound if no other features of malignancy are present.
Perform computed tomography if associated features of malignancy are present (perceptible thickened wall, multiple or thick septations, extensive septal calcification).

Septations
Follow-up with ultrasound if few and thin (≤ 1 mm).
Perform computed tomography if there is septal irregularity and nodularity, multiple complex septations or solid elements at septal wall attachment.

Calcification
Follow-up with ultrasound if small amount of calcium or milk of calcium without associated soft tissue mass.
Perform computed tomography if thick, irregular, or amorphous calcification.
Perform computed tomography if calcification obscures adequate sonographic visualization.

Perceptible defined wall or mural nodularity
Presumed malignant, perform computed tomography.

Use a combination of ultrasound and computed tomography to analyze the internal features of a complex renal cyst to determine if more likely benign or malignant. Benign-type lesions can be followed with serial imaging, whereas malignant-type lesions will require surgical removal.

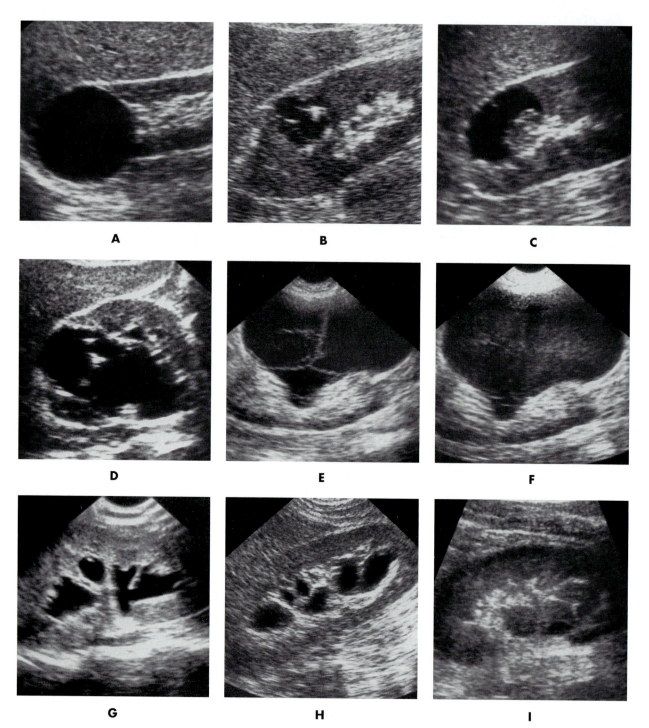

FIG. 9-62. Simple, complex, and parapelvic renal cysts A, Simple renal cyst with posterior acoustic enhancement. B, Complex benign renal cyst with septations and small insignificant echogenic foci with ring-down. C, Cyst with a nondependent mural nodule indicative of malignancy. D, Complex benign cyst with a few scattered echogenic foci on the septa representing calcifications. E, Complex benign cyst with a few thin septations. F, Same cyst as E, following hemorrhage into the cyst. Multiple internal echoes are now seen. G, H, and I, Central cystic structures. G, Central cysts join and show a calyceal pattern indicative of hydronephrosis. H, Multiple, haphazard noncommunicating central cystic spaces representing parapelvic cysts. I, Multiple hemorrhagic parapelvic cysts containing internal echoes.

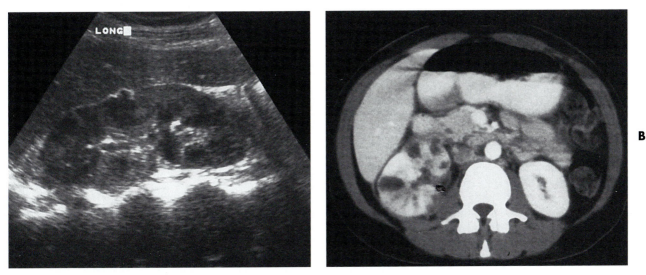

FIG. 9-63. Localized cystic disease. A, Sagittal sonogram shows multiple renal cysts in the right kidney. **B,** Confirmatory computed tomography shows multiple right renal cysts and a normal left kidney.

CT will help to determine whether or not a complex cystic lesion is more likely benign or malignant.

Internal echoes within a cyst are usually the result of hemorrhage or infection. Approximately 6% of cysts are complicated by hemorrhage.[185] Infection of a cyst may occur by hematogenous seeding, vesico-ureteric reflux, or iatrogenically following cyst puncture or surgical manipulation. Sonographically, infected cysts usually also demonstrate a thickened wall with a debris-fluid or gas-fluid level. Hemorrhagic cysts may be followed with serial ultrasound if other imaging features of malignancy are absent (Fig. 9-62). Infected cysts will require aspiration and drainage for diagnosis and treatment.

Septations may be seen within a renal cyst and they often occur following hemorrhage, infection and percutaneous aspiration. Occasionally, two adjacent cysts sharing a wall may appear as a large septated cyst. If septae are thin (≤ 1 mm), smooth, and attach to the cyst wall without thickened elements, a benign cyst can be diagnosed (Fig. 9-62).[186] If septal irregularity, thickness greater than 1 mm or solid elements at the wall attachment are present, the lesion must be presumed malignant. Cyst aspiration is not indicated in these multiseptated cystic lesions.[186] Ultrasound is often better than CT in defining the internal characteristics of a cystic lesion.

Calcification of renal cysts may be fine and linear or amorphous and thick. If all other ultrasound and CT criteria for cyst are met, the presence of a small amount of calcium or thin, fine areas of calcification in the wall or on a septae, without associated soft tissue mass or enhancement, likely represents a complicated cyst rather than malignancy (Fig. 9-62).

However, thick, irregular, amorphous calcification is more worrisome and likely requires surgical removal to determine if the lesion is benign or malignant.[186] Calcium may also be present as milk of calcium with layering present (Fig. 9-64). Bright, echogenic foci with ringdown are seen frequently on septae and cyst walls. These foci are of no consequence and do not correspond with calcification on CT (Fig. 9-62, *B*).

Perceptible, defined, thickened wall or mural nodularity essentially excludes a diagnosis of benign cyst (Fig. 9-62). These lesions will all require surgical removal to exclude malignancy.

Parapelvic Cysts

Parapelvic cysts do not communicate with the collecting system and likely are lymphatic in origin or develop from embryologic rests.[187] Most are asymptomatic, although they may cause hematuria, hypertension, hydronephrosis, or become infected.[188] **On sonography,** parapelvic cysts appear as well defined anechoic renal sinus masses (Fig. 9-62). It may be difficult to differentiate multiple parapelvic cysts from hydronephrosis. When hydronephrosis is present, the anechoic fluid-filled calyces and renal pelvis can be seen to communicate, whereas multiple parapelvic cysts often have haphazard orientation and are seen as noncommunicating renal sinus cystic masses (Fig. 9-62). If differentiation between the two is not possible with sonography, either IVP or contrast-enhanced CT will easily resolve the dilemma (Fig. 9-65).

Medullary Cysts

Medullary Sponge Kidney. Medullary sponge kidney (MSK) is defined as dilated, ectatic collecting

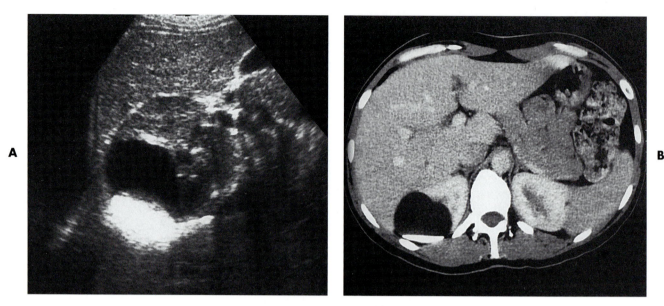

FIG. 9-64. **Renal cyst with milk of calcium.** **A,** Transverse sonogram shows a large renal cyst with dependent echogenic material which was mobile on real-time examination. **B,** Computed tomography demonstrates milk of calcium layering in the dependent portion of the cyst.

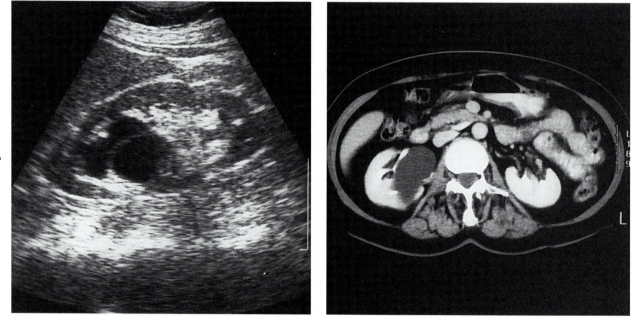

FIG. 9-65. **Parapelvic cysts.** **A,** Sagittal sonogram shows hypoechoic masses in the renal sinus simulating a duplex collecting system with upper-moiety hydronephrosis. **B,** Confirmatory computed tomography shows a large central parapelvic cyst.

tubules. It may be **focal** or **diffuse.** The etiology is unknown. The incidence in the general population is not known, but is found in up to 12% of patients with renal stones.[189] It usually occurs in the third to fourth decade.[190] There is an association with hemihypertrophy, Ehlers-Danlos syndrome, congenital hypertrophic pyloric stenosis, hyperparathyroidism, Caroli's

disease, and autosomal recessive polycystic disease.[190] Uncomplicated MSK is usually not associated with symptoms; however, with stone formation renal colic, hematuria, dysuria, and flank pain may occur.[190] **On sonography,** tubular ectasia may be difficult to recognize. When nephrocalcinosis is present, multiple echogenic shadowing foci are seen localized to the medullary pyramids (Fig. 9-42). If a focus of calcification has eroded into the collecting system, a stone will be seen which may or may not be obstructing.

Medullary Cystic Disease. **Medullary cystic disease of the kidney** occurs as a result of progressive renal tubular atrophy. The kidneys are small or normal sized with tubulointerstitial fibrosis and cysts in the medulla or at the corticomedullary junction.[191] The pathogenesis is unknown. There is a **childhood form** inherited as an autosomal recessive disorder and an **adult form** inherited as an autosomal dominant disorder. **On sonography,** small echogenic kidneys with medullary cysts (0.1 to 1.0 cm) are seen.

Polycystic Kidney Disease

Autosomal Recessive. Autosomal recessive polycystic kidney disease (ARPCK) is divided into four types, depending on the individual's age at onset of clinical manifestations and include: **perinatal, neonatal, infantile, and juvenile.** The disease is characterized pathologically by dilatation of renal collecting tubules, hepatic cysts, and periportal fibrosis. Younger patients present predominantly with renal abnormality, whereas older patients have predominantly hepatic abnormality. It occurs in 1 in 6000 to 1 in 14,000 live births. Perinatal disease will demonstrate massive renal enlargement, hypoplastic lungs, and oligohydramnios. Death usually occurs as a result of renal failure and pulmonary hypoplasia. Older children will present with manifestations of portal hypertension. **On sonography,** massively enlarged, echogenic kidneys with lack of corticomedullary differentiation are seen. Occasionally, macroscopic cysts will be noted (Fig. 9-66).

Autosomal Dominant. Autosomal dominant polycystic kidney disease (ADPCK) is a disorder resulting in a large number of bilateral cortical and medullary renal cysts. The cysts may vary considerably in size and are often asymmetric. ADPCK is the most common hereditary renal disorder with no gender predilection. It is found in 1:500 to 1:1000 and accounts for 10% to 15% of patients on dialysis.[192] Up to 50% of patients will have no family history as the disease is characterized by variable expression and also occurs as a result of spontaneous mutation. Signs and symptoms of palpable mass(es), pain, hypertension, hematuria, and urinary tract infection usually do not develop until the fourth or fifth decade. Renal failure develops in 50% of patients and is usually present by 60 years of age.[192] Complications of ADPCK include infection, hemorrhage, stone formation, cyst rupture, and obstruction. Associated anomalies occur including: (1) liver cysts (30% to 60%); (2) pancreatic cysts (10%); (3) splenic cysts (5%); (4) cysts in thyroid, ovary, endometrium, seminal vesicles, lung, brain, pituitary gland, breast, and epididymis; (5) cerebral berry

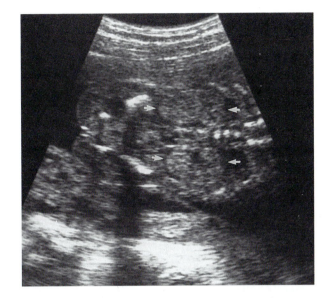

FIG. 9-66. Autosomal recessive polycystic kidney disease. *In utero* coronal sonogram showing bilateral large echogenic kidneys (*arrows*).

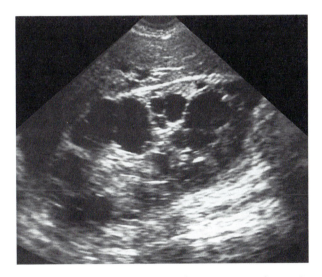

FIG. 9-67. Autosomal dominant polycystic kidney disease. Sagittal sonogram shows multiple cysts enlarging the kidney.

aneurysms (18% to 40%); (6) abdominal aortic aneurysm; (7) cardiac lesions; and (8) colonic diverticula. Patients with ADPCK, not on dialysis, do not have an increased incidence of renal cell carcinoma.[192]

On sonography, the kidneys are enlarged with multiple bilateral asymmetric cysts of varying size (Fig. 9-67). Cysts complicated by hemorrhage or infection will demonstrate thick walls, internal echoes and/or fluid-debris levels (Fig. 9-68). Dystrophic calcification on cyst walls or stones may be seen as echogenic foci with distal sharp acoustic shadowing. Renal cysts in patients under the age of 30 are rare.

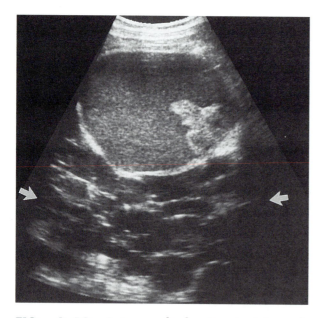

FIG. 9-68. Autosomal dominant polycystic kidney disease with large, hemorrhagic cyst. Sagittal sonogram showing a polycystic kidney (*arrows*) with a large complex cyst containing internal echoes and adherent clot.

Ravine et al.[193] modified the Bear[194] criteria, and state that patients less than or equal to 30 years of age with a family history of ADPCK require two renal cysts (unilateral or bilateral) to make the diagnosis of ADPCK disease. For patients 30 to 59 years of age, two cysts in both kidneys are required and for those 60 years of age or older, four cysts in each kidney are needed. Ultrasound is the best imaging modality available for screening families of known affected individuals as well as for routine follow-up of those patients with known disease.

Multicystic Dysplastic Kidney

Multicystic dysplastic kidney (MCDK) is a nonhereditary developmental anomaly also known as renal dysplasia, renal dysgenesis, and multicystic kidney. The kidney is small, malformed, and composed of multiple cysts with little if any normal renal parenchyma. It therefore functions poorly if at all. The dysplastic change is usually **unilateral** and involves the entire kidney; however, it rarely may be **bilateral, segmental, or focal.** If unilateral the condition is asymptomatic, if bilateral, it is incompatible with life. Men and women are equally affected as are both sides. Up to 30% will have contralateral UPJ obstruction. The exact pathogenesis is obscure; however, 90% are associated with some form of urinary tract obstruction during embryogenesis. The severity of the malformation affects the spectrum of findings which range from a large multicystic mass present at birth to a kidney with smaller cysts not discovered until adulthood.

On sonography, the findings include: (1) multiple noncommunicating cysts; (2) absence of both normal parenchyma and normal renal sinus; and (3) focal echogenic areas representing primitive mesenchyma or tiny cysts (Fig. 9-69).[195] In adults, the cystic renal fossa mass is not large and cyst wall calcification is appreciated as echogenic foci with shadowing (Fig. 9-70). Calcification may be so extensive that ultrasound visualization is impossible and CT is required to make the diagnosis. Segmental disease is usually seen in duplex kidneys and, if the cysts are very tiny, the mass may appear solid and echogenic.

Multilocular Cystic Nephroma

Multilocular cystic nephroma (MLCN) is an uncommon benign cystic neoplasm composed of multiple, noncommunicating cysts contained within a well-defined capsule. Occasionally, sarcomatous stroma is present making this a more malignant lesion. MLCN has no predilection for side and occasionally bilateral tumors are seen. These tumors are found in males less than 4 years of age and females between the ages of 4 and 20 or 40 and 60.[196] Most children present with an abdominal mass, whereas adults can be asymptomatic or present with abdominal pain, hematuria, hypertension, and urinary tract infection.

On sonography, the appearance of MLCN is quite variable depending on the number and size of the locules. If the locules are large, multiple, noncommunicating cysts will be seen within a well-defined mass (Fig. 9-71). If the locules are tiny, a more solid-appearing nonspecific echogenic mass will be present. Calcification of the capsule and septae is uncommon. With either appearance, it is impossible with imaging to differentiate it from cystic renal cell carcinoma.

Renal Cystic Disease Associated with Neoplasms

Acquired Cystic Kidney Disease. Acquired cystic kidney disease (ACKD) occurs in the native kidneys of patients with renal failure undergoing either hemodialysis or peritoneal dialysis with a frequency of 90% after 5 years of dialysis.[98,99,197] Renal cell carcinoma occurs in 4% to 10% of patients with ACKD.[197] The pathogenesis of ACKD is speculative. Epithelial hyperplasia causing tubular obstruction occurring as a result of toxic substances plays some role in the development of both cysts and tumors.[197] Pathologically multiple small cysts (0.5 to 3 cm) involving both renal cortex and medulla are found. Hemorrhage into cysts is common. Ultrasound, CT, and MRI are useful in the evaluation and follow-up of patients with ACKD and its complications.[98,99,198] Current data suggest that ACKD and tumor development persist even after successful renal transplantation. As well, ACKD and tumors may develop in renal allografts during dialysis therapy.[199]

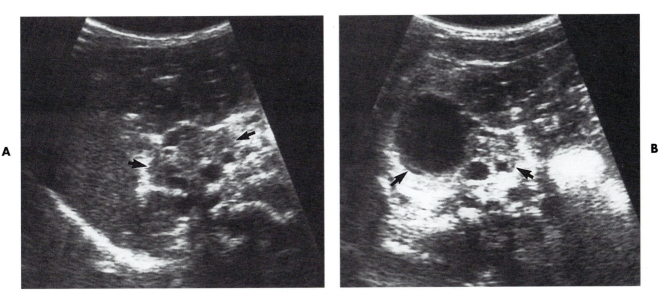

FIG. 9-69. Multicystic dysplastic kidney in a child. A, Sagittal and B, transverse sonograms demonstrate multiple, noncommunicating cysts, absence of normal parenchyma and renal sinus, and focal echogenic areas representing primitive mesenchyme (*arrows*).

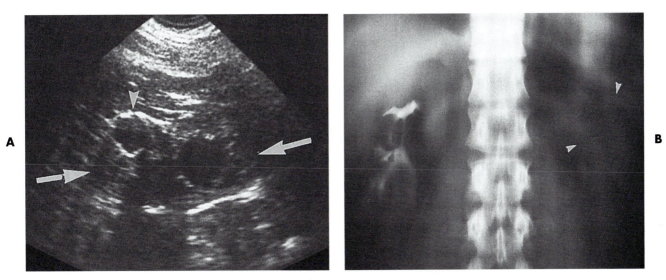

FIG. 9-70. Multicystic dysplastic kidney in an adult. A, Sagittal sonogram reveals a small kidney (*arrows*) with cysts. Some cysts have ringlike calcification (*arrowhead*). B, Tomogram from an intravenous pyelogram demonstrates a small, nonfunctioning left kidney with multiple, grapelike calcifications (*arrowheads*).

On sonography, three to five cysts in each kidney in a patient with chronic renal failure are diagnostic.[199] The cysts are usually small as are the kidneys which usually are quite echogenic (Fig. 9-72). Internal echoes will be seen in cysts that have hemorrhaged. Tumors will be solid or cystic with mural nodules.

von Hippel-Lindau Disease. von Hippel-Lindau disease (VHL) is transmitted as an autosomal dominant gene with variable expression and moderate penetrance. Its incidence is 1:35,000.[192] The predom-inant significant abnormalities include **retinal angiomatosis, CNS hemangioblastomas, pheochromocytomas,** and **renal cell carcinoma** (40%). Renal cell carcinoma in patients with VHL usually is multifocal (75% to 90%) and bilateral (75%). These patients are often offered nephron sparing surgery. In addition, **renal cysts,** which are the most common finding in this disease, are found in 76% of patients.[200] Cysts range in size from 0.5 to 3.0 cm and are mostly cortical in location. **Sonography** is good

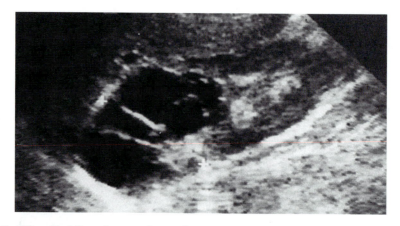

FIG. 9-71. Multilocular cystic nephroma. Sagittal sonogram demonstrates a multiseptated upper-pole renal mass with noncommunicating locules.

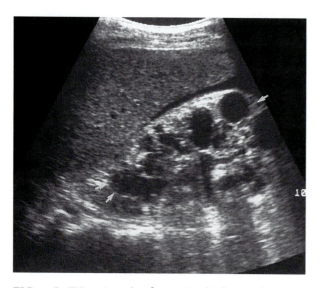

FIG. 9-72. Acquired cystic kidney disease. Sagittal sonogram demonstrates an echogenic kidney (*arrows*) with parenchymal loss and multiple cysts. A small amount of intraperitoneal dialysate fluid is seen.

for screening these patients; however, CT is better for detection of the small multifocal bilateral tumors found in this disease.

Tuberous Sclerosis. Tuberous sclerosis (TS) is a genetically transmitted disease characterized by **mental retardation, seizures, and adenoma sebaceum.** Some cases are transmitted in an autosomal dominant fashion though many cases result from spontaneous mutation. The incidence ranges from 1:9,000 to 1:170,000.[201] Associated renal lesions include **cysts, angiomyolipomas (AML),** and **renal cell carcinoma** (1% to 2%).[192] The renal cysts vary in size from microscopic to 3 cm. **On sonography,** if cysts only are present it may be difficult to differentiate from ADPCK disease. If cysts and multiple AMLs are present and confirmed with CT, tuberous sclerosis can be suggested (Fig. 9-73). Periodic CT screening is recommended to assess for AML growth and tumor development.

TRAUMA

Kidney

Traumatic injury to the kidney may be either **blunt** or **penetrating.** Most forms of blunt trauma to the kidney are relatively minor and heal without treatment. Penetrating injuries are usually the result of gunshot or stab wounds. Kidneys with cysts, tumors, and hydronephrosis are more prone to injury. Renal injuries are classified into **four categories** and include:

I)   Minor injury (75% to 85%); contusions and lacerations
II) Major injury (10%); renal fracture
III) Catastrophic injury (5%); vascular pedicle injury and shattered kidney
IV) UPJ Avulsion

Category I lesions are treated conservatively while category III and IV lesions require urgent surgery. Category II lesions will be treated conservatively or surgically depending on severity.[202]

Computed tomography is regarded as the premier imaging modality for the evaluation of suspected renal trauma. As renal trauma is frequently accompanied by injuries to other organs, CT has the advantage of multiorgan imaging. Theoretically, sonography has the capability of evaluating traumatized kidneys but realistically, technical limitations usually hinder an adequate examination. Sonography does not provide information regarding renal function and is probably best used in the follow-up of patients with known renal parenchymal traumatic injury. **Renal hematomas** may be hypoechoic, hyperechoic, or heterogeneous. **Lacerations** will be seen as linear defects which may extend through the kidney if a fracture is present (Fig. 9-74). Associated perirenal collections consisting of blood and urine will be present if the kidney is fractured. **Subcapsular hematoma** may be seen as a perirenal fluid collection that flattens the underlying renal contour (Fig. 9-75). **A shattered kidney** will consist of multiple fragments of disorganized tissue

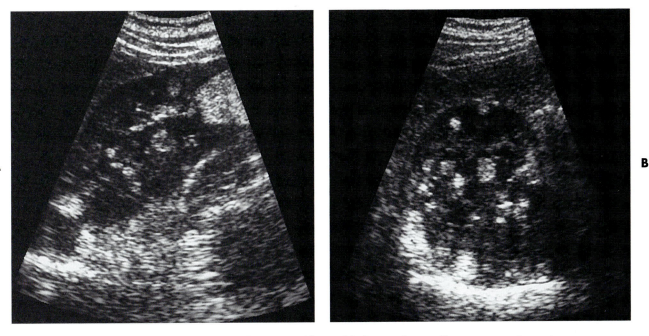

FIG. 9-73. Tuberous sclerosis with multiple angiomyolipomas. A, Sagittal and **B,** transverse sonograms demonstrate multiple, well-defined echogenic tumors throughout the kidney.

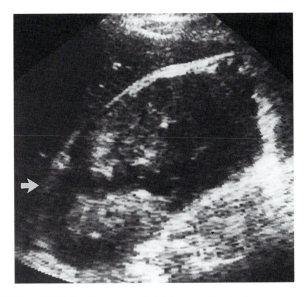

FIG. 9-74. Fractured kidney. Sagittal sonogram demonstrates a linear hypoechoic tear through the renal sinus (*arrow*).

with associated hemorrhage and urine collection in the renal bed. Color Doppler may be helpful in the assessment of **vascular pedicle injuries.**

Ureter

Traumatic injury of the ureter is most commonly **iatrogenic** related to gynecological (70%) or urologic (30%) surgery.[203] Blunt and penetrating injuries are far less common. Sonography is not useful in the assessment of these injuries, except to detect sizable fluid collections and/or hydronephrosis.

Bladder

Bladder injury may be the result of **blunt, penetrating,** or **iatrogenic trauma.** Bladder injury may result in extra or intraperitoneal rupture or a combination of the two. Sonography is usually not helpful in the assessment of these injuries.

VASCULAR

Renal Vascular Doppler

The number and size of arteries supplying a kidney are quite variable. Duplex and color-imaging Doppler are able to demonstrate both normal and abnormal renal blood flow. Flow in the renal artery demonstrates a low resistance perfusion pattern on duplex Doppler indicative of continuous forward blood flow during diastole. The measurement of resistance index (RI = peak systolic frequency − end diastolic frequency/ peak systolic frequency) on duplex Doppler is used to assess arterial resistance. Keogan et al.[204] recommend averaging a number of RI measurements in a kidney before a single representative average is reported. The RI of native kidneys is normally 0.60 to 0.92.[205] Mostbeck et al.[206] reported that the RI, however, varies with heart rate and can range from 0.57 ± 0.06 (pulse 120/min) to 0.70 ± 0.06 (pulse 70/min). **Variation in RI** has been described, in both native and transplant kidneys, with: (1) obstruction; (2) medical renal disease; (3) renal vein thrombosis; (4) renal artery stenosis; and (5) transplant rejection and dysfunction.

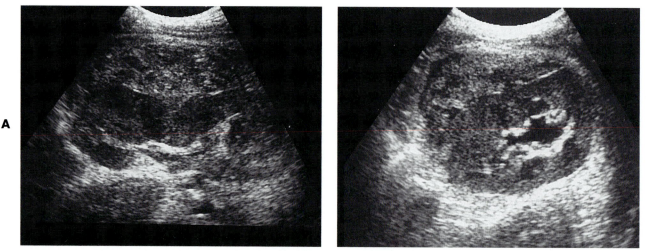

FIG. 9-75. Acute subcapsular renal hematoma. A, Sagittal and **B,** transverse sonograms show a large, postbiopsy echogenic collection compressing the renal parenchyma. Acute hematomas may be echogenic or isoechoic relative to the parenchyma. Indentation of the renal cortex may be the only clue to their presence.

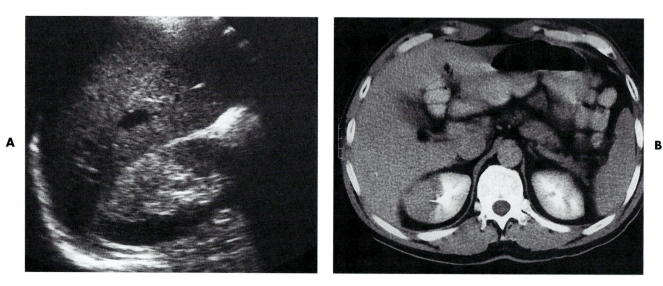

FIG. 9-76. Renal infarct. A, Sagittal sonogram shows a wedge-shaped echogenic mass in the anterolateral renal cortex. **B,** Confirmatory computed tomography shows segmental infarction.

Color Doppler sonography is based on mean Doppler frequency shift, whereas power Doppler relies on the integrated Doppler power spectrum which is related to the number of erythrocytes producing the Doppler shift. At the present time, power Doppler is subject to significant flash artifact however, Bude et al.[207] demonstrated that in normal co-operative individuals, power Doppler is superior to conventional color Doppler in the demonstration of normal intrarenal vessels. Power Doppler also has the advantage of not being subject to aliasing and angle dependence; however, direction and velocity of motion are only apparent with color Doppler imaging.

Renal Arterial Occlusion and Infarction

Renal artery occlusion may occur with **embolus** or **thrombosis.** The degree of renal insult depends on the size and location of the occluded vessel. If the main renal artery is occluded, the entire kidney will be affected, whereas segmental and focal infarction may occur with peripherally located vascular occlusion. **On sonography,** acute complete renal arterial occlusion may demonstrate a normal kidney. Duplex and color Doppler will not demonstrate flow to the kidney. Segmental or focal infarction may appear as a hypoechoic, wedge-shaped mass indistinguishable from acute pyelonephritis (Fig. 9-76). With time, an echogenic mass[208] or scar may form. With chronic occlusion, an end-stage, small, scarred kidney will be seen.

Arteriovenous Fistula and Malformations

Abnormal **arteriovenous communications** may be **acquired** (75%) or **congenital** (25%). **Acquired lesions** are usually iatrogenic, although spontaneous abnormal arteriovenous communications may occur with eroding tumors. Most acquired lesions consist of a single, dominant feeding artery and a single, dominant draining vein. **Congenital malformations** consist of a tangle of small abnormal vessels. Gray-scale sonography may reveal no abnormality. The addition of duplex and color Doppler has been helpful in defining these lesions.[209] Duplex Doppler demonstrates increased flow velocity, decreased resistivity (0.3 to 0.4), and turbulent diastolic flow in the arterial limb. Arterial pulsations in the draining vein are also observed. Spectral broadening is present. Color Doppler may demonstrate a tangle of tortuous vessels with multiple colors indicative of the haphazard orientation and turbulent flow within the malformation.

Renal Artery Stenosis

Hypertension may be primary (95% to 99%) or secondary (1% to 5%). The vast majority of patients with secondary hypertension suffer from renovascular disease. Renovascular disease is most commonly due to atherosclerosis (66%) with the majority of the remaining cases due to fibromuscular dysplasia.[210] Many different imaging techniques have been used in an effort to detect patients with renovascular hypertension and include: (1) IV and intra-arterial digital subtraction angiography; (2) captopril renal scintigraphy; (3) duplex and color Doppler ultrasound; and (4) magnetic resonance angiography.

There has been significant effort over the past 10 years to use duplex and color Doppler to diagnose renal artery stenosis reliably. Despite this, use of this method remains controversial. The approach is twofold: (1) detection of abnormal Doppler signals at or just distal to the stenosis; or (2) detection of abnormal Doppler signals in the intrarenal vasculature. Evaluation of the main renal arteries in their entirety is usually impossible. It is estimated that the main renal arteries are not seen in up to 42% of patients.[211] As well, approximately 14% to 24% of patients will have accessory renal arteries which are usually not detected sonographically. Therefore, evaluation of the main renal arteries as a screening technique for renal artery stenosis has failed. The second approach is to interrogate the intrarenal vasculature which can be identified in virtually all patients. Normally, there is a steep upstroke in systole with a second small peak in

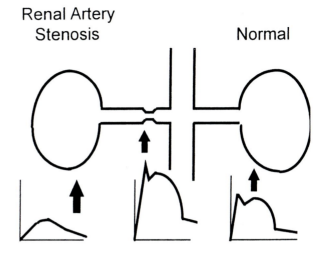

FIG. 9-77. **Schematic diagram of renal artery Doppler tracings.** The tracing on the right side of the diagram is a normal renal artery. The tracing in the middle shows high-velocity flow measured at the stenosis. The tracing on the left side of the diagram shows the dampened tardus-parvus waveform downstream from the stenosis. (From Mitty HA, Shapiro RS, Parsons RB, et al: Renovascular hypertension. *Radiol Clin North Am* 1996;34(5): 1017-1036.)

early systole. A **tardus-parvus waveform** seen downstream from a stenosis refers to a slowed systolic acceleration with a low amplitude of the systolic peak. To evaluate the delayed upstroke, two measurements are taken:

- **acceleration time**—time from start of systole to peak systole
- **acceleration index**—slope of the systolic upstroke

An acceleration time greater than 0.07 seconds and a slope of systolic upstroke less than 3 m/s^2 are suggested as thresholds to assess for renal artery stenosis.[211] Simple recognition of the change in pattern may be adequate (Fig. 9-77).[212] Pharmacologic manipulation with captopril[213] may enhance the waveform abnormalities in patients with renal artery stenosis. At the present time however, Doppler sonography remains a controversial technique for the detection of native renal artery stenosis.

Renal Artery Aneurysm

Renal artery aneurysm is a **saccular** or **fusiform** dilatation of the renal artery or one of its branches and occurs with an incidence of 0.09% to 0.3%.[214] The etiology may be **congenital, inflammatory, traumatic, atherosclerotic, or related to fibromuscular disease.** If large (> 2.5 cm), noncalcified, or associated with pregnancy, the possibility of rupture increases and treatment is recommended. **On gray-scale sonography,** a cystic mass may be seen. The addition of duplex and color Doppler will readily demonstrate arterial flow within the cystic mass.

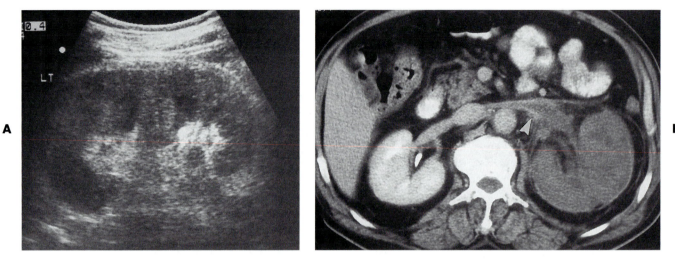

FIG. 9-78. Renal vein thrombosis. A, Sagittal sonogram demonstrates a diffusely enlarged edematous left kidney with loss of corticomedullary differentiation. **B,** Confirmatory computed tomography shows a poorly functioning inhomogeneous kidney with thrombus in the left renal vein (*arrowhead*).

Renal Vein Thrombosis

Renal vein thrombosis (RVT) usually occurs because of underlying abnormality of the kidney, hydration, or coagulation status. Tumors of the kidney and left adrenal gland may grow into the veins resulting in RVT. Extrinsic compression related to tumors, retroperitoneal fibrosis, pancreatitis, and trauma may cause RVT by attenuating the vessel and slowing flow. In adults, the most common etiology is membranous glomerulonephritis, and 50% of patients with this disease will have RVT. If thrombosis is acute, signs and symptoms of flank pain and hematuria will occur. With a more chronic onset, and development of venous collaterals, symptoms are usually insignificant. The **sonographic features** of **acute RVT** are nonspecific and include an enlarged, edematous, hypoechoic kidney with loss of normal corticomedullary differentiation (Fig. 9-78).[215,216] Occasionally, thrombus will be seen within the renal vein, but acutely, it may be anechoic and invisible. The use of duplex and color Doppler may help; however, lack of detectable flow in a patent renal vein is possible, especially if the flow is of low velocity. Absent or reversed end diastolic flow in the intraparenchymal native renal arteries may be a secondary sign of RVT. Platt et al.[217] evaluated 20 native kidneys in 12 patients with clinical findings suggestive of acute RVT. They found that normal arterial Doppler studies should not prevent further work-up if RVT is suspected, nor should absent or reversed diastolic signals be considered highly suggestive of RVT. If equivocal, MRI should be performed. **Chronic RVT** usually results in a small, end-stage, echogenic kidney.

Ovarian Vein Thrombosis

Ovarian vein thrombosis is seen in postpartum women but may also be seen as a result of pelvic inflammatory disease, Crohn disease, or following gynecologic surgery. The right side is more commonly affected than the left. **Gray-scale, duplex, and color Doppler sonography** may reveal a long, tubular structure filled with thrombus extending from the region of the renal vein to deep within the pelvis. Patients are usually treated with anticoagulation and antibiotics.

MEDICAL DISEASES OF THE GENITOURINARY TRACT

Acute Tubular Necrosis

Acute tubular necrosis (ATN) is the most common cause of acute reversible renal failure and is related to deposition of cellular debris within the renal collecting tubules. Both ischemic and toxic insults will cause tubular damage. Some of the initiating factors include **hypotension, dehydration, drugs, heavy metals, and solvent exposure. The sonographic appearance** of ATN depends on the underlying etiology. Hypotension-causing ATN will often produce no sonographic abnormality, whereas drugs, metals, and solvents will cause enlarged echogenic kidneys.

Prerenal disease and ATN account for 75% of all cases presenting with acute renal failure. Platt et al.[218] evaluated the usefulness of duplex Doppler in trying to differentiate these two common causes and found that most cases of acute renal failure will have elevated resistance index (RI >0.7). At the initial exam-

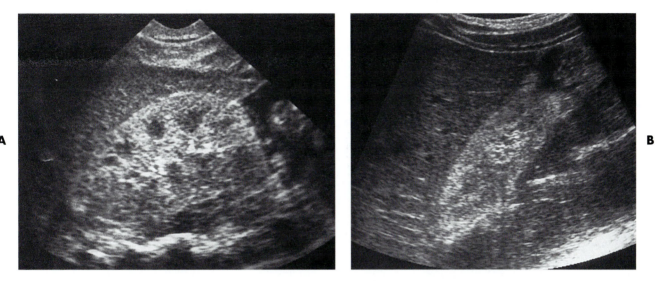

FIG. 9-79. Medical renal disease, two different patients. Sagittal sonograms showing A, Enlarged kidney with echogenic cortex and prominent medullary pyramids. These changes are seen with acute medical renal disease. **B,** Small kidney with the parenchyma as echogenic as the renal sinus. This is a more chronic appearance.

ination, duplex Doppler with elevated RI ($>$0.75) may be helpful in differentiating ATN from prerenal failure, because most patients with prerenal failure will have RI less than 0.75. The exception are patients with prerenal failure combined with severe liver disease (hepatorenal syndrome) who also exhibit elevated RI ($>$0.75).

Acute Cortical Necrosis

Acute cortical necrosis (ACN) is a rare cause of acute renal failure caused by ischemic necrosis of the cortex with sparing of the medullary pyramids. The outermost aspect of cortex remains viable as a result of capsular blood supply. ACN occurs in association with **sepsis, burns, severe dehydration, snake bites, and pregnancy complicated by placental abruption or septic abortion.** The exact etiology is uncertain, although it is likely related to a transient episode of intrarenal vasospasm, intravascular thrombosis, or glomerular capillary endothelial damage. **On sonography,** the renal cortex is initially hypoechoic.[219] With time (mean = 2 months) calcification of the cortex becomes apparent.

Glomerulonephritis

Acute glomerulonephritis is a disease of the glomerulus with proliferative and necrotizing abnormality. Systemic diseases that also have acute glomerulonephritis as a feature include **polyarteritis nodosa, systemic lupus erythematosus, Wegener's granulomatosis, Goodpasture's syndrome, thrombocytopenic purpura, and hemolytic uremic syndrome.** Patients often present with hematuria, hyper-

tension, and azotemia. **On sonography,** both kidneys are affected and the size may range from normal to markedly enlarged. The echopattern of the cortex is altered with medullary sparing and may be normal, hypoechoic, or hyperechoic (Fig. 9-79). With treatment, the kidneys may revert to normal size and echopattern. **Chronic glomerulonephritis** occurs with progression of acute disease and occurs over a period of weeks to months following an acute episode. Profound global symmetric parenchymal loss occurs. The calyces and papillae are normal, and there is an increase in the amount of peripelvic fat. Small, smooth, echogenic kidneys are seen with prominence of the central echo complex (Fig. 9-79).

Acute Interstitial Nephritis

Acute interstitial nephritis (AIN) is an acute hypersensitivity reaction of the kidney most commonly related to drugs. **Penicillin, methicillin, rifampin, sulfa-based drugs, nonsteroidal anti-inflammatory drugs (NSAIDs), cimetidine, furosemide, and thiazide drugs** have been implicated. Usually, renal failure will resolve with cessation of drug therapy. **On sonography,** enlarged echogenic kidneys are noted.

Diabetes Mellitus

Diabetes mellitus is the most common cause of chronic renal failure. Diabetic nephropathy is believed to be related to glomerular hyperfiltration. Renal hypertrophy occurs. With time, diffuse intercapillary glomerulosclerosis develops,[220] causing progressive decrease in renal size. On sonography, the kidneys are enlarged and, with time, reduction in size and increase

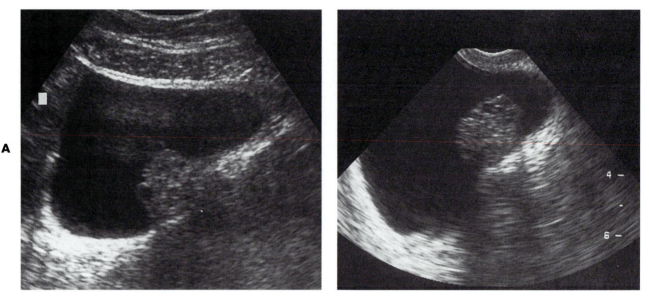

A

B

FIG. 9-80. Bladder endometriosis. A, Suprapubic transvesicle sagittal ultrasound reveals a solid mass at the bladder base. **B,** Transvaginal sagittal scan demonstrates cystic components in the mass which is typical for endometriosis.

in cortical echogenicity with preservation of the corticomedullary junction are noted. With end-stage disease, the kidneys become smaller and more echogenic, and the medulla becomes as echogenic as the cortex.[220]

Amyloidosis

Amyloidosis may be **primary** or **secondary** and usually is a systemic disease. Ten percent to 20% of cases may be localized to one organ system.[221] Patients with amyloidosis often present with renal failure. Patients with primary disease are more often men with a mean age of 60 years. Causes of secondary amyloidosis include **multiple myeloma** (10% to 15%); **rheumatoid arthritis** (20% to 25%); **tuberculosis** (50%); **familial Mediterranean fever** (26% to 40%); **renal cell carcinoma,** and **Hodgkin disease.**[221] On sonography, acutely the kidneys may be symmetrically enlarged. With disease progression, the kidneys shrink in size and demonstrate cortical atrophy with increased cortical echogenicity. Focal renal masses, amorphous calcification, a central renal pelvic mass which may be a hemorrhage or amyloid deposit, and perirenal soft tissue masses may be seen. Similarly, involvement of the ureter and bladder may be localized or diffuse. Wall thickening or masses with or without calcification may be seen. The diagnosis is made with biopsy.

Endometriosis

Endometriosis occurs when endometrial tissue is found outside the uterus in women during the reproductive years. Patients typically present with pain, infertility, dysmenorrhea, dyspareunia, and menorrhagia. Approximately 1% of women with pelvic endometriosis will have urinary tract involvement most frequently in the bladder. Most present with hematuria. **Bladder endometriosis** may be **focal** or **diffuse.** Less commonly, the ureter and rarely the kidney are affected. **On sonography,** bladder endometriosis may present as a mural or intraluminal cyst, or a complex or solid lesion. Diagnosis is usually made cystoscopically with biopsy (Fig. 9-80).

Interstitial Cystitis

Interstitial cystitis is a chronic inflammation of the bladder wall of unknown etiology. It usually affects middle-aged women and has been associated with other systemic diseases including **systemic lupus, rheumatoid arthritis, and polyarteritis.**[61] Irritative voiding symptoms predominate. **On sonography,** a small capacity, thick-walled bladder is seen. Ureteric obstruction may be present (Fig. 9-81).

NEUROGENIC BLADDER

Voiding is a well-coordinated neurologic process controlled by areas within the cerebral cortex. These areas control the detrusor muscle of the bladder as well as both the internal and external urethral sphincters. For simplicity, lesions causing neurogenic bladder may be divided into those causing:
- **detrusor areflexia**—lower motor neuron lesion
- **detrusor hyperreflexia**—lesions above the sacral reflux arc

On sonography, detrusor areflexia results in a smooth, large-capacity, thin-walled bladder. The blad-

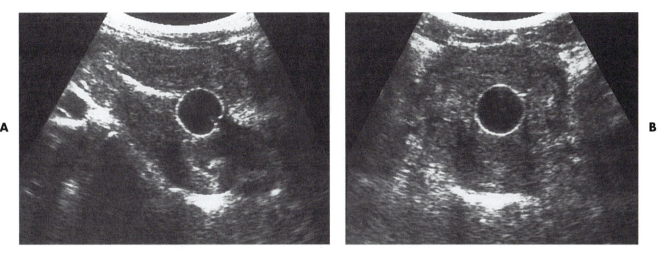

FIG. 9-81. Interstitial cystitis. A, Sagittal and B, transverse sonograms demonstrate marked circumferential bladder wall thickening with a centrally placed Foley catheter.

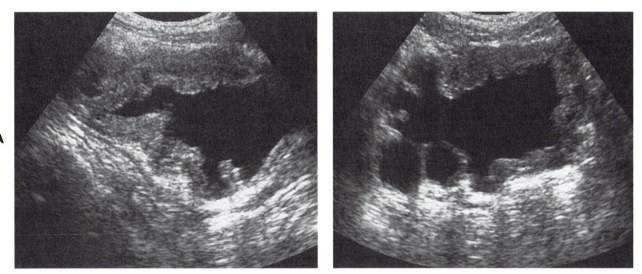

FIG. 9-82. Neurogenic bladder. Detrusor hyperreflexia. A, Sagittal and B, transverse sonograms reveal marked bladder wall thickening and trabeculation giving a Christmas tree appearance.

der may extend high into the abdomen. **Detrusor hyperreflexia** produces a thick-walled, vertical, trabeculated bladder often with associated upper-tract dilatation. A large, postvoid residual will be seen (Fig. 9-82).[222] If neurogenic bladder dysfunction is not properly diagnosed and treated, rapid deterioration of renal function may occur.

BLADDER DIVERTICULA

Bladder diverticula may be **congenital** or **acquired. Congenital diverticula** are known as **Hutch diverticula** and are located near the ureteral orifice. Most **acquired diverticula** result from bladder outlet obstruction. Bladder mucosa herniates through weak

areas in the wall which are typically located posterolaterally near the ureteral orifices. The diverticular neck may be either narrow or wide. It is the narrow neck diverticula that lead to urinary stasis and give rise to complications including **infection, stones, tumors, and ureteral obstruction. On sonography,** an outpouching from the bladder is noted. Its internal echogenicity varies depending on the diverticular content. The neck is often easily appreciated (Fig. 9-83).

RENAL TRANSPLANT

Normal

Morphology. Sonographic evaluation of a renal transplant is usually easily performed because of its

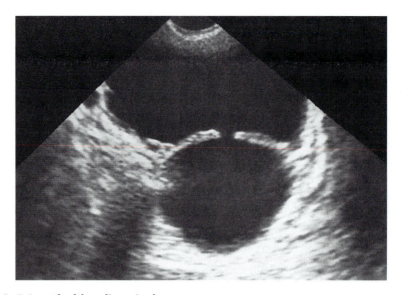

FIG. 9-83. **Bladder diverticulum.** Transverse sonogram demonstrates a large posterior bladder diverticulum with a narrow neck.

superficial, extraperitoneal location in the right or left lower quadrant. Corticomedullary differentiation and the central echogenic renal sinus are often more optimally visualized than in a native kidney. Following surgery, the transplant graft will undergo hypertrophy. There can be a 5% to 15% volume increase in the first 2 weeks, and this may eventually increase up to 20%.[223,224]

Doppler. Duplex Doppler of the intra- and extraparenchymal transplant arteries demonstrates a low-resistance flow pattern. Evaluation of the intra- and extraparenchymal transplant veins shows nonpulsatile continuous flow. The use of color Doppler allows rapid localization of the vessels for duplex Doppler interrogation thus decreasing examination time. Both color and duplex Doppler should be performed with a low-filter setting, maximal gain without background noise, and the smallest scale demonstrating peak velocities without aliasing. In our laboratory, normal peak systolic velocity of the main renal artery is less than or equal to 180 cm/sec. Resistance index range of 0.6 to 0.8 is normal, 0.8 to 0.9 is equivocal, and greater than 0.9 suggests increased vascular resistance.

Urologic Complications

Obstruction. **Obstruction** may occur at any level but most frequently occurs at the ureteric-bladder anastomosis. Immediately postoperatively, edema at the anastomotic site may cause transient pelvicaliectasis and hydroureter. Anastomotic stricture may result from ischemia or iatrogenic injury. Intraluminal and extrinsic masses including stones, blood clot, sloughed papilla, fungus balls, peritransplant collections, and an overly distended bladder may give rise to dilatation of the intrarenal collecting system and ureter (Fig. 9-84). Unlike

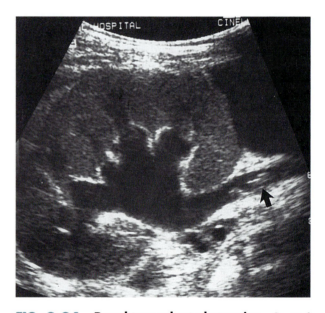

FIG. 9-84. **Renal transplant obstruction.** Sagittal sonogram demonstrates moderate hydronephroureterosis with echogenic mobile blood clot in the distal ureter *(arrow)*.

native kidneys, the renal transplant is denervated, thus obstruction is manifested only by deteriorating renal function parameters. Dilation of the renal transplant collecting system and ureter does not always indicate obstruction. Platt et al.[225] evaluated the role of combining the findings of elevated RI (≥ 0.75) and a dilated collecting system in predicting true obstruction. They found an elevated RI in 85% of their obstructed kidneys. Approximately 10% with obstruction had normal RI, although they were also associated with a urine leak. Many other processes may elevate RI including rejection

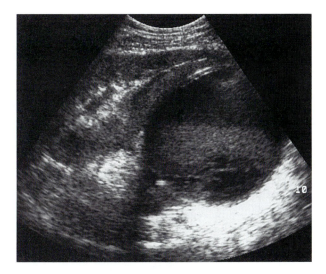

FIG. 9-85. Renal transplant with postoperative hematoma. Sagittal sonogram demonstrates a large hematoma with a fluid-fluid level posterior to the inferior pole of the transplant kidney.

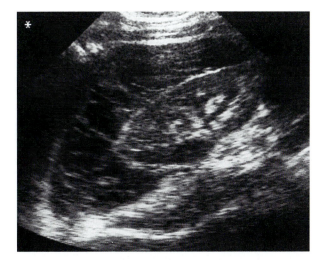

FIG. 9-86. Renal transplant with postoperative lymphocoele. Sagittal sonogram shows a large, multiseptated, peritransplant fluid collection.

and ATN. They conclude that in the setting of pyelocaliectasis and transplant dysfunction, elevated RI should increase suspicion for obstruction. On the other hand, a normal Doppler waveform with dilatation of the collecting system suggests that the dilatation is not caused by obstruction if a leak has also been excluded.

Collections. Up to 50% of graft recipients will demonstrate perirenal fluid collections.[226,227] The most common collections include **hematoma, urinoma, lymphocoele, and abscess. Hematomas** are common in the immediate postoperative period. They usually are small, insignificant, and resolve spontaneously. Occasionally, they are large and may cause obstruction. Hematoma may occur following renal graft biopsy. On sonography, the hematoma will vary in appearance depending on patient age. Acutely, they tend to be echogenic becoming more complex and hypoechoic with time. Hematomas may be extracapsular, subcapsular, or intraparenchymal (Fig. 9-85).

Urinomas usually develop within the first 2 weeks following transplantation. Urine leak commonly occurs from the ureter related to ischemic necrosis or from the region of the anastomosis. On sonography, they tend to be well-defined, anechoic fluid collections. If large leaks are present, widespread extravasation and ascites will be seen.

Lymphocoeles result from surgical disruption of the iliac chain lymphatics. They are the most common collection, giving rise to transplant collecting system obstruction. On sonography, a hypoechoic fluid collection is seen often with multiple internal septations (Fig. 9-86). Small collections can often be followed but larger collections often require drainage which can be accomplished percutaneously or surgically.

An **abscess** may develop if any of the previously mentioned collections become infected, or it may arise on its own. On sonography, a complex peritransplant collection is seen. The abscess may demonstrate a fluid-fluid level or air within. Immediate percutaneous drainage is recommended in these immunocompromised patients.

Vascular Complications. Renal artery stenosis will occur in up to 10% of transplanted kidneys, usually within the first year. It may arise as a result of surgical complication, rejection, or intrinsic vascular disease. Three types of stenoses may occur: (**1**) **anastomotic;** (**2**) **distal donor;** and (**3**) **recipient artery. Anastomotic strictures** occur most frequently in end-to-end anastomosis, **distal stenoses** occur more frequently in end-to-side anastomoses, and **recipient artery stenoses** occur equally in both types.[228] Technical difficulty or rejection may give rise to anastomotic or distal donor stenoses. Recipient artery stenoses are rare and usually the result of intrinsic atherosclerotic disease or intraoperative clamp injury.[228]

Duplex and color Doppler are extremely reliable as a screening tool in the detection of RAS. The most reliable finding is that of a high-velocity jet at the stenosis (>7.5 KHz) and distal turbulent flow.[229] Velocity measurements greater than 180 cm/sec are suggestive of stenosis (Fig. 9-87). These findings may also be seen with vascular kinking. With color, focal areas of aliasing at the stenosis will be seen (Fig. 9-87). If duplex and color Doppler imaging of the renal artery is normal, significant stenosis can be excluded.

Renal artery thrombosis occurs acutely usually within the first month of transplantation and usually results in loss of the graft. It occurs in less than 1% of

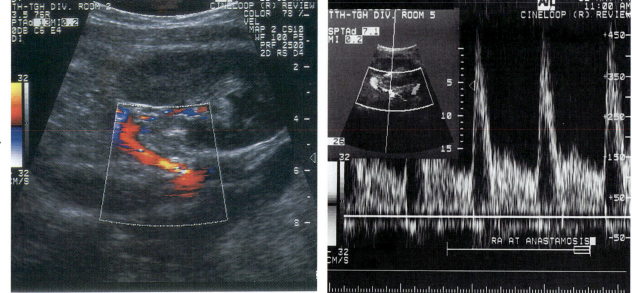

FIG. 9-87. Renal transplant with renal artery stenosis. A. Sagittal color Doppler sonogram demonstrates a focal area of aliasing at the stenosis. **B.** Duplex Doppler demonstrates a high-velocity jet at the stenosis.

renal transplant patients.[228] The most common cause is **hyperacute** and **acute rejection,** resulting in occlusion of small arterioles with retrograde thrombosis of the main renal artery. Other causes include: **(1) intraoperative intimal vascular trauma; (2) technically poor intimal anastomosis; (3) end-to-end anastomoses; (4) hypotension; (5) hypercoagulable states; (6) vascular kinking; (7) cyclosporin; (8) atherosclerotic emboli; and (9) with acquired renal artery stenosis.**[228] If **thrombosis is complete,** duplex and color Doppler will not detect arterial or venous flow distal to the occlusion. If **occlusion is incomplete** but progressive, serial duplex Doppler may demonstrate decreased, reversed, or absent diastolic flow which eventually progresses to complete absence of both systolic and diastolic flow. Absent arterial flow does not necessarily indicate complete occlusion and may be caused by poorly calibrated Doppler equipment or rarely by high-grade stenosis with minimal flow.[228]

Renal vein thrombosis (RVT) and stenosis is rare (0% to 4%) and usually occurs early in the postoperative period. Etiologies include **hypovolemia, surgical or technical difficulty, propagation of femoral or iliac deep-vein thrombosis, and compression by fluid collections.**[228] It is important to diagnose **RVT** early as thrombectomy improves graft survival. Duplex and color Doppler reveal absent renal venous flow with reversed diastolic arterial flow (Fig. 9-88).

Renal vein stenosis will reveal a normal or enlarged kidney with decreased parenchymal echo-

genicity on gray-scale sonography. Color Doppler will reveal focal aliasing. Duplex Doppler will demonstrate increased velocities (three to four times greater in the stenosis than in the prestenotic segment).[228]

Intrarenal arteriovenous fistula (AVF) and pseudoaneurysms are usually iatrogenic in origin resulting from renal biopsy. **AVFs** develop when both artery and vein are injured, and pseudoaneurysms develop with arterial injury only. Most AVFs are small and resolve spontaneously, whereas large ones will decrease renal perfusion caused by the large shunt, cause persistent hematuria or high-output cardiac failure. Treatment is usually percutaneous embolization. Gray-scale imaging may not reveal small AVFs. Duplex Doppler will demonstrate high-velocity, low-resistance arterial waves with arterialized venous tracings.[228] Color imaging will reveal a prominent feeding artery, draining vein, and a tangle of abnormal vessels, appearing as focal areas of color aliasing. Flow turbulence will result in vibration of the vessel wall and perivascular tissues. Therefore, these moving tissues are assigned a color (Fig. 9-89).[205]

Pseudoaneurysms will appear on gray scale as a cystic area. Duplex Doppler reveals turbulent pulsatile flow centrally with to-and-fro motion at the aneurysm neck. With color, disorganized central flow, with a change in color at the neck as flow comes in and out of the aneurysm, will be seen (Fig. 9-90). With both AVFs and pseudoaneurysms, flow in the remainder of the unaffected parenchymal vessels will be normal.

Extrarenal AVFs and pseudoaneurysms are usually the result of surgical difficulty at the time of

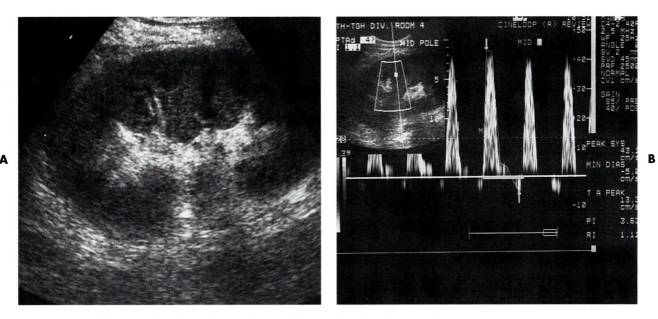

FIG. 9-88. Renal transplant with renal vein thrombosis. A, Sagittal sonogram shows an enlarged swollen kidney with loss of corticomedullary differentiation. **B,** Duplex Doppler shows increased intrarenal arterial resistance (RI = 1.11) with retrograde diastolic arterial flow.

reconstruction. Spontaneous rupture of an extrarenal pseudoaneurysm is catastrophic and its discovery requires urgent surgical intervention. The findings on gray scale, duplex, and color Doppler are similar to their intrarenal counterparts.

Tumors. Renal transplant patients that are immunosuppressed have an increased incidence of developing malignancy including lymphoma and Kaposi sarcoma.

Medical Complications

Rejection. Graft rejection can be classified into **four types:** (1) hyperacute rejection (during surgery); (2) accelerated acute rejection (2 to 3 days); (3) acute rejection (1 to 10 weeks); and (4) chronic rejection (months to years).

Hyperacute rejection usually does not require imaging because the diagnosis is evident during surgery. **Accelerated acute rejection and acute rejection** demonstrate similar imaging findings. Gray scale will reveal a swollen kidney with loss of corticomedullary differentiation. The central renal sinus may become compressed or less echogenic because of edema. Thickening of the urothelium may occur (Fig. 9-91). Total renal blood flow is decreased with rejection but also occurs with acute tubular necrosis (ATN) and cyclosporin-induced toxicity. RI is often increased, but is relatively nonspecific, because it is also increased with arterial stenosis, renal vein thrombosis, acute ureteral obstruction, severe ATN, severe cyclosporin toxicity, pyelonephritis, and compression of

> **RENAL TRANSPLANT**
>
> **Causes of elevated resistance index**
> *Rejection
>   Acute tubular necrosis
>   Cyclosporin toxicity
> *Ureteral obstruction
> *Transplant compression by surrounding collections
>   Renal artery occlusion
>   Renal artery stenosis
>   Renal vein thrombosis
>   Pyelonephritis
>
> *Most commonly encountered

the transplant by surrounding collections. Renal biopsy is usually required to determine the cause of graft dysfunction. **Chronic rejection** often reveals a small kidney with increased cortical echogenicity. The findings are similar to other processes, resulting in chronic disease such as chronic cyclosporin toxicity or changes related to superimposed hypertension or diabetes. RI values may be normal.

Acute Tubular Necrosis. Acute tubular necrosis (ATN) is the result of donor ischemia prior to vascular anastomosis. It usually occurs in the immediate posttransplant period and usually is self-limiting (days to weeks) with little effect on graft survival.

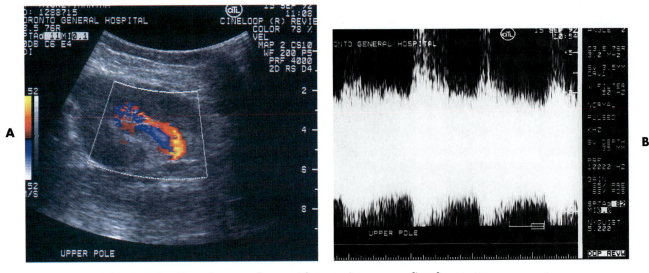

FIG. 9-89. Renal transplant with arteriovenous fistula. A, Transverse color Doppler sonogram showing a prominent feeding artery, draining vein, and a tangle of abnormal vessels. **B,** Duplex Doppler reveals high-velocity, low-resistance arterial waves.

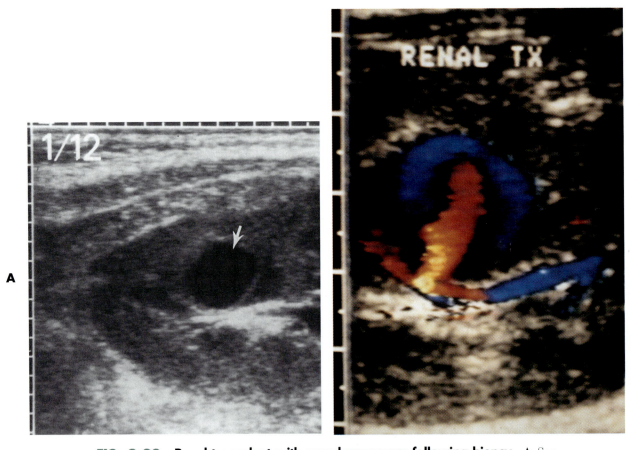

FIG. 9-90. Renal transplant with pseudoaneurysm following biopsy. A, Sagittal sonogram shows a cystic mass in the kidney (*arrow*). **B,** Color Doppler reveals flow within the mass and a jet through the pseudoaneurysm neck. (From Lewis BD, James EM, Charboneau JW, et al: Current applications of color Doppler imaging in the abdomen and extremities. *RadioGraphics* 1989;9(4):599-631.)

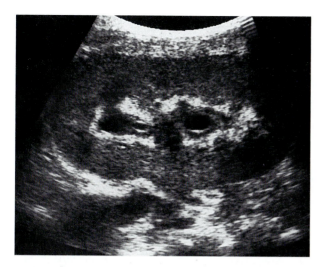

FIG. 9-91. Renal transplant rejection. Sagittal sonogram shows granular parenchyma with loss of corticomedullary differentiation. Urothelial thickening is present centrally.

Imaging cannot differentiate ATN from rejection or cyclosporin-induced nephrotoxicity.

Cyclosporin-Induced Nephropathy. Cyclosporin-induced nephropathy does not usually cause an elevation in the RI or an alteration in graft appearance.[230] However, cyclosporin toxicity may cause graft enlargement, increased cortical echogenicity, and increased RI.[231]

ULTRASOUND-GUIDED INTERVENTION

Intraoperative Ultrasound
At the present time, nephron-sparing surgery is being performed on patients with bilateral renal tumors, tumor in a solitary kidney, small renal tumors, indeterminate masses, and tumors in patients with underlying renal insufficiency. Real-time intraoperative ultrasound is useful, because it can provide valuable information regarding the location and extent of the lesion being resected. As well, intraoperative color Doppler sonography is useful for detecting renal artery complications (intimal flaps, thromboses, and anastomotic stenosis) during transaortic renal endarterectomy or bypass grafting.[232]

Biopsy
Biopsy of a native kidney, renal transplant, or renal mass can safely be performed with ultrasound guidance. If visualization with ultrasound is suboptimal, CT guidance may be used. Ultrasound guidance is preferable, because it is quicker and allows real-time visualization of needle placement. Generally, an 18-gauge core biopsy is sufficient, however, for mass lesions a cytologic sample is also obtained. Potential complications include hemorrhage and pneumothorax. Needle tract seeding with 18-gauge needles or smaller is extremely rare and has been reported in a single case only.[233]

Abscess Drainage
The use of ultrasound and CT has greatly improved our ability to detect, characterize, and accurately localize intra-abdominal and retroperitoneal abscesses. The use of percutaneous drainage is well established as a mechanism to deal with these collections and is often curative obviating the need for surgery. Ultrasound guidance is a quick, effective way to guide needle placement using either ultrasound or fluoroscopy for final tube placement. It has the advantage of portability and can, therefore, be performed at the bedside in critically ill intensive care unit patients.

Nephrostomy
Nephrostomy tube insertion is a relatively common procedure performed in patients for ureteric obstruction, urine leaks, access for percutaneous stone removal and percutaneous endopyelotomy. The use of ultrasound to allow real-time guidance of the needle tip into a selected calyx will save time as well as decrease radiation exposure to both the patient and the operator. If necessary, the procedure could be performed entirely with ultrasound guidance in critically ill, nonmobile, intensive care unit patients.

POSTSURGICAL EVALUATION

Kidney
When small tumors are wedged out during surgery, vascularized retroperitoneal fat is wedged into the defect. Postoperative appearance by both ultrasound and CT may simulate a focal renal mass. **On ultrasound** the mass may be hyperechoic or isoechoic (Fig. 9-92).[234,235] Being aware of this appearance will prevent unnecessary work-up.

Conduits
Urinary diversion is created for patients with nonfunctioning bladders or those patients who have had cystectomy. Recently, the trend has been to form continent urinary diversions. A portion of bowel is used to create a pouch that can mimic normal bladder function. The pouch may attach to the abdominal wall (**cutaneous pouch**) or urethra (**orthotopic pouch**). Postoperative complications are similar for both and include urine extravasation, reflux, fistula formation, abscess, urinoma, hematoma, deep-vein thrombosis,

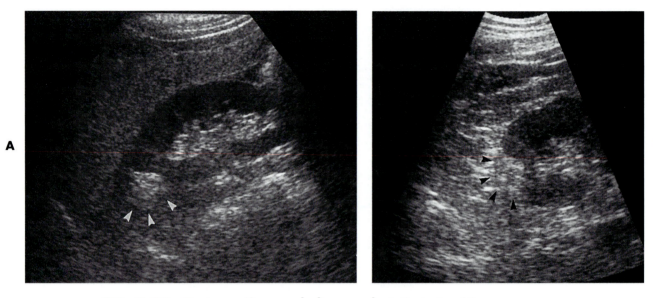

A   B

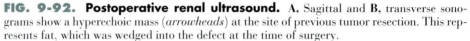

FIG. 9-92. **Postoperative renal ultrasound.** **A,** Sagittal and **B,** transverse sonograms show a hyperechoic mass (*arrowheads*) at the site of previous tumor resection. This represents fat, which was wedged into the defect at the time of surgery.

ileus and small bowel obstruction.[236] The role of sonography is mostly in detecting complications rather than evaluating the pouch itself. If the pouch is urine filled, sonographic assessment is possible. Often, thickened or irregularly shaped bowel wall, pseudomasses, intraluminal mucus collections, and intussuscepted bowel segments can be seen.[236]

ACKNOWLEDGEMENT

The authors would like to thank Marie McInnis for typing the manuscript and Dr. Jenny Tomashpolskaya for her wonderful illustrations.

REFERENCES

1. The kidney. In: Cotran RS, Kumar V, Robbins SL, editors. *Pathologic Basis of Disease.* 5th ed. Philadelphia: WB Saunders Co; 1994:927-989.

Embryology
2. The urogenital system. In: Moore KL, Persaud TVN, editors. *The Developing Human.* 5th ed. Philadelphia: WB Saunders Co; 1993:265-303.

Anatomy
3. Anatomy, structure, and embryology. In: Netter FH. *The CIBA Collection of Medical Illustrations. Vol 6.* Kidneys, Ureters, and Urinary Bladder. CIBA Pharmaceutical Co; 1987: 2-35.
4. Emamian SA, Nielsen MB, Pedersen JF et al: Kidney dimensions at sonography: correlation with age, sex, and habitus in 665 adult volunteers. *AJR* 1993;160:83-86.

5. Platt JF, Rubin JM, Bowerman RA et al: The inability to detect kidney disease on the basis of echogenicity. *AJR* 1988; 151:317-319.
6. Carter AR, Horgan JG, Jennings TA et al: The junctional parenchymal defect: a sonographic variant of renal anatomy. *Radiology* 1985;154:499-502.
7. Yeh HC, Halton KP, Shapiro RS et al: Junctional parenchyma: revised definition of hypertrophied column of Bertin. *Radiology* 1992;185:725-732.
8. Leekam RN, Matzinger MA, Brunelle M et al: The sonography of renal columnar hypertrophy. *J Clin Ultrasound* 1983;11: 491-494.
9. Middleton W, Lelan Melson G: Renal duplication artifact in US imaging. *Radiology* 1989;173:427-429.
10. Chesbrough RM, Burkhard TK, Martinez AJ et al: Gerota versus Zuckerkandl: the renal fascia revisited. *Radiology* 1989;173:845-846.
11. Bechtold RE, Dyer RB, Zagoria RJ et al: The perirenal space: relationship of pathologic processes to normal retroperitoneal anatomy. *RadioGraphics* 1996;16:841-854.

Genitourinary Tract Sonography
12. Mortensson O, Duchek M: Translabial sonography in evaluating the lower female urogenital tract. *AJR* 1996;166:1327-1331.

Congenital Anomalies of the Genitourinary Tract
13. Congenital and hereditary disorders. In: Netter FH. *The CIBA Collection of Medical Illustrations. Volume 6.* Kidneys, Ureters, and Urinary Bladder. CIBA Pharmaceutical Co; 1987: 223-249.
14. Congenital anomalies of the urinary tract. In: Elkin M, editor. *Radiology of the Urinary System 1st edition.* Boston: Little, Brown and Company; 1980:62-147.
15. Friedland GW, Devries PA, Nino-Murcia M et al: Congenital anomalies of the urinary tract. In: Pollack HM, editor. *Clinical Urography. An Atlas and Textbook of Urologic Imaging.* Philadelphia: WB Saunders Co; 1990:559-787.

16. Horgan JG, Rosenfield NS, Weiss RM et al: Is renal ultrasound a reliable indicator of a nonobstructed duplication anomaly? *Pediatric Radiology* 1984;14:388-391.

17. Talner LB: Specific causes of obstruction. In: Pollack HM editor. *Clinical Urography. An Atlas and Textbook of Urologic Imaging*. Philadelphia: WB Saunders Co; 1990:1629-1751.

18. Vargas B, Lebowitz RL: The coexistence of congenital megacalyces and primary megaureter. *AJR* 1986;147:313.

19. Tortora FL Jr, Lucey DT, Fried FA et al: Absence of the bladder. *J Urol* 1983;129(6):1235-1237.

20. Spataro RF, Davis RS, McLachlan MSF, et al: Urachal abnormalities in the adult. *Radiology* 1983;149:659-663.

21. Schnyder PA, Candarjia G: Vesicourachal diverticulum. CT diagnosis in two adults. *AJR* 1981;137:1063-1065.

Infections of the Genitourinary Tract

22. Piccirillo M, Rigsby CM, Rosenfield AT: Sonography of renal inflammatory disease. *Urol Radiol* 1987;9:66-78.

23. Papanicolaou N, Pfister RC: Acute renal infections. *Radiologic Clinics of North America* 1996;34(5):965-995.

24. Talner LB, Davidson AJ, Lebowitz RL, et al: Acute pyelonephritis: can we agree on terminology? *Radiology* 1994;192:297-305.

25. Lowe LH, Zagoria RJ, Baumgartner BR et al: Role of imaging and intervention in complex infections of the urinary tract. *AJR* 1994;163:363-367.

26. Brun-Buisson C, Doyon F, Carlet J et al: Incidence, risk factors and outcome of severe sepsis and septic shock in adults. *JAMA* 1995;274:968.

27. Yoder IC, Pfister RC, Lindfors KK et al: Pyonephrosis imaging and intervention. *AJR* 1983;141:735-740.

28. Patel NP, Lavengood RW, Ernande SM et al: Gas-forming infections in the genitourinary tract. *Urology* 1992;39:341-345.

29. Michaeli J, Mogle P, Perlberg S et al: Emphysematous pyelonephritis. *J Urol* 1984;131:203-208.

30. Wan YL, Lee TY, Bullard MJ et al: Acute gas- producing bacterial renal infection: Correlation between imaging findings and clinical outcome. *Radiology* 1996;198:433-438.

31. Joseph RC, Amendola MA, Artze M et al: Genitourinary tract gas: Imaging evaluation. *RadioGraphics* 1996;16:295-308.

32. Bhathena DB, Weiss JH, Holland NH et al: Focal and segmental glomerular sclerosis in reflux nephropathy. *Am J Med* 1980;68:886.

33. Kay CJ, Rosenfield AT, Taylor KJW et al: Ultrasonic characteristics of chronic atrophic pyelonephritis. *AJR* 1979;132:47-49.

34. Hartman DS, Davis CJ, Goldman SM et al: Xanthogranulomatous pyelonephritis: sonographic-pathologic correlation of the 16 cases. *J Ultrasound Med* 1984;3:481-488.

35. Anhalt MA, Cawood CD, Scott R: Xanthogranulomatous pyelonephritis: a comprehensive review with report of 4 additional cases. *J Urol* 1971;105:10-17.

36. Gammil S, Rabinowitz JG, Peace R et al: New thoughts concerning xanthogranulomatous pyelonephritis. *AJR* 1975;125:154-163.

37. Cousins C, Somers J, Broderick N et al: Xanthogranulomatous pyelonephritis in childhood: ultrasound and CT diagnosis. *Pediatr Radiol* 1994;24:210-212.

38. Davidson AJ: Chronic parenchymal disease. In: Pollack HM, editor. *Clinical Urography. An Atlas and Textbook of Urologic Imaging*. Philadelphia: WB Saunders Co; 1990:2277-2288.

39. Hoffman JC, Schnur MJ, Koenigsburg M: Demonstration of renal papillary necrosis by sonography. *Radiology* 1982;145:785-787.

40. Elkin M: Urogenital tuberculosis. In: Pollack HM, editor. *Clinical Urography. An Atlas and Textbook of Urologic Imaging*. Philadelphia: WB Saunders Co; 1990:1020-1052.

41. Das KM, Indudhara R, Vaidyanathan S: Sonographic features of genitourinary tuberculosis. *AJR* 1992;158:327-329.

42. Pollack HM, Banner MP, Martinez LO et al: Diagnostic considerations in urinary bladder wall calcification. *AJR* 1981; 136:791.

43. Premkumar A, Lattimer J, Newhouse JH: CT and sonography of advanced urinary tract tuberculosis. *AJR* 1987;148:65-69.

44. Das KM, Vaidyanathan, Rajwanshi A et al: Renal tuberculosis: diagnosis with sonographically guided aspiration cytology. *AJR* 1992;158:571-573.

45. Spring D: Fungal diseases of the urinary tract. In: Pollack HM, editor. *Clinical Urography. An Atlas and Textbook of Urologic Imaging*. Philadelphia: WB Saunders Co; 1990:987-998.

46. Shirkhoda A: CT findings in hepatosplenic and renal candidiasis. *J Comput Assist Tomogr* 1987;11:795.

47. Mindell HJ, Pollack HM: Fungal disease of the ureter. *Radiology* 1983;146:46.

48. Boldus RA, Brown RC, Culp DA: Fungus balls in the renal pelvis. *Radiology* 1972;102:555.

49. Stuck KJ, Silver TM, Jaffe HM et al: Sonographic demonstration of renal fungus balls. *Radiology* 1981;142:473.

50. Palmer PES, Reeder MM. Parasitic disease of the urinary tract. In: Pollack HM, editor. *Clinical Urography. An Atlas and Textbook of Urologic Imaging*. Philadelphia: WB Saunders Co; 1990:999-1019.

51. Buchanan WM, Gelfand M: Calcification of the bladder in urinary schistosomiasis. *Trans R Soc Trop Med Hyg* 1970;64:593-596.

52. Diamond HM: Echinococcal disease of the kidney. *J Urol* 1976;115:742-744.

53. King DJ: Ultrasonography of echinococcal cysts. *J Clin Ultrasound* 1976;1:64-67.

54. Sabnis RB, Punekar SV, Desai RM et al: Instillation of silver nitrate in the treatment of chyluria. *Br J Urolog* 1992;70:660-662.

55. Hamper UM, Goldblum LE, Hutchins GM et al: Renal involvement in AIDS: sonographic-pathologic correlation. *AJR* 1988;150:1321-1325.

56. Schaffer RM, Schwartz GE, Becker JA et al: Renal ultrasound in acquired immune deficiency syndrome. *Radiology* 1984; 153:511-513.

57. Pastor-Pons E, Martinez-Lon M, Alvarez-Bustos G et al: Isolated renal mucomycosis in two patients with AIDS. *AJR* 1996;166:1282-1284.

58. Spouge AR, Wilson S, Gopinath N, et al: Extrapulmonary *Pneumocystis carinii* in a patient with AIDS. Sonographic findings. *AJR* 1990;155:76-78.

59. Towers MJ, Withers CE, Hamilton PA et al: Visceral calcification in patients with AIDS may not always be due to *Pneumocystis carinii*. *AJR* 1991;156:745-747.

60. Falkoff GE, Rigsby CM, Rosenfield AT: Partial, combined cortical and medullary nephrocalcinosis: US and CT patterns in AIDS associated MAI infection. *Radiology* 1987;162:343-344.

61. Clayman RV, Weyman PJ, Bahnson RR: Inflammation of the bladder. In: Pollack HM, editor. *Clinical Urography. An Atlas and Textbook of Urologic Imaging* Philadelphia. WB Saunders Co; 1990:902-924.

62. Stark GL, Feddersen R, Lowe BA et al: Inflammatory pseudotumor (pseudosarcoma) of the bladder. *J Urol* 1989; 141:610-612.

63. Kenney PJ, Breatnach ES, Stanley RJ: Chronic Inflammation. In: Pollack HM, editor. *Clinical Urography. At Atlas and Textbook of Urologic Imaging*. Philadelphia. WB Saunders Co; 1990:822-843.

64. Lewin KJ, Fair WR, Steigbigel RT et al: Clinical and laboratory studies into the pathogenesis of malacoplakia. *J Clin Pathol* 1976;29:354-363.

65. Curran FT: Malakoplakia of the bladder. *Br J Urol* 1987; 59:559.

66. Kauzlauric D, Barmeir E: Sonography of emphysematous cystitis. *J Ultrasound Med* 1985;4:319-320.

67. Weiner DP, Koss LG, Sablay B et al: The prevalence and significance of Brunn's nests, cystitis cystica and squamous metaplasia in normal bladders. *J Urol* 1977;122:317.

68. Lang EK, Fritzsche P: Fistulas of the genitourinary tract. In: Pollack HM, editor. *Clinical Urography. An Atlas and Textbook of Urologic Imaging.* Philadelphia: WB Saunders Co; 1990:2579-2593.

69. Wilson S: The Gastrointestinal Tract. In: Rumack CM, Wilson SR, Charboneau JW, editors. *Diagnostic Ultrasound.* St. Louis. Mosby-Year Book Inc., Co. 1991:181-207.

70. Damani N, Wilson S: Non-gynecologic applications of transvaginal sonography. Submitted to *RadioGraphics* August 1997.

Genitourinary Tract Stones and Nephrocalcinosis

71. Sierakowski R, Finlayson B, Landes RR et al: The frequency of urolithiasis in hospital discharge in the United States. *Invest Urol* 1978;15:438.

72. Spirnak JP, Resnick M, Banner MP: Calculus disease of the urinary tract, general considerations. In: Pollack HM, editor. *Clinical Urography. An Atlas and Textbook of Urologic Imaging.* Philadelphia. WB Saunders Co; 1990:1752-1758.

73. Middleton WD, Dodds WJ, Lawson TL et al: Renal calculi: sensitivity for detection with US. *Radiology* 1988;167:239-244.

74. Kimme-Smith C, Perrella RR, Kaveggia LP et al: Detection of renal stones with real-time sonography: effect of transducers and scanning parameters. *AJR* 1991;157:975-980.

75. Sinclair D, Wilson S, Toi A, Greenspan L: The evaluation of suspected renal colic: ultrasound scan versus excretory urography. *Ann Emerg Med* 1989;18:556-559.

76. Erwin BC, Carroll BA, Sommer FG: Renal colic: the role of ultrasound in initial evaluation. *Radiology* 1984;152:147-150.

77. Haddad MC, Sharif HS, Shahed MS et al: Renal colic: diagnosis and outcome. *Radiology* 1992;184:83-88.

78. Haddad MC, Sharif HS, Samihan AM, et al: Management of renal colic: redefining the role of the urogram. *Radiology* 1992;184:35-36.

79. LeRoy A: Diagnosis and treatment of nephrolithiasis: current perspectives. *AJR* 1994;163:1309-1313.

80. Cronan JJ, Tublin ME: Role of the resistance index in the evaluation of acute renal obstruction. *AJR* 1995;164:377-378.

81. Laing FC, Benson CB, DiSalvo DN et al: Distal ureteral calculi: detection with vagina US. *Radiology* 1994;192:545-548.

82. Hertzberg BS, Kliewer MA, Paulson EK et al: Distal ureteral calculi: detection with transperineal sonography. *AJR* 1994; 163:1151-1153.

83. Burge HJ, Middleton WD, McClennan BL et al: Ureteral jets in healthy subjects and in patients with unilateral ureteral calculi: comparison with color Doppler US. *Radiology* 1991; 180:437-442.

84. Price CI, Adler RS, Rubin JM: Ultrasound detection of differences in density: explanation of ureteric jet phenomenon and implications for new ultrasound applications. *Invest Radiol* 1989;24:876-883.

85. Baker S, Middleton WD: Color Doppler sonography of ureteral jets in normal volunteers: importance of relative specific gravity of urine in the ureter and bladder. *AJR* 1992; 159:773-775.

86. Platt JF, Rubin JM, Ellis JH: Acute renal obstruction: evaluation with intrarenal duplex Doppler and conventional US. *Radiology* 1993;186:685-688.

87. Tublin ME, Dodd GD, Verdile VP: Acute renal colic: diagnosis with duplex Doppler US. *Radiology* 1994;193:697-701.

88. Katz DS, Lane MJ, Sommer FG: Unenhanced helical CT of ureteral stones: incidence of associated urinary tract findings. *AJR* 1996;166:1319-1322.

89. Smith RC, Rosenfield AT, Choe KA et al: Acute flank pain: comparison of non-contrast-enhanced CT and intravenous urography. *Radiology* 1995;194:789-794.

90. Smith RC, Verga M, McCarthy S et al: Diagnosis of acute flank pain: value of unenhanced helical CT. *AJR* 1996;166: 97-101.

91. Banner M: Nephrocalcinosis. In: Pollack HM, editor. *Clinical Urography. An Atlas and Textbook of Urologic Imaging.* Philadelphia. WB Saunders Co; 1990:1768-1775.

92. Patriquin H, Robitaille P: Renal calcium deposition in children: sonographic demonstration of the Anderson-Carr progression. *AJR* 1986;146:1253-1256.

Tumors of the Genitourinary Tract

93. Bennington JL, Beckwith JB: *Atlas of tumor pathology, 2nd series*, Fascicle 12. Tumors of the kidney, renal pelvis and ureter. Washington, DC: Armed Forces Institute of Pathology, 1975:25-162.

94. Bennington JL, Laubscher FA: Epidemiologic studies on carcinoma of the kidney. I. Association of renal adenocarcinoma with smoking. *Cancer* 1968;21:1069.

95. Cohen AJ, Li FP, Berg S et al: Hereditary renal cell carcinoma associated with a chromosomal translocation. *N Engl J Med* 1979;301:592.

96. Choyke PL, Glenn GM, Walther MM et al: von Hippel-Lindau disease: genetic, clinical, and imaging features. *Radiology* 1995;194:629-642.

97. Choyke PL, Glenn GM, Walther MM et al: The natural history of renal lesions in von Nippel-Lindau disease: a serial CT imaging study in 28 patients. *AJR* 1992;159:1229-1234.

98. Takase K, Takahashi S, Tazawa S et al: Renal cell carcinoma associated with chronic renal failure: evaluation with sonographic angiography. *Radiology* 1994;192:787-792.

99. Levine E, Grantham J, Slusher S et al: CT of acquired cystic kidney disease and renal tumors in long-term dialysis patients. *AJR* 1984;142:125-131.

100. Skinner DG, Colvin RB, Vermillion CD et al: Diagnosis and management of renal cell carcinoma. A clinical and pathologic study of 309 cases. *Cancer* 1971;28:1165.

101. Sufrin G, Murphy GP: Renal adenocarcinoma. *Urol Surv* 1980;30:129.

102. Raval B, Lamki N: Computed tomography in detection of occult hypernephroma. *CT* 1983;7:199-207.

103. Curry N: Small renal masses (lesions smaller than 3 cm): imaging evaluation and management. *AJR* 1995;164:355-362.

104. Warshauer DM, McCarthy SM, Street L et al: Detection of renal masses: sensitivities and specificities of excretory urography/linear tomography, US and CT. *Radiology* 1988;169: 363-365.

105. Jamis-Dow CA, Choyke PL, Jennings SB et al: Small ($\leq$ 3 cm) renal masses: detection with CT versus US and pathologic correlation. *Radiology* 1996;198:785-788.

106. Szolar DH, Kammerhuber F, Altziebler S et al: Multiphasic helical CT of the kidney: increased conspicuity for detection and characterization of small (< 3 cm) renal masses. *Radiology* 1997;202:211-217.

107. Urban B: The small renal mass. What is the role of multiphasic helical scanning? *Radiology* 1997;202:22-23.

108. Birnbaum BA, Jacobs JE, Ramchandani P: Multiphasic renal CT: comparison of renal mass enhancement during the corticomedullary and nephrographic phases. *Radiology* 1996; 200:753-758.
109. Zeman R, Zeiberg A, Hayes W et al: Helical CT of renal masses: the value of delayed scans. *AJR* 1996;167:771-776.
110. Campeau NG, Johnson CD, Felmlee JP et al: MR Imaging of the abdomen with a phased-array multicoil: prospective clinical evaluation. *Radiology* 1995;195:769-776.
111. Semelka RC, Hricak H, Stevens S et al: Combined gadolinium-enhanced and fat-saturation MR imaging of renal masses. *Radiology* 1991;178:803-809.
112. Bosniak MA, Birnbaum BA, Krinsky GA et al: Small renal parenchymal neoplasms: further observations on growth. *Radiology* 1995;194:589-597.
113. Charboneau JW, Hattery RR, Ernst EC et al: Spectrum of sonographic findings in 125 renal masses other than benign simple cyst. *AJR* 1983;140:87-94.
114. Forman HP, Middleton WD, Melson GL et al: Hyperechoic renal cell carcinomas: increase in detection at US. *Radiology* 1993;188:431-434.
115. Yamashita Y, Takahashi M, Watanable O et al: Small renal cell carcinoma: pathologic and radiologic correlation. *Radiology* 1992;184:493-498.
116. Yamashita Y, Ueno S, Makita O et al: Hyperechoic renal tumors: anaechoic rim and intratumoral cysts in US differentiation of renal cell carcinoma from angiomyolipoma. *Radiology* 1993;188:179-182.
117. Sniderman KW, Kreiger JN, Seligson GR et al: The radiologic and clinical aspects of calcified hypernephroma. *Radiology* 1979;131:31-35.
118. Phillips TL, Chin FG, Palubinskas AJ: Calcifications in renal masses: an eleven year survey. *Radiology* 1963;80:786-794.
119. Kikkawa K, Lasser EC: "Ring-like" or "rim-like" calcification in renal cell carcinoma. *AJR* 1969;107:737-742.
120. Daniels WW, Hartman GW, Witten DM et al: Calcified renal masses: a review of ten years' experience at the Mayo Clinic. *Radiology* 1972;103:503-508.
121. Onitsuka H, Murakami J, Naito S et al: Case Report. Diffusely calcified renal cell carcinoma: CT Features. *J Comp Asst Tomog* 1992;16(4):654-656.
122. Weyman PJ, McClennan BL, Lee J et al: CT of calcified renal masses. *AJR* 1982;138:1095-1099.
123. Press GA, McClennan BL, Melson GL et al: Papillary renal cell carcinoma: CT and sonographic evaluation. *AJR* 1984; 143:1005-1009.
124. Mancilla-Jimenez R, Stanley RJ, Blath RA: Papillary renal cell carcinoma. *Cancer* 1976;38:2469-2480.
125. Yamashita Y, Watanabe O, Miyazaki H et al: Cystic renal cell carcinoma. *Acta Radiologica* 1994;35(1):19-24.
126. Hartman DS, Davis CJ, Johns T et al: Cystic renal cell carcinoma. *Urology* 1986;28(2):145-153.
127. Silverman SG, Lee BY, Seltzer SE et al: Small (≤ 3 cm) renal masses: correlation of spiral CT features and pathologic findings. *AJR* 1994;163:597-605.
128. Vanderburgh L, Thurston W: Imaging features of cystic renal cell carcinoma. In press.
129. Taylor KJW, Ramos I, Carter D et al: Correlation of Doppler US tumor signals with neovascular morphologic features. *Radiology* 1988;166:57-62.
130. Taylor KJW, Ramos I, Morse SS et al: Focal liver masses: differential diagnosis with pulsed Doppler US. *Radiology* 1987; 164:643-647.
131. Kier R, Taylor KJW, Feyock AL et al: Renal masses: characterization with Doppler US. *Radiology* 1990;176:703-707.
132. Ramos IM, Taylor KJW, Kier R et al: Tumor vascular signals in renal masses: detection with Doppler US. *Radiology* 1988; 168:633-637.

133. Kuijpers D, Jaspers R: Renal masses: differential diagnosis with pulsed Doppler US. *Radiology* 1989;270:59-60.
134. McNichols DW, Segura JW, DeWeerd JH: Renal cell carcinoma: long-term survival and late recurrence. *J Urol* 1981; 126:17.
135. Zagoria RJ, Bechtold RE, Dyer RB: Staging of renal adenocarcinoma: role of various imaging procedures. *AJR* 1995; 164:363-370.
136. Habboub HK, Abu-Yousef MM, Williams RD et al: Accuracy of color Doppler sonography in assessing venous thrombus extension in renal cell carcinoma. *AJR* 1997;168:267-271.
137. Fritzsche PJ, Millar C: Multimodality approach to staging renal cell carcinoma. *Urol Radiol* 1992;14:3-7.
138. Buckley JA, Urban BA, Soyer P et al: Transitional cell carcinoma of the renal pelvis: a retrospective look at CT staging with pathologic correlation. *Radiology* 1996;201:194-198.
139. Leder RA, Dunnick NR: Transitional cell carcinoma of the pelvicalices and ureter. *AJR* 1990;155:713-722.
140. Yousem DM, Gatewood OM, Goldman SM et al: Synchronous and metachronous transitional cell carcinoma of the urinary tract: prevalence, incidence and radiographic detection. *Radiology* 1988;167:613-618.
141. Ramji F, Thurston W, Wilson S: Transitional cell carcinoma of the kidney: sonographic features. In press.
142. Dinsmore BJ, Pollack HM, Banner MP: Calcified transitional cell carcinoma of the renal pelvis. *Radiology* 1988;167:401-404.
143. Hartman DS, Pyatt RS, Daily E: Transitional cell carcinoma of the kidney with invasion into the renal vein. *Urol Radiol* 1983;5:83-87.
144. Winalski CS, Lipman JC, Tumeh SS: Ureteral neoplasms. *RadioGraphics* 1990;10:271-283.
145. Dershaw DD, Scher HI: Sonography in evaluation of carcinoma of the bladder. *Urology* 1987;29:454.
146. Dondalski M, White EM, Ghahremani G et al: Carcinoma arising in urinary bladder diverticula: imaging findings in six patients. *AJR* 1993;161:817-820.
147. Barentsz JO, Ruijs SHJ, Strijk SP: The role of MR Imaging in carcinoma of the urinary bladder. *AJR* 1993;160:937-947.
148. Narumi Y, Sato T, Hori S et al: Squamous cell carcinoma of the uroethelium: CT evaluation. *Radiology* 1989;173:853-856.
149. Blacher EJ, Johnson DE, Abdul-Karim FW et al: Squamous cell carcinoma of the renal pelvis. *Urology* 1985;25:124.
150. Mirone V, Prezioso D, Palombini S et al: Mucinous adenocarcinoma of the renal pelvis. *Eur Urol* 1984;10:284.
151. Merino MJ, Livolsi VA: Oncocytomas of the kidney. *Cancer* 1982;50:1852.
152. Honda H, Bonsib S, Barloon T et al: Unusual renal oncocytomas: pathologic and CT correlations. *Urol Radiol* 1992; 14:148-154.
153. Hartman GW, Hattery RR: Benign neoplasms of the renal parenchyma. In: Pollack HM, editor. *Clinical Urography. An Atlas and Textbook of Urologic Imaging.* Philadelphia: WB Saunders Co; 1990:1193-1215.
154. Davidson AJ, Hayes WS, Hartman DS et al: Renal oncocytoma and carcinoma: failure of differentiation with CT. *Radiology* 1993;186:693-696.
155. Goiney RC, Goldenberg L, Cooperberg P et al: Renal oncocytoma: sonographic analysis of 14 cases. *AJR* 1984;143:1001-1004.
156. Tikkakoski T, Paivansalo M, Alanen A et al: Radiologic findings in renal oncocytoma. *Acta Radiologica* 1991;32(5):363-367.
157. Curry NS, Schabel SI, Garvin AJ et al: Intratumoral fat in a renal oncocytoma mimicking angiomyolipoma. *AJR* 1190; 154:307-308.

158. Gentry LR, Gould HR, Alter AJ et al: Hemorrhagic angiomyolipoma: demonstration by CT. *J Comp Asst Tomography* 1981;5(6):861-865.

159. Oesterling JE, Fishman EK, Goldman SM et al: The management of renal angiomyolipoma. *J Urol* 1986;135:1121-1124.

160. Silverman SG, Pearson GD, Seltzer SE et al: Small (161. Siegel CL, Middleton WD, Teefey SA et al: Angiomyolipoma and renal cell carcinoma: US differentiation. *Radiology* 1996; 198:789-793.

162. Arenson AM, Graham RT, Shaw P et al: Angiomyolipoma of the kidney extending into the inferior vena cava: sonographic and CT findings. *AJR* 1988;151:1159-1161.

163. Earthman WJ, Mazer MJ, Winfield AC: Angiomyolipomas in tuberous sclerosis: selective embolotherapy with alcohol with long-term follow-up study. *Radiology* 1986;160:437.

164. Richmond J, Sherman RS, Diamond HD et al: Renal lesions associated with malignant lymphomas. *Am J Med* 1962; 32:184.

165. Horii SC, Bosniak MA, Megibow AJ et al: Correlation of computed tomography and ultrasound in the evaluation of renal lymphoma. *Urol Radiol* 1983;5:69-76.

166. Heiken JP, Gold RP, Schnur MJ et al: Computed tomography of renal lymphoma with ultrasound correlation. *J Comp Asst Tomography* 1983;7(2):245-250.

167. Gregory A, Behan M: Lymphoma of the kidneys: unusual ultrasound appearances due to infiltration of the renal sinus. *J Clin Ultrasound* 1981;9:343-345.

168. Jafri SZ, Bree RL, Amendola MA et al: CT of renal and perirenal non-Hodgkin lymphoma. *AJR* 1982;138:1101-1105.

169. Deuskar V, Martin LFW, Leung W: Renal lymphoma: an unusual example. *J Canadian Assoc Radiol* 1987;38:133-135.

170. Binkovitz LA, Hattery RR, LeRoy AJ: Primary lymphoma of the bladder. *Urol Radiol* 1988;9:231-233.

171. Kirshbaum JD, Preuss FS: Leukemia: a clinical and pathological study of 123 fatal cases in 14,400 necropsies. *Arch Int Med* 1943;71:777.

172. Sternby NH: Studies in enlargement of leukemic kidneys. *Acta Haemat* 1955;14:354.

173. Kumari-Subaiya S, Lee WJ, Festa R et al: Sonographic findings in leukemic renal disease. *J Clin Ultrasound* 1984; 12:465-472.

174. Araki T: Leukemic involvement of the kidney in children: CT features. *J Comput Assist Tomogr* 1982;6:781.

175. Mitnick JS, Bosniak MA, Rothberg M et al: Metastatic neoplasm to the kidney studied by computed tomography and sonography. *J Comput Assist Tomogr* 1985;9:43.

176. Pace K, Thurston W: Unusual presentation of metastatic breast cancer to the kidney. In press.

177. Choyke PC, White EM, Zeman RK et al: Renal metastases: clinicopathologic and radiologic correlation. *Radiology* 1987; 162:359-363.

178. Ambos MA, Bosniak MA, Megibow AJ et al: Ureteral involvement by metastatic disease. *Urol Radiol* 1979;1:105.

179. Rao BK, Scanlan KA, Hinke ML: Abdominal case of the day. *AJR* 1986;146:1074-1079.

180. Brick SH, Friedman AC, Pollack HM et al: Urachal carcinoma: CT findings. *Radiology* 1988;169:377-381.

181. Dunnick NR, Hartman DS, Ford KK et al: The radiology of juxtaglomerular tumors. *Radiology* 1983;147:321-326.

182. McKeown DK, Nguyen GK, Rudrick B et al: Carcinoid of the kidney: radiologic findings. *AJR* 1988;150:143-144.

183. Chen M, Lipson SA, Hricak H: MR imaging evaluation of benign mesenchymal tumors of the urinary bladder. *AJR* 1997; 168:399-403.

184. Kogan MG, Koenigsberg M, Laor E et al: US case of the day. *RadioGraphics* 1996;16:443-447.

Renal Cystic Disease

185. Jackman RJ, Stevens GM: Benign hemorrhagic renal cyst. Nephrotomography, renal arteriography and cyst puncture. *Radiol* 1974;110:7-13.

186. Bosniak M: The current radiological approach to renal cysts. *Radiol* 1986;158:1-10.

187. Hidalgo H, Dunnick NR, Rosenberg ER et al: Parapelvic cysts: appearance on CT and sonography. *AJR* 1982; 138:667-671.

188. Chan JCM, Kodroff MB: Hypertension and hematuria secondary to parapelvic cyst. *Pediatrics* 1980;65:821-822.

189. Ginalski JM, Portmann L, Jaeger PH: Does medullary sponge kidney cause nephrolithiasis? *AJR* 1990;155:299-302.

190. Goldman S, Hartman DS: Medullary sponge kidney. In: Pollack HM, editor. *Clinical Urography. An Atlas and Textbook of Urologic Imaging.* Philadelphia: WB Saunders Co; 1990:1167-1177.

191. Resnick JS, Hartman DS: Medullary cystic disease of the kidney. In: Pollack HM, editor. *Clinical Urography. An Atlas and Textbook of Urologic Imaging.* Philadelphia: WB Saunders Co; 1990:1178-1184.

192. Choyke PL: Inherited cystic diseases of the kidney. *Radiologic Clinics of North America* 1996;34(5):925-946.

193. Ravine D, Gibson RN, Walker RG: Evaluation of ultrasonographic diagnostic criteria. *Lancet* 1994;343:824.

194. Bear JC, McManamon P, Morgan J et al: Age at clinical onset and at ultrasound detection of adult polycystic kidney disease. Data for genetic counselling. *Am J Med Genet* 1984; 18:45.

195. Sanders RC, Hartman DS: The sonographic distinction between neonatal multicystic kidney and hydronephrosis. *Radiology* 1984;151:621-625.

196. Madewell JE, Goldman SM, Davis CJ et al: Multilocular cystic nephroma: a radiographic-pathologic correlation of 58 patients. *Radiology* 1983;146:309-321.

197. Master V, Cruz C, Schmidt R et al: Renal malignancy in peritoneal dialysis patients with acquired cystic kidney disease. *Advances in Peritoneal Diagnosis* 1989;5:145-149.

198. Taylor AJ, Cohen EP, Erickson SJ et al: Renal imaging in long-term dialysis patients: a comparison of CT and sonography. *AJR* 1989;153:765-767.

199. Levine E: Acquired cystic kidney disease. *Radiologic Clinics of North America.* 1996;34(5):947-964.

200. Levine E, Collins DL, Horton WA et al: CT screening of the abdomen in von Hippel-Lindau disease. *AJR* 1982;139:505-510.

201. Kuntz N: Population studies. In: Gomez MR: *Tuberous Sclerosis, 2nd edition.* New York, Raven Press; 1988:214.

Trauma

202. Federle MP: Evaluation of renal trauma. In: Pollack HM, editor. *Clinical Urography. An Atlas and Textbook of Urologic Imaging.* Philadelphia: WB Saunders Co; 1990:1472-1494.

203. Lang EK: Ureteral injuries. In: Pollack HM, editor. *Clinical Urography. An Atlas and Textbook of Urologic Imaging.* Philadelphia: WB Saunders Co; 1990:1495-1504.

Vascular

204. Keogan MT, Kliewer MA, Hertzberg BS, et al: Renal resistance indexes: variability in Doppler US measurement in a healthy population. *Radiology* 1996;199:165-169.

205. Middleton WD, Kellman GM, Leland Melson GL, et al: Post biopsy renal transplant arteriovenous fistulas: color Doppler US characteristics. *Radiology* 1989;171:253-257.

206. Mostbeck GH, Gossinger HD, Mallek R et al: Effect of heart rate on Doppler measurements of resistive index in renal arteries. *Radiology* 1990;175:511-513.

207. Bude RO, Rubin JM, Adler RS: Power versus conventional color Doppler sonography: comparison in the depiction of normal intrarenal vasculature. *Radiology* 1994;192:777-780.

208. Erwin BC, Carroll BA, Walter JF et al: Renal infarction appearing as an echogenic mass. *AJR* 1982;138:759-761.

209. Takebayashi S, Aida N, Matsui K: Arteriovenous malformations of the kidneys: diagnosis and follow-up with color Doppler sonography in six patients. *AJR* 1991;157:991-995.

210. Hillman BJ: Imaging advances in the diagnosis of renovascular hypertension. *AJR* 1989;15:4-14.

211. Mitty HA, Shapiro RS, Parsons RB et al: Renovascular hypertension. *Radiol Clin North Am* 1996;34(5):1017-1036.

212. Stavros AT, Parker SH, Yakes WF et al: Segmental stenosis of the renal artery: pattern recognition of tardus and parvus abnormalities with duplex sonography. *Radiology* 1992;184:487-492.

213. Rene PC, Oliva VL, Bui BT et al: Renal artery stenosis: evaluation of Doppler US after inhibition of angiotensin-converting enzyme with captopril. *Radiology* 1995;196:675-679.

214. Fleshner N, Johnston KW: Repair of an autotransplant renal artery aneurysm: case report and literature review. *J Urol* 1992;148:389-391.

215. Rosenfield AT, Zeman RK, Cronan JJ et al: Ultrasound in experimental and clinical renal vein thrombosis. *Radiology* 1980;137:735-741.

216. Braun B, Weilemann LS, Weigand W: Ultrasonographic demonstration of renal vein thrombosis. *Radiology* 1981;138:157-158.

217. Platt JF, Ellis JH, Rubin JM: Intrarenal arterial Doppler sonography in the detection of renal vein thrombosis of the native kidney. *AJR* 1994;162:1367-1370.

Medical Diseases of the Genitourinary Tract

218. Platt JF, Ruben JM, Ellis JH: Acute renal failure: possible role of duplex Doppler US in distinction between acute prerenal failure and acute tubular necrosis. *Radiology* 1991;179:419-423.

219. Sty JR, Starshak RJ, Hubbard AM: Acute renal cortical necrosis in hemolytic uremic syndrome. *J Clin Ultrasound* 1983;11:175-178.

220. Rodriguez-de-Velasquez A, Yoder IC, Velasquez P et al: Imaging the effects of diabetes on the genitourinary system. *RadioGraphics* 1995;15:1051-1068.

221. Urban BA, Fishman EK, Goldman SM et al: CT evaluation of amyloidosis: spectrum of disease. *RadioGraphics* 1993;13:1295-1308.

Neurogenic Bladder

222. Amis ES, Blavas JG: Neurogenic bladder simplified. *Radiol Clin North Am* 1991;29(3):571-580.

Renal Transplant

223. Lachance SL, Adamson D, Barry JM: Ultrasonically determined kidney transplant hypertrophy. *J Urol* 1988;139:497.

224. Babcock DS, Slovis TL, Han BK et al: Renal transplants in children: Long-term follow-up using sonography. *Radiology* 1985;156:165.

225. Platt JF, Ellis JH, Rubin JM: Renal transplant pyelocaliectasis: role of duplex Doppler US in evaluation. *Radiology* 1991;179:425-428.

226. Letourneau JG, Day DL, Ascher NL et al: Imaging of renal transplants. *AJR* 1988;150:833-838.

227. Silver TM, Campbell D, Wicks JD et al: Peritransplant fluid collections. *Radiology* 1981;138:145-151.

228. Dodd GD, Tublin ME, Shah A et al: Imaging of vascular complications associated with renal transplants. *AJR* 1991;157:449-459.

229. Taylor KJW, Morse SS, Rigsby CM et al: Vascular complications in renal allografts: detection with duplex Doppler US. *Radiology* 1987;162:31-38.

230. Pozniak MA, Kelcz F, D'Alessandro A et al: Sonography of renal transplants in dogs: the effect of acute tubular necrosis, cyclosporin nephrotoxicity and acute rejection on resistive index and renal length. *AJR* 1992;158:791-797.

231. Buckley AR, Cooperberg PL, Reeve CE et al: The distinction between acute renal transplant rejection and cyclosporin nephrotoxicity: value of duplex sonography. *AJR* 1987;1:525.

Ultrasound Guided Intervention

232. Lantz EJ, Charboneau JW, Halle HJW et al: Intraoperative color Doppler sonography during renal artery revascularization. *AJR* 1994;162:859-863.

233. Bush WH, Burnett LL, Gibbons RP: Needle tract seeding of renal cell carcinoma. *AJR* 1977;129:725-727.

Post Surgical Evaluation

234. Papanicolaou N, Harbury OL, Pfister RC: Fat-filled post operative renal cortical defects: sonographic and CT appearance. *AJR* 1988;151:503-505.

235. Millward SF, Lanctin HP, Lewandowski BJ et al: Fat-filled post-operative renal pseudotumor: variable appearance in ultrasonography images. *Can Assoc Radiol J* 1992;43:116-119.

236. Ng C, Amis ES: Radiology of continent urinary diversion. *Radiol Clin North Am* 1991;29(3):557-570.

CHAPTER 10

The Prostate

•

Robert L. Bree, M.D.

After its confusing and controversial beginnings, the applications of transrectal ultrasound (TRUS) of the prostate have become better defined, particularly as they relate to the diagnosis of prostate cancer.[1-3] Up to 5 years ago, ultrasound was considered a primary screening test for prostate cancer. This role has now been replaced by prostate specific antigen (PSA) and digital rectal examination.[4,5] In the hands of the office practitioner, TRUS is used as a guide to performing a systematic biopsy of the prostate.[6] In departments with color Doppler capabilities, TRUS can act as a diagnostic and staging technique for prostate cancer, as well as a modality to evaluate a number of benign and inflammatory prostate and seminal vesicle abnormalities.[7,8]

HISTORY OF PROSTATE ULTRASOUND

The prostate is located deep in the pelvis and, when enlarged, is sonographically accessible from a transabdominal, transvesicle approach. Correlative studies have shown that volumetric evaluation of the prostate with suprapubic ultrasound is accurate and that a gram of prostate tissue is equivalent to 1 cm³. The usefulness of the transvesicle examination for detection of prostate tumors is limited because most prostate cancers occur posteriorly and their small size makes identification difficult. Most of the current interest in prostatic imaging relates to transrectal techniques. In 1974 Japanese[9] investigators were the first to publish their experience with a radial scanner situated on a chair. The technique has evolved slowly since that time, with significant advances occurring with the development of gray-scale, real-time imaging, improved transducer crystal design, and, most recently, biplane probes that allow for prostatic assessment in both axial and longitudinal planes.[10-12] The newest innovation with application to the prostate is color Doppler.[7]

Many early investigators enthusiastically undertook studies to evaluate the role of transrectal ultrasound in patients with prostate cancer. Their reports suggested that even small cancers produced areas of hyperechogenicity.[13-15] Further studies suggested that prostate cancer was difficult to detect, particularly in its early stages.[16,17] With the evolution of higher-frequency probes, larger series of prostate cancer were reported. Authors have sparked a continuing debate concerning the sonographic appearance of prostate cancer, with some series describing small hypoechoic lesions[18] and others describing large hyperechoic cancers.[19]

ANATOMY

Original textbook anatomic descriptions of the prostate use **lobar anatomy,** describing anterior, posterior, and median lobes. Although the concept of a median lobe may be useful in the evaluation of patients with benign prostatic hypertrophy, this lobar anatomy has not been useful in identification of carcinoma of the prostate.[20] Detailed anatomic dissections of the prostate reveal **zonal anatomy,** whereby the prostate is divided into four glandular zones surrounding the prostatic urethra: the peripheral zone, transition zone, central zone, and the periurethral glandular area (Figs. 10-1 to 10-5). In the normal gland, however, sonography can rarely identify these zones unless a pathologic condition is present. On **sonography,** it is more useful to separate the prostate into a peripheral zone and the inner gland, which encompasses the transition and central zones and the periurethral glandular area. A nonglandular re-

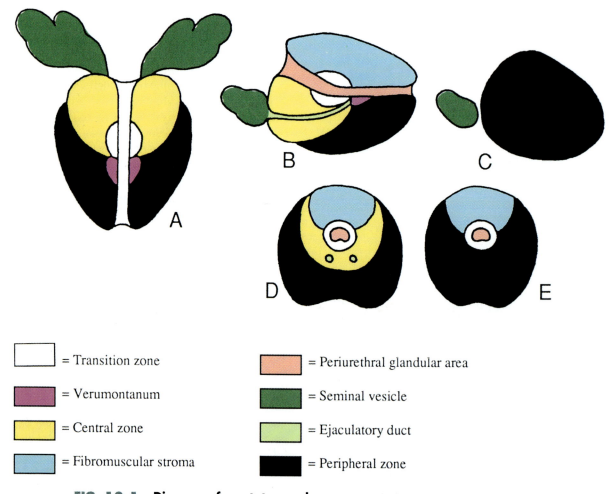

Transition zone

Verumontanum

Central zone

Fibromuscular stroma

Periurethral glandular area

Seminal vesicle

Ejaculatory duct

Peripheral zone

FIG. 10-1. **Diagram of prostate zonal anatomy.** **A,** Coronal section, midprostate. **B,** Sagittal midline section. **C,** Sagittal section, lateral prostate and seminal vesicle. **D,** Axial section, prostatic base. Paired ejaculatory ducts are seen posterior to urethra and periurethral glandular area. Peripheral zone encompasses most of posterior and lateral aspect of gland. **E,** Axial section, apex of gland showing mostly peripheral zone, and urethral and periurethral glandular area.

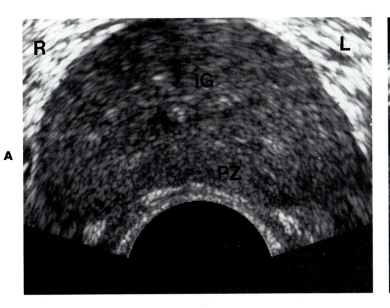

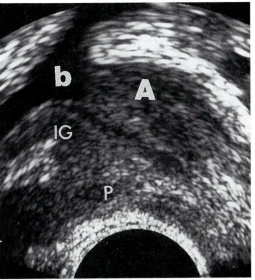

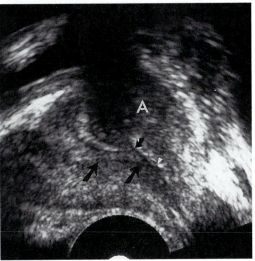

FIG. 10-2. Normal prostate anatomy. A, Axial image, midprostate gland. Peripheral zone, *PZ,* and inner gland, *IG,* are of same echogenicity. Patient's left, *L,* and right, *R,* are indicated. Probe is near anterior rectal wall, allowing for excellent resolution of entire prostate gland. **B,** Midline (true) parasagittal scan. Inner gland, *IG,* and peripheral zone, *P,* are isoechoic. Anterior fibromuscular stroma, *A,* is hypoechoic. Periurethral glandular area and anterior urethra lie between anterior fibromuscular stroma and inner gland; *b* = bladder. **C,** Additional sagittal image from a different patient demonstrates the ejaculatory duct *(straight arrows)* joining the urethra *(curved arrow)* at the verumontanum *(arrowhead).* The anterior fibromuscular stroma, *A,* is also identified.

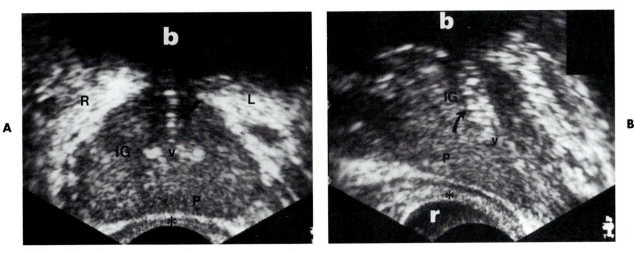

FIG. 10-3. Normal prostate with corpora amylacea. A, Oblique coronal view. **B,** Oblique sagittal view. Images show that corpora amylacea in periurethral glandular tissue produce multiple bright echoes *("Eiffel tower")* surrounding urethra *(arrows)* extending down to verumontanum, *V. R,* Right; *L,* left; *b,* bladder; *IG,* inner gland; *P,* peripheral zone; *r,* rectum; *,* rectal wall.

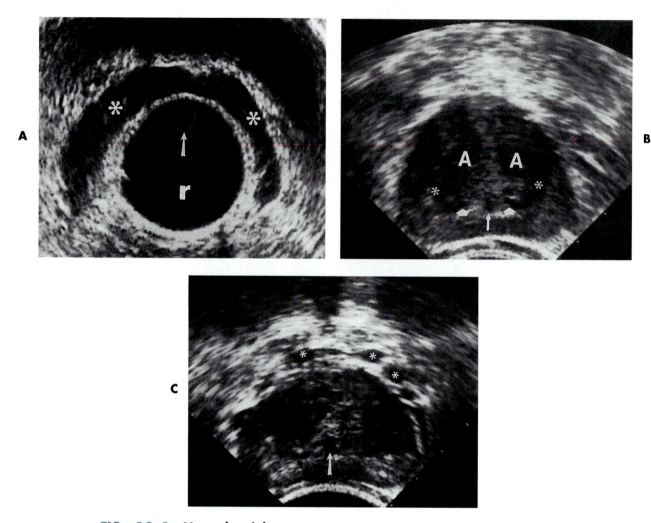

FIG. 10-4. Normal axial anatomy in patient with benign prostatic hyperplasia (BPH). **A,** Seminal vesicles, *, are seen as paired hypoechoic multiseptated structures surrounding rectum, *r;* arrow, rotating radial probe. **B,** Base of prostate gland. *A,* Adenoma; *, surgical capsule; short arrows, ejaculatory ducts; long arrow, urethra. **C,** Caudal to verumontanum, urethra *(arrow)* is seen posteriorly as a result of BPH. *, Prominent periprostatic vessels.

gion on the anterior surface of the prostate is termed the anterior fibromuscular stroma. Other fibromuscular structures in the prostate include the preprostatic sphincter, postprostatic sphincter, and longitudinal smooth muscle of the proximal urethra.[21-23]

The **peripheral zone,** the largest of the glandular zones, contains approximately 70% of the prostatic glandular tissue and is the source of most prostate cancer. It surrounds the distal urethral segment and is separated from the transition zone and central zone by the surgical capsule, which is often hyperechoic as a result of corpora amylacea or calcification. The peripheral zone occupies the posterior, lateral, and apical regions of the prostate, extending somewhat anteriorly (Figs. 10-1 to 10-5). The ducts of the peripheral zone enter the distal urethra.

The **transition zone** in the normal patient contains approximately 5% of the prostatic glandular tissue. It is seen as two small glandular areas located adjacent to the proximal urethral segment. It is the site of origin of benign prostatic hyperplasia. The ducts of the transition zone end in the proximal urethra at the level of the verumontanum, which bounds the transition zone caudally (Figs. 10-1 to 10-5).

The **central zone** constitutes approximately 25% of the glandular tissue. It is located at the prostatic base. The ducts of the vas deferens and seminal vesicles enter the central zone, and the ejaculatory ducts pass through it (Figs. 10-1 to 10-5). The central zone is relatively resistant to disease processes and is the site of origin of only 5% of prostate cancers. Central zone ducts terminate in the proximal urethra near the

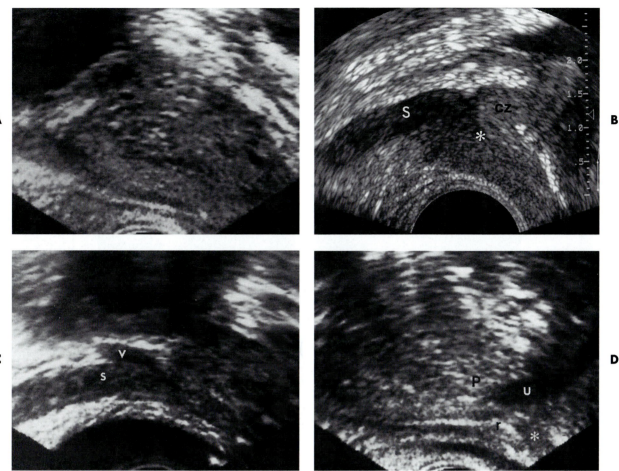

FIG. 10-5. Normal sagittal anatomy. A, Lateral scan of mildly enlarged gland with sector side-firing probe. Peripheral zone is isoechogenic. Linear inhomogeneities seen in central gland represent cystic dilation of ducts, a normal variant. **B,** Midline sagittal image. Seminal vesicle, *S,* extends into prostate, creating beak, *; *cz,* central zone. **C,** Lateral scan through junction of prostate gland and seminal vesicle shows vas deferens, *v,* entering seminal vesicle, *s,* as it joins with prostate. **D,** Apex of prostate centers around trapezoid area. Boundaries are membranous urethra, *u,* peripheral zone, *P,* rectum, *r,* and rectourethralis muscle, *.

verumontanum. The **periurethral glands** form about 1% of the glandular volume. They are embedded in the longitudinal smooth muscle of the proximal urethra, also known as the internal prostatic sphincter (Figs. 10-1 to 10-5).[20-22]

Vascular Anatomy

Blood flow to the prostate is supplied by the prostaticovesical arteries arising from the internal iliac arteries on each side. This vessel then gives rise to the prostatic artery and inferior vesical artery. The prostatic artery gives rise to the urethral and capsular arteries. The inferior vesicle artery supplies the bladder base, seminal vesicles, and ureter. The urethral artery supplies about one third of the prostate while the capsular branches supply the remainder of the gland.[23]

With color Doppler, particularly using the power mode, the prostate is a very vascular structure. The capsular and urethral arteries are easily seen, and branches to the inner gland and peripheral zone are usually very prominent (Fig. 10-6). When searching for pathology, it has been most useful to decrease the color gain to allow improved perception of pathologic vessels, often a hallmark of cancer.[7]

Scan Orientation

Using a transrectal approach, various scanning orientations have been proposed. The most commonly used convention illustrated is similar to that for transabdominal sonography (Fig. 10-1). As if standing at the foot of a supine patient, looking up, the rectum is displayed at the bottom of the screen with the ultrasound beam em-

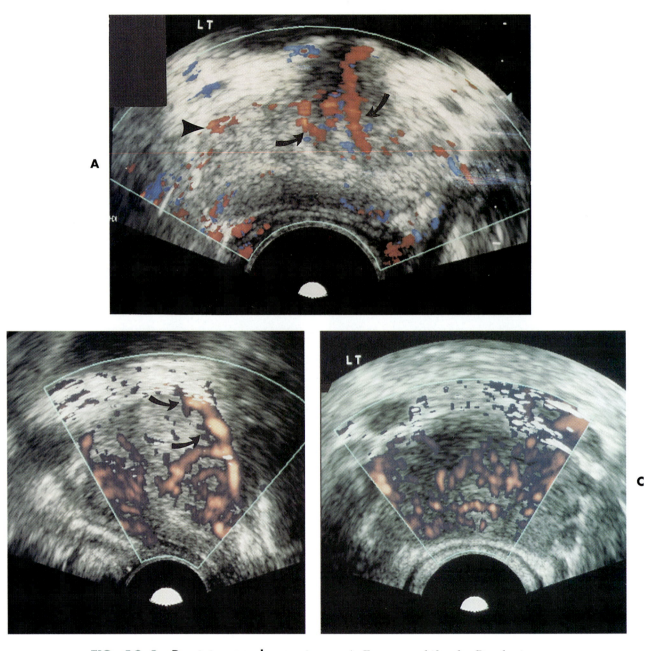

FIG. 10-6. Prostate vascular anatomy. A, Frequency shift color Doppler images demonstrate normal periurethral arteries *(curved arrows)* and capsular arteries. One capsular artery is designated *(arrowhead)*. In this color image, flow also is seen in the periprostatic region, peripheral zone, and rectal wall. **B,** Power Doppler image in sagittal plane demonstrates periurethral vessels *(curved arrows)* and increased number of vessels compared with frequency shift image. **C,** Coronal image using power Doppler demonstrates diffuse vascularity throughout the prostate. This is a normal finding using power Doppler.

anating from within the rectum. On transverse imaging, the anterior abdominal wall is at the top of the screen with the right side of the patient on the left side of the image. In a sagittal plane, the anterior abdominal wall is again located at the top of the screen, and the head of the patient is on the left side of the image (Fig. 10-2).

The most commonly used commercially available probes fire from the end and can be used for both transrectal and transvaginal imaging; longitudinal

and axial scans are obtained by rotating the probe through a 180-degree axis. The sagittal and axial images are relatively more oblique than those obtained with side-firing probes. Therefore axial images near the base of the gland are considered semicoronal in orientation. In addition, the prostate appears more elongated when imaged with a end-firing probe than when a true axial orientation is presented (Figs. 10-1, *A*, and 10-3). With end-firing probes, the top of the

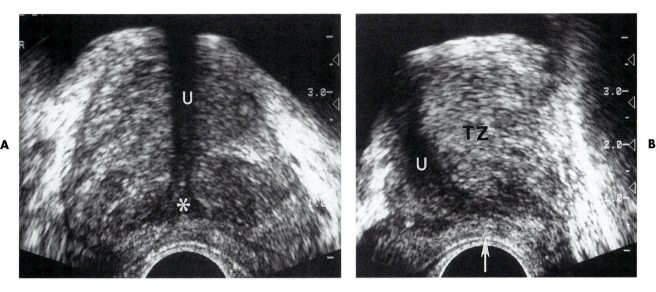

FIG. 10-7. Benign prostatic hyperplasia. A. Coronal image of prostate in patient with significant hyperplasia. Surrounding the urethra, *U*, is extensive transition zone hyperplasia. The base of the urethra broadens in this plane, *, to create the "Eiffel Tower" appearance. **B,** Sagittal view demonstrates extensive hyperplasia in the transition zone, *tz*, deviating the urethra, *U*, superiorly. This urethral deviation creates voiding symptoms. The peripheral zone *(arrow)* is compressed posteriorly and is quite thin.

image is in an oblique direction toward the head, and the bottom of the image is in an oblique direction toward the feet. Because of these differences in probe design, the anatomy that is depicted may vary from machine to machine.

Axial and Coronal Anatomy

The seminal vesicles are seen as paired, relatively hypoechoic, multiseptated structures surrounding the rectum cephalad to the base of the prostate gland (see Figs. 10-1, 10-4, *A*, and 10-5, *B* and *C*). In the axial plane, the anterior urethra and its surrounding smooth muscle and glandular area appear relatively hypoechoic (Fig. 10-6, *B*). On coronal images, the junction of the hypoechoic periurethral area with the verumontanum creates an appearance resembling the Eiffel Tower (Fig. 10-7, *A*).[20] The inner gland is separated from the peripheral zone by the surgical capsule. This can be seen occasionally in the normal gland. More often corpora amylacea, seen as echogenic foci, develop at the level of the surgical capsule (Figs. 10-4, *B*, and 10-6, *B*). Frequently the separation between the zones on transverse imaging is only positional, and no distinct structures will be present to clarify the anatomy (Fig. 10-2).

Sagittal Anatomy

The most lateral images of the gland in the sagittal plane show peripheral zone tissue with uniform echogenicity. With glandular hyperplasia, the transition zone may extend laterally, compressing the peripheral zone posteriorly (Fig. 10-7, *B*). At the base of the

gland, the seminal vesicles immediately adjoin the central and peripheral zone (Fig. 10-5, *B*). When corpora amylacea fill the periurethral glands, they may form a linear hyperechoic configuration (Fig. 10-5, *B*). The entrance of the seminal vesicles and vas deferens into the central zone produces an invaginated extraprostatic space, which is a pathway for a neoplasm to extend from the prostate gland into the seminal vesicle. A hypoechoic beaklike configuration is formed by the entrance of the seminal vesicles and vas deferens into the central zone (Fig. 10-5, *B* and *C*). The ejaculatory ducts can occasionally be seen coursing through the central zone from the seminal vesicles and joining the urethra at the verumontanum as it extends from an anterior to a more posterior position (Fig. 10-2, *C*). The urethra and surrounding glands and smooth muscle are most often hypoechoic (Figs. 10-2, *B*, and 10-7, *B*), but when corpora amylacea are present, may be hyperechoic (Figs. 10-3, *B*, and 10-5, *B*). The anterior fibromuscular stroma can be easily seen on sagittal imaging anterior to the urethra (Fig. 10-2, *C*).

Prostate Capsule

On transverse and sagittal imaging, the border of the prostate with the periprostatic fat may be sharply defined or, occasionally, less sharply defined, particularly in areas far from the transducer or on the edge of the imaging field. Histologically, the prostatic capsule is not well defined, and vessels and nerves course through the periprostatic tissue, which includes smooth muscle, skeletal muscle, and loose connective tissue. Posteriorly, the periprostatic tissue is fibroadipose, and no true surrounding capsule exists (Figs. 10-2 and 10-3).[23] In addition to the absence of a well-defined capsule, the presence of prominent vessels in the periprostatic soft tissues may make assessment of capsular integrity difficult in patients with prostate cancer (Fig. 10-4). At the apex of the gland, a trapezoid area is formed by the rectourethralis muscle, the rectum, the urethra, and the prostate gland. This area of potential weakness is a site of extraprostatic spread of cancer (Fig. 10-5).[21]

Normal Prostatic Echo Patterns

Normal prostate sonograms often contain isoechoic structures most characteristically in the peripheral, transition, and central zones. Smooth muscle produces a hypoechoic appearance, although an enlarged transition zone is also able to produce such echogenicity. Hyperechoic structures are most characteristic of fat, corpora amylacea, or calculi.

EQUIPMENT AND TECHNIQUES

Most modern ultrasound machines have transrectal probes, which have been developed to perform ultrasound of the prostate and rectum. Probe design and biopsy attachments vary. Probes should be at least 5 MHz, and most are as high as 7 or 8 MHz.

Transducer Design

Following the initial development of linear array and rotating radial probe designs, manufacturers have now developed probes for biplane transrectal prostate scanning with either a single probe or multiple probes on the same machine.[24] A convenient probe design is an **end-viewing transducer,** which allows for multiplanar imaging in semicoronal and axial projections (Fig. 10-8). Other probe designs include **360-degree radial** scanners paired with end-viewing probes for a sagittal image and **paired side-viewing axial and sagittal probes.** The advantages of end-viewing probe designs include patient convenience, ease of use, and biopsy capability at the time of the diagnostic examination. It probably makes little difference to the patient, however, if a single probe is in place for the same length of time as two individual probes. The only difference is the discomfort of a round probe insertion.

Probes must be covered during the examination (Fig. 10-8, *B*). Condoms, which have been developed to fit individual probes, are often made of latex. Since patients may have significant latex allergies, they should be questioned to determine if this condition exists, in which case alternate covers should be used. Between uses, the probes should be washed and then soaked in an antiseptic solution. Recommendations

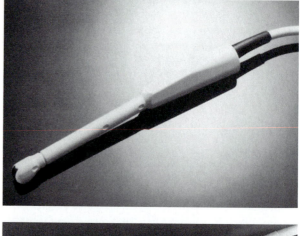

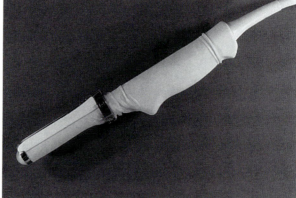

FIG. 10-8. Transrectal probe. A, Curved linear end-firing design. (Courtesy of General Electric Medical Systems, Milwaukee, Wis.) **B,** Probe fitted with biopsy guide, which snaps onto probe handle. (Courtesy of ATL, Bathel, Wa.)

from the manufacturer should be followed, particularly concerning the depth of insertion of the probe into the solution.

Some probes require a water path between the crystal and the rectal mucosa. This decreases the near-field artifact and allows for better visualization of the peripheral zone, which may be very close to the rectal wall. The amount of water necessary depends on the focal zone of the probe and the probe frequency. Careful attention should be paid to correctly positioning the probe to take advantage of the focal zone. A disadvantage of the water-path design is the occasional inadvertent introduction of air into the water path, creating an artifact.

Scanning Technique

Most clinicians who perform prostate ultrasound prefer that the patient lie in a left lateral decubitus position for the scan. Others prefer a lithotomy position, particularly if the examination is done in conjunction with other urologic procedures. A self-administered enema is routinely used before scanning.

It is routine to perform a rectal examination before probe insertion to correlate the imaging with any abnormalities on physical examination and to ensure that there are no rectal abnormalities that could interfere with the scan. Following adequate lubrication, the probe is gently inserted into the rectum. Insertion is often painless, particularly in older men with decreased rectal sphincter tone. Hard-copy images are obtained on a multiimage camera at multiple levels throughout the prostate gland.

When examining the prostate gland, a systematic approach is necessary. If one begins in the transverse or semicoronal plane, the seminal vesicles are seen at the cephalad portion of the prostate gland above the prostatic base. These paired structures may be different in size and shape, depending on age and sexual activity. They are generally hypoechoic and irregular and usually symmetrical (Fig. 10-4, *A*). Continuing in the transverse or semicoronal plane, the base of the prostate is then examined with demonstration of the central zone, transition zone, and periurethral glandular area. The anterior fibromuscular stroma is hypoechoic. In a semicoronal plane, the periurethral area may be very hypoechoic and simulate a transurethral resection defect (Fig. 10-7, *A*). The urethra and the ejaculatory ducts may be identified. At the level of the verumontanum, the ejaculatory ducts and urethra merge. Near the apex of the gland, most of the tissue is the peripheral zone. It is often difficult in the normal gland to separate the peripheral zone from the inner gland. Only when the surgical capsule is identified can these two areas be separated.

In the sagittal plane, rotating from right to left will assess glandular symmetry and confirm any suspicious abnormalities seen on axial or coronal imaging. The seminal vesicles and periurethral area are better evaluated in the sagittal plane.

Color Doppler is routinely used, particularly when cancer is suspected and biopsy is contemplated. The color sensitivity and gain is set so that normal peripheral zone vessels are not seen. Thus when increased vascularity is seen, an abnormality is suspected (Fig. 10-9).

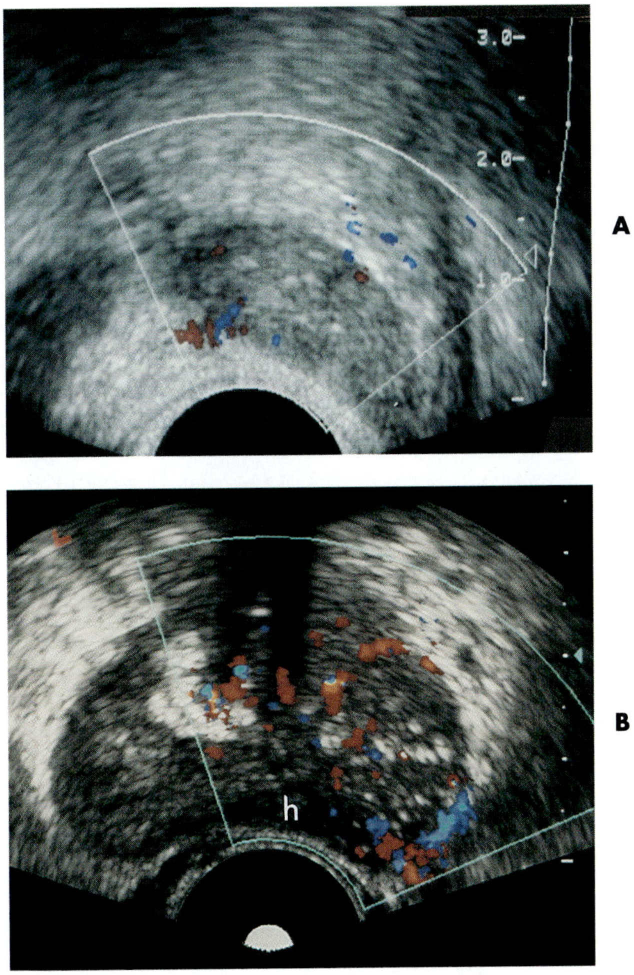

Biopsy Techniques

The addition of ultrasound-guided biopsy procedures to the diagnostic examination adds an important dimension to prostate ultrasound. Conventional prostate biopsy uses the examining finger in the rectum and transperineal or transrectal needle placement. The use of transrectal ultrasound for biopsy guidance was first performed with a transperineal approach using an axial rotating scanner.[25] Many investigators have described their experiences with transrectal and transperineal ultrasound-guided biopsy techniques.[20,26,27]

Currently, sonography-guided prostate biopsy is performed with a **transrectal approach.** Needle-

FIG. 10-9. Prostate color Doppler. A, Color Doppler image of small prostate cancer. The cancer is at the prostatic base and is isoechoic. The increased number of small vessels denotes the presence of possible cancer, and a biopsy demonstrated a Gleason 7 cancer. Note that the remainder of the peripheral zone is avascular, which helps to better appreciate the hypervascular tumor. **B,** Color Doppler image through the midprostate, demonstrating hypervascularity in the left peripheral zone with an associated hypoechoic mass, *h,* representing Gleason 6 comedocarcinoma. No other areas of increased vascularity are seen. Note background of increased echoes consistent with comedocarcinoma.

guidance systems that clamp onto the side of the probe are available for end-firing and side-firing probes (Fig. 10-8; Fig. 10-10). Electronic guidelines show the needle path (Fig. 10-11), facilitating the procedure.

Transrectal prostate biopsies are routinely performed with an **automatic biopsy gun** with 18-gauge needles. Thus a type of core biopsy specimen is obtained with minimal manipulation and with remarkable patient acceptance and safety.[20,26,28] The needle advances approximately 2 to 3 cm with the push of a button. The inner needle advances, and the outer needle cuts the tissue core and fixes it into the beveled

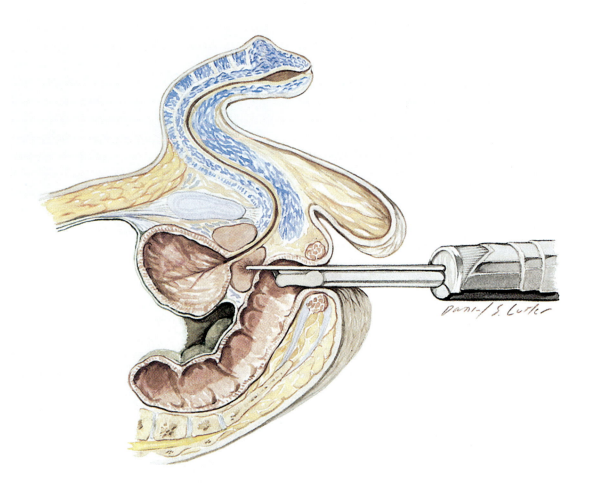

FIG. 10-10. Transrectal biopsy procedure. End-firing probe is in rectum. Electronic guidelines denote direction of needle path, which should be aligned with lesion. Needle is placed against the rectal wall before obtaining specimen.

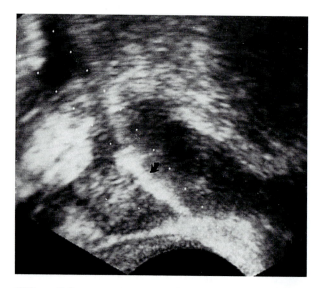

FIG. 10-11. Prostate biopsy 1 cm dots. Guidelines denote path that needle will traverse. Needle echo *(arrow)* obscures lesion.

chamber of the inner needle (Fig. 10-12). Some clinicians advocate the use of cytologic examinations in the prostate, although the ease of obtaining histologic cores has made cytologic techniques less popular.

Prostate biopsy may be performed in an ambulatory setting with little or no patient preparation. Patients on anticoagulants or aspirin should not undergo biopsy until these drugs have been discontinued for several days. It has become standard practice to administer a rapidly absorbed antibiotic such as ciprofloxacin in one dose just before and in several doses following the biopsy.[29-31] Informed consent should be obtained as with other biopsy procedures.

Transrectal biopsy is often performed immediately following the diagnostic examination. The patient remains in the left lateral decubitus position and the biopsy attachment is placed on the probe (see Fig. 10-8, *B*). Although no great attempt is made to provide a sterile field, some advocate the use of antiseptic enemas before performing the biopsy.

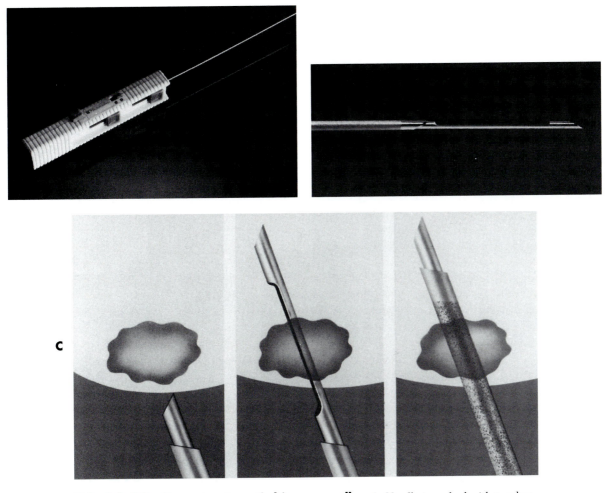

FIG. 10-12. Tru-cut automatic biopsy needle. **A,** Needle is cocked with two buttons on side and fired with button on top. **B,** Side view of needle shows beveled chamber of inner needle and outer needle, which cuts tissue. **C,** Tru-cut technique with automatic needle. Inner needle traverses lesion, and outer needle cuts biopsy core into beveled chamber. (Courtesy Microvasive, Watertown, Mass.)

Two major lesion localization methods are currently practiced. The first, **the systematic, sextant biopsy,** requires the operator to simply identify the prostate and divide it into six segments, obtaining a random sample from each segment.[6,30-34] This technique has become standard now that the number of prostate biopsies has increased, primarily due to widespread use of PSA as a screening test for prostate cancer. Because of the current prevalence of sonographic isoechoic cancer, the second localization method, **lesional directed biopsy,** is infrequently used, since the current patient population is primarily a PSA-screened population, as opposed to those suspected of having cancer because of symptoms or an abnormal digital rectal examination. With the advent of **color Doppler lesion detection,** however, those operators who use color Doppler may be at an advantage over those using a random, systematic approach when gray-scale abnormalities are either present or absent (Fig. 10-13).[8, 35-37]

When a gray-scale or color Doppler lesion is localized, the needle is placed into the guidance system and moved to a position so that the needle tip is approximately 1 cm proximal to the lesion (see Fig. 10-12). The lesion can then be sampled one or more times. Usually some random or systematic biopsies are performed, even when a lesion is detected and biopsied. This allows for complete evaluation of the gland and some staging information.[33,34,38]

Significant **complications** from prostate biopsy—regardless of the mode of guidance, needle size, or approach—have been relatively low. Minor complications, primarily related to bleeding, are common and may be seen in at least 30% to 40% of patients undergoing transrectal biopsy. Major complications include sepsis, large hematomas, and tumor seeding. With the use of prophylactic antibiotics, the incidence of septic complications requiring therapy should be less than 1%.[28,29,39]

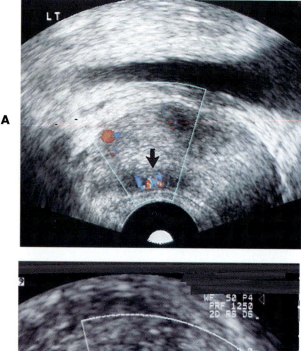

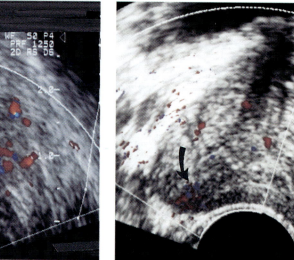

FIG. 10-13. **Prostate Color Doppler.** **A,** Prostate cancer. A hypoechoic mass in the peripheral zone demonstrates increased color with multiple small vessels seen within this peripheral zone mass *(arrow)*. Biopsy demonstrated Gleason 7 cancer. **B,** Granulomatous prostatitis. A large hypoechoic mass, *G*, was avascular with color Doppler. At biopsy this proved to be granulomatous prostatitis. **C,** Isoechoic cancer only demonstrated with color Doppler. The *arrow* denotes an area of increased vascularity that had no corresponding gray-scale abnormality. Biopsy demonstrated Gleason 7 cancer.

Sonographic-guided **biopsy results** depend directly on the index of suspicion of the lesion that is biopsied. If all palpable and nonpalpable abnormalities are sampled with ultrasound guidance, higher positive results for cancer will be found than if only nonpalpable lesions undergo ultrasound-guided biopsy and the remainder undergo conventional biopsy techniques. In a large study series, 52% of lesions that were biopsied were adenocarcinoma. An additional 11% were diagnosed as prostatic intraepithelial neoplasia, a premalignant disorder.[27] In general, positive biopsy result rates, when using ultrasound criteria for selection, range from 40% to 60%.[39-41] Color Doppler has increased the sensitivity and specificity regardless of whether a gray-scale lesion is detected[8, 35-37] (Fig. 10-13).

The most important decision made in the course of the prostate ultrasound examination is the **decision to perform a biopsy.** A number of factors can influence this decision, including the wishes of the

patient. Patients who do not wish to be treated for prostate cancer should not even receive a PSA determination. Patients in the eighth decade of life and beyond who suffer from more life-threatening diseases should not be screened for prostate cancer, which can have a long natural history before becoming clinically important.[42,43] Other important tools available to help make the decision are absolute **PSA levels** and PSA levels related to patient age (Table 10-1),[44] PSA density determination,[45,46] PSA velocity,[47] and color Doppler.[8]

PSA density is determined by dividing the PSA by the volume of the gland. Volumes can be measured by using a stepping device whereby areas of the prostate are cumulatively added to create a volume, or by using volume formulas, depending on the prostatic shape. Most often the prostate is elliptical in shape, and using the formula for a prolate ellipse ($L \times W \times H \times 0.523$) gives an accurate volume measurement. For a sphere, use $4/3 \ \pi r^3$, and for a cylinder, use $\pi r^2 \times$ Height

TABLE 10-1
PSA DETERMINATIONS

Normal PSA Levels (Monoclonal Assay)	
0-4 ng/ml	Normal
4-10 ng/ml	Intermediate
>10 ng/ml	Abnormal

Age-Specific PSA Levels	
Age	**Normal Range**
40-49	0-2.5
50-59	0-3.5
60-69	0-4.5
70-79	0-6.5

(r = radius). A PSA density of greater than 0.12 to 0.15 is considered abnormal. **PSA velocity** measures the increase in PSA. An increase of greater than 20% over 1 year is a strong indication for biopsy.[47]

There is debate over whether ultrasound guidance is necessary in the biopsy of **palpable prostatic nodules.** Some researchers believe that an ultrasound-guided biopsy has no advantage as compared with a digitally directed prostatic biopsy. Some palpable lesions may be better sampled with digital guidance because they may not be seen at all with ultrasound. When a palpable abnormality is not discovered sonographically, biopsy with digital technique is appropriate. Conversely, when a digitally guided biopsy yields negative results in a suspicious gland, repeat biopsy with ultrasound guidance is important.[48]

BENIGN DISEASES

Benign Prostatic Hyperplasia

Enlargement of the prostate gland is common in older men. The gland size, however, does not always correlate with symptoms of prostatism. There does appear to be a correlation between these symptoms (difficult initiation of voiding, nocturia, and small stream) and growth of the gland as it relates to the anterior urethra. Glandular volumes can be determined accurately by volumetric techniques performed sonographically.[49] These formulas can also be used to calculate the volume of tumor in the gland. Volume can be converted to weight because 1 cc of prostate tissue is equivalent to 1 g. Glandular weight and volume are age related. The weight of the gland in a younger patient is approximately 20 g. Beginning at age 50, the doubling time of the weight of the prostate is approximately 10 years. Prostate glands weighing more than 40 g are generally considered enlarged in older men.[50]

The **sonographic appearance** of benign prostatic hyperplasia (BPH) is varied and depends on the

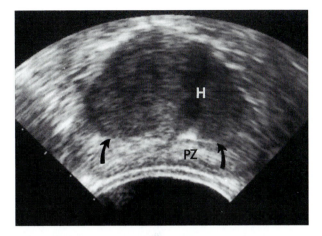

FIG. 10-14. Benign prostatic hyperplasia, typical appearance. Transverse image shows echogenic peripheral zone, *PZ*, is separated from hypoechoic hyperplastic inner gland, *H*, by surgical capsule *(arrows)*, which contains calcification in corpora amylacea.

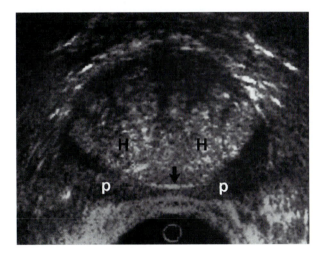

FIG. 10-15. Benign prostatic hyperplasia, BPH, atypical appearance. Transverse image shows isoechoic peripheral zone, *p*, hyperechoic inner gland with transition zone hyperplasia, *H*, and surgical capsule *(arrow)*.

histopathologic changes. Distinct nodules or diffuse enlargement can be present in the transition zone, the periurethral glandular tissue, or both.[20,22] The typical sonographic feature of BPH is enlargement of the inner gland, which remains relatively hypoechoic to the peripheral zone (Fig. 10-14). The echo pattern depends on the admixture of glandular and stromal elements because nodules may be fibroblastic, fibromuscular, muscular, hyperadenomatous, and fibroadenomatous.[20,51] This combination may result in either an isoechoic or hyperechoic appearance (Fig. 10-7; Fig. 10-15).

Other sonographic features of BPH include calcifications and rounded hyperechoic nodules (Fig. 10-16). The occasional hypoechoic nodule that simulates carcinoma and that histologically represents hy-

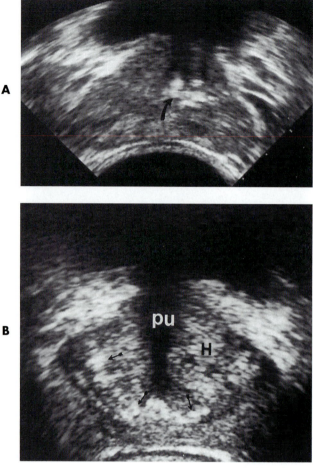

A

B

FIG. 10-16. Benign prostatic hyperplasia.
A, Prostatic calcifications, common feature in hyperplasia, are seen in transition zone *(arrow)*. Acoustic shadowing is anterior because probe is in rectum. **B,** Hyperplastic echogenic nodule, *H,* and corpora amylacea *(arrows)* are seen in this oblique coronal image. Elongated periurethral glandular area, *pu,* is hypoechoic because of glandular and smooth muscular tissue.

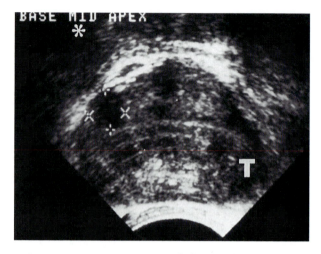

FIG. 10-17. Tumor and hyperplasia. Transverse image shows large tumor on left side of gland, *T.* Well-defined hypoechoic nodule of hyperplasia is seen in right transition zone *(cursor marks)*.

perplasia may also be seen (Fig. 10-17). Because of the distortion of the gland in patients with BPH, these nodules may appear to be in the peripheral zone when they actually lie in the transition zone. The surgical capsule can be a distinct demarcation between the inner gland and peripheral zone. When in the transition zone, hypoechoic nodules will be hyperplastic in approximately 80% to 90%.[52,53]

In the patient with symptoms of prostatism, ultrasound can be useful to determine prostatic volume. Because the growth of the gland is primarily anterior, particularly in patients with symptoms, the volume or weight cannot be estimated well by digital palpation. Ultrasound can analyze the effect of the hyperplasia on the anterior urethra and assess "median lobe" enlargement (Fig. 10-7). In fact, very large glands may often be seen in asymptomatic patients whereas pa-

tients with severe voiding difficulties have only enlargement anteriorly and centrally. Ultrasound can monitor gland size in patients undergoing drug therapy for prostatism.

In patients who have had transurethral resections, ultrasound is useful in evaluating the anterior urethra, extending from the bladder to the verumontanum. It is interesting to note that, although urologic surgeons may believe they have removed a large amount of the prostate, scans done relatively soon after transurethral resection show small- to moderate-sized defects in the periurethral glandular tissue and transition zone. There may be some redistribution of prostatic tissue to account for the large amount of prostate mass remaining. Patients, however, are uniformly symptom free following these procedures, suggesting that the amount of prostatic tissue removed does not necessarily correlate with the success of the procedure (Fig. 10-18).

Patients with benign prostatic hypertrophy often have glands that are abnormal to palpation. The role of ultrasound in these patients is to separate benign from malignant lesions and to guide biopsies when this distinction cannot be made sonographically. A patient with a hard nodule that is felt by digital rectal examination and that contains calcification with shadowing can be spared an unnecessary biopsy if the palpable lesion corresponds to that seen with ultrasound.

Hyperplastic nodules are the most common cause of false-positive prostate ultrasound examination results. However, a small number of patients with BPH may harbor prostatic intraepithelial neoplasia (PIN) (atypical hyperplasia), which is a premalignant lesion. When follow-up biopsies are done, these lesions may develop into prostatic carcinoma. Also, prostate cancer may coexist adjacent to or within the same

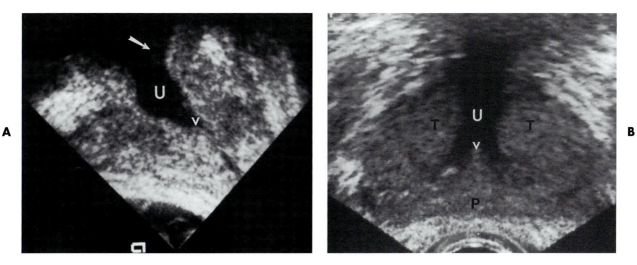

FIG. 10-18. Posttransurethral prostatectomy (TURP). A, Sagittal midline image shows small nodule of tissue *(arrow)* that commonly protrudes into urethral lumen following resection. Anterior urethra is dilated to verumontanum, *v*, allowing posterior urethra and prostate to act as sphincter. **B,** Oblique coronal scan through base of gland shows dilated urethra, *U*, and verumontanum, *v*. Some hyperplasia is seen in transition zone, *T*, on either side of urethra. Peripheral zone, *P*, is isoechoic.

gland as PIN. Close follow-up, subsequent biopsies, and correlation with prostate specific antigen are helpful when evaluating these patients further. In over 10% of patients with benign or PIN lesions, a subsequent biopsy will yield cancer.[51,54-56]

Inflammation of the Prostate and Seminal Vesicles

With the major emphasis of transrectal ultrasound on diagnosis of carcinoma of the prostate, there have been few studies analyzing its usefulness in inflammatory diseases. There is a significant incidence of acute and chronic prostatitis with varied symptoms. **Chronic prostatitis** may be associated with specific pathogens such as *Chlamydia* or *Mycoplasma* organisms. If no known etiologic factor can be found, the condition is then termed **prostatodynia.**[57,58] **Sonographic findings** that can be seen with chronic prostatitis include focal masses of different degrees of echogenicity, ejaculatory duct calcifications, capsular thickening or irregularity, and periurethral glandular irregularity. Dilation of periprostatic veins and distended seminal vesicles have been described with chronic prostatitis or prostatodynia.[58] Sonographic-guided biopsy has been used to identify chronic prostatitis and to confirm the presence of bacteria.[59]

Chronic prostatitis or seminal vesiculitis can lead to **hematospermia.** Transrectal ultrasound may be useful to rule out neoplasm and also to guide aspiration and injection of steroids and antibiotics to treat the infection.[60] Many possible causes of hematospermia, including prostatic and seminal vesicle cysts, seminal vesicle or ejaculatory calculi, and vascular

---

> **SONOGRAPHIC FINDINGS OF CHRONIC PROSTATITIS**
>
> Focal masses of different degrees of echogenicity
> Ejaculatory duct calcifications
> Capsular thickening or irregularity
> Periurethral glandular irregularity
> Dilation of periprostatic veins
> Distended seminal vesicles

malformations can be detected with gray-scale and color Doppler sonography (Fig. 10-19).[61] Ultrasound should be an initial procedure performed in patients with this distressing symptom.

Chronic granulomatous prostatitis can mimic the sonographic features of prostatic carcinoma. Diffuse large and small hypoechoic zones or a solitary hypoechoic lesion may be seen. Patients undergoing bacillus Calmette-Guérin (BCG) therapy for bladder cancer are at risk of development of granulomatous prostatitis (Fig. 10-13, *B*; Fig. 10-20).[62]

In patients with **acute prostatitis,** the role of ultrasound is limited. Physical examination and placing a probe in the rectum are often difficult because of pain, and ultrasound may demonstrate significant abnormality, mimicking carcinoma. In general the glands are hypoechoic. Color Doppler, as with other infections, shows a very vascular focus in areas of prostatitis, mimicking carcinoma (Fig. 10-21). Ultrasound can lead to an early diagnosis of a prostatic abscess. In a patient

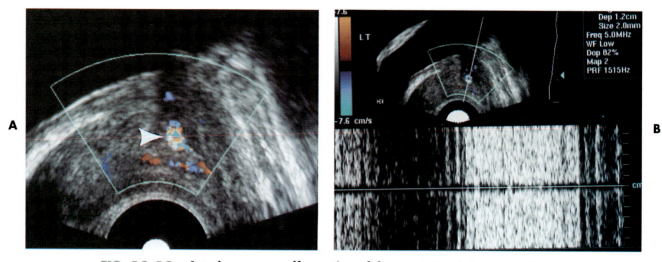

FIG. 10-19. **Arteriovenous malformation of the prostate.** **A,** Longitudinal image through the midline in a 30-year-old man with massive hematospermia. Gray-scale examination was normal. Color Doppler demonstrates marked increased flow with aliasing *(arrow)* in the posterior periurethral area. **B,** Spectral Doppler demonstrates turbulent multidirectional flow through the arteriovenous malformation. Transurethral laser therapy obliterated this lesion.

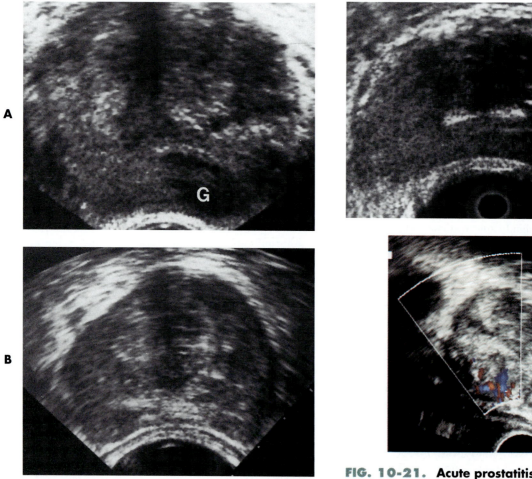

FIG. 10-20. **Granulomatous prostatitis, biopsy proven.** **A,** Focal pattern. Patient with benign prostatic hyperplasia has large hypoechoic mass on left side of peripheral zone, *G.* **B,** Diffuse pattern. Inhomogeneity throughout gland and large and small hypoechoic and hyperechoic nodules are seen.

FIG. 10-21. **Acute prostatitis.** **A,** Transverse scan shows large hypoechoic area on left side of gland, which could mimic carcinoma. Follow-up examination was normal. **B,** Color Doppler image of a different patient demonstrates hypervascularity in the peripheral zone. This patient had acute symptoms and biopsy demonstrated acute prostatitis. This cannot be separated from the color Doppler appearance of cancer.

with acute prostatitis refractory to treatment, the development of an anechoic mass with or without internal echoes suggests the presence of an abscess (Fig. 10-22). Sonographic-guided aspiration and installation of antibiotic into the abscess may be performed using a transrectal or transperineal approach.[63,64]

Prostatic and Seminal Vesicle Cysts

Most patients with cystic lesions in the prostate and seminal vesicle will be asymptomatic. Occasionally, these cysts can cause symptoms or become infected, particularly if they are large.

Congenital abnormalities are common in and around the prostate and seminal vesicles. The Müllerian tubercle gives rise to the prostatic utricle, a midline, small, blind-ending pouch that is situated near the summit of the colliculus seminalis, which is a mound on the poste-

rior wall of the prostatic urethra. **Prostatic utricle cysts** are caused by dilation of the prostatic utricle. Utricle cysts can be associated with unilateral renal agenesis and rarely contain spermatozoa. Utricle cysts are always in the midline and are usually small (Fig. 10-23). **Müllerian duct cysts** may arise from remnants of the Müllerian duct. Müllerian duct cysts may extend lateral to the midline and can be large. They have no other associations and never contain spermatozoa.[65,66] **Ejaculatory duct cysts** are usually small and probably represent cystic dilation of the ejaculatory duct possibly as a result of obstruction (Fig. 10-24). Alternatively, they may be diverticula of the duct. These cysts contain spermatozoa when aspirated. They can be associated with infertility and may be diagnosed in patients with a low sperm count. They may cause perineal pain.[65,67] Cysts occurring within the prostate gland may be caused

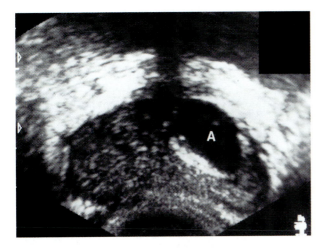

FIG. 10-22. Prostate abscess, abscess in patient with incompletely treated urinary tract infection. Cystic mass with internal echoes is present in transition zone, *A*. Aspiration of mass yielded purulent material.

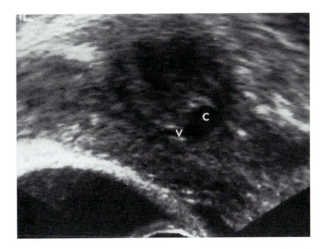

FIG. 10-23. Utricle cyst, an isolated congenital anomaly. Sagittal scan shows small midline cyst, *c*, extending from verumontanum, *v*.

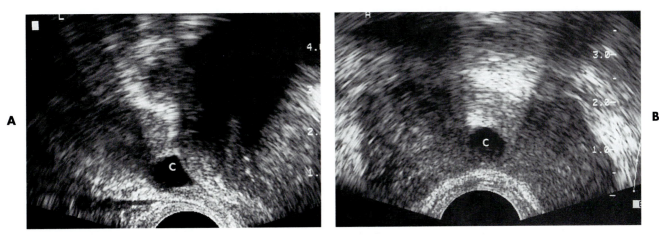

FIG. 10-24. Ejaculatory duct cyst. Patient with oligospermia is scanned for evidence of obstruction. Sagittal, **A**, and coronal, **B**, scans demonstrate dilated ejaculatory duct indicative of an ejaculatory duct cyst, **C**, causing obstruction of flow from the seminal vesicle to the urethra.

by benign prostatic hyperplasia or may be **retention cysts. Seminal vesicle cysts,** when large and solitary, may be associated with ipsilateral renal agenesis. This is the result of a wolffian duct anomaly (Fig. 10-25). Affected patients may benefit from aspiration when cysts are large and symptomatic.[66,67]

PROSTATE CANCER

Clinical Aspects

The epidemiology of prostate cancer has changed dramatically since the advent of PSA screening programs. The incidence of prostate cancer in the United States has risen to about 300,000 new cases per year, up from 100,000 five years ago. The incidence is higher in African-American men and in men with a strong personal family history for the disease. It has become the most commonly diagnosed cancer in men, leading lung and colorectal cancer by a factor of two to three times. The death rate from prostate cancer has risen slightly, probably because of longer lifespans, and less likely because of increased virulence of the disease. It is the second leading cause of cancer deaths in men at about 45,000 per year in the United States. The lifetime probability of death from prostate cancer is about 1 in 40.[68]

Clinical Stage and Grade

Prostate cancer is most commonly staged by the Jewett and Whitmore classification (Fig. 10-26 and Table 10-2).[69] In recent years the TNM classification has gained popularity because of its international uniformity and ability to integrate clinical, imaging, and pathologic staging information.[70] In addition to clinical staging, the Gleason histologic scoring system analyzes the degree of glandular differentiation and dedifferentiation microscopically; grade 1 is well differentiated and

grade 5 is poorly differentiated. The cancers are graded by evaluating the most representative histologic pattern and a less representative area and adding the grades of the two areas together to obtain a number between 2 and 10.[71] Most clinicians now use a combination of PSA, the stage, and Gleason scoring system to define the tumor and assign prognosis[2,72,73] (Table 10-3).

TABLE 10-2

JEWETT AND WHITMORE CLASSIFICATION OF PROSTATIC TUMORS

Stage	Definition
A	Nonpalpable cancers
A1	<5% of tissue and Gleason grade >7
A2	>5% of tissue or Gleason grade >7
B	Palpable nodule
B1	Palpable nodule <1.5 cm in diameter
B2	Palpable nodule >1.5 cm in diameter, confined within the prostatic capsule
C	Extension beyond the prostatic capsule without distant metastases
D	Metastases
D1	Metastases to regional lymph nodes
D2	Metastases to bone or viscera

TABLE 10-3

AJCC STAGING OF PROSTATE CANCER

Primary Tumor (T) Stage	Definition
T1	Clinically inapparent tumor not palpable or visible by imaging
T1a	Tumor incidental histologic finding in more than 5% of tissue resected
T1b	Tumor incidental histologic finding in more than 5% of tissue resected
T1c	Tumor identified by needle biopsy (e.g., because of elevated PSA)
T2	Tumor confined within the prostate
T2a	Tumor involves half of a lobe or less
T2b	Tumor involves more than half of a lobe, but not both lobes
T2c	Tumor involves both lobes
T3	Tumor extends through the prostatic capsule
T3a	Unilateral extracapsular extension
T3b	Bilateral extracapsular extension
T3c	Tumor invades the seminal vesicle(s)
T4	Tumor is fixed or invades adjacent structures other than the seminal vesicle(s)
T4a	Tumor invades any of bladder neck, external sphincter, or rectum
T4b	Tumor invades muscles and/or is fixed to the pelvic wall

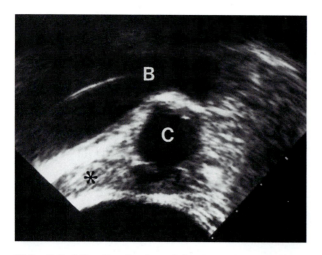

FIG. 10-25. Seminal vesicle cyst. Transverse scan shows large cyst, *C*, extending anteriorly from left seminal vesicle and indenting bladder, *B*. Normal right seminal vesicle, *.

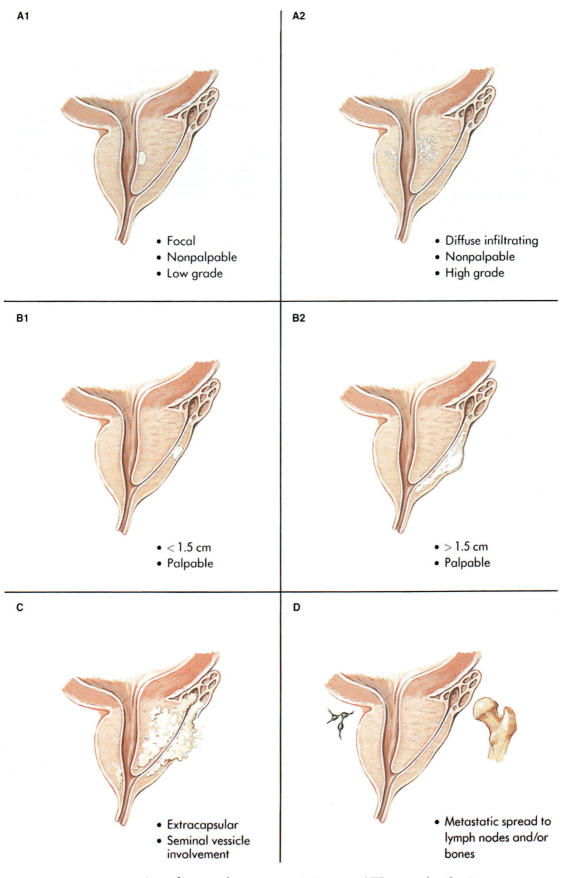

A1
- Focal
- Nonpalpable
- Low grade

A2
- Diffuse infiltrating
- Nonpalpable
- High grade

B1
- < 1.5 cm
- Palpable

B2
- > 1.5 cm
- Palpable

C
- Extracapsular
- Seminal vessicle involvement

D
- Metastatic spread to lymph nodes and/or bones

FIG. 10-26. Staging of prostatic tumors. The Jewett and Whitmore classifications.

INDICATIONS FOR TRANSRECTAL ULTRASOUND OF THE PROSTATE

Abnormal digital rectal examination
Abnormal laboratory test results indicative of prostate cancer
- PSA
- Acid phosphatase
- Other evidence of metastatic disease

Guidance for directed sonographic biopsy
Monitoring response to treatment for prostate cancer

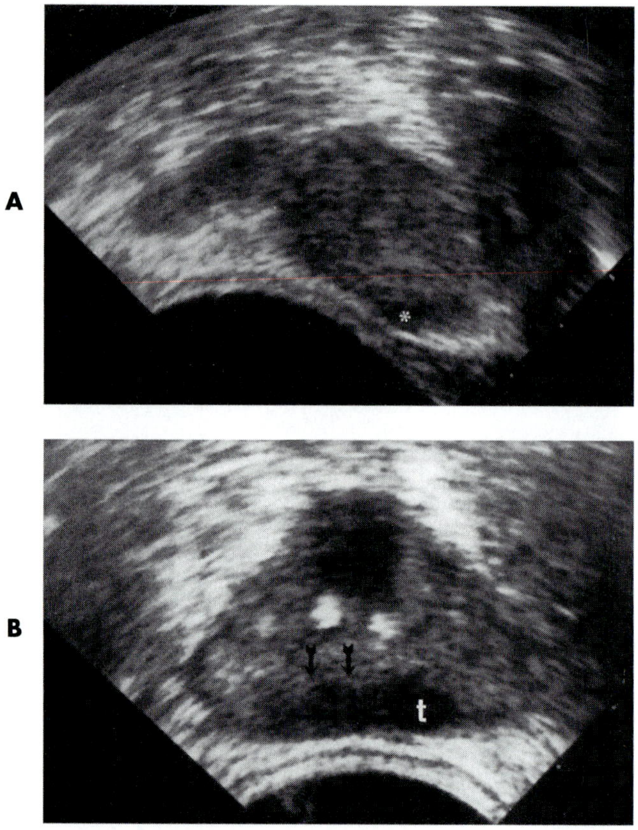

FIG. 10-27. Small, typical, palpable hypoechoic prostate cancer. **A,** Sagittal image shows 8 mm, nonpalpable, oval-shaped hypoechoic mass, *, in peripheral zone near apex of gland. **B,** Solid anechoic portion of tumor, *t*, is located at left with infiltration into peripheral zone toward midline *(arrows)*.

Stage A or T1 tumors are nonpalpable clinically. The tumors are typically located in the inner gland, having developed in the transition zone or periurethral glandular tissue (T1). If a T1 tumor is extensive (T1b), it may extend into the peripheral zone from the inner gland or it may be diffuse in the peripheral zone and extend into the inner gland so that it is not detectable by digital rectal examination. Most T1 tumors found today are small and only discovered because of an elevated PSA or PSA density and an ultrasound-guided biopsy yielding cancer. These are clinical stage T1c.[74] It is difficult to predict whether these cancers are significant and require treatment.[75] One model suggests that at least 85% of T1c cancers are significant, will behave as biologically active tumors, and deserve treatment.[76]

Stages B (T2) and C (T3) tumors are often palpable by digital rectal examination and represent local cancer, typically in the peripheral zone. T3 tumors extend into the seminal vesicles or periprostatic soft tissue. Patients with clinical stages T1 to T3 have no evidence of metastatic disease by available testing.[70] **Stage D (T4) tumors** represent cancer that, at the time of presentation, is present either in lymph nodes or distant organs or bones. With TNM staging the local tumor stage is modified with N (node status) and M (non–lymph node distant metastasis).

When initially discovered, most prostate cancers are small or widely metastatic, with the minority of patients being discovered with stages T2 or T3. With the current use of prostate ultrasound along with PSA, this may change as cancers, particularly those present in both lobes, are discovered at an earlier stage.

Indications for Transrectal Ultrasound of the Prostate

The indications for transrectal ultrasound of the prostate in patients with known or suspected prostate cancer are: (1) evaluation of the patient with an abnormal digital rectal examination; (2) evaluation of the patient with abnormal laboratory test results indicative of prostate cancer, including PSA, acid phosphatase, or other evidence of metastatic disease; (3) guidance for directed sonographic biopsy; and (4) monitoring response to treatment for prostate cancer.

Sonographic Appearance

The sonographic appearance of prostate cancer has been debated extensively. Early investigators felt that most prostate cancers were hyperechoic.[19] With the development of higher-frequency transducers, the concept of the hypoechoic and mixed appearance of prostate cancer evolved.[18,52,77]

With currently available high-frequency transrectal probes, prostate cancer may have varied appearances, depending on the size and background of the prostate in which it is growing. Small prostate cancers are generally **hypoechoic** because of the nodular cellular appearance of the carcinoma against the background of normal peripheral zone glandular tissue (Fig. 10-27).[55] When attempting to correlate the echogenicity of neoplasms with the amount of stromal fibrosis, it was found that hypoechoic lesions had less stromal fibrosis

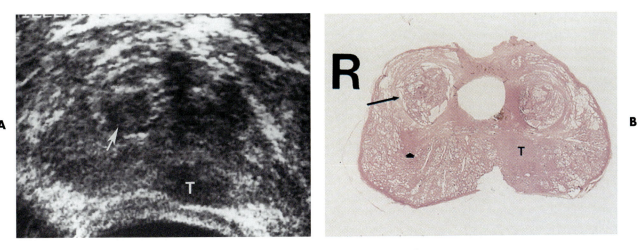

FIG. 10-28. Sonographic pathologic correlation of prostate cancer. A, Preoperative sonogram in axial plane shows palpable hypoechoic lesion, *T,* in left peripheral zone and second hypoechoic area *(arrow)* in right transition zone. **B,** Whole-mount specimen following radical prostatectomy shows peripheral zone tumor, *T,* as solid area surrounded by glandular tissue. Second focus of tumor *(thick arrow)* in anterior peripheral zone *(less than 5 mm)* could not be appreciated on preoperative sonogram. Second hypoechoic area in transition zone *(thin arrow)* is area of nodular hyperplasia. *R,* right side.

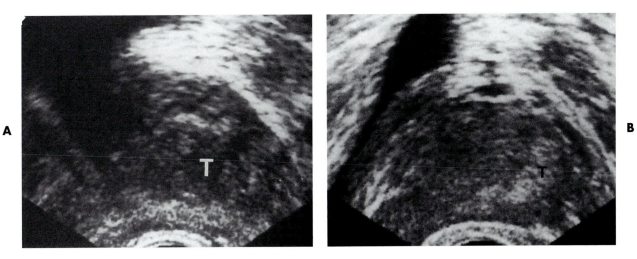

FIG. 10-29. Hyperechoic cancers. A, Sagittal image shows large hyperechoic tumor, *T,* with multiple hyperechoic foci. Histologically, there was significant desmoplasia with tumor intermixed with hyperplasia. **B,** Sagittal scan in lateral aspect of this gland shows small hyperechoic focus of tumor, *T,* in peripheral zone. Biopsy demonstrated significant desmoplastic response to this high-grade neoplasm.

than did their more echogenic counterparts (Fig. 10-28). In addition, the hypoechoic lesions tended to be better differentiated with lower Gleason grades.[78] Another report, however, found the opposite information in a correlative study with pathologic states, suggesting that the hypoechoic tumors were poorly differentiated and that the poorly differentiated tumors were better seen with ultrasound.[79] Further research suggests that echogenicity varies with the presence of tumor glands with enlarged lumina as well as residual prostatic glands and stroma.[80]

Hyperechoic cancer, although seen infrequently, has been identified. With large cancers, the appearance may be caused by a **desmoplastic response** of the surrounding glandular tissue to the presence of the tumor or to infiltration of neoplasm into a background of benign prostatic hyperplasia[78,81-83] (Fig. 10-29). Other histologic types of cancer, including the **cribriform pattern and comedonecrosis,** also correlate with echogenic cancer (Fig. 10-30). Rarely are prostate cancers associated with deposits of intraluminal crystalloid material, which also can produce increased echogenicity[84] (Fig. 10-31). It has been our experience that a few extensive large cancers have a hyperechoic appearance, probably as a result of the infiltration of the neoplasm into a background of benign prostatic hyperplasia (Fig. 10-32). Biopsy of hyperechoic lesions with sonographic guidance is the only way in which it can be proved that the lesion seen represents a neoplasm (Figs. 10-29 to 10-32).

A significant number of prostate cancers are difficult or impossible to detect with transrectal ultrasound because they are **isoechoic** with the surrounding prostate gland. When an isoechoic tumor is present, it can be detected only if **secondary signs** are appreciated, including glandular asymmetry, capsular bulging, and areas of attenuation.[75,85] When isoechoic tumors are

subjected to histopathologic correlation, it can be seen grossly that they are larger and tend to blend into the background of hyperplasia (Fig. 10-33).

The ability to define prostate cancer with both the digital rectal examination and with sonography is determined by the ability to differentiate the cancer from the background of normal or hyperplastic tissue. When the cancer totally replaces an entire zone or the entire gland, this distinction becomes more difficult. This **diffuse** type of cancer must be identified based on the expected echogenicity of the area examined rather than its relation to surrounding structures. When the tumor replaces the entire peripheral zone, it will often be less echogenic than the inner gland, which is a reversal of the normal sonographic relation (Fig. 10-34).

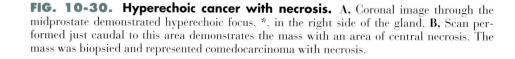

FIG. 10-30. Hyperechoic cancer with necrosis. A, Coronal image through the midprostate demonstrated hyperechoic focus, *, in the right side of the gland. **B,** Scan performed just caudal to this area demonstrates the mass with an area of central necrosis. The mass was biopsied and represented comedocarcinoma with necrosis.

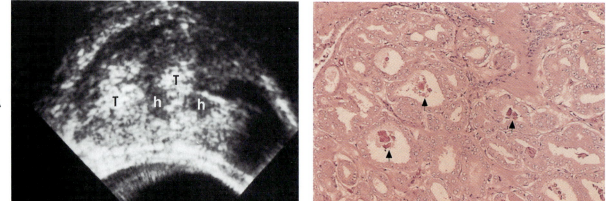

FIG. 10-31. Hyperechoic cancer with crystals. A, Transverse scan shows transurethral resection defect and extensive stage A2 cancer with multiple hyperechoic foci, *T,* intermixed with hypoechoic foci, h, in inner gland. **B,** Histologic specimen demonstrates multiple intraluminal crystalloid deposits in tumor acini *(arrows)*.

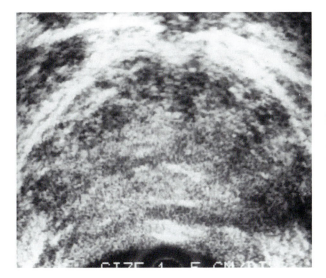

FIG. 10-32. Diffuse hyperechoic cancer. A diffusely inhomogeneous, primarily hyperechoic cancer is illustrated. A Gleason 9 cancer was found at surgery. This appearance is unusual.

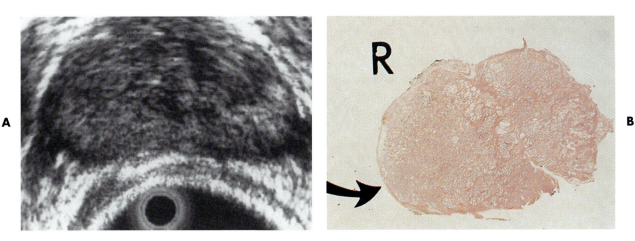

A   B

FIG. 10-33. Isoechoic cancer, sonographic and histologic correlation. A. Transverse scan shows subtle asymmetry of gland with enlarged right side. Biopsy proved palpable carcinoma. **B.** Radical prostatectomy specimen shows diffuse glandular hyperplasia throughout both lobes. Tumor *(arrow)* infiltrating glandular hyperplasia cannot be identified at this magnification and was only seen microscopically. *R,* right side.

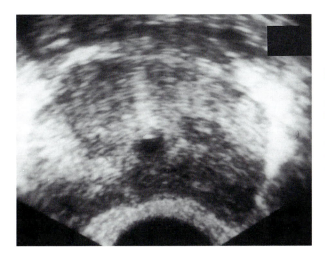

FIG. 10-34. Diffuse peripheral zone cancer. A transverse scan demonstrates extensive involvement of the peripheral zone, which is diffusely hypoechoic. There is extension anteriorly into the inner gland on the left side. This appearance may be more difficult to appreciate when the entire peripheral zone is replaced by tumor. The normal relationship of the peripheral zone to the inner gland is reversed.

When the entire gland is replaced with tumor, on a background of hyperplasia, the gland may be diffusely inhomogeneous (Fig. 10-32). A very hypoechoic appearance is expected with diffuse cancer when the gland is not enlarged and the hyperplastic background is totally replaced (Fig. 10-35).

Recently, **color Doppler** has been added to transrectal ultrasound in an attempt to further increase the sensitivity and specificity of prostate ultrasound and ultrasound-guided biopsy. Initial reports on color Doppler were disappointing, showing only a minimum advantage for adding color Doppler to gray-scale imaging, but suggesting that in isoechoic areas, color Doppler may add useful information. These initial reports did not evaluate the biopsies individually but only evaluated the information on a case-by-case basis. Additionally, no information about the specificity of color Doppler could be obtained.[35-37]

In a recent study, our group reported on the use of **color Doppler** in patients with **suspected prostate cancer,** correlating the color Doppler findings with each biopsy site.[8] In this study, 220 separate biopsy sites, including 27 focal lesions, were evaluated and graded on a scale of 0 to 2, with grade 2 representing markedly increased vascularity. Each biopsy specimen was separated and evaluated histopathologically and correlated with a color Doppler image from that site. Of 34 grade 2 biopsy sites, 29 were either carcinoma or prostatitis (Figs. 10-9 and 10-13, *A* and *C;* Fig. 10-36). In 7 prostate cancer patients with no gray-scale abnormality, color Doppler demonstrated at least one grade

2 site. Importantly, 93% of sites that did not contain grade 2 color information did not contain cancer or prostatitis, even when a lesion was identified with ultrasound (Fig. 10-13, *B*). In this preliminary study we also suggested that if avoidance of detection of low-grade cancer is clinically important, color Doppler might be a useful adjunct to define areas of neovascularity that correlate with higher-grade cancers. We will be doing further study in this area, correlating newer color Doppler and three-dimensional ultrasound techniques with radical prostatectomy specimens.

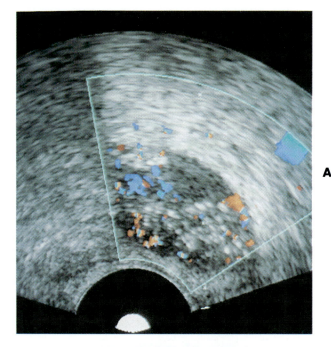

A

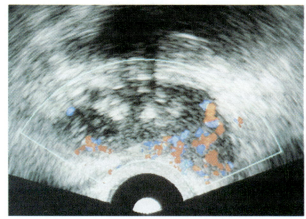

B

FIG. 10-36. **Color Doppler of prostate cancer.** **A,** Sagittal image demonstrates a hypoechoic mass in the peripheral zone with increased vascularity within it. Biopsy demonstrated Gleason 7 prostate cancer. Note background of focal echoes compatible with cribriform carcinoma. **B,** Isoechoic cancer with hypervascularity. Gray-scale imaging failed to reveal focal mass. Color Doppler demonstrates diffuse increased vessels suggestive of cancer. Biopsy revealed Gleason 7 carcinoma.

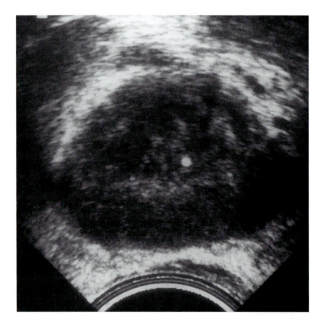

FIG. 10-35. **Diffuse cancer.** Axial scan shows diffusely inhomogeneous gland with loss of definition of zonal anatomy.

More recent studies evaluating the role of color Doppler in the isoechoic cancer also confirm the ability of color Doppler to identify higher-grade cancers in the isoechoic gland.[86,87] Importantly, investigators are now studying the cause of hypervascular color Doppler images as a function of neovascularity that has been identified in prostate and other cancers.[88-90] These studies indicate that increased microvessel density is higher in cancer than in benign tissue. In addition, angiogenesis-associated growth factors have been implicated in angiogenesis seen in malignant tumors, including the prostate. It is further suggested that angiogenesis and its associated hypervascularity seen by color Doppler may have stage and grade implications for prostate cancer.[90]

Location of Prostate Cancer
About 70% of prostate cancers arise in the peripheral zone, 20% in the transition zone, and 10% in the central zone.[91] With ultrasound, peripheral zone cancers are the most commonly detected, and the clinician must strongly suspect cancer to identify and biopsy lesions outside of the peripheral zone with gray-scale imaging. With color Doppler, any area seen with small, irregular vessels should be biopsied (Fig. 10-36). Occasionally a patient may need a second biopsy when the PSA level is elevated above 10 ng/ml and the initial biopsy was negative. In that instance, biopsies of the inner gland are warranted.

Prostate cancer that begins in the peripheral zone often grows longitudinally in that zone before extending into the inner gland. The surgical capsule acts as an anatomic barrier to inner gland spread (Fig. 10-34). In a large series of patients undergoing ultrasound and ultrasound-guided biopsy, 13% of lesions in the transition zone were malignant as opposed to 41% in the peripheral zone. In this series, however, only hypoechoic lesions underwent biopsy and color Doppler was not yet available.[92]

Results of Prostate Ultrasound in Cancer Detection
Because there is no gold standard by which to measure the accuracy of prostate ultrasound in the detection of prostate cancer, there is uniform lack of agreement on the accuracy of the technique. Only those studies that correlate sonographic findings with ultrasound-guided biopsy or radical prostatectomy can be used to determine the sensitivity of the procedure. In a National Institutes of Health (NIH) trial using gray-scale imaging only, lesion detection was poor, but detection of cancer in individual patients was not assessed because all patients had known cancer.[93] In general, prostate ultrasound has been relegated to prove the presence or absence of cancer, primarily by biopsy guidance. Its role in detecting cancer has been diminished.

Screening for Prostate Cancer
Several screening studies have been published in the literature. A study of 784 self-referred men revealed 22 cancers, of which 20 were detected with TRUS and 10 by digital examination. This suggested that ultrasound was twice as effective as digital examination for detection of unsuspected prostate cancer.[94] It was found that there was a cost of $6500 per diagnosed cancer with the use of TRUS with a slightly higher cost for diagnosing early cancer. This is less than the cost of diagnosing breast cancer with mammography screening programs.[95] In another study using PSA and TRUS, 225 men with negative rectal examination results were followed in a urology office. Because of suspicious TRUS, elevated PSA, or both, biopsies were performed. Thirty percent of the biopsies were positive for carcinoma. As with other screening studies, no proof of negative examination findings was obtained.[96] Even though ultrasound was used extensively for screening in the past, currently all screening is done with PSA.

Studies evaluating digital rectal examination, prostate ultrasound, and PSA conclude that all men over age 50 should have routine yearly PSA and digital rectal examinations. This age decreases to 40 in African-American men and men with a positive family history.[70] Universal screening leading to biopsy could detect prostate cancer in 5.3% of men over age 50 who will develop clinical prostate cancer sometime in their lifetime.[20] Unfortunately, early detection of cancer may not add years to patient lives. Also, patients with the best prognosis may be the ones identified with screening. Therefore the possibility of overdetection with screening is raised. A new randomized controlled trial has been initiated to study whether watchful waiting or treatment changes the natural history of this disease.[97]

Staging of Prostate Cancer
Following the diagnosis of prostate cancer, definitive therapeutic decisions cannot be made unless the stage of prostate cancer is determined. In general, incidental prostate cancer found on transurethral prostatectomy (TURP) (stage T1a) only needs follow-up examinations without further therapy. Prostate sonography with ultrasound-guided biopsy has been suggested to evaluate these patients in addition to or instead of a repeat transurethral resection or blind needle biopsy. For example, if a minimal amount of cancer were found on a transurethral resection as the result of resection sampling of the edge of a large cancer, ultrasound could properly assess and determine the stage of cancer.[98]

Clinical stages T1 and T2 can be treated with radical prostatectomy or radiation therapy. Controversy exists concerning the best therapy for locally invasive prostate cancer (stage T3). If microscopic invasion is found, surgery followed by radiation seems to be an acceptable approach. With macroscopic invasion there appears to be no advantage to surgery, and radiation therapy is recommended. Sonographic staging allows for separation of those patients with macroscopic local extension into the periprostatic fat, seminal vesicles, or local lymph nodes from those with disease confined to the prostate gland (Fig. 10-37).

The **role of ultrasound** in **local staging** has been assessed. Investigators have found sensitivities for local extension into the capsule or seminal vesicles to be as high as 90% and as low as 40% to 60%. More importantly, specificities for invasion ranged from 46% to 90%, depending on the size of the primary tumor.[93,99] Large tumors can be easily seen to extend outside of the capsule as a result of the loss of symmetry and capsular irregularity (Figs. 10-35 and 10-37). Anatomically, however, the prostate does not contain a true capsule but a fibromuscular band. This creates a dilemma for the pathologist and urologist in determining the exact significance of the depth of invasion outside this band and into the periprostatic soft tissues.[23]

Seminal vesicle extension can be defined sonographically by enlargement, cystic dilation, asymmetry, anterior displacement, hyperechogenicity, and loss of the seminal vesicle beak (Figs. 10-38 to 10-40).[21,100] This phenomenon is best appreciated when comparing the normal with the abnormal side.[93] Tumors that extend into the seminal vesicle can also obstruct the seminal vesicle, causing diffuse enlargement (Fig. 10-39). Hemorrhage into the seminal vesicle following biopsy can simulate obstruction.

There is a potential role for **staging biopsies** in patients with known prostate cancer. Almost one half of patients who are treated surgically with radical prostatectomy for clinical organ-confined prostate cancer are found to have invasion outside of the gland, a situation leading to treatment failure in a significant number of patients.[4,7,8] Anecdotal reports suggest that some of these patients will do well when there is only minimal extracapsular spread, but this hypothesis has not been well tested. Only a few reports have described the role of direct staging biopsies for prostate cancer, and these have been directed toward the seminal vesicles.[101-103]

When routine preoperative seminal vesicle biopsy is performed and tumor is found, there is 100% incidence of capsular penetration and 50% have positive lymph nodes (Fig. 10-40). In patients with low PSA

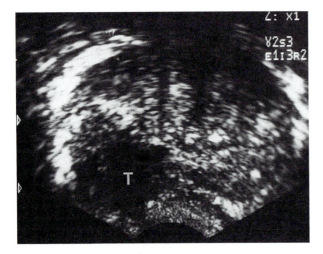

FIG. 10-37. Incidentally discovered prostate cancer in a patient with rectal cancer. A prostate mass, *T*, was discovered at the time of endorectal sonography for a rectal cancer. The rectal cancer was an early-stage cancer, but the prostate cancer required radiation therapy. It was staged as T3. (From Bree RL. Ultrasound imaging of rectal and perirectal abnormalities. In Thrall JH, ed. *Current Practice of Radiology.* St Louis: Mosby-Year Book; 1993.

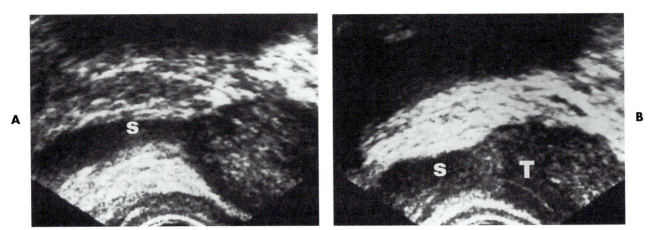

FIG. 10-38. Seminal vesicle invasion. A, Right sagittal scan shows normal right seminal vesicle, *S*. B, Left sagittal scan shows large tumor, *T*, with extension into large left seminal vesicle, *S*, with loss of seminal vesicle beak.

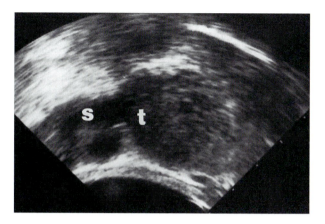

FIG. 10-39. Seminal vesicle obstruction. Right sagittal scan shows seminal vesicle, *s*, is dilated because of obstruction by extensive prostatic tumor, *t*, at base. This cannot be separated from direct seminal vesicle tumor extension or hemorrhage following biopsy.

levels and a negative biopsy, gross capsular penetration is uniformly absent.[103] Seminal vesicle biopsy prior to radiation therapy is recommended to more appropriately plan the therapeutic fields and select patients for lymph node sampling.[102]

Direct biopsy of the prostatic capsule has not been routinely performed. We have occasionally purposely performed staging pericapsular biopsies to attempt to prove extracapsular spread. When the pathologist sees tumor intermixed with fat, there is extracapsular invasion, probably of the macroscopic type.

Both seminal vesicle invasion and local periprostatic invasion have been studied with CT and MRI and compared with ultrasound. CT is a poor staging technique for involvement of both local periprostatic structures and lymph nodes.[104,105] MRI is slightly more advantageous than ultrasound in detecting local invasion and involvement of the seminal vesicles.[93] Use of endorectal surface coils may further enhance the ability of MRI of the prostate, but even then its role may be limited to selected patients where decisions about radiation therapy or hormonal therapy are crucial.[106,107]

Monitoring for Treatment and Response to Therapy

Ultrasound has been used as a guidance technique for placement of iodine-125 seed implantations for interstitial therapy of prostate cancer. Follow-up examinations have shown significant volume reduction, although biopsy of lesions in these patients revealed residual cancer in 50% (Fig. 10-41).[108-111] In advanced cancer, prostate volume decrease in patients following orchiectomy of at least 50% was a good

A

B

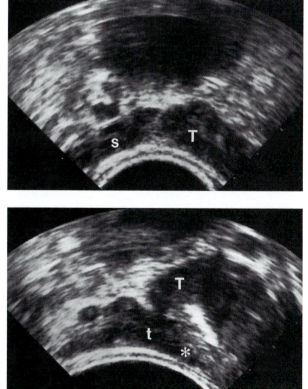

FIG. 10-40. Seminal vesicle extension of carcinoma. A, Axial image shows normal right seminal vesicle, *s*, and tumor invasion of left seminal vesicle, *T*. **B,** Sagittal scan shows extensive prostate tumor, *T*, with tumor extension into seminal vesicle, *t*. Invaginated extraprostatic space, ***, is route by which tumor extends into seminal vesicle. Ultrasound-guided biopsy of seminal vesicle revealed carcinoma.

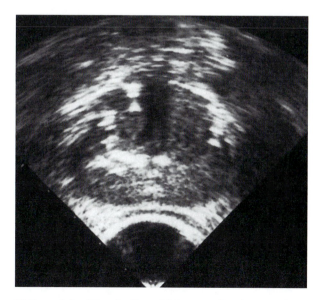

FIG. 10-41. Iodine-125 seeds in patient treated previously for prostate cancer. Axial scan shows multiple very bright echoes with reverberation artifacts beyond. No abnormal masses are seen in this gland.

prognostic sign.[112] Patients with sonographic abnormalities following radiation therapy for prostate cancer had positive biopsy findings in a high percentage of hypoechoic lesions, particularly when the PSA was elevated (Fig. 10-42). As with the preradiation prostate, a significant number of patients underwent random biopsies, which also yielded positive results for cancer, particularly when there was a high suspicion of recurrence.[113,114] We have not found color Doppler useful in postradiation patients. The radiation appears to interfere with the ability to develop neovascularity. The sextant biopsy technique has been adequate to find recurrent tumor in patients following radiation therapy (Fig. 10-43).

Patients examined for tumor recurrence following radical prostatectomy typically present with a detectable PSA. If a mass is seen in the prostate bed or there is loss of the retroanastomotic fat plane, there is strong evidence for recurrence. Careful biopsy of the recurrent mass can be done with ultrasound guidance.[115]

Ultrasound is used to monitor interstitial therapy such as cryotherapy. The ultrasound probe is placed in the rectum while the cryoablation procedure is performed with a transperineal approach.[116] It has been suggested that ultrasound can determine the extent of the ablation process and help to decrease complications. Planning with ultrasound has been used with transperineal prostate brachytherapy. This technique can help quantify the isodose calculation and decrease the subjectivity of the treatment procedure.[117]

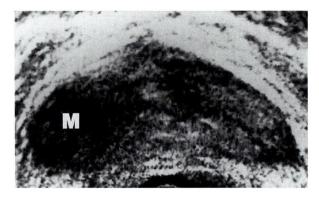

FIG. 10-42. Radiation fibrosis *(biopsy proven)* in a patient previously treated with external beam radiation. Palpable and sonographically identifiable mass, *M*, suggestive of carcinoma is seen in right lobe.

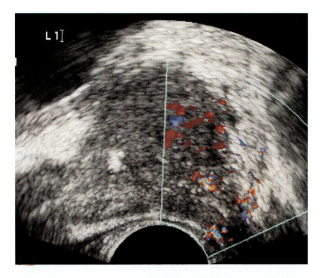

FIG. 10-43. Color Doppler following radiation therapy with tumor recurrence. A patient with elevated PSA was examined 2 years following radiation therapy. Vascularity is mildly increased but not typical for newly diagnosed prostate cancer. Biopsies revealed diffuse recurrent cancer. Appearance of cancer following radiation therapy appears to be different from untreated tumors.

REFERENCES

1. Choyke PL. Imaging of prostate cancer. *Abdom Imag* 1995;20:505-515.
2. Huch Boni RA, Boner JA, Debatin JF et al. Optimization of prostate carcinoma staging: comparison of imaging and clinical methods. *Clin Radiol* 1995;50:593-600.
3. Flanigan RC, Catalona WJ, Richie JP et al. Accuracy of digital rectal examination and transrectal ultrasonography in localizing prostate cancer. *J Urol* 1994;152:1506-1509.
4. Babaian RJ, Camps JL. The role of prostate-specific antigen as part of the diagnostic triad and as a guide when to perform a biopsy. *Cancer* 1991;68:2060-2063.
5. Catalona WJ, Smith DS, Ratliff TL et al. Detection of organ-confined prostate cancer is increased through prostate specific antigen based screening. *JAMA* 1993;270:948-954.
6. Spencer JA, Alexander AA, Gomella L et al. Ultrasound-guided four quadrant biopsy of the prostate: efficacy in the diagnosis of isoechoic cancer. *Clin Radiol* 1994;49:711-714.
7. Newman JS, Bree RL, Rugin JM. Prostate cancer: diagnosis with color Doppler sonography with histologic correlation of each biopsy site. *Radiology* 1995;195:86-90.
8. Neumaier CE, Martinoli C, Derchi LE et al. Normal prostate gland: examination with color Doppler US. *Radiology* 1995;196:453-457.

History of Prostate Ultrasound

9. Watanabe H, Igari D, Tanahasi Y et al. Development and application of new equipment for transrectal ultrasonography. *J Clin Ultrasound* 1974;2:91-98.
10. Gammelgaard J, Holm HH. Transurethral and transrectal ultrasonic scanning in urology. *J Urol* 1980;124:863-868.
11. Rifkin MD, Kurtz AB, Goldberg BB. Sonographically guided transperineal prostatic biopsy: preliminary experience with a longitudinal linear-array transducer. *AJR* 1983;140:745-747.
12. Sekine H, Oka K, Takehara Y. Transrectal longitudinal ultrasonotomography of the prostate by electronic linear scanning. *J Urol* 1982;127:62.
13. Boyce WH, McKinney WM, Resnick MI et al. Ultrasonography as an aid in the diagnosis and management of surgical diseases of the pelvis. *Ann Surg* 1976;184:477-489.
14. King WW, Wilkiemeyer RM, Boyce WH et al. Current status of prostatic echography. *JAMA* 1973;226:444-447.

15. Watanabe H. History and applications of transrectal sonography of the prostate. *Urol Clin North Am* 1989;16:617-622.

16. Fritzsche PJ, Axford PD, Ching VC et al. Correlation of transrectal sonographic findings in patients with suspected and unsuspected prostatic disease. *J Urol* 1983;130:272-274.

17. Spirnak JP, Resnick MI. Transrectal ultrasonography. *Urology* 1983;23:461-467.

18. Lee F, Gray JM, McLeary RD et al. Prostatic evaluation by transrectal sonography: criteria for diagnosis of early carcinoma. *Radiology* 1986;158:91-95.

19. Rifkin MD, Friedland GW, Shortliffe L. Prostatic evaluation by transrectal endosonography: detection of carcinoma. *Radiology* 1986;158:85-90.

Anatomy

20. Lee F, Torp-Pedersen ST, Siders DB et al. Transrectal ultrasound in the diagnosis and staging of prostatic carcinoma. *Radiology* 1989;170:609-615.

21. Kaye KW, Richter L. Ultrasonographic anatomy of normal prostate gland: reconstruction by computer graphics. *Urology* 1990;35:12-17.

22. McNeal JE. The zonal anatomy of the prostate. *Prostate* 1981;2:35-49.

23. Ayala AG, Ro JY, Babaian R et al. The prostatic capsule: does it exist? *Am J Surg Pathol* 1989;13:21-27.

Equipment and Scanning Techniques

24. Rifkin MD. Endorectal sonography of the prostate: clinical implications. *AJR* 1987;148:1137-1142.

25. Holm HH, Gammelgaard J. Ultrasonically guided precise needle placement in the prostate and seminal vesicles. *J Urol* 1981;125:385-387.

26. Parker SH, Hopper KD, Yakes WF et al. Image-directed percutaneous biopsies with a biopsy gun. *Radiology* 1989;171:663-669.

27. Torp-Pedersen S, Lee F, Littrup PJ et al. Transrectal biopsy of the prostate guided with transrectal ultrasound: longitudinal and multiplanar scanning. *Radiology* 1989;170:23-27.

28. Clements R, Aideyan OU, Griffiths GJ et al. Side effects and patient acceptability of transrectal biopsy of the prostate. *Clin Radiol* 1993;47:125-126.

29. Bree RL. Prostate and other transrectally guided biopsies. In: McGahan JP, ed. *Interventional Ultrasound.* Baltimore: Williams & Wilkins; 1990:221-237.

30. Dyke CH, Toi A, Sweet JM. Value of random ultrasound-guided transrectal prostate biopsy. *Radiology* 1990;176:345-349.

31. Hodge KK, McNeal JE, Terris MK, et al. Random systematic versus directed ultrasound guided transrectal core biopsies of the prostate. *J Urol* 1989;142:71-75.

32. Olson MC, Posniak HV, Fisher SG, et al. Directed and random biopsies of the prostate: indications based on combined results of transrectal sonography and prostate-specific antigen density determinations. *AJR* 1994;163:1407-1411.

33. Peller PA, Young DC, Marmaduke DP et al. Sextant prostate biopsies: a histopathologic correlation with radical prostatectomy specimens. *Cancer* 1995;75(2):530-538.

34. Slonim SM, Cuttino JT, Johnson CJ et al. Diagnosis of prostatic carcinoma: value of random transrectal sonographically guided biopsies. *AJR* 1993;161:1003-1006.

35. Kelly IMG, Lees WR, Rickards D. Prostate cancer and the role of color Doppler US. *Radiology* 1993;189:153-156.

36. Patel U, Rickards D. The diagnostic value of color Doppler flow in the peripheral zone of the prostate with histological correlation. *Brit J Urol* 1994;74:590-595.

37. Rifkin MD, Sudakoff GS, Alexander AA. Prostate: techniques, results and potential applications of color Doppler US-scanning. *Radiology* 1993;186:509-513.

38. Narayan P, Gajendran V, Taylor SP et al. The role of transrectal ultrasound-guided biopsy-based staging, preoperative serum prostate-specific antigen, and biopsy gleason score in prediction of final pathological diagnosis in prostate cancer. *Urology* 1995;46:205-212.

39. Cooner WH, Mosley BR, Rutherford CL Jr et al. Prostate cancer detection in a clinical urological practice by ultrasonography, digital rectal examination and prostate specific antigen. *J Urol* 1990;143:1146-1154.

40. Spencer JA, Alexander AA, Gomella L et al. Clinical and US findings in prostate cancer: patients with normal prostate-specific antigen levels. *Radiology* 1993;189:389-393.

41. Littrup PJ, Kane RA, Mettlin CJ et al. Cost-effective prostate cancer detection: reduction of low-yield biopsies. *Cancer* 1994;74:3146-3158.

42. Fleming C, Wasson JH, Albertsen PC et al. A decision analysis of alternative treatment strategies for clinically localized prostate cancer. Prostate patient outcomes. *JAMA* 1993;269(20):2650-8.

43. Barry MJ, Fleming C, Coley CM et al. Should Medicare provide reimbursement for prostate-specific antigen testing for early detection of prostate cancer? IV. Estimating the risks and benefits of an early detection program. *Urology* 1995;46(4):445-461.

44. Oesterling JE, Jacobsen SJ, Cooner WH. The use of age-specific reference ranges for serum prostate specific antigen in men 60 years old or older. *J Urol* 1995;153(4):1160-1163.

45. Benson MC, Whang IS, Olsson CA et al. The use of prostate specific antigen density to enhance the predictive value of intermediate levels of serum prostate specific antigen. *J Urol* 1992;147:817-821.

46. Lee F, Littrup PJ, Loft-Christensen L et al. Predicted prostate specific antigen results using transrectal ultrasound gland volume. *Cancer* 1992;70:211-220.

47. Brawer MK, Beatie J, Wener MH et al. Screening for prostatic carcinoma with prostate specific antigen: results of the second year. *J Urol* 1993;150:106-109.

48. Hodge KK, McNeal JE, Stamey TA. Ultrasound guided transrectal core biopsies of the palpably abnormal prostate. *J Urol* 1988;142:66-70.

Benign Abnormalities of the Prostate and Seminal Vesicles

49. Hendrikx AJ, van Helvoort, van Dommelen CA et al. Ultrasonic determination of prostatic volume: a cadaver study. *Urology* 1989;34(3):123-125.

50. Jacobsen H, Torp-Pedersen S, Juul N. Ultrasonic evaluation of age-related human prostatic growth and development of benign prostatic hyperplasia. *Scand J Urol Nephrol* 1988;107(suppl):26-31.

51. Shinohara K, Scardino PT, Carter S et al. Pathologic basis of the sonographic appearance of the normal and malignant prostate. *Urol Clin North Am* 1989;16:675-691.

52. Burks DD, Drolshagen LF, Fleischer AC et al. Transrectal sonography of benign and malignant prostatic lesions. *AJR* 1986;146:1187-1191.

53. Oyen RH, Van de Voorde QM, Van Poppel HP et al. Benign hyperplastic nodules that originate in the peripheral zone of the prostate gland. *Radiology* 1993;189:707-711.

54. Brawer MK, Rennels MA, Nagle RB et al. Prostatic intraepithelial neoplasia: a lesion that may be confused with cancer on prostatic ultrasound. *J Urol* 1989;142:1510-1512.

55. Lee F, Torp-Pedersen S, Carroll JT et al. Use of transrectal ultrasound and prostate-specific antigen in diagnosis of prostatic intraepithelial neoplasia. *Urology* 1989;34(suppl):4-8.

56. Fogarty KT, Arger PH, Shibutani Y et al. Follow-up benign hypoechoic peripheral zone lesions of the prostate gland: US

characteristics and cancer prevalence. *Radiology* 1994;191: 69-74.

57. Doble A, Carter S. Ultrasonographic findings in prostatitis. *Urol Clin North Am* 1989;16(4):763-772.

58. Di Trapani D, Pavone C, Serretta V et al. Chronic prostatitis and prostatodynia: ultrasonographic alterations of the prostate, bladder neck, seminal vesicles and periprostatic venous plexus. *Eur Urol* 1988;15:230-234.

59. Doble A, Thomas BJ, Furr PM et al. A search for infectious agents in chronic abacterial prostatitis using ultrasound guided biopsy. *Br J Urol* 1989;64:297-301.

60. Fuse H, Sumiya H, Ishii H et al. Treatment of hemospermia caused by dilated seminal vesicles by direct drug injection guided by ultrasonography. *J Urol* 1988;140:991-992.

61. Worischeck JH, Parra RO. Chronic hematospermia: assessment by transrectal ultrasound. *Urology* 1994;43(4):515-520.

62. Bude R, Bree RL, Adler RS et al. Transrectal ultrasound appearance of granulomatous prostatitis. *J Ultrasound Med* 1990;9:677-680.

63. Cytron S, Weinberger M, Pitlik S et al. Value of transrectal ultrasonography for diagnosis and treatment of prostatic abscess. *Urology* 1988;32(5):454-458.

64. Papanicolaou N, Pfister R, Stafford S et al. Prostatic abscess: imaging with transrectal sonography and magnetic resonance. *AJR* 1987;149:981-982.

65. Nghiem HT, Kellman GM, Sandberg SA et al. Cystic lesions of the prostate. *RadioGraphics* 1990;10:635-650.

66. Shabsigh R, Lerner S, Fishman IJ et al. The role of transrectal ultrasonography in the diagnosis and management of prostatic and seminal vesicle cysts. *J Urol* 1989;141:1206-1209.

67. Littrup PJ, Lee F, McLeary RD et al. Transrectal ultrasound of the seminal vesicles and ejaculatory ducts: clinical correlation. *Radiology* 1988;168:625-628.

Prostate Cancer

68. Jacobsen SJ, Katusic SK, Bergstralh EJ et al. Incidence of prostate cancer diagnosis in the eras before and after serum prostate-specific antigen testing. *JAMA* 1995;274(18):1445-1449.

69. Whitmore WF Jr. Natural history staging of prostate cancer. *Urol Clin North Am* 1984;11:205-220.

70. Garnick MB. Prostate cancer: screening, diagnosis, and management. *Ann Intern Med* 1993;118:804-818.

71. Gleason DF, Veterans Administration Cooperative Urological Research Group. *Histologic Grading and Clinical Staging of Prostatic Carcinoma.* Philadelphia: Lea & Febiger; 1977.

72. Epstein JI, Walsh PC, Carmichael M et al. Pathologic and clinical findings to predict tumor extent of nonpalpable *(stage T1c)* prostate cancer. *JAMA* 1994;271:368-374.

73. Partin AW, Yoo J, Carter HB et al. The use of prostate specific antigen, clinical stage and Gleason score to predict pathological stage in men with localized prostate cancer. *J Urol* 1993;15:110-114.

74. Austenfeld MS. Preoperative estimate of extent of disease in T1c: how well can we predict. *Semin Urol Oncol* 1995;13(3):176-180.

75. Ellis WJ, Brawer MK. The significance of isoechoic prostatic carcinoma. *J Urol* 1994;152:2304-2307.

76. Dugan JA, Bostwick DG, Myers RP et al. The definition and preoperative prediction of clinically insignificant prostate cancer. *JAMA* 1996;275:288-294.

77. Dahnert WF, Hamper UM, Eggleston JC et al. Prostatic evaluation by transrectal sonography with histopathologic correlation: the echogenic appearance of early carcinoma. *Radiology* 1986;158:97-102.

78. Rifkin MD, McGlynn ET, Choi H. Echogenicity of prostatic cancer correlated with histologic grade and stromal fibrosis: endorectal ultrasound studies. *J Urol* 1989;170:549-552.

79. Shinohara K, Wheeler TM, Scardino PT. The appearance of prostate cancer on transrectal ultrasonography: correlation of imaging and pathological examinations. *J Urol* 1989;142:76-82.

80. Hasegawa Y, Sakamoto N. Relationship of ultrasonographic findings to histology in prostate cancer. *Eur Urol* 1994;26(1):10-17.

81. Rifkin MD, Dahnert W, Kurtz AB. State of the art: endorectal sonography of the prostate gland. *AJR* 1990;154:691-700.

82. Dahnert WF, Hamper UM, Walsh PC et al. The echogenic focus in prostatic sonograms, with xeroradiographic and histopathologic correlation. *Radiology* 1986;159:95-100.

83. Lee F. Transrectal ultrasound: diagnosis and staging of prostatic carcinoma. *Urology* 1989;33(suppl):5-10.

84. Hamper UM, Sheth S, Walsh PC et al. Bright echogenic foci in early prostatic carcinoma: sonographic and pathologic correlation. *Radiology* 1990;176:339-343.

85. Dahnert WF. Ultrasonography of carcinoma of the prostate: a critical review. *Appl Radiol* 1988;17:39-44.

86. Decarvalho V, Kuligowska E. The role of color Doppler for improving the detection of cancer in the isoechoic prostate gland. Presented at the Annual Meeting of the American Institute of Ultrasound in Medicine; March 1996; New York.

87. Littrup PJ, Klein RM, Gross ML et al. Color Doppler guides prostate biopsies of higher grade cancers: racial implications. Presented at the Annual Meeting of the American Institute of Ultrasound in Medicine; March 1996; New York.

88. Bigler SA, Deering RE, Brawer MK. A quantitative morphometric analysis of the microcirculation in prostate carcinoma. *Hum Pathol* 1993;24:220-226.

89. Brawer MK, Deering RE, Brown M et al. Predictors of pathologic stage in prostatic carcinoma: the role of neovascularity. *Cancer* 1994;73(3):678-687.

90. Louvar E, Littrup PJ, Uyu L et al. The pathophysiology of increased color Doppler flow in the prostate. Presented at the Annual Meeting of the American Institute of Ultrasound in Medicine; March 1996; New York.

91. McNeal JE, Redwine EA, Freiha FS et al. Zonal distribution of prostatic adenocarcinoma. *Am J Surg Pathol* 1988;12:897-906.

92. Lee F, Torp-Pedersen S, Littrup PJ et al. Hypoechoic lesions of the prostate: clinical relevance of tumor size, digital rectal examination, and prostate-specific antigen. *Radiology* 1989;170:29-32.

93. Rifkin MD, Zerhouni EA, Gastsonis CA. Comparison of magnetic resonance imaging and ultrasound in staging early prostate cancer. *N Engl J Med* 1990;323(10):621-626.

94. Lee F, Littrup PJ, Torp-Pedersen S et al. Prostate cancer: comparison of transrectal ultrasound and digital rectal examination. *Radiology* 1988;168:389-394.

95. Torp-Pedersen S, Littrup PJ, Lee F et al. Early prostate cancer: diagnostic costs of screening transrectal ultrasound and digital rectal examination. *Radiology* 1988;169:351-354.

96. Cooner WH, Mosley BR, Rutherford CL et al. Clinical application of transrectal ultrasonography and prostate specific antigen in the search for prostate cancer. *J Urol* 1988;139:758-761.

97. Wilt TJ, Brawer MK. The prostate cancer intervention versus observation trial: a randomized trial comparing radical prostatectomy versus expectant management for the treatment of clinically localized prostate cancer. *J Urol* 1994;152:1910-1914.

98. Parra RO, Gregory JG. Transrectal ultrasound in stage A1 prostate cancer. *Urology* 1989;34:344-346.
99. Hamper UM, Sheth S, Walsh PC et al. Carcinoma of the prostate: value of transrectal sonography in detecting extension into the neurovascular bundle. *AJR* 1990;155:1015-1019.
100. Terris MK, McNeal JE, Stamey TA. Invasion of the seminal vesicles by prostatic cancer: detection with transrectal sonography. *AJR* 1990;155:811-815.
101. Bastacky SI, Walsh PC, Epstein JI. Relationship between perineural tumor invasion on needle biopsy and radical prostatectomy capsular penetration in clinical stage B adenocarcinoma of the prostate. *Am J Surg Pathol* 1993;17(4):336-341.
102. Stock RG, Stone NN, Ianuzzi C et al. Seminal vesicle biopsy and laparoscopic pelvis lymph node dissection: implications for patient selection in the radiotherapeutic management of prostate cancer. *Int J Radiat Oncol Biol Phys* 1995;33(4):815-821.
103. Vallancien G, Prapotnich D, Beillon B et al. Seminal vesicle biopsies in the preoperative staging of prostatic cancer. *Eur Urol* 1991;19:196-200.
104. Platt J, Bree RL, Schwab RE. Accuracy of computed tomography in the staging of carcinoma of the prostate. *AJR* 1987;149:315-318.
105. Salo JO, Kivisaari L, Rannikko S et al. Computerized tomography and transrectal ultrasound in the assessment of local extension of prostatic cancer before radical retropubic prostatectomy. *J Urol* 1987;137:435-438.
106. Jager GJ, Ruijter ETG, van de Kaa CA et al. Local staging of prostate cancer with endorectal MR imaging: correlation with histopathology. *AJR* 1996;166:845-852.
107. D'Amico AV, Whittington R, Malkowicz SB et al. A multivariable analysis of clinical factors predicting for pathological features associated with local failure after radical prostatectomy for prostate cancer. *Int J Radiat Oncol Biol Phys* 1994;30(2):293-302.
108. Iversen P, Bak M, Juul N et al. Ultrasonically guided 125 iodine seed implantation with external radiation in management of localized prostatic carcinoma. *Urology* 1989;34:181-186.
109. Broseta E, Boronat F, Domimguez C et al. Modification del patron ecografico del carcinoma de prostata tratado mediante agonistas Lh-rh. *Arch Esp de Urol* 1989;42:125-128.
110. Clements R, Griffiths GJ, Peeling WB et al. Transrectal ultrasound in monitoring response to treatment of prostate disease. *Urol Clin North Am* 1989;16:735-740.
111. Egender G, Pirker E, Rapf C et al. Transrectal ultrasonography as follow-up method in prostatic carcinoma after external beam and interstitial radiotherapy. *Eur J Radiol* 1988;8:37-43.
112. Carpentier P, Schroeder FH, Schmitz PIM. Transrectal ultrasonometry of the prostate: the prognostic relevance of volume changes under endocrine management. *World J Urol* 1986;4:159-162.
113. Egawa S, Wheeler TM, Greene DR et al. Detection of residual prostate cancer after radiotherapy by sonographically guided needle biopsy. *Urology* 1992;39(4):358-363.
114. Kabalin JN, Hodge KK, McNeal JE et al. Identification of residual cancer in the prostate following radiation therapy: role of transrectal ultrasound guided biopsy and prostate specific antigen. *J Urol* 1989;142:326-333.
115. Salomon CG, Flisak ME, Olson MC et al. Radical prostatectomy: transrectal sonographic evaluation to assess for local recurrence. *Radiology* 1993;189:713-719.
116. Wieder J, Schmidt JD, Casola G et al. Transrectal ultrasound-guided transperineal cryoablation in the treatment of prostate carcinoma: preliminary results. *J Urol* 1995;154(2 pt 1):435-441.
117. Edmundson GK, Yan D, Martinez AA. Intraoperative optimization of needle placement and dwell times for conformal prostate brachytherapy. *Int J Radiat Oncol Biol Phys* 1995;33(5):1257-1263.

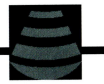

CHAPTER 11

The Adrenal Glands

•

Wendy Thurston, M.D., B.Sc., F.R.C.P.C.
Stephanie R. Wilson, M.D., F.R.C.P.C.

The adrenal glands are the smallest paired organs found in the abdomen, weighing about 4 g each in a normal nonstressed adult.[1] Though small and tucked anteromedial to the upper pole of the kidneys, the adrenal glands play a significant role in the maintenance of homeostasis through hormone secretion.

Computed tomography (CT) has been regarded as the premier imaging modality to identify adrenal gland disease. However, sonography can be efficient and economical in the work-up of patients with suspected adrenal gland pathology. Because the adrenal glands may be involved with both local and systemic disease, a thorough understanding of the applications and limitations of all imaging techniques is necessary to direct the most appropriate imaging strategy.

EMBRYOLOGY

The adrenal gland is composed of two parts, a **cortex** and **medulla,** which have different embryologic origins. The cortex develops from **mesoderm** tissue and the medulla from **neuroectodermal** tissue.

During the sixth week of fetal development there is rapid proliferation of mesenchymal cells, originating from the posterior abdominal wall peritoneal epithelium near the cranial end of the mesonephros (primitive kidney). These cells penetrate the retroperitoneal mesenchyme to become the **primitive adrenal cortex.**[2] Further mesenchymal cell proliferation occurs, and these cells envelope the primitive cortex more compactly to become the **permanent adrenal cortex.** By the end of the eighth gestational week the cortical mass separates from the posterior peritoneal surface and becomes surrounded by retroperitoneal connective tissue.

During the seventh week of development, cells originating from neuroectoderm migrate and invade the medial aspect of the developing primitive adrenal cortex. These cells differentiate into the chromaffin cells of the **adrenal medulla.**

At birth the gland is comprised predominantly of primitive fetal cortex and adrenal medulla. Immediately after birth the primitive cortex begins to involute and disappears by 1 year of age. Simultaneously, the thin, compact, **permanent adrenal cortex** further differentiates into the three zones of the adult gland: **glomerulosa, fasciculata,** and **reticularis** (Fig. 11-1).[3]

NORMAL ANATOMY, MORPHOLOGY, AND PHYSIOLOGY

Anatomy

The adrenal glands are found at the level of the eleventh or twelfth thoracic rib, lateral to the first lumbar vertebrae. Each measures from 2 to 3 cm in width, 4 to 6 cm in length, and 3 to 6 mm in thickness.[2] Each gland is composed of an **anteromedial ridge** and a **medial** and **lateral wing.** The glands are surrounded by fatty areolar tissue that has a thin, fibrous capsule and many fibrous extensions into the adrenal glands.[2] With their fascial support the adrenals are relatively fixed, unlike the kidney, which is not anchored to the perinephric fascia. Thus the adrenal glands have a more constant relationship with the abdominal great vessels than they do with the kidneys. The adrenal gland and kidney will separate during deep inspiration or in the upright position. This may allow differentiation between renal and adrenal masses, particularly during sonographic examination.[4,5]

The **right adrenal gland** is located posterior to the inferior vena cava. Medially the crus of the diaphragm runs parallel to the medial wing of the gland while the lateral wing is adjacent to the posteromedial aspect of the liver (Fig. 11-2; Fig. 11-3). The medial wing may extend caudally along the medial aspect of the upper pole of the kidney. The tip of the gland always terminates cephalad to the renal vessels.[6]

The **left adrenal gland** is positioned anteromedially to the kidney (see Fig. 11-2). It may extend from above the superior pole of the kidney to the level of the renal hilum in 10% of persons.[7,8] The aorta and crus of the diaphragm are on the medial aspect of the adrenal. The cephalic two thirds of the gland is posterior to the stomach and therefore covered by peritoneum of the lesser sac. The caudal one third of the gland is related to the posterior aspect of the pancreatic body and splenic vasculature (see Fig. 11-3).[9]

On sonography, the adrenal gland is less echogenic than the surrounding perirenal fat while the medulla is evident as a highly echogenic central linear structure. The echogenic linear medulla is most prominent in the fetus and newborn; however, it can be identified in thin adults (Fig. 11-4).

Oppenheimer et al.[10] proposed that the medullary echogenicity in newborn infants is due to an increased amount of collagen around the central vessels and haphazard orientation of its cell population, resulting in multiple reflective interfaces.

Morphology

The **medial wing** of the adrenal gland is larger superiorly and smaller or absent inferiorly while the **lateral wing** is larger inferiorly and smaller superiorly.[7] Complete visualization of the adrenal gland in a single sonographic plane is virtually impossible because of the complex shape of the organ.[11]

Physiology

The **adrenal cortex** secretes **steroid hormones** and the **medulla** secretes **catecholamines.**

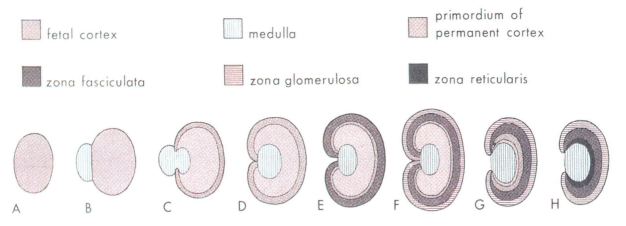

FIG. 11-1. Adrenal gland embryology. A, Six weeks. **B,** Seven weeks. **C,** Eight weeks. **D** and **E,** Later stages of encapsulation of the medulla by the cortex. **F,** Newborn. **G,** One year showing fetal cortex has almost disappeared. **H,** Four years showing the adult pattern of the cortical zones. (Modified from Moore KL. *The Developing Human: Clinically Oriented Embryology.* 5th ed. Philadelphia: WB Saunders Co: 1993.)

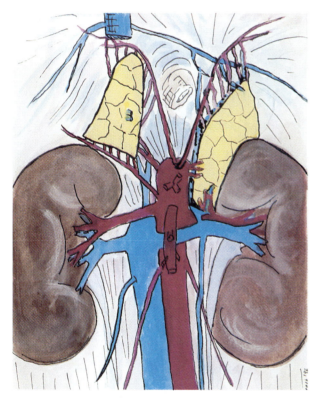

FIG. 11-2. Anatomy and blood supply of the adrenal glands. (Courtesy of Jenny Tomash.)

The **cortex** is subdivided into **three distinct zones.** The **zona glomerulosa,** which is the outermost layer, produces and secretes the **mineralocorticoid aldosterone.** This hormone is part of a coordinated hormonal system (renin-angiotensin-aldosterone) involved in the homeostasis of fluid volume and blood pressure. The principal action of aldosterone is on the renal tubules, causing sodium retention. The **zona fasciculata** and **reticularis** act as a single unit and secrete **cortisol (glucocorticoid)** and **androgens.** The adrenal cortex in a nonstressed adult secretes about 20 mg per day of cortisol and with stressful stimuli may increase secretion up to 150 to 200 mg per day.[12] The physiologic significance of the adrenal androgens is not known. In excess, they may cause hirsutism or virilization in females and precocious pseudopuberty in males.[12]

The **adrenal medulla** is responsible for the synthesis and secretion of **catecholamines (epinephrine and norepinephrine).** These hormones play an important role in an individual's response to actual or anticipated stress though they are not essential to life.[12]

ADRENAL SONOGRAPHY

Technical Aspects

Ability to visualize the adrenal glands sonographically is multifactorial related to body habitus, operator experience, and type of equipment. With the introduction of high-resolution, real-time sector scanners, the adrenal glands have become easier to examine. Ideally the patient should fast for 6 to 8 hours prior to the exam in an attempt to reduce the amount of intervening bowel gas.

Marchal et al.[11] reported that the normal right and left adrenal glands were visualized by high-resolution real-time sonography in 92% and 71% of patients, respectively. Cortex and medulla was differentiated in 13% of patients. Alternatively, Günther et al.[13] studied 60 healthy subjects with high-resolution real-

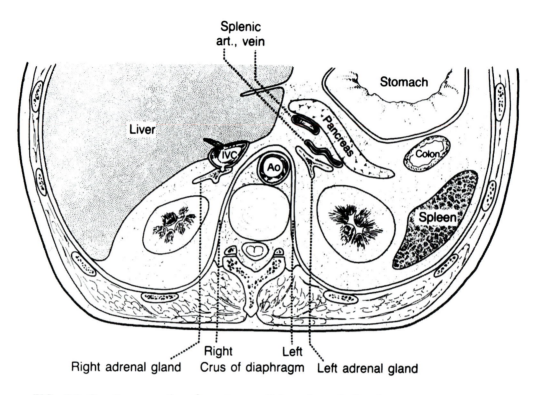

FIG. 11-3. Cross-sectional anatomy of the adrenal glands. (From Mitty HA, Yeh HC. *Radiology of the Adrenals with Sonography and CT.* Philadelphia: WB Saunders Co; 1982.)

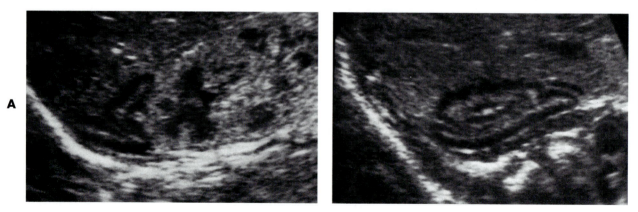

FIG. 11-4. Normal newborn adrenal gland. **A,** Sagittal and, **B,** transverse sonograms demonstrate the linear echogenic medulla with the surrounding hypoechoic cortex.

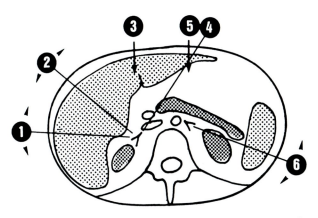

FIG. 11-5. Scan planes for sonographic visualization of the adrenal glands. *1, 2* = Lateral approach (right): 1 = midaxillary line; 2 = anterior axillary line. *3, 5* = Ventral approach (right and left): paramedian or midclavicular line. *4* = Ventral approach (right adrenal through the left liver lobe): longitudinal oblique scan. *6* = Lateral approach (left): posterior axillary line. (Modified from Günther RW, Kelbel C, Lenner V. Real-time ultrasound of normal adrenal glands and small tumors. *J Clin Ultrasound* 1984;12:211-217. Reprinted by permission of John Wiley & Sons, Inc.)

time sonography and identified adrenal glands in only 1 thin female. In newborn infants, real-time high-frequency scanning identified the right and left adrenal glands in 97% and 83% of patients, respectively.[10]

Scanning Techniques

Because of the complex shape of the adrenal gland, a comprehensive, systematic, multiplanar approach is necessary to fully evaluate it. The gland should be assessed in the transverse, coronal, and longitudinal plane as well as in the supine, oblique, and lateral decubitus positions.

Right Adrenal Gland. The right adrenal gland is best evaluated intercostally at the midaxillary or anterior axillary line.[7,11,13] The liver provides a good acoustic window. Alternatively, a subcostal oblique approach parallel to the rib cage at the midclavicular line can be used. Scanning from a direct anterior or posterior approach is typically poor because of overlying bowel gas or intervening muscle and fat interfaces (Fig. 11-5).

Left Adrenal Gland. The left adrenal gland is best evaluated intercostally at the posterior axillary or midaxillary line through the spleen or kidney.[7,13] As with the right adrenal gland, a direct posterior approach is usually not helpful. Sometimes, visualization of the left adrenal bed through the epigastrium is possible (Fig. 11-6). Occasionally, filling the stomach with fluid may help while using a direct ventral approach.

Pitfalls

When the scan plane is parallel to the anterior surface of the lateral wing, false enlargement may be ob-

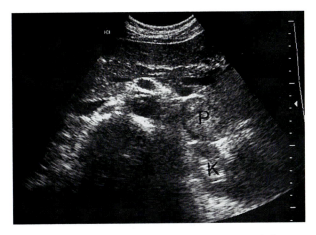

FIG. 11-6. Left adrenal gland enlarged due to tumor. Visualization of this pheochromocytoma, *P*, via a ventral epigastric approach. *K*, Kidney.

ADRENAL PSEUDOMASSES

Thickened diaphragmatic crus
Accessory spleen
Gastric fundus
Gastric diverticulum
Renal vein
Retrocrural and retroperitoneal adenopathy
Upper pole renal cysts and tumors
Pancreatic tumors
Hypertrophied caudate lobe of the liver
Fluid-filled colon interposed between stomach and kidney

---

served.[4] This could lead to erroneous diagnosis of hyperplasia or a small mass. If this occurs, changing the angle of the insonating sound beam by altering the intercostal space should allow differentiation between real and false enlargement.

Structures that may **simulate adrenal masses** include: a thickened diaphragmatic crus, an accessory spleen, the gastric fundus, a gastric diverticulum, the renal vein, retrocrural and retroperitoneal lymphadenopathy, upper pole renal cysts and tumors, pancreatic tumors, a hypertrophied caudate lobe of the liver, and interposition of a fluid-filled colon (see the box on this page).[7,13]

CONGENITAL ABNORMALITIES

Agenesis

Bilateral adrenal agenesis is extremely rare and incompatible with life. Unilateral adrenal agenesis does occur, with the contralateral gland demonstrating compensatory hypertrophy.[9]

Accessory Glands and Heterotopia

Accessory glands develop from "rests" of adrenal tissue. Typically they are found close to the parent gland; however, they have been described in many locations, including: the region of the celiac plexus, the kidney, along the course of the spermatic and ovarian veins, the testes, the ovary, the broad ligament, near the tail of the epididymis, the canal of Nuck, hernia sacs, hydrocele sacs, and the mesentery of the appendix.[14] Graham[15] described a 32% incidence of accessory adrenal tissue in 100 consecutive autopsies. The majority of accessory glands contain cortical tissue only. Heterotopia, on the other hand, consists of an adrenal gland containing both medullary and cortical tissue and has been described in many locations, including the brain and lung.[9]

Congenital Adrenal Hypoplasia

This condition is rare and the exact etiology unknown. If recognized early, treatment with replacement therapy may allow long survival.

Congenital Adrenal Hyperplasia

Congenital adrenal hyperplasia is an **autosomal recessive** disorder due to an inborn error of metabolism in the enzymatic production of cortisol or aldosterone. Males and females are affected equally.[14] Deficiency in a hormone results in overproduction of adrenocorticotropic hormone (ACTH) and/or renin/angiotensin. **Six distinct clinical syndromes** have been identified.

The specific clinical syndrome and its manifestations depend on which hormone has impaired synthesis as well as the biologic properties of the intermediate hormones that are overproduced.[16] The two most common syndromes include:

- **Virilizing form:** partial 21-hydroxylase deficiency; and
- **Salt-losing form:** more complete 21-hydroxylase deficiency.

These demonstrate the clinical manifestation of virilism and have thus been termed the **adrenogenital syndromes.**

Pathologically, all demonstrate **diffuse cortical hyperplasia** most markedly in the **zona reticularis.**[14] The glands may weigh up to 10 to 15 times their normal weight.[1]

Bryan et al.[17] found sonography helpful in the evaluation of infants born with ambiguous genitalia. Sonography was able to assess the size of the adrenal glands as well as confirm the presence of a uterus. They found in eight infants with proven metabolic abnormality that the adrenal glands were enlarged in three, at the upper limit of normal in three, and within

normal limits in two. Normal size was taken from the literature as 2 to 5 mm in thickness.[10] In nine infants with ambiguous genitalia due to other causes, adrenal gland enlargement was not noted. Bryan et al.[17] concluded that when enlarged adrenal glands are seen, the diagnosis of congenital adrenal hyperplasia is likely; however, the demonstration of normal adrenal glands does not exclude the diagnosis. Early diagnosis and treatment with appropriate hormones can allow normal sexual and physical development (Fig. 11-7).

Vanzulli et al.[18] performed scrotal ultrasound on 30 pubertal and postpubertal patients with adrenogenital syndrome to assess for the presence of testicular lesions. These lesions are known as **testicular tumors of adrenogenital syndrome.**[19] Their exact cell of origin is uncertain, but they occur as a result of elevated ACTH. Similar testicular lesions can be found in other disease states with elevated ACTH such as Addison's disease and Cushing's syndrome.[20] The testicular lesions are typically solid, multifocal (100%), bilateral (75%), hypoechoic (100%), and well defined (75%). They remain stable or decrease in size during hormonal therapy.[18]

INFECTIOUS DISEASES

Tuberculosis, histoplasmosis, blastomycosis, meningococcus, echinococcus, cytomegalovirus, herpes, and pneumocystis are the most frequent infectious organisms that affect the adrenal gland.[21-23]

Tuberculosis has a variable appearance, depending on the stage of infection. Acutely, there is bilateral diffuse enlargement, often inhomogeneous, due to caseous necrosis. Punctate calcification is a feature. Chronically, the glands become atrophic and cal-

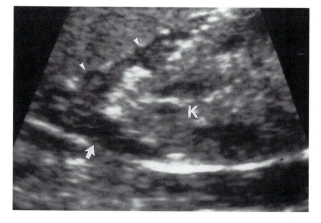

FIG. 11-7. Congenital adrenal hyperplasia.
Sagittal sonogram demonstrating nodularity *(arrowheads)* and thickening *(arrow)* of the adrenal gland. *K,* Kidney. (Courtesy of A. Daneman, M.D., Hospital for Sick Children, Canada.)

cified.[22,24] Tuberculosis and histoplasmosis are the two most common agents responsible for adrenal calcification in the adult population (Fig. 11-8).[24] Calcification in the absence of a soft tissue mass should suggest infection rather than neoplasm. When the adrenal glands are involved with tuberculosis, chest radiographs and sputum cultures may be negative. Prior to development of antituberculous therapy, tuberculosis was the most common cause of Addison's disease (adrenal insufficiency). Today, autoimmune disorders predominate as the most common cause of adrenal insufficiency.

In association with **acquired immunodeficiency syndrome (AIDS),** both infectious and neoplastic involvement of the adrenal gland are being found with increased frequency at autopsy. The most common offending organisms include fungi (histoplasmosis), mycobacteria, cytomegalovirus (CMV), herpes, pneumocystis, human immunodeficiency virus (HIV), and toxoplasmosis.[22,23] Grizzle et al.[23] described focal or diffuse damage of the glands by cytomegalovirus in 70% of patients who die with AIDS. Sonographically, these lesions are usually hypoechoic masses that may be heterogeneous and gas containing if abscess formation occurs.

Bacterial adrenal abscesses are found more commonly in the neonate and are relatively uncommon in adults.[25,26] In the neonate, hematogeneous seeding of normal glands or those affected by hemorrhage can result in abscess formation.[26]

As **organ transplantation** becomes more popular, patients receiving exogenous steroid for immunosuppression are also at increased risk for developing adrenal infection. Patients with **endogenous excess steroid production** also have an increased risk of developing adrenal infection.[23]

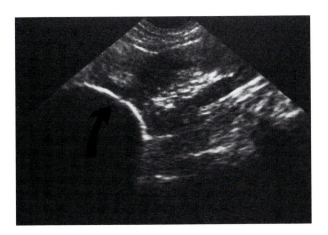

FIG. 11-8. Adrenal gland calcification. Sagittal sonogram shows calcification with distal acoustic shadowing of the adrenal gland *(arrow)*.

BENIGN ADRENAL NEOPLASMS

Adenoma

Adrenal adenomas can be regarded as either **hyperfunctioning** or **nonhyperfunctioning.** Adrenal adenomas are found in about 3% of adult autopsies and most are nonhyperfunctioning.[27] Ten percent of patients will have bilateral adrenal adenomas.[21] The incidence increases with advancing age.[28] Adenomas have been reported in patients with hypertension, diabetes, hyperthyroidism, renal cell carcinoma,[29] and hereditary adenomatosis of the colon and rectum.[30] Patients with hyperfunctioning adrenal adenomas will present with the manifestations of excess hormone secretion whereas nonhyperfunctioning adenomas are typically detected incidentally. Hyperfunctioning adrenal adenomas most commonly give rise to **Cushing's syndrome** or **Conn's disease.**

Cushing's Syndrome. Cushing's syndrome was described in 1932 by Harvey Cushing and consists of truncal obesity, hirsutism, amenorrhea, hypertension, weakness, and abdominal striae. This results from **excessive cortisol secretion,** which may occur with adrenal hyperplasia (70%), adenoma (20%), carcinoma (10%),[27] or from exogenous corticosteroid administration. **Cushing's disease,** on the other hand, is the result of hyperplastic adrenal glands excreting excessive cortisol due to elevated ACTH production from a pituitary adenoma. Biochemical profile with high plasma cortisol and urinary 17-hydroxycorticoid levels and low serum ACTH suggests an autonomous adrenal tumor (adenoma/carcinoma) as the source of excessive hormone.

Conn's Disease. Conn's disease results from **excessive secretion of aldosterone** and was first described in 1955.[31] Primary aldosteronism can result from adrenal adenoma (70%),[14] adrenal hyperplasia (30%),[14] and, rarely, adrenal carcinoma.[32] Clinically, hyperaldosteronism causes hypertension, muscular weakness, tetany, and ECG abnormalities. Patients with unexplained hypertension and hypokalemia should suggest excess secretion of aldosterone. Patients with hyperaldosteronism from an adenoma most typically are female[33] whereas those with hyperaldosteronism from hyperplasia more commonly are male.[34] These tumors tend to be small, usually less than 2 cm in size. Biochemically, elevated urine and serum aldosterone levels, hypokalemia, hypernatremia, and elevated bicarbonate and low plasma pH levels are found. A suppressed renin level indicates primary hyperaldosteronism.

Pathologically, it may be difficult to differentiate nodules of hyperplasia from adrenal adenomas. Nodules greater then 1 cm are likely to be adenomas.[1] As well, it may be impossible histologically to differentiate adenoma from carcinoma with biologic behavior as the only defining feature. Histologically, nonhyperfunctioning adenomas are composed of lipid-filled cells indicative of their secretory inactivity.[1]

Patients with a small adrenal mass and evidence of excess hormone production usually require resection, which is often done laparoscopically. Size criteria are often used to direct further management with nonhyperfunctioning adrenal masses. A size of 3 to 6 cm is usually considered for a nonfunctioning adrenal mass to be potentially malignant.[35,36]

Imaging of Adrenal Adenoma. The majority of adrenal masses are discovered as an incidental finding on CT examination or as an isolated finding during the staging work-up in a patient with a known primary tumor. The **intracytoplasmic lipid** of adrenal adenomas has directed interest in the use of unenhanced CT attenuation values and opposed phase chemical shift MRI to potentially allow their diagnosis.[37] Korobkin et al.[38] assessed the percentage of lipid-rich cortical cells histologically in 20 resected adrenal adenomas. They found an inverse linear relationship between the amount of lipid in adrenal adenomas and their unenhanced CT number. Many accumulated series have demonstrated that if an adrenal mass has unenhanced CT attenuation values of 10 HU or less, the overall sensitivity and specificity for the diagnosis of adrenal adenoma are 75% and 96%, respectively.[39] At 0 HU or less, the sensitivity and specificity are 47% and 100%, respectively.[39] It has also been shown that loss of signal in an adrenal mass on opposed phase chemical shift MRI is also related to the amount of intracytoplasmic lipid.[37,38,40] An optimal algorithm for characterizing an adrenal mass has not been firmly established; however, it appears that the use of unenhanced CT attenuation values or opposed phase chemical shift MRI allows characterization of an adrenal mass as benign without the need for other invasive procedures.[41]

On sonography, adrenal adenomas are solid, small, round, and well defined (Fig. 11-9). Sonography is often better than CT in determining organ of origin of a large mass, particularly in the right upper quadrant. Gore et al.[42] demonstrated that the right upper quadrant retroperitoneal fat reflection is displaced posteriorly by hepatic and subhepatic masses, whereas kidney and adrenal masses displace it anteriorly. This is best appreciated using a parasagittal plane (Fig. 11-10).

Myelolipoma

Adrenal myelolipomas are rare, benign, **nonhyperfunctioning** tumors composed of varying proportions of fat and bone marrow elements. The etiology and pathogenesis of these lesions are not known, though they are felt to arise in the **zona fasciculata** of the adrenal cortex.

Males and females are equally affected as are both glands. Tumors most commonly occur during the fifth or sixth decade of life.

Myelolipomas are typically discovered incidentally in asymptomatic individuals with a frequency at autopsy of 0.08% to 0.2%.[43] Although tumors can range in size from microscopic to 30 cm, most are less than 5 cm in diameter.[44] If these tumors undergo hemorrhage, necrosis, or compress surrounding structures, symptoms may occur.

Imaging features of myelolipoma depend on the varying proportion of **fat, myeloid element, hemorrhage,** and **calcification/ossification** present.

On sonography, these tumors are typically seen as an echogenic mass in the adrenal bed if a significant amount of fat is present. When small, they may be hard to differentiate from the adjacent echogenic retroperitoneal fat. **Propagation speed artifact** occurs as a result of decreased sound velocity through fatty masses. Originally described by Richman et al.[45] with an adrenal myelolipoma, apparent diaphragmatic disruption was noted as a result of this velocity change. The presence of this artifact is good evidence as to the fatty nature of a mass.[43,45] Musante et al.[43] found this artifact only when tumors were larger than 4 cm. The tumors may be homogeneous or heterogeneous and, if composed predominantly of myeloid component, will be isoechoic or hypoechoic. The heterogeneity may be due to internal hemorrhage, which is common. Focal areas of calcification may be seen.

CT is very sensitive for the diagnosis of adrenal myelolipomas and should be performed to confirm the presence of fat suspected sonographically. Musante et al.[43] found that unenhanced CT could explain confusing sonographic signs, including the demonstration of fat within sonographically isoechoic/hypoechoic myeloid predominant myelolipomas (Fig. 11-11).

The **differential diagnosis** of a suprarenal fatty mass includes myelolipoma, renal angiomyolipoma, lipoma, retroperitoneal liposarcoma, lymphangioma, increased fat deposition, and teratoma.[46] If the adrenal origin of a fatty mass can be ascertained with imaging (US, CT, or MRI), the most likely diagnosis is adrenal myelolipoma. When large or atypical, fine-needle aspiration may be necessary to establish the diagnosis. The presence of **mature fat cells** and **megakaryocytes** is characteristic for adrenal myelolipoma.[46-48]

Pheochromocytoma

Pheochromocytoma was first described by Frankel in 1886. Pheochromocytomas are usually **hyperfunctioning tumors** that secrete **norepinephrine** and **epinephrine** into the blood. It is the excess secretion of these catecholamines that gives rise to the clinical manifestations of hypertension, pounding or severe headache, palpitations often with tachycardia, and excessive inappropriate perspiration.[49] These symptoms are often episodic.

These tumors typically arise from the **neuroectodermal tissue** of the **adrenal medulla.** They are usually solitary but 10% are bilateral. Ectopic extraadrenal pheochromocytomas occur in 10% of patients and have been described in the organ of Zuckerkandl, the sympathetic nerve chains, the aortic and carotid chemoreceptors, the bladder, the prostate, and the chest. Multiple or extraadrenal pheochromocytomas are more common in children.[50] Ten to thirteen percent of intraadrenal pheochromocytomas and 40% of extraadrenal pheochromocytomas are malignant.[21] Metastatic disease is the only reliable indicator of malignancy. Pheochromocytomas are associated

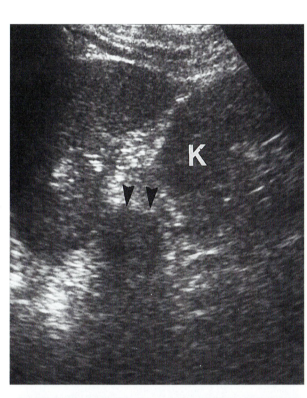

A

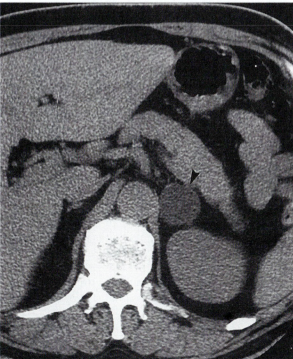

B

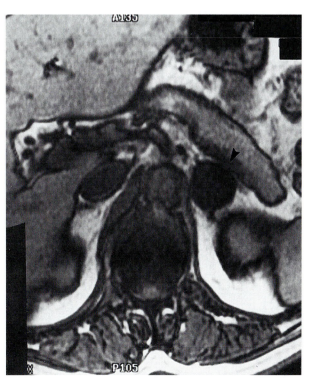

C

FIG. 11-9. **Adrenal adenoma.** A, Sagittal sonogram shows small, solid left adrenal mass *(arrowheads)* between the spleen and the upper pole of the left kidney, *K.* B, Confirmatory CT scan showing low attenuation (HU = 0) of the left adrenal adenoma *(arrowhead).* C, Opposed phase chemical shift gradient-echo imaging demonstrates signal loss in this lipid-rich mass *(arrowhead).*

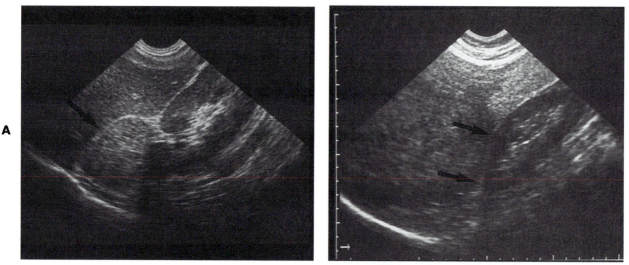

FIG. 11-10. Retroperitoneal fat stripe displacement. Parasagittal sonograms demonstrating, **A,** anterior displacement of the retroperitoneal fat stripe *(arrow)* by a right adrenal cortical cancer, and **B,** posterior displacement of the retroperitoneal fat stripe *(arrows)* by a large hepatic adenoma.

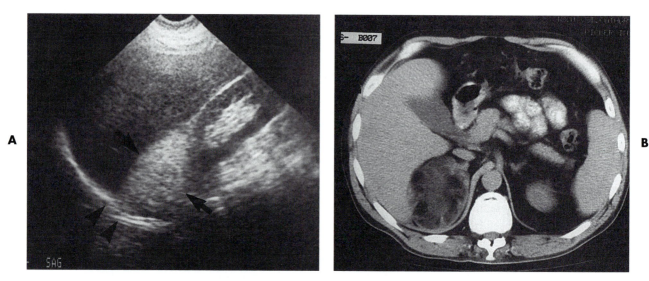

FIG. 11-11. Myelolipoma. A, Sagittal sonogram shows a large echogenic adrenal mass *(arrows)* with apparent diaphragmatic disruption *(arrowheads)* as a result of propagation speed artifact. **B,** Confirmatory CT demonstrates the presence of fat within the right adrenal mass.

with many **neuroectodermal disorders,** including tuberous sclerosis, neurofibromatosis, Hippel-Lindau disease, and multiple endocrine neoplasia (MEN) IIa (50%) and IIb (90%).[21] The autopsy incidence of pheochromocytomas is about 0.1%, and the frequency in hypertensive patients is 0.4% to 2%.[51] This rare tumor occurs most commonly in adults between the fourth and sixth decade of life and is a curable cause of hypertension.

Biochemical screening is essential to confirm the diagnosis of pheochromocytoma. This is accomplished by measuring the level of **urinary catecholamines** and its metabolites **vanillylmandelic acid (VMA)** and **total metanephrines.**

Pathologically, pheochromocytomas are well encapsulated, weigh 90 to 100 g, and measure 5 to 6 cm in diameter.[51] The right gland is affected twice as frequently as the left gland.[14] These tumors have a

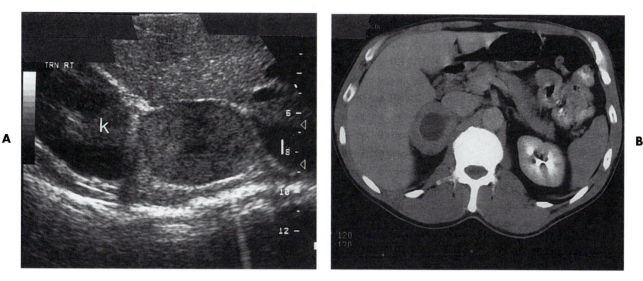

FIG. 11-12. Pheochromocytoma. **A,** Transverse sonogram shows a solid right adrenal mass situated between the kidney, *k,* and inferior vena cava, *I.* A central hypoechoic area corresponds to an area of necrosis. **B,** CT scan shows the large, partially necrotic tumor intimate to the posterior aspect of the inferior vena cava.

red to brown color on cut surface and microscopically demonstrate large pleomorphic cells with abundant cytoplasm and irregular nuclei. Calcification may be seen. Neurosecretory granules are seen ultrastructurally.[49]

Sonography has proved accurate in detecting adrenal pheochromocytomas, particularly since most are large and well marginated. Bowerman et al.[51] found in a series of eight surgically confirmed cases of pheochromocytoma that most were either heterogeneous or homogeneously solid. Those that were heterogeneous had areas of necrosis or hemorrhage. Two tumors were predominantly cystic, which corresponded to old blood and necrotic debris, and one of these demonstrated a fluid-fluid level (Fig. 11-12).

Extraadrenal pheochromocytoma thought to lie in the retroperitoneum may be more difficult to localize with sonography because of body habitus and overlying bowel gas. In these patients, CT or MRI may be extremely useful for localization. For patients with suspected recurrent or metastatic disease, iodine-131-MIBG scintigraphy can play a significant role in screening.[52]

Multiple Endocrine Neoplasia

Multiple endocrine neoplasia (MEN) is **familial** and is categorized into **three types:**
- **MEN I** affects pancreatic islets, the adrenal cortex, and pituitary and parathyroid gland;
- **MEN IIa (Sipple's syndrome)** shows medullary thyroid carcinoma, parathyroid hyperplasia, and pheochromocytoma; and

- **MEN IIb (III)** includes all features of IIa with marfanoid facies, mucosal neuromas, and gastrointestinal ganglioneuromatosis.

MEN II is inherited as an **autosomal dominant trait** and believed to be caused by a genetic defect in the neural crest.[53] **Pheochromocytomas** in **MEN syndromes** most typically are:
- in the adrenal gland;
- usually bilateral (65%)[54];
- multicentric within the gland;
- more often malignant; and
- frequently asymptomatic.

Patients diagnosed with MEN II should be screened biochemically and with imaging on a routine basis as they will eventually develop bilateral adrenal pheochromocytomas.

Rare Benign Adrenal Neoplasms

Ganglioneuromas are benign tumors occurring most frequently in adults.[55] They are composed of **ganglion** and **Schwann cells** and arise most frequently in the sympathetic chain with 30% arising in the adrenal gland.[55] They are slow growing and usually clinically silent unless pressure phenomenon occurs. Rarely, they increase urinary catecholamine levels with symptoms of diarrhea, hypertension, and sweating.[56] Sonographically, they are solid and homogeneous and, because of their soft consistency, are pliable and change shape rather than displace organs.[56] The diagnosis can only be made histologically.

Hemangiomas of the adrenal gland are rare, benign, **nonhyperfunctioning** tumors. Most are small

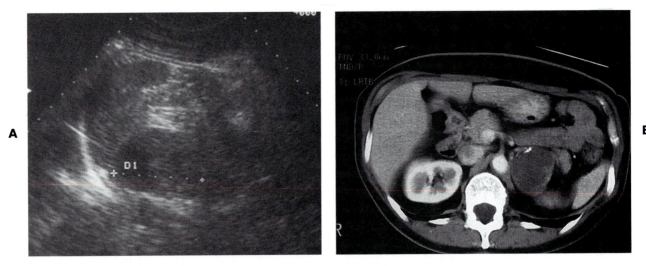

FIG. 11-13. Adrenal gland hemangioma. A, Sagittal sonogram shows calipers marking a nonspecific solid mass in the left adrenal gland. **B,** CT shows a nonspecific enhancing heterogeneous left adrenal mass with focal calcification.

and discovered incidentally at autopsy. They may grow large and range from 2 to 15 cm in diameter.[57] Histologically, these hemangiomas resemble hemangiomas elsewhere in the body and consist of **multiple dilated, endothelial-lined, blood-filled channels.**[58] Sonographically, they have a nonspecific structural pattern with cystic, solid, and complex appearances. Calcification in the form of phleboliths may be seen (Fig. 11-13).[59] MRI has been useful in the differentiation of liver hemangiomas and perhaps may play a role here if the diagnosis is suspected. With time and growth, these lesions often hemorrhage; therefore treatment is surgical.

Other rare adrenal gland tumors such as **teratomas, lipomas, fibromas, leiomyomas, osteomas,** and **neurofibromas** have been reported. Radiologic findings are nonspecific. Most typically the diagnosis is made histologically.

MALIGNANT ADRENAL NEOPLASMS

Adrenal Cortical Cancer

Primary adrenal cortical cancer is a rare malignancy and accounts for only 0.2% of all deaths from cancer.[60] It may arise from any of the layers in the adrenal cortex. Tumors may be **hyperfunctioning (54%)** or **nonhyperfunctioning (46%).**[60] Hyperfunctioning tumors are detected earlier because of their clinical manifestations of excess hormone production, which include:

- Cushing's syndrome (most common);
- adrenogenital syndrome (virilization or feminization);
- precocious puberty; and
- Conn's syndrome (rare).

Hyperfunctioning tumors occur more commonly in females while nonhyperfunctioning tumors are more common in males. Overall, adrenal cortical cancer occurs more commonly in females. These tumors occur most commonly in the fourth decade with equal frequency on both sides. Tumors range in size from small to very large at the time of presentation. On cut surface they are predominantly yellow with larger lesions exhibiting areas of hemorrhage and necrosis. Adrenal cortical cancer is a highly malignant tumor and has a tendency to invade the adrenal vein, inferior vena cava, and lymphatics[61] and to recur following surgery.

The **sonographic appearance** is variable, depending on the size of the mass. Hyperfunctioning tumors tend to be smaller when discovered and usually demonstrate a homogeneous echo pattern similar to renal cortex. The larger, nonhyperfunctioning lesions are more heterogeneous, with central areas of necrosis and hemorrhage. Nineteen percent will demonstrate calcification. All lesions tend to be well defined with a lobulated border (Fig. 11-14). Occasionally, a surrounding echogenic, capsulelike, thin rim is seen (27%).[60] Fishman et al.[62] have suggested that this may represent a well-vascularized portion of the adrenal cortical cancer and may be specific for this diagnosis.

Unfortunately, the sonographic appearance of adrenal masses does not allow differentiation between adenoma, carcinoma, pheochromocytoma, and metastases. Smaller lesions are more likely benign, and larger masses with hemorrhage, necrosis, and calcifi-

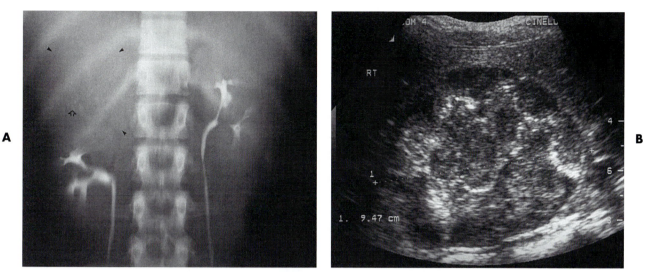

FIG. 11-14. Adrenal cortical cancer. A, Intravenous pyelogram shows a large right adrenal mass *(arrowheads)* with central dystrophic calcification *(open arrow)*. **B,** Sagittal sonogram shows a large heterogeneous solid mass with multiple linear echogenic foci corresponding to the calcification.

cation are more likely malignant. If a large, necrotic, calcified adrenal mass is noted as an isolated finding, in the absence of a known primary tumor, adrenal cortical cancer should be suspected. Sonography is an excellent screening method that allows rapid, noninvasive confirmation and localization of a lesion in patients suspected of having an adrenal tumor on clinical grounds. Duplex and color Doppler may be helpful to interrogate the veins for venous tumor extension. Ultrasound can be used to assess for metastatic spread as well as guided fine-needle aspiration. Fine-needle aspiration can be difficult when trying to differentiate adenoma from well-differentiated carcinoma.

Lymphoma

Primary lymphoma of the adrenal gland is rare but may occur. It may arise from heterotrophic lymphoid elements that are occasionally found in normal adrenal glands.[63] More commonly, however, adrenal gland involvement is due to **contiguous spread** from bulky retroperitoneal disease. **Non-Hodgkin disease** is the most common cell type with 4% of patients exhibiting discrete adrenal masses, often bilateral (46%).[64,65] At autopsy, adrenal involvement will be seen in 24%.[64] Following therapy, isolated adrenal gland recurrence may be seen. Necrosis and calcification within adrenal gland lymphoma are rare without prior treatment.[64]

On sonography, intranodal and extranodal lymphoma most typically appears as a discrete or conglomerate hypoechoic mass. This is likely related to the internal monotonous cell population within the tumor. Masses may be so hypoechoic as to simulate

cysts; however, lack of appropriate through-transmission will indicate their solid nature (Fig. 11-15).

Kaposi's Sarcoma

The adrenal glands of patients with **acquired immunodeficiency syndrome (AIDS)** demonstrate an increased incidence of both **opportunistic infection** (CMV, histoplasmosis, candida, cryptococcus, herpes, pneumocystis, mycobacterium avium intracellulare, HIV, and toxoplasmosis)[22,23,66,67] and **neoplasm** (Kaposi's sarcoma and lymphoma). If 90% or more of adrenal tissue is damaged by infection or tumor, frank adrenal insufficiency occurs.[68] This is often a late manifestation in AIDS patients.[66,67]

Sonographically, Kaposi's sarcoma of the adrenal gland is not well documented in the literature. A nonspecific solid mass with or without necrosis may be seen in the adrenal bed. Biopsy is necessary for confirmation (Fig. 11-16).

Metastases

The adrenal gland is the **fourth** most frequent site of metastatic disease after lung, liver, and bone. The most common **primary tumors** giving rise to adrenal metastases include lung, breast, melanoma, kidney, thyroid, and colon cancer. Most are clinically silent. The discovery of an adrenal mass in a patient with a known primary malignancy is equally likely to be an adenoma or metastasis.

Adrenal metastases may be unilateral or bilateral and are variable in size, ranging from microscopic deposits to enormous masses. Central necrosis and hemorrhage may occur. Calcification in metastases is rare.[41]

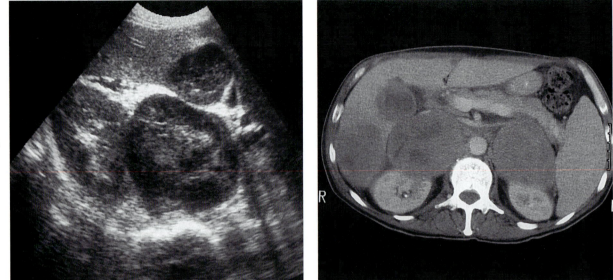

FIG. 11-15. Adrenal lymphoma. A, Transverse sonogram shows a large, solid right adrenal mass as well as a large, solid hepatic mass in this AIDS patient. **B,** CT shows bilateral solid adrenal masses, hepatic masses, and splenomegaly.

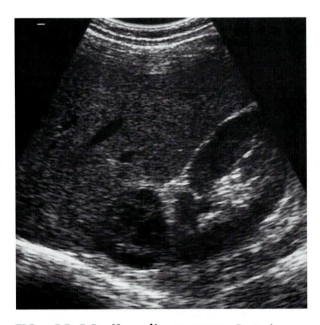

FIG. 11-16. Kaposi's sarcoma. Sagittal sonogram shows a heterogeneous, predominantly solid right adrenal mass.

The use of unenhanced CT attenuation values and opposed phase chemical shift MRI has shown promise in the ability to differentiate adrenal adenomas from metastatic lesions.[37-41,69] Unenhanced CT attenuation values of 20 or greater and lack of signal loss on opposed phase chemical shift imaging indicate a non-lipid-rich mass, favoring a metastasis. Percutaneous biopsy is necessary to confirm or exclude metastases.

Sonographically, the masses are solid and may demonstrate inhomogeneity due to necrosis or hemorrhage (Figs. 11-17 and 11-18). Percutaneous needle biopsy may be performed with either ultrasound or CT guidance.

ADRENAL CYSTS

Adrenal cysts are rare benign lesions and are discovered most frequently as an incidental finding at autopsy with a frequency of 0.06%.[70] They are found with equal frequency on both sides and are typically unilateral. They may be bilateral in up to 15%.[71] They may occur at any age but most commonly are found in the third through fifth decade. There is a 3:1 female preponderance.[72]

Most adrenal cysts are asymptomatic but with growth may cause symptoms related to displacement or compression of adjacent structures. These include abdominal pain or discomfort, nausea, vomiting, and back pain.

Adrenal cysts are classified into **four types** based on origin[58,73-75]:

1. **Endothelial (45%):** angiomatous, lymphangiectatic, and hamartomatous;
2. **Pseudocysts (39%):** secondary to hemorrhage into a normal adrenal gland or tumor;
3. **Epithelial (9%);** and
4. **Parasitic (7%):** most commonly echinococcal infection.

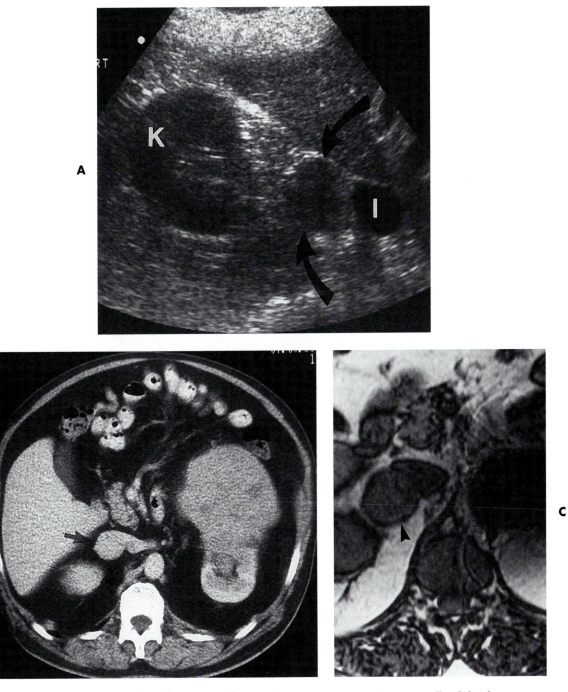

FIG. 11-17. Adrenal metastasis. A, Transverse sonogram shows a small, solid right adrenal mass between the inferior vena cava and kidney *(arrows)*. *K*, Kidney; *I*, inferior vena cava. B, CT scan shows a solid right adrenal mass *(arrow)* and a large left renal cell carcinoma. C, Opposed phase chemical shift gradient-echo imaging demonstrates a lack of signal loss in this nonlipid-rich mass *(arrowhead)*. Artifact in the left renal bed is from clips following left nephrectomy.

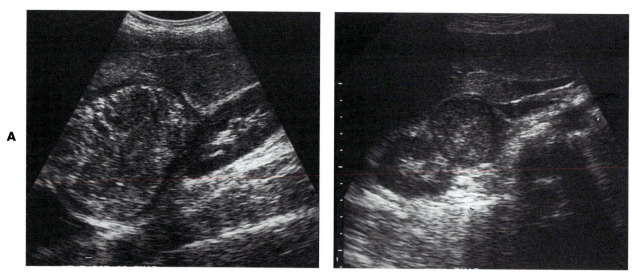

FIG. 11-18. Adrenal metastases. A, Sagittal sonogram shows a large, solid right adrenal mass. **B,** Transverse sonogram shows the adrenal mass between the kidney and inferior vena cava.

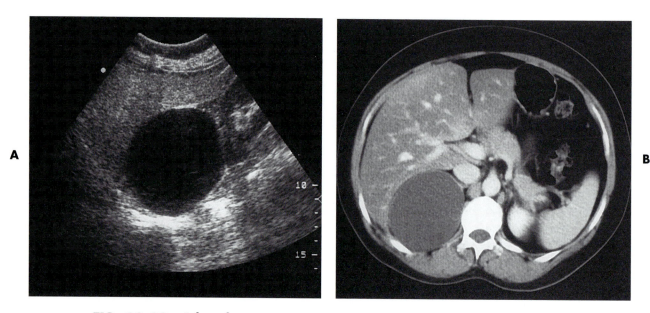

FIG. 11-19. Adrenal cyst. A, Sagittal sonogram shows a large, well-defined anechoic cyst with through transmission. **B,** CT shows a low attenuation lesion in the right adrenal gland.

Sonographically, these cysts have the same characteristics as cysts elsewhere in the body. They are usually round or oval with a thin smooth wall. Good through-transmission is present, but often internal debris is noted. Fifteen percent will display peripheral curvilinear wall calcification usually in the pseudocysts and parasitic adrenal cysts (Fig. 11-19).

Percutaneous cyst aspiration showing **adrenal steroids** or **cholesterol** may be helpful to determine an adrenal origin if imaging techniques fail to do so.[72]

Adrenal cysts are benign and can be followed with serial imaging. If large and symptomatic, percuta-

neous aspiration with or without sclerosis or surgery may be necessary.

ADRENAL HEMORRHAGE

Spontaneous Hemorrhage

Spontaneous adrenal hemorrhage in the adult population is uncommon. It is usually associated with **severe stress,** including septicemia, burns, trauma, and hypotension. It may also occur in patients with **hematologic abnormalities,** including thrombocy-

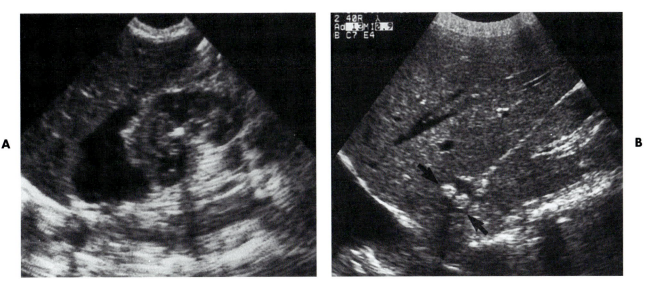

FIG. 11-20. Spontaneous adrenal hemorrhage. A, Sagittal sonogram in a neonate shows enlargement of the entire adrenal gland with internal fluid-containing septations. **B,** Sagittal sonogram in an adult shows two echogenic masses representing clotted blood in an enlarged right adrenal gland *(arrows).*

topenia and disseminated intravascular coagulation (DIC) (Fig. 11-20). Patients on **anticoagulation therapy** are also susceptible to adrenal hemorrhage, which usually occurs within the first 3 weeks following initiation of therapy.[58] It has also been recently recognized that ligation and division of the right adrenal vein during **orthotopic liver transplantation** may cause venous congestion and hemorrhagic infarction or hematoma formation in the right adrenal gland.[76] The resulting congested gland may rupture, causing excessive hemorrhage requiring reoperation.

Posttraumatic Hemorrhage

Posttraumatic adrenal hemorrhage may be present in up to 25% of severely injured patients.[77] Most patients will have ipsilateral thoracic, abdominal, or retroperitoneal injury.[78] The right adrenal gland is affected more often than the left. **Three mechanisms** have been proposed to explain traumatic adrenal hemorrhage:

- Direct compression of the gland with rupture of sinusoids and venules;
- Inferior vena cava (IVC) compression elevating right adrenal venous pressure as its vein drains directly into the IVC; and
- Deceleration forces causing shearing of small vessels perforating the adrenal capsule.[77,78]

Most typically, the **sonographic appearance** of acute adrenal hemorrhage is a bright echogenic mass in the adrenal bed, which becomes smaller and anechoic with time. Occasionally, an adrenal hemorrhage will initially appear as an anechoic mass becoming more echogenic with time. This likely is due to the fact that the initial hemorrhage consists of unclotted blood (Fig. 11-20). With resolution of an adrenal hematoma, focal areas of calcification may develop. Most traumatic adrenal hematomas (83%) have a round or oval appearance and occur predominantly in the **medulla.**[78] The central hemorrhage may stretch or disrupt the cortex, resulting in periadrenal hemorrhage (Fig. 11-21).

Unilateral adrenal hemorrhage has little clinical significance; however, patients with bilateral hemorrhage are at increased risk for development of acute adrenal insufficiency. It is crucial to exclude hemorrhage into a preexisting underlying neoplasm and therefore serial follow-up studies are necessary to document resolution of the adrenal hemorrhage. Most hematomas will resolve with time, requiring no intervention.

DISORDERS OF METABOLISM

Hemochromatosis

Hemochromatosis may be **primary (idiopathic)** or **secondary** following repeated blood transfusions. Patients with **idiopathic hemochromatosis** have a defect in their intestinal mucosa, which allows increased iron absorption and subsequent excess deposition in liver, pancreas, heart, spleen, kidneys, lymph nodes, endocrine glands, and skin. Clinically they present with cirrhosis, diabetes mellitus, and hyperpigmentation.[79] Patients with **secondary hemochromatosis** have increased iron deposition in the

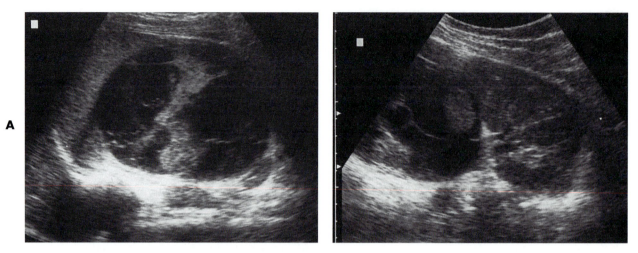

FIG. 11-21. Adrenal hemorrhage following trauma. A, Sagittal sonogram shows a large, complex left adrenal mass. **B,** Sagittal sonogram shows the large mass displaces the kidney inferior and anterior.

reticuloendothelial cells of the spleen, liver, and bone marrow. Organ dysfunction does not usually occur.[79]

Excessive iron deposition in the adrenal glands often leads to mild adrenocortical insufficiency, but Addison's disease is rare.[80] The adrenal glands are usually small and may show increased attenuation on CT scan.

Wolman's Disease

Wolman's disease is a rare **autosomal recessive lipid storage disease** due to deficiency of liposomal acid lipase. Most patients die within 6 months of birth. The disease is characterized by marked hepatosplenomegaly and massive adrenal gland enlargement. The adrenal glands demonstrate diffuse punctate calcification.

ULTRASOUND-GUIDED ADRENAL INTERVENTION

Biopsy

Welch et al.[81] reviewed their experience of adrenal biopsy over a 10-year time period, which included 277 percutaneous biopsies in 270 patients. Sensitivity was 81%, specificity 99%, and accuracy 90%. Positive predictive value was 99%, and negative predictive value was 80%. Complication rate was 2.8%. Potential complications of percutaneous adrenal biopsy depend on the approach and include hematoma (0.05% to 2.5%),[82] pneumothorax (most common),[82] pancreatitis (6%),[83] sepsis, and needle tract seeding. Needle biopsy of a pheochromocytoma may precipitate a hypertensive crisis and should be avoided.[84]

Most commonly, biopsies of the adrenal glands are performed with CT guidance. However, if the lesion is visible and readily accessible, ultrasound may be used to guide the procedure. Often a transhepatic approach is chosen on the right to avoid the pleural space (Fig. 11-22). On the left a posterior, lateral, or anterior approach is chosen, depending on the lesion size and available safe access. A posterior approach is preferable to an anterior approach on the left in an attempt to avoid development of acute pancreatitis.

Drainage

Percutaneous drainage of an adrenal abscess or drainage and sclerosis of an adrenal cyst is possible provided safe access for catheter placement exists. Choice of catheter size depends on the viscosity of the material to be drained. Because of the deep location of the adrenal gland, these procedures are most frequently performed with CT guidance.

INTRAOPERATIVE ULTRASOUND

Intraoperative ultrasound with a 7.5 MHz transducer may be helpful when partial adrenalectomy is being performed. The exposed adrenal gland is scanned to allow precise localization of the pathology, which therefore allows the surgeon to obtain clear resection margins.

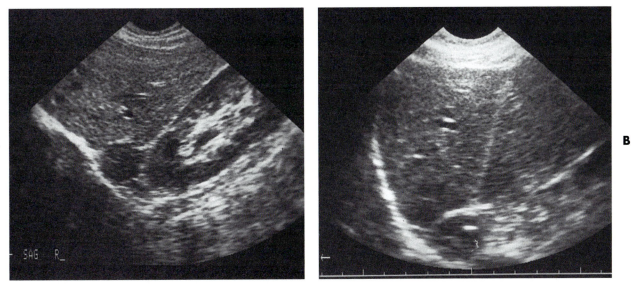

FIG. 11-22. Adrenal biopsy. A, Sagittal sonogram shows a small adrenal metastasis in a patient with lung cancer. **B,** Sonographic guidance for transhepatic placement of a needle (echogenic line) into the adrenal mass for percutaneous biopsy.

REFERENCES

1. The endocrine system. In: Cotran RS, Kumar V, Robbins SL, eds. *Pathologic Basis of Disease.* 5th ed. Philadelphia: WB Saunders Co; 1994:1149-1165.

Embryology

2. The suprarenal glands (adrenal glands). In: Netter FH. *The CIBA Collection of Medical Illustrations. Vol 4: Endocrine System and Selected Metabolic Diseases.* Summit, NJ: CIBA Pharmaceutical; 1981:77-108.
3. The urogenital system. In: Moore KL, eds. *The Developing Human: Clinically Oriented Embryology.* 5th ed. Philadelphia: WB Saunders Co; 1993:265-303.

Normal Anatomy, Morphology, and Physiology

4. Yeh HC. Sonography of the adrenal glands: normal glands and small masses. *AJR* 1980;135:1167-1177.
5. Yeh HC, Mitty HA, Rose JR et al. Ultrasonography of adrenal masses—usual features. *Radiology* 1978;127:467.
6. Brownlie K, Kreel L. Computer assisted tomography of normal suprarenal glands. *J Comput Assist Tomogr* 1978;2:1-20.
7. Yeh H. Ultrasonography of the adrenals. *Semin Roentgenol* 1988;23:250-258.
8. Yeh H. Adrenal and retroperitoneal sonography. In: Leopold GR, ed. *Ultrasound in Breast and Endocrine Disorders.* New York: Churchill Livingstone; 1984.
9. Mitty HA. Adrenal embryology, anatomy, and imaging techniques. In: Pollack HM, ed. *Clinical Urography: An Atlas and Textbook of Urologic Imaging.* Philadelphia: WB Saunders Co; 1990:2291-2305.
10. Oppenheimer DA, Carroll BA, Yousem S. Sonography of the normal neonatal adrenal gland. *Radiology* 1983;146:157-160.
11. Marchal G, Gelin J, Verbeken E et al. High resolution real-time sonography of the adrenal glands: a routine examination. *J Ultrasound Med* 1986;5:65-68.
12. Lurie SN, Neelon FA. Physiology of the adrenal gland. In: Pollack HM, ed. *Clinical Urography: An Atlas and Textbook of Urologic Imaging.* Philadelphia: WB Saunders Co; 1990:2306-2312.
13. Günther RW, Kelbel C, Lenner V. Real-time ultrasound of normal adrenal glands and small tumors. *J Clin Ultrasound* 1984;12:211-217.

Congenital Abnormalities

14. Rosai J. Adrenal gland and other paraganglia. In: Rosai J, ed. *Ackerman's Surgical Pathology.* 8th ed. St Louis: Mosby-Year Book; 1996:1015-1058.
15. Graham LS. Celiac accessory adrenal glands. *Cancer* 1953;6:149-152.
16. White PC, New M, Dupont B. Congenital adrenal hyperplasia. *N Engl J Med* 1987;316:1519-1524, 1580-1586.
17. Bryan PJ, Caldamone AA, Morrison SC et al. Ultrasound findings in the adreno-genital syndrome (congenital adrenal hyperplasia). *J Ultrasound Med* 1988;7:675-679.
18. Vanzulli A, DelMaschio A, Paesano P et al. Testicular masses in association with adrenogenital syndrome: US findings. *Radiology* 1992;183:425-429.
19. Rutgers LJ, Young RH, Scully RE. The testicular "tumor" of the adrenogenital syndrome. *Am J Surg Pathol* 1988;12:503-513.
20. Seidenwurm D, Smathers RL, Kan P et al. Intratesticular adrenal rests diagnosed by ultrasound. *Radiology* 1985;155:479-481.

Infectious Diseases

21. Shumam WP, Moss AA. The adrenal glands. In: Moss AA, Gamsu G, Genant HK, eds. *Computed Tomography of the Body with Magnetic Resonance Imaging.* Philadelphia: WB Saunders Co; 1992:1021-1057.
22. Rezneck RH, Armstrong P. The adrenal gland. *Clin Endocrinol* 1994;40:561-576.
23. Grizzle WE. Pathology of the adrenal gland. *Semin Roentgenol* 1988;23:323-331.
24. Dunnick NR. The adrenal gland. In: Taveras JM, Ferrucci T, eds. *Radiology.* Philadelphia: JB Lippincott Co; 1990:4.
25. O'Brien WM, Coyke PL, Copeland PL et al. Computed tomography of adrenal abscesses. *J Comput Assist Tomograph* 1987;11:550-551.

26. Atkinson GO, Kodroff MB, Gay BB et al. Adrenal abscess in the neonate. *Radiology* 1985;155:101-104.

Benign Adrenal Neoplasms

27. Dunnick NR. Adrenal imaging: current status. *AJR* 1990; 154:927-936.

28. Commons RR, Callaway CP. Adenomas of the adrenal cortex. *Arch Intern Med* 1948;81:37-41.

29. Ambos MA, Bosniak MA, Lefleur RS et al. Adrenal adenoma associated with renal cell cancer. *AJR* 1981;136:81-84.

30. Painter TA, Jagelman DG. Adrenal adenomas in association with hereditary adenomatosis of the colon and rectum. *Cancer* 1985;55:2001-2004.

31. Conn JW. Primary aldosteronism. *J Lab Clin Med* 1955; 45:661.

32. Slee PH, Schaberg A, van Brummelen P. Carcinoma of the adrenal cortex causing primary aldosteronism. *Cancer* 1983;51:2341-2345.

33. Conn JW, Knopf RF, Nesbit RM. Clinical characteristics of primary aldosteronism from an analysis of 145 cases. *Am J Surg* 1964;107:159-172.

34. Grant CS, Carpenter P, van Heerden JA et al. Primary aldosteronism. *Arch Surg* 1984;119:585-589.

35. Hubbard MM, Husami TW, Abumrad NN. Non-functioning adrenal tumors: dilemmas in management. *Am J Surg* 1989;5:516-522.

36. Bitter DA, Ross DS. Incidentally discovered adrenal masses. *Am J Surg* 1989;158:159-161.

37. McNicholas MMJ, Lee MJ, Mayo-Smith WW et al. An imaging algorithm for the differential diagnosis of adrenal adenomas and metastases. *AJR* 1995;165:1453-1459.

38. Korobkin M, Giordano TJ, Brodeur FJ et al. Adrenal adenomas: relationship between histologic lipid and CT and MR findings. *Radiology* 1996;200:743-747.

39. Korobkin M, Brodeur FJ, Yutzy GG et al. Differentiation of adrenal adenomas from nonadenomas using CT attenuation values. *AJR* 1996;166:531-536.

40. Outwater EK, Siegelman ES, Huang AB et al. Adrenal masses: correlation between CT attenuation value and chemical shift ratio at MR imaging with in-phase and opposed phase sequences. *Radiology* 1996;200:749-752.

41. Dunnick NR, Korobkin M, Frances I. Adrenal radiology: distinguishing benign from malignant adrenal masses. *AJR* 1996;167:861-867.

42. Gore RM, Callen PW, Filly RA. Displaced retroperitoneal fat: sonographic guide to right upper quadrant mass localization. *Radiology* 1982;142:701-705.

43. Musante F, Derchi LE, Zappasodi F et al. Myelolipoma of the adrenal gland: sonographic and CT features. *AJR* 1988; 151:961-964.

44. Nobel MJ, Montague DK, Levin HS. Myelolipoma: an unusual surgical lesion of the adrenal gland. *Cancer* 1982;49:952-958.

45. Richman TS, Taylor KJW, Kremkau FW. Propagation speed artifact in a fatty tumor (myelolipoma): significance for tissue differential diagnosis. *J Ultrasound Med* 1983;2:45-47.

46. Vick CW, Zeman RK, Mannes E et al. Adrenal myelolipoma: CT and ultrasound findings. *Urol Radiol* 1984;6:7-13.

47. de Blois GG, DeMay RM. Adrenal myelolipoma diagnosis by computed-tomography-guided fine-needle aspiration. *Cancer* 1985;55:848-850.

48. Galli L, Gaboardi F. Adrenal myelolipoma: report of diagnosis by fine needle aspiration. *J Urol* 1986;136:655-657.

49. Korobkin M. Pheochromocytoma. In: Pollack HM, ed. *Clinical Urography: An Atlas and Textbook of Urologic Imaging*. Philadelphia: WB Saunders Co; 1990:2347-2361.

50. Manger W, Gifford R Jr. Pheochromocytoma: diagnosis and management. *NY State J Med* 1980;80:216.

51. Bowerman RA, Silver TM, Jaffe MH et al. Sonography of adrenal pheochromocytomas. *AJR* 1981;137:1227-1231.

52. Quint LE, Glazer GM, Francis IR et al. Pheochromocytoma and paraganglioma: comparison of MR imaging with CT and I-131 MIBG scintigraphy. *Radiology* 1987;165:89-93.

53. Cho KJ, Freier DT, McCormick TL et al. Adrenal medullary disease in multiple endocrine neoplasia type II. *AJR* 1980; 134:23-29.

54. Brunt LM, Wells SA Jr. The multiple endocrine neoplasia syndromes. *Invest Radiol* 1985;20:916-927.

55. Silverman ML, Lee AK. Anatomy and pathology of the adrenal glands. *Urol Clin North Am* 1989;16(3):417-432.

56. Bosniak M. Neoplasms of the adrenal medulla. In: Pollack HM, ed. *Clinical Urography: An Atlas and Textbook of Urologic Imaging*. Philadelphia: WB Saunders Co; 1990:2344-2346.

57. Vergas AD. Adrenal hemangioma. *Urology* 1980;16:389-390.

58. Rumanick WM, Bosniak MA. Miscellaneous conditions of the adrenals and adrenal pseudotumors. In: Pollack HM, ed. *Clinical Urography: An Atlas and Textbook of Urologic Imaging*. Philadelphia: WB Saunders Co; 1990:2399-2412.

59. Derchi L, Rapaccini GL, Banderali A et al. Ultrasound and CT findings in two cases of hemangioma of the adrenal gland. *J Comput Assist Tomogr* 1989;13(4):659-661.

Malignant Adrenal Neoplasms

60. Hamper UM, Fishman EK, Harman DS et al. Primary adrenocortical carcinoma: sonographic evaluation with clinical and pathologic correlation in 26 patients. *AJR* 1987;148:915-919.

61. Ritchey ML, Kinard R, Novicki DE. Adrenal tumors: involvement of the inferior vena cava. *J Urol* 1987;138:1134-1136.

62. Fishman EK, Deutch BM, Hartman DS et al. Primary adrenal cortical carcinoma: CT evaluation with clinical correlation. *AJR* 1987;148:531-535.

63. Glazer HS, Lee JKT, Balfe DM et al. Non-Hodgkin lymphoma: computed tomographic demonstration of unusual extranodal involvement. *Radiology* 1983;149:211-217.

64. Vicks BS, Perusek M, Johnson J et al. Primary adrenal lymphoma: CT and sonographic appearances. *J Clin Ultrasound* 1987;15:135-139.

65. Feldberg MAM, Hendriks MJ, Klinkhamer AC. Massive bilateral non-Hodgkin's lymphoma of the adrenals. *Urol Radiol* 1986;8:85-88.

66. Freda PU, Wardlaw SL, Brudney K et al. Clinical case seminar: Primary adrenal insufficiency in patients with the acquired immunodeficiency syndrome: a report of five cases. *J Clin Endocrinol Metab* 1994;79(6):1540-1545.

67. Donovan DS, Dluhy RG. AIDS and its effect on the adrenal gland. *Endocrinologist* 1991;1(4):227-232.

68. Findling JW, Buggy BP, Gilson IH et al. Longitudinal evaluation of adrenocortical function in patients infected with the human immunodeficiency virus. *J Clin Endocrinol Metab* 1994;79(4):1091-1096.

69. Schwartz LH, Panicek DM, Koutcher JA et al. Adrenal masses in patients with malignancy: prospective comparison of echoplanar, fast spin-echo and chemical shift MR imaging. *Radiology* 1995;197:421-425.

Adrenal Cysts

70. Wahl HR. Adrenal cysts. *Am J Pathol* 1951;27:758.

71. Scheible W, Coel M, Siemers PT et al. Percutaneous aspiration of adrenal cysts. *AJR* 1977;128:1013-1016.

72. Tung TA, Pfister RC, Papanicolaou N et al. Adrenal cysts: imaging and percutaneous aspiration. *Radiology* 1989;173: 107-110.

73. Kearney GP, Mahoney EM. Adrenal cysts. *Urol Clin North Am* 1977;4:273-283.

74. Abeshouse GA, Goldstein RB, Abeshouse BS. Adrenal cysts: review of the literature and report of three cases. *J Urol* 1959;81:711.

75. Barron SH, Emanual B. Adrenal cysts: case report and review of pediatric literature. *J Pediatr* 1961;59:592.

Adrenal Hemorrhage

76. Bowen A, Keslar P, Newman B et al. Adrenal hemorrhage after liver transplantation. *Radiology* 1990;176:85-88.

77. Murphy BJ, Casillas J, Yrizarry JM. Traumatic adrenal hemorrhage: radiologic findings. *Radiology* 1988;169:701-703.

78. Burks DW, Mirvis SE, Shanmuganathan K. Acute adrenal injury after blunt abdominal trauma: CT findings. *AJR* 1992;158:503-507.

Disorders of Metabolism

79. Baron RL, Freeny PC, Moss AA. The liver. In: Moss AA, Gamsu G, Genant HK, eds. *CT of the Body with Magnetic Resonance Imaging.* Philadelphia: WB Saunders Co; 1992:735-821.

80. Doppman JL. Adrenal cortical hypofunction. In: Pollack HM, ed. *Clinical Urography: An Atlas and Textbook of Urologic Imaging.* Philadelphia: WB Saunders Co; 1990:2338-2343.

Ultrasound-Guided Adrenal Intervention

81. Welch TJ, Sheedy PF II, Stephens DH et al. Percutaneous adrenal biopsy: review of a 10-year experience. *Radiology* 1994;193:341-344.

82. Zornoza J. Fine-needle biopsy of lymph nodes, adrenal glands and periureteral tissues. In: Pollach HM, ed. *Clinical Urography: An Atlas and Textbook of Urologic Imaging.* Philadelphia: WB Saunders Co; 1990:2854-2860.

83. Kane NM, Korobkin M, Francis IR et al. Percutaneous biopsy of left adrenal masses: prevalence of pancreatitis after anterior approach. *AJR* 1991;157:777-780.

84. Casola G, Nicolet V, van Sonnenberg E et al. Unsuspected pheochromocytoma: risk of blood-pressure alterations during percutaneous adrenal biopsy. *Radiology* 1986;159:733-735.

CHAPTER 12

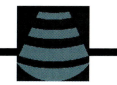

The Retroperitoneum and Great Vessels

•

Dónal B. Downey, M.B., B.Ch., F.R.C.P.C.

The **retroperitoneum,** which contains the **great vessels,** is a large, posterior abdominal area[1-3] that is clinically challenging because symptoms of retroperitoneal disease are usually nonspecific; physical examination is difficult; it reacts less severely and less acutely to insults than do most other anatomical re-gions; and many retroperitoneal masses, fluid collections, and inflammatory and vascular disorders are large at the time of diagnosis.[2]

Ultrasound is extremely useful in evaluating the retroperitoneum. It can be used to diagnose and characterize many lesions and can guide diagnostic and therapeutic interventions.[4-6] It is highly accurate in assessing great-vessel aneurysms.[7]

Several anatomic and physiologic factors combine to make sonography of the retroperitoneum and the great vessels challenging. Sonographic images are frequently degraded by bowel gas, thick muscles, fat, and sometimes by the lungs and uterus.[8] The area is large[2] and deep and cannot be seen in its entirety from any one perspective. The thin renal fascia, which divides the area into compartments (Fig. 12-1 through Fig. 12-3), is often not seen directly so its location must be deduced. Some disease processes destroy the retroperitoneal fascial planes (e.g., pancreatic pseudo-cysts[9,10]). Also, the fascia may be severely attenuated and displaced by large masses or fluid collections.[11]

These difficulties can usually be overcome by optimizing patient factors, choosing the best ultrasound machine and set-up, and selecting the optimum scanning technique.

SCANNING TECHNIQUE

When possible, patients should be scanned following an overnight fast. Giving patients water or oral ultra-

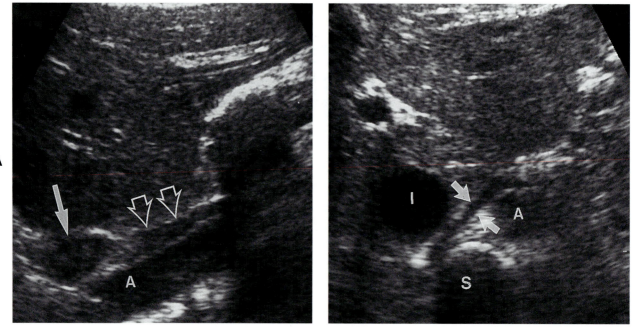

FIG. 12-1. Normal right diaphragmatic crus. A, Midline longitudinal scan showing the gastroesophageal junction *(closed arrow)*, the upper abdominal aorta (A), and the crus of the right diaphragm *(open arrows)*. **B,** Transverse upper abdominal scan shows the crus of the right diaphragm *(arrows)* between the aorta (A) and the inferior vena cava (I). S, spine.

sound contrast material[12] may enhance visibility of the pancreas and other retroperitoneal structures.

The ultrasound machine that gives the best visibility of deep structures should be used—if the examiner has a choice of machines. One scanning technique that helps to insure that the entire retroperitoneum is scanned involves dividing the area into subsegments based on easily identifiable **sonographic landmarks.** These include the **kidneys,** the **aorta,** the **iliac arteries,** the **superior mesenteric artery** (SMA), the **inferior vena cava** (IVC), the **crura,** the **psoas muscles,** and the **common femoral vessels** at the inguinal ligament. The landmark organ or blood vessel is completely evaluated in at least two different planes, preferably orthogonal to each other.

Next, the fibrous and fatty tissue in the neighboring anatomical spaces and structures adjacent to that organ in the retroperitoneum are scanned. If one gets lost, orientation may be regained by returning to the sonographic landmark. One must adopt a very flexible approach to patient movement, transducer position, and respiration, as visibility is extremely variable.

A firm, slow, **graded compression technique** similar to that used for the diagnosis of appendicitis[13] often allows improved retroperitoneal visibility because it moves bowel loops out of the way. In the upper abdomen, the area between the rectus adominis muscles usually provides a good acoustic window when the patient is supine (Fig. 12-1). A coronal perspective

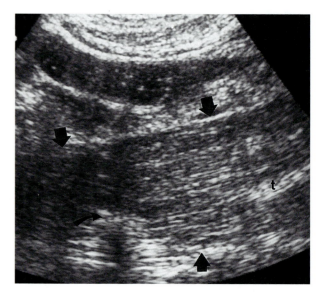

FIG. 12-2. Left flank coronal sonogram shows the psoas muscle *(arrows)*, the vertebral transverse process *(curved arrow)*, and the psoas tendon (t) which is an echogenic structure in the caudal third of the muscle.

through the flank, with the patient in a supine or decubitus position, is often most useful in the middle and lower retroperitoneum (Fig. 12-2). A good acoustic window is also found in many patients along the lateral aspect of the rectus abdominis muscle.

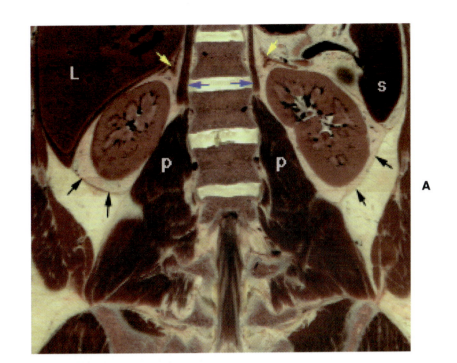

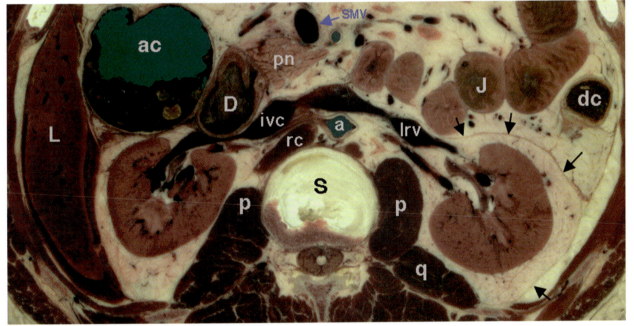

FIG. 12-3. Normal retroperitoneal anatomy. A, Coronal slice through the "visible human"* at the level of the kidneys. **B,** Transaxial slice through the visible human at the level of the renal vein. Arrows, Gerota's fascia and lateral conal fascia. Blue arrows, crura of diaphragm. Yellow arrow, adrenal glands. L, liver. s, spleen. p, psoas. ivc, inferior vena cava. a, aorta. lrv, left renal vein. smv, superior mesenteric vein. dc, descending colon. ac, ascending colon. J, jejunum. q, quadratus lumborum. pn, pancreas. rc, right crus of diaphragm. S, spine. D, duodenum. (Courtesy of Dr. Victor Spitzer, *Visible Human Project, University of Colorado School of Medicine.)

RETROPERITONEUM

Anatomy of the Retroperitoneum

The retroperitoneum is a posterior abdominal segment that lies between the transversalis fascia and the parietal peritoneum (Fig. 12-3) and contains a vari-able amount of fibrous and fatty tissue. It is limited cranially by the diaphragm and caudally by the pelvic brim.[1-3]

Two layers of renal fascia divide the retroperi-toneum coronally into **three separate compart-ments**[3] (Fig. 12-3). The **anterior pararenal space** lies between the posterior parietal peritoneum and the anterior perirenal fascia (Gerota's facia or Toldt's facia)[3,14] (Fig. 12-3). It contains the ascending and descending colon, the second, third, and fourth parts of the duodenum, the pancreas, the inferior vena cava, the aorta, the proximal superior mesenteric artery and vein, and the hepatic and splenic vessels.[1,3]

The **posterior pararenal space** lies between the posterior perirenal fascia (Zuckerkandl's fascia)[3,14] and the fascia covering the quadratus lumborum and the psoas muscle.[8] It contains no solid organs.[3] The posterior pararenal space communicates with the properitoneal space anterolaterally, and caudally it communicates with the posterior pelvis. It may also communicate with the anterior pararenal space near the pelvic brim.[1,3]

The **perirenal space** lies between the two layers of perirenal fascia and contains the kidney, adrenal gland, and proximal ureter. Its superior end is open; caudally, it is cone-shaped and filled with fat. Its caudal tip communicates with the pelvic extraperitoneal space. Laterally, the two renal fascial layers fuse to form the lateral conal fascia.[2]

The **retrofascial space** contains the **psoas** and **quadratus lumborum** muscles (Figs. 12-3 and 12-4) which are frequently included in descriptions of the retroperitoneum.[8] They lie posterior to the retroperitoneum and are covered by their own fascia. The quadratus lumborum is roughly quadrilateral in shape, being wider cranially than caudally.[15] It arises from the medial part of the twelfth rib and attaches to the vertebral transverse process before fusing into the iliac crest and the iliolumbar ligament. The psoas muscle is frequently made up of two conjoined muscles, the dominant psoas major and the smaller psoas minor, which is present in 60% of people. They take origin from the lumbar vertebrae and transverse process and insert into the lesser trochanter of the femur.[16] Near the inguinal ligament they receive fibers from the iliacus muscle.[16]

The **diaphragmatic crura** are the linear muscular portions of the diaphragm that border the aortic hiatus and attach to the lateral aspect of the lumbar vertebrae[17] (Fig. 12-1). The right crus is bigger, longer, and more lobular. It attaches to the anterior bodies and intervertebral discs from L1 to L3. The left crus attaches to L1 and L2 and that intervertebral disc.[2,17] The right crus lies posterior to the inferior vena cava, right renal artery, right adrenal, and liver (Figs. 12-1 and 12-3, *A*).[17]

Sonographic Appearance of the Retroperitoneum

The kidneys, inferior vena cava, pancreas, duodenum, aorta, and hepatic and splenic vessels are readily identified on ultrasound (Figs. 12-1, 12-2, and 12-4) and occasionally, the perirenal fascial planes may be directly identified (Fig. 12-4).

The **diaphragmatic crura** are useful anatomical landmarks, but they may be mistaken for pathology, especially if they are thickened.[18] On transverse scanning, the right crus is identified in about 90% of cases, the left in about 50%. They are usually hypoechoic and surrounded by echogenic tissue[18] (Fig. 12-1). On longitudinal scanning, the right crus is seen in about 50% of cases. The **quadratus lumborum** (Figs. 12-3 and 12-4) is usually hypoechoic relative to the adjacent fat and can mimic fluid collections, especially in obese patients.[19] Scanning the opposite side is often helpful, as the muscles are usually symmetrical. The **psoas muscles** are usually easy to see by scanning coronally through the flanks and angling the upper portion of the transducer posteriorly to follow the plane of the muscle[20] (Fig. 12-2). The caudal part of the psoas is usually easy to see in a transverse plane, while its upper portions are often obscured by gas.[20] The muscles are hypoechoic with vertically oriented echogenic lines in them; caudally, they have an echogenic central tendon (Fig. 12-2).

The **mesentery** extends anteriorly from the retroperitoneum and contains the **splanchnic blood vessels** and the attached small bowel.[2] The leaves of this mesentery are shown as echogenic lines (Fig. 12-5).

Retroperitoneal Pathology

The most common manifestation of retroperitoneal pathology is the presence of a mass[21] (Figs. 12-6 and

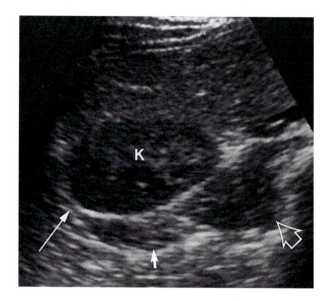

FIG. 12-4. Normal posterior pararenal space. Transverse sonogram through the right kidney (K) shows the quadratus lumborum muscle *(closed arrow)*, the psoas muscle *(open arrow)*, and the posterior renal fascia *(narrow arrow)*.

12-7). Other sonographic signs of disease include the displacement of normal structures to an abnormal location (Fig. 12-8), direct invasion of adjacent organs (Fig. 12-7), asymmetry of normal structures (Fig. 12-8), silhouetting of normal structures by disease (Fig. 12-9), and loss of retroperitoneal detail (Fig. 12-7).[8]

On finding a mass the examiner should:
- assess it in two dimensions and insure it is real;
- trace its entire circumference and measure it;
- assess for the presence of air or calcium;
- determine its relationship to other organs, blood vessels, and structures and seek its origin;
- assess whether it is fixed or free;
- determine its internal echogenicity and blood flow; and
- discover whether it is cystic, solid, or vascular.

Solid Masses. These are usually classified into lymphadenopathy, primary malignancies, secondary malignancies, infections, and other lesions that masquerade as solid masses on sonography.

Lymphadenopathy. The aim of ultrasound is to detect enlarged retroperitoneal lymph nodes, characterize them, and measure them accurately.[22] Although ultrasound is superior to computed tomography (CT) in some thin patients for detecting retroperitoneal adenopathy, CT is usually the imaging procedure of choice because it provides a standard and repeatable view of the retroperitoneum that is not degraded by bowel gas. Retroperitoneal node-size measurement is more easily repeatable on CT, and enlarged intraperitoneal nodes, which are present in 50% of non-Hodgkin's lymphoma patients at presentation,[22,23] are easier to appreciate on CT.

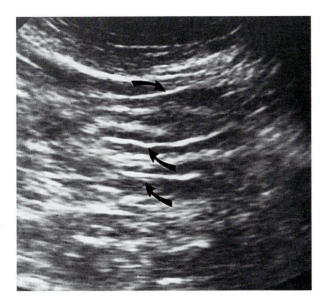

FIG. 12-5. Normal mesenteric folds. Transverse midline, midabdominal scan showing the echogenic lines of the normal folds of the mesentery *(arrows)*.

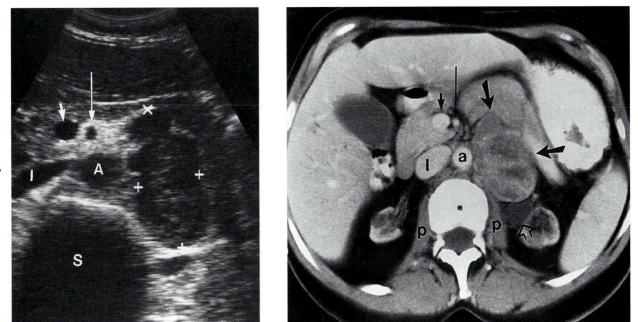

A   B

FIG. 12-6. Metastatic sarcomatoid renal cell carcinoma originating in a left lower quadrant transplant kidney with spread cephalad in the retroperitoneum. Transverse ultrasound **A,** and contrast enhanced computed tomography scan **B,** showing a large left retroperitoneal, anterior pararenal space, lobulated mass *(big arrows* or +) displacing the stomach, pancreas, and bowel anteriorly. It displaces the aorta (a) slightly to the right. The native kidneys are small and the left one is hydronephrotic *(open arrow).* Long thin arrow, superior mesenteric artery. I, inferior vena cava. a, aorta. p, psoas. Short arrow, SMV.

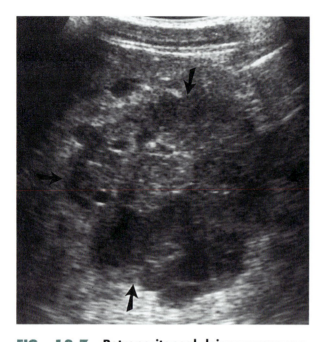

FIG. 12-7. Retroperitoneal leiomyosarcoma.
Longitudinal sonogram of the left retroperitoneum shows an extensive complex tumor *(arrows)* that is more solid anteriorly and cystic posteriorly.

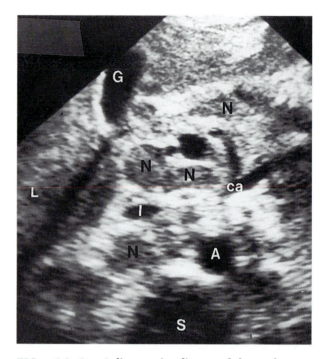

FIG. 12-8. Celiac axis distorted by adenopathy. AIDS patient with multiple upper abdominal nodes distorting the normal configuration the celiac axis. Transverse scan just below celiac axis. N, nodes. I, IVC. A, aorta. ca, celiac artery. L, liver. G, gallbladder. S, spine.

CRITERIA FOR ASSESSING NODAL DISEASE

Abdomen	< 1.0 cm	= normal
	> 1.0 cm, single	= suspicious
	> 1.5 cm, single	= abnormal
	>1.0 cm, multiple	= abnormal
Retrocrural	> 0.6 cm	= abnormal
Pelvic	> 1.5 cm	= abnormal

In the abdomen, the most useful criterion for assessing nodal disease is **node size.**

Lesions that occur in normal-sized nodes will be missed using these criteria; approximately 10% of lymphoma patients are found to have disease in normal-sized nodes.[8] At sonography, **malignant nodes** are usually round or oval and have a longitudinal/transverse ratio of < 2. Eccentric cortical widening and a narrow or absent echogenic hilus also suggest malignancy.[24] Malignancy is suggested on color Doppler when avascular intranodal regions are shown and intranodal vessels are displaced or distorted.[25]

While needle biopsy of nodal disease will rarely give the pathologist all the information required to make a full histologic diagnosis in patients with lymphoma, ultrasound-guided biopsy is useful for distin-guishing lymphoma from other diseases, for assessing the response to treatment of known disease, and for diagnosing some infections.[4,5,26] A variety of different approaches can be used (Fig. 12-10). In general, it is best to choose the shortest, least obstructed path to the lesion in order to facilitate good sonographic visibility, and to use a standard technique.[27]

Retroperitoneal adenopathy is most commonly seen in **lymphoma**; para-aortic adenopathy is present in 25% of patients newly diagnosed with Hodgkin's disease and in 50% of patients with non-Hodgkin's lymphoma.[23,28] Ultrasound is between 80% and 90% accurate in detecting retroperitoneal nodal lymphoma and it can also detect extranodal disease.[22,29] Its **sonographic appearance** is variable. Most commonly, discrete hypoechoic masses or anechoic masses are seen both anterior and posterior to the great vessels (Figs. 12-8 and 12-10).[29] These nodes have poor sound transmission and, unlike cysts, they do not have increased through-transmission.[22] Sometimes the nodes fuse to form a hypoechoic mantle of tissue that surrounds the aorta and that may elevate it from the spine (Fig. 12-9). **Extranodal lymphoma** is also typically hypoechoic and may spread directly from the nodes to the solid organs or may arise de novo in the retroperitoneal space and retrofascial muscles. The sonographic morphology has not been found to correlate with any particular histologic pattern.[30] If the

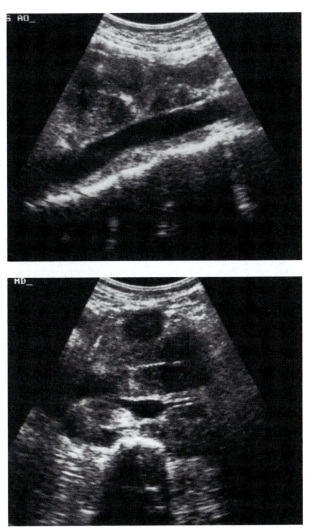

A

B

FIG. 12-9. Para-aortic lymph nodes. Multiple hypoechoic masses surround aorta and aortic branches. Aorta is displaced slightly anteriorly from spine by retroaortic nodes. **A,** sagittal and, **B,** transverse scans.(Courtesy of Stephanie R. Wilson, M.D., University of Toronto.)

Ultrasound Guided Retroperitoneal Biopsy

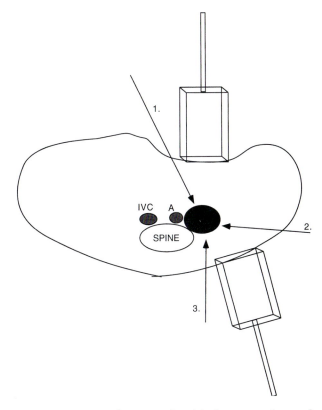

FIG. 12-10. Ultrasound-guided retroperitoneal biopsies. Line diagram showing different approaches: 1. Transducer and needle approach mass from the front. It is necessary to apply firm pressure to displace bowel out of the way with this approach. 2. and 3. Transducer is placed posteriorly and needle is inserted posteriorly or laterally.

mass silhouettes the aortic border as opposed to coming close to it (Fig. 12-11), it is reasonable to assume that the nodes are truly retroperitoneal, and radiation ports may be adjusted accordingly.[22]

Retroperitoneal metastases occur either by lymphatic or hematogenous spread or by direct extension from other solid organs or the adjacent peritoneal cavity. They may stay confined within the node or spread beyond its confines. Metastatic deposits from testicular tumors and pelvic tumors are most common, though lung, melanoma, and gastrointestinal metastases also occur.

Sonographic appearances of nonlymphomatous malignant nodal disease are variable, although such nodes are less likely to be as intensely hypoechoic as those with lymphoma, and they are often more echogenic and

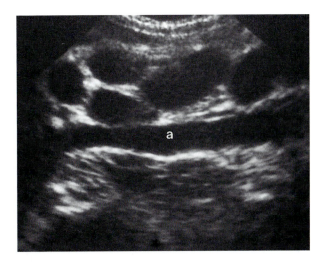

FIG. 12-11. Non-Hodgkin's lymphoma. Longitudinal scan showing multiple very hypoechoic, discrete, enlarged para-aortic nodes and mesenteric nodes. No posterior echo enhancement is seen. a, aorta.

PRIMARY RETROPERITONEAL NEOPLASMS

Mesenchymal	**Neurogenic**
Lipoma/liposarcoma	Neurilemmoma,
Leiomyoma/	neurofibroma
leiomyosarcoma	Malignant schwannoma
Hemangiopericytoma/	Neuroblastoma
angiosarcoma	ganglioneuroblastoma
Fibroma/fibrosarcoma	Ganglioneuroma
Rhabdomyoma/	Paraganglioma/
rhabdomyosarcoma	pheochromocytoma
Malignant fibrous	
histiocytoma	**Embryonic rest**
Mesothelioma	Teratoma
Chondrosarcoma	Seminoma
Osteosarcoma	Yolk sac tumor
Hemangioma	Wilm's tumor

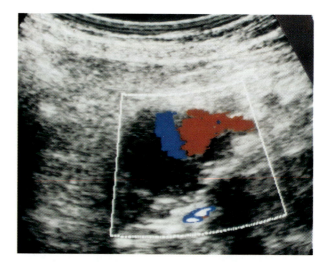

FIG. 12-12. Gastroduodenal artery pseudo-aneurysm, post-acute pancreatitis. Color Doppler image shows the aneurysm arising from the gastroduodenal artery just at its origin from the hepatic artery seen on the right.

heterogeneous.[8] Ultrasound is less accurate in assessing metastatic nodal disease than in assessing lymphoma; a 31% sensitivity and an 87% specificity were reported in patients with testicular tumors.[31]

Infection can also cause lymphadenopathy, as can **AIDS** (Fig. 12-8) and AIDS-related lymphoma. Sonographic appearances are, again, nonspecific.

One of the more important, though rare, tumors that occurs in the retroperitoneum is the **germ cell tumor.**[32,33] Most of them are secondary lesions. When a retroperitoneal primary germ cell tumor is thought to have been found, it is essential to check the scrotum carefully.[32,33] The lesions can be benign or malignant; they are generally heterogeneous. **Teratomas** may be suspected in the pediatric population if a fat-fluid level or a large area of calcification is seen.[34]

Primary retroperitoneal tumors. Primary retroperitoneal tumors are rare neoplasms that arise and develop in the retroperitoneal space but are not attached to the adjacent retroperitoneal organs.[11] Most are of mesenchymal origin (see box above) and between 70% and 90% of those that occur in adults are malignant. Three times as many men as women are affected, and the 5-year survival varies between 22% and 50%.[35,36] **Liposarcoma, leiomyosarcoma, and malignant fibrous histiocytoma** are the most common (Fig. 12-7).[1,35,36] Fixation of the tumor and invasion of adjacent structures are the worst prognostic features. Complete surgical excision offers the best hope of cure, though this is often technically very difficult.[11,35,36]

Ultrasound rarely produces a specific diagnosis, as there is considerable overlap in the sonographic ap-

pearances of retroperitoneal tumors, with most lesions being large and heterogeneous and many containing cysts (Fig. 12-7). Increased echogenicity within the retroperitoneal masses may be related to fat, calcification,[34] increased vascularity,[37] or hemorrhage.[38,39] Tumors of **muscle origin** are more likely to be hypoechoic, while isoechoic masses may represent lipomas in which the fat is indistinguishable from adjacent retroperitoneal fat.

While CT will often give a better overview of a retroperitoneal lesion, ultrasound may give a better appreciation of whether the lesion is fixed or has invaded adjacent structures, both important features for prognosis and surgical planning.[35,36] Ultrasound also allows rapid and accurate biopsy of retroperitoneal masses (Fig. 12-10). It is prudent to evaluate with Doppler all retroperitoneal masses prior to biopsy to avoid biopsying or draining an aneurysm (Fig. 12-12).[40]

Retroperitoneal fibrosis. Retroperitoneal fibrosis (**Ormond's disease**) is idiopathic in 68% of cases. In 8% it is associated with **malignancy** (infiltrating secondary neoplasia of the stomach, lung, breast, colon, prostate, and kidney) and in 12% it is associated with methisergide use. Less frequent associations include Crohn's disease, Reidel's struma, sclerosing cholangitis, radiation therapy, aneurysm surgery or leakage, retroperitoneal infection, and urine leakage.[41-44]

When the process occurs around the aorta it is called an **inflammatory aneurysm** and its exact cause is unknown (Fig. 12-13).[45,46] Pathologic changes seen in both conditions include clumps of fibrous tissue with

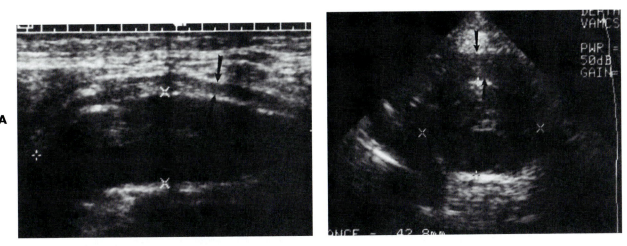

A

B

FIG. 12-13. Inflammatory abdominal aortic aneurysm. A, Longitudinal and, B, transverse scans show aneurysm with thin layer *(arrows)* of fibrous tissue, anterior and adjacent to aortic wall.

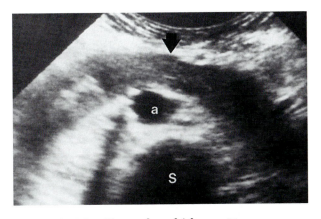

FIG. 12-14. Horseshoe kidney. Transverse scan shows the isthmus *(arrow)* of a horseshoe kidney lying over the distal aorta (a); spine (s).

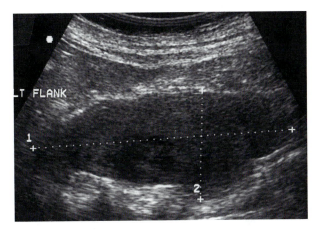

FIG. 12-15. Postangiogram hematoma. Linear isoechoic mass on L psoas. Longitudinal scan in a patient 3 hours following an angiographic procedure. The extensive retroperitoneal hematoma *(cursors)* is of medium echogenicity.

associated inflammatory infiltrate on the anterior aspect of the aorta, IVC, and psoas muscles.[43,44] It is an important diagnosis to make as, unrecognized, it can lead to renal failure or can be mistaken for more serious pathology. It usually responds well to medical therapy.

Sonographically, the appearances are nonspecific. The fibrous clumps are mostly hypoechoic, smoothly marginated, and homogeneous masses that often appear as plaque around the distal aorta. In cases where the clumps of fibrosis are not obvious, the characteristic medial deviation of the ureters may suggest the diagnosis. Whereas CT is the diagnostic modality of choice,[44] ultrasound can be used to follow the response of the ureters and the masses to steroid and other interventions.

Other masses and pseudomasses. Benign masses such as **horseshoe kidneys** (Fig. 12-14), **ptotic kidneys, bowel duplication cysts**, and a **low-lying pancreas** should be considered as possible explanations for a retroperitoneal mass.[8] Perhaps the most frequent problem with sonography occurs when a loop of aperistaltic bowel mimics a true mass. The distinction can usually be made by changing the patient's position during the exam and watching the area while the patient drinks. **Acute retroperitoneal hemorrhage,** a potentially lethal condition,[47] may be quite echogenic and may appear to be a focal mass[38] (Fig. 12-15). **Varices** can also mimic solid lesions[48] as can **extramedullary hematopoiesis.**

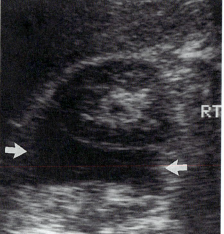

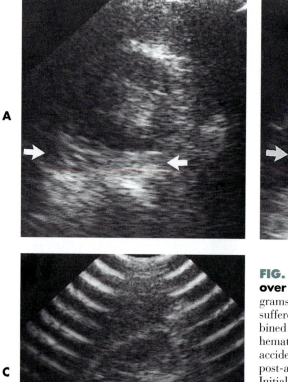

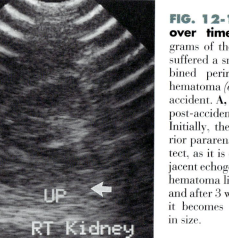

FIG. 12-16. Retroperitoneal bleed over time. Sequential transverse sonograms of the right kidney in a patient who suffered a small renal laceration and a combined perirenal and posterior pararenal hematoma *(arrows)* following a motor vehicle accident. **A,** 2 days post-accident; **B,** 12 days post-accident; **C,** 22 days post-accident. Initially, the combined perirenal and posterior pararenal hematoma is very hard to detect, as it is echogenic and similar to the adjacent echogenicity of the perirenal fat. As the hematoma liquefies, **B,** it is easily detectable, and after 3 weeks, **C,** with increasing fibrosis, it becomes more echogenic and decreases in size.

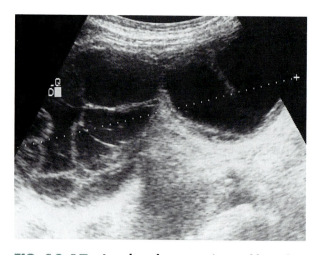

FIG. 12-17. Loculated retroperitoneal lymphocele occurring just above a transplant kidney in the left lower quadrant. The wall is thick and there are septations of various sizes.

Fluid Collections. These are commonly found in the retroperitoneum. They include hematomas[49] (Figs. 12-15 and 12-16), lymphoceles[50-52] (Fig. 12-17), abscesses, urinomas, cystic tumors,[34] germ cell tumors,[33] primary retroperitoneal cysts,[53] exophytic renal cysts, lymphangiomas,[54-56] cystic hamartomas,[57] venous varices,[48,58] and dilated renal collecting systems. Many of these pathologies are similar on sonography, and localization of the fluid to a given compartment is helpful in diagnosing both their nature and their origin.

Primary cysts and lymphangiomas. Primary retroperitoneal cysts are frequently large and usually have the sonographic appearance of simple cysts.[53] **Lymphangiomas** are congital malformations of the lymphatic system and are seen as elongated unilocular or multilocular[56,59] cysts with thick septations; 44% contain some debris. The diagnosis is important, as incompletely removed lesions can give rise to severe chylous ascites or local recurrence.[59]

Lymphoceles. Lymphoceles (Fig. 12-17) are common following surgical procedures. They have been reported in between 10% and 27% of patients following staging lymphadenectomy[50] and are frequently found adjacent to transplanted kidneys.[50,51] Most are small, develop within 10 to 21 days after surgery, and resolve spontaneously. Treatment of larger lesions includes surgery, percutaneous drainage, and the injection of sclerosing agents.[52]

Most lymphoceles are anechoic and resemble simple cysts (Fig. 12-10).[50,51] Between 20% and 50% present as complex masses with septations that are usually not of clinical significance (Fig. 12-17). Most lymphoceles occur lateral to the bladder and within 3 cm of the abdominal wall, but they can occur anywhere in the abdomen and pelvis.[50,51] Their differentiation from abscess, hematoma, or urinoma is often difficult, especially if debris is present. Localized tenderness and increasing size should make one suspicious of infection.[51]

Urinomas. In many medical centers, urinomas most often arise following iatrogenic intervention, although they also occur following high-grade ureteric obstruction and trauma.[60] Persisting urinomas may induce fibrosis or become infected. They usually resolve following drainage of the collecting system with or without ureteric stenting.[60] Classically, they present as hypoechoic retroperitoneal collections often conforming to the shape of the compartment in which they are located.

Varices may appear quite cystic on B-mode exam or quite echoic. Doppler usually confirms the diagnosis, but it is important to the use the correct frequency transducer and to set up the machine appropriately to show slow flow.

Pancreatic pseudocysts. Pseudocysts are well-demarcated pockets of fluid that develop around the pancreas following pancreatitis. The anterior pararenal space is most frequently involved,[61] although the other retroperitoneal spaces may be involved too, especially if pancreatic fluid dissolves the fascia.[9,10] Diagnostic aspiration is often very helpful in differentiating them from other clear fluid collections and may help in the treatment.

Retroperitoneal hemorrhage. Retroperitoneal hemorrhage occurs through a defect in the patient's coagulation process,[49] spontaneous vascular rupture,[62] traumatic vascular rupture, or medical intervention,[47,63,64] or it occurs secondary to tumor bleeding or vessel invasion. It has also been reported following lithotripsy.[65] Common sites of bleeding include the psoas muscle and the perinephric space (Figs. 12-15 and 12-16). Psoas hematoma may be very difficult to diagnose, especially in early stages.

Acute retroperitoneal hemorrhage may be catastrophic,[47] but often it is confined by the fascial layers, which may tamponade the process and obviate the need for surgery. In the acute situation it is essential that the patient be stable before any imaging is undertaken. CT is preferable to ultrasound, as it is both more sensitive and more specific in identifying the presence and extent of disease.[66]

The **sonographic appearances of retroperitoneal hemorrhage** are variable (Figs. 12-15 and 12-16). Solid or cystic masses are the most common sonographic findings. Cystic lesions vary from being entirely sonolucent, like a urinoma, to being markedly echogenic and indistinguishable from adjacent fat in the acute or chronic state (Fig. 12-16, *A* and *C*). Cellular debris may layer dependently in a hematoma, making its differentiation from an abscess difficult. The character of blood clots changes over time. Some work suggests that the age of the clot can be crudely estimated based on its echogenicity,[38,67] as dense fibrin clots, which occur later in disease processes, are more echogenic than are loose fibrin clots,[67] which are more common at the start of the coagulation process.[38]

Retroperitoneal Infections. These infections may be primary or may be caused by spread from an adjacent organ, such as the kidney, bowel, or spine. A preexisting fluid collection such as a **pancreatic pseudocyst** may also be secondarily infected. Paraspinal infections may arise with disc or vertebral body infection. Diverticulitis and Crohn's disease are the major antecedent bowel conditions that spread inflammatory processes into the retroperitoneum. Predisposing factors include **diabetes mellitus, ureteral obstruction, AIDS, trauma,** or **surgery,** and **alcohol** and **drug abuse.**

Percutaneous drainage is an important diagnostic test and is also the treatment of choice in most cases of retroperitoneal infection. In many cases it may be the only treatment required.

The **appearances on ultrasound** are rarely specific, so distinguishing abscesses from other collections or masses is challenging. Air within an abscess may be difficult to discern on sonography, and where suspected, a plain film or a CT scan of the abdomen should be performed. Also, distinguishing aperistaltic bowel loops, dilated ureters, thrombosed aneurysms (Fig. 12-12), and vessels from abscesses is often challenging, as these conditions may produce **pseudocollections.**

Xanthogranulomatous pyelonephritis. Xanthogranulomatous pyelonephritis is an unusual chronic renal infection that results in enlargement of the kidney, destruction of the normal parenchyma, and severe infiltration of the kidney by lipid-laden macrophages.[68,69] Stones are present in over 80% of cases, and obstruction is common. It usually involves a whole kidney and there is an intense surrounding fibrotic reaction. The perirenal and pararenal spaces are usually involved; the kidney often contains a staghorn calculus. The enlarged kidney is usually clearly seen on ultrasound, as are adjacent abscesses, when present. The calculi are often not as obvious as one might expect, because the perirenal fibrosis attenuates the ultrasound beam. Ill-defined hypoechoic areas may be seen in the collecting systems.[68]

GREAT VESSELS

Aorta

The abdominal aorta is a compliant tube[70] that supplies blood to the digestive organs, the kidneys, the adrenals, the gonads, the abdominal and paraspinal musculature, and the pelvis and lower limbs.[71] It contributes significantly to the continuous forward flow of blood during diastole by acting as a reservoir of fluid during systole when it has a very pulsatile inflow. It decreases in size during diastole by discharging blood into the rest of the circulation in a much less pulsatile manner.[72]

The abdominal aorta tapers from its cranial to its caudal extent in 95% of people and usually measures less than 2.3 cm in diameter for men and 1.9 cm for women.[73,74] It increases in diameter by approximately 24% between ages 25 and 71, and both the overall diameter and the rate of increase in diameter are greater in men than in women.[70,75] The upper limit of normal for aortic diameter varies with age, as the diameter normally increases by up to 25% in the seventh and eighth decades. In one study, the maximum normal diameter was 2.4 cm for a 60-year-old and 3.7 cm for a 75-year-old.[74]

Anatomy. The abdominal aorta (Figs. 12-1, 12-3, *B*, 12-18, and 12-19) enters the abdomen through the aortic hiatus of the diaphragm, immediately anterior to the twelfth dorsal vertebra. It descends along the anterior part of the vertebral bodies. The upper abdominal aorta lies posterior and slightly to the left of the gastroesophageal junction. The median arcuate ligament of the diaphragm abuts its anterior surface, and it is flanked on either side by the diaphragmatic crura. To its right lies the azygous vein and thoracic duct; on its left lies the hemiazygous vein.[71] Below the level of the crura, it lies immediately to the left of the IVC and posterior to the celiac artery, superior mesenteric artery, inferior mesenteric artery, left renal vein, gonadal vessels, and root of the mesentery. At the L4 level, it bifurcates into the paired **common iliac arteries,**[71] which are about 5 cm long and generally run slightly anterior to the corre-

sponding veins. The maximum diameter of the common iliac artery is 1.4 to 1.5 cm for men and 1.2 cm for women.[73,75] The **common iliac arteries** bifurcate into the **external** and the **internal iliac arteries.** The external iliac artery lies just on the medial aspect of the psoas.

The **main aortic branches**[71] that are frequently seen on ultrasound are the **celiac artery** (Fig. 12-19), the **paired renal arteries,** the **superior mesenteric artery** (Fig. 12-18, *B*), and the **common iliac arteries.** The **celiac artery** is the first major abdominal aortic branch and typically it bifurcates into the hepatic and splenic arteries within 3 cm of its origin. It has a

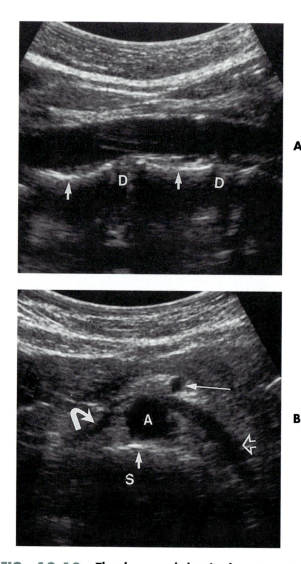

FIG. 12-18. The lower abdominal aorta. A, Longitudinal and **B,** transverse sonograms. The intervertebral discs (d) posterior to the aorta. The anterior surfaces of the vertebral bodies are echogenic *(short straight arrow).* Curved arrow, IVC. Open arrow, left renal vein. A, aorta. S, spine. Narrow arrow, superior mesenteric artery.

T-shaped or a Y-shaped configuration in the transverse plane (Fig. 12-20). The **left gastric artery** is given off superiorly and is sometimes seen. The **internal iliac arteries** have numerous branches immediately after the common iliac artery bifurcation but they are rarely seen on routine sonograms. The **external iliac artery** gives off the inferior epigastric artery and the deep circumflex iliac artery before continuing below the inguinal ligament as the common femoral artery.[71]

Other aortic branches not usually identified include the paired inferior diaphragmatic (inferior phrenic) branches, the paired middle suprarenal arteries, the paired gonadal arteries, the inferior mesenteric artery, and the paired first to fourth lumbar arteries. At the aortic termination, the middle sacral artery is given off posteroinferiorly.

Aortic Sonography. The **indications** for an aortic sonogram include a pulsatile abdominal mass, hemodynamic compromise in the lower limb arterial system, abdominal pain, and an abdominal bruit.

Objectives of aortic sonography include:

- Visualization of the entire aorta and its main branches;
- Detection of atheromatous stenoses, aneurysms, dissections, or other pathology; and
- Evaluation of adjacent organs and structures.

At sonography the aorta is shown as a hypoechoic tubular structure with echogenic walls (Figs. 12-18, *A* and 12-1, *A*). It is usually located just to the left of the midline, although it is variable in position when it becomes ectatic. The midabdominal aorta, at the level of the origin of the renal arteries, is frequently difficult to visualize well because of overlying bowel gas.

The normal flow pattern in the aorta is classified as **plug flow**, a situation in which most of the blood is moving at the same velocity[72] (Figs. 12-19 and 12-21). In the aorta and iliac arteries, flow is typically of the **high-resistance type** (Figs. 12-19 and 12-21), with a sharp increase in antegrade velocity

---

INDICATIONS FOR AN AORTIC SONOGRAM

Pulsatile abdominal mass
Hemodynamic compromise in the lower limb arterial system
Abdominal pain
Abdominal bruit

Abdominal Aortic Branches

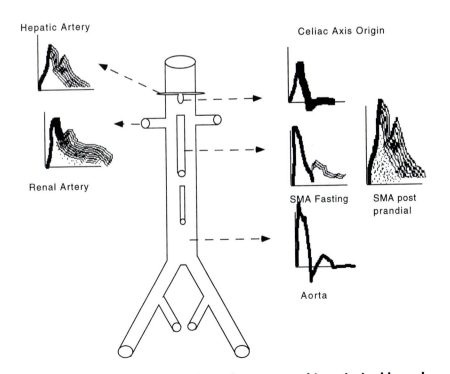

FIG. 12-19. Doppler tracings from the aorta and its principal branches.

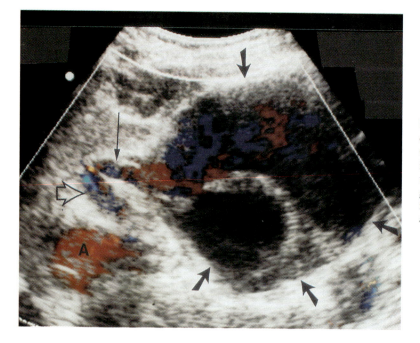

FIG. 12-20. Splenic artery mycotic aneurysm (partially thrombosed). One of 4 mycotic aneurysms that developed in a 17-year-old female following a tooth extraction. Transverse sonogram through epigastrium shows the aneurysm *(arrows)* arises from the splenic artery *(thin arrow)*. Celiac axis *(open arrow)*. A, aorta.

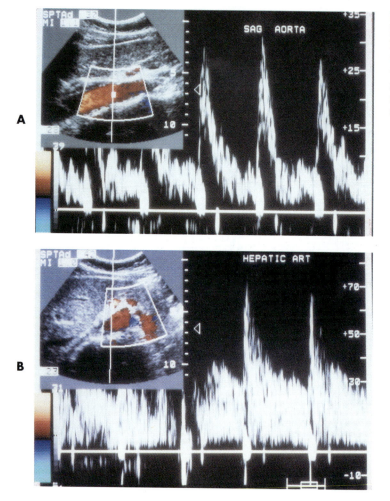

FIG. 12-21. Normal Doppler tracings. A, Upper abdominal aorta shows a high resistance pattern and a narrow spectrum. There may be a small amount of reverse flow in early diastole. **B,** Hepatic artery shows a low resistance pattern and a narrow systolic spectrum with a wider diastolic spectrum.

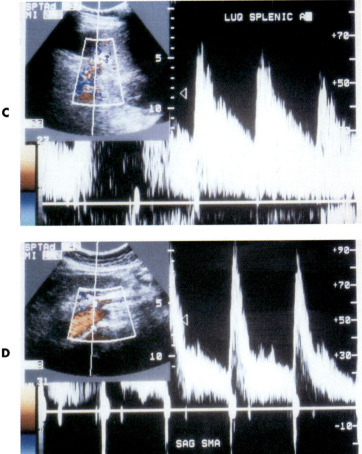

C

D

FIG. 12-21, cont'd. C, Splenic artery shows a similar spectrum but with more spectral broadening. **D,** SMA shows a higher resistance pattern and a narrower spectrum.

during systole, followed by a rapid decrease in velocity and culminating in a brief period of reversed flow. During the remainder of diastole there is some low velocity, antegrade flow. Spectral Doppler analysis shows the peak antegrade velocity decreases, and the amount of retrograde flow increases as one progresses from the proximal aorta to the iliac system. The main aortic branches supply numerous low-resistance areas and as such, these have a lower resistive index and a lower pulsatility index (Fig. 12-21, C). These smaller vessels show a more variable velocity pattern across the blood vessel and so the thickness of the spectral line is broadened.

Good **acoustic windows** for scanning the abdominal aorta include:

- The midline in the upper abdomen;
- The left flank, with the patient supine (or right lateral decubitus); and
- Along the lateral aspect of the lower rectus abdominis muscle for evaluating the iliac vessels.

The entire aorta should be visualized in transverse and longitudinal planes and its maximum anteroposterior (AP) and transverse diameter measured accurately[7] (Fig. 12-22).

Patency of the aorta and its branch vessels can be confirmed with color Doppler analysis and where aliasing occurs, a Doppler spectral tracing helps to determine whether a true stenosis is present or not.[7] Angle-corrected spectral Doppler analysis at stenosis typically shows increased pulsatility (increased pulsatility index and resistive index) proximal to the stenosis, increased peak systolic and peak diastolic velocity immediately at the stenosis, turbulence immediately poststenosis, and dampening of the waveform further distal to the stenoses (Fig. 12-23).[76,77]

SPECTRAL DOPPLER OF STENOSIS EVIDENCE

Increased pulsatility proximal to the stenosis
Increased pulsatility index and resistive index
Increased peak systolic velocity at the stenosis
Increased peak diastolic velocity at the stenosis
Turbulence immediately poststenosis
Dampening of the waveform further distal to the stenosis

Aneurysm Measurement Technique

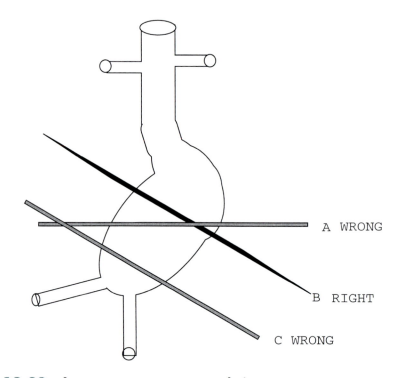

FIG. 12-22. **Aneurysm measurement technique.** Line diagram showing a typical infrarenal abdominal aortic aneurysm. Three scan planes are shown. A is incorrect, as it is not perpendicular to the main axis of the vessel. B is correct. C is in the correct plane but not in the widest part of the aneurysm.

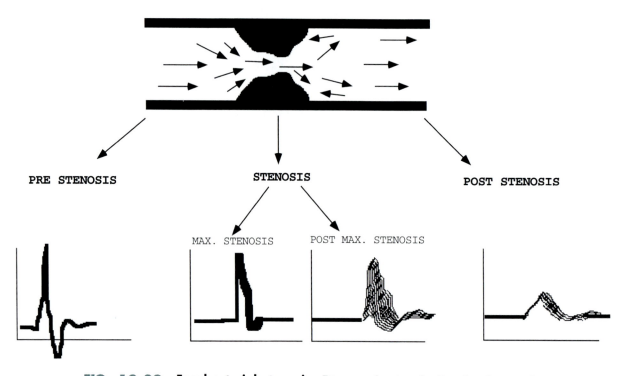

FIG. 12-23. **Focal arterial stenosis.** Diagram showing the Doppler changes that occur before, at, and beyond a focal stenosis anywhere in the arterial system. Before the stenosis, the pulsatility increases. Immediately at the stenosis, the velocity increases but the spectral tracing remains narrow. Just beyond the area of maximum stenosis, there is marked spectral broadening. The waveform is markedly dampened distally.

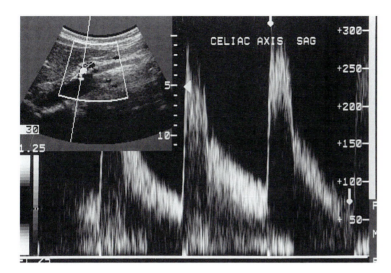

FIG. 12-24. Celiac artery stenosis. Doppler tracing showing spectral broadening and increased peak systolic velocity to 305 cm/second.

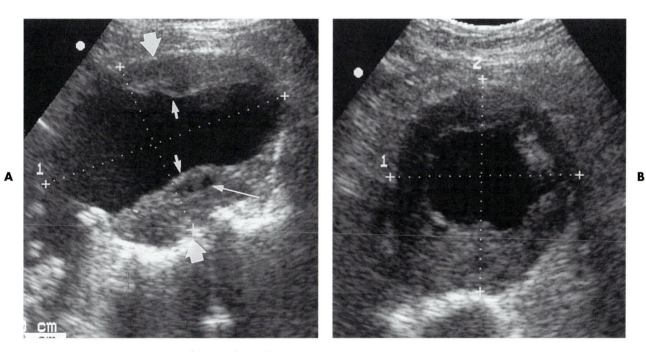

FIG. 12-25. Infrarenal aortic aneurysm. A, Longitudinal and B, transverse image show extensive atheromatous plaque and thrombus with an area of ulceration *(narrow arrow)* in the intima with some cystic change in the wall. Combined plaque and mural thrombus, bigger arrows. Gradicules are on the margins of the aneurysm, which measures 11 × 7.3 cm.

Stenoses should be mapped and waveform and peak systolic velocity documented (Fig. 12-24).

Aortic Pathology. The abdominal aorta and its main branches are affected by atheroma,[78] aneurysm formation,[7] connective tissue disorders,[79,80] rupture,[62,81] thrombosis, infections,[82] and displacement by and invasion from diseases in adjacent structures.

Atheromatous disease. Atheroma or **arteriosclerosis** is a vascular wall disorder characterized by the presence of lipid deposits in the intima (Fig. 12-25). The atheromatous plaque is a soft, porridge-like material which may discharge into the vessel lumen, causing a **distal embolus** or a **thrombus** or both at the donor site. Plaques cause mural irregularity and frequently narrow the vessel lumen, with resulting distal ischemia.[78] Stenotic or occlusive disease most often occurs in the infrarenal portion of the aorta. Atheroma may also be associated with mural weakening and aneurysm formation.[78]

The incidence of atheromatous disease increases with age, and it affects more men than women.[78] It affects both the aorta, the iliac arteries, and the other aortic branch arteries and is most common on the pos-

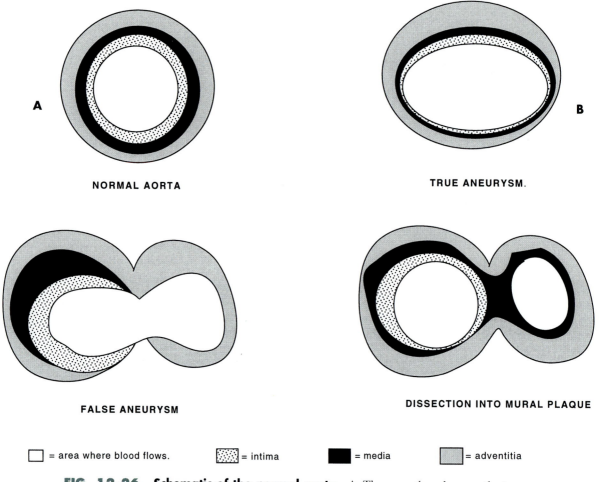

NORMAL AORTA

TRUE ANEURYSM.

FALSE ANEURYSM

DISSECTION INTO MURAL PLAQUE

☐ = area where blood flows.　▦ = intima　■ = media　▨ = adventitia

FIG. 12-26. Schematic of the normal aorta. A, There are three layers—the inner intima (dots), the middle media (black), and the outer adventitia (gray). **B, True aneurysm:** the vessel enlarges, as do all three mural layers. **C, False aneurysm:** the vessel enlarges but part of the protruding portion is covered only by adventitia. **D, Dissecting aneurysm:** while the outer diameter of the aorta has increased, the diameter of the true lumen is unchanged. However, a new lumen, or "false lumen," has opened within the media and is not lined by intima.

terior wall in the aortoiliac area.[78] It is associated with cigarette smoking, diabetes mellitus, hypertension, and increased levels of the low density lipoprotein (LDL) fraction of serum cholesterol.[76]

If significant lower limb pain is present, it is prudent to assess the entire lower limb arterial tree to rule out emboli and to look for further stenoses.[7] Similarly, in lower limb analysis the presence of a dampened waveform in the common femoral artery should provoke a search for a stenotic lesion more proximal in the arterial tree.

Aneurysms. An aneurysm is any swelling in a blood vessel, either focal or diffuse.[83] Histologically, they are classified into **true** aneurysms, which are lined by all three layers of the aorta (Fig. 12-26, *B*), and **false** aneurysms (Fig. 12-26, *C*) (**pseudoaneurysms**), which are not. True aneurysms form when the tensile strength of the wall decreases. A mi-

nority of true aneurysms are due to clearly identified underlying diseases that predispose affected patients to aneurysm formation such as **Ehlers-Danlos** syndrome[79,80] a rare disease typically affecting young African-American women that is associated with hypertension and is characterized by the absence of clot in the lumen of the vessel. Most true aneurysms, however, are idiopathic.

In **false**, or **pseudoaneurysms**, blood escapes through a hole in the innermost vessel lining (the intima) but is contained by the deeper layers of the aorta or by the adjacent tissue (Fig. 12-26, *C*). Most pseudoaneurysms are round or oval-shaped protuberances from the artery; blood circulates into them in systole and out of them in diastole (Fig. 12-27). They can be caused by infection (mycotic) (Fig. 12-20) or can result from trauma, surgery, or interventional radiology procedures (Fig. 12-27). A **dissecting aneurysm** is a

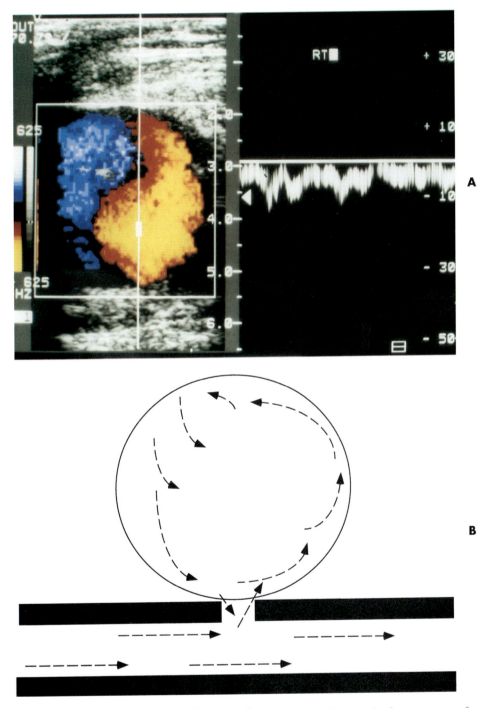

FIG. 12-27. Postangiographic pseudoaneurysm. Longitudinal sonograms of the right groin. **A,** Initial color Doppler shows the typical ying/yang appearance and the relatively low-velocity flow within the lesion. **B,** Diagram demonstrates how blood circulates in these pseudoaneurysms. The entry jet is invariably pulsatile. The blood swirling in the pseudoaneurysm may have variable waveforms and is often monophasic, nonpulsatile.

special type of pseudoaneurysm in which blood leaves the lumen through an intimal defect, courses a variable distance in the wall, and reenters the aorta further distal in the arterial system (Fig. 12-26, *D*).

Idiopathic abdominal aortic aneurysms (AAAs) are true aneurysms (Fig. 12-26, *B*), 95% of which are infrarenal in location.[84] Of patients with AAAs, 30% to 60% are asymptomatic and the rest present with abdominal, back, or leg pain.[7] They may also present following leakage or rupture. While AAAs are strongly associated with atherosclerosis, their origin is likely to be multifactorial[81,85-88] because

- Most people with atheroma do not develop aneurysms;[7,87]
- AAA patients frequently have arteriomegaly, with vessels 40% to 50% bigger than those with atheromatous aortic occlusive disease (Fig. 12-28);[81,85]
- There is a definitely increased risk of the disease in close relatives[84,87] (an estimated 11% to 18% increased risk in a first-degree relative); and
- It also appears that proper innervation of the aorta may also help to stop aneurysm formation, as the aorta is bigger in spinal injury patients.[88]

The true **incidence** of AAAs is unknown but studies suggest a 5% to 10% prevalence in men over 60.[7,89-92] The incidence is highest in elderly men, with between 70% and 90% of AAAs occurring in men over 65.[7] Various cases have been made for screening entire groups of elderly people or subgroups at high risk,[93-95] but as yet there is no consensus.

The recognized **complications** of idiopathic abdominal aortic aneurysms include **rupture, thrombosis, dissection, distal embolism, infection,** and **obstruction** and **invasion of adjacent structures.**[81]

The most common complications of abdominal aortic aneurysms are **branch artery occlusions or stenoses**[7] which have more to do with the atheroma than with the aneurysm. They can occur anywhere but are most commonly seen in the inferior mesenteric artery (IMA) and the renal arteries.

AORTIC RUPTURE. The most catastrophic of aortic aneurysm complications is aortic rupture, which has a mortality rate of at least 50%. Most aneurysms that rupture have not been recognized prior to rupture.[85] Natural history indicates a cumulative incidence of rupture of 25% over 8 years for aneurysms greater than 5 cm in AP diameter.[85] There is a 5% cumulative incidence of rupture over the same time period for abdominal aortic aneurysms with AP diameter between 3.5 and 4.9 cm and a 0% incidence for aneurysms less than 3.5 cm in anteroposterior diameter.[85] Other studies support these findings.[96-98] The average rate at which an aneurysm enlarges varies between 0.2 to 0.4 or 0.5 cm per year, depending on the study.[81,85,99-101] However, there is considerable interpersonal variation, so the optimal time interval for screening these patients is unclear. One protocol is to scan larger aneurysms at 6-month intervals and smaller ones at 12-month intervals.

Aortic rupture is a surgical emergency, and if any imaging is done, computed tomography is the test of choice.[7] It is better at detecting acute bleeds, is not hampered by bowel gas, and provides a greater overall perspective. Some aortic ruptures may be contained in the retroperitoneum; they are referred to as chronic ruptures.[102] If patients with this condition do come to ultrasound, retroperitoneal complex fluid collections are the most common findings.[7,103]

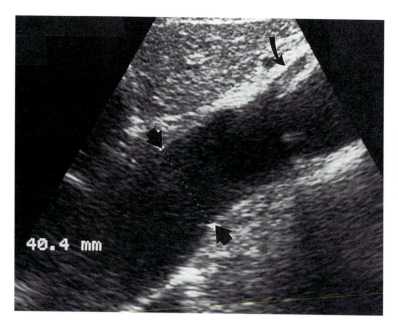

FIG. 12-28. Arteriomegaly with associated atheroma and distal aneurysm formation. Longitudinal midline scan shows a diffusely widened upper abdominal aorta *(fat arrows)*. Superior mesenteric artery *(curved arrow)*.

The aneurysm may compress, displace, or invade the ureter, the bowel, the inferior vena cava, and the kidney and renal arteries.[81,103,104] The left kidney is more frequently affected than the right.[81] Iliac aneurysms may rupture into the ureter, the rectosigmoid colon, and the iliac vein.[104]

MURAL THROMBUS. Mural thrombus in AAAs is prevalent in most large lesions and is frequently circumferential but eccentric (Figs. 12-25 and 12-29). This thrombus is often poorly attached and friable and is an important source of distal emboli (Fig. 12-20).[7] The thrombus within an aneurysm is usually not organized and therefore adds no tensile strength to the vessels. The volume of thrombus has no bearing on the risk of rupture.[104]

ILIAC/SUPRARENAL ANEURYSMS. Of patients with distal aortic aneurysms, 5% will have an associated iliac artery aneurysm (Fig. 12-30).[86,103] Most occur in the common iliac segment, with the next most common area being the external iliac just beyond the bifurcation. Patients with iliac artery aneurysms have a much higher incidence of aneurysms elsewhere in the body.[84,86] Such aneurysms are of great concern if they exist independently, as they are very difficult to diagnose.[7]

Trauma, syphilis, and mycotic disease should all be considered potential causes if aneurysms are discovered suprarenally.

INFLAMMATORY AORTIC ANEURYSMS. Inflammatory aortic aneurysms (Fig. 12-13) are a variant of atherosclerotic abdominal aortic aneurysms in which the wall of the aneurysm is thickened and surrounded by fibrosis and adhesions of a type similar to those

seen in retroperitoneal fibrosis.[45,105] Their surgical repair is associated with a higher mortality and morbidity than is standard aneurysm surgery, so diagnosis prior to surgery is desirable.[45,46,106] Of abdominal aortic aneurysms, 4% to 23% are estimated to be inflammatory in origin.[46,106] They are very difficult to diagnose, as they often present with pain and may mimic a retroperitoneal bleed.[106] While less than 25% of idiopathic AAAs present with pain, pain was present in 84% of patients with inflammatory aneurysms.

SONOGRAPHIC APPEARANCES OF ABDOMINAL AORTIC ANEURYSMS. In experienced hands, the diagnosis of aortic aneurysms on sonography is close to 100%.[93] The diagnosis is made by finding a **focal dilatation** of the aorta or a **generalized dilatation** bigger than 3 cm.[7] Aneurysms elongate as they grow, and as the lower end of the aorta rarely moves significantly caudally, most AAAs deflect to the left side or kink anteriorly, or both, as they enlarge (Fig. 12-22). The anterior and posterior borders of the aneurysm are usually better seen than its lateral borders which may be indistinct (Fig. 12-25, *B*). The adventitia is usually continuous with adjacent fibrofatty tissue and is echogenic. **Mural thrombus,** which frequently makes up most of the wall, is usually of low to medium echogenicity (Fig. 12-25) and it may or may not have a lamellated appearance. The intimal lining may be smooth or irregular, and calcification may also be present (Fig. 12-31).

Sonographic measurement of these AAAs may be challenging and it is important to get an accurate outer-layer-to-outer-layer measurement in a plane perpendicular to the long axis of the vessels[7] (Fig. 12-22). The

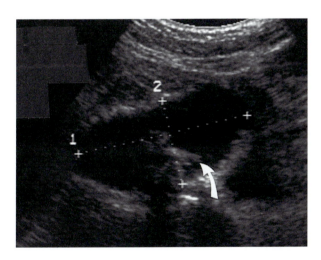

FIG. 12-29. Aortic aneurysm with eccentric plaque. A focal area of plaque has developed some thrombus around it and protrudes into the lumen. This is seen to "flutter" in the lumen during real-time scanning and is a potential source of emboli.

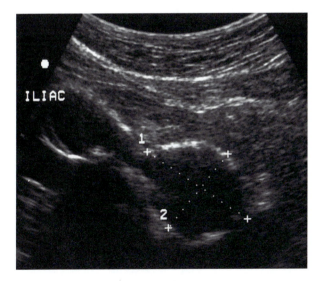

FIG. 12-30. Common iliac artery aneurysm. Longitudinal sonogram showing a left common iliac artery aneurysm (gradicules). The distal AAA seen on the left of the sonogram has a smaller size.

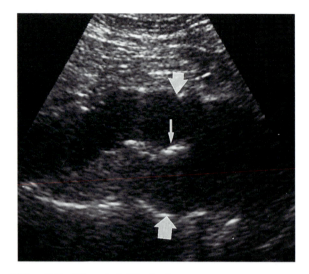

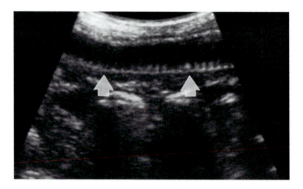

FIG. 12-32. Vascular graft. Longitudinal scan along the patient's left flank region subcutaneous vascular axillofemoral graft *(arrows)*.

FIG. 12-31. Calcified plaque. Longitudinal view of an AAA with posterior thrombus. Adventitia (fat arrows). Calcified plaque (narrow arrow).

mean difference between the aortic diameter as measured at surgery and as measured by ultrasound was 2.9 mm in one study.[107]

Analysis of an AAA would include its maximum true length, width, and transverse dimensions; documentation of its **shape**; and documentation of its **location,** including suprarenal extension or involvement of the common iliac vessels. This analysis is of great practical importance, as different surgical approaches are used with the different types of aneurysms. The etiology, complication rate, and post-procedure morbidity are also quite distinct. The nature and type of the **wall thickening** should be assessed: is it calcified plaque, flowing blood, soft plaque, or well-established plaque? The patent channel should be found and the flow pattern characterized. An effort should be made to detect any dissection and to evaluate hypoechoic channels for flow with Doppler. Both kidneys should always be examined, their size measured, and pelvicaliectasis excluded.[7] Doppler evaluation of the renal artery is not part of a "routine" aortic scan, but it should be considered if there is a shrunken kidney or if the patient has hypertension.[7]

The following **descriptive terms** and sonographic criteria are commonly used for **idiopathic abdominal aortic aneurysms.**

- **Bulbous:** sharp junction between normal and abnormal;
- **Fusiform:** gradual transition between normal and abnormal;
- **Saccular:** sharp, sudden transition between normal and abnormal;
- **Dumbbell:** figure eight appearance to the aneurysm.

The aims of the examiner of a patient with an AAA should be to:
- Diagnose the aneurysm;
- Diagnose any complications;
- Provide information that will allow the surgeon to decide whether to intervene surgically; and
- Monitor the effects of any therapy given for the AAA.

The decision to operate on an aneurysm is based on:
- The absolute size, especially when the diameter is over 6 cm;
- Documented enlargement over time;
- Associated pain or tenderness;
- Associated distal emboli;
- Renal obstruction or vascular compromise;
- Gastrointestinal bleeding; and
- Suspected rupture.

This decision must be carefully considered in each patient, as these patients are often at risk for concomitant disease. One study reported a 73% 5-year survival of patients with small aneurysms, with most mortality coming from diseases not directly related to the aneurysm.[108]

AORTIC GRAFTS. At sonography arterial grafts are quite echogenic and have a textured appearance (Fig. 12-32).[7] They are usually named after the vessels they are hooked up with (Fig. 12-33) and can be anastomosed in either an end-to-side or an end-to-end manner. The native aorta is usually wrapped around the graft and fluid frequently accumulates between the graft and the vessel wall. The vessel wall is often thickened at the anastomotic site as a result of puckering at the site of the sutures.

Some surgeons are using intraoperative ultrasound to assess the vessels during surgery, as ultrasound has been shown to be ideally suited to monitoring vascular reconstructions.[109]

COMMON AORTIC GRAFTS

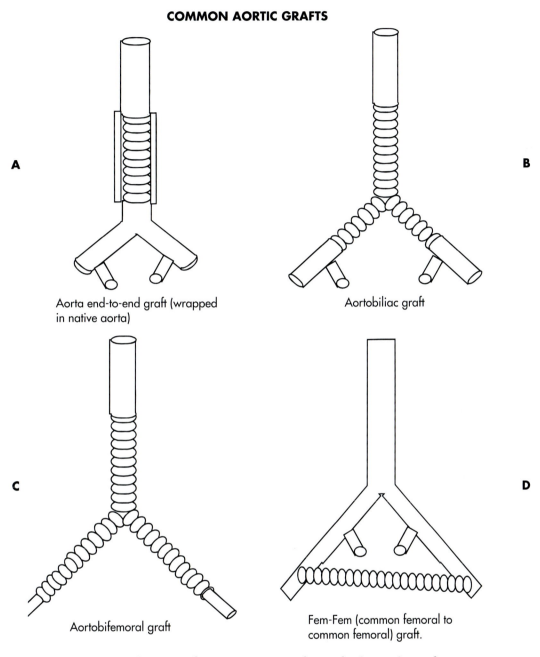

Aorta end-to-end graft (wrapped in native aorta)

Aortobiliac graft

Aortobifemoral graft

Fem-Fem (common femoral to common femoral) graft.

FIG. 12-33. **Diagram of common types of prosthetic aortic grafts.**

When **scanning postprocedurally** it is essential:
- to assess the upper and lower anastomoses;
- to check these sites for stenoses, aneurysms, and pseudoaneurysm formations with Doppler;
- to identify and measure fluid collections around the graft and elsewhere in the abdomen; and
- to check blood flow distally.

The most common finding sonographically is fluid collections around the grafts (Fig. 12-34).[7] These may be **hematomas, lymphoceles, seromas, or abscesses.** Distinguishing among the different etiologies

is difficult. If the collection is large or echogenic or increasing in size or far away from the graft, then infection must be considered,[7] and fine-needle aspiration is indicated.[110] Lymphocele around the graft may be very hypoechoic and may simulate a dissection.[111] Color and spectral Doppler are very useful in these instances.

Dissection. For an **aortic dissection** to occur, a defect must exist in the intima and an internal weakness must exist in the wall[7] (Fig. 12-25, *D*). Most are idiopathic, but some are related to Marfan's disease, pregnancy, bicuspid aortic valve, trauma, focal

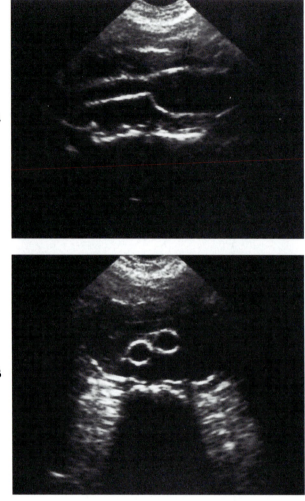

FIG. 12-34. Perigraft fluid. A, Sagittal and **B,** transverse sonograms show aortobifemoral graft surrounded by hypoechoic fluid collection. On aspiration, this was seroma. (Courtesy of Stephanie R. Wilson, M.D., University of Toronto.)

stenoses, or hypertension.[112] Aortic dissection typically commences in the thorax and extends into the abdomen, with less than 5% occurring primarily in the abdomen. It may extend into the iliac vessels and the other aortic branch vessels. It may also occlude aortic branch vessels. Dissection may also occur within the thickened wall of an atheromatous AAA.

A special type of dissection is the iatrogenic, postangiographic type where the dissection is more localized and the amount of blood flow in the false lumen is usually much less.

Aortic dissection is easily recognized on **sonography**, with the classical appearance being a thin membrane "fluttering" in the lumen at different phases of the cardiac cycle (Fig. 12-35). Color Doppler shows blood flow in both channels, although flow rates frequently differ between the channels.

Every effort should be made to distinguish a true dissection from a **pseudodissection** (Fig. 12-36) which is caused by liquefaction of aneurysm thrombus.[113] The distinguishing features include no fluttering of the intravascular membrane, no flow in one lumen, and a thick membrane in pseudolesions.

Infection. This rare condition is difficult to diagnose and often results in **mycotic aneurysms** (Fig. 12-20). Septic emboli, which are frequently associated with valvular heart disease or other cardiac anomalies and group D streptococci,[5] often cause the disease. Infection may also result from the hematogenous spread of organisms, especially staphylococci and salmonella.[85] Staphylococci or streptococci may invade a preceding idiopathic aneurysm and produce a focal abscess. Infection may also be secondary to previous surgery or other intervention[114] or may result from the spread of an infection in adjacent structures. Sonography alone will rarely indicate a diagnosis, but by combining the findings with clinical information, one can suggest the diagnosis in many cases. The disease itself can result in thrombosis, arterial rupture, distal ischemia, and invasion into adjacent structures.[115]

Pseudoaneurysms/arteriovenous fistula. While these may occur postinfection (Fig. 12-20) and posttrauma, most pseudoaneurysms result from problems at the site of angiographic puncture (Fig. 12-27) or at the site of a surgical anastomosis. They have a spectacular **sonographic appearance** on color Doppler examination (Fig. 12-27) where a pulsatile jet is seen as blood enters the aneurysm during systole, with turbulent blood flow in diastole. Recently there has been interest in **treating pseudoaneurysms** with ultrasound-guided compression. The neck of the pseudoaneurysm is identified by sonography and compressed, blocking blood flow into the region. If compressed long enough, a clot will form and the defect will be healed.[116,117] The procedure is well tolerated and works effectively in the majority of patients.

Occasionally, postangiography, postsurgery, or spontaneously, an arteriovenous fistula may form. It is also possible for one to arise in association with a tumor.

Aortic Branches
Celiac/mesenteric arteries. Classically, the celiac artery has a high-resistive pattern at its origin, with a small amount of reversed early diastolic flow (Fig. 12-19). As one goes more distally, it loses the reversed early diastolic flow component, and the hepatic and splenic arteries usually have a low-resistive type of pattern (Figs. 12-14 and 12-21, *B*). The celiac artery has continuous forward flow throughout the cardiac cycle of the low-resistance type. The **hepatic artery** arises solely from the celiac axis 72% of the time. The superior mesenteric artery gives off the common hepatic artery in 4% of cases, the right hepatic artery in 11% of cases, and the left hepatic artery

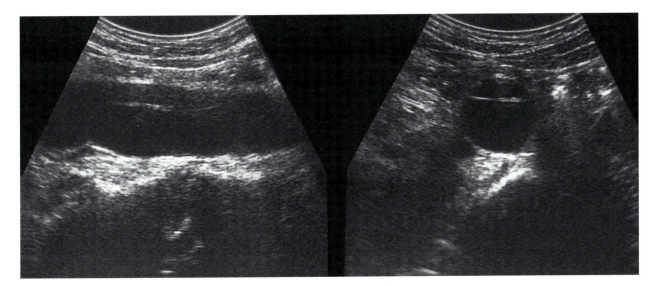

FIG. 12-35. Dissection of abdominal aorta. A, Sagittal and B, transverse sonograms show the intimal flap anteriorly separating the true lumen from the false lumen. (Courtesy of Stephanie R. Wilson, M.D., University of Toronto.)

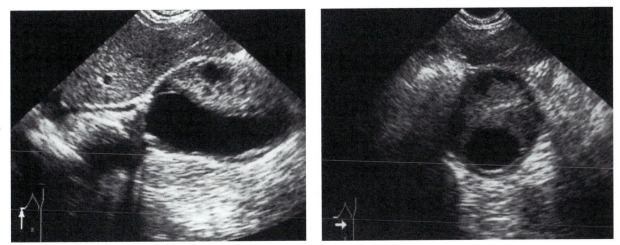

FIG. 12-36. Aortic pseudodissection due to hypoechoic thrombus mimicking dissection. A, Sagittal and B, transverse sonograms show hypoechoic zone near outer margin of laminated thrombus. Clot in this area is recent, as compared with more echogenic laminated thrombus closer to liver. (Courtesy of Stephanie R. Wilson, M.D., University of Toronto.)

in 10% of cases. The **splenic artery** is frequently tortuous, producing spectral broadening without any increase in peak systolic velocity[77] (Fig. 12-21, C).

The **superior mesenteric artery** (SMA) (Fig. 12-21, D) commences about 1 cm caudal to the celiac axis, has a short component that proceeds anteriorly, and then has a long portion that extends inferiorly. The flow pattern and the Doppler spectral trace pattern in the SMA vary depending on whether or not the patient is fasting. In the **fasting state**, the pattern is of high resistance with a small amount of reversed flow in early diastole. **Following eating**, in a normal

person the peak systolic and diastolic velocities increase dramatically (Fig. 12-19). The reversed diastolic flow disappears, a low-resistive pattern develops, and the systolic spectral peaks become broadened. This pattern is most prominent 45 minutes postprandially and is dependent on the type and amount of food ingested.[118]

Intestinal ischemia is a clinical disease with a variety of different symptoms, so it is difficult to diagnose. It is caused by a deficiency of blood delivery to the bowel and usually requires significant narrowing or obstruction of both the celiac axis and the superior mesenteric artery (Fig. 12-24). While sonography helps with the diagnosis in many cases, the exact sensitivity and specificity of ultrasound are unknown.[118] Some authors have devised complex protocols to assess the pattern postprandially in greater detail by scanning at standard intervals after standardized meals.[118]

Splanchnic aneurysms may be congenital, atherosclerotic, posttraumatic, mycotic, or inflammatory. About 10% of patents with **chronic pancreatitis** develop these pseudoaneurysms, which occur in the hepatic artery, splenic artery, SMA, gastroduodenum, or IMA. They may be saccular or fusiform and usually have no reverse flow within them. They may have layers of thrombus on the walls (Fig. 12-20). They present a significant risk to the interventional radiologist, as they may be mistaken for simple abscesses.[40] It is probably prudent to evaluate with Doppler all collections prior to drainage.

Renal arteries. The renal arteries arise within 1.5 cm of the origin of the SMA[7] and can be sonographically identified in 86% of cases.[119] Twenty-two percent of patients have two renal arteries, and 2% have three or more.[120] Doppler tracings should be obtained from within the renal artery and also from within the kidney. The Doppler tracings are typically of a low-resistance type, with the peak systolic and diastolic readings decreasing as one goes farther into the kidney.[77]

RENAL ARTERY STENOSIS (RAS). This produces a rare (2%)[121] but treatable cause of hypertension and may be due to atherosclerotic disease or fibromuscular hyperplasia, a rare disease typically affecting young women.[122] While both are treatable with angioplasty, the latter has a much better prognosis.

Significant **controversy** persists about the **role of Doppler** ultrasound in the **diagnosis of RAS**.[123] While most people agree that Doppler scanning techniques are challenging and have a long learning curve, controversy remains as to its true specificity and sensitivity. The best scanning technique is also unclear.[123] Sensitivities from 71% to 99% and specificities from 62% to 99% have been reported.[123] The renal arteries can be insonated directly and a spectral tracing taken along their course while looking for the characteristic changes of a stenosis (Fig. 12-23). Although previously, peak-systolic velocities greater than 100 cm/sec were reported to be abnormal,[123] we now know that a **threshold of 180 cm/sec** is probably more accurate.[124,125]

The **ratio** of the **peak velocities** in the aorta and the stenotic renal segment is also helpful; **a 3.5 ratio indicates a greater than 60% chance of RAS**.[123,124]

Another useful Doppler technique evaluates the **spectral Doppler waveform intrarenally**.[122,123,126] This technique is faster and has a lower failure rate.[123] The shape of the systolic upstroke is evaluated, and **the acceleration time and acceleration index** are calculated (Fig. 12-38). The acceleration index is the ratio of the maximum systolic velocity to the length of the time to peak systole. An acceleration index of 3 m/sec^2 or greater is normal. Sensitivities of 78% to 87% and specificities of 83% to 98% have been reported.[122,123,126]

Stavros, in looking at the segmental renal arteries, noted that the **lack of the normal early systolic peak** in the renal artery tracing was the best predictor of renal artery stenosis with luminal narrowing greater than 60% (95% sensitivity and 97% specificity)[122] (Fig. 12-37).

ANEURYSMS AND ARTERIOVENOUS FISTULA. Most of these are acquired problems and may be posttraumatic or post-large-bore needle biopsy. The aneurysms are usually pseudoaneurysms and sonographically, they resemble those that arise from the external iliac artery or the common femoral artery. One quarter of arteriovenous fistulas are congenital and less than 5% result from malignancy. On sonography, they usually produce a mosaic of color in the kidney.

Inferior Vena Cava

Anatomy. The inferior vena cava is a large vein that returns blood from the lower limbs, pelvis, and abdomen to the right atrium. It is formed by the paired common iliac veins on the anterior surface of the L5 vertebral body and lies anteriorly and slightly to the right of the spine.[127] It transverses the diaphragm and enters the right atrium at the level of the eighth thoracic vertebra. Its main branches are the hepatic veins, the renal veins, and the common iliac veins.[127] The walls of the IVC are much thinner than those of the aorta and the pressure of blood it deals with is also much lower.

Sonography. The intrahepatic portion of the IVC is routinely viewed by using the liver as an acoustic window (Figs. 12-40 and 12-41). The remainder of the vessel is inconsistently seen because it is intermittently flat and oval-shaped and may be obscured by overlying bowel gas and pannus. Common iliac veins and external iliac veins are seen inconsistently with their corresponding arteries on the lateral aspect of the pelvic brim. The IVC lumen is usually anechoic, although with slow-flowing blood, it becomes more echogenic and may show swirling. This is seen with right heart failure, fluid overload, and caudal to an IVC obstruction. The appearance varies with respiration. With **deep inspiration,** venous return decreases and the IVC dilates. With **deep expiration,** venous return improves and the IVC diameter decreases. By doing a **valsalva,** venous return is blocked and flow temporarily reversed in the IVC, causing it to bulge. The IVC transmits both cardiac and respiratory pulsations; the transmissions are more noticeable sonographically the closer one comes to the heart (Fig. 12-41, *A*). The classical tracing has a saw-

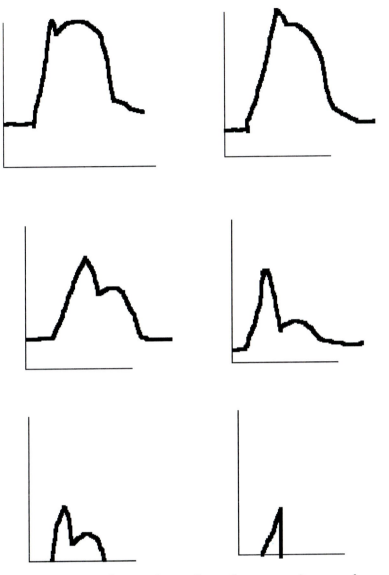

FIG. 12-37. **Patterns of normal systolic peaks as seen in normal segmental renal arteries.** Patients without renal artery stenosis, after Stavros et al.[122] The main feature of all these is the early systolic "spike," or early systolic compliance peak. Lack of the early systolic peak often indicates renal artery stenosis.

tooth pattern. Most distally and in the common iliac veins there is a more phasic pattern similar to the pattern in the proximal limbs.

Pathology

Congenital abnormalities. Most abnormalities occur at or below the level of the renal veins.[128] The IVC, azygous, and hemiazygous vessels form in the embryo from the paired cardinal veins. The most frequent congenital anomalies are duplication (0.2% to 3%) and transposition (0.2% to 0.5%) (Fig. 12-42).[77,128] Both of these form a normal vein at the level of the renal hilum. Interruption of the IVC by azygous or hemiazygous continuation is caused by the failure of the hepatic veins to form; that occurs in about 0.6% of cases.[77] In these instances the hepatic veins drain

directly into the right atrium. These IVC anomalies are often associated with other cardiac malformations.

Thrombosis. The most commonly encountered intraluminal anomaly of the IVC is thrombus, which usually spreads from another vein in the pelvis, lower limb, liver, or kidney.[129] IVC thrombis is sonographically diagnosed as an intraluminal filling defect that usually expands the diameter of the vessel (Figs. 12-39 and 12-40). The echogenicity of a thrombus depends on its age; chronic thrombi may calcify. If a thrombus is hypoechoic or isoechoic with the liver, color Doppler is very helpful in making the diagnosis, for color frequently surrounds the thrombus.

Spectral Doppler analysis produces no signal from uncomplicated thrombus. Arterial-type tracing may

Systolic acceleration ratio $\triangle V / \triangle T$

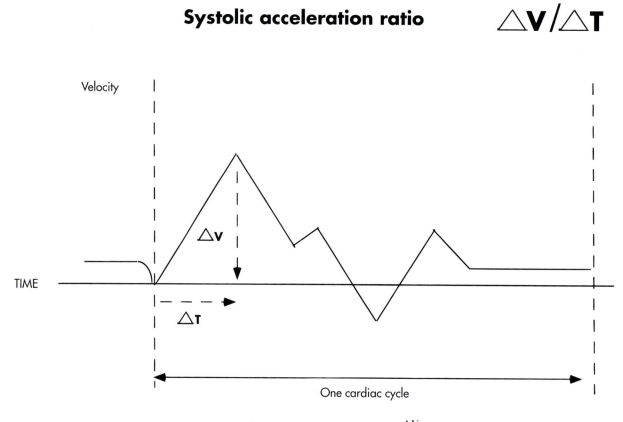

FIG. 12-38. Systolic acceleration index is $\dfrac{\Delta V}{\Delta T}$.

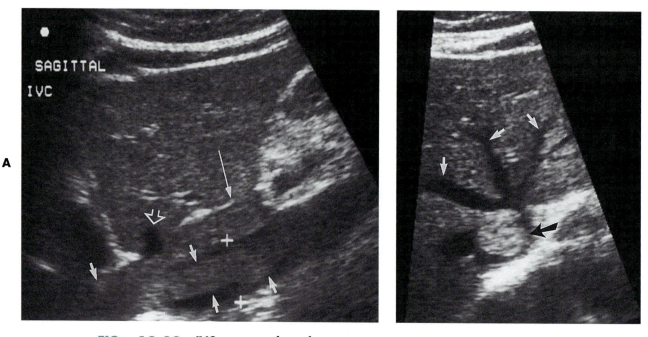

FIG. 12-39. IVC tumor thrombus. A, Longitudinal sonogram shows tumor thrombus *(arrow)* extending up the inferior vena cava and into the right atrium. Middle hepatic vein *(open arrow)*. Fissure for the ligamentum venosum *(narrow arrow)*. **B,** Transverse scan showing the tumor thrombus occupying most of the lumen of the inferior vena cava *(black arrow)*. Patent hepatic veins *(white arrows)*.

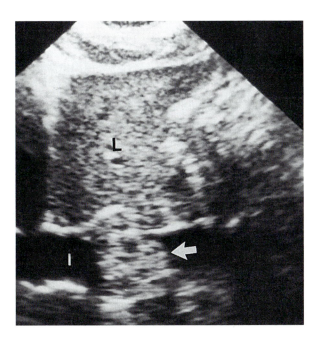

FIG. 12-40. Large breast metastasis (*arrow*) in the inferior vena cava (I). Sagittal image, liver (L).

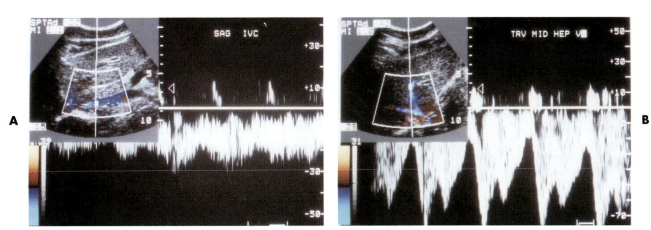

FIG. 12-41. Normal Doppler tracing in the **A,** inferior vena cava and **B,** hepatic vein.

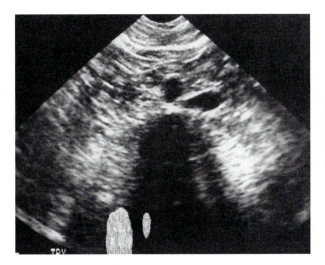

FIG. 12-42. Persistent left inferior vena cava. Transverse scan just above umbilicus shows normal round aorta on the right and more flattened inferior vena cava on the left. (Courtesy of Stephanie R. Wilson, M.D., University of Toronto.)

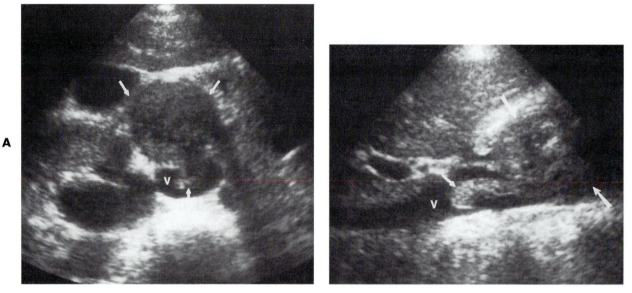

FIG. 12-43. Ovarian vein thrombosis. A tubular hypoechoic, inhomogeneous mass was seen arising out of the pelvis in a patient after cesarean delivery. **A,** Transverse and **B,** longitudinal sonograms show the superior extent of this large thrombus *(arrows)* which extends into the IVC (V) from its anterior aspect.

be seen within tumor thrombi. In obese patients, B-mode artifact may produce a pseudolesion on the images. In these patients, color Doppler is very helpful in confirming vessel patency.

The presence of IVC tumor thrombus is usually diagnosed readily. The kidney is the most likely site of origin (Fig. 12-39).

A variety of **vena caval filters** are now being inserted in the IVC to prevent distal venous thrombi from going on to pulmonary embolism. Ultrasound can sometimes see these as echogenic structures within the IVC and can also monitor complications that may occur at their site of insertion.[130]

Mural lesions/IVC rupture. Mural-based lesions include adherent thrombus and tumor (Fig. 12-40). Primary tumors are rare, but of them, the **leiomyosarcoma** is the most common. Leiomyosarcoma of the wall of the IVC is the most common type and location of mural tumor in the venous system (60%).[131] It occurs most commonly in older women, and surgery is the treatment of choice. The location and extent of the disease determine the resectability of the lesion, so every effort should be made to document it accurately.[131] Metastatic lesions include direct spread from **lymphoma, hepatocellular carcinoma, breast** (Fig. 12-40), and **renal cell carcinoma** (Fig. 12-39).

Mural IVC lesions can exert mass effect and affect structures like the ureter (retrocaval ureter), or the lesions can spread into IVC branches such as the renal veins and the hepatic veins.

IVC rupture usually follows severe abdominal trauma or surgical or interventional therapy. It frequently results in large retroperitoneal bleeds and it is associated with damage to other structures from the same preceding cause.

Cardiac failure/fluid overload. Cardiac failure and fluid overload increase the diameter of the IVC and hepatic veins and exaggerate the normal Doppler flow pattern.

IVC Branches and Tributaries

Renal Veins. The right renal vein is very short, while the left renal vein has a much longer course as it travels between the aorta and the SMA to reach the IVC. Both are usually best scanned on the transverse plane.[132] The renal veins (especially the left) frequently collect blood from varices in portal hypertension patients.

Circumaortic veins are rare. The left renal vein retroaortic variant, which occurs in about 2% of patients, is of great importance when contemplating surgery.[132]

Renal veins may be displaced and compromised by retroperitoneal hemorrhage, aortic aneurysms, tumors, and aberrant vessels. Malignant extension into the renal veins can occur in renal cell carcinoma (Fig. 12-39), renal lymphoma, transitional cell carcinoma, Wilms' tumor, and adrenal carcinoma.[133]

Renal vein thrombosis is associated with acute glomerulonephritis, lupus, amyloidosis, hypercoagulable states, sepsis, trauma, and dehydration.[133] Of those who have undergone renal transplants, 1%

develop this problem. On sonography, one may see dilation of the vein proximal to the occlusion. The kidney enlarges and there is decreased echogenicity secondary to edema in the kidney.[134] In the neonate, chronic cases may go on to calcify.[135] Doppler study shows no renal vein flow and a high-resistive arterial pattern.

Hepatic veins. There are usually three hepatic veins, which lie between the hepatic segments and drain posteriorly into the IVC close to the diaphragm. In most people the middle and left hepatic veins fuse just before joining the IVC,[136] and other congenital variants are possible but infrequently recognized sonographically.[136] Hepatic vein Doppler spectral tracings are usually triphasic and pulsatile, reflecting transmitted cardiac pulsations (Fig. 12-41, *B*). This pattern is abolished in about 20% of cases of cirrhosis and hypertension, and it is exaggerated in right heart failure.[137]

Iliac/ovarian veins. The common and external iliac veins run with the adjacent arteries. They are predominantly medial and anterior at the inguinal ligament, and they become posterior and lateral to the accompanying arteries close to the IVC. They have a respiratory phasicity and can be compressed by adjacent structures and pathology, including lymphoceles, hematoma, transplant kidneys, abscess, and aneurysm. They collapse with a valsalva maneuver because of their intra-abdominal position but increase in diameter following augmentation by a squeezing of the leg or by elevation.[138] It occurs most often on the right side, and sonographic detection should include evaluation of the expected entry of the vein directly into the IVC.

Ovarian vein thrombosis (Fig. 12-43) usually occurs postpartum and is associated with endometritis and surgery. Sonography frequently shows massive enlargement of all or part of the ovarian vein, often with an echogenic thrombus within it.[138] It usually occurs on the right side. Sonographic detection should include evaluation of the expected entry of the vein directly into the IVC.

REFERENCES

1. Davidson AJ. *Radiology of the Kidney.* Philadelphia: WB Saunders Co; 1985:629-659.
2. Meyers MA. The extraperitoneal spaces: normal and pathologic anatomy. In: *Dynamic Radiology of the Abdomen: Normal and Pathologic Anatomy.* 2nd ed. New York: Springer-Verlag; 1982:105-185.
3. Dunnick R, McCallum RW, Sandler CM. *Textbook of Uroradiology.* Baltimore: Williams & Wilkins Co; 1991:1-14.
4. Damgaard-Pedersen K, von der Maase H. Ultrasound and ultrasound-guided biopsy, CT and lymphography in the diagnosis of retroperitoneal metastases in testicular cancer. *Scand J Urol Nephrol Suppl* 1991;137:139-144.
5. Nobrega J, dos Santos G. Aspirative cytology with fine needle in the abdomen, retroperitoneum and pelvic cavity: a seven-year experience of the Portuguese Institute of Oncology, Center of Porto. *Eur J Surg Oncol* 1994;20:37-42.
6. Jeffrey RB Jr. Imaging of the peritoneal cavity. *Curr Opin Radiol* 1991;3:471-473.
7. Zwiebel WJ. Aortic and iliac aneurysm. *Semin Ultrasound CT MR* 1992;13:53-68.
8. Carroll B. The retroperitoneum. In: Sarti DA, ed. *Diagnostic Ultrasound: Text and Cases.* 2nd ed. Chicago: Year Book; 1987:456-462.
9. Dodds WJ, Darweesh RM, Lawson TL et al. The retroperitoneal spaces revisited. *AJR* 1986;147:1155-1161.
10. Rubenstein WA, Whalen JP. Extraperitoneal spaces. *AJR* 1986;147:1162-1164.
11. Hartman DS, Hayes WS, Choyke PL, Tibbetts GP. From the archives of the AFIP. Leiomyosarcoma of the retroperitoneum and inferior vena cava: radiologic-pathologic correlation. *Radiographics* 1992;12:1203-1220.

Scanning Technique

12. Langer JE, Nisenbaum HL, Coleman BG et al. Improved visualization of upper abdominal anatomy with SonoRx, an orally administered ultrasound contrast agent. *JUM* 1996;15,3(S):86.
13. Puylaert JB. Acute appendicitis: Ultrasound evaluation using graded compression. *Radiology* 1986;158:355-360.

Retroperitoneum

14. Chesbrough RM, Burkhard TK, Martinez AT. Gerota versus Zuckerkandl: the renal fascia revisited. *Radiology* 1989;173:845-846.
15. Gray H. *Gray's Anatomy.* 31st ed. London: Longmans; 1954:589-590.
16. Gray H. *Gray's Anatomy.* 31st ed. London: Longmans; 1954:640-642.
17. Gray H. *Gray's Anatomy.* 31st ed. London: Longmans; 1954:572-576.
18. Callen PW, Filly RA, Sarti DA. Ultrasound of the diaphragmatic crura. *Radiology* 1979;130:721-724.
19. Callen PW, Filly RA, Marks WM. The quadratus lumborum muscle: a possible source of confusion in sonographic evaluation of the abdomen. *JCU* 1979;7:349-352.
20. Creagh-Barry M, Adam EJ, Joseph AE. The value of oblique scans in the ultrasonic examination of the abdominal aorta. *Clin Radiol* 1986;37:239-241.
21. Filly RA, Margalin S, Castellino RA. The ultrasonographic spectrum of abdominal and pelvic Hodgkins disease and non-Hodgkins lymphoma. *Cancer* 1976;38:2143-2148.
22. Jing BS. Diagnostic imaging of abdominal and pelvic lymph nodes in lymphoma. *Rad Clin North Am* 1990;28:801-831.
23. Castellino RA. The non-Hodgkin's lymphomas: practical concepts for the diagnostic radiologist. *Radiology* 1991;178:315-321.
24. Vassallo P, Wernecke K, Roos N, Peters PE. Differentiation of benign from malignant superficial lymphadenopathy: the role of high-resolution US. *Radiology* 1992;183:215-220.
25. Tschammler A, Ott G, Kumpfleins P et al. Differentiation of malignant from reactive lymphadenopathy using color Doppler flow imaging. *J Ultrasound Med* 1996;15:86.
26. Al-Mofleh IA. Ultrasound-guided fine-needle aspiration of retroperitoneal, abdominal and pelvic lymph nodes: Diagnostic reliability. *Acta Cytol* 1992;36:413-415.
27. Downey DB, Wilson SR. Sonographically guided biopsy of small intra-abdominal masses. *Can Assoc Radiol J* 1993;44:350-353.
28. Castellino RA, Billingham M, Dorfman RF. Lymphographic accuracy in Hodgkin's disease and malignant lymphoma with

a mote on the "reactive" lymph node as a cause of most false-positive lymphograms. *Invest Radiol* 1990;25:412-422.

29. Carroll BA. Ultrasound of lymphoma. *Semin Ultrasound* 1982;3:114-122.

30. Hillman BJ, Haber K. Echographic characteristics of malignant lymph nodes. *J Clin Ultrasound* 1980;8:213-215.

31. Bussar-Maatz R, Weissbach L. Retroperitoneal lymph node staging of testicular tumours. TNM Study Group. *Br J Urol* 1993;72:234-240.

32. Bohle A, Studer UE, Sonntag RW. Primary or secondary extra-gonadal germ cell tumors. *J Urol* 1986;135:939-943.

33. Choyke PL, Hayes WS, Sesterhenn IA. Primary extragonadal germ cell tumors of the retroperitoneum: differentiation of primary and secondary tumors. *Radiographics* 1993;13:1365-1375.

34. Davidson AJ, Hartman DS, Goldman SM. Mature teratoma of the retroperitoneum: radiologic, pathologic, and clinical correlation. *Radiology* 1989;172:421-425.

35. Dalton RR, Donohue JH, Mucha P. Management of retroperitoneal sarcomas. *Surgery* 1989;106:725-733.

36. Solla JA, Reed K. Primary retroperitoneal sarcoma. *Am J Surg* 1986;152:496-498.

37. Koci TM, Worthen NJ, Phillips JJ. Perirenal hemangioendothelioma in a newborn. *J Comput Assist Tomogr* 1989;13:145-147.

38. Siegal B, Swami V, Justin J et al. Ultrasonic tissue characterization of blood clots. *Surg Clin North Am* 1990;70:13-29.

39. Goldman SM, Davidson AJ, Neal J. Retroperitoneal and pelvic hemangiopericytomas: clinical, radiologic, and pathologic correlation. *Radiology* 1988;168:13-17.

40. Lee MJ, Saini S, Geller SC et al. Pancreatitis with pseudoaneurysm formation: a pitfall for the interventional radiologist. *AJR* 1991;156:97-98.

41. Degesys GE, Dunnick NR, Silverman PM. Retroperitoneal fibrosis: use of computed tomography in distinguishing among possible causes. *AJR* 1986;146:57-60.

42. Baker LRI, Mallinson WJW, Gregory MC. Idiopathic retroperitoneal fibrosis: a retrospective study of 60 cases. *Br J Urol* 1988;160:497-503.

43. Sanders RC, Duff T, McLoughlin MG. Sonography in the diagnosis of retroperitoneal fibrosis. *J Urol* 1977;118:944-946.

44. Fagan CJ, Amparo EG, Davis M. Retroperitoneal fibrosis. *Semin Ultrasound* 1982;3:123-138.

45. Fitzgerald EJ, Blackett RL. "Inflammatory" abdominal aortic aneurysms. *Clin Radiol* 1988;39:247-251.

46. Cullenward MJ, Scanlan KA, Pozniak MA, Acher CA. Inflammatory aortic aneurysm (periaortic fibrosis): radiologic imaging. *Radiology* 1986;159:75-82.

47. Lodge JP, Hall R. Retroperitoneal haemorrhage: a dangerous complication of common femoral arterial puncture. *Eur J Vasc Surg* 1993;7:355-357.

48. Kedar RP, Cosgrove DO. Case report: retroperitoneal varices mimicking a mass: diagnosis on colour Doppler. *Br J Radiol* 1994;67:661-662.

49. Graif M, Martinovitz U, Strauss S. Sonographic localization of hematomas in hemophilic patients with positive iliopsoas sign. *AJR* 1996;148:121-123.

50. Spring DB, Schroder D, Babu S. Ultrasonic evaluation of lymphocele formation after staging lymphadenectomy for prostate carcinoma. *Radiology* 1981;141:479-483.

51. Rifkin MD, Needleman L, Kurtz AB. Sonography of nongynecologic cystic masses of the pelvis. *AJR* 1984;142:1169-1174.

52. Akhan O, Cekirge S, Ozmen M. Percutaneous transcatheter ethanol sclerotherapy of postoperative pelvic lymphoceles. *Cardiovasc Intervent Radiol* 1992;15:224.

53. Derchi LE, Rizzatto G, Banderali A. Sonographic appearance of primary retroperitoneal cysts. *J Ultrasound Med* 1989;8:381-384.

54. Breidahl WH, Mendelson RM. Retroperitoneal lymphangioma. *Australas Radiol* 1995;39:187-191.

55. Iyer R, Eftekhari F, Varma D, Jaffe N. Cystic retroperitoneal lymphangioma: CT, ultrasound and MR findings. *Pediatr Radiol* 1993;23:305-306.

56. Davidson AJ, Hartman DS. Lymphangioma of the retroperitoneum: computed tomography and sonographic appearances. *Radiology* 1990;175:507-510.

57. DeLange EE, Black WC, Mills SE. Radiologic features of retroperitoneal cystic hamartoma. *Gastrointest Radiol* 1988;13:266-270.

58. Sussman SK, Jacobs JE, Glickstein MF, Foley LC. Cross-sectional imaging of idiopathic solitary renal vein varix: report of two cases. *Urol Radiol* 1991;13:98-102.

59. Reading CC. Palpable neck masses. In: Bluth EI, Arger PH, Hertzberg BS et al., eds. Syllabus: A Special Course in Ultrasound. Oak Brook: Radiological Society of North America; 1996:351-362.

60. Dunnick NR. Genitourinary tract trauma. In: McClennan BL, ed. Syllabus: A Categorical Course in Genitourinary Radiology. Oak Brook: Radiological Society of North America; 1994:95-102.

61. Jeffrey RB, Laing FC, Wing VW. Extraperitoneal spread of acute pancreatitis: new observations with real-time ultrasound. *Radiology* 1986;159:707-711.

62. Graham M, Chan A. Ultrasound screening for clinically occult abdominal aortic aneurysm. *Can Med Assoc J* 1988;138:627-629.

63. Castoldi MC, Del Moro RM, D'Urbano ML et al. Sonography after renal biopsy: assessment of its role in 230 consecutive cases. *Abdom Imaging* 1994;19:72-77.

64. Lumsden AB, Miller JM, Kosinski AS et al. A prospective evaluation of surgically treated groin complications following percutaneous cardiac procedures. *Am Surg* 1994;60:132-137.

65. Papanicolaou N, Stafford SA, Pfister RC. Significant renal hemorrhage following extracorporeal shock wave lithotripsy: imaging and clinical features. *Radiology* 1987;163:661-664.

66. Belville JS, Morgentaler A, Loughlin KR. Spontaneous periniphric and subcapsular renal hemorrhage: evaluation with computer tomography, ultrasound and angiography. *Radiology* 1989;172:733-738.

67. Tomaru T, Uchidi Y, Masuo M. Experimental canine arterial thrombus formation and thrombolysis: a fibreoptic study. *Am Heart J* 1987;114:63.

68. Kenney PJ. Chronic renal infections. In: McClennan BL, ed. Syllabus: A Categorical Course in Genitourinary Radiology. Oak Brook: Radiological Society of North America; 1994:51-54.

69. Hayes WS, Hartman DS, Sesterhenn IA. From the archives of the AFIP: xanthogranulomatous pyelonephritis. *Radiographics* 1991;11:485-498.

Great Vessels

70. Sonesson B, Hansen F, Stale H, Lanne T. Compliance and diameter in the human abdominal aorta—the influence of age and sex. *Eur J Vasc Surg* 1993;7:690-697.

71. Gray H. *Gray's Anatomy*. 31st ed. London: Longmans; 1954:783-805.

72. Burns PN. Hemodynamics. In: Taylor KJW, Burns PN, Wells PNT, eds. *Clinical Applications of Doppler Ultrasound*. 2nd ed. New York: Raven Press; 1995:35-53.

73. Pedersen OM, Aslaksen A, Vik-Mo H. Ultrasound measurement of the luminal diameter of the abdominal aorta and iliac arteries in patients without vascular disease. *J Vasc Surg* 1993;17:596-601.

74. Grimshaw GM, Thompson JM. The abnormal aorta: a statistical definition and strategy for monitoring change. *Eur J Vasc Endovasc Surg* 1995;10:95-100.

75. Lanne T, Sonesson B, Bergqvist D et al. Diameter and compliance in the male human abdominal aorta: influence of age and aortic aneurysm. *Eur J Vasc Surg* 1992;6:178-184.

76. Polak JF. Pathophysiology. In: Polak JF, ed. *Peripheral Vascular Sonography: A Practical Guide*. Baltimore: Williams & Wilkins; 1992:59-72.

77. Zwiebel WJ, Fracto D. Basics of abdominal and pelvic Doppler: instrumentation, anatomy, and vascular Doppler signatures. *Semin Ultrasound CT MR* 1992;13:3-21.

78. Allison DJ. Arteriography. In: Grainger RG, Allison DJ, eds. *Diagnostic Radiology: An Anglo-American Textbook of Imaging*. Vol 3. Edinburgh: Churchill Livingstone; 1986: 2014-2015.

79. Recchia D, Sharkey AM, Bosner MS et al. Sensitive detection of abnormal aortic architecture in Marfan syndrome with high-frequency ultrasonic tissue characterization. *Circulation* 1995;91:1036-1043.

80. Abdool-Carrim AT, Robbs JV, Kadwa AM et al. Aneurysms due to intimomedial mucoid degeneration. *Eur J Vasc Endovasc Surg* 1996;11:324-329.

81. Ballard DJ, Hallett JW. Natural History of aneurysms. In: Strandness DE, vanBreda A, eds. *Vascular Diseases: Surgical and Interventional Therapy*. New York: Churchill Livingstone; 1994;565-569.

82. Lobe TE, Richardson CJ, Boulden TF et al. Mycotic thromboaneurysmal disease of the abdominal aorta in preterm infants: its natural history and its management. *J Pediatr Surg* 1992;27:1054-1059.

83. Durham JD, Kaufman JA. Imaging of acquired thoracic and abdominal aortic disease. In: Strandness DE, vanBreda A, eds. *Vascular Diseases: Surgical and Interventional Therapy*. New York: Churchill Livingstone; 1994:258-263.

84. Cohen JR, Hallett JW. Pathophysiology of arterial aneurysm development. In: Strandness DE, vanBreda A, eds. *Vascular Diseases, Surgical and Interventional Therapy*. New York: Churchill Livingstone; 1994:559-564.

85. Nevitt MP, Ballard DJ, Hallett JW Jr. Prognosis of abdominal aortic aneurysms: a population-based study. *N Engl J Med* 1989;321:1009-1014.

86. Dent TL, Lindenauer SM, Ernst E et al. Multiple arteriosclerotic arterial aneurysms. *Arch Surg* 1972;105:338.

87. Johansen K, Koepsell T. Familial tendency for abdominal aortic aneurysms. *JAMA* 1986;256:1934.

88. Gordon IL, Kohl CA, Arefi M et al. Spinal cord injury increases the risk of abdominal aortic aneurysm. *Am Surg* 1996;62:249-252.

89. Lucarotti M, Shaw E, Poskitt K et al. The Gloucestershire aneurysm screening programme: the first 2 years' experience. *Eur J Vasc Surg* 1993;7:397-401.

90. Krohn CD, Kullmann G, Kvernebo K et al. Ultrasonographic screening for abdominal aortic aneurysm. *Eur J Surg* 1992; 158:527-530.

91. Lederle FA, Walker JM, Reinke DB. Selective scanning for abdominal aortic aneurysms with physical examination and ultrasound. *Arch Int Med* 1988;148:1783.

92. Joyce JW. Preoperative evaluation of aneurysms. In: Strandness DE, vanBreda A, eds. *Vascular Diseases: Surgical and Interventional Therapy*. New York: Churchill Livingstone; 1994;579-588.

93. Quill DS, Colgan MP, Summer DS. Ultrasonic screening for the detection of abdominal aortic aneurysms. *Surg Clin North Am* 1989;69:713-720.

94. Collin J, Araujo L, Walton J, Lindsell D. Oxford screening programme for abdominal aortic aneurysm in men aged 65 to 74 years. *Lancet* 1988;2:613-615.

95. Russell JG. Is screening for abdominal aortic aneurysm worthwhile? *Clin Radiol* 1990;41:182-184.

96. Guirguis EM, Barber GG. The natural history of abdominal aortic aneurysms. *Am J Surg* 1991;162:481-483.

97. Kaufman JA, Bettmann MA. Prognosis of abdominal aortic aneurysms: a population-based study. *Invest Radiol* 1991; 26:612-614.

98. Glimaker H, Holmberg L, Elvin A et al. Natural history of patients with abdominal aortic aneurysm. *Eur J Vasc Surg* 1991;5:125-130.

99. Bernstein EF, Chan EL. Abdominal aortic aneurysm in high-risk patients: outcome of selective management based on size and expansion rate. *Ann Surg* 1984;200:255-263.

100. Cronenwett JL, Murphy TF, Zelenock GB et. Actuarial analysis of variables associated with rupture of small abdominal aortic aneurysms. *Surgery* 1985;98:462-483.

101. Sterpetti AV, Shultz RD, Feldhaus RJ et al. Abdominal aortic aneurysm in elderly patients: selective management based on clinical status and aneurysm expansion rate. *Am J Surg* 1985; 150:772-776.

102. Moran KT, Persson AV, Jewell ER. Chronic rupture of abdominal aortic aneurysms. *Am J Surg* 1989;55:485-487.

103. Richardson JW, Greenfield LJ. Natural history and management of iliac aneurysms. *J Vasc Surg* 1988;8:165-171.

104. Scott RA, Wilson NM, Ashton HA et al. Is surgery necessary for abdominal aortic aneurysm less than 6 cm in diameter? *Lancet* 1993;342:1395-1396.

105. Fiorani P, Bondanini S, Faraglia V et al. Clinical and therapeutic evaluation of inflammatory aneurysms of the abdominal aorta. *Int Angiol* 1986;5:49-53.

106. Pennell RC, Hollier LH, Liu JT et al. Inflammatory aortic aneurysms: a thirty-year review. *J Vasc Surg* 1985;2:859.

107. Maloney JD, Pairolero PC, Smith SF et al. Ultrasound evaluation of abdominal aortic aneurysms. *Circulation* 1977; 56:80-85.

108. Zollner N, Zoller WG, Spengel F et al. The spontaneous course of small abdominal aortic aneurysms: aneurysmal growth rates and life expectancy. *Klin Wochenschr* 1991; 69:633-639.

109. Okuhn SP, Stoney RJ. Intraoperative use of ultrasound in arterial surgery. *Surg Clin North Am* 1990;70:61-70.

110. Guinet C, Buy JN, Ghossain MA et al. Aortic anastomotic pseudoaneurysms: US, CT, MR, and angiography. *J Comput Assist Tomogr* 1992;16:182-188.

111. Puyau FA, Adinolfi MF, Kerstein MD. Lymphocele around aortic femoral grafts simulating a false aneurysm. *Cardiovasc Intervent Radiol* 1985;8:195-198.

112. Hillman BJ. Disorders of the renal artery circulation and renal vascular hypertension. In: Pollack HM, ed. *Clinical Urography*. Philadelphia: WB Saunders Co; 1990:2127-2185.

113. King PS, Cooperberg PL, Madigan SM. The anechoic crescent in abdominal aortic aneurysms: not a sign of dissection. *AJR* 1986;146:345-348.

114. Wilson SE, Van Wagenen P, Panaro E. Arterial infection. *Curr Prob Surg* 1978;15:5.

115. Calligaro KD, Bergen WS, Savarese RP et al. Primary aortoduodenal fistula due to septic aortitis. *J Cardiovasc Surg (Torino)* 1992;33:192-198.

116. Fellmeth BD, Roberts AC, Bookstein JJ et al. Postangiographic femoral artery injuries: non-surgical repair with ultrasound-guided compression. *Radiology* 1991;178:671-675.

117. Feld R, Patton GM, Carabasi RA et al. Treatment of iatrogenic femoral artery injuries with ultrasound-guided compression. *J Vasc Surg* 1992;16:832-840.

118. Flinn WR, Rizzo RJ, Park JS et al. Duplex scanning for the assessment of mesenteric ischemia. *Surg Clin North Am* 1990;70:99-108.

119. Avasthi PS, Voyles WF, Greene ER. Non-invasive diagnosis of renal artery stenosis by echo-Doppler velocimetry. *Kidney International* 1984;25:824-829.

120. Boijsen E. Angiographic studies of the anatomy of single and multiple renal arteries. *Acta Radiol* 1959;183:1-135.

121. Desberg AL, Paughter DM, Lammert GK et al. Renal artery stenosis: evaluation with color Doppler flow imaging. *Radiology* 1990;177:749-753.

122. Stavros AT, Parker SH, Yakes WF et al. Segmental stenosis of the renal artery: pattern recognition of tardus and parvus abnormality with duplex sonography. *Radiology* 1992;184:487-492.

123. Needleman L. Hypertension and bruit. In: Bluth EI, Argon PH, Hertzberg BS, Middleton WD, eds. Syllabus: A Special Course in Ultrasound. Oak Brook: Radiological Society of North America; 1996:217-225.

124. Olin JW, Piedmonte MR, Young JR et al. The utility of duplex ultrasound scanning of the renal arteries for diagnosing significant renal artery stenosis. *Ann Intern Med* 1995;122:833-838.

125. Hoffman U, Edwards JM, Carter S et al. Role of duplex scaning for the detection of atherosclerotic renal artery disease. *Kidney Int* 1991;39:1232-1239.

126. Martin RL, Nanra RS, Wlodarczyk J et al. Renal hilar Doppler analysis in the detection of renal artery stenosis. *J Vasc Technol* 1991;15:173-180.

127. Gray H. *Gray's Anatomy*. 31st ed. London: Longamans, Green and Co., 1954:859-862.

128. Kellerman GH, Alpern MB, Sandler MA et al. Computed tomography of vena caval abnormalities with embryologic correlation. *Radiographics* 1988;8:533-556.

129. Goiney R. Ultrasound imaging of inferior vena caval thrombosis. *JUM* 1985;4:387-389.

130. Mewissen MW, Erickson SJ, Foley WD et al. Thrombosis at venous insertion sites after inferior vena caval filter placement. *Radiology* 1989;173:155-157.

131. Van Rooij WJ, Martens F, Vebeeton B et al. CT and MR imaging of leiomyosarioma of the inferior vena cava. *JCAT* 1988;12:415-419.

132. Beckman CF, Abrams HL. Renal venography: anatomy, technique, applications, analysis of 132 venograms, and a review of the literature. *AJR* 1982;138:339-341.

133. Mellins HZ. Renal vein obstruction. In: Pollack HM, ed. *Clinical Urolgraphy*. Philadelphia: WB Saunders Co; 1990: 2119-2126.

134. Rosenberg ER, Trought WS, Kirks DR et al. Ultrasonic diagnosis of renal vein thrombosis in neonates. *AJR* 1980;134:35-38.

135. Brill PW, Mitty HA, Straus L. Renal vein thrombosis: a cause of intrarenal calcification in the newborn. *Pediatr Radiol* 1977;6:172-175.

136. Patriquin HB, Lafortune MA. Doppler sonography of the child's abdomen. In: Taylor KJW, Burns PN, Wells PNT, eds. *Clinical Applications of Doppler Ultrasound*. 2nd ed. New York: Raven Press, 1995.

137. Bolondi L, Gaiani S, Simoncelli S et al. Changes in hepatic venous flow in liver disease assessed by Doppler US: Relationship with histology. *J Hepatol* 1991;13(suppl):98.

138. Adkins J, Wilson SR. Unusual course of the gonadol vein: a case report of postpartum avoniem vein thrombosis mimicking acute appendicitis clinically and sonographically. *JUIM* 1996;15:409-412.

C H A P T E R   1 3

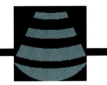

The Abdominal Wall

•

Khanh T. Nguyen, M.Sc., M.D., F.R.C.P.C.
Eric E. Sauerbrei, B.Sc., M.Sc., M.D., F.R.C.P.C.
Robert L. Nolan, B.Sc., M.D., F.R.C.P.C.
Bernard J. Lewandowski, M.D.

A common indication for scanning the abdominal wall is the presence of a palpable mass. Is the mass in the wall or inside the abdominal cavity? Is it cystic or solid? Sonography can readily give the answer to these questions. Occasionally, an abnormality is found in the abdominal wall during routine scanning of the intraabdominal organs.

SCANNING TECHNIQUES

Because the skin is "out of focus" with even the highest-frequency transducers, scanning the skin requires various stand-off techniques to obtain the best resolution and to avoid the "bang effect" of direct transducer placement on the skin. Flotation pads that are liquid-filled microcell sponges,* synthetic polymer blocks,† and silicone elastomer blocks‡ are commercially available. These substances are dense enough to stand unsupported and have a uniform consistency to minimize artifacts.

Scanning the abdominal wall requires no special patient preparation. The examination can be performed over surgical wounds by applying an adhesive plastic membrane§ over the wound after removing the dressing.[1] The adhesive is sterile and prevents both

*Reston flotation pad, 3M Company, Minneapolis, Minn.
†Kitecko, 3M Company, St. Paul, Minn.
‡Echomould, AHS/Belgium, Steenweg op Zellick 30, B-1080, Brussels, Belgium.
§Op-site, Smith and Nephew, Welwyn Garden City, Hertfordshire, England.

contamination of the wound by the transducer and contamination of the transducer by an infected wound or draining sinus. Gentle pressure with the transducer is applied, but excessive pressure should be avoided over wounds and other tender areas. The highest frequency possible that allows penetration to the area of interest should be used; this usually is accomplished with a high-frequency linear array probe.

ANATOMY

The abdominal wall is divided into anterior, anterolateral, and posterior parts, and is best appreciated on

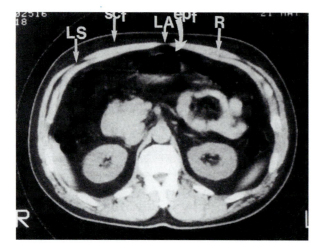

FIG. 13-1. **CT of abdomen showing the normal anatomy of anterior abdominal wall.** *LA*, linea alba; *LS*, linea semilunaris; *R*, rectus muscle; *scf*, subcutaneous fat; *epf*, extraperitoneal fat.

a transverse computed tomography (CT) scan (Fig. 13-1) or in schematic form (Fig. 13-2). The anterior abdominal wall is a laminated structure. From the outermost layer working in, the wall includes the skin, the superficial fascia, the subcutaneous fat, the muscle layers, the transversalis fascia, and a layer of extraperitoneal fat. The anterior muscle layer is composed of the paired midline rectus muscles and the anterolaterally situated external oblique, the internal oblique, and transversus abdominis muscles. The rectus abdominis muscles insert superiorly into the fifth, sixth, and seventh ribs and extend inferiorly to the pubic crest. They are enclosed anteriorly and posteriorly by the rectus sheath, which is formed by the aponeuroses of the internal oblique, external oblique, and transversus muscles. The posterior caudal aspect of the sheath ends at the arcuate line, which is situated usually midway between the umbilicus and the symphysis pubis. Distal to the arcuate line, the aponeuroses of all three muscles pass in front of the rectus muscle, which is then separated posteriorly from the peritoneum only by the transversalis fascia.[2] At the medial border of the rectus, the aponeuroses fuse to form the linea alba, which separates the rectus muscles in the midline.

The normal epidermis is a highly reflective layer measuring 1 to 4 mm in thickness.[3] The subcutaneous fat layer is of variable thickness. A significant amount of work has been done to determine the usefulness of this sonographic measurement to predict total body density and to compare the ability of ultrasound assessment with traditional caliper techniques in measuring subcutaneous fat. Real-time sonography has

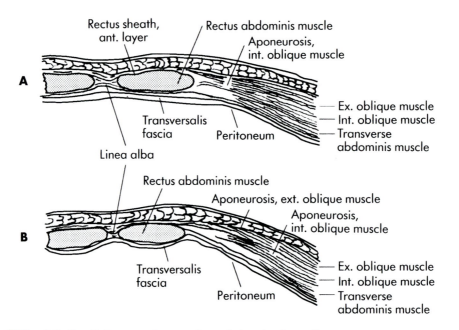

FIG. 13-2. **Schema of anterior abdominal wall,** **A,** above arcuate line and, **B,** below arcuate line.

proven as effective as caliper techniques in cadaver experiments[4] as well as in young male and obese subjects whereas A-mode scanning is less effective but probably more convenient than CT scanning.[5-8] One report, however, concluded that total abdominal circumference provides a better estimate of body fat in obese women than does ultrasound measurement of subcutaneous fat because ultrasound did not measure the deep fat. Nonetheless, these measurements are important in sports medicine and in obesity clinics.

Over the years there have been conflicting reports concerning the echogenicity of fat. Some fatty tissues (e.g., breast lipomas) are relatively anechoic, and subcutaneous fat is relatively hypoechoic; however, fat in the liver is echogenic.[9] The spectrum of echogenicity displayed by fat and fatty tissues can be explained by the water content within the fat. In an in vitro experiment, margarine (containing 85% vegetable oil and 15% water) scanned in a water bath was echogenic and attenuated sound whereas when the margarine melted, floating echogenic globules were seen. When the margarine was heated until the water vaporized and then rescanned after cooling, the substance was anechoic.[9] The authors concluded that not only is pure fat anechoic, but that a mixture of fat and water is echogenic.

Because water and fat are immiscible, there are multiple fat/water and water/fat interfaces, each with a significant acoustic impedance mismatch that causes the marked echogenicity.[10]

The musculofascial layer is usually more echogenic than the subcutaneous fat layer (Fig. 13-3, A). With high-resolution probes, individual muscle bundles can be identified that show fairly uniform texture and orientation (Fig. 13-3, B). Because the muscles of the back are thicker, they are more difficult to visualize in detail than the muscles of the anterolateral walls.

The extraperitoneal fat collection posterior to the muscles appears thick in many people, particularly those who are obese, at the level of the linea alba and linea semilunaris (see Fig. 13-3, A). This acts as the source of the split image artifact, which will be discussed later in this chapter. It should not be mistaken for a tumor.

PATHOLOGY

Cutaneous Lesions

Sonographic evaluation of the skin has been used to detect clinically occult foci of recurrent or metastatic melanoma and has been used to guide fine-needle aspiration biopsies of these lesions.[11,12] Pigmented nevi and malignant melanomas are clearly demarcated from normal skin (Fig. 13-4). Most melanomas are hypoechoic and demonstrate enhancement through transmission. Although malignant melanoma is rarely found on the anterior abdominal wall, almost 75% of patients with melanoma develop cutaneous or subcutaneous metastases.[12] More importantly, the nodules may be found in unexpected locations.

Hernias

Ventral Hernia. Ventral hernias may be acquired or congenital. Acquired hernias are more frequently seen in patients who are obese or elderly or in

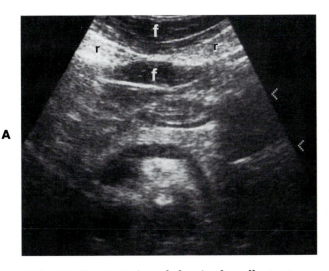

A

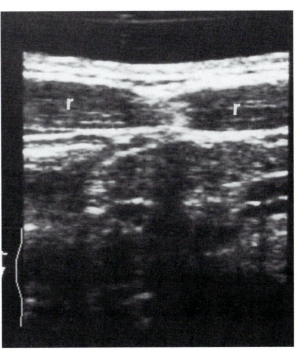

B

FIG. 13-3. Anterior abdominal wall. **A,** Transverse scan. The muscles appear echogenic. The fat, *f,* appears hypoechoic. Note the prominent extraperitoneal fat collection that appears lens-shaped. **B,** Sagittal scan. The individual muscle bundles, *r,* appear hypoechoic in this thin patient.

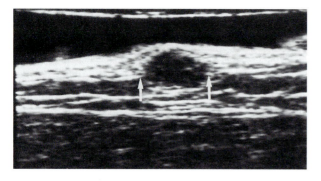

FIG. 13-4. Subcutaneous metastatic melanoma. The nodule appears hypoechoic. Note disruption of the skin layer *(arrows)*.

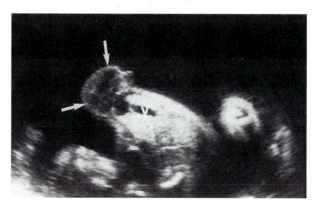

FIG. 13-6. Omphalocele seen in utero at 18 weeks' menstrual age. Note the umbilical vein, *v*, running into the omphalocele *(arrows)*, which is covered by a membrane.

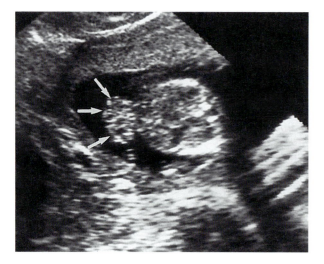

FIG. 13-5. Gastroschisis seen in utero at 17 weeks' menstrual age. Note the mass of herniated bowel *(arrows)* in this transverse view of the fetus.

those with previous trauma or surgery. The typical locations are at points of weakness where no muscle is present, along the linea alba in the midline or the linea semilunaris on each side (spigelian hernia), and in the inferior lumbar space.[13-15] The fascial defect and the herniated contents (omental fat or bowel) are usually identified by careful scanning with a 7.5 MHz linear array transducer. Seen in cross section, herniated bowel loops appear as target lesions with strong reflective central echoes representing air in the lumen. When obstructed, they appear as tubular, fluid-filled structures containing valvulae conniventes (small bowel) or fecal material (colon). Congenital ventral hernias consist of gastroschisis and omphalocele. **Gastroschisis** (Fig. 13-5) occurs in about 1 per 174,000 births and usually as an isolated anomaly. The abdominal wall defect is usually on the right side of the umbilical cord insertion, with herniation of small bowel not covered by a membrane. In contrast, **omphalocele** (Fig. 13-6) occurs directly at the site of

the umbilical cord insertion. It is three times more common than gastroschisis and is associated with other organ malformations. The hernia sac usually contains liver and/or bowel. Both conditions may be detected by sonography in the fetus in utero as early as 18 weeks' menstrual age.[16]

Spigelian Hernia. Spigelian hernia, the only spontaneous hernia of the lateral abdominal wall, was first described in the year 1721.[17,18] It consists of a defect in the aponeurosis of the transversus abdominis muscle lateral to the rectus sheath. The most common location of spigelian hernias is at or near the junction of linea semilunaris and the arcuate line. Before the use of high-resolution sonography, the diagnosis of spigelian hernia was missed in 50% of cases preoperatively because the classic findings are often missing.[19,20] The sonographic diagnosis of a spigelian hernia depends on the demonstration of a defect at any point in the linea semilunaris that represents the hernial orifice[21] (Fig. 13-7). If associated with protrusion of deep tissues, the hernia is usually bounded anteriorly by the external oblique aponeurosis. The external aponeurosis is so thick at this level that only 15 of 876 patients have been reported to have a subcutaneous hernial sac. More than 280 articles and 5 medical theses have been published on spigelian hernias, yet a review of the literature by Spangen revealed that only 876 patients had undergone surgery.[22] It should be noted that all patients with a spigelian hernia have tenderness over the orifice on palpation.

Lumbar Hernia. Lumbar hernias are uncommon and are most often acquired rather than congenital.[23,24] Spontaneous hernias occur in two areas of weakness in the flank: the inferior (Petit's hernia) and superior (Grynfeltt hernia) lumbar triangles. Acquired lumbar hernias are usually posttraumatic or iatrogenic.[25,26]

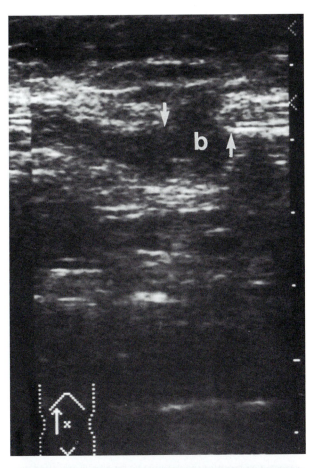

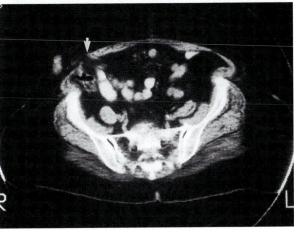

FIG. 13-7. Spigelian hernia. A, Ultrasound appearance. Bowel, *b,* is seen herniating through the fascial defect *(arrows).* **B,** CT appearance. Note the hernia orifice *(arrow).*

Lumbar hernias are usually asymptomatic. Since the neck of the hernia is wide, strangulation is uncommon, occurring in about 10% of cases. It is postulated that they are more common in females because of the wider pelvis.[27] The diagnosis depends on cross-sectional imaging, usually CT.[28-30] There has been, however, at least one case report in which the diagnosis was made sonographically.[31] In this case, sonography showed fluid-filled loops of small bowel extending from the peritoneal cavity into a mid-flank mass.

Incisional Hernia. Incisional hernias are delayed complications of abdominal surgery and occur in 0.5% to 14% of patients[32-34]; the current rate is about 4%. Since almost 2 million abdominal operations are performed in the United States every year, the problem is not a trivial one.[35,36] Enlargement of these hernias will usually manifest within the first year; however, 5% to 10% will remain silent.[37] Clinically unsuspected incisional hernias are often detected by CT scanning.[38] Sonography may occasionally identify a herniated bowel loop at the incision site.

Inguinal Hernia. The inguinal canal extends from the deep inguinal ring to the superficial inguinal ring. The deep inguinal ring is a defect in the transversalis fascia anterior to the femoral vessels and above the inguinal ligament. The superficial inguinal ring is an opening in the aponeurosis of the external oblique muscle. Hesselbach's triangle is formed by the lateral border of the rectus sheath medially, the inferior epigastric artery laterally, and the inguinal ligament inferiorly. Direct inguinal hernias protrude through a weakened inguinal canal floor medial to the inferior epigastric artery whereas an indirect hernia exits via the deep inguinal ring (i.e., lateral to the inferior epigastric artery) and courses through the inguinal canal. Both direct and indirect inguinal hernias can extend into the scrotum.

Since both the superficial inguinal ring and the inferior epigastric artery are not easily seen sonographically, ultrasound has not been helpful in distinguishing direct from indirect inguinal hernias. However, sonography can distinguish hernias from other inguinal canal masses such as undescended testicles or varicoceles.[39] Inguinal sonography can be useful in delineating the superior aspect of a scrotal mass[40] and defining the presence of intestine and/or omentum in a hernial sac.

Sonography can detect complications of inguinal herniorrhaphy. The most common acute complication is hematoma extending from the inguinal canal into the scrotum. Less common complications include epididymitis and ischemic orchitis. Delayed scrotal swelling (several months after surgery) is usually secondary to a small hydrocele.[41] One theory is that inguinal herniorrhaphy aggravates an existing hydrocele by disturbing the lymphatic drainage.[42]

Femoral Hernia. Sonography is recommended in patients with groin pain and no palpable mass,[43] questionable palpable masses, and elderly obese patients with unexplained abdominal pain.[44] Up to 70% of nonobstructed femoral hernias are misdiagnosed by nonsurgical practitioners,[45] and 25% of femoral hernias are misdiagnosed surgically because they can be incarcerated and yet be impalpable.[46] The boundaries of the femoral canal are the femoral vein laterally, the superior pubic ramus posteriorly, and the ileopubic tract anteromedially. The sonographic detection of a femoral hernia depends on the demonstration of a mass medial to the femoral vein (Fig. 13-8). The mass must then be differentiated from other masses found in the femoral triangle, which include hematomas, pseudoaneurysms, arteriovenous (AV) fistulae, lipomas, lymph nodes, hydroceles, saphenous varices, and inguinal hernias.

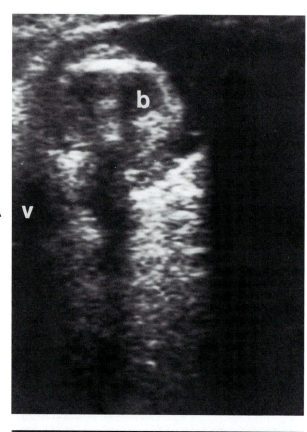

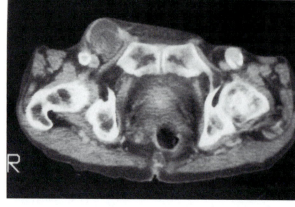

FIG. 13-8. Strangulated femoral hernia. A, Transverse scan. Note the target appearance typical of a dilated bowel loop, *b*, medial to the vessels, *v*. B, CT scan. The mass in the right groin is indistinguishable from a vascular or nodal lesion.

Rectus Sheath Hematoma

Rectus sheath hematomas are either posttraumatic or spontaneous. The traumatic causes include direct trauma, surgery, or sudden vigorous abdominal contractions that may occur with seizures, paroxysms of coughing,[47] sneezing, defecation, urination, and intercourse.[48,49] Recently a single case of rectus sheath hematoma as a complication of tetanus has been reported.[50] Anticoagulant therapy is the most common cause of spontaneous rectus sheath hematoma. Other less common associations include collagen diseases, steroid therapy, pregnancy,[51] and bleeding disorders.[52] Bleeding is usually secondary to either the rupture of the epigastric artery or veins or a primary tear of the muscle fibers.[53] The bleeding is usually intramuscular but may be extramuscular and confined by the rectus sheath. The tamponade effect of the sheath usually limits the size of the hematomas; however, there is a case report of a massive hematoma where the bleeding site was identified sonographically.[54] Clinical findings include abdominal pain, palpable mass, ecchymosis, and the Fothergill sign,[55,56,57] which involves palpating the suspected abdominal mass while the patient tenses the abdominal muscles. An abdominal wall mass will remain fixed whereas an intraabdominal mass will become less apparent. The sonographic appearance depends on the location of bleed with respect to the arcuate line, its age, and the transducer frequency. Above the arcuate line, the linea alba prevents the spread of hematoma across the midline; thus the hematomas are ovoid transversely and biconcave in the long axis.[58,59] Below the arcuate line, blood can spread to the pelvis or cross the midline, forming a large mass that indents on the dome of the urinary bladder (Fig. 13-9).

Fluid Collections

Fluid collections are usually seromas, liquefying hematomas, or abscesses related to previous surgery or trauma. Occasionally, a urachal cyst may be seen extending from the umbilicus to the dome of the urinary bladder.[39] A urachal cyst may be complicated by hemorrhage or infection (urachal abscess).[59] Uncommonly, tumors may arise in the urachus in children or young adults.[60]

Sterile fluid collections are usually echo-free. When complicated by hemorrhage or infection, they appear more complex, with septations and/or layering low-level echoes representing blood cells or debris (Fig. 13-10). Fluid collections may be aspirated percutaneously under sonographic guidance, with the specimen sent for Gram's stain and culture and sensitivity.

Vascular Lesions
Subcutaneous Arterial Bypass Grafts.
High-resolution sonography is ideal in imaging sub-

cutaneous axillofemoral and femorofemoral arterial bypass grafts.[61-64] Postoperatively, the grafts demonstrate transient, small, perigraft fluid collections at the level of the surgical tunnels, which disappear as the graft is incorporated into the subcutaneous tissues. Persistent perigraft fluid collections or localized collections are abnormal and are usually seromas or abscesses.[65] Any abnormal perigraft fluid collection should be followed until it resolves or a definitive diagnosis is made. Although loss of pulsatility within the graft may indicate thrombosis,[66] duplex Doppler and color flow Doppler imaging make the diagnosis easier. Other reported complications include graft aneurysms due to failure of the graft and pseudoaneurysms.

Pseudoaneurysms and Arteriovenous Fistulas.
Most femoral artery pseudoaneurysms involve the common femoral artery and are secondary to vascular reconstruction.[67,68] Pseudoaneurysm is also a well-known but uncommon complication of femoral artery catheterization, with an incidence of 0.1%.[69] Arteriovenous (AV) fistulas are considerably rarer. A pseudoaneurysm is a pulsatile hematoma secondary to bleeding into the soft tissue, with fibrous encapsulation and a persistent communication between the vessel and the fluid space. The vessel wall does not heal, and the blood flows back and forth between the two spaces during the cardiac cycle.[70-72] Most hematomas and pseudoaneurysms are within 2 cm of the arterial injury. The real-time criteria of pseudoaneurysm include echogenic swirls within a cystic cavity, expansile pulsatility, hypoechoic mass, and a visible tract.[73] When present, echogenic swirls are diagnostic of a pseudoaneurysm. Unfortunately, they are not often seen. Similarly, expansile pulsatility is difficult to evaluate and has not always been helpful.[74] A fistulous tract is the least observed sonographic finding (Fig. 13-11). Thus the ultrasound findings alone may not be sufficient to distinguish a hematoma from a pseudoaneurysm.[75] Duplex Doppler and color flow Doppler imaging have increased our ability to distinguish these entities.[76] The Doppler characteristics of a pseudoaneurysm include arterial flow within a mass separate from the artery and to-and-fro flow between the artery and the mass. One author states that demonstration of to-and-fro flow at the neck of the pseudoaneurysm is not a necessary condition for the diagnosis of a pseudoaneurysm and reports sensitivities of 94% and specificities of 97%, with an accuracy of 96% using the first criterion alone.[77] With duplex Doppler imaging the sample volume should interrogate the cavity and not an adjacent small vessel whereas with color flow Doppler imaging, a perivascular color flow artifact should not be interpreted as representing abnormal flow within a pseudoaneurysm.[78] A false-positive diagnosis using color has been reported in a case of necrotizing lymphadenitis

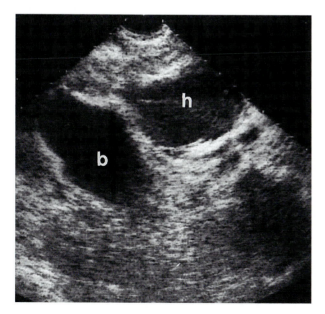

FIG. 13-9. Rectus sheath hematoma. Sagittal scan of the pelvis shows a collection, *h*, with a fluid-fluid level. Distal to the arcuate line, it dips down into the pelvis to compress the urinary bladder, *b*.

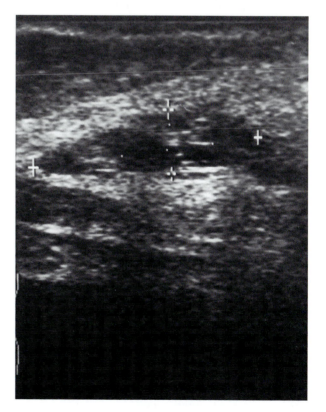

FIG. 13-10. Infected seroma. Pus was obtained from this irregular septated collection beneath a recent surgical incision.

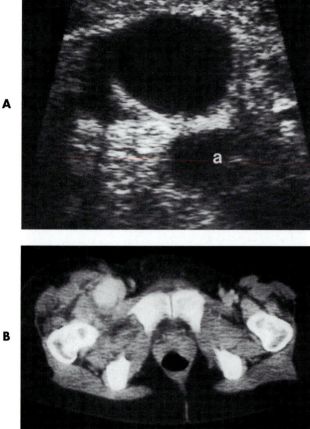

A

B

FIG. 13-11. Pseudoaneurysm. A, Transverse scan of right groin shows a cystic pulsatile mass anterior to the femoral artery, *a.* **B,** CT scan through the level of the right groin shows contrast material in the pseudoaneurysm.

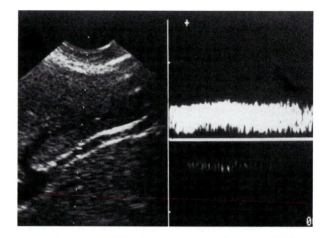

FIG. 13-12. Recanalized paraumbilical vein (sagittal scan). Typical venous Doppler signal was obtained from this tubular structure running from the left portal vein to the umbilicus.

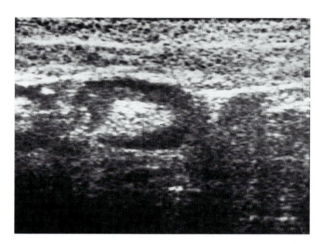

FIG. 13-13. Lymphomatous nodes in the groin showing reactive morphology with a hypoechoic rim and an echogenic center. The majority of lymphomatous nodes are hypoechoic or even anechoic. Biopsies are required to confirm the diagnosis.

after arteriography where the mass was mistaken for a false aneurysm on the basis of a jet within the hilum of the inflamed inguinal lymph node.[79]

Varices. A recanalized umbilical vein seen in portal hypertension (Fig. 13-12), saphenous varices, and varicoceles found in the femoral triangle and inguinal area are easily identified since they are characteristically compressible and have typical venous Doppler characteristics.

Lymph Nodes

Ultrasound can be used to detect lymphadenopathy when there is no palpable mass, or it can be used to categorize a palpable groin mass as lymphadenopathy. Although it was originally thought that normal lymph nodes are not detected sonographically because they are indistinguishable from subcutaneous fat,[80] high-resolution sonography can detect pathologically proven normal superficial lymph nodes. Most nodes are ovoid in shape and are variable in size. Very few are homogeneous. They vary in echogenicity, de-

pending on the degree of central lipomatosis.[81] Thus the center of the node is echogenic, and the periphery is hypoechoic. With extensive lipomatosis, the node may become indistinguishable from the surrounding subcutaneous tissue. Ultrasound is more effective in demonstrating lymphadenopathy than is clinical palpation,[82-84] and it is useful for staging lymphoma and for monitoring therapy.[85] There is no criterion to distinguish malignant from inflammatory lymphadenopathy, and the metastatic inference must be confirmed by biopsy. Although not all enlarged nodes are malignant and not all malignant nodes are enlarged, there are some sonographic clues available to help distinguish malignant from inflamed nodes. Lymphomatous nodes are extremely hypoechoic (Fig. 13-13) and may even be anechoic, especially in non-

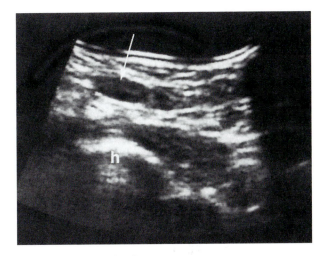

FIG. 13-14. Undescended testicle. Sagittal scan of the right groin reveals an ovoid hypoechoic mass *(arrow)* anterior to the hip, *h.*

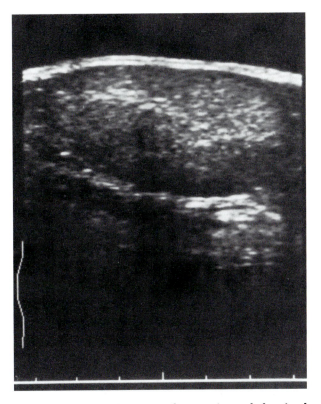

FIG. 13-15. Lipoma of anterior abdominal wall. The lesion is well encapsulated and highly echogenic.

Hodgkin's lymphoma.[80] A recent study of patients with palpable lymph nodes suggests that a 1 to 3 mm central artery can be seen centrally within enlarged lymphomatous nodes whereas in lymph nodes with carcinomatous involvement the central artery is not seen sonographically because it is infiltrated and destroyed on microscopy.[86] As discussed in the section on pseudoaneurysms, this central artery has been identified in one case of lymphadenitis.

Undescended Testicles

Cryptorchidism is the most common congenital anomaly of the male reproductive system, with an incidence of between 0.23% and 0.8% in the adult population.[87] It is bilateral in 10% to 25% of all cases.[88,89] Testicular descent can stop at any point between the hilum of the ipsilateral kidney to the external inguinal ring.[90,91] Of all undescended testicles, 80% are palpable and 20% are not palpable. Of those that are not palpable, 80% are in the inguinal canal and the remaining 20% are intraabdominal[92,93]; the testicle is absent in 4% of cases when it is not palpable. Sonography is useful in the detection of undescended testicles (Fig. 13-14). The undescended testis often appears smaller than the normal testis. It usually appears ovoid, and its long axis is usually parallel to the inguinal canal. Visualization of the echogenic hilum of the lymph node should distinguish the structure from a testicle. Unfortunately, although sonography can often detect testicles that are in the inguinal canal, it is less successful in detecting intraabdominal testicles.[94-96]

Neoplasms

The abdominal wall is an uncommon site for neoplastic disease. The most common primary neoplasms are **desmoid tumors,** which arise from fascia or aponeurosis of muscles. The most common location is in the anterior abdominal wall. Desmoid tumors are usually seen in patients with previous abdominal surgery and often occur at the site of the previous laparotomy scar. They also occur in patients with familial polyposis and are often associated with pregnancy. Of patients with desmoid tumors, 70% are between 20 to 40 years of age. There is a 3:1 female preponderance.[97-102] CT and ultrasound are ideal methods to demonstrate both the site and extent of the mass.[99] Lipoma (Fig. 13-15), neuroma, and neurofibroma are occasionally seen.

The most frequent malignant subcutaneous nodules are **metastatic melanoma.** Secondary malignancies from lymphoma or carcinoma of the lung, breast, ovary, and colon are less frequent.[39,59] The metastasis may occur as an isolated finding (Fig. 13-16), but more often it is seen in patients with widespread metastatic disease elsewhere. The abdominal wall may also be locally invaded by malignancies arising from the pleura, peritoneum, diaphragm (mesothelioma, rhabdomyosarcoma, fibrosarcoma), or intraabdominal organs such as the colon.

ARTIFACTS

The anatomic arrangement of the lower abdominal wall has been implicated in an important artifact observed deep in the pelvis. It has been called a "ghost artifact" (named after the "ghosting" seen in television images) or, more appropriately, the split-image artifact.[103-105]

The split-image artifact arises because of the presence of extraperitoneal fat deep to the linea alba and rectus abdominis muscles. In transverse scan planes at the midline, sound rays are refracted at the muscle/fat interfaces in such a way that smaller structures in the abdomen or pelvis may be completely duplicated. For example, a small gestational sac may appear as two sacs, one small embryo may appear as two embryos, one aorta may appear as two aortas, and so on. The effect is usually seen only when the collection of fat beneath the linea alba is large (and thus the muscle/fat interfaces lie in an oblique orientation) and the structure of interest is deep below the abdominal wall.

Scanning in sagittal and oblique scan planes will fail to demonstrate the duplicated images seen in the transverse scans and thus resolve the ambiguity (Fig. 13-17).

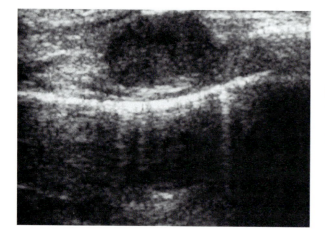

FIG. 13-16. Metastasis in anterior abdominal wall. A hypoechoic nodule, a metastatic tumor from renal cell carcinoma, is seen superficial to the peritoneum, which shows as a strong white line. (Courtesy of Stephanie R. Wilson, M.D., University of Toronto.)

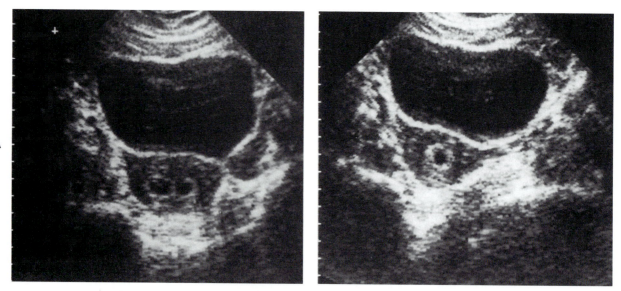

A

B

FIG. 13-17. Split-image artifact. A, Two gestational sacs were seen in this transverse scan of the pelvis. B, In fact, only one gestational sac was present. When the transducer is angled or the parasagittal plane is scanned, the artifact will disappear. In the upper abdomen, a double aorta or double superior mesenteric artery may be seen because of this artifact.

REFERENCES
Scanning Techniques
1. Fataar S, Goodman H, Tuft R et al. Postoperative abdominal sonography using a transsonic sealing membrane. *AJR* 1983;141:565-566.

Anatomy
2. Warwick R, Williams PL, eds. *Gray's Anatomy*. Edinburgh: Longman Group Ltd; 1978:519-527.
3. Shafir R, Itzchak Y, Heymen Z et al. Preoperative ultrasonic measurements of the thickness of cutaneous malignant melanoma. *J Ultrasound Med* 1984;3:205-208.
4. Jones PR, Davies PS, Norgan NG. Ultrasonic measurements of subcutaneous adipose tissue in man. *Am J Phys Anthropol* 1986;73:359-363.
5. Weits T, van der Beek EJ, Wedel M. Comparison of skinfold caliper measurements of subcutaneous fat tissue. *Int J Obesity* 1986;10:161-168.
6. Kuczmarski RJ, Fanelli MT. Ultrasonic assessment of body composition in obese adults: overcoming the limitations of the skinfold caliper. *Am J Clin Nutr* 1987;45:717-724.
7. Chumlea WC, Roche AF. Ultrasonic and skinfold caliper measures of subcutaneous adipose tissue thickness in elderly men and women. *Am J Phys Anthropol* 1986;71:351-357.
8. Black D, Vora J, Hayward M et al. Measurement of subcutaneous fat thickness with high frequency pulsed ultrasound: comparison with a caliper and a radiographic technique. *Clin Phys Physiol Measure* 1988;9:57-64.
9. Behan M, Kazam E. The echogenic characteristics of fatty tissues and tumors. *Radiology* 1978;129:143-151.
10. Errabolu RL, Sehgal CM, Bahn RC et al. Measurement of ultrasonic nonlinear parameter in excised fat tissue. *Ultrasound Med Biol* 1988;14:137-146.

Pathology
11. Fornage BD. Fine-needle aspiration biopsy with a vacuum test tube. *Radiology* 1988;169:553.
12. Fornage BD, Lorigan JG. Sonographic detection and fine-needle aspiration biopsy of nonpalpable recurrent or metastatic melanoma in subcutaneous tissues. *J Ultrasound Med* 1989;8:421-424.
13. Thomas JL, Cunningham JJ. Ultrasonic evaluation of ventral hernias disguised as intra-abdominal neoplasms. *Arch Surg* 1978;113:589-590.
14. Rubio PA, Del Castillo H, Alvaraz A. Ventral hernia in a massively obese patient: diagnosis by computed tomography. *South Med J* 1981;10:1307-1308.
15. Spangen L. Ultrasound as a diagnostic aid in ventral abdominal hernia. *J Clin Ultrasound* 1975;3:211-213.
16. Sauerbrei EE, Nguyen TK, Nolan RL. The fetus. In: Sauerbrei EE, ed. *A Practical Guide to Ultrasound in Obstetrics and Gynecology*. New York: Raven Press; 1987:111-159.
17. La Chausse BI. De hernia ventrali 1746. In: Haller: *Disputations Chirurgicales*. Bosquet (Lausanne) 1755;3:181-211.
18. LeDran HF. Observation de Chirurgie. Paris: C. Osmont; 1771:143.
19. Weiss Y, Lernau O, Nissan S. Spigelian hernia. *Ann Surg* 1974;180:836-839.
20. Deitch EA, Engel JM. Spigelian hernia: an ultrasound diagnosis. *Arch Surg* 1980;115:93.
21. Spangen L. Spigelian hernia. *Acta Chir Scand (Suppl)* 1976;462.
22. Spangen L. Spigelian hernia. *World J Surg* 1989;13:573-580.
23. Swartz WT. Lumbar hernia. In: Nyhus LM, Condon RE, eds. *Hernia*, 2nd ed. Philadelphia: JB Lippincott Co; 1978:409-426.

24. Ponka JL. Lumbar hernia. In: Ponka JL. *Hernias of the Abdominal Wall*. Philadelphia: WB Saunders Co; 1980:465-477.
25. Quick CR. Traumatic lumbar hernia. *Br J Surg* 1982;69:160-162.
26. Castelein RM, Sauter AJ. Lumbar hernia in an iliac bone graft. *Acta Orthop Scand* 1985;56:2273-2274.
27. Light HG. Hernia of the inferior lumbar space: a cause of back pain. *Arch Surg* 1983;118:1077-1080.
28. Lawdahl R, Moss CN, Van Dyke JA. Inferior lumbar (Petit's) hernia. *AJR* 1986;147:744-745.
29. Baker ME, Weinerth JL, Andriani RT et al. Lumbar hernia: diagnosis by CT. *AJR* 1987;148:565-567.
30. Chenoweth J, Vas W. Computed tomography demonstration of inferior lumbar (Petit's) hernia. *Clin Imag* 1989;13:164-166.
31. Siffring PA, Forrest TS, Frick MP. Hernia of the inferior lumbar space: diagnosis with US. *Radiology* 1989;170:190.
32. Fischer JD, Turner FW. Abdominal incisional hernias—a 10 year review. *Can J Surg* 1974;17:202-204.
33. Bucknall TE, Cox PJ, Ellis H. Burst abdomen and incisional hernia: a prospective study of 1129 major laparotomies. *Br Med J* 1982;284:931-933.
34. Baker RJ. Incisional hernia. In: Nyhus LM, Condon RE, eds. *Hernia*. 2nd ed. Philadelphia: JB Lippincott Co; 1978:329-341.
35. Larson GM, Vandertoll DJ. Approaches to repair of ventral hernia and full thickness losses of the abdominal wall. *Surg Clin North Am* 1984;64:335-349.
36. Ghahremani GG, Meyers MA. Iatrogenic abdominal hernias. In: Meyers MA, Ghahremani GG. *Iatrogenic Gastrointestinal Complications*. New York: Springer-Verlag; 1981:269-278.
37. Ellis H, Gajraj H, George CD. Incisional hernias: when do they occur? *Br J Surg* 1983;70:290-291.
38. Ghahremani GG, Jimenez MA, Rosenfeld M et al. CT diagnosis of occult incisional hernias. *AJR* 1987;148:139-142.
39. Engel JM, Deitch EE. Sonography of the anterior abdominal wall. *AJR* 1981;137:73-77.
40. Subramanyam BR, Balthazar EJ, Raghavendra BN et al. Sonographic diagnosis of scrotal hernia. *AJR* 1982;139:535-538.
41. Archer A, Choyke PL, O'Brien W et al. Scrotal enlargement following inguinal herniorrhaphy: ultrasound evaluation. *Urol Radiol* 1988;9:249-252.
42. Wantz GE. Complications of inguinal hernia repair. *Surg Clin North Am* 1984;64:287-298.
43. Ekberg O, Abrahamsson P, Kesek P. Inguinal hernia in urological patients: the value of herniography. *J Urol* 1988;139:1253-1255.
44. Deitch EA, Soncrant M. The value of ultrasound in the diagnosis of nonpalpable femoral hernias. *Arch Surg* 1981;116:185-187.
45. Waddington RT. Femoral hernia: a recent appraisal. *Br J Surg* 1971;59:920-922.
46. Ponka PL, Brush BE. Problem of femoral hernia. *Arch Surg* 1971;102:411-413.
47. Lee TM, Greenberger PA, Nahrwold DL et al. Rectus sheath hematoma complicating an exacerbation of asthma. *J Allergy Clin Immunol* 1986;78:290-292.
48. Lee PWR, Bark M, Macfie J et al. The ultrasound diagnosis of rectus sheath haematoma. *Br J Surg* 1977;64:633-634.
49. Manier JW. Rectus sheath haematoma. Six case reports and a literature review. *Am J Gastroenterol* 1972;54:433-435.
50. Suhr GM, Green AE. Rectus abdominis sheath hematoma as a complication of tetanus: diagnosis by computed tomography scanning. *Clin Imag* 1989;13:82-86.

51. Torpin R, Coleman J, Handkins JR. Hematoma of the rectus abdominis muscle in pregnancy, labor, or puerperium: report of three cases. *J Med Assoc Ga* 1969;58:158-159.

52. DeLaurentis DA, Rosemond GP. Hematoma of the rectus abdominis muscle complicated by anticoagulant therapy. *Am J Surg* 1966;112:359.

53. Henzel JH, Pories WJ, Smith JL et al. Pathogenesis and management of abdominal wall haematomas. *Arch Surg* 1966; 93:929-935.

54. Savage PE, Joseph AEA, Adam EJ. Massive abdominal wall hematoma: real-time ultrasound localization of bleeding. *J Ultrasound Med* 1985;4:157-158.

55. Gocke JE, MacCarty RL, Faulk WT. Rectus sheath hematoma: diagnosis by computed tomography scanning. *Mayo Clin Proc* 1981;56:757-761.

56. Fisch AE, Brodey PA. Computed tomography of the anterior abdominal wall: normal anatomy and pathology. *J Comput Assist Tomogr* 1981;5:728-733.

57. Tromans A, Campbell N, Sykes P. Rectus sheath haematoma. Diagnosis by ultrasound. *Br J Surg* 1981;68:518-519.

58. Kaftori JK, Rosenberger A, Pollack S et al. Rectus sheath hematoma: ultrasonographic diagnosis. *AJR* 1977;128:283-285.

59. Diakoumakis EE, Weinberg B, Seife B. Unusual case studies of anterior wall mass as diagnosed by ultrasonography. *J Clin Ultrasound* 1984;12:351-354.

60. Kwok-Liu JP, Zikman JM, Cockshott WP. Carcinoma of the urachus: the role of computed tomography. *Radiology* 1980; 137:731-734.

61. Gooding GAW, Herzog KA, Hedgecock NW et al. B-mode ultrasonography of prosthetic vascular grafts. *Radiology* 1978;127:763-766.

62. Gooding GAW, Effeney DJ, Goldstone J. The aortofemoral graft: detection and identification of healing complications by ultrasonography. *Surgery* 1981;89:949-1001.

63. Clifford PC, Skidmore R, Bird DR et al. Pulsed Doppler and real-time "duplex" imaging of Dacron arterial grafts. *Ultrasonic Imag* 1980;2:381-390.

64. Wolson AH, Kaupp HA, McDonald K. Ultrasound of arterial graft surgery complications. *AJR* 1979;133:869-875.

65. Gooding GAW, Effeney DJ. Sonography of axillofemoral and femorofemoral subcutaneous arterial bypass grafts. *AJR* 1985;144:1005-1008.

66. Gooding GAW, Effeney DJ. Static and real-time scanning B-mode sonography of arterial occlusions. *AJR* 1982;139:949-952.

67. Lang EK. A survey of the complications of percutaneous retrograde arteriography: Seldinger technique. *Radiology* 1973; 81:257-263.

68. Szilagyi DE, Smith RE, Elliot JP et al. Anastomotic aneurysms after vascular reconstruction problems of incidence, etiology and treatment. *Surgery* 1975;78:800-816.

69. Brener BJ, Couch NP. Peripheral arterial complications of left heart catheterization and their management. *Am J Surg* 1973;125:521-525.

70. Rapoport S, Sniderman KW, Morse SS et al. Pseudoaneurysm: complication of faulty technique in femoral arterial puncture. *Radiology* 1985;154:529-530.

71. Quera LA, Flinn WR, Yao JST et al. Management of peripheral arterial aneurysms. *Surg Clin North Am* 1979;59:693-706.

72. Perl S, Wener L, Lyon WS. Pseudoaneurysms after angiography. *Med Ann DC* 1973;42:173-175.

73. Abu-Yousef MM, Wiese JA, Shamma AR. Case report. The "to-and-fro" sign: duplex Doppler evidence of femoral artery pseudoaneurysm. *AJR* 1988;150:632-634.

74. Mitchell DG, Needleman L, Bezzi M et al. Femoral artery pseudoaneurysm: diagnosis with conventional duplex and color Doppler US. *Radiology* 1987;164:687-690.

75. Sandler MA, Alpern MB, Madrazo BL et al. Inflammatory lesions of the groin: ultrasonic evaluation. *Radiology* 1984;151:747-750.

76. Sacks D, Robinson MD, Perlmutter GS. Femoral arterial injury following catheterization duplex evaluation. *J Ultrasound Med* 1989;8:241-246.

77. Coughlin BF, Paushter DM. Peripheral pseudoaneurysms: evaluation with duplex US. *Radiology* 1988;168:339-342.

78. Middleton WD, Erickson S, Melson GL. Perivascular color artifact: pathologic significance and appearance on color Doppler US images. *Radiology* 1989;171:647-652.

79. Morton MJ, Charboneau JW, Banks PM. Inguinal lymphadenopathy simulating a false aneurysm on color-flow Doppler sonography. *AJR* 1988;151:115-116.

80. Hillman BJ, Haber K. Echographic characteristics of malignant lymph nodes. *J Clin Ultrasound* 1980;8:213-215.

81. Marchal G, Oyen R, Verschakelen J et al. Sonographic appearance of normal lymph nodes. *J Ultrasound Med* 1985;4:417-419.

82. Bruneton JN, Roux P, Caramella E et al. Ear, nose, and throat cancer: ultrasound diagnosis of metastasis to cervical lymph nodes. *Radiology* 1984;142:771-773.

83. Bruneton JN, Normand F. Cervical lymph nodes. In: Bruneton JN, ed. *Ultrasonography of the Neck.* Berlin: Springer-Verlag; 1987:81-92.

84. Bruneton JN, Caramella E, Hery M et al. Axillary lymph node metastasis in breast cancer: preoperative detection with US. *Radiology* 1986;158:325-326.

85. Bruneton JN, Normand F, Balu-Maestro C et al. Lymphomatous superficial lymph nodes: US detection. *Radiology* 1987;165:233-235.

86. Majer MC, Hess CF, Kolbel G et al. Small arteries in peripheral lymph nodes: a specific sign of lymphomatous involvement. *Radiology* 1988;168:241-243.

87. Martin DC. The undescended testis—evolving concepts in management. *J Cont Ed Urol* 1977;1:17-31.

88. Glickman MG, Weiss RM, Itzchak Y. Testicular venography for undescended testicles. *AJR* 1977;129:67-70.

89. Pinch L, Aceto T, Meyer-Bahlburg HF. Cryptorchidism: a paediatric review. *Urol Clin North Am* 1974;1:573-592.

90. Diamond AB, Meng CH, Kodroff M et al. Testicular venography in the nonpalpable testis. *AJR* 1977;129:71-75.

91. Levitt SB, Kogan SJ, Schneider KM et al. Endocrine tests in phenotypic children with bilateral impalpable testes can reliably predict "congenital" anorchism. *Urology* 1978;11: 11-14.

92. Kogan SJ, Gill B, Bennett B et al. Human monorchism: a clinicopathological study of unilateral absent testes in 65 boys. *J Urol* 1986;135:758-761.

93. Madrazo BL, Klugo RC, Parks JA et al. Ultrasonographic demonstration of undescended testes. *Radiology* 1979;133: 181-183.

94. Wolverson MK, Jagannadharao B, Sundaram M et al. CT in localization of impalpable cryptorchid testes. *AJR* 1980; 134:725-729.

95. Wolverson KW, Houttuin E, Heiberg H et al. Comparison of computed tomography with high-resolution real-time ultrasound in the localization of the impalpable undescended testis. *Radiology* 146:133-136.

96. Weiss RM, Carter AR, Rosenfield AT. High-resolution real-time ultrasonography in the location of the undescended testis. *J Urol* 1986;135:936-938.

97. Pasciak RM, Kozlowski JM. Mesenteric desmoid tumor presenting as an abdominal mass following salvage cystectomy for invasive bladder cancer. *J Urol* 1987;138:145-146.

98. McAdam WAF, Golinger JC. The occurrence of desmoids in patients with familial polyposis coli. *Br J Surg* 1970;57:618.

99. Baron RL, Lee JK. Mesenteric desmoid tumours: sonographic and computed tomographic appearance. *Radiology* 1981; 140:777-779.

100. Brasfield RD, Das Gupta TK. Desmoid tumours of the anterior abdominal wall. *Surgery* 1969;65:241-246.

101. Mantello MT, Haller JO, Marquis JR. Sonography of abdominal desmoid tumors in adolescents. *J Ultrasound Med* 1989;8:467-470.

102. Magid D, Fishman EK, Bronwyn J et al. Desmoid tumors in Gardner's syndrome: use of computed tomography. *AJR* 1984;142:1141-1145.

Artifacts

103. Buttery B, Davison G. The ghost artifact. *J Ultrasound Med* 1984;3:49-52.

104. Muller N, Cooperberg PL, Rowley VA et al. Ultrasonic refraction by the rectus abdominis muscles: the double image artifact. *J Ultrasound Med* 1984;3:515-519.

105. Sauerbrei EE. The split image artifact in pelvic sonography: the anatomy and physics. *J Ultrasound Med* 1985;4:29-34.

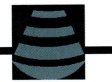

C H A P T E R   1 4

The Peritoneum and the Diaphragm

•

Khanh T. Nguyen, M.Sc., M.D., F.R.C.P.C.
Eric E. Sauerbrei, B.Sc., M.Sc., M.D., F.R.C.P.C.
Robert L. Nolan, B.Sc., M.D., F.R.C.P.C.

The peritoneum is the largest serous membrane of the body. It consists of a single layer of flattened mesothelial cells covering a layer of loose connective tissue. The mesothelium forms a dialyzing membrane across which substances in complete solution (solutes) are absorbed directly into the blood capillaries. Particulate matters in suspension pass into the lymphatic circulation probably with the aid of phagocytes. The parietal peritoneum is the membrane lining the inside of the abdominal wall; the visceral peritoneum is reflected over the intraabdominal organs to which it is firmly attached; it is an integral part of the organ that it covers. The peritoneal cavity is the potential space between the parietal and visceral membranes.

The diaphragm, in addition to its function as an active muscle of respiration, is a musculofibrous sheet separating the thoracic from the abdominal cavity. It is innervated by the phrenic and lower intercostal nerves; it is vascularized by the phrenic arteries, which are branches of the aorta.

SCANNING TECHNIQUES

No special patient preparation is required for scanning. Routinely, a 3.5 or 5 MHz sector probe is used. If a superficial lesion is detected, a higher-frequency linear array probe may be used for better visualization.

The patient is usually scanned in the supine position. Decubitus or erect positions will help to determine whether a fluid collection is free or loculated. When scanning a collection with an air-fluid level, it is helpful to scan from a posterior approach, through the fluid-filled dependent portion. In this way, scanning through the air, which reflects all the sound, is avoided.[1]

Scanning the diaphragm is performed with the patient in the supine or sitting position, in quiet respiration. Coughing or sniffing tests may be used to evaluate diaphragmatic motion. Measurements for normal diaphragmatic excursion have been established for newborns.[2] On sagittal scans of neonates, the average normal excursion of the right hemidiaphragm measures 2.6 cm (+0.1) for the anterior third, 3.6 cm (+0.2) for the middle third, and 4.5 cm (+0.2) for the posterior third. Measurements for adults are not available.

ANATOMY

Peritoneum

Multiple peritoneal ligaments and folds connect the viscera to each other and to the abdominal and pelvic walls. The lesser omentum is the fold connecting the liver to the stomach (hepatogastric ligament) and to the duodenum (hepatoduodenal ligament). The lesser omentum contains the portal vein, hepatic artery, and common bile duct at its free margin. The greater omentum is the largest fold, extending inferiorly from the greater curvature of the stomach to cover the anterior aspect of the transverse colon and hanging down like a curtain in front of the small bowel. The right border of the greater omentum extends as far as the proximal duodenum; its left border is continuous with the gastrosplenic ligament. In addition to functioning as a storehouse for fat, the greater omentum may limit the spread of disease in the peritoneal cavity. The mesenteries refer to peritoneal folds, which suspend the small bowel and colon from the posterior abdominal and pelvic wall. They include the mesentery of the small bowel, the mesoappendix, the transverse mesocolon, and the sigmoid mesocolon. The transverse mesocolon divides the peritoneal cavity into the supramesocolic and inframesocolic compartments.[3,4]

The **supramesocolic** compartment is in turn divided into two spaces by the falciform ligament, which runs in the midline from the umbilicus to the diaphragm and suspends the liver from the diaphragm and anterior abdominal wall. The two

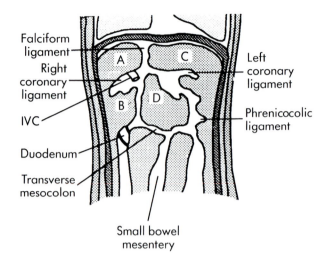

FIG. 14-1. Frontal diagram of peritoneal compartments. *A*, Right subphrenic space; *B*, right subhepatic space; *C*, left subphrenic space; *D*, lesser sac; *IVC*, inferior vena cava. (Adapted from Halvorsen RA, Jones MA, Rice RP et al. Anterior left subphrenic abscesses: characteristic plain film and CT appearance. *AJR* 1982;139:233-289.)

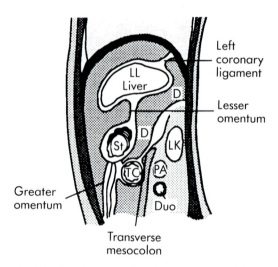

FIG. 14-2. Parasagittal diagram of left subphrenic spaces. *D*, Lesser sac; *St*, stomach; *TC*, transverse colon; *PA*, pancreas; *LK*, left kidney; *Duo*, duodenum. (Adapted from Halvorsen RA, Jones MA, Rice RP et al. Anterior left subphrenic abscesses: characteristic plain film and CT appearance. *AJR* 1982;139:233-289.)

spaces are the **right** and **left** supramesocolic spaces (Figs. 14-1 to 14-3).

The right supramesocolic space consists of the **lesser sac** and the **right perihepatic space.** The lesser sac has a superior recess that lies on the right side adjacent to the caudate lobe of the liver and an inferior recess on the left side separating the stomach anteriorly from the pancreas posteriorly. It communicates with the greater peritoneal sac through the foramen of Winslow (epiploic foramen), which is located inferior

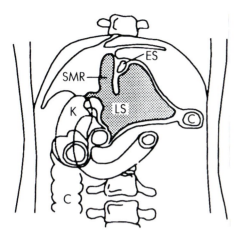

FIG. 14-3. Frontal diagram of lesser sac. *SMR,* Superomedial recess; *LS,* lateral recess; *ES,* esophagus; *C,* colon; *K,* kidney. (Adapted from Halvorsen RA, Jones MA, Rice RP et al. Anterior left subphrenic abscesses: characteristic plain film and CT appearance. *AJR* 1982;139:233-289.)

to the caudate lobe and posterior to the free edge of the lesser omentum. The right perihepatic space consists of the **right subphrenic** and **right subhepatic** spaces. The subphrenic space is immediately inferior to the diaphragm; it is bounded posteromedially by the right superior coronary ligament. Medial to this ligament is the bare area of the liver not covered by the peritoneum and in direct contact with the retroperitoneal space. The right subhepatic space lies inferior to the liver. It has an anterior component adjacent to the gallbladder fossa and a posterior compartment that is the hepatorenal recess or Morrison's pouch.

The **left** supramesocolic space consists of four compartments: the **left perihepatic** spaces (anterior and posterior) and the **left subphrenic** spaces (anterior perigastric and posterior perisplenic). The left anterior subphrenic space is separated from the lesser sac posteriorly by the left coronary ligament that suspends the left lobe of the liver from the diaphragm. It extends over the liver to the most superior left upper quadrant.

The oblique root of the mesentery extending from the duodenojejunal flexure (ligament of Treitz) to the ileocecal junction divides the **inframesocolic** compartment into a smaller right space and a larger left space. The right space is bounded laterally by the ascending colon and inferiorly by the ileocecal junction; the left space is bounded laterally by the descending colon and inferiorly by the sigmoid colon. The two spaces open inferiorly to the pelvic cavity, which is the most dependent part of the peritoneal cavity in both the erect and recumbent positions. The pelvic recesses communicate freely with the right supramesocolic compartment via the right paracolic gutter lateral to the ascending colon; on the left side, the phrenocolic ligament at the cephalad end of the left paracolic gutter prevents communication with the left supramesocolic compartment.[3,4]

When the peritoneal spaces are filled with fluid or tumor or when the membranes are thickened by disease, they may be identified by using sonography. The normal small bowel mesentery, which usually contains fat and blood vessels, is better seen by computed tomography (CT) than by ultrasound.

Diaphragm

The diaphragm consists of a central, crescent-shaped, tendinous plate connected by peripheral muscular bundles to the lower sternum and lower six ribs anteriorly and to the lumbar spine posteriorly. The anterior muscular fibers are shorter than the posterior ones. Because of this, the diaphragm has a dome-shaped configuration with convexity toward the thorax. The two crura anchoring the diaphragm to the spine join in the midline to form the arcuate ligament; posterior to this and in front of the spine at the level of the twelfth dorsal vertebra is the aortic hiatus. The esophageal hiatus is usually at the level of the tenth dorsal vertebra, slightly to the left of the midline, between the decussating mitral fibers of the right crux. The inferior vena cava passes through the right side of the central tendon, usually at the level of the eighth or ninth dorsal vertebra (Fig. 14-4).

Sonographically, the muscles of the diaphragm are seen as a thin, hypoechoic band. The interface between diaphragm and liver (or spleen) appears as a thin echogenic line. The interface between diaphragm and lung appears as a stronger and thicker echogenic band. Occasionally, another thin echogenic line is present cephalad to the diaphragm/lung interface.[5] This is a mirror-image artifact of the diaphragm/liver interface (Figs. 14-5 and 14-6). The term "diaphragmatics slips" refers to normal, prominent muscular insertions. In cross section they may appear as focal echogenic masses of various shapes (round, triangular, oval) that may be mistaken for focal liver or peritoneal lesions.[6] By rotating the transducer and scanning in their long axis, they appear elongated and become larger in inspiration (Figs. 14-7 and 14-8). The diaphragmatic crura may be seen as thin hypoechoic bands anterior to the upper abdominal aorta and posterior to the inferior vena cava. They also become thicker in deep inspiration.[6]

PERITONEAL PATHOLOGY

Ascites

Accumulation of fluid in the peritoneal cavity is termed **ascites.** The fluid may be a transudate or an

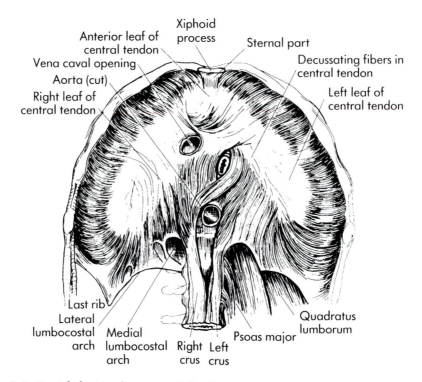

FIG. 14-4. **Abdominal aspect of diaphragm.** (Adapted from *Gray's Anatomy*. 35th ed. Edinburgh: Longman Group Ltd; 1973.)

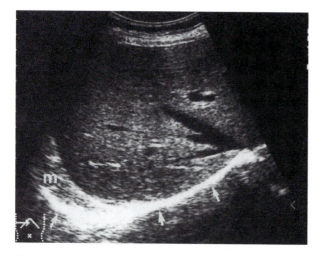

FIG. 14-5. **The right hemidiaphragm in transverse scan.** The echogenic curved line *(arrows)* represents the diaphragm/lung interface. The triangular hypoechoic band, *m*, represents the peripheral muscular bundles.

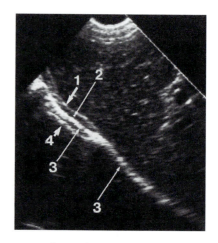

FIG. 14-6. **The right hemidiaphragm in parasagittal view.** *1*, Diaphragm/liver interface; *2*, muscles of diaphragm; *3*, diaphragm/lung interface; *4*, mirror-image of diaphragm/liver interface.

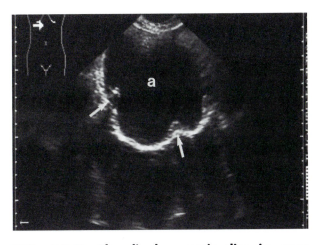

FIG. 14-7. The diaphragmatic slips in cross section. Transverse scan. They appear as small hypoechoic masses *(arrows)*. Note the large ascites, *a*.

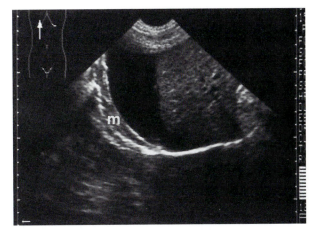

FIG. 14-8. The diaphragmatic slips in deep inspiration. When scanned in their long axis, these slips appear elongated, *m*, and become thicker.

exudate; it may be blood, pancreatic juice, chyle, pus, or urine.

The anatomic compartmentalization together with the action of gravity and variation in intraabdominal pressure during respiration determine the distribution of fluid and its contents throughout the peritoneal cavity. Gravity causes fluid to flow along peritoneal reflections: the fluid tends to pool in the lower end of the mesenteric root at the ileocecal junction and in the sigmoid mesocolon (Fig. 14-9). From there it spills into the pelvic cul-de-sac and paravesical recesses. In the recumbent position, fluid flows preferentially cephalad along the right paracolic gutter and collects in the right subphrenic and perihepatic spaces. On the left side, flow is weak and limited cephalad by the phrenicocolic ligament.[7] Because of this, minimal ascites is most frequently found in the hepatorenal recess (Morrison's pouch) and in the pelvic cul-de-sac, which are the most dependent spaces of the peritoneal cavity (Fig. 14-10). It is possible to detect with real-time sonography as little as a few milliliters of free fluid in these locations.[8-10] It is also apparent from the above discussion that the abdominal and pelvic cavities form an anatomic continuum. If fluid is seen in the abdomen, it should also be looked for in the pelvis and vice versa. This should be remembered when evaluating certain conditions such as blunt abdominal trauma, ruptured ectopic pregnancy, and intraperitoneal abscesses. A small amount of fluid in the pelvic cul-de-sac may be the only sign of injury to the upper abdominal viscera. Similarly, fluid in the hepatorenal recess may be seen in a ruptured ectopic pregnancy. A right subphrenic collection may originate from a pelvic source.

Ultrasound performs better than CT in localizing ascitic fluid in relation to the peritoneal spaces because it allows instant visualization in different planes. It is

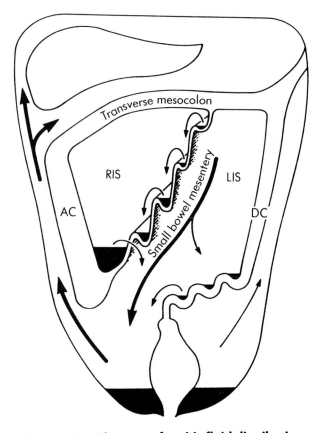

FIG. 14-9. Diagram of ascitic fluid distribution. *RIS,* Right inframesocolic space; *LIS,* left inframesocolic space; *AC,* ascending colon; *DC,* descending colon. (From Siegel MJ. Spleen and peritoneal cavity. In: Siegel MJ, ed. *Pediatric Sonography.* New York: Raven Press; 1991.)

worthwhile to note that fluid in the bare area of the liver is not intraperitoneal; it is either pleural or subcapsular. A right subphrenic collection does not extend posterior to the inferior vena cava, as a right pleural effusion often does.[11] In massive ascites, the liver, spleen,

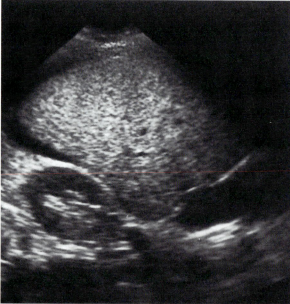

FIG. 14-10. Minimal ascites around liver.

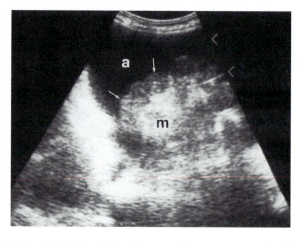

FIG. 14-11. Massive ascites surround the bowel. Bowel loops *(arrows)* are displaced medially by ascites, *a*, and arranged around the periphery of the mesentery, *m*.

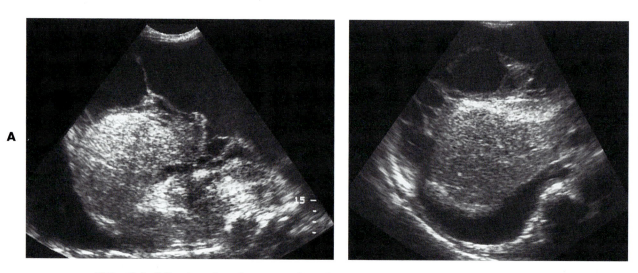

A **B**

FIG. 14-12. Loculated septated ascites. A. Longitudinal scan around the liver. B. Transverse scan.

and bowel are displaced medially and toward the center of the abdomen.[12] The bowel may appear as echogenic structures distributed around the periphery of the fan-shaped mesentery (Fig. 14-11). Loculated ascites as an isolated finding simulates mesenteric or omental cyst, lymphocele, abscess, or a cystic neoplasm (Fig. 14-12). Diagnosis often requires fine-needle percutaneous aspiration, which is frequently performed under ultrasound guidance.

The sonographic appearance of the fluid is variable. In general, simple ascites or a transudate is usually sonolucent. Fluid collections complicated by hemorrhage, infection, or an exudate may contain septations or floating debris.[13]

Intraperitoneal Abscess

Intraperitoneal abscesses may develop following spillage of contaminated material from perforated bowel; or they may occur as the result of direct contamination during surgery; or they may be seen as a complication of trauma, pancreatitis, or in conditions associated with decreased immune response. The majority of intraperitoneal abscesses occur in the upper abdomen between the transverse colon and diaphragm: 60% are found on the right side, 25% occur on the left, and about 15% are bilateral. The most common offending organisms are *Escherichia coli*, **streptococci**, **staphylococci**, and *Klebsiella*. Mixed infections are also common.[14] Clinical findings typi-

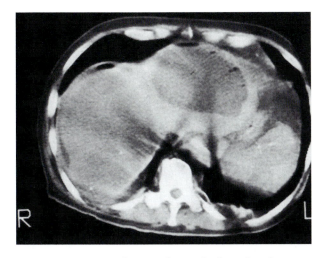

FIG. 14-13. Left anterior subphrenic abscess.
CT scan of upper abdomen. There is a well-defined fluid collection in the midabdomen, which may be in the left lobe of the liver.

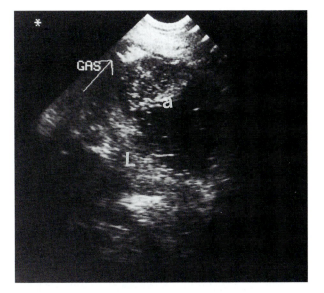

FIG. 14-14. Left anterior subphrenic abscess.
On the ultrasound scan, the left lobe of the liver, *L*, appears compressed and displaced posteriorly by the collection, *a*. The midline location high under the diaphragm anterior to the liver suggests an anterior left subphrenic abscess. This was successfully drained via a percutaneous approach. Note the gas collection floating on the top of the abscess.

cally include fever, leukocytosis, abdominal pain, and tenderness.

It is generally accepted that sonography performs better than CT in the detection of subphrenic and perihepatic abscesses, although the left upper quadrant may present some difficulties.[15,16] Ultrasound is also the screening modality of choice for thin patients and for patients with vague clinical findings. CT performs better in detecting interloop abscesses and those located in the lower abdomen and pelvis. CT is also the best imaging technique for obese patients and for patients with recent surgery.[15,16] Therefore the choice of the initial imaging modality should be tailored to the patient's size and clinical status. Most often the best results are obtained with the appropriate use of more than one imaging technique (ultrasound, CT, nuclear medicine, and magnetic resonance imaging).

An air-fluid collection in the midupper abdomen may be in the lesser sac or in the left anterior subphrenic space. Both spaces may extend across the midline.[17] Most lesser sac abscesses usually originate from disease processes in contiguous organs, particularly the pancreas. They are seen posterior to the stomach and at a lower plane than the subphrenic abscesses, which are anterior to the stomach and may simulate abscesses in the left lobe of the liver (Figs. 14-13 and 14-14).

A loculated fluid collection containing gas bubbles is strongly suggestive of an abscess. This is not often seen. More frequently one finds a fluid collection ovoid or spherical or irregular in shape, which may or may not contain septations or debris. Occasionally a fluid-fluid level may be detected (Figs. 14-15 and 14-16). Some abscesses may simulate an echogenic solid mass or a simple cystic lesion. Others show a

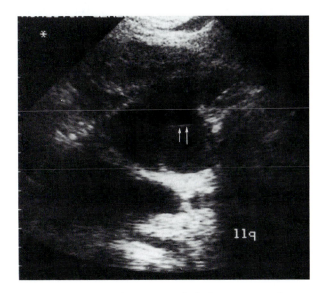

FIG. 14-15. Abscess in left lower quadrant.
Parasagittal scan reveals a fluid collection on the left side of the abdomen. A faint fluid-fluid level is seen *(arrows)*. It is not possible to say whether this is sterile or infected.

complex appearance, partly cystic, partly solid (Figs. 14-17 and 14-18). Diagnosis and drainage are established by using the percutaneous approach.[18] Ultrasound or CT guidance may be used, depending on the location of the abscess.

A few authors claim an accuracy approaching 90% in the sonographic detection of intraabdominal ab-

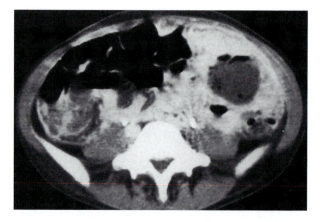

FIG. 14-16. Abscess in left lower quadrant. CT scan shows the presence of gas bubbles in the abscess, which is partially surrounded by bowel and is successfully drained via a percutaneous approach. CT performs better in detecting small gas bubbles. Sonography detects fluid levels and septation more easily.

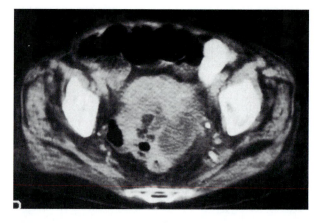

FIG. 14-18. Diverticular abscess. CT scan of pelvis. There is a mass of inhomogeneous density adjacent to bowel. This proved to be a diverticular abscess that was drained transrectally under ultrasound guidance.

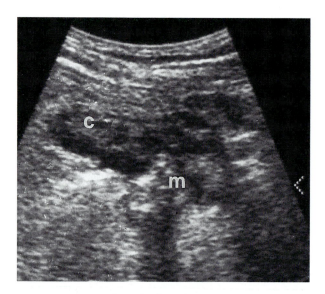

FIG. 14-17. Diverticular abscess. Transverse scan of pelvis. A complex mass, *m*, is seen adjacent to a loop of sigmoid colon, *c*.

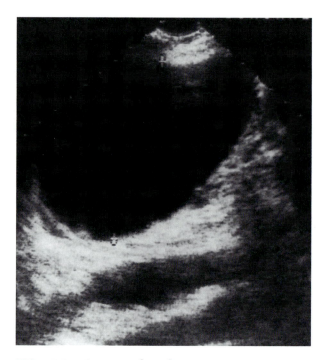

FIG. 14-19. Lymphocele. This appears as a large, simple, fluid collection on the left side of the abdomen in this patient who had previous nodal dissection.

scesses.[15,16] This includes abscesses affecting the solid viscera. In practice, the results are probably in the range of 40% to 50%, as published by Lundstedt et al., for the sonographic detection of abscesses occurring in the peritoneal cavity.[19] The ultrasound examination is often severely limited by the presence of open wounds, drainage tubes, large dressings, and bowel gas.

Lymphoceles

Disruption of lymphatic vessels following surgery (lymphadenectomy, kidney transplant) or trauma results in the development of lymphoceles, which are lymph-containing collections that occur most com-

monly in the pelvis, in the abdominal peritoneal recesses, or in the retroperitoneum.[20]

Lymphoceles are usually small. However, some may attain considerable size, measuring many centimeters in diameter and causing pressure symptoms or hydronephrosis of the transplanted kidney. Small lymphoceles frequently resorb over time. Large and symptomatic lymphoceles (Fig. 14-19) are usually decompressed percutaneously or surgically.[21] Some success has been obtained with sclerotherapy using instillation of tetracycline into the cyst.[22]

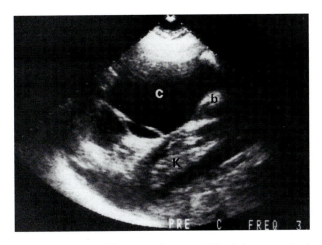

FIG. 14-20. Mesenteric cyst. This left parasagittal scan reveals a cystic lesion, *c*, adjacent to bowel, *b*. *K*, Kidney.

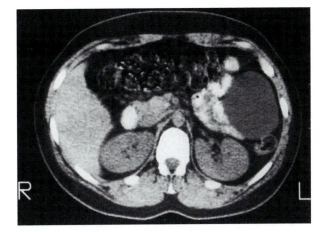

FIG. 14-21. Mesenteric cyst. CT appearance. The lesion is closely adjacent to the small bowel.

Uncomplicated lymphoceles appear as echo-free collections mimicking loculated ascites or mesenteric and omental cysts or pancreatic pseudocysts. Septation and floating debris are usually seen when they are complicated by hemorrhage or infection. Diagnosis requires percutaneous aspiration under ultrasound or CT guidance. Fat globules are found in the fluid.

Omental and Mesenteric Cysts

Omental and mesenteric cysts are lesions of obscure etiology. Some authors consider them to be hamartomas, part of lymphangiomatosis; others believe they are caused by congenital lymphatic obstruction.[23] Mesenteric cysts are usually found in the root of the mesentery; omental cysts occur adjacent to the bowel. The fluid they contain may be serous, bloody or mixed, or a "cheesy white" material thought to be inspissated chyle.[24] The majority of the patients present with a palpable abdominal mass.

Sonographically, omental and mesenteric cysts often appear as unilocular cystic lesions (Figs. 14-20 and 14-21) that may be septated.[25,26] Rarely, a fat-fluid level may be seen; this is thought to be because of the presence of chyle associated with an inflammatory exudate.[27] In contrast to bowel duplication cysts, they are not lined with a mucosal layer. Differentiation from other cystic lesions of the abdomen is often difficult without percutaneous needle aspiration. The rare cystic teratoma and lymphangioma of the mesentery have been reported.[28,29]

Meconium Peritonitis

Prenatal bowel perforation results in aseptic chemical inflammation of the peritoneum termed meconium peritonitis. **Intestinal stenosis** or **atresia** and **meco-**

nium ileus (cystic fibrosis) are the most common causes, accounting for 65% of cases. Other causes include perforated **Meckel's diverticulum** or **appendix, bowel perforation** related to volvulus, **internal hernia,** and **vascular thrombosis.**[30]

Extravasated meconium causes an intense foreign body reaction. This results in a fibroadhesive peritonitis that may calcify over time. A fibrous wall may develop around the mass of spilled meconium, producing a pseudocyst that may appear echogenic (Figs. 14-22 and 14-23). Antenatal detection of meconium peritonitis has been made by showing a mass in the fetal abdomen that may be complex or cystic with an echogenic wall.[30-33] Calcified peritoneal thickening may be seen as scattered linear echoes with or without acoustic shadowing. After birth, there may be a diffuse echogenicity throughout the abdomen described as a "snowstorm" appearance. Other findings include fetal ascites, dilated bowel loops, and polyhydramnios.[31-34]

Peritoneal Tuberculosis

Inflammation of the peritoneum caused by ***Mycobacterium tuberculosis*** is now a rare occurrence, particularly in the Western world. This is usually caused by direct spread from gastrointestinal tuberculosis or following hematogenous dissemination from a lung focus. Only a few reports exist in the sonographic literature, describing ascites, enlarged necrotic mesenteric nodes, and echogenic epigastric masses representing caseating granulomas (Fig. 14-24).[35,36] The greater omentum may be thickened by granulomatous deposits and adhesions. This may appear on sonography as an "omental cake" indistinguishable from peritoneal carcinomatosis or mesothelioma,[37] which will be described later in this chapter. Diagnosis requires peritoneoscopy and biopsies.

Mesenteritis

Inflammation and thickening as well as fat necrosis of the mesentery may develop in a number of conditions, including Crohn's disease, pancreatitis, trauma, surgery, or as part of retroperitoneal fibrosis. Occasionally, this may appear as a focal echo-poor mass simulating a neoplasm.[38,39] Diagnosis may be suspected in the appropriate clinical setting but may require percutaneous fine-needle biopsy.

Retained Surgical Sponges

Surgical sponges may be lost in the abdomen during surgery. Without opaque markers, they cannot be detected by radiography.

Surgical sponges may be seen in abdominal sonography and may cause diagnostic confusion if one is not aware of and familiar with their appearance. The ones surrounded by an abscess usually appear as infected

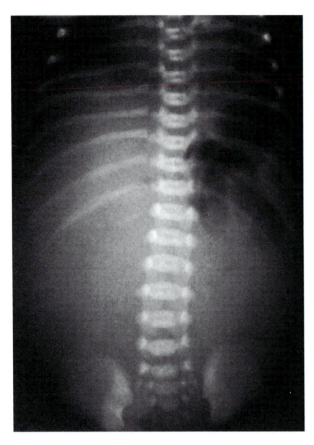

FIG. 14-22. Meconium pseudocyst. A large, soft-tissue, pelvoabdominal mass is seen in this abdominal radiograph of a newborn.

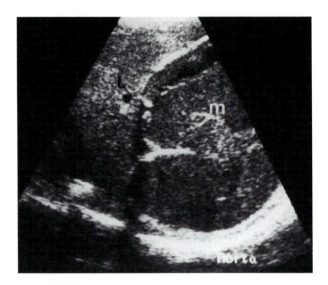

FIG. 14-23. Meconium pseudocyst. Abdominal sonogram reveals an echogenic mass, *m*, filling the abdomen. *L*, Liver. At surgery, this proved to be a meconium pseudocyst resulting from ileal atresia.

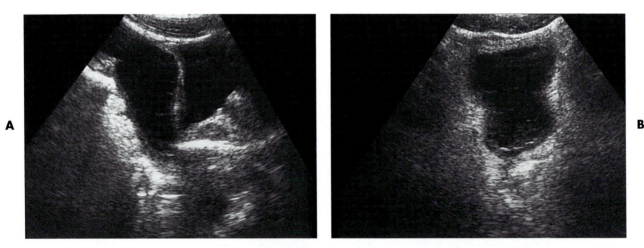

FIG. 14-24. Peritoneal tuberculosis in a 33-year-old black man with an 80-pound weight loss. **A,** Sagittal and, **B,** transverse sonograms of the pelvis show a large, loculated fluid collection located just above the bladder dome. (From Hanbridge A, Wilson SR. Sonography: a valuable tool for assessment of the peritoneum. *RadioGraphics.* In press.)

collections or masses.[40] The ones not associated with abscess usually show a clean, clear-cut, acoustic shadow in relation to a palpable mass.[41] The abdominal radiograph helps to exclude residual barium in the bowel or a calcified neoplasm.

Peritoneal Neoplasms

Mesenteric and omental neoplasms are rare. The most common benign primary mesenteric neoplasm is desmoid tumor. Common peritoneal malignancies include lymphoma, mesothelioma, and carcinomatosis.

Desmoid Tumors. Desmoid tumors arise from fascia and aponeuroses. They occur most commonly in the abdominal wall. Mesenteric desmoid tumors usually appear as hypoechoic masses that may contain areas of acoustic shadowing thought to arise from fibrotic collagenous tissue and not from calcification.[42]

Lymphoma. The most common primary mesenteric malignancy is lymphoma. Fifty percent of patients with non-Hodgkin's lymphoma and only 5% of patients with Hodgkin's lymphoma have mesenteric involvement.[43]

Isolated, enlarged lymph nodes measuring more than 1.5 cm in maximal diameter may be detected around the celiac axis, the superior mesenteric artery, or in the porta hepatis. They are often hypoechoic, but they may be echogenic. More frequently, mesenteric lymphoma appears as a lobulated mass encasing the mesenteric vessels that manifest as linear echoes within the mass (Figs. 14-25 and 14-26). This has been described as the "sandwich sign" more commonly seen in lymphoma than in metastatic disease.[44]

Mesothelioma. Mesothelioma is a sarcoma arising from a serous membrane. Closely related to asbestos exposure, it affects the pleura (65% of cases) more often than the peritoneum (33% of cases); both pleura and peritoneum are affected in 2% of cases.[45] Clinical signs and symptoms are usually vague. The latent period may be as long as 40 years following the initial exposure to asbestos.

The disease typically causes thickening of the omentum, which appears sonographically as sheetlike, superficial masses described as "omental mantle or cake."[46,47] The anterior surface follows the contour of the abdominal cavity; the posterior surface is adjacent to bowel loops and is often outlined by a thin collection of fluid (Figs. 14-27 and 14-28). However, this appearance may also be seen with peritoneal carcinomatosis and tuberculosis. The surrounding bowel may be invaded and become fixed, not changing location with different patient position. Ascites, when present, is usually minimal, although massive ascites may sometimes occur. Liver metastases, pleural plaques, and effusions are readily identified by sonography. CT scanning performs better than ultrasound in detecting small nodules attached to the peritoneal surface or buried in the mesenteric fat, focal peritoneal thickening, and calcified pleural plaques. Gallium uptake by pleural and peritoneal mesotheliomas has been reported.[48] Diagnosis may be made by fine-needle aspiration biopsies, which should be performed at different sites in order to obtain adequate samples.[49] In most cases peritoneoscopy or laparotomy is required. The extremely rare cystic mesothelioma of the peritoneum is a separate entity that has no relation to previous exposure to asbestos.[50,51]

Carcinomatosis. Metastases to the peritoneum and mesentery arise from a variety of sources, the most common being carcinoma of the ovaries and of the gastrointestinal tract.[43] Four mechanisms determine the spread of metastatic disease in the abdomen: mesenteric pathways, intraperitoneal seeding, and lymphatic and hematogenous spread.

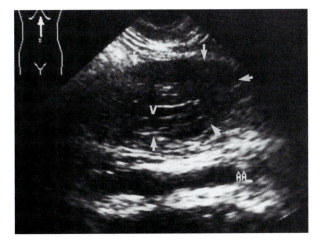

FIG. 14-25. Mesenteric lymphoma. The mesenteric vessels, *v*, are surrounded by a hypoechoic mass *(arrows)*. The appearance has been described as the "sandwich" sign. This is also seen with metastatic disease. *AA*, Abdominal aorta.

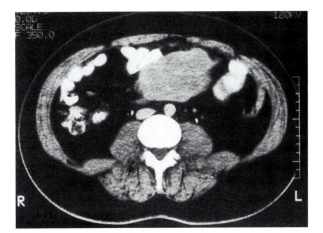

FIG. 14-26. Mesenteric lymphoma CT scan.

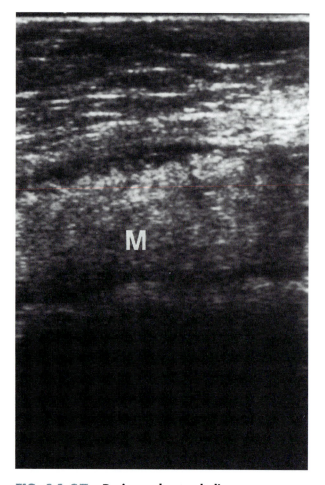

FIG. 14-27. Peritoneal mesothelioma. Sonogram shows typical "omental cake," *M*, resulting from thickening of the omentum. The lobulated posterior contour is due to adjacent bowel.

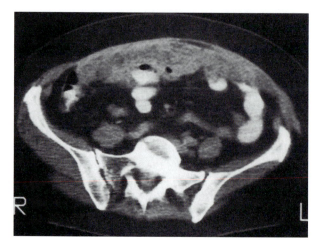

FIG. 14-28. Peritoneal mesothelioma. CT appearance of "omental cake." Note absence of ascites.

Gastrointestinal malignancies often invade surrounding viscera by growing along mesenteric and ligamentous attachments. This has been well illustrated by Meyers et al.[52] Carcinoma of the stomach spreads along the gastrocolic ligament to affect the transverse colon; conversely, carcinoma of the transverse colon may extend cephalad along the same ligament to affect the stomach. The transverse mesocolon may serve as a conduit for spread of pancreatic carcinoma, which tends to invade the posteroinferior border of the transverse colon.

The natural flow of ascitic fluid and its contents determine the intraperitoneal seeding of malignancies in the peritoneal cavity. Malignant cells that shed in the fluid grow at specific sites where fluid tends to collect. These sites are the pelvic cul-de-sac, the root of the mesentery at the ileocecal junction, the sigmoid mesocolon, and the right paracolic gutter. They are locations where peritoneal metastases are commonly found, and these can be detected by barium studies and sonography.[53] When the greater omentum is thickened by secondary infiltration, it may be detected by ultrasound or CT scanning as sheetlike masses described as "omental mantle or cake" seen in mesothelioma or tuberculosis (Fig. 14-29). When ascites is present, small nodules attached to the abdominal wall or peritoneal surface are easily identified (Fig. 14-30).

Lymphatic spread results in enlarged mesenteric nodes that may be isolated or may appear as conglomerated, lobulated, hypoechoic masses indistinguishable from lymphoma.

Hematogenous dissemination occurs via the mesenteric arteries, which carry the metastatic emboli to the vasa recta on the antimesenteric border of the bowel, where they grow submucosally into large masses that can be detected by sonography. Melanoma and carcinoma of the breast and lung commonly disseminate this way.[54]

In the search for metastatic disease in the abdomen, it should be stressed that a negative ultrasound scan does not preclude other imaging tests, including barium studies, CT, MRI, and intraperitoneal injection of I-131 labeled B72.3 antibody.[55] Ultrasound may also be used to guide percutaneous biopsy and to monitor response to treatment.

Pseudomyxoma Peritonei. Pseudomyxoma peritonei is characterized by mucinous peritoneal implants and gelatinous ascites. It is most often caused by secondary metastases from mucin-producing adenocarcinoma of the ovary, appendix, colon, and rectum, although a few benign neoplasms of the ovary and appendix may be responsible for the condition.[56] It is not frequently seen in ultrasound practice. A few reports describe nodular masses ranging from hypoechoic to strongly echogenic distributed throughout the peritoneal cavity[57-59] (Fig. 14-31). The masses correspond to calcified lesions seen on abdominal radiographs.

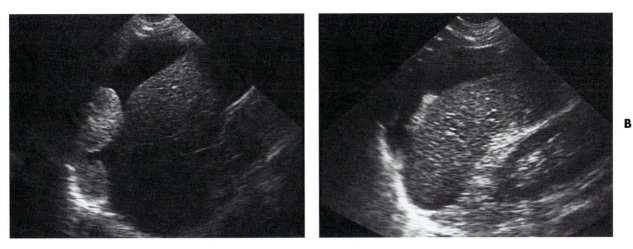

FIG. 14-29. Peritoneal metastases, parietal and visceral. A, Sagittal sonogram of right upper quadrant shows ascites over the convexity of the liver. Two echogenic tumor deposits are seen on the parietal peritoneum of the lateral abdominal wall, which did not move with the liver with respiration. **B,** Sagittal sonogram of the same region shows the kidney and part of the right lobe of the liver. A visceral metastasis shows as a plaquelike area of increased echogenicity on the surface of the liver, which moves with the liver with respiration. (From Hanbridge A, Wilson SR. Sonography: a valuable tool for assessment of the peritoneum. *RadioGraphics*. In press.)

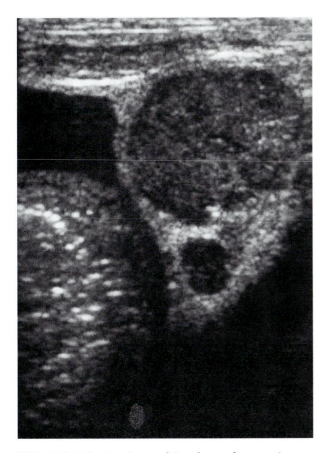

FIG. 14-30. Peritoneal implants from primary carcinoma of colon. Two hypoechoic, round, peritoneal seeds of colon are shown adjacent to a gas-containing loop of bowel. Ascites makes their identification easier as does the selection of a high-frequency linear array transducer. (From Hanbridge A, Wilson SR. Sonography: a valuable tool for assessment of the peritoneum. *RadioGraphics*. In press.)

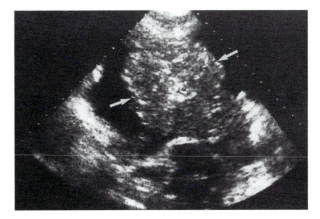

FIG. 14-31. Pseudomyxoma peritonei. Large, calcified, peritoneal mass *(arrows)* surrounded by ascites. A number of similar lesions are seen throughout the abdomen of this patient with ovarian cancer.

Leiomyomatosis Peritonealis Disseminata. Leiomyomatosis peritonealis disseminata is an extremely rare condition that should be included in the differential diagnosis of peritoneal mesothelioma and carcinomatosis. It affects pregnant women or women of childbearing age. It is characterized by the presence of peritoneal masses that are disseminated benign leiomyoma. Ascites is usually not present.[60]

Diffuse Infiltrative Lipomatosis. Diffuse infiltrative lipomatosis is a rare condition that usually affects young patients. It is characterized by extensive overgrowth of fatty tissue in the mesentery. Sonography shows a strongly echogenic mass; the fatty

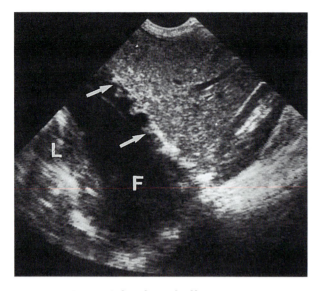

FIG. 14-32. Right pleural effusion, parasagittal scan. Fluid. *F*, is seen outlining the diaphragmatic slips *(arrows)*. Atelectatic lung. *L*, appears as echogenic mass floating in the pleural effusion.

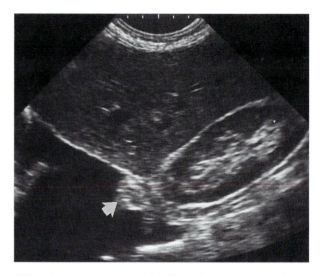

FIG. 14-33. Parietal pleural metastasis from bronchogenic carcinoma. Sagittal sonogram of the right upper quadrant shows normal liver and kidney. There is a large right pleural effusion. A metastasis interrupts the smooth contour of the diaphragm *(arrow)*. (Courtesy of Stephanie R. Wilson, M.D., University of Toronto.)

nature of the mass is apparent on CT scanning. Differentiation from a liposarcoma is difficult.[61]

DIAPHRAGMATIC PATHOLOGY

Paralysis

Sonography is increasingly used instead of fluoroscopy in the evaluation of the diaphragm. The technique offers several advantages:

- It is free of ionizing radiation, therefore more suitable for children and pregnant women;
- It can be easily performed at the patient's bedside with portable equipment;
- It can identify the diaphragm even when the latter is obscured by peridiaphragmatic abnormalities such as effusion or tumor (Figs. 14-32 and 14-33); and
- For patients on a respirator, scanning may be done with the respirator disconnected for a few seconds in order to evaluate unassisted ventilation.

The examination is made with the patient in the parasagittal and transverse position in quiet respiration; scanning transversely over the xiphoid usually allows simultaneous visualization of both hemidiaphragms. Paradoxical motions may be elicited by the coughing and sniffing tests. Paralysis of one hemidiaphragm can be detected by showing absent or paradoxical motion on the affected side compared with the usual or exaggerated excursion on the opposite side.[62,63]

Eventration

Eventration accounts for 5% of all diaphragmatic defects. Traditionally, it is considered a congenital mal-

formation resulting from incomplete muscularization of the membranous diaphragm. Others suggest that it may be acquired secondary to focal ischemia, infarct, or neuromuscular weakness.[6]

Eventration may be complete or partial. The complete form occurs more commonly on the left and in males. The partial form more commonly affects the anterior portion of the right hemidiaphragm. Eventration may be bilateral: in this case, it is frequently seen in trisomies 13-15 and 18 and in Beckwith-Wiedemann syndrome.[64,65] Diaphragmatic eventration has been diagnosed prenatally.[66]

Partial eventration is usually of no clinical significance and should not be subject to multiple investigations. Complete eventration may cause respiratory distress in the newborn or in the obese and may require surgical plication.[64] Chest radiographs in partial eventration may suggest a mass in the lower thorax or in the liver. Ultrasound helps clarify the issue by showing absence of a mass and the typical diaphragmatic bulge filled by the liver.[6] Complete eventration has not been described in the ultrasound literature.

Inversion

Normally, the convexity of the diaphragmatic dome is toward the thorax. A large pleural effusion or neoplasm may push the diaphragm such that its convexity is toward the abdomen (Fig. 14-34). This is called diaphragmatic inversion and occurs more commonly on the left side. Only part or the entire hemidiaphragm may be affected.[6,67] The inverted hemidiaphragm shows little or asynchronous motion, resulting in paradoxical ventilation and air exchange

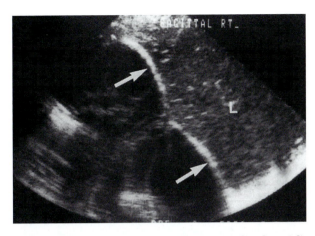

FIG. 14-34. Inversion of the right hemidiaphragm *(arrows)* by a septated pleural effusion. Parasagittal scan. *L,* Liver.

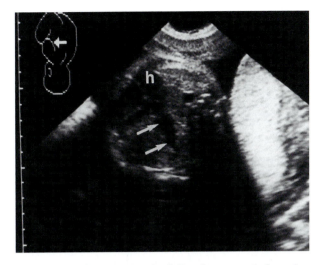

FIG. 14-35. Congenital diaphragmatic hernia. Scan through the fetal thorax reveals herniated, fluid-filled stomach *(arrows)* in the thorax adjacent to and displacing the heart, *h.*

between the two lungs, thus causing respiratory distress. It may stimulate a mass on CT scanning because of its inverted cone shape. Parasagittal and transverse sonographic scan planes help to clarify the situation.

Hernia

Acquired defects in the diaphragm are less common than congenital ones, which occur in about 1 in 2000 to 1 in 12,500 live births. Of congenital diaphragmatic hernias (CDH), 50% are associated with other malformations.[68] Two major types are recognized: the posterior Bochdalek hernia and the anterior Morgagni hernia.

Posterior Bochdalek hernias are the most common congenital diaphragmatic defect, resulting from defective closure of the pleuroperitoneal canal during fetal development. There is a left-sided preponderance ranging from 9:1 to 2:1. On the left side there may be herniation of the stomach, spleen, or kidney into the lower thorax; on the right side, part of the liver or right kidney may herniate through the defect; most frequently, however, omental fat is found above the diaphragm. Chest radiographs usually show a focal posterior hump corresponding to the herniated organ in the diaphragmatic contour.[69]

The rare anterior Morgagni hernias are due to maldevelopment of the septum transversum. They are often associated with a pericardial defect. There may be herniation of an abdominal organ or fat into the pericardial sac or herniation of the heart into the upper abdomen.[70] Morgagni hernia usually appears as a triangular mass in the right cardiophrenic angle anteriorly and medially, posterior to the sternum. Diaphragmatic hernias are best demonstrated by CT scanning.[68]

Antenatal detection of CDH by ultrasound has been reported.[71,72] The diagnosis should be suspected

when the fetal heart is displaced either by an intrathoracic solid mass (liver, kidney) or by a fluid-filled structure (stomach, bowel) (Fig. 14-35). Pulmonary hypoplasia often results from compression of the fetal lung by the herniated viscera. Over 50% of infants with CDH die from respiratory failure.[73]

Rupture

Diaphragmatic rupture is usually caused from penetrating injury and blunt trauma and rarely occurs because of infection such as liver amebiasis. The left side is more commonly affected in blunt trauma.[74-76]

The diagnosis of diaphragmatic rupture is often difficult without using multiple imaging modalities, which include chest radiographs, contrast studies of the bowel, CT, and MRI scanning. Chest radiography may offer a clue to the diagnosis that is often obscured by life-threatening conditions associated with multiple injuries.[77] Ultrasound usually offers a limited contribution, but may detect a large rent (over 10 cm long) showing disruption of diaphragmatic echoes and herniation of abdominal viscera into the thorax.[78,79]

Neoplasms

Diaphragmatic neoplasms, either primary or secondary, are rare. Primary tumors include various types of sarcomas. Secondary involvement is often due to local invasion by adjacent pleural, peritoneal, or thoracic and abdominal wall malignancies. Distant metastases from bronchogenic or ovarian carcinoma, Wilms' tumor, and osteogenic sarcoma are less common.[80]

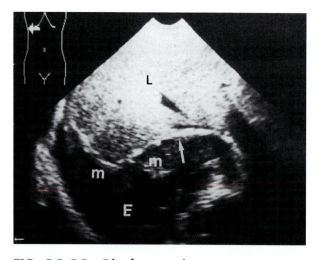

FIG. 14-36. Diaphragmatic metastases. Transverse scan shows multiple solid masses, *m*, causing segmental inversion and disruption of the right hemidiaphragm *(arrow)*. E, Pleural effusion. Metastases from bronchogenic carcinoma. L, Liver.

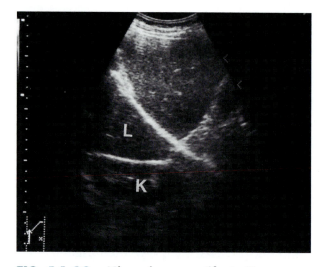

FIG. 14-38. Mirror-image artifact. Phantom images of liver, *L*, and kidney, *K*, at the base of the thorax, caused by reflection of sound beam at the diaphragm.

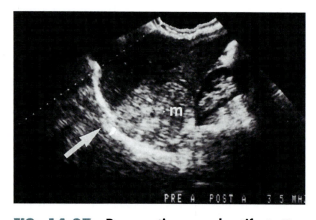

FIG. 14-37. Propagation speed artifact. Note apparent disruption and posterior displacement of the right hemidiaphragm *(arrow)*. This is caused by the difference in velocity of the sound beam through the liver and the fatty mass, *m*, in the liver.

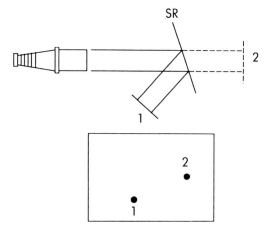

FIG. 14-39. Mirror-image artifact. Schema of mechanism. (From Kremkau FW. Imaging artifacts. In: Kremkau FW, ed. *Diagnostic Ultrasound—Principles, Instruments and Exercises.* Philadelphia: WB Saunders Co; 1989.)

The metastatic deposits usually cause disruption or interruption of the diaphragmatic echoes seen on sonography.[81] They may produce partial or complete inversion of the involved hemidiaphragm (Fig. 14-36).

ARTIFACTS

Disruption and Displacement of Diaphragmatic Echoes

A fatty mass in the liver or right adrenal gland or a cystic lesion in the liver may cause apparent interruption and displacement of the right diaphragmatic echoes (Fig. 14-37). This artifact has been referred to as the propagation speed artifact and has been used to suggest the tissue characteristic of the mass causing the artifact.[82,83] It is caused by the difference in velocity of the sound beam through the liver and through the fatty or cystic mass; Cooperberg et al. suggested that refraction at the edge of the lesion may also play a role in the production of the artifact.[84]

Mirror-Image Artifact

Mirror-image artifact is caused by scattered reflection of sound. The right lung/diaphragm interface acts as an acoustic mirror resulting from the presence of air in the lung, which is a strong reflector of sound. When two or more reflectors are in the way of the sound beam, objects that are on one side of a strong reflector may be artificially reproduced on the other side (Fig. 14-38). The formation of this artifact can be explained as follows[85,86]: when the incident sound beam hits the diaphragm/lung interface, some of the beam is reflected away from the incident path into the abdomen. This reflected beam is in turn reflected back from various structures to the diaphragm and then back to the probe along the incident path. It takes longer for the reflected beam to reach the transducer. The longer time is translated into a printed signal that appears to originate from the other side of the diaphragm along the direction of the beam (Fig. 14-39).

REFERENCES

Scanning Techniques

1. Golding RH, Li DKB, Cooperberg PL. Sonographic demonstration of air-fluid levels in abdominal abscesses. *J Ultrasound Med* 1982;1:151-155.
2. Laing IA, Teele RL, Stark AR: Diaphragmatic movements in newborn infants. *J Pediatr* 1988;112:638-643.

Anatomy

3. Heiken JP. Abdominal wall and peritoneal cavity. In: Leek TL, Sagel SS, Stanley RJ, eds. *Computed Tomography with MRI Correlation.* New York: Raven Press; 1988:661-705.
4. Whalen JP. Anatomy and radiologic diagnosis of perihepatic abscesses. *Radiol Clin North Am* 1976;14:406-428.
5. Lewandowski BJ, Winsberg F. Echographic appearance of the right hemidiaphragm. *J Ultrasound Med* 1983;2:243-249.
6. Yeh H-C, Halton KP, Gray CE. Anatomic variations and abnormalities in the diaphragm seen with ultrasound. *Radio-Graphics* 1990;10:1019-1030.

Peritoneal Pathology

7. Myers MA, ed. *Dynamic Radiology of the Abdomen: Normal and Pathologic Anatomy.* 3rd ed. New York: Springer-Verlag; 1988.
8. Gooding GAW, Cummings SR. Sonographic detection of ascites in liver disease. *J Ultrasound Med* 1984;3:169-172.
9. Proto AV, Lane EJ, Marangola JA. A new concept of ascitic fluid distribution. *AJR* 1976;126:974.
10. Meyers MA. The spread and localization of acute intraperitoneal effusions. *Radiology* 1970;95:547-554.
11. Halvorsen RA, Fedyshin PJ, Korobkin M et al. CT differentiation of pleural effusion from ascites: an evaluation of four signs using blinded analysis of 52 cases. *Invest Radiol* 1986;21:391-395.
12. Yeh H-C, Wolf BS. Ultrasonography in ascites. *Radiology* 977;124:783-790.
13. Edell SL, Geften WB. Ultrasonic differentiation of types of ascitic fluid. *AJR* 1979;133:111-114.
14. Magilligan DJ Jr. Suprahepatic abscess. *Arch Surg* 1968; 96:14-19.
15. Taylor KJW, Wasson JFM, de Graaf C et al. Accuracy of grey-scale ultrasound in the diagnosis of abdominal and pelvic abscesses in 220 patients. *Lancet* 1978;1:83-84.
16. Mueller PR, Simeone JF. Intra-abdominal abscess: diagnosis by sonography and computed tomography. *Radiol Clin North Am* 1983;21:425-443.
17. Halvorsen RA, Jones MA, Rice RP et al. Anterior left subphrenic abscesses: characteristic plain film and CT appearance. *AJR* 1982;139:283-289.
18. van Sonnenberg E, Mueller PR, Ferrucci JT. Percutaneous drainage of 250 abdominal abscesses and fluid collections. Pt I. Results, failures and complications. *Radiology* 1984;151:337-341.
19. Lundstedt C, Hederström E, Holmin T et al. Radiological diagnosis in proven intra-abdominal abscesses formation: a comparison between plain films of the abdomen, ultrasonography and computed tomography. *Gastrointest Radiol* 1983;8:261-266.
20. Spring DB, Schroeder D, Babu S et al. Ultrasonic evaluation of lymphocele formation after staging lymphadenectomy for prostatic cancer. *Radiology* 1981;141:479-483.
21. Lessner AM, Lempert N, Pietrocola DM et al. Diagnosis and treatment of pelvic lymphoceles in the renal transplant patient. *NY State J Med* 1984;84:491-494.
22. White M, Mueller PR, Ferrucci JT Jr et al. Percutaneous drainage of postoperative abdominal and pelvic lymphoceles. *AJR* 1985;145:1065-1069.
23. Fragoyamis SG, Anagnostopoulos G. Hemangiolymphomatous hamartoma of the mesentery. *AJDC* 1974;128:233-234.
24. Walker AR, Putnam TC. Omental, mesenteric and retroperitoneal cysts: a clinical study of 33 new cases. *Ann Surg* 1973;178:13-19.
25. Geer LL, Mittelstaedt CA, Staab EV et al. Mesenteric cyst: sonographic appearance with CT correlation. *Pediatr Radiol* 1984;14:102-104.
26. Mittelstaedt C. Ultrasonic diagnosis of omental cysts. *Radiology* 1975;114:673-676.
27. van Mil JBC, Lameris JS. Unusual appearance of a mesenteric cyst. *Diagn Imag* 1983;52:28-32.
28. Pricto ML, Casanova A, Delgado J et al. Cystic teratoma of the mesentery. *Pediatr Radiol* 1989;19:439.
29. Nicolet V, Gagnon A, Filiatrault D et al. Sonographic appearance of an abdominal cystic lymphangioma. *J Ultrasound Med* 1984;3:85-86.
30. Brugman SM, Bjelland JJ, Thomasson JE et al. Sonographic findings with radiographic correlation in meconium peritonitis. *J Clin Ultrasound* 1979;7:305-306.
31. Garb M, Riseborough J. Meconium peritonitis presenting as fetal ascites on ultrasound. *Br J Radiol* 1980;53:602-604.
32. Blumenthal D, Rushorich AM, Williams RK et al. Prenatal sonographic findings of meconium peritonitis with pathologic correlation. *J Clin Ultrasound* 1982;10:350-352.
33. Hartung RW, Kilcheski TS, Greaney RC et al. Antenatal diagnosis of cystic meconium peritonitis. *J Ultrasound Med* 1983;2:49-50.
34. Laver JD, Cradock TV. Meconium pseudocyst: prenatal sonographic and antenatal radiologic correlation. *J Ultrasound Med* 1982;1:333-335.
35. Borgia G, Ciampi R, Nappa S et al. Tuberculous mesenteric lymphadenitis clinically presenting as abdominal mass: CT and sonographic findings. *J Clin Ultrasound* 1985;13:491-493.
36. Epstein BM, Mann JH. CT of abdominal tuberculosis. *AJR* 1982;139:861-866.
37. Wu C-C, Chow K-S, Lü T-N et al. Sonographic features of tuberculous omental cakes in peritoneal tuberculosis. *J Clin Ultrasound* 1988;16:195-198.
38. Marshak RH, Lindner AE, Maklansky D et al. Mesenteric fat necrosis simulating a carcinoma of the cecum. *Am J Gastroenterol* 1980;5:459-462.
39. Kordan B, Payne SD. Fat necrosis simulating a primary tumor of the mesentery: sonographic diagnosis. *J Ultrasound Med* 1988;7:345-347.

40. Sekiba K, Akamatsu N, Niwa K. Ultrasound characteristics of abdominal abscesses involving foreign bodies *(gauze)*. *J Clin Ultrasound* 1979;7:284-285.

41. Barriga P, Garcia C. Ultrasonography in the detection of intraabdominal retained surgical sponges. *J Ultrasound Med* 1984;3:173-176.

42. Baron RL, Lee JK. Mesenteric desmoid tumors. *Radiology* 1981;140:777-779.

43. Levitt RG, Koehler RE, Sagel SS et al. Metastatic disease of the mesentery and omentum. *Radiol Clin North Am* 1982;20:501-510.

44. Mueller PR, Ferrucci JT Jr, Harbin WP et al. Appearance of lymphomatous involvement of the mesentery by ultrasonography and body computed tomography: the "sandwich sign." *Radiology* 1980;134:467-473.

45. Moertel CG. Peritoneal mesothelioma. *Gastroenterology* 1972;63:346-350.

46. Yeh H-C, Chahinian AP. Ultrasonography and computed tomography of peritoneal mesothelioma. *Radiology* 1980;135:705-712.

47. Cooper C, Jeffrey RB, Silverman PM et al. Computed tomography of omental pathology. *J Comp Assist Tomogr* 1986;10:62-66.

48. Dach J, Patel N, Patel S et al. Peritoneal mesothelioma: CT, sonography and gallium-67 scan. *AJR* 1980;135:614-616.

49. Reuter K, Raptopoulos V, Reale F et al. Diagnosis of peritoneal mesothelioma: computed tomography, sonography and fine needle aspiration biopsy. *AJR* 1983;140:1189-1194.

50. O'Neil JD, Ros PR, Storm BL et al. Cystic mesothelioma of the peritoneum. *Radiology* 1989;170:333-337.

51. Schneider JA, Zelnick EJ. Benign cystic peritoneal mesothelioma. *J Clin Ultrasound* 1985;13:190-192.

52. Meyers MA. Metastatic disease along the small bowel mesentery: roentgen features. *AJR* 1975;123:67-73.

53. Meyers MA. Distribution of intra-abdominal malignant seeding: dependency on dynamics of flow and ascitic fluid. *AJR* 1973;119:198-206.

54. Meyers MA, McSweeney J. Secondary neoplasms of the bowel. *Radiology* 1979;133:419-424.

55. Carrasquillo JA, Sugarbaker P, Colcher D et al. Peritoneal carcinomatosis: imaging with intraperitoneal injection of I-131 labelled B72.3 monoclonal antibody. *Radiology* 1988;167:34-40.

56. Fernandez R, Daly JM. Pseudomyxoma peritonei. *Arch Surg* 1980;115:409-414.

57. Merritt CB, Williams SM. Ultrasound findings in a patient with pseudomyxoma peritonei. *J Clin Ultrasound* 1978;6:417-418.

58. Seshill MB, Coulam CM. Pseudomyxoma peritonei: computed tomography and sonography. *AJR* 1981;136:803-806.

59. Seale WB. Sonographic findings in a patient with pseudomyxoma peritonei. *J Clin Ultrasound* 1982;10:441-443.

60. Remigers SA, Michael AS, Bardawil WWA et al. Sonographic findings in leiomyomatosis peritonealis disseminata. A case report and literature review. *J Ultrasound Med* 1985;4:497-500.

61. Siegel MJ. Spleen and peritoneal cavity. In: Siegel MJ, ed. *Pediatric Sonography*. New York: Raven Press; 1991;6:161-178.

Diaphragmatic Pathology

62. Haber K, Asher WM, Freimann AK. Echographic evaluation of diaphragmatic motion in intra-abdominal disease. *Radiology* 1975;114:141-144.

63. Diament MJ, Boerhat MI, Kangarloo H. Real-time sector ultrasound in the evaluation of suspected abnormalities of diaphragmatic motion. *J Clin Ultrasound* 1985;13:539-543.

64. Symbas PN, Hatcher CR Jr, Waldo W. Diaphragmatic eventration in infancy and childhood. *Ann Thorac Surg* 1977;24:113-119.

65. Weller MH. Bilateral eventration of the diaphragm. *West J Med* 1976;124:415-419.

66. Jurcak-Zaleski S, Comstock C, Kirk JS. Eventration of the diaphragm—prenatal diagnosis. *J Ultrasound Med* 1990;9:351-354.

67. Subramanyam BR, Raghavendra BN, LeFleur RS. Sonography of the inverted right hemidiaphragm. *AJR* 1981;136:1004-1006.

68. Panicek DM, Benson CB, Gottlieb RH et al. The diaphragm: anatomic, pathologic and radiologic considerations. *RadioGraphics* 1988;8:385-424.

69. Gale ME. Bochdalek hernia: prevalence and CT characteristics. *Radiology* 1985;156:449-452.

70. Gale ME. Anterior diaphragm: variations in the CT appearance. *Radiology* 1986;161:635-639.

71. Chinn DH, Filly RA, Callen PW et al. Congenital diaphragmatic hernia diagnosed prenatally by ultrasound. *Radiology* 1983;148:119-123.

72. Comstock CH. The antenatal diagnosis of diaphragmatic anomalies. *J Ultrasound Med* 1986;5:391-396.

73. Benacaraff BK, Adzick NS. Fetal diaphragmatic hernia: ultrasound diagnosis and clinical outcome in 19 cases. *Am J Obstet Gynecol* 1987;156:573-575.

74. Landay MJ, Setiawan H, Hirsch G et al. Hepatic and thoracic amebiasis. *AJR* 1980;135:449-454.

75. Ball T, McCrory R, Smith JO et al. Traumatic diaphragmatic hernia: errors in diagnosis. *AJR* 1988;138:633-637.

76. Bergqvist D, Dahlgren S, Hedelin H. Rupture of the diaphragm in patients wearing seatbelts. *J Trauma* 1978;18:781-783.

77. Gelman R, Mirris SE, Gens D. Diaphragmatic rupture due to blunt trauma: sensitivity on plain chest radiographs. *AJR* 1991;156:51-57.

78. Rao KG, Woodlief RM. Grey-scale ultrasonic documentation of ruptured right hemidiaphragm. *Br J Radiol* 1980;53:812-814.

79. Ammann AM, Brewer WH, Mauhl KI et al. Traumatic rupture of the diaphragm: real-time sonographic diagnosis. *AJR* 1983;140:915-916.

80. Kangarloo H, Sukor R, Sample WF et al. Ultrasonographic evaluation of juxtadiaphragmatic mass in children. *Radiology* 1977;125:785-787.

81. Worthen NJ, Worthen WF II. Disruption of the diaphragmatic echoes: a sonographic sign of diaphragmatic disease. *J Clin Ultrasound* 1982;10:43-45.

82. Pierce G, Golding RH, Cooperberg PI. The effects of tissue velocity on acoustical interfaces. *J Ultrasound Med* 1982;1:185-187.

Artifacts

83. Richman TS, Taylor KJW, Kremkase FW. Propagation speed artifact in a fatty tumor (myelolipoma): significance for tissue differential diagnosis. *J Ultrasound Med* 1983;2:45-47.

84. Mayo J, Cooperberg PL. Displacement of the diaphragmatic echo by hepatic cysts: a new explanation with computer simulation. *J Ultrasound Med* 1984;3:337-340.

85. Kremkau FW. Imaging artifacts. In: Kremkau FW, ed. *Diagnostic Ultrasound—Principles, Instruments and Exercises*. Philadelphia: WB Saunders Co; 1989:147-176.

86. Zagzebski JA. Images and artifacts. In: Hagen-Ansert SL, ed. *Textbook of Diagnostic Sonography*. St Louis: Mosby–Year Book; 1983:44-60.

CHAPTER 15

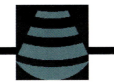

The Uterus and Adnexa

•

Shia Salem, M.D., F.R.C.P.C.

Sonography plays an integral role in the evaluation of gynecologic disease. Both the transabdominal and transvaginal approaches are now well established techniques for assessing the female pelvic organs. Color and spectral Doppler sonography have evolved to play a role in assessing normal and pathologic blood flow. Doppler can also distinguish vascular structures from nonvascular structures such as dilated fallopian tubes or fluid-filled bowel loops. The more recent addition of sonohysterography has provided more detailed evaluation of the endometrium, allowing differentiation among intracavitary, endometrial, and submucosal lesions. Sonography also plays an important role in guiding interventional procedures. Computed tomography (CT) and magnetic resonance imaging (MRI) have supplementary roles when sonography is inconclusive and in the staging of pelvic malignancies.

NORMAL PELVIC ANATOMY

The **uterus** is a hollow, thick-walled muscular organ. Its internal structure consists of a muscular layer, or **myometrium,** which forms most of the substance of the uterus, and a mucous layer, the **endometrium,** which is firmly adherent to the myometrium. The **uterus** is located between the two layers of the broad ligament laterally, the bladder anteriorly, and the rectosigmoid colon posteriorly. It is divided into two major portions, the **body** and the **cervix,** by a slight narrowing at the level of the internal os. The **fundus** is the superior area of the body above the entrance of the fallopian tubes. The area of the body where the tubes enter the uterus is called the **cornua.** The anterior surface of the uterine fundus and body is covered by peritoneum. The peritoneal space anterior to the uterus is the **vesicouterine pouch** or **anterior cul-de-sac.** This space is usually empty, but may contain bowel loops. Posteriorly, the peritoneal reflection extends to the posterior fornix of

the vagina, forming the **rectouterine recess,** or **posterior cul-de-sac.** Laterally, the peritoneal reflection forms the **broad ligaments,** which extend from the lateral aspect of the uterus to the lateral pelvic sidewalls. The **round ligaments** arise from the uterine cornua anterior to the fallopian tubes in the broad ligaments, extend anterolaterally, and course through the inguinal canals to insert into the fascia of the labia majora.

The **cervix** is located posterior to the angle of the bladder and is anchored to the bladder angle by the parametrium. The cervix opens into the upper vagina through the external os. The **vagina** is a fibromuscular canal that lies in the midline and runs from the cervix to the vestibule of the external genitalia. The cervix projects into the proximal vagina, creating a space between the vaginal walls and the surface of the cervix called the **vaginal fornix.** Although the space is continuous, it is divided into anterior, posterior, and two lateral fornices.[1]

The two **fallopian tubes** run laterally from the uterus in the upper free margin of the broad ligament. Each tube varies from 7 to 12 cm in length and is divided into intramural, isthmic, ampullary, and infundibular portions.[2] The **intramural** portion, which is approximately 1 cm long, is contained within the muscular wall of the uterus and is the narrowest part of the tube. The **isthmus,** constituting the medial third, is slightly wider, round, cordlike, and continuous with the **ampulla,** which is tortuous and forms approximately one half the length of the tube.[1] The ampulla terminates in the most distal portion, the **infundibulum,** or fimbriated end, which is funnel-shaped and opens into the peritoneal cavity (Fig. 15-1).

The **ovaries** are elliptical in shape, with the long axis usually oriented vertically. The surface of the ovary is not covered by peritoneum but by a single layer of cuboidal or columnar cells called the **germinal epithelium** that becomes continuous with the peritoneum at the hilum of the ovary. The internal structure of the

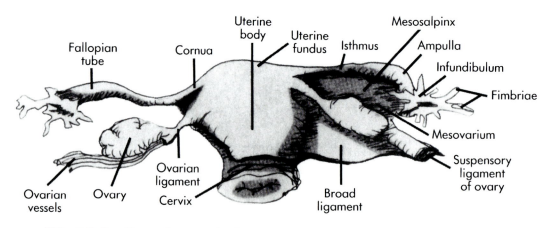

FIG. 15-1. **Normal gynecologic organs.** Diagram of uterus, ovaries, tubes, and related structures. On left side, broad ligament has been removed. (Courtesy of Jocelyne Salem.)

ovary is divided into an outer cortex and inner medulla. The cortex consists of an interstitial framework, or stroma, which is composed of reticular fibers and spindle-shaped cells and which contains the ovarian follicles and corpus lutea. Beneath the germinal epithelium, the connective tissue of the cortex is condensed to form a fibrous capsule, the **tunica albuginea.** The medulla, which is smaller in volume than the cortex, is composed of fibrous tissue and blood vessels, especially veins. In the nulliparous female, the ovary is located in a depression on the lateral pelvic wall called the **ovarian fossa,** which is bound anteriorly by the obliterated umbilical artery, posteriorly by the ureter and the internal iliac artery, and superiorly by the external iliac vein.[1] The fimbriae of the fallopian tube lie superior and lateral to the ovary. The anterior surface of the ovary is attached to the posterior surface of the broad ligament by a short mesovarium. The lower pole of the ovary is attached to the uterus by the ovarian ligament, whereas the upper pole is attached to the lateral wall of the pelvis by the lateral extension of the broad ligament known as the suspensory (infundibulopelvic) ligament of the ovary. The suspensory ligament contains the ovarian vessels and nerves. These ligaments are not rigid, and therefore the ovary can be quite mobile, especially in women who have had pregnancies.

The **arterial blood supply** to the uterus comes primarily from the **uterine artery,** a major branch of the anterior trunk of the internal iliac artery. The uterine artery ascends along the lateral margin of the uterus in the broad ligament and, at the level of the uterine cornua, runs laterally to anastomose with the ovarian artery. The uterine arteries anastomose extensively across the midline through the anterior and posterior arcuate arteries, which run within the broad ligament and then enter the myometrium.[1,2] The uterine plexus of veins accompanies the arteries.

The **ovarian artery** arises from the aorta laterally, slightly inferior to the renal arteries. It crosses the external iliac vessels at the pelvic brim and runs medially within the suspensory ligament of the ovary. After giving off branches to the ovary, it continues medially in the broad ligament to anastomose with the uterine artery. The **ovarian veins** leave the ovarian hilum and form a plexus of veins in the broad ligament that communicate with the uterine plexus of veins. The right ovarian vein drains into the inferior vena cava inferior to the right renal vein, whereas the left ovarian vein drains directly into left renal vein.[1]

The **lymphatic drainage** of the pelvic organs is variable but tends to follow recognizable patterns. The lymph vessels of the ovary accompany the ovarian artery to the lateral aortic and periaortic lymph nodes. The lymphatics of the fundus and upper uterine body and fallopian tube accompany those of the ovary. The lymphatics of the lower uterine body course laterally to the external iliac lymph nodes, whereas those of the cervix course in three directions—laterally, to the external iliac lymph nodes; posterolaterally, to the internal iliac lymph nodes; and posteriorly, to the lateral sacral lymph nodes. The lymphatics of the upper vagina course laterally with the branches of the uterine artery to the external and internal iliac lymph nodes, whereas those of the midvagina follow the vaginal artery branches to the internal iliac lymph nodes. The lymphatic vessels of the lower vagina near the orifice join those of the vulva and drain to the superficial inguinal lymph nodes.[1]

SONOGRAPHIC TECHNIQUE

The standard **transabdominal sonogram** is performed with a distended urinary bladder, which provides an acoustic window to view the pelvic organs and serves as a reference standard for evaluating cystic structures. The distended bladder displaces the bowel out of the pelvis and displaces the pelvic organs 5 to 10 cm from the anterior abdominal wall. The highest frequency transducer possible should be used. In practice, most sonograms are performed using a 3.5-MHz transducer. However, a 5.0-MHz transducer should be used whenever possible. The urinary bladder is considered ideally filled when it covers the entire fundus of the uterus. Overdistension may distort the anatomy by compression and may also push the pelvic organs beyond the focal zone of the transducer, limiting detail.

Imaging of the uterus and adnexa is performed in both sagittal and transverse planes. The long axis of the uterus is identified in the sagittal plane, and a somewhat oblique angulation is often necessary to visualize the entire uterus and cervix. The adnexa may be imaged by scanning obliquely from the contralateral side, although in many instances visualization can be achieved by scanning directly over the adnexa, especially when an overdistended bladder pushes the adnexa beyond the focal zone of the transducer. Gentle pressure on the transducer may be necessary to bring the area of interest within the focal zone.

For **transvaginal sonography,** the bladder must be empty to bring the pelvic organs into the focal zone of the transvaginal transducer. An empty bladder also provides patient comfort during the examination. Transvaginal transducers range in frequency from 5.0 to 7.5 MHz. The transducer is prepared with ultrasound gel and then covered with a protective rubber sheath, usually a condom. Air bubbles should be eliminated to avoid artifacts. An external lubricant is then applied to the outside of the protective covering. The transducer is inserted into the vagina with the patient supine, knees gently flexed and hips elevated slightly on a pillow. The elevated hips allow free movement of the transducer by the operator. A **slightly reversed Trendelenburg position** may be helpful in lowering the pelvic organs. It is important to avoid placing the patient in the Trendelenburg position, as small amounts of pelvic fluid may be missed.

With gentle rotation and angulation of the transducer, both sagittal and coronal images can be obtained. Slight anterior angulation of the transducer will bring the fundus of an anteverted uterus into view. To visualize the cervix, the transducer must be pulled slightly outward, away from the external os. Extreme angulation may be needed to visualize the entire adnexa and cul-de-sac. Abdominal palpation may be helpful in

bringing adnexal structures closer to the transducer.

Image orientation may be confusing initially as the sagittal images are displayed 90 degrees counterclockwise from their actual orientation, whereas the coronal scans are similarly rotated in their craniocaudad direction but correctly displayed as to right-left orientation (Fig. 15-2).

Sonohysterography involves the instillation of sterile saline into the endometrial cavity. A sterile speculum is inserted and the cervix is cleansed with an antiseptic solution. A catheter, usually a 5-F pediatric feeding tube, is inserted into the uterine cavity to the level of the uterine fundus. The catheter should be

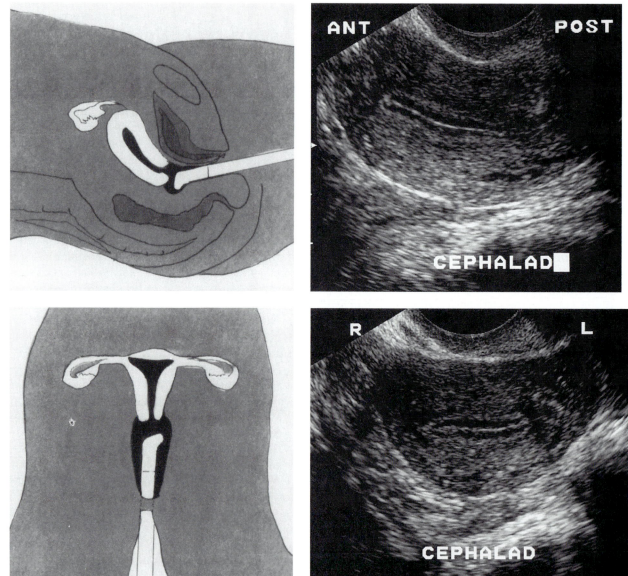

FIG. 15-2. Transvaginal sonography orientation. A, Illustration of transvaginal scanning in sagittal plane. B, Corresponding sagittal sonogram of uterus. C, Illustration of transvaginal scanning in coronal plane. D, Corresponding coronal sonogram of uterus. R indicates right; L, left. (A and C, courtesy of Jocelyne Salem.)

prefilled with saline prior to insertion to minimize air artifact. A hysterosalpingography catheter with a balloon may also be used and is necessary in women with a patulous or incompetent cervix to prevent retrograde leakage of saline into the vagina. The balloon should be placed as close to the internal os as possible and inflated with saline, not air.

The speculum is then removed and the transvaginal transducer is inserted into the vagina. The catheter position in the endometrial cavity is confirmed and sterile saline is then injected slowly through the catheter under continuous sonographic control. The uterus is scanned systematically in sagittal and coronal planes to delineate the entire endometrial cavity. The examination is not performed in women with acute pelvic inflammatory disease. Prophylactic antibiotics are given to women with chronic pelvic inflammatory disease and to women with a history of mitral valve prolapse or other cardiac disorders.[3]

Transabdominal versus Transvaginal Scanning

Transabdominal and transvaginal sonography are complementary techniques; both are used extensively in evaluation of the female pelvis. The **transabdominal approach** visualizes the entire pelvis and gives a global overview. Its main **limitations** include the examination of patients who are unable to fill their bladders, the examination of obese patients, the evaluation of a retroverted uterus in which the fundus may be located beyond the focal zone of the transducer, and less optimal characterization of adnexal masses. Because of the proximity of the transducer to the uterus and adnexa, **transvaginal sonography** allows the use of higher-frequency transducers, producing much better resolution. However, because of the higher frequencies, the **field of view is limited**, and that is the **major disadvantage** of this technique. Large masses may fill or extend out of the field of view, making orientation difficult, and superiorly or laterally placed

ovaries or masses may not be visualized. Transvaginal sonography better distinguishes adnexal masses from bowel loops and provides greater detail of the internal characteristics of a pelvic mass because of its improved resolution. Thus, the two techniques complement each other.

Several studies **comparing the two techniques** in a variety of pelvic disorders have shown that transvaginal sonography provides better anatomic detail and image quality.[4-8] This is not surprising because of the higher-frequency transducers used. Only a few studies have compared sonographic findings with surgical outcome. Andolf and Jörgensen found no significant difference in diagnostic outcome between the two techniques, despite the better image quality of transvaginal sonography.[9] DiSantis et al., using only transvaginal sonography within 72 hours of elective pelvic surgery, detected 16 of 21 (76%) histologically normal ovaries in premenopausal women and only 12 of 59 (20%) in postmenopausal women. Only 13 of 22 (59%) and 6 of 11 (54%) of adnexal masses were identified in premenopausal and postmenopausal women, respectively.[10]

Most laboratories, including my own, use **transabdominal** sonography as the **initial** pelvic examination, with **transvaginal** sonography reserved for a more **detailed evaluation,** if necessary. If the patient arrives with an empty bladder, the transvaginal study may be performed initially, but transabdominal scanning also should be done, even with an empty bladder, to exclude a large pelvic mass. Many women will require both studies; however, if the transabdominal study is completely normal or a well-defined abnormality is detected, no further study is usually necessary. Transvaginal sonography should be done if the transabdominal findings are uncertain or inconclusive or to better characterize a lesion. In patients who have a high risk of disease, such as a strong family history of ovarian cancer, transvaginal sonography should also be performed, even if the transabdominal study appears normal. Similarly, transvaginal sonography should also be performed in women with suspected endometrial disorders. For follow-up examinations, only the more efficiently diagnostic technique is needed.

ADVANTAGES OF TRANSVAGINAL SONOGRAPHY

Use of higher-frequency transducers with better resolution

Examination of patients who are unable to fill their bladders

Examination of obese patients

Evaluation of a retroverted uterus

Better distinction between adnexal masses and bowel loops

Greater detail of the internal characteristics of a pelvic mass

---

INDICATIONS FOR TRANSVAGINAL SONOGRAPHY

Uncertain transabdominal findings

Better characterization of a lesion

Strong family history of ovarian cancer

Suspected endometrial disorders

Assessment of a retroverted or retroflexed uterus

UTERUS

Normal Sonographic Anatomy

The uterus lies in the true pelvis between the urinary bladder anteriorly and the rectosigmoid colon posteriorly (Fig. 15-3). Uterine position is variable and changes with varying degrees of bladder and rectal distention. The cervix is fixed in the midline, but the body is quite mobile and may lie obliquely on either side of the midline. **Flexion** refers to the axis of the uterine body relative to the cervix, whereas **version** refers to the axis of the cervix relative to the vagina. The uterus is usually anteverted and anteflexed, but it may appear straight or slightly retroflexed on transabdominal sonograms due to posterior displacement by the distended bladder. The uterus may also be retroflexed when the body is tilted posteriorly (relative to the cervix) or retroverted when the entire uterus is tilted backwards (relative to the vagina) (Fig. 15-4). The fundus of a retroverted or retroflexed uterus is frequently difficult to assess by transabdominal sonography. As this portion of the uterus is situated at a distance from the transducer, it may appear hypoechoic and simulate a fibroid. Transvaginal sonography has proved to be excellent for assessing the retroverted or retroflexed uterus because the transducer is in close proximity to the posteriorly located fundus.[8]

The **size** and **shape** of the normal uterus vary throughout life and are related to age, hormonal status, and parity. The infantile or **prepubertal uterus** ranges from 2.0 to 3.3 cm in length, with the cervix accounting for two thirds of the total length, and 0.5 to 1.0 cm in anteroposterior (AP) diameter.[11] The prepubertal uterus has a tubular or inverse pear-shaped appearance, with the AP diameter of the cervix being greater than that of the fundus.[12] In the immediate neonatal period, because of residual maternal hormone stimulation, the **neonatal uterus** is approximately 0.6 to 0.9 cm longer and 0.7 to 0.8 cm greater in AP diameter than the prepubertal uterus.[13] Also because of residual ma-

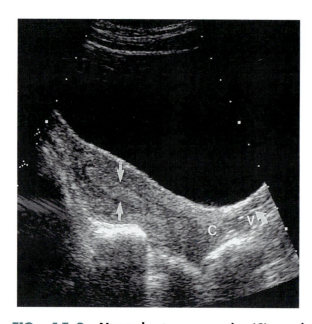

FIG. 15-3. Normal uterus, cervix (C), and vagina (V). Sagittal scan. Note endometrium *(arrows)* and central linear echo, representing apposed surfaces of vaginal mucosa *(curved arrow).*

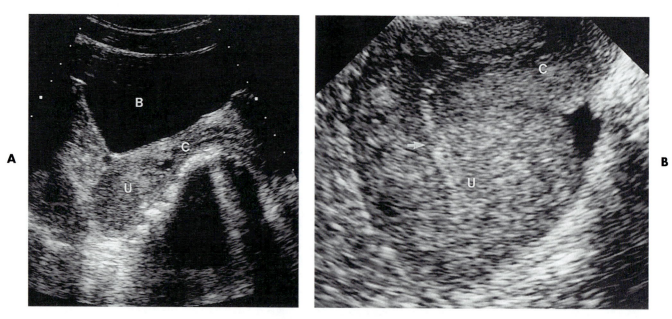

FIG. 15-4. Retroverted and retroflexed uterus. A, Sagittal transabdominal scan shows retroverted uterus. **B,** Sagittal transvaginal scan shows retroflexed uterus. Note endometrium *(arrow).* U, Uterus. C, Cervix. B, Bladder.

ternal hormone stimulation, an echogenic endometrium is seen in nearly all neonatal uteri, and a small amount of endometrial fluid may also be present (Fig. 15-5).[14]

After 7 years of age, the uterus gradually increases in size until puberty. At this time, there is a more dramatic increase in size, with more pronounced growth in the body until it reaches the eventual adult, pear-shaped appearance, with the diameter and length of the body being approximately double that of the cervix.[12] The normal postpubertal, or **adult, uterus** varies considerably in size. The maximum dimensions of the nulliparous uterus are approximately 8 cm in length by 5 cm in width by 4 cm in AP diameter. Multiparity increases the normal size by more than 1 cm in each dimension.[15,16] After menopause, the uterus atrophies, with the most rapid decrease in size occurring in the first 10 years following cessation of menstruation.[15] In patients over the age of 65 years, the uterus ranges from 3.5 to 6.5 cm in length and 1.2 to 1.8 cm in AP diameter.[16]

The normal **myometrium** consists of three layers that can be distinguished by sonography. The **intermediate layer** is the thickest and has a uniformly homogeneous texture of low to moderate echogenicity. The **inner layer** of myometrium is thin, compact, and relatively hypovascular.[17,18] This inner layer, which is hypoechoic and surrounds the relatively echogenic endometrium, has also been referred to as the subendometrial halo. The thin **outer layer** is slightly less echogenic than the intermediate layer and is separated from it by the arcuate vessels.

The **arcuate arteries** lie between the outer and intermediate layers of the myometrium and branch into the radial arteries which run in the intermediate layer to the level of the inner layer. The radial arteries then branch into the spiral arteries, which enter the endometrium. The uterine veins are larger than the accompanying arcuate arteries and are frequently identified as small focal anechoic areas by both trans-abdominal and transvaginal sonography.[19] This can be confirmed by Doppler examination (Fig. 15-6). **Calcification** may be seen in the arcuate arteries in postmenopausal women because of Monkeberg's sclerosis.[20,21] On sonography, such calcification appears as peripheral linear echogenic areas with shadowing; they should be distinguished from calcified leiomyomas (Fig. 15-7). This is a normal aging process; it may be accelerated in diabetic patients.

Small, highly echogenic foci in the inner layer of myometrium may be seen in normal women (Fig. 15-8). These foci, measuring only a few millimeters, may be single or multiple and are usually nonshadowing. They are thought to represent dystrophic calcification related to previous instrumentation such as dilatation and curettage or endocervical biopsy.[22] They are of no clinical significance.

Uterine perfusion can be assessed by duplex Doppler or color Doppler sonography of the uterine arteries. In normal women, the Doppler waveform usually shows a high-velocity, high-resistance pattern.

The normal **endometrial cavity** is seen as a thin echogenic line as a result of specular reflection from the interface between the opposing surfaces of the endometrium.[23] The sonographic appearance of the **endometrium** varies during the menstrual cycle (Figs. 15-9, A, B, and C) and has been correlated with histology.[17,24,25] The endometrium is composed of a **superficial functional layer** and a **deep basal layer.** The functional layer thickens throughout the menstrual cycle and is shed with each menses. The basal layer remains intact during the cycle and contains the spiral arteries, which elongate to supply the functional layer as it thickens. The proliferative phase of the cycle before ovulation is under the influence of estrogen, whereas progesterone is mainly responsible for maintenance of the endometrium in the secretory phase following ovulation. The **menstrual phase** endometrium

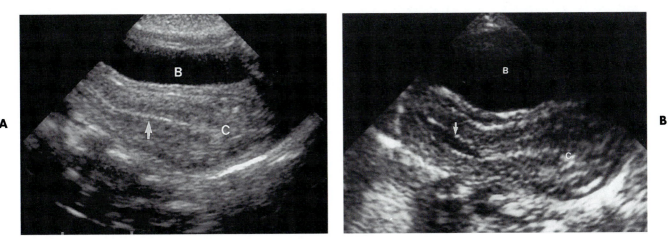

FIG. 15-5. Normal neonatal uterus. Sagittal scans. Note inverse pear shape with cervix (C) having greater AP diameter and length than body. **A,** The endometrium *(arrow)* is thin and normal. **B,** There is a small amount of fluid within endometrial canal *(arrow)*. B, Bladder.

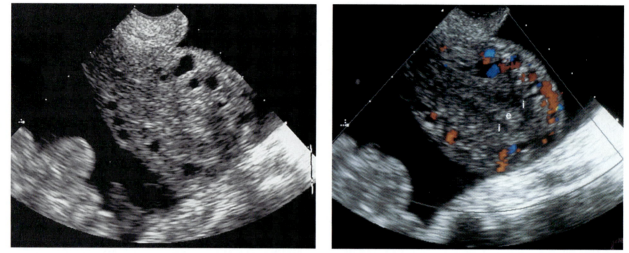

FIG. 15-6. Uterine veins. A, Transvaginal sagittal scan of uterus surrounded by ascites shows multiple peripheral anechoic areas. B, Confirmation by color Doppler. Endometrium (e), hypoechoic inner layer of myometrium (i). The outer layer of myometrium is separated from the intermediate layer by the arcuate veins.

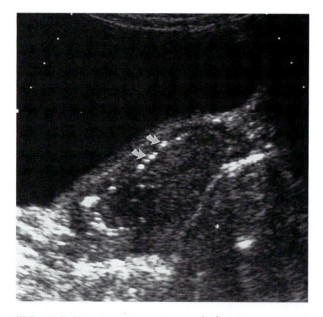

FIG. 15-7. Arcuate artery calcification. Sagittal scan shows multiple small peripheral linear hyperechoic foci (curved arrows).

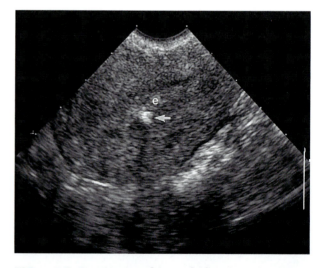

FIG. 15-8. Dystrophic calcification in inner layer of myometrium. Transvaginal scan shows echogenic focus (arrow) with shadowing located in hypoechoic inner layer of myometrium, which surrounds the endometrium (e).

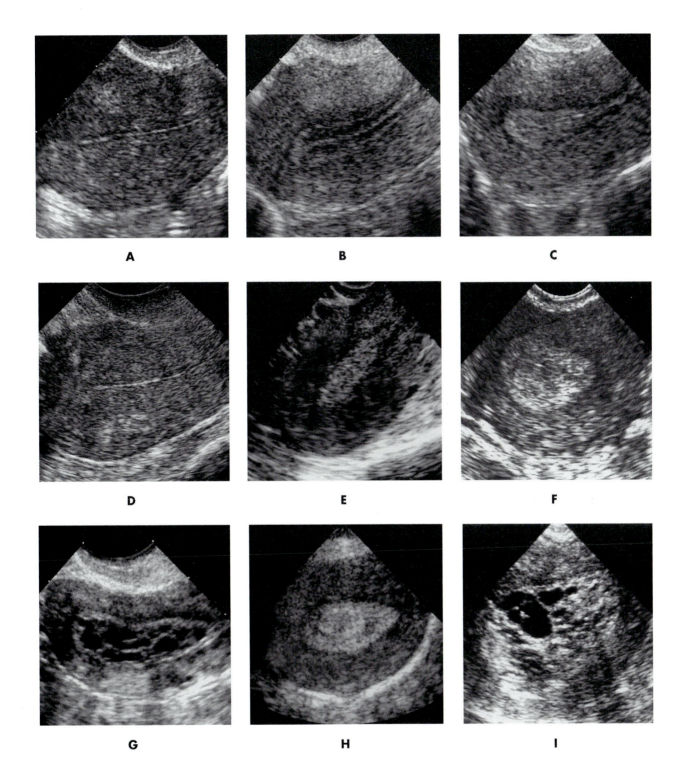

FIG. 15-9. **Endometrial changes.**   Transvaginal scans. **A,** Normal, thin early prolifer-ative endometrium. **B,** Normal late proliferative endometrium with triple-layer appearance. Central echogenic line due to opposed endometrial surfaces surrounded by thicker hypoechoic functional layer, bounded by outer echogenic basal layer. **C,** Normal, thick hyperechoic secre-tory endometrium. **D,** Normal, thin postmenopausal endometrium. **E,** Thickened, well-defined hyperechoic postmenopausal endometrium due to hyperplasia. **F,** Thickened endometrium shown on sonohysterogram to be due to multiple small polyps. **G,** Thick, cystic endometrium due to hyperplasia in patient on tamoxifen. **H,** Rounded, well-defined polyp which is slightly more hyperechoic than surrounding secretory endometrium. **I,** Thick, cystic endometrium due to large polyp in patient on tamoxifen.

consists of a thin, broken echogenic line. During the **proliferative phase,** the endometrium thickens, reaching 4 to 8 mm. The endometrium is best measured on a midline sagittal scan of the uterus and should include both anterior and posterior portions of the endometrium. It is important not to include the thin hypoechoic inner layer of myometrium in this measurement. A relatively hypoechoic region that represents the functional layer can be seen around the central echogenic line. In the early proliferative phase, this hypoechoic area is thin, but it increases and becomes more clearly defined in the later proliferative phase, probably as a result of edema. The hypoechoic appearance of the proliferative endometrium has been related to the relatively homogeneous histologic structure because of the orderly arrangement of the glandular elements. Following ovulation, the functional layer of the endometrium changes from hypoechoic to hyperechoic as the endometrium progresses to the **secretory**

phase.[24,25] The endometrium in this phase measures 7 to 14 mm in thckness. The hyperechoic texture in the secretory endometrium is related to increased mucus and glycogen within the glands as well as to the increased number of interfaces caused by the tortuosity of the spiral arteries. Acoustic enhancement may be seen posterior to the secretory endometrium, but it is not specific because it has also been seen with the proliferative endometrium, although not as frequently.[25]

Following menopause, the endometrium becomes **atrophic** as it is no longer under hormonal control. Sonographically, the endometrium is seen as a thin echogenic line measuring no more than 8 mm (Fig. 15-9, *D*).

Congenital Abnormalities

Congenital uterine abnormalities occur in approximately 0.5% of females and are associated with an increased incidence of spontaneous abortion and other obstetric complications.[26] The fused caudal ends of the two Müllerian (paramesonephric) ducts form the uterus, cervix, and upper vagina, whereas the unfused cranial ends form the paired fallopian tubes. Fusion occurs in a cephalad direction, and the median septum formed by the medial walls of the Müllerian ducts resorbs, leaving a single uterine cavity.[2]

Uterine malformations (Fig. 15-10) may be due to
- Arrested development of the Müllerian ducts;
- Failure of fusion of the Müllerian ducts; or
- Failure of resorption of the median septum.

THE PREMENOPAUSAL ENDOMETRIUM	
Menstrual phase	Thin broken echogenic line
Proliferative phase	Hypoechoic thickening 4 to 8 mm
Secretory phase	Hyperechoic thickening 7 to 14 mm

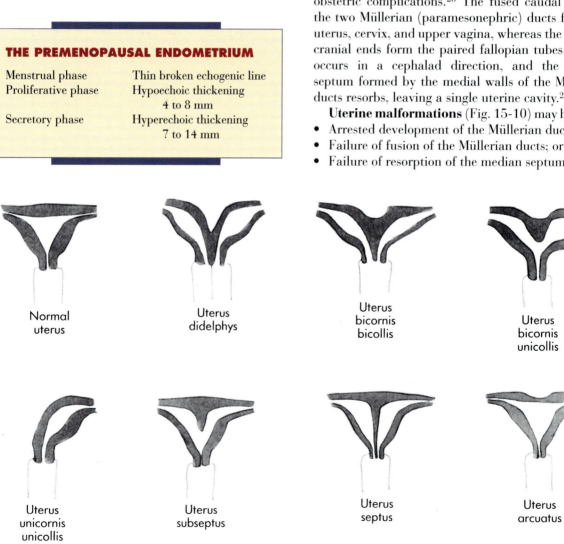

FIG. 15-10. Congenital uterine abnormalities. Diagram of common types. (Courtesy of Jocelyne Salem.)

Arrested development of the Müllerian ducts may be either unilateral or bilateral. Arrested bilateral development is extremely rare and results in congenital absence of the uterus or **uterine aplasia.** Arrested unilateral development results in a uterus unicornis unicollis (one uterine horn and one cervix). Hypoplasia of one Müllerian duct may result in a rudimentary uterine horn. Most rudimentary horns are noncommunicating and are connected to the opposite cornua by fibrous bands. If the endometrium in a rudimentary horn is nonfunctional, no clinical symptoms occur, but if a functional endometrium is present, retention of menstrual blood in the rudimentary horn may occur.

Failure of fusion of the Müllerian ducts may be complete, resulting in a **uterus didelphys** (two vaginas, two cervices, and two uteri), or partial, which may result in either a **uterus bicornis bicollis** (one vagina, two cervices, and two uterine horns) or a **uterus bicornis unicollis** (one vagina, one cervix, and two uterine horns). **Uterus arcuatus** is the mildest fusion anomaly, resulting in a partial indentation of the uterine fundus with a relatively normal endometrial cavity and is considered either a very mild form of the bicornuate uterus or a normal variant.

Failure of resorption of the median septum results in a **septate** or **subseptate uterus,** depending on whether the failure is complete or partial, respectively. This results in complete or partial duplication of the uterine cavities without duplication of the uterine horns and is the most common uterine abnormality. The septate or subseptate uterus can be distinguished from the bicornuate uterus by looking at the external contour of the uterus.

There is a high association between **uterine malformations** and **congenital renal abnormalities,** especially renal agenesis and ectopia.[27] The most common uterine anomaly associated with renal agenesis is the uterus bicornis bicollis with a partial vaginal septum in which one side has no outlet for menstrual blood, resulting in a unilateral hematometrocolpos.[28] In all patients with uterine malformations, the kidneys should be evaluated sonographically. Also, in females with an absent or ectopic kidney, the uterus should be scanned for malformations. The abnormalities are always on the same side.

Most uterine anomalies can be detected by sonography.[29] Two endometrial echo complexes may be seen in the bicornuate or septate uterus. Sonography can also outline the external contour of the uterus. In the **didelphys** and **bicornuate uterus,** the endometrial cavities are widely separated and there is a deep indentation on the fundal contour (Fig. 15-11, A). The **septate uterus,** in contrast, has a relatively normal outline, and the two endometrial cavities are closer together and are separated by a thin, fibrous septum (Fig. 15-11, B). The septum has a poor blood supply and contains little if any myometrium.[30] Sonography combined with hysterosalpingography has a high level of accuracy in distinguishing between the septate and the bicornuate uterus.[31] It is important to differentiate these two conditions, as the septate uterus can be treated by outpatient hysteroscopic incision of the fibrous septum, but because the bicornuate uterus consists of two separate uterine horns, each containing a full complement of myometrium and endometrium, correction requires abdominal surgery.

The unicornuate uterus is difficult to differentiate from the normal uterus by sonography. It may be suspected when the uterus appears small and laterally positioned. Hydometra in the opposite rudimentary horn may be seen and mistaken for a uterine or adnexal mass. The bicornuate uterus may also be confused with a uterine or adnexal mass if the central endometrial echo complex is not seen in one horn. In many instances, the bicornuate uterus is first diagnosed incidentally in early pregnancy when a gestational sac is present in one horn and there is decidual reaction in the other (Fig. 15-11, C).

MRI is highly accurate in demonstrating uterine anomalies.[32] However, because of the relatively high cost of MRI, it is usually reserved for the more complicated anomalies.

Uterine abnormalities have also been seen in patients who have had **in utero exposure to diethylstilbestrol.** Diethylstilbestrol given during the first trimester crosses the placenta and exerts a direct effect on the Müllerian system of the fetus. Sonography may demonstrate a diffuse decrease in the size of the uterus and an irregular T-shaped uterine cavity.[33,34]

Abnormalities of the Myometrium

Leiomyoma (Fibroid).
Leiomyomas are the most common neoplasms of the uterus. They occur in approximately 20% to 30% of females over the age of 30 years,[35] and they are more common in black women. They are usually multiple and are the most common cause of enlargement of the nonpregnant uterus. Although frequently asymptomatic, women with leiomyomas can experience pain and uterine bleeding. Leiomyomas may be classified as **intra-**

LEIOMYOMA CLASSIFICATION

Intramural
    Confined to the myometrium
Submucosal
    Projecting into the uterine cavity
Subserosal
    Projecting from the peritoneal surface

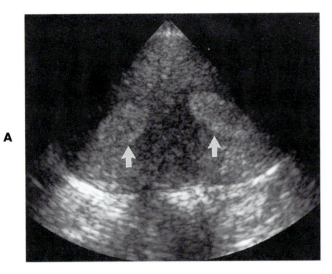

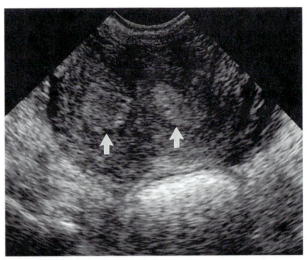

FIG. 15-11. Uterine anomalies. A, Coronal transvaginal scan through fundus of a bicornuate uterus shows two endometria *(arrows)* widely separated by uterine musculature. **B,** Coronal transvaginal scan through fundus of a septate uterus shows two endometria *(arrows)* separated only by a small amount of tissue. These endometria fused in lower uterus. **C,** Transverse transabdominal scan through fundus of a bicornuate uterus shows gestational sac (G) in left horn and decidual reaction *(arrow)* in right horn.

mural, confined to the myometrium; **submucosal,** projecting into the uterine cavity and displacing or distorting the endometrium; or **subserosal,** projecting from the peritoneal surface of the uterus.

Intramural fibroids are the most common. Submucosal fibroids, although less common, produce symptoms most frequently. Subserosal fibroids may be pedunculated and present as an adnexal mass. They may also project between the leaves of the broad ligament, where they are referred to as intraligamentous. Cervical fibroids account for approximately 8% of all fibroids.

Fibroids are **estrogen dependent** and may increase in size during anovulatory cycles as a result of unopposed estrogen stimulation[36] and during pregnancy, although about half of all fibroids show little significant change during pregnancy.[37] Large fibroids do not interfere with pregnancy or normal vaginal delivery, except when they are located in the lower uterine segment or the cervix. They rarely develop in postmenopausal women, and most stabilize or de-

crease in size following menopause. However, they may increase in size in postmenopausal patients undergoing hormone replacement therapy. Tamoxifen has also been reported to cause growth in leiomyomas.[38] A rapid increase in size, especially in a postmenopausal patient, should raise the possibility of sarcomatous change.[2]

Pathologically, leiomyomas are composed of spindle-shaped, smooth muscle cells arranged in whorl-like patterns separated by variable amounts of fibrous connective tissue. The surrounding myometrium may become compressed to form a pseudocapsule. As they enlarge, leiomyomas may outgrow their blood supply, resulting in ischemia and cystic degeneration.

Sonographically, leiomyomas have **variable** appearances (Fig. 15-12). The uterus may be enlarged, with a globular outline and heterogeneous echotexture resulting from small, diffuse leiomyomas. Localized leiomyomas are most commonly **hypoechoic** or **heterogeneous** in echotexture. They frequently distort the external contour of the uterus.

Minimal contour irregularity at the interface between the uterus and bladder may be a subtle diagnostic sign.[39] Many leiomyomas demonstrate areas of **acoustic attenuation** or **shadowing** without a discrete mass, making it impossible to estimate size. The attenuation is thought to be due to dense fibrosis within the substance of the tumor. Kliewer et al. have recently suggested that posterior shadowing arising from within the substance of a leiomyoma (but not from echogenic foci) originates from transitional zones between apposed tissues.[40] Histologically, the transitional zones included the margins of the leiomyoma with adjacent normal myometrium, the borders between fibrous tissue and smooth muscle, and the edges of whorls and bundles of smooth muscle.[40] **Calcification** may occur in older females, frequently appearing as focal areas of increased echogenicity with shadowing or as a curvilinear echogenic rim, which may simulate the outline of a fetal head.[41] **Degeneration** and **necrosis** produce areas of decreased echogenicity or cystic spaces within the fibroid. This tends to occur more commonly during pregnancy, affecting approximately 7% to 8% of pregnant patients with fibroids, who may present with pain over this area.[37] Giant leiomyomas with multiple cystic spaces due to edema have been described.[42]

Submucosal fibroids may impinge on the endometrium, distorting the lumen. Transvaginal sonography allows better differentiation between a submucosal and an intramural lesion and its relationship to the endometrial cavity.[43] In some cases, sonohysterography may be necessary to distinguish a submucosal leiomyoma from an endometrial lesion. Transvaginal sonography can detect very small leiomyomas and may be diagnostic in showing the uterine origin of large, pedunculated, subserosal leiomyomas that simulate adnexal masses. However, subserosal or pedunculated fibroids may be missed if the transvaginal approach alone is used, because of the limited field of view.[44] Leiomyomas in the fundus of a retroverted uterus are much better delineated by transvaginal sonography.

Lipomatous Uterine Tumors (Lipoleiomyoma).

Lipomatous uterine tumors are uncommon, benign neoplasms consisting of variable portions of mature lipocytes, smooth muscle, or fibrous tissue. Histologically, these tumors comprise a spectrum including pure lipomas, lipoleiomyomas, and fibrolipomyomas. **Sonographically,** the finding of a highly echogenic, attenuating mass within the myometrium is virtually diagnostic of this condition (Fig. 15-13).[45] Color Doppler shows complete absence of flow within the mass.[46] It is important to identify the lesion within the uterus so as not to con-

fuse it with the more common, similar-appearing, fat-containing ovarian dermoid.[47] Because lipomatous uterine tumors are usually asymptomatic, they do not require surgery.

Leiomyosarcoma.
Leiomyosarcoma is rare, accounting for 1.3% of uterine malignancies, and may arise from a preexisting uterine leiomyoma.[35] Frequently, patients are asymptomatic, although uterine bleeding may occur. This condition is rarely diagnosed preoperatively. Sonographically, the appearance is similar to that of a rapidly growing or degenerating leiomyoma, except when there is evidence of local invasion or distant metastases (Fig. 15-14).

Adenomyosis.
Adenomyosis is a condition characterized pathologically by the presence of endometrial glands and stroma within the myometrium. It is usually more extensive in the posterior wall.[35] The endometrial glands arise from the basal layer and are typically resistant to hormonal stimulation. Adenomyosis can occur in both diffuse and nodular forms. The more common diffuse form is composed of widely scattered adenomyosis foci within the myometrium, whereas the nodular form is composed of circumscribed nodules called adenomyomas. The clinical presentation is usually nonspecific, consisting of pelvic pain, dysmenorrhea, and menorrhagia.

Sonographically, the diagnosis has been considered to be difficult. Using transabdominal sonography, this diagnosis may be suggested if there is **diffuse uterine enlargement** with a normal contour, normal endometrial texture, and normal myometrial texture.[48] **Thickening of the posterior myometrium,** with the involved area being slightly more anechoic than normal myometrium, has also been described.[49] More recent reports have suggested that transvaginal sonography is more accurate in diagnosing this condition (Fig. 15-15).[50,51] **Inhomogeneous hypoechoic areas within the myometrium,** having indistinct margins, have been described. **Small myometrial cysts** may also be present within these inhomogeneous areas and have been shown histologically to represent dilated glands in ectopic endometrial tissue.[51] Adenomyosis is the most common cause of myometrial cysts, although cysts within the myometrium may also be congenital in origin or may be seen in leiomyomas undergoing cystic degeneration. Localized adenomyomas may be seen by transvaginal sonography as inhomogeneous, circumscribed areas in the myometrium, having indistinct margins and containing anechoic lacunae.[52] However, they are usually difficult to distinguish from leiomyomas, and these two conditions frequently occur together.

MRI is highly accurate in demonstrating adenomyosis, which appears as ill-defined areas of decreased signal intensity within the myometrium or dif-

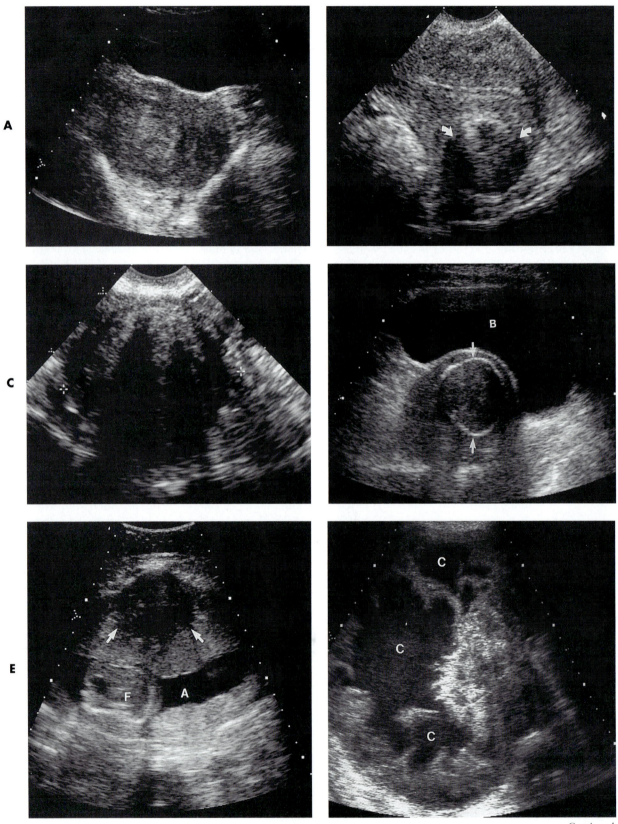

Continued.

FIG. 15-12. For legend see opposite page.

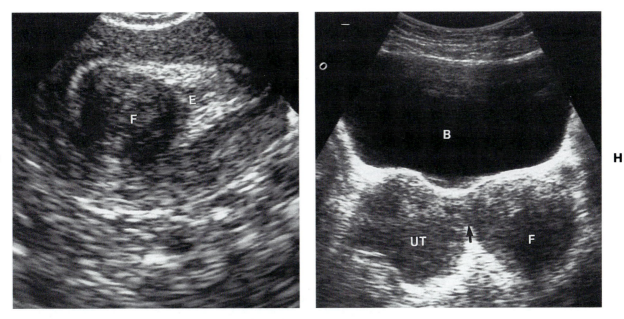

G   H

FIG. 15-12, cont'd. Uterine fibroids, varying appearances. A, D, E, F, H. Transabdominal scans. **B, C, G,** transvaginal scans. **A,** Enlarged uterus with lobulated contour and inhomogenous texture. **B,** Localized hypoechoic fibroid *(curved arrows)*. **C,** Marked attenuation of sound beam by fibroid (outlined by cursors). **D,** Calcified fibroid with curvilinear calcification *(arrows)* mimicking a fetal head. B, Bladder. **E,** Fibroid with cystic degeneration *(arrows)* in pregnancy. Patient presented with pain and tenderness over degenerating fibroid. F, fetus. A, amniotic fluid. **F,** Giant fibroid with multiple large cystic areas. This large fibroid seen during pregnancy showed marked increase in size and cystic areas (C) postpartum, suggesting possibility of leiomyosarcoma. **G,** Hypoechoic submucosal fibroid (F) distorting and displacing endometrium (E). **H,** Transverse scan shows pedunculated subserosal fibroid (F) presenting as solid left adnexal mass. Note communication *(arrow)* with uterus (UT). B, Bladder.

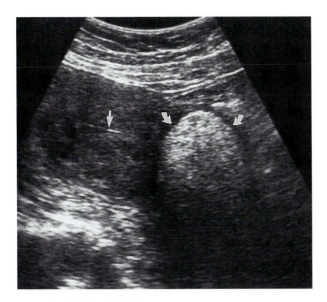

FIG. 15-13. Lipoleiomyoma. Transabdominal sagittal scan shows highly echogenic mass *(curved arrows)* with marked posterior attenuation within myometrium. *Arrow,* Endometrium.

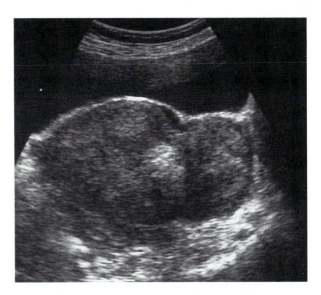

FIG. 15-14. Leiomyosarcoma. Transabdominal transverse scan shows enlarged lobulated uterus with diffusely inhomogeneous echo texture.

fuse or focal thickening of the juctional zone on T2 weighted images.[53-55]

Arteriovenous Malformations (AVM). Uterine AVMs (Fig. 15-16) consist of a vascular plexus of arteries and veins without an intervening capillary network. They are rare lesions, usually involving the myometrium and at times the endometrium. Although they may be congenital, most cases are acquired due to pelvic trauma, surgery, and gestational trophoblastic neoplasia. Patients, typically young women in the child-bearing years, present with metrorrhagia with hemoglobin-dropping blood loss. Diagnosis is critical, as dilatation and curettage may lead to catastrophic hemorrhage.

On sonography, uterine AVMs may be nonspecific, with minimal findings. They may be seen as multiple serpiginous, anechoic structures within the pelvis and may be confused with multiloculated ovarian cysts, fluid-filled bowel loops, and hydrosalpinx.[56] Color Doppler is diagnostic, showing **abundant blood flow within the anechoic structures.**[57,58] There is a florid color mosaic which is more extensive than the gray-scale abnormality. Spectral Doppler shows high-velocity, low-resistance arterial flow with high-velocity venous flow often being indistinguishable from the arterial signal.[58]

Treatment and confirmation include angiography with embolic therapy.

Abnormalities of the Endometrium

Because of its improved resolution, transvaginal sonography is better able to image and depict subtle abnormalities within the endometrium and to clearly define

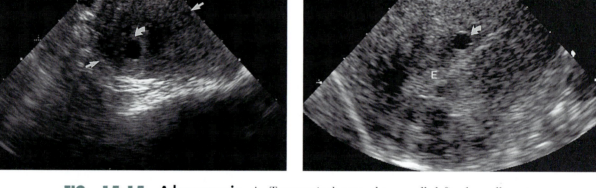

FIG. 15-15. Adenomyosis. A, Transvaginal scan shows well-defined small cyst *(curved arrow)* within an inhomogeneous hypoechoic area with indistinct margins *(arrows)* in fundal myometrium. **B,** Transvaginal scan in another patient shows a well-defined cyst *(curved arrow)* in the inner layer of myometrium. E, Endometrium.

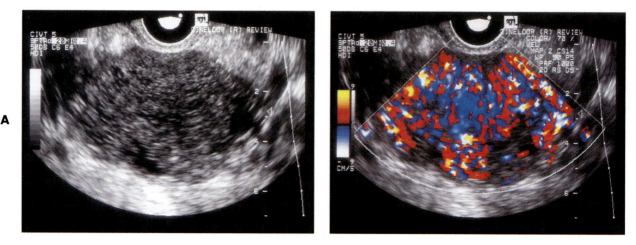

FIG. 15-16. Uterine arteriovenous malformation. A, Transverse transvaginal sonogram shows a textural inhomogeneity in the uterine fundus. **B,** Color Doppler image shows a floridly colored mosaic pattern with apparent flow reversals and areas of color aliasing. (From Huang M, Muradali D, Thurston WA et al. Uterine arteriovenous malformations (AVMs): ultrasound and Doppler features with MRI correlation. *Radiology* 1997. In press.)

the endometrial-myometrial border.[59] Knowledge of the normal sonographic appearance of the endometrium allows for earlier recognition of endometrial pathologic conditions manifested by endometrial thickening with well defined or poorly defined, irregular margins (see box). Many endometrial pathologies, such as **hyperplasia, polyps, and carcinoma,** can cause abnormal bleeding, especially in the postmenopausal patient. All of these conditions can have similar sonographic appearances.

Postmenopausal Endometrium. Several studies have shown that in patients with **postmenopausal bleeding** who have had endometrial sampling, an endometrial measurement of less than 5 mm can be considered normal.[60-65] The bleeding in these patients is usually due to an **atrophic endometrium.** In a recent large study of 1168 women with postmenopausal bleeding, in which 114 endometrial cancers were found, no women with endometrial cancer had an endometrium measuring less than 5 mm.[65]

Further studies have assessed the endometrium in **asymptomatic postmenopausal patients,** and it is felt that an endometrium of less than 9 mm can be considered normal.[66-69] Most reports have included a mixed group of patients, some of whom were undergoing hormone replacement therapy and some of whom were not. Many postmenopausal patients are now on hormone replacement therapy, as estrogen replacement decreases the risk of osteoporosis and relieves menopausal symptoms. However, unopposed estrogen replacement is associated with an increased risk of endometrial hyperplasia and carcinoma. Therefore, estrogen therapy is frequently combined with progesterone, in continuous combined or in sequential regimens. Patients on sequential hormone therapy have a changing endometrial appearance on sonography similar to the premenopausal endometrium. If noncyclic bleeding occurs, endometrial hyperplasia, polyps, and malignancy must be considered. In these patients, it is important that sonography be done either at the beginning or the end of the hormone cycle when the endometrium is at its thinnest.[69]

An endometrial thickness greater than 4 mm and 8 mm in the bleeding and asymptomatic postmenopausal woman, respectively, requires endometrial sampling. However, if the patient is on a sequential hormone regimen, the sonogram must be done early or late in the cycle (see box below).

A small amount of **fluid within the endometrial canal,** detected by transvaginal sonography, may be a

---

CAUSES OF ENDOMETRIAL THICKENING

Early intrauterine pregnancy
Incomplete abortion
Ectopic pregnancy
Retained products
Trophoblastic disease
Endometritis
Adhesions
Hyperplasia
Polyps
Carcinoma

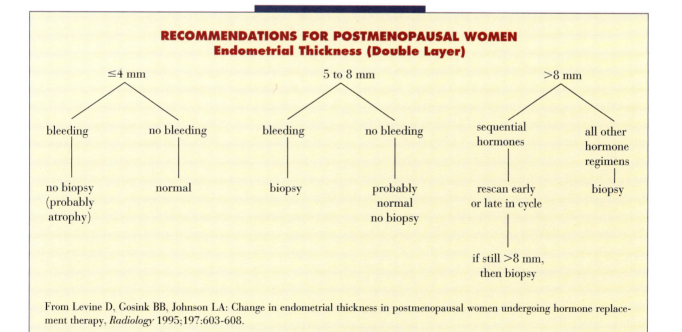

RECOMMENDATIONS FOR POSTMENOPAUSAL WOMEN
Endometrial Thickness (Double Layer)

≤4 mm
  bleeding → no biopsy (probably atrophy)
  no bleeding → normal

5 to 8 mm
  bleeding → biopsy
  no bleeding → probably normal no biopsy

>8 mm
  sequential hormones → rescan early or late in cycle → if still >8 mm, then biopsy
  all other hormone regimens → biopsy

From Levine D, Gosink BB, Johnson LA: Change in endometrial thickness in postmenopausal women undergoing hormone replacement therapy, *Radiology* 1995;197:603-608.

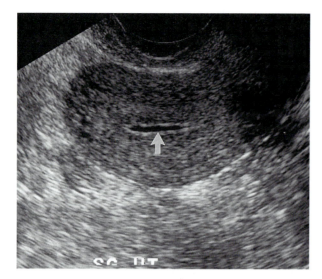

FIG. 15-17. Small amount of fluid (arrows) in postmenopausal endometrial canal. Transvaginal scan.

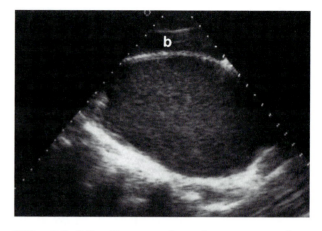

FIG. 15-18. Hematocolpos in young patient with imperforate hymen. Sagittal scan shows distended vagina filled with echogenic material compressing bladder (b) anteriorly.

normal finding in asymptomatic patients (Fig. 15-17).[70] Larger amounts of fluid may be associated with benign conditions, most often related to cervical stenosis, or with malignancy.[71,72] The fluid should be excluded when measuring the endometrium. As the fluid allows better detail of the endometrium, it is extremely important to assess the endometrium carefully for irregularities and polypoid masses.[73]

Hydrometrocolpos and Hematometrocolpos. Obstruction of the genital tract results in the accumulation of secretions, blood, or both in the uterus and/or vagina, with the location depending on the amount of obstruction. Before menstruation, the accumulation of secretions in the vagina and uterus is referred to as hydrometrocolpos. Following menstruation, hematometrocolpos results from the presence of retained menstrual blood. The obstruction may be congenital and is most commonly due to an **imperforate hymen.** Other congenital causes include a **vaginal septum, vaginal atresia,** or a **rudimentary uterine horn.**[74] Hydrometra and hematometra may also be acquired as a result of cervical stenosis from **endometrial or cervical tumors** or from **postirradiation fibrosis.**[71,75]

Sonographically, if the obstruction is at the vaginal level, there is marked distention of the vagina and endometrial cavity with fluid. If seen before puberty, the accumulation of secretions is anechoic. Following menstruation, the presence of old blood results in echogenic material in the fluid (Fig. 15-18). There may also be layering of the echogenic material, resulting in a fluid-fluid level.

Acquired hydrometra or hematometra usually shows a distended, fluid-filled endometrial cavity which may contain echogenic material (Fig. 15-19). Superimposed infection (**pyometra**) is difficult to dis-

tinguish from hydrometra on sonography, and this diagnosis is usually made clinically in the presence of hydrometra.[75]

Endometrial Hyperplasia. Hyperplasia of the endometrium is defined as a proliferation of glands of irregular size and shape, with an increase in the gland/stroma ratio when compared with the normal proliferative endometrium.[35] The process is diffuse but may not involve the entire endometrium. Histologically, endometrial hyperplasia can be divided into hyperplasia without cellular atypia and hyperplasia with cellular atypia (atypical hyperplasia). Long-term follow-up studies have shown that about one quarter of atypical hyperplasia will progress to carcinoma, as opposed to less than 2% of hyperplasia without cellular atypia.[35] Each of these types may be further subdivided into simple (cystic) or complex (adenomatous) hyperplasia, depending on the amount of glandular complexity and crowding. In simple (cystic) hyperplasia, the glands are cystically dilated and surrounded by abundant cellular stroma, whereas in complex (adenomatous) hyperplasia, the glands are crowded together, with little intervening stroma.

Endometrial hyperplasia is a common cause of abnormal uterine bleeding. Hyperplasia develops from unopposed estrogen stimulation; in postmenopausal and perimenopausal women, it is usually due to **unopposed estrogen hormone replacement therapy.** Hyperplasia is less commonly seen during the reproductive years, but it may occur in women with **persistent anovulatory cycles, polycystic ovarian disease,** and in **obese women** with increased production of endogenous estrogens. Hyperplasia may also be seen in women with estrogen-producing tumors, such as **granulosa cell tumors** and **thecomas of the ovary.**

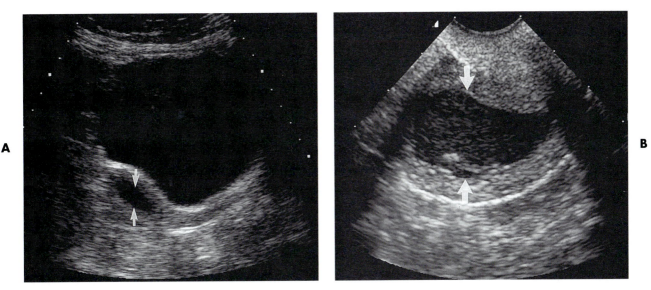

FIG. 15-19. Hematometra in patient with cervical stenosis secondary to cervical carcinoma. A, Transabdominal sagittal scan shows small postmenopausal uterus with fluid-filled endometrial canal *(arrows)*. B, Transvaginal scan shows distended endometrial canal *(arrows)* filled with fluid containing echogenic material of varying intensity as a result of blood and debris.

Sonographically, the endometrium is usually thick and echogenic, with well-defined margins (Fig. 15-9, *E*). Small cysts may be seen within the endometrium in **cystic hyperplasia;** however, a similar appearance may be seen in **cystic atrophy,** and cystic changes can also be seen in **endometrial polyps.** These cystic areas have been shown to represent the dilated cystic glands seen at histology.[76,77] Although cystic changes within a thickened endometrium are more frequently seen in benign conditions, they can also be seen in **endometrial carcinoma.**[78]

Endometrial Atrophy. The majority of women with postmenopausal uterine bleeding have endometrial atrophy.[61-65,79] On transvaginal sonography, an atrophic endometrium is usually thin, measuring less than 5 mm, and in these patients, no further investigation or therapy is necessary. Histologically, the endometrial glands may be dilated, but the cells are cuboidal or flat and the stroma is fibrotic. A thin endometrium with cystic changes on transvaginal sonography is consistent with a diagnosis of cystic atrophy, but when the endometrium is thick, the appearance is indistinguishable from that of cystic hyperplasia.[78]

Endometrial Polyps. Endometrial polyps are common lesions that are more frequently seen in perimenopausal and postmenopausal women. They may cause uterine bleeding, although most are asymptomatic. In the menstruating woman, they may present with intermenstrual bleeding or menometrorrhagia and may be a cause of infertility. Histologically, polyps are localized overgrowths of endometrial tissue covered by epithelium and they contain a variable

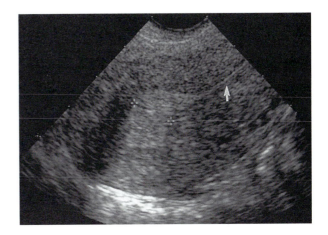

FIG. 15-20. Endometrial polyp. Transvaginal scan shows localized endometrial thickening in uterine fundus (outlined by cursors). This appearance is nonspecific and can also be seen with localized hyperplasia and carcinoma. Endometrium in the uterine body *(arrow)* is thin and normal.

number of glands, stroma, and blood vessels.[35] They may be pedunculated or broad-based or have a thin stalk. Approximately 20% of endometrial polyps are multiple. Malignant degeneration is uncommon. Occasionally, a polyp will have a long stalk, allowing it to protrude into the cervix or even into the vagina.

On sonography, polyps may appear as nonspecific echogenic endometrial thickening, which may be diffuse or localized (Fig. 15-9, *F* and Fig. 15-20). However, they may also appear as a focal, round, echogenic mass within the endometrial cavity

(Fig. 15-9, *H*),[80] and this appearance is much more easily identified when there is fluid within the endometrial cavity outlining the mass. Because fluid is instilled into the endometrial cavity during **sonohysterography**, this technique is ideal for demonstrating polyps (Figs. 15-21, *A* through *F*).[81,82] Sonohysterography is also a valuable technique when transvaginal sonography is unable to differentiate an **endometrial polyp** from a **submucosal leiomyoma** (Figs. 15-21, *G* and *H*). The polyp can be seen arising from the endometrium, whereas a normal layer of endometrium is seen overlying the submucosal fibroid.[83]

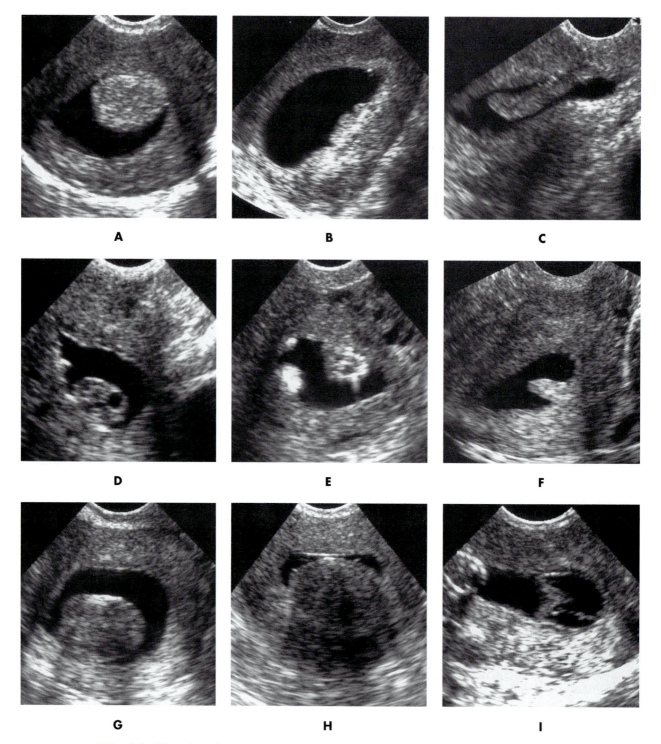

FIG. 15-21. Sonohysterograms. A, Well-defined, round echogenic polyp. **B,** Carpet of small polyps. **C,** Polyp on a stalk. **D,** Polyp with cystic areas. **E,** Small polyp. **F,** Small polyp. **G,** Hypoechoic submucosal fibroid. **H,** Hypoechoic attenuating submucosal fibroid. **I,** Endometrial adhesions. Note bridging bands of tissue within fluid-filled endometrial canal. (Courtesy of Stephanie R. Wilson, M.D., University of Toronto.)

Cystic areas may be seen within a polyp (Fig. 15-9, *I*), representing the histologically dilated glands.[76,77] Occasionally, a **feeding artery** in the pedicle may be seen with color Doppler.

Endometrial polyps may not be diagnosed on dilatation and curettage, as a polyp on a pliable stalk may be missed by the curette. If abnormal bleeding persists after a nondiagnostic dilatation and curettage in a postmenopausal woman with an endometrial thickness greater than 8 mm, then hysteroscopy with direct visualization of the endometrial cavity is recommended.[84]

Endometrial Carcinoma. Endometrial carcinoma is the most common gynecologic malignancy in North America, and its incidence has been rising. It occurs in approximately 3% of women yet accounts for less than 1.5% of cancer deaths because more than 75% of the carcinomas are confined to the uterus at the time of clinical presentation. Most—75% to 80%—endometrial carcinomas occur in postmenopausal women. The most common clinical presentation is uterine bleeding, although only 10% of women with postmenopausal bleeding will have endometrial carcinoma. There is a strong association with replacement estrogen therapy. In the premenopausal woman, anovulatory cycles and obesity are also considered risk factors, as in endometrial hyperplasia. Approximately 25% of patients with atypical endometrial hyperplasia will progress to well-differentiated endometrial carcinoma.[35]

Sonographically, a thickened endometrium must be considered cancer until proven otherwise. The thickened endometrium may be well-defined, uniformly echogenic, and indistinguishable from hyperplasia and polyps. Cancer is more likely when the endometrium has an inhomogeneous echotexture with irregular or poorly defined margins (Fig. 15-22).

Cystic changes within the endometrium are more commonly seen in **endometrial atrophy, hyperplasia,** and **polyps** but can also be seen with carcinoma.[78] Endometrial carcinoma may also obstruct the endometrial canal, resulting in hydrometra or hematometra. Although certain sonographic appearances tend to favor a benign or malignant etiology, there are overlapping features, and endometrial biopsy is usually required for a definite diagnosis.

Tamoxifen, a nonsteroidal antiestrogen compound, is widely used for adjuvant therapy in pre- and postmenopausal women with breast cancer. Tamoxifen acts by competing with estrogen for estrogen receptors. In premenopausal women it has an antiestrogen effect, but in postmenopausal women it may have weak estrogenic effects. An **increased risk of endometrial carcinoma** has been reported in patients on tamoxifen therapy,[85] as well as an increased risk of **endometrial hyperplasia** and **polyps.**[86,87] On sonography, tamoxifen-related endometrial changes are nonspecific and similar to those described in hyperplasia, polyps, and carcinoma.[87-89] Cystic changes within the thickened endometrium are frequently seen (Fig. 15-9, *F, I* and Fig. 15-23, *A*).

In some patients on tamoxifen therapy, the cystic changes have actually been shown to be **subendometrial** in location (Fig. 15-23, *B*) and may represent abnormal adenomyomatous-like changes in the inner layer of myometrium.[90]

The role of color and spectral Doppler in the diagnosis of endometrial carcinoma is still controversial. Initial studies using transvaginal color and spectral Doppler suggested that endometrial carcinoma could be differentiated from a normal or benign postmenopausal endometrium by the presence of

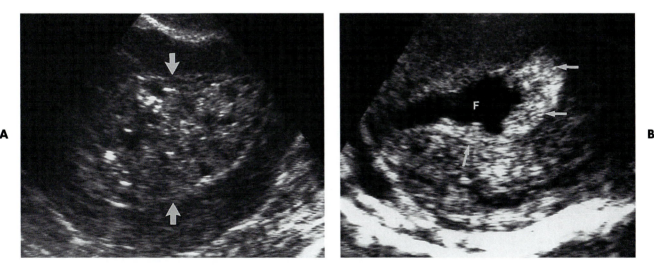

A **B**

FIG. 15-22. Endometrial carcinoma, varying appearances. Transvaginal scans. **A,** Thickened inhomogenous endometrium *(arrows)* with multiple small cystic areas. **B,** Localized irregular endometrial thickening *(arrows)* with echogenic polypoid projections into fluid-filled endometrial canal (F).

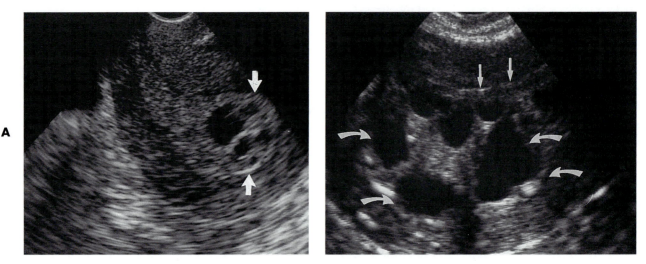

FIG. 15-23. Tamoxifen effect, varying appearances. Transvaginal scans. **A,** Cystic polyp *(arrows)* in patient on long-term tamoxifen therapy. **B,** Multiple cystic areas *(curved arrows)* adjacent to thin endometrium *(arrows)* in postmenopausal woman on long-term tamoxifen therapy. Sonographic appearance did not change over a 9-month interval, and endometrial sampling on two separate occasions showed only endometrial atrophy. Changes probably result from adenomyosis in inner layer of myometrium.

low-resistance flow in the uterine arteries in women with endometrial cancer, as compared with high-resistance flow in women with normal or benign endometria.[91,92] Subsequent reports, however, have shown no significant difference in uterine blood flow between benign and malignant endometrial processes.[93-95] Low-resistance flow in the uterine artery has also been reported in association with uterine fibroids.[92] More recent reports have assessed subendometrial and endometrial blood flow, as well, and some investigators have found a significant difference between benign and malignant endometrial lesions, with malignancies demonstrating low-resistance flow in the subendometrial and endometrial arteries.[68,96] Others, in evaluating these arteries, have found no statistically significant difference.[94,95,97] Blood flow is difficult to detect in the normal endometrium. Sladkevicius et al. felt endometrial thickness to be a better method for discriminating between normal and pathologic or benign and malignant endometrium than Doppler of the uterine, subendometrial, or intraendometrial arteries.[95] Further studies with large numbers of patients are necessary to determine whether Doppler will play a role in differentiating benign from malignant endometrial processes.

Sonography may be used in the preoperative evaluation of a patient with endometrial carcinoma by determining myometrial invasion.[98-100] Intactness of the subendometrial halo (the inner layer of myometrium) usually indicates superficial invasion, whereas obliteration of the halo is indicative of deep invasion.[98] MRI may also be helpful in assessing myometrial invasion. Transvaginal sonography and unenhanced T2-weighted MRI have been reported to have similar ac-

curacy,[101] but contrast-enhanced MRI is believed to be superior to both in demonstrating myometrial invasion.[102] MRI can also assess cervical extension. Sonography may be helpful in staging carcinoma and distinguishing between tumors limited to the uterus (stages I and II) and those with extrauterine extension (stages III and IV).[99] CT may also be helpful in staging by demonstrating lymphadenopathy and distant disease (stages III or IV).

Endometritis. Endometritis may occur postpartum, following dilatation and curettage, or in association with pelvic inflammatory disease. **Sonographically,** the endometrium may appear thick, irregular, or both and the cavity may or may not contain fluid (Fig. 15-24). Gas with distal acoustic shadowing may be seen within the endometrial canal. However, gas can be seen in up to 21% of clinically normal women following uncomplicated vaginal delivery in the first 3 weeks postpartum.[103] Therefore, clinical correlation is necessary when endometrial gas is seen in the postpartum patient.

Endometrial Adhesions (Synechiae). Endometrial adhesions may be a cause of infertility or recurrent pregnancy loss. The sonographic diagnosis is difficult unless fluid is distending the endometrial cavity. The endometrium usually appears normal on transabdominal and transvaginal sonograms, although adhesions may be seen transvaginally as irregularities or a hypoechoic bridge-like band within the endometrium.[104] This is best seen during the secretory phase when the endometrium is more hyperechoic. **Sonohysterography** is an excellent technique for demonstrating adhesions, as fluid is instilled into the

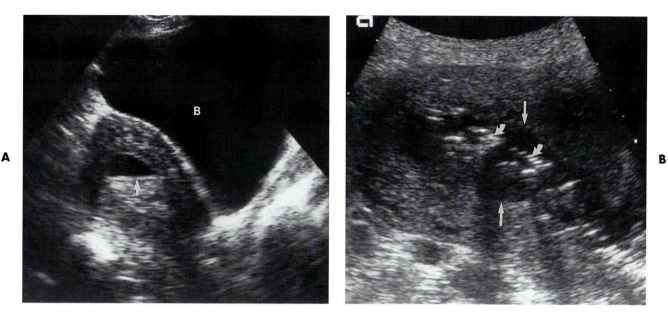

FIG. 15-24. Endometritis, varying appearances. Transabdominal sagittal scans. **A,** Fluid-fluid level *(arrow)* within endometrial canal in patient with pelvic inflammatory disease. This resolved following antibiotic therapy. B, Bladder. **B,** Multiple linear hyperechogenic foci *(curved arrows)* with shadowing due to gas within distended endometrial canal *(arrows)* in a febrile postpartum patient.

endometrial cavity. Adhesions appear as bridging bands of tissue that distort the cavity (Fig. 15-21, *I*) or as thin, undulating membranes best seen on real time.[3] Thick, broad-based adhesions may prevent distension of the uterine cavity.[81] The adhesions can be divided under hysteroscopy.

Intrauterine Contraceptive Devices. Intrauterine contraceptive devices (IUDs) are readily demonstrated on sonography (Fig. 15-25). They appear as highly echogenic linear structures in the endometrial cavity in the body of the uterus. Several types of IUDs demonstrate a characteristic appearance on sonography, reflecting their gross appearance. One must be able to distinguish the IUD from the normal, high-amplitude central endometrial cavity echo. Acoustic shadowing from the IUD is usually demonstrated, and two parallel echoes (entrance-exit reflections), representing the anterior and posterior surfaces of the IUD, may also be observed.[105] Sonography can demonstrate malposition, perforation, and incomplete removal of an IUD. Eccentric position of an IUD suggests myometrial penetration. If the IUD is not seen on sonography, a radiograph should be taken to assess whether the IUD is lying free in the peritoneal cavity or is not present, having been previously expelled. The IUD may be hidden by coexisting intrauterine abnormalities such as blood clots or an incomplete abortion. When an IUD is present in the uterus in association with an intrauterine pregnancy, the IUD can be seen reliably early in the first trimester,

but it is rarely identified thereafter. In the first trimester, the IUD can usually be removed safely under ultrasound guidance.

Abnormalities of the Cervix

The cervix may be difficult to assess adequately by transabdominal sonography, as it lies low in the pelvis, posterior to the bladder. Better visualization is obtained by transvaginal sonography, especially if the probe is partially withdrawn and angled either posteriorly, if the uterus is anteverted, or anteriorly, if the uterus is retroverted.

Cervical abnormalities are usually diagnosed clinically. **Nabothian (inclusion) cysts** of the cervix are commonly seen during routine sonography (Fig. 15-26). They may vary in size from a few millimeters to 4 cm. They may be single or multiple and are usually diagnosed incidentally, but they may be associated with healing chronic cervicitis. Occasionally, Nabothian cysts may have internal echoes that may be caused by hemorrhage or infection. Multiple cysts may be a cause of benign enlargement of the cervix.[106]

Cervical polyps are a frequent cause of vaginal bleeding and may be seen on sonography (Fig. 15-27). However, the diagnosis is usually made clinically. Approximately 8% of **leiomyomas** arise in the cervix. They may be pedunculated and prolapse into the vagina. In patients who have had a hysterectomy, the cervical stump may occasionally simulate a mass. Transvaginal sonography is usually diagnostic; it can

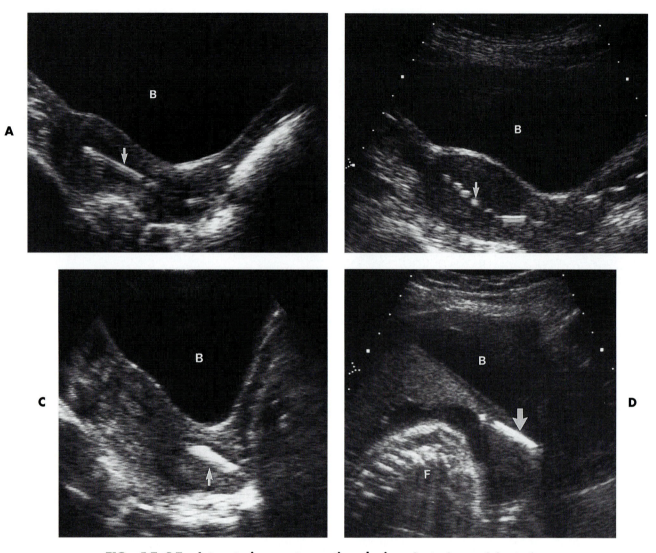

FIG. 15-25. **Intrauterine contraceptive device.** Sagittal transabdominal scans. **A,** Highly echogenic linear structure *(arrow)* in normal location within endometrial canal in body of uterus. **B,** Interrupted echogenic foci *(arrow)* in endometrial canal in body of uterus. Typical appearance of Lippes loop. **C,** Intrauterine contraceptive device *(arrow)* in cervical canal. **D,** Intrauterine contraceptive device *(arrow)* in a 30-week gravid uterus. F, Fetus. B, Bladder.

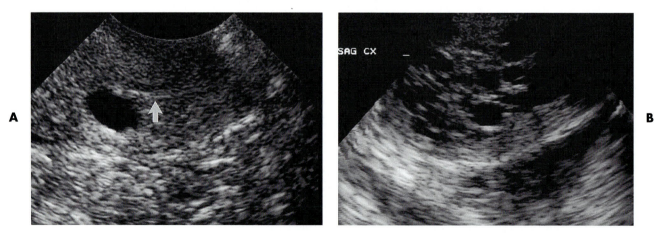

FIG. 15-26. **Nabothian cysts.** Transvaginal scans. **A,** Single Nabothian cyst in the cervix. Endocervical canal *(arrow)*. **B,** Multiple nabothian cysts in cervix.

demonstrate a normal cervix. **Cervical stenosis** may be secondary to previous radiation therapy, previous cone biopsy, postmenopausal cervical atrophy, or cervical carcinoma.

Cervical carcinoma is usually diagnosed clinically, and patients are rarely referred for sonographic evaluation. Sonography may demonstrate a solid retrovesical mass, which may be indistinguishable from a cervical fibroid (Fig. 15-28). Sonography may be used for staging, but CT and MRI are preferable.

VAGINA

The vagina runs anteriorly and caudally from the cervix between the bladder and rectum. It is best seen sonographically on midline sagittal sections with a slight caudal angulation of the transducer. It appears as a collapsed hypoechoic tubular structure with a central, high-amplitude, linear echo representing the apposed surfaces of the vaginal mucosa (Fig. 15-2). The most common congenital abnormality of the female genital tract is an **imperforate hymen** resulting in hematocolpos. Occasionally, sonography is used to characterize a vaginal mass. **Gartner's duct cysts** are mesonephric duct remnants that form single or multiple cysts along the lateral or anterolateral wall of the vagina (Fig. 15-29). These are the most common cystic lesions of the vagina and are usually found incidentally during sonographic examination. **Solid masses** of the vagina are rare (Fig. 15-30). Two cases of neurofibroma of the vagina that appear as solid masses have been described.[107] As in carcinoma of the cervix, sonography is not used for diagnosis of carcinoma of the vagina, but it may play a role in staging.

In patients who have had a hysterectomy, a **vaginal cuff** should not be mistaken for a mass. The upper limit of normal for the anteroposterior diameter of the vaginal cuff is 2.1 cms.[108] A cuff that is larger than 2.1 cm or that contains a definite mass suggests malignancy. Nodular areas may be due to postirradiation fibrosis.[108]

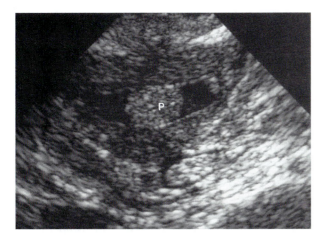

FIG. 15-27. Cervical polyp. Transvaginal scan shows echogenic polyp (P) outlined by fluid in cervical canal.

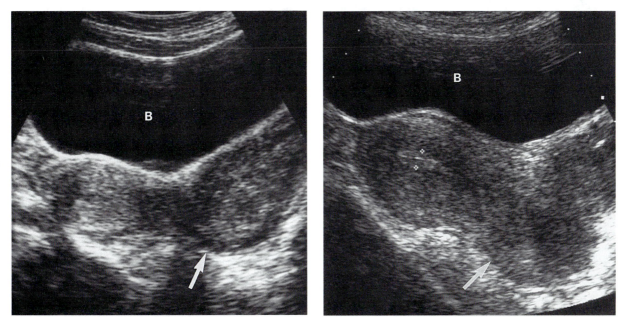

FIG. 15-28. **Cervical fibroid and carcinoma in two different patients with a similar appearance.** Transabdominal sagittal scans. **A,** Enlarged inhomogeneous cervix *(arrow)* due to cervical fibroid. **B,** Enlarged inhomogeneous cervix *(arrow)* due to cervical carcinoma. Endometrium outlined by cursors. B, Bladder.

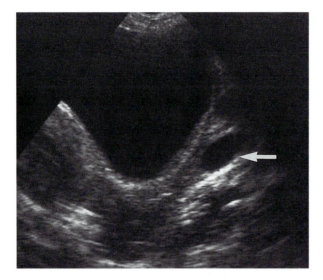

FIG. 15-29. Gartner's duct cyst. Sagittal scan shows cystic mass *(arrow)* in vaginal wall.

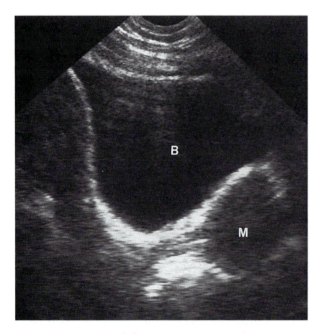

FIG. 15-30. Solid mass **(M) in vagina.** Sagittal scan. At surgery, this was located along anterior wall of vagina and, pathologically, was uterine fibroid. B, Bladder.

RECTOUTERINE RECESS (POSTERIOR CUL-DE-SAC)

The **posterior cul-de-sac** is the most posterior and inferior reflection of the peritoneal cavity. It is located between the rectum and vagina and is also known as the *pouch of Douglas.* The posterior fornix of the vagina is closely related to the posterior cul-de-sac and is separated by the thickness of the vaginal wall and the peritoneal membrane. The posterior cul-de-sac is a potential space, and because of its location, it

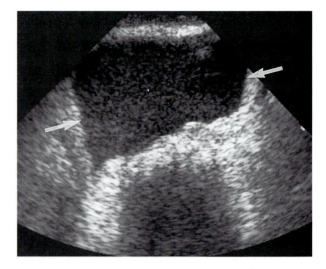

FIG. 15-31. Echogenic fluid in cul-de-sac *(arrows)* **due to blood.** Transvaginal scan.

is frequently the initial site for intraperitoneal fluid collection. As little as 5 cc of fluid have been detected by transvaginal sonography.[109]

Fluid in the cul-de-sac is a normal finding in asymptomatic women and can be seen during all phases of the menstrual cycle. Possible sources have been postulated, including blood or fluid caused by follicular rupture, blood caused by retrograde menstruation, and increased capillary permeability of the ovarian surface caused by the influence of estrogen.[110,111]

Pathologic fluid collections in the pouch of Douglas may be seen in association with generalized ascites, blood resulting from a ruptured ectopic pregnancy or hemorrhagic cyst, or pus resulting from infection. Sonography may aid in differentiating the type of fluid because blood, pus, mucin, and malignant exudates usually contain echoes within the fluid, whereas serous fluid (either physiologic or pathologic) is usually anechoic. Clotted blood may be very echoic.[112] Transvaginal sonography can demonstrate echoes within the fluid more frequently because of its improved resolution (Fig. 15-31).[113]

Pelvic abscesses and hematomas can occur in the cul-de-sac, and the sonographic appearance is similar to these conditions elsewhere in the body.

OVARY

Normal Sonographic Anatomy

Uterine location influences the position of the ovaries. The normal ovaries are usually identified laterally or posterolaterally to the anteflexed midline uterus. When the uterus lies to one side of the midline (a normal variant), the ipsilateral ovary often lies supe-

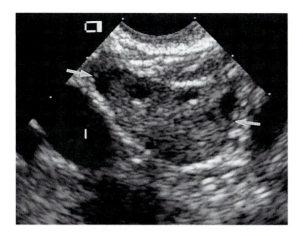

FIG. 15-32. Normal ovary. Transvaginal scan in menstruating woman shows ovary *(arrows)* with a few peripheral follicles. Internal iliac vein (I) is seen posterior to ovary.

rior to the uterine fundus. In a retroverted uterus, the ovaries tend to be located laterally and superiorly, near the uterine fundus. When the uterus is enlarged, the ovaries tend to be displaced more superiorly and laterally. Following hysterectomy, the ovaries tend to be located more medially and directly superior to the vaginal cuff.

Because of the laxity of the ligamentous attachments, the ovary can be quite variable in position and may be located high in the pelvis or in the cul-de-sac. Because of their **variable position,** superiorly or extremely laterally placed ovaries may not be visualized by the transvaginal approach, as they are out of the field of view. The ovaries are ellipsoid in shape, with their craniocaudad axes paralleling the internal iliac vessels, which lie posteriorly and serve as a helpful reference (Fig. 15-32). In patients with uterine leiomyomas, some investigators have been able to visualize the ovaries more frequently by transvaginal sonography than by the transabdominal method.[7,8]

On **sonography,** the normal ovary has a relatively homogeneous echotexture with a central, more echogenic medulla. Well-defined, small anechoic or cystic follicles may be seen peripherally in the cortex. The appearance of the ovary changes with age and with the phase of the menstrual cycle. During the early proliferative phase, many follicles that are stimulated by both follicle-stimulating hormone (FSH) and luteinizing hormone (LH) develop and increase in size until about day 8 or 9 of the menstrual cycle. At that time one follicle becomes dominant, destined for ovulation, and increases in size, reaching up to 2.0 to 2.5 cm at the time of ovulation. The other follicles become atretic. A **follicular cyst** develops if the fluid in one of these nondominant follicles is not resorbed. Following ovulation, the corpus luteum develops and may be

identified sonographically as a small hypoechoic or isoechoic structure peripherally within the ovary. The corpus luteum involutes before menstruation.

Because of the variability in shape, ovarian **volume** has been considered the best method for determining ovarian size. The volume measurement is based on the formula for a prolate ellipse (0.523 × length × width × height). Recent studies have shown that ovarian volumes are larger than previously thought. In the first 2 years of life, the mean ovarian volume is slightly greater than 1 cc in the first year and 0.7 cc in the second year.[114] The upper limit of normal has been reported as 3.6 cc in the first 3 months, 2.7 cc from 4 to 12 months, and 1.7 cc in the second year.[114] Ovarian volume remains relatively stable up to 5 years of age and then gradually increases up to menarche when the mean volume is 4.2 ± 2.3 cc, with an upper limit of 8.0 cc.[12] Small follicles or cysts are frequently seen in neonatal and premenarchal ovaries. These usually measure less than 9 mm but may be as large as 17 mm.[115]

In the adult menstruating female, a normal ovary may have a volume as large as 22 cc. Cohen et al. assessed 866 normal ovaries by transabdominal sonography and reported a mean ovarian volume of 9.8 ± 5.8 cc, with an upper limit of 21.9 cc.[116] Another study of 406 patients with normal ovaries used transvaginal sonography and reported a mean ovarian volume of 6.8 cc, with an upper limit of 18.0 cc.[117]

Focal calcification may occasionally be seen in an otherwise normal-appearing ovary and is thought to represent stromal reaction to previous hemorrhage or infection.[118] However, the calcification may be the initial or early manifestation of a neoplasm, so follow-up sonography is recommended.

Postmenopausal Ovary

Following menopause, the ovary atrophies and the follicles disappear over the subsequent few years, with the ovary decreasing in size with increasing age.[119-121] Due to its smaller size and lack of follicles, the postmenopausal ovary may be difficult to visualize sonographically (Fig. 15-33). A stationary loop of bowel may be mistaken for a normal ovary; therefore, scanning must be done slowly to look for peristalsis. **Sonographic visualization** of normal postmenopausal ovaries varies greatly in the literature, from a low of 20% to a high of 99%, using either the transabdominal or transvaginal approach.[10,116,119-123] The variation is likely to be due to differences in technique and length of time since menopause, as ability to see the ovaries has been shown to decrease with lengthening time since menopause.[124] Also, the absence of the uterus may play a role, as the ovaries are less likely to be seen following hysterectomy because of the loss

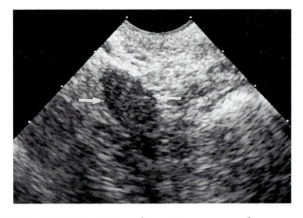

FIG. 15-33. Normal postmenopausal ovary.
Transvaginal scan shows normal postmenopausal ovary *(arrows)*. Note small size and lack of follicles.

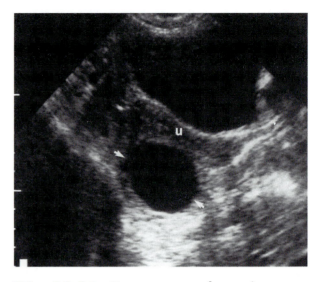

FIG. 15-34. Postmenopausal ovarian cyst.
Sagittal scan in 75-year-old-woman shows 4-cm ovarian cyst *(arrows)* posterior to uterus (u). Cyst contains no internal echoes or septations and had not changed in size over two years.

of normal anatomical landmarks. Wolf et al., in a study of 290 postmenopausal ovaries known to be present, using both transabdominal and transvaginal sonography, visualized only 41% of ovaries transvaginally and 58% transabdominally. Using both techniques resulted in their visualizing more ovaries than when they used either technique alone (68%).[124] Highly placed ovaries may be out of the field of view of transvaginal transducers, and transabdominal sonography may not be sensitive enough to image very small ovaries. Nonvisualization of an ovary does not exclude the possibility of an ovarian lesion.

Various studies of size have shown a mean ovarian volume ranging from 1.2 cc to 5.8 cc.[116,117,119-123] The mean values in these studies may be somewhat high, as nonvisualized ovaries were not included. One study assessing 563 patients with normal postmenopausal ovaries by transvaginal sonography reported a mean ovarian volume of 2.0 cc with an upper limit of normal of 8.0 cc.[117] **An ovarian volume of more than 8.0 cc is definitely considered abnormal.** Some authors have suggested that an ovarian volume more than twice that of the opposite side should also be considered abnormal, regardless of the actual size.[120,122]

Postmenopausal Cysts. Small anechoic **cysts** (less than 3 cm in diameter) may be seen in up to 15% of postmenopausal ovaries and are not related to age, length of time since menopause, or hormone use (Fig. 15-34).[124] These cysts are more frequently seen by transvaginal sonography due to its improved resolution, but in some women, especially those who have had a hysterectomy or those with highly placed ovaries, the cysts may be seen only by transabdominal sonography. These cysts can disappear or change in size over time.[125]

Several studies have shown a very low incidence of malignancy in unilocular postmenopausal cysts that measure less than 5 cm in diameter and are without septation or solid components.[126-129] It is recommended that these patients be followed by serial sonographic examinations without surgical intervention unless there is an increase in size or change in the characteristics of the lesion.[129] Surgery is recommended for postmenopausal cysts greater than 5 cm and for those containing internal septations and/or solid nodules.

Nonneoplastic Lesions

Functional Cysts. Functional cysts of the ovary include follicular, corpus luteum, and theca-lutein cysts. A **follicular cyst** occurs when a mature follicle fails to ovulate or to involute. Follicular cysts range from 1.0 cm to 20.0 cm in size. However, because normal follicles can vary from a few millimeters to 2.0 cm and can reach up to 2.5 cm at maturity, a follicular cyst cannot be diagnosed with certainty until it is greater than 2.5 cm.[130] They are usually unilateral, asymptomatic, and frequently detected incidentally on sonographic examination. Follicular cysts usually regress spontaneously.

The **corpus luteal cyst** results from failure of absorption or from excess bleeding into the corpus luteum. They are less common than follicular cysts but tend to be larger and more symptomatic. Pain is the major symptom. These cysts are usually unilateral and more prone to hemorrhage and rupture. If the ovum is fertilized, the corpus luteum continues as the corpus luteum of pregnancy, which may become en-

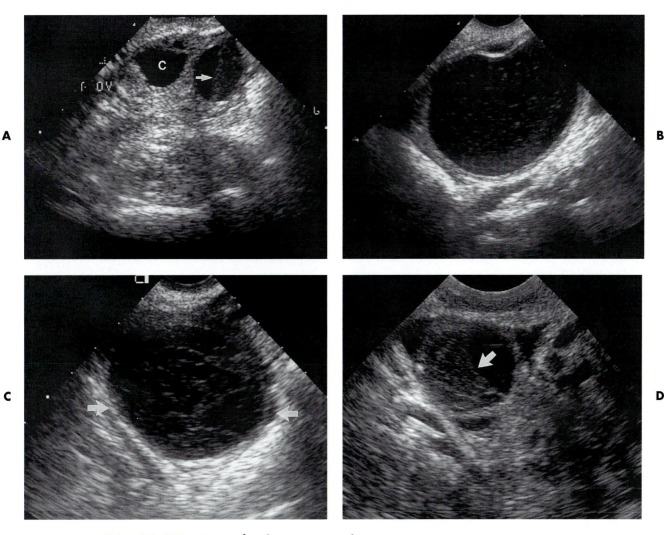

FIG. 15-35. Hemorrhagic cysts, varying appearances. Transvaginal scans. **A,** Small hemorrhagic corpus luteum contains echogenic material with a fluid-fluid level *(arrow)*. Small adjacent anechoic cyst (C). **B,** Large cyst containing multiple internal low-level echoes. **C,** Reticular pattern of internal echoes and septations within cyst *(arrows)*. **D,** Echogenic thrombus showing clot retraction *(arrow)* within cyst.

larged and cystic. Maximum size is reached at 8 to 10 weeks and by 16 weeks the cyst has usually resolved.

Sonographically these functional cysts are typically unilocular, anechoic structures with well-defined thin walls and posterior acoustic enhancement.

Hemorrhagic Cysts. Internal hemorrhage may occur in both types of functional cysts, although it is much more frequently seen in corpus luteal cysts. Women with hemorrhagic cysts frequently present with acute onset of pelvic pain. Hemorrhagic cysts show a spectrum of findings as a result of the variable sonographic appearance of blood (Fig. 15-35). The sonographic appearance depends on the amount of hemorrhage and the time of the hemorrhage relative to the time of the sonographic examination.[131,132] The internal characteristics are much better appreciated on transvaginal sonography because of its improved

resolution. An acute hemorrhagic cyst is usually hyperechoic and may mimic a solid mass. However, it usually has a smooth posterior wall and shows posterior acoustic enhancement, indicating the cystic nature of the lesion. As the clot hemolyses, the internal pattern becomes more complex, with a reticular-type pattern containing internal echoes and septations. A demarcation line or fluid-fluid level between the clot and the fluid component may be seen. The echogenic clot may also settle to the dependent portion of the cyst. The presence of echogenic free intraperitoneal fluid in the cul-de-sac can help confirm the diagnosis of a leaking or ruptured hemorrhagic cyst. Rupture of a hemorrhagic cyst may mimic a ruptured ectopic pregnancy, both clinically and sonographically.

Functional cysts are the **most common cause of ovarian enlargement in young women.**[130] Because most functional cysts typically resolve within one to two menstrual cycles, follow-up is usually not required for small, simple cysts. However, follow-up of larger or hemorrhagic cysts can be performed at a different time of the menstrual cycle, usually in 6 weeks, to show a changing appearance or resolution.

Theca-luteal cysts are the largest of the functional cysts and are associated with high levels of human chorionic gonadotropin (HCG). These cysts typically occur in patients with gestational trophoblastic disease but can also be seen in the ovarian hyperstimulation syndrome as a complication of drug therapy for infertility. Sonographically, theca-luteal cysts are usually bilateral, multilocular, and very large. They may undergo hemorrhage, rupture, and torsion.

Ovarian Remnant Syndrome.
Infrequently, a cystic mass may be encountered in a patient who has undergone bilateral oophorectomy in which a small amount of residual ovarian tissue has been left behind. The surgery has usually been technically difficult because of adhesions from endometriosis, pelvic inflammatory disease, or tumor. The residual ovarian tissue has been hormonally stimulated, and that results in a functional hemorrhagic cyst.[133]

Parovarian (Paratubal) Cysts.
Parovarian cysts account for about 10% of all adnexal masses. They are found in the broad ligament and are usually of mesothelial or paramesonephric origin, or rarely of mesonephric origin.[134] They may occur at any age but are most common in the third and fourth decades of life. They vary in size, and sonographically have the typical appearance of cysts (Fig. 15-36). They are frequently located superior to the uterine fundus[134] and may contain internal echoes as a result of hemorrhage.[135] The cyst may undergo torsion and rupture

similar to other cystic masses. Parovarian cysts show no cyclic changes. A specific diagnosis is possible only by demonstrating a normal ipsilateral ovary close to, but separate from, the cyst.[136]

Peritoneal Inclusion Cysts.
Peritoneal inclusion cysts occur predominantly in premenopausal women with a history of previous abdominal surgery, but they may also be seen in patients with a history of trauma, pelvic inflammatory disease, or endometriosis. The ovaries are the main producers of peritoneal fluid in women.[111] In patients with peritoneal adhesions, fluid may accumulate within the adhesions and entrap the ovaries, resulting in a large adnexal mass.[137,138] Peritoneal inclusion cysts are lined with mesothelial cells; this condition has also been referred to as *benign cystic mesothelioma* or *benign encysted fluid*. Clinically, most patients present with pain and/or a pelvic mass.

On sonography, peritoneal inclusion cysts are multiloculated cystic adnexal masses (Fig. 15-37). The diagnostic finding is the presence of an **intact ovary amid septations and fluid**.[138] This indicates the extraovarian origin of the mass. The ovary may be located centrally or displaced peripherally, and although it may appear distorted, it is easily identified. The septations represent the mesothelial and fibrous strands seen pathologically. The fluid is usually anechoic but may contain echoes in some compartments as a result of hemorrhage or proteinaceous fluid. Conservative therapy is recommended, as peritoneal inclusion cysts have no malignant potential.

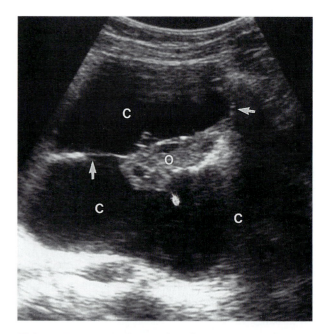

FIG. 15-37. Peritoneal inclusion cyst. Transabdominal scan shows multiple fluid-filled cystic areas (C) with linear septations *(arrows)* representing adhesions attached to normal ovary (O).

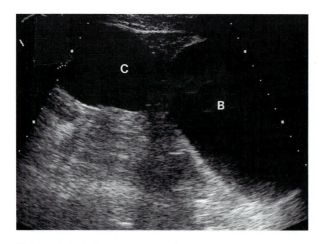

FIG. 15-36. Parovarian cyst. Transabdominal sagittal scan shows large cyst (C) located superior and to right of uterus and bladder (B). Transvaginal scan showed cyst to be separate from both ovaries.

Endometriosis. Endometriosis is defined as the presence of functioning endometrial tissue outside the uterus. Endometriosis most commonly occurs in the ovary, fallopian tube, broad ligament, and posterior cul-de-sac, but it can also occur almost anywhere else in the body, including the bladder and bowel. Two forms have been described: **diffuse** and **localized (endometrioma).** The diffuse form, which is more common, consists of minute endometrial implants involving the pelvic viscera and their ligamentous attachments. The ectopic endometrium is hormonally responsive and undergoes bleeding during the menses, resulting in a local inflammatory reaction with adhesions. This diffuse form is rarely diagnosed by sonography because the implants are too small to be imaged.[139] Endometriosis commonly affects women during the reproductive years, and clinical symptoms include dysmenorrhea, dyspareunia, and infertility.

The localized form consists of a discrete mass referred to as an **endometrioma,** or chocolate cyst. Although endometriosis is frequently associated with infertility, an endometrioma may occasionally be seen in a pregnant patient. Endometriomas are usually asymptomatic and are frequently multiple. The characteristic sonographic appearance is that of a well-defined unilocular or multilocular, predominately cystic mass containing diffuse homogeneous, low-level, internal echoes (Fig. 15-38). This is much better appreciated on transvaginal sonography.[140] These low-level internal echoes may be seen diffusely throughout the mass or in the dependent portion. Occasionally, a fluid-fluid level can be seen.

The appearance may be similar to a hemorrhagic ovarian cyst because both are cystic masses that contain blood of variable age.[141] However, a hemorrhagic cyst more frequently demonstrates a reticular internal pattern and is more frequently associated with free fluid in the cul-de-sac. A hemorrhagic cyst will resolve or show a significant decrease in size over the next few menstrual cycles, whereas endometriomas tend to show little change in size and internal echo pattern. Endometriomas or hemorrhagic cysts showing less typical features may be confused with an ovarian neoplasm or tubo-ovarian abscess. Clinically, most women with an acute hemorrhagic cyst present with acute pelvic pain, whereas women with an endometrioma are asymptomatic or have more chronic discomfort associated with their menses.

Polycystic Ovarian Disease. Polycystic ovarian disease (PCOD) is a complex endocrinologic disorder resulting in chronic anovulation. An imbalance of LH and FSH results in abnormal estrogen and androgen production.[130] The serum LH level is elevated and the FSH level is depressed; an elevated LH/FSH ratio is a characteristic finding. Pathologically, the ovaries contain an increased number of follicles in various stages of maturation and atresia, and there is an increased local concentration of androgens, producing stromal abnormality. PCOD is a common cause of infertility. The classic Stein-Leventhal syndrome (oligomenorrhea, hirsutism, obesity) is only one form in the spectrum of clinical manifestations of PCOD.

The typical sonographic findings are those of bilaterally enlarged ovaries containing multiple small

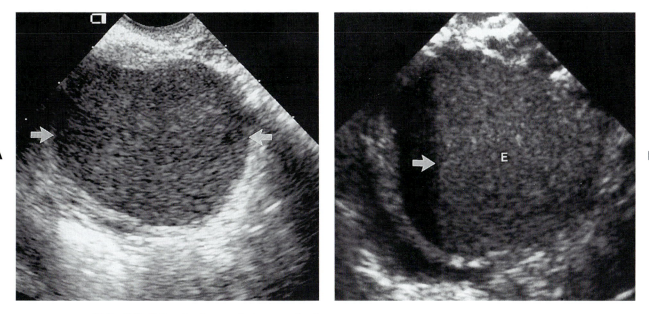

FIG. 15-38. Endometrioma, typical appearances. Transvaginal scans. **A,** Typical appearance of endometrioma with diffuse, homogeneous, low-level echoes throughout cystic mass *(arrows)* with mild acoustic enhancement. **B,** Homogeneous internal echo pattern (E) with fluid-fluid level *(arrow).*

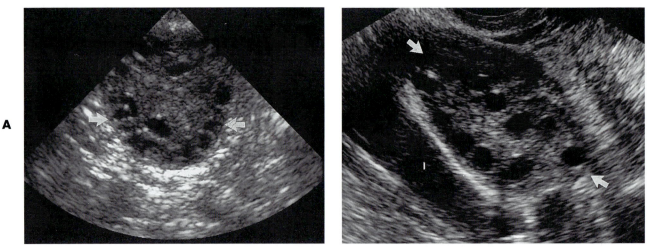

FIG. 15-39. Polycystic ovarian disease, typical appearances. Transvaginal scans. **A,** Enlarged round ovary *(arrows)* with increased stromal echogenicity and multiple peripheral cysts; "string of pearls" sign. **B,** Enlarged ovary *(arrows)* with multiple peripheral and central cysts. I, Internal iliac vein.

follicles and increased stromal echogenicity (Fig. 15-39). The ovaries have a more rounded shape, with the follicles usually located peripherally, although they can also occur randomly throughout the ovarian parenchyma. Transvaginal sonography, because of its superior resolution, is more sensitive in detecting the small follicles. The follicles measure from 0.5 to 0.8 cm in size with more than five in each ovary.[142] However, these typical findings are seen in fewer than half the patients with this condition. Ovarian volume is normal in approximately 30%.[142,143] A combination of mean follicular size and ovarian volume has been found to be more sensitive and specific than either feature alone.[144] Using transvaginal sonography, increased stromal echogenicity is believed to be the most sensitive and specific sign of PCOD.[144,145] The diagnosis is usually made biochemically, but sonography is useful in cases in which the diagnosis is uncertain or in the clinically unsuspected patient. Because ovulation does not occur, the follicles will persist on serial studies. Long-term follow-up is recommended in these patients because the unopposed high estrogen levels appear to be associated with an increased risk of endometrial and breast carcinoma.[130]

Ovarian Torsion. Torsion of the ovary is an acute abdominal condition requiring prompt surgical intervention. It is caused by partial or complete rotation of the ovarian pedicle on its axis. This results in compromise of the lymphatic and venous drainage, causing congestion and edema of the ovarian parenchyma and leading to eventual loss of arterial perfusion and resultant infarction. Torsion may occur in normal ovaries or in association with a preexisting ovarian cyst or mass. The mass is almost always benign.[146] Torsion of a normal ovary usually occurs in children and younger females with especially mobile adnexa, allowing torsion at the mesosalpinx.[147] Torsion usually occurs in childhood and during the reproductive years. There is an increased risk during pregnancy. Clinically, there is severe pelvic pain, nausea, and vomiting. A palpable mass may be present. If the pain is right-sided, ovarian torsion may clinically mimic acute appendicitis.

The sonographic findings are variable, depending on the degree of vascular compromise and whether an adnexal mass is present (Fig. 15-40). The ovary is enlarged. Multiple cortical follicles in an enlarged ovary are considered a specific sign, although they are not always present.[147] The multifollicular enlargement is the result of transudation of fluid into the follicles from the circulatory impairment. Color and spectral Doppler examination may show absent flow in the affected ovary. However, Doppler findings may vary depending on the degree and chronicity of the torsion and whether or not there is an associated adnexal mass.[148] The presence of Doppler arterial waveforms and color flow has been reported in surgically proven cases of torsion.[149,150] The possible explanations proposed are that venous thrombosis leads to symptoms before arterial occlusion occurs and that persistent adnexal arterial flow is related to the dual ovarian arterial blood supply (from the ovarian artery and ovarian branches of the uterine artery).[150]

Massive Edema of the Ovary. This is a rare condition resulting from partial or intermittent torsion of the ovary, causing venous and lymphatic obstruction but not arterial occlusion. This results in ovarian enlargement due to marked stromal edema. The few cases described sonographically show a large, predominantly multicystic adnexal mass.[151-153]

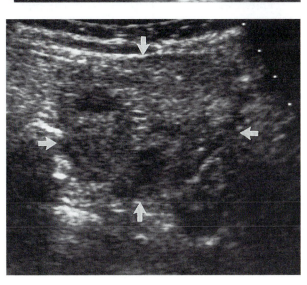

A

B

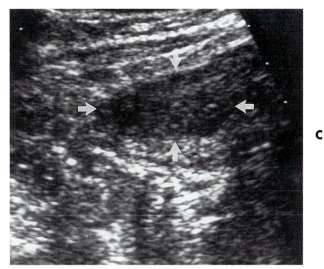

C

FIG. 15-40. Ovarian torsion. A, Transabdominal sagittal scan in 16-year-old girl presenting with acute left-sided lower abdominal pain shows large adnexal mass containing multiple peripheral anechoic follicles *(arrows)*. B, Bladder. **B,** Transabdominal scan in patient with 28-week twin pregnancy presenting with acute right lower abdominal pain shows markedly enlarged right ovary *(arrows)* with a few peripheral anechoic follicles. Doppler showed no flow. **C,** Normal left ovary *(arrows)* of patient in B.

Neoplasms

Ovarian Cancer. Ovarian cancer is the fourth leading cause of cancer death among women in the United States. In 1995, there were an estimated 26,000 new cases of ovarian cancer diagnosed in the United States, and there were about 14,500 deaths.[154] Ovarian cancer comprises 25% of all gynecologic malignancies, with its peak incidence occurring in the sixth decade of life. Although only the third most common gynecologic malignancy, it has the highest mortality rate as a result of late diagnosis. As there are few clinical symptoms, approximately 60% to 70% of women have advanced disease (stages III or IV) at the time of diagnosis. The overall 5-year survival rate is 20% to 30%, but with early detection in stage I, the rate rises to 80%. Therefore, efforts have been directed at developing methods of early diagnosis of this condition.

Increasing age, nulliparity, a history of breast, endometrial, or colon cancer, or a family history of ovarian cancer have been associated with a higher risk of developing ovarian cancer. **Family history** is considered to be the most important risk factor. The lifetime risk of a woman's developing ovarian cancer is 1 in 70 (1.4%). However, if a woman has a first-degree relative (mother, daughter, sister) or second-degree relative (aunt or grandmother) who has had ovarian cancer, the risk is 5%. With two or more relatives, the lifetime risk increases to 7%.[155] About 3% to 5% of women with a family history of ovarian cancer will have a hereditary ovarian cancer syndrome. The three main hereditary syndromes associated with ovarian cancer are the **breast-ovarian cancer syndrome,** the most common, in which there is a high frequency of both cancers; the **hereditary nonpolyposis colorectal cancer syndrome** (Lynch II) in which ovarian cancer occurs in association with nonpolyposis colorectal cancer or endometrial cancer or both; **site-specific ovarian cancer syndrome** without an excess of breast or colorectal cancer, the least common.[156]

Heredity ovarian cancer syndromes are thought to have an autosomal dominant inheritance, and the lifetime risk of ovarian cancer in these patients is approximately 40% to 50%. They have an earlier age of onset (10 to 15 years) than do other ovarian cancers.[156]

A number of clinical **screening trials** of asymptomatic, predominantly postmenopausal women have been reported.[157-160] These trials have focused on biological tumor markers such as CA 125 and on sonography, initially transabdominal and more recently transvaginal. CA 125 is a high-molecular-weight glycoprotein recognized by the OC 125 monoclonal antibody. It has proven extremely useful in following the clinical course of patients undergoing chemotherapy and in detecting recurrent subclinical disease.[161,162] Although serum CA 125 is elevated in approximately 80% of women with epithelial ovarian cancer, it detects less than 50% of stage I disease and is insensitive to mucinous and germ-cell tumors.[162] Also, other malignancies as well as several benign conditions may be associated with elevated serum CA 125.[162,163] Therefore, the use of serum CA 125 as a screening test has been disappointing. Studies combining CA 125 with sonography have been more encouraging.[158] More recent screening trials have included color and pulsed Doppler sonography in addition to transvaginal sonography in asymptomatic women,[164] in women with a family history of ovarian or other cancer,[165,166] and in women with previous breast cancer.[167] At present, the use of

sonography for ovarian cancer screening must be considered to be in the research stage and cannot be recommended for routine clinical use. An NIH consensus conference on ovarian cancer held in 1994 concluded that "there is no evidence available yet that the current screening modalities of CA 125 and TVS can be effectively used for widespread screening to reduce mortality from ovarian cancer nor that their use will result in decreased rather than increased morbidity and mortality. Routine screening has resulted in unnecessary surgery with its attendant potential risks."*

Histologically, epithelial neoplasms comprise 65% to 75% of ovarian tumors and 90% of ovarian malignancies.[35] The remaining neoplasms consist of germ cell tumors (15% to 20%), sex cord-stromal tumors (5% to 10%), and metastatic tumors (5% to 10%) (Table 15-1).

Sonographically, ovarian cancer usually presents as an adnexal mass. Sonography reflects the gross morphologic condition of the tumor but not the histology. Therefore, it has been difficult to distinguish benign from malignant ovarian tumors by sonography. Well-defined anechoic lesions are more likely to be benign, whereas lesions with irregular walls, thick, irregular septations, mural nodules, and solid echogenic elements favor malignancy.[168,169] Scoring systems based

---

*NIH Consensus Conference. Ovarian cancer: screening, treatment and follow-up. JAMA 1995;273:491-497.

TABLE 15-1
HISTOLOGIC OUTLINE OF OVARIAN NEOPLASMS

Type	Incidence	Example
I Surface epithelial-stromal tumors	65% to 75%	Serous cystadenoma (carcinoma)
		Mucinous cystadenoma (carcinoma)
		Endometrioid carcinoma
		Clear cell carcinoma
		Transitional cell tumor
II Germ cell tumors	15% to 20%	Teratoma
		Dermoid
		Immature
		Dysgerminoma
		Yolk sac tumor
III Sex cord-stromal tumors	5% to 10%	Granulosa cell tumor
		Sertoli-Leydig cell tumor
		Thecoma and fibroma
IV Metastatic tumors	5% to 10%	Genital primary
		Uterus
		Extragenitial primary
		Stomach
		Colon
		Breast
		Lymphoma

on the morphologic characteristics have been proposed.[170-172] These systems assign a numeric value for individual sonographic findings; the higher the score, the higher the likelihood of malignancy. However, different authors have assigned different numerical values to the abnormal findings, making it difficult to compare the systems. Also, benign lesions such as hemorrhagic cysts and teratomas may contain irregular wall thickening, mural nodules, and solid elements, giving a high score and, thus, a false diagnosis of malignancy.

Doppler Findings in Ovarian Cancer.

More recently, color and pulsed Doppler sonography have been advocated for distinguishing benign from malignant ovarian masses. Support is based on the premise that malignant masses, because of internal neovascularization, will have high diastolic flow that can be detected on spectral Doppler waveforms (Fig. 15-41). Malignant tumor growth is dependent upon angiogenesis with the development of abnormal tumor vessels.[173] These abnormal vessels lack smooth muscle within their walls which, along with arteriovenous shunting, leads to decreased vascular resistance and thus higher diastolic flow velocity. Two angle-independent indexes, the pulsatility index (PI) and the resistive index (RI) are used to analyze the Doppler waveform pattern. The PI is the peak systolic velocity minus the end-diastolic velocity divided by the mean velocity; the RI is the peak systolic velocity minus the end-diastolic velocity divided by the peak systolic velocity.

Initial studies using transvaginal color and pulsed Doppler reported both high sensitivity and high specificity in distinguishing benign from malignant ovarian masses, with malignant masses having a PI of less than 1.0 or an RI of less than 0.4.[174-177] However, numerous subsequent articles have been unable to reproduce such high sensitivity and specificity and have shown considerable overlap between benign and malignant lesions.[178-187] In categorizing lesions, most authors have used the lowest PI or RI obtained, assuming the worst-case value, as this may correspond to the only histologic evidence of malignancy.[177,178]

In menstruating women, the ovarian arterial waveform varies according to the phase of the menstrual cycle. During the menstrual and proliferative phase, there is a high-resistance flow pattern. With development of the corpus luteum at midcycle, a low-resistance waveform pattern is seen because of newly formed vessels along the wall of the corpus luteum. These vessels also lack smooth muscle and demonstrate low-resistance, high-diastolic flow similar to tumor neovascularity. Therefore, in menstruating women, it is recommended that Doppler studies be done between days 3 and 10 of the menstrual cycle to avoid confusion with normal luteal flow.

Although most reports have found a tendency for both PI and RI to be lower in malignant lesions, there has been too much overlap to differentiate reliably between benign and malignant lesions in the individual patient. Some authors have found no specific cut-off value for either PI or RI that had both high sensitivity and high specificity.[179-181] Absence of flow within a lesion usually indicates a benign lesion, but several reports have shown absent flow within malignant lesions, as well.[175,176,179-182]

Other parameters, such as vessel location and the presence of a diastolic notch, have been suggested to improve the specificity of Doppler assessment of ovarian masses.[188] Malignant lesions tend to have more central flow, whereas benign lesions tend to have more peripheral flow. Stein et al., however, found considerable overlap, with 21% of malignant lesions having only peripheral flow and 31% of benign lesions having central flow.[181] The presence of a diastolic notch indicates normal smooth muscle within the arterial wall that is absent in malignant lesions. However, this finding is frequently absent in benign lesions as well, so its absence has no diagnostic significance.

Some reports have compared the morphologic features on sonography with the Doppler findings and found that Doppler did not add any more diagnostic information than did morphologic assessment alone.[182-184] Others have found that Doppler, when added to sonographic morphologic assessment, improves specificity and positive predictive value.[186,187,189] Doppler is probably not needed if the mass has a characteristic benign morphology, as sonography is highly accurate in this group of lesions.[181,185] Doppler may be of value in assessing the mass that is morphologically indeterminant or suggestive of malignancy. However, the Doppler findings should not be used in isolation but should be combined with morphologic assessment, clinical findings, patient age, and phase of menstrual cycle to best evaluate an adnexal mass.[190]

Surface Epithelial-Stromal Tumors.

Surface epithelial-stromal tumors are generally considered to arise from the surface epithelium that covers the ovary and the underlying ovarian stroma. These tumors can be divided into five broad categories based on epithelial differentiation: **serous, mucinous, endometrioid, clear cell,** and **transitional cell (Brenner)**.[35] This group of tumors accounts for 65% to 75% of all ovarian neoplasms and 80% to 90% of all ovarian malignancies. There is an intermediate group of approximately 10% to 15% of serous and mucinous tumors that are histologically categorized as borderline or of low malignant potential. These tumors have cytologic features of malignancy but do not invade the stroma and, although malignant, have a much better prognosis. The mode of spread of the malignant tumors is primarily intraperitoneal, although direct extension to

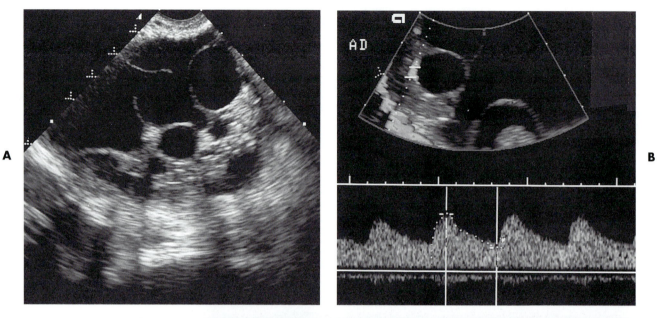

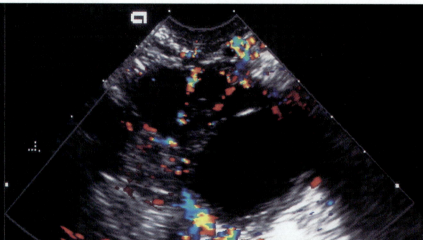

FIG. 15-41. **Ovarian cancer,** contribution of Doppler in different patients. **A,** Transvaginal scan shows large multiseptated predominantly cystic mass with solid echogenic components. **B,** Same patient as **A.** Spectral Doppler through area of vascularity in echogenic component *(cursors)* shows increased diastolic flow. Lowest PI obtained was 0.59 and RI 0.40. **C,** Transvaginal color Doppler shows vascular septae in a multicystic mass. **D,** Transabdominal color Doppler shows vascularity in a predominantly solid mass (M).

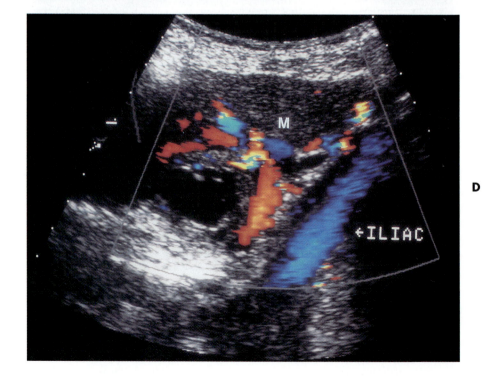

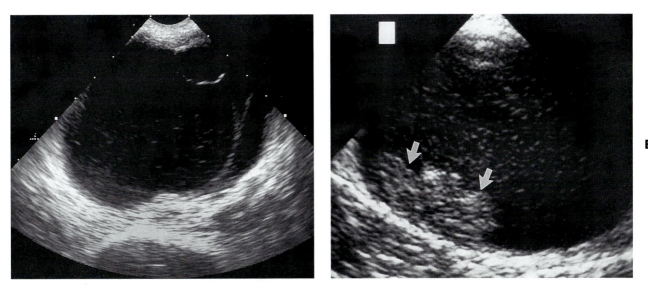

FIG. 15-42. Serous cystadenoma, varying appearances. Transvaginal scans. **A,** Large cystic ovarian mass with thin septations and low-level internal echoes. **B,** Large cystic mass with solid echogenic material *(arrows)* and multiple low-level internal echoes. Sonographic appearance indistinguishable from malignancy.

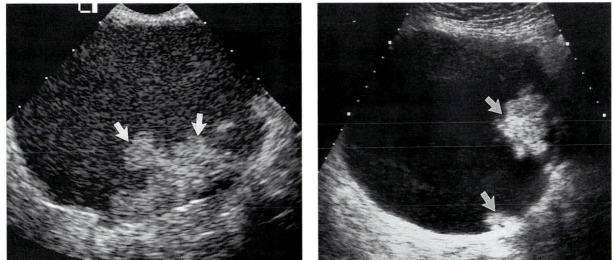

FIG. 15-43. Serous cystadenocarcinoma, varying appearances. A, Transvaginal scan shows large cystic mass containing multiple low-level internal echoes and solid echogenic components *(arrows)*. **B,** Transabdominal scan shows large cystic mass with irregular solid echogenic mural nodules *(arrows)* and low-level internal echoes.

contiguous structures and lymphatic spread are not uncommon. Lymphatic spread is predominantly to the paraortic nodes. Hematogenous spread usually occurs late in the course of the disease.

Serous cystadenoma and cystadenocarcinoma. Serous tumors are the most common, comprising 30% of all ovarian neoplasms. Approximately 50% to 70% of serous tumors are benign. Serous cystadenomas account for 20% to 25% of all benign ovarian neoplasms, and serous cystadenocarcinomas account for 40% to 50% of all malignant ovarian neoplasms.[35] The peak incidence of serous cystadenomas is in the fourth and fifth decades, whereas serous cys-

tadenocarcinomas most frequently occur in perimenopausal and postmenopausal women. Approximately 20% of benign serous tumors and 50% of malignant serous tumors are bilateral. Their sizes vary greatly, but in general, they are smaller than mucinous tumors.

Sonographically, serous cystadenomas are usually large, thin-walled, unilocular cystic masses that may contain thin septations (Fig. 15-42). Papillary projections are occasionally seen. Serous cystadenocarcinomas may be quite large and usually present as multilocular cystic masses containing multiple papillary projections arising from the cyst walls and septae (Fig. 15-43). The

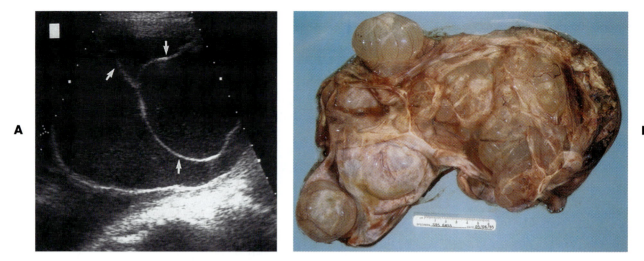

FIG. 15-44. Mucinous cystadenoma. A, Transabdominal scan shows large cystic mass with multiple thin septations *(arrows)* and fine low-level internal echoes. B, Gross pathologic specimen shows multiple cystic loculations.

septae and walls may be thick. Echogenic solid material may be seen within the loculations. Papillary projections may form on the surface of the cyst and surrounding organs, resulting in fixation of the mass. Ascites is frequently seen.

Mucinous cystadenoma and cystadenocarcinoma. Mucinous tumors are the second most common ovarian epithelial tumor, accounting for 20% to 25% of ovarian neoplasms. Mucinous cystadenomas constitute 20% to 25% of all benign ovarian neoplasms, and mucinous cystadenocarcinomas make up 5% to 10% of all primary malignant ovarian neoplasms.[35] They are less frequently bilateral than are their serous counterparts, with only 5% of the benign and 15% to 20% of the malignant lesions occurring on both sides. Approximately 85% of mucinous tumors are benign.

On sonographic examination, mucinous cystadenomas can be huge cystic masses, measuring up to 15 to 30 cm and filling the entire pelvis and abdomen. Multiple thin septae are present and low-level echoes caused by the mucoid material may be seen in the dependent portions of the mass (Fig. 15-44). Papillary projections are less frequently seen than in the serous counterpart. Mucinous cystadenocarcinomas are usually large, multiloculated cystic masses containing papillary projections and echogenic material; they generally have a sonographic appearance similar to that of serous cystadenocarcinomas.

Penetration of the tumor capsule or rupture may lead to intraperitoneal spread of mucin-secreting cells that fill the peritoneal cavity with a gelatinous material. This condition, known as **pseudomyxoma peritonei,** may be similar sonographically to ascites or may contain multiple septations in the fluid that fills much of the pelvis and abdomen (Fig. 15-45). Low-level echogenic material may be seen within the fluid. This condition may occur in mucinous cystadenomas and in mucinous cystadenocarcinomas. A ruptured mucocele of the appendix and metastatic colon carcinoma can also lead to pseudomyxoma peritonei.

Endometrioid tumor. Nearly all endometrioid tumors are malignant. They are the second most common epithelial malignancy, comprising 20% to 25% of ovarian malignancies.[35] Approximately 25% to 30% are bilateral. Their histologic characteristics are identical to those of endometrial adenocarcinoma, and 30% of patients with this condition have associated endometrial adenocarcinoma, which is thought to represent an independent primary tumor. The endometrioid tumor has a better prognosis than do other epithelial malignancies, which is probably related to diagnosis at an earlier stage. Sonographically, it usually presents as a cystic mass containing papillary projections, although in some cases there is a predominantly solid mass that may contain areas of hemorrhage or necrosis.[191,192]

Clear cell tumor. This tumor is considered to be of Müllerian duct origin and to be a variant of endometrioid carcinoma. It is nearly always malignant and constitutes 5% to 10% of primary ovarian carcinomas. It is bilateral in about 20% of patients. Sonographically, it usually presents as a nonspecific, complex, predominantly cystic mass.[191,192]

Transitional cell (Brenner) tumor. This tumor is derived from the surface epithelium that undergoes metaplasia to form typical uroepithelial-like components.[35] It is uncommon, accounting for 1% to 2% of all ovarian neoplasms, and is nearly always benign; 6% to 7% are bilateral. Most patients are

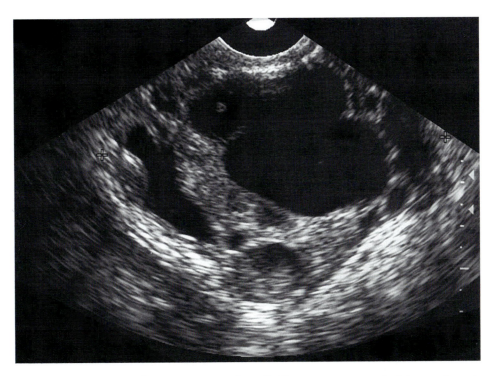

FIG. 15-45. Pseudomyxoma peritonei. Transverse transvaginal image through the pouch of Douglas shows no identifiable landmarks. There is a complex cystic and solid appearance. Some pockets of fluid are clear or echo-free and others are particulate. (Courtesy of Stephanie R. Wilson, M.D., University of Toronto.)

asymptomatic, and the tumor is discovered incidentally on sonographic examination or at surgery. Thirty percent are associated with cystic neoplasms, usually serous or mucinous cystadenomas or cystic teratomas, frequently in the ipsilateral ovary (Fig. 15-46).[193] Sonographically, Brenner tumors are hypoechoic solid masses. Calcification may occur in the outer wall. Cystic areas are unusual and when present are usually due to a coexistent cystadenoma.[192] Pathologically, they are solid tumors composed of dense fibrous stroma. They appear similar to ovarian fibromas and thecomas and to uterine leiomyomas, both sonographically and pathologically.

Germ Cell Tumors. Germ cell tumors are derived from the primitive germ cells of the embryonic gonad. They account for 15% to 20% of ovarian neoplasms, with approximately 95% being benign cystic teratomas. The others, including dysgerminomas and endodermal sinus (yolk sac) tumors, occur mainly in children and young adults and are nearly always malignant. Germ cell tumors are the most common ovarian malignancies in children and young adults. When a large, predominantly solid ovarian mass is present in a girl or young woman, the diagnosis of a malignant germ cell tumor should be strongly considered.[194]

Cystic teratoma. Cystic teratomas make up approximately 15% to 25% of ovarian neoplasms; 10% to 15% are bilateral. They are composed of well-differen-

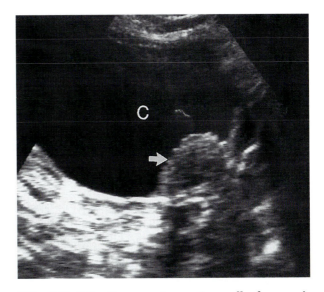

FIG. 15-46. Brenner tumor in wall of a mucinous cystadenoma. Transabdominal scan shows a large, well-defined cystic mass (C) with a solid hypoechoic mural nodule *(arrow)*. Pathology showed a Brenner tumor within wall of a large mucinous cystadenoma.

tiated derivatives of the **three germ layers**—ectoderm, mesoderm, and endoderm. Because **ectodermal elements** generally predominate, cystic teratomas are virtually always benign and are also called **dermoid cysts.** Cystic teratomas and serous cystadenomas are the two most common ovarian neoplasms. In contrast to surface epithelial-stromal tumors, cystic teratomas are more commonly seen in the active reproductive years, but they can occur at any age and are not infrequently seen in postmenopausal women. Complications include torsion and rupture. Torsion is the most common complication, whereas rupture is uncommon; occurring in approximately 1% of cases and causing a secondary chemical peritonitis. Malignant transformation is also uncommon, occurring in approximately 2% of cases, usually in older women.[35]

Sonographically, cystic teratomas have a variable appearance ranging from completely anechoic to completely hyperechoic. However, certain features are considered specific (Fig. 15-47 and Fig. 15-48). These include a predominantly cystic mass with an echogenic mural nodule, the **"dermoid plug.**[195]**"** The dermoid plug usually contains hair, teeth, or fat and frequently casts an acoustic shadow. Correlation with CT images has shown that in many cases the cystic component is pure sebum (which is liquid at body temperature) rather than fluid.[196]

A mixture of matted hair and sebum is highly echogenic because of multiple tissue interfaces, and it produces ill-defined acoustic shadowing that obscures the posterior wall of the lesion. This has been termed the **"tip-of-the-iceberg"** sign.[197] Highly echogenic foci with well-defined acoustic shadowing may arise from other elements, including teeth and bone. Multiple linear hyperechogenic interfaces may be seen floating within the cyst and have been shown to be hair fibers.[198] This is also considered a specific sign and has been referred to as the **"dermoid mesh.**[199]**"** A **fat-fluid** or **hair-fluid** level may be seen, and that is also considered specific. An echogenic dermoid may appear similar to bowel gas and may be overlooked. If a definite pelvic mass is clinically palpable and the sonogram appears normal, the patient should be re-examined, with the intention of looking carefully for a dermoid.

Struma ovarii is a teratoma that is composed entirely or predominantly of thyroid tissue. It occurs in 2% to 3% of teratomas. Although associated hormonal effects are rare, sonography may be valuable in identifying a pelvic lesion in a hyperthyroid patient when there is no evidence of a thyroid lesion in the neck.[200]

Immature teratomas represent less than 1% of all teratomas and contain immature tissue from all three germ-cell layers. They are rapidly growing malignant tumors that most commonly occur in the first two decades of life. Sonographically, these tumors present as solid masses.

Dysgerminoma. Dysgerminomas are malignant germ cell tumors that constitute approximately 1% to 2% of primary ovarian neoplasms and 3% to 5% of ovarian malignancies.[35] They are composed of undifferentiated germ cells and are morphologically identical to the male testicular seminoma. They are highly radiosensitive and have a 5-year survival rate of 75% to 90%. This tumor occurs predominantly in women under 30 and is bilateral in approximately 15% of cases. The dysgerminoma and the serous cystadenoma are the two most common ovarian neoplasms seen in pregnancy.[191] Sonographically, they are solid masses that are predominantly echogenic but may contain small anechoic areas caused by hemorrhage or necrosis (Fig. 15-49).[194] CT and MR have shown these solid masses to be lobulated with fibrovascular septa between the lobules.[201] A recent report using color Doppler in three dysgerminomas showed prominent arterial flow within the fibrovascular septa of a multilobulated, solid, echogenic mass.[202]

Yolk sac (endodermal sinus) tumor. This rare, rapidly growing tumor with a poor prognosis is the second most common malignant ovarian germ cell neoplasm after dysgerminoma. It is thought to arise from the undifferentiated and multipotential embryonal carcinoma by selective differentiation toward yolk sac and vitelline structures.[35] It usually occurs in females under 20 years old and is almost always unilateral. Increased levels of serum alpha-fetoprotein (AFP) may be seen in association with this tumor. The sonographic appearance is similar to that of the dysgerminoma.[191,194]

Sex Cord-Stromal Tumors. Sex cord-stromal tumors arise from the sex cords of the embryonic gonad and/or from the ovarian stroma. The main tumors in this group include the granulosa cell tumor, Sertoli-Leydig cell tumor (androblastoma), thecoma, and fibroma. This group accounts for 5% to 10% of all ovarian neoplasms and 2% of all ovarian malignancies.

Granulosa cell tumor. This tumor makes up approximately 1% to 2% of ovarian neoplasms and has a low malignancy potential. The majority occur in postmenopausal women; nearly all are unilateral. They are the most common estrogenically active ovarian tumor,[35] and clinical signs of estrogen production can occur. Approximately 10% to 15% of patients with this tumor eventually develop endometrial carcinoma. Sonographically, these tumors vary from small to very large masses. The small masses are predominantly solid, having an echogenicity similar to that of uterine fibroids. The larger masses are multiloculated and cystic, having an appearance similar to that of cystadenomas.[191]

Sertoli-Leydig cell tumor (androblastoma). This is a rare tumor that constitutes less than 0.5% of ovarian neoplasms. It generally occurs in women under 30 years of age; almost all occurrences are unilateral. Malignancy occurs in 10% to 20% of these tumors.

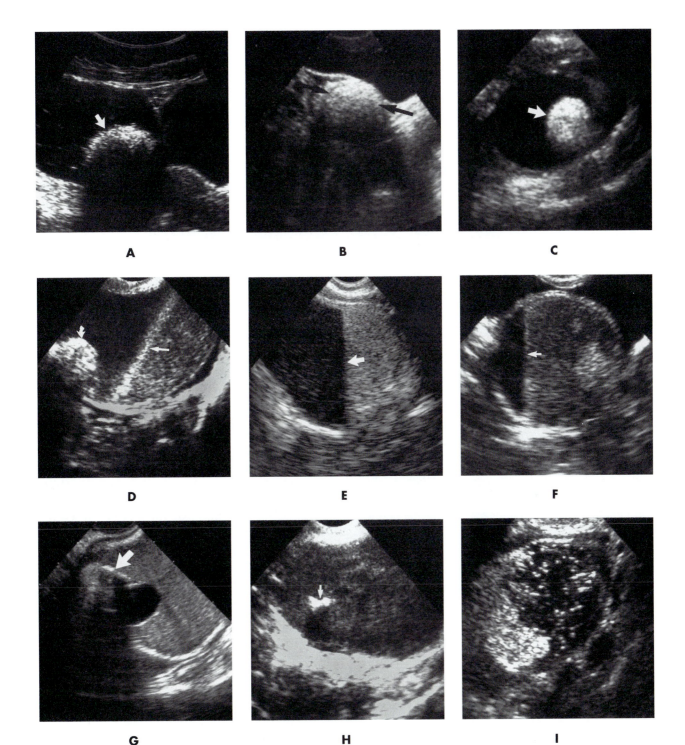

FIG. 15-47. Cystic teratomas (dermoid cysts). A and B, Transabdominal scans. C-I, *Transvaginal scans.* A, Cystic mass with area of high-amplitude echogenicity with posterior acoustic shadowing. B, "Tip of the iceberg," highly echogenic mass with ill-defined posterior shadowing. C, "Dermoid plug," cystic mass with solid echogenic mural nodule. D, Mass of varying echogenicity with hair-fluid level and highly echogenic fat-containing dermoid plug with shadowing. E, Mass with fat-fluid level. F, Predominantly echogenic mass with fat-fluid level. G, Mass containing uniform echoes, small cystic area, and calcification with shadowing. H, Uniform echogenic mass containing high-amplitude echogenic focus due to tooth with shadowing. I, "Dermoid mesh," multiple linear hyperechogenic interfaces floating within cystic mass.

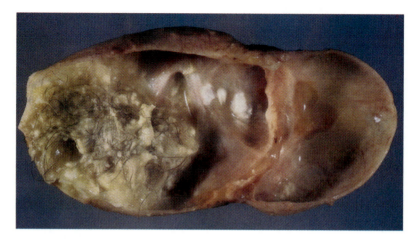

FIG. 15-48. Cystic teratoma. Pathologic specimen shows large ovarian mass containing fluid, fat, hair, and teeth.

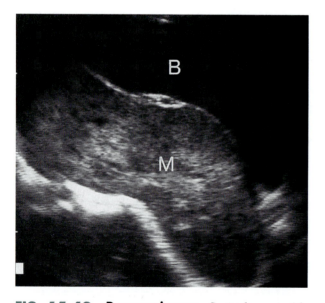

FIG. 15-49. Dysgerminoma. Sagittal scan in 16-year-old girl shows large echogenic solid pelvic mass (M) posterior to bladder (B).

Clinically, signs and symptoms of masculinization occur in many patients, although about half will have no endocrine manifestations.[35] Occasionally, these tumors may be associated with estrogen production. Sonographically, they have an appearance similar to that of granulosa cell tumors.

Thecoma and fibroma. Both these tumors arise from the ovarian stroma and may be difficult to distinguish from each other pathologically. Tumors with an abundance of thecal cells are classified as thecomas, whereas those with fewer thecal cells and abundant fibrous tissue are classified as thecofibromas and fibromas. **Thecomas** comprise approximately 1% of all ovarian neoplasms and 70% occur in postmenopausal females. They are unilateral, al-most always benign, and frequently show clinical signs of estrogen production. **Fibromas** comprise approximately 4% of ovarian neoplasms, are benign, usually unilateral, and occur most commonly in menopausal and postmenopausal women. Unlike thecomas, they are rarely associated with estrogen production and therefore are frequently asymptomatic, despite reaching a large size. Ascites has been reported in half the patients with fibromas larger than 5 cm in diameter.[203] **Meigs' syndrome** (associated ascites and pleural effusion) occurs in 1% to 3% of patients with ovarian fibromas but is not specific, having been reported in association with other ovarian neoplasms as well. Sonographically, these tumors have a characteristic appearance (Fig. 15-50). A hypoechoic mass with marked posterior attenuation of the sound beam is seen as a result of the homogeneous fibrous tissue in these tumors.[203] The main differential diagnosis is that of a Brenner tumor or pedunculated uterine fibroid. Not all fibromas and thecomas show this characteristic appearance, and a variety of sonographic appearances have been noted, probably as a result of the tendency for edema and cystic degeneration to occur within these tumors (Fig. 15-51).[204]

Metastatic Tumors. Approximately 5% to 10% of ovarian neoplasms are metastatic in origin. The most common primary sites of ovarian metastases are tumors of the breast and gastrointestinal tract. The term *Krukenberg tumor* should be reserved for those tumors containing the typical mucin-secreting "signet ring" cells, usually of gastric or colonic origin. Endometrial carcinoma frequently metastasizes to the ovary, but it may be difficult to distinguish from primary endometrioid carcinoma, as discussed earlier. Sonographically, ovarian metastases are usually bilateral solid masses, but they may become necrotic and have a

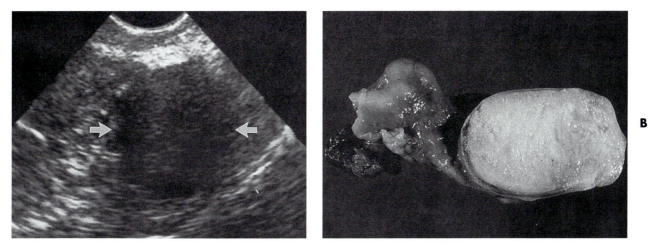

FIG. 15-50. Ovarian fibroma. A, Transvaginal scan shows hypoechoic solid mass *(arrows)* with some posterior attenuation. **B,** Pathologic specimen shows homogeneous solid nature of fibroma.

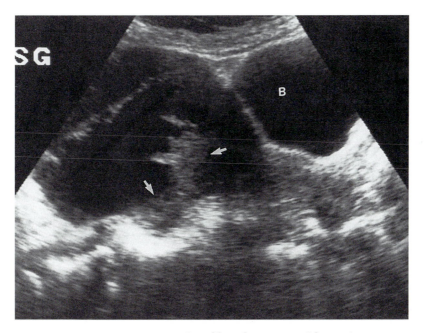

FIG. 15-51. Ovarian fibrothecoma with cystic degeneration. Transabdominal sagittal scan shows large, predominantly cystic mass with solid echogenic areas *(arrows)* located superior to bladder (B). Pathology showed fibrothecoma with multiple areas of cystic degeneration.

complex, predominantly cystic appearance that simulates primary cystadenocarcinoma (Fig. 15-52).[205,206] Ascites may be seen in either primary or metastatic tumors. Lymphoma may involve the ovary, usually in a diffuse, disseminated form that is frequently bilateral. The sonographic appearance is that of a solid hypoechoic mass similar to lymphoma elsewhere in the body.

FALLOPIAN TUBE

The normal fallopian tube is difficult to identify by transabdominal or transvaginal sonography unless it is surrounded by fluid. The normal fallopian tube is an undulating echogenic structure of approximately 8 to 10 mm in width, running posterolaterally from the uterus

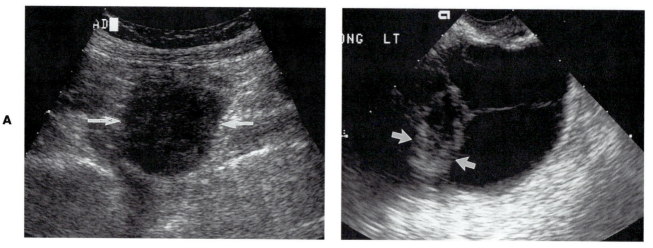

A

B

FIG. 15-52. Ovarian metastasis, varying appearances. A, Transabdominal scan shows solid hypoechoic ovarian mass *(arrows)*, metastatic from primary breast carcinoma. **B,** Transvaginal scan shows complex, predominantly cystic mass with septations and solid echogenic areas *(arrows)*. Although sonographic appearance is similar to primary ovarian carcinoma, pathologic diagnosis was ovarian metastasis from primary colon cancer.

to lie within the cul-de-sac near the ovary. The lumen is not seen unless it is fluid-filled.[207] Developmental abnormalities of the tube are rare. Abnormalities of the tube include pregnancy, infection, and neoplasm.

Pelvic Inflammatory Disease

Pelvic inflammatory disease (PID) is a common condition that is increasing in frequency. It is usually due to sexually transmitted diseases, most commonly associated with gonorrhea and chlamydia. The infection commonly spreads by ascent from the cervix and endometrium. Less common causes include direct extension from appendiceal, diverticular, or postsurgical abscesses that have ruptured into the pelvis as well as puerperal and post-abortion complications. Hematogeneous spread is rare but can occur from tuberculosis. PID is usually bilateral, except when it is caused by direct extension of an adjacent inflammatory process, when it is most commonly unilateral. The presence of an intrauterine contraceptive device increases the risk of PID. Long-term sequelae include chronic pelvic pain, infertility, and an increased risk of ectopic pregnancy.

Sexually transmitted PID spreads along the mucosa of the pelvic organs, initially infecting the cervix and uterine endometrium (endometritis), the fallopian tubes (acute salpingitis), and finally the region of both ovaries and the peritoneum. A pyosalpinx develops as a result of occlusion of the tube. The patients usually present clinically with pain, fever, pelvic tenderness, and vaginal discharge. A pelvic mass may be palpated.

Sonographic Finds of PID. The sonographic findings may be normal early in the course of the disease.[208] As the disease progresses or becomes chronic, a spectrum of findings may occur (Fig. 15-53, Fig. 15-54, and Fig. 15-55). Endometrial thickening or

> ### SONOGRAPHIC FINDINGS OF PID
>
> **Endometritis**
> Endometrial thickening or fluid
> **Pus in cul-de-sac**
> Particulate fluid
> **Periovarian inflammation**
> Enlarged ovaries with multiple cysts and indistinct margins
> **Pyosalpinx or hydrosalpinx**
> Fluid-filled fallopian tube with or without internal echoes
> **Tubo-ovarian complex**
> Fusion of the inflamed dilated tube and ovary
> **Tubo-ovarian abscess**
> Complex multiloculated mass with variable septations, irregular margins and scattered internal echoes

fluid may indicate **endometritis.** Pus may be demonstrated in the cul-de-sac; it contains echogenic particles, which distinguish it from serous fluid in this region. Enlarged ovaries with multiple cysts and indistinct margins may be seen as a result of periovarian inflammation.[208] On transabdominal sonography, dilated tubes appear as complex, predominantly cystic masses that are often indistinguishable from other adnexal masses. However, transvaginal sonography recognizes the fluid-filled tube by its tubular shape, somewhat folded configuration, and well-defined echogenic walls.[209] The dilated tube can be distinguished from a fluid-filled bowel loop by the lack of peristalsis. Occasionally, color Doppler may be necessary to differentiate hydrosalpinx

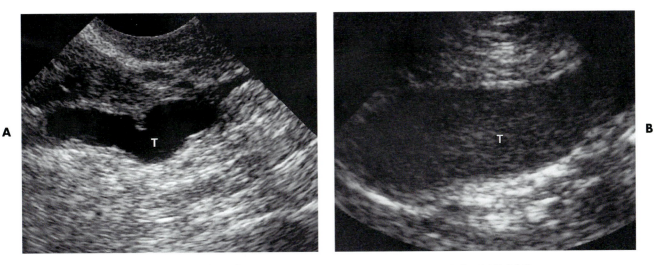

FIG. 15-53. Hydrosalpinx. A, Transvaginal scan shows dilated, fluid-filled fallopian tube (T). **Pyosalpinx. B,** Transvaginal scan shows dilated fallopian tube (T) filled with low-level internal echoes due to pus.

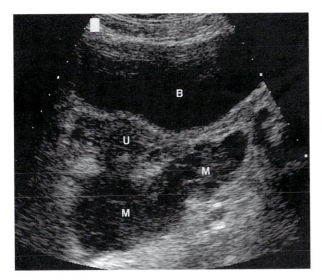

FIG. 15-54. Pelvic inflammatory disease. Transabdominal scan shows large, predominantly hypo-echoic mass (M) with ill-defined margins posterior and to the left of the uterus (U). B, Bladder.

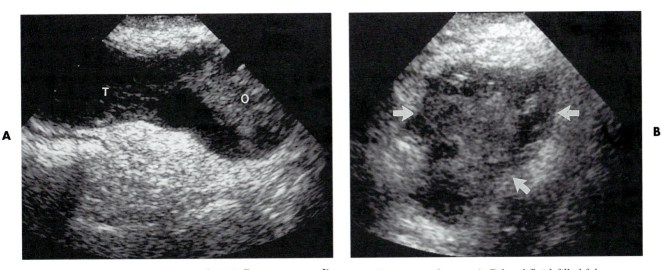

FIG. 15-55. Pelvic inflammatory disease. Transvaginal scans. **A,** Dilated fluid-filled fal-lopian tube (T) adjacent to enlarged ovary (O). **B,** Magnified view of ovary with somewhat indistinct margins *(arrows)* and multiple ill-defined peripheral follicles. Appearance typical of perioophoritis.

from a prominent pelvic vein. Low-level internal echoes may be seen within the fluid-filled tube as a result of pus (**pyosalpinx**), and a fluid-pus level may occasionally be seen. Anechoic fluid within the tube indicates hydrosalpinx which suggests that the infection is chronic. As the infection worsens, periovarian adhesions may form, with fusion of the inflamed dilated tube and ovary which is called the **tubo-ovarian complex.** Further progression results in a **tubo-ovarian abscess** which appears sonographically as a complex multiloculated mass with variable septations, irregular margins, and scattered internal echoes. There is usually posterior acoustic enhancement, and a fluid-debris level or gas may occasionally be seen within the mass. The sonographic appearance may be indistinguishable from other benign and malignant adnexal masses, and clinical correlation is necessary for suggesting the correct diagnosis. Because the ovaries are relatively resistant to infection, areas of recognizable ovarian tissue may be seen within the inflammatory mass by transvaginal sonography.[109]

Both transabdominal and transvaginal sonography are useful in assessing patients with PID. The transabdominal approach is helpful in assessing the extent of the disease, whereas the transvaginal approach is sensitive to detecting dilated tubes, periovarian inflammatory change, and the internal characteristics of tubo-ovarian abscesses.[208,210] Sonography is also useful in following the response to antibiotic therapy. Tubo-ovarian abscesses may be treated by sonographically guided transvaginal aspiration and drainage.[211,212] Catheter drainage is used if the aspirate is frankly purulent, whereas complete aspiration without catheter drainage may be done if the aspirate is not purulent.[212]

In **chronic PID**, extensive fibrosis and adhesions may obscure the margins of the pelvic organs, which blend into a large, ill-defined mass. Isolated torsion of the fallopian tube is uncommon, but it occurs in association with chronic hydrosalpinx.[213] The patient presents with abrupt onset of severe pelvic pain. Hydrosalpinx and tubal torsion have also been reported as a late complication in patients undergoing tubal ligation.[214]

Carcinoma

Carcinoma of the fallopian tube is the least common (less than 1%) of all gynecologic malignancies, with adenocarcinoma being the most common histologic type. It occurs most frequently in postmenopausal women in their sixth decade who present clinically with pain, vaginal bleeding, and a pelvic mass. It usually involves the distal end, but it may involve the entire length of the tube. Sonographically, carcinoma of the fallopian tube has been described as a sausage-shaped, solid, or cystic mass with papillary projections.[215,216]

SONOGRAPHIC EVALUATION OF A PELVIC MASS

Sonography is commonly used to evaluate a pelvic mass (Table 15-2). When a mass is found on sonography, it should be characterized by:

- location (uterine or extrauterine);
- size;
- external contour (well-defined, ill-defined, or irregular borders); and
- internal consistency (cystic, complex predominantly cystic, complex predominantly solid, or solid).

TABLE 15-2
OVARIAN MASSES

Sonographic Characteristics	Suggestive of Benign Disease	Suggestive of Malignant Disease
Size	Small: <5 cm	Large: >10 cm
External Contour	Thin Wall Well-Defined Borders	Thick Wall Ill-Defined or Irregular Borders
Internal Consistency	Purely Cystic Thin Septations	Solid or Complex Thick or Irregular Septations Papillary Projections Echogenic Solid Nodules
Doppler	High-Resistance or No Flow Avascular Nodules	Low-Resistance Flow Vascular Nodules
Associated Findings		Ascites Peritoneal Implants

Generally, uterine masses are mainly solid as opposed to ovarian masses which are mainly cystic. If the mass can be shown to arise from the uterus it is usually a benign leiomyoma. Leiomyomas are common causes of solid adnexal masses, in which case showing their origin from the uterus is diagnostic. Occasionally, it may be impossible to determine the exact origin of the mass by sonography, and MRI may be helpful.

The vast majority of ovarian masses are functional in nature. The size of the mass is important, as masses of less than 5 cm are usually benign, whereas larger masses have a higher incidence of malignancy. Ovarian masses that are purely cystic and have well-defined borders are nearly always benign. Solid ovarian masses are usually malignant, except for teratomas, fibromas, and transitional cell (Brenner) tumors, which frequently have a specific sonographic appearance. Complex masses may be either benign or malignant and should be further assessed for wall contour, septations, and mural nodules. Irregular borders, thick irregular septations, papillary projections, and echogenic solid nodules favor malignancy. Color and spectral Doppler may also be of value. Vascularity may be demonstrated within the septae or nodules. High-resistance flow strongly suggests benign disease, whereas low-resistance flow suggests malignancy, although it can also be seen with benign disease. Although ascites may be associated with benign masses, it is much more frequently seen with malignant disease. Malignant ascites frequently contains echogenic particulate matter.

If a pelvic mass is suspected of being malignant, the abdomen should also be evaluated for evidence of ascites and peritoneal implants, obstructive uropathy, lymphadenopathy, and hepatic and splenic metastases. Hepatic and splenic metastases are uncommon in ovarian carcinoma, but when they occur, they are usually peripheral on the surface of the liver or spleen as a result of peritoneal implantation. Hematogenous metastases within the liver or splenic parenchyma may occur late in the course of the disease.

NONGYNECOLOGIC PELVIC MASSES

Pelvic masses and pseudomasses may be of nongynecologic origin. To make this diagnosis, it is important to visualize the uterus and ovaries separately from the mass (Fig. 15-56). This is frequently not possible because of displacement of the normal pelvic structures by the mass. Nongynecologic pelvic masses most commonly originate from the gastrointestinal or urinary tract or may develop after surgery.

Postoperative Pelvic Masses

Postoperative masses may be **abscesses, hematomas, lymphoceles, urinomas,** or **seromas.** Sono-

graphically, **abscesses** are ovoid-shaped, anechoic masses with thick, irregular walls and posterior acoustic enhancement. Variable internal echogenicity may be seen and high-intensity echoes with shadowing caused by gas may be demonstrated. **Hematomas** show a spectrum of sonographic findings, varying with time.[217] During the initial acute phase, hematomas are anechoic. Following organization and clot formation, they become highly echogenic. With lysis of the clot, hematomas become more complex, until finally, with complete lysis, they are again anechoic. It is frequently not possible to distinguish an abscess from a hematoma sonographically, and clinical correlation is usually necessary.

Pelvic lymphoceles occur following surgical disruption of lymphatic channels, usually after pelvic lymph node dissection or renal transplantation. Sonographically, lymphoceles are cystic, having an appearance similar to that of **urinomas,** which are localized collections of urine, or **seromas,** which are collections of serum. Sonography-guided aspiration may be necessary to differentiate these conditions.

Gastrointestinal Tract Masses

The most frequent pelvic **pseudomasses** are fecal material in the rectum simulating a complex mass in the cul-de-sac and a fluid-filled rectosigmoid colon presenting as a cystic adnexal mass. Transvaginal sonography can usually distinguish the pseudomass from a true mass, but when it cannot, a repeat examination with a water enema may be necessary.[218] **Bowel neoplasms,** especially those involving the rectosigmoid, cecum, and ileum may simulate an adnexal mass. These tumors frequently show the characteristic

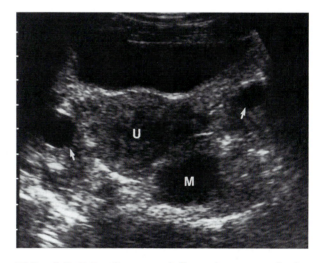

FIG. 15-56. Extramedullary hematopoiesis. Transverse scan in 44-year-old asymptomatic woman with thalassemia shows anechoic mass (M) to left and separate from uterus (U) and both ovaries, which contain cysts *(arrows)*. Diagnosis made by percutaneous biopsy under computed tomography guidance.

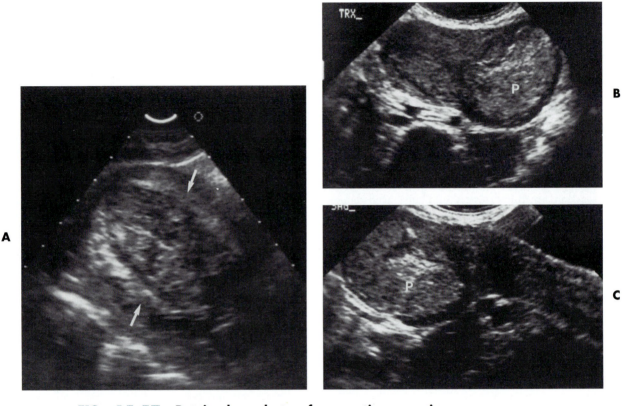

FIG. 15-57. Retained products of conception, varying appearances. **A,** Sagittal scan in patient 3 days after therapeutic abortion shows thickened endometrial cavity *(arrows)* filled with echoes of varying intensity. **B,** Transverse scan in patient with persistent bleeding two weeks postpartum shows retained placental tissue (P). **C,** Sagittal scan of same patient. (B and C, courtesy of Stephanie R. Wilson, M.D., University of Toronto.)

target sign of a gastrointestinal mass, consisting of a central echogenic focus caused by air within the lumen, surrounded by a thickened hypoechoic wall.[219] **Abscesses** related to inflammatory disease of the gastrointestinal tract may also present as an adnexal mass. On the right side, this is most frequently caused by appendicitis or Crohn's disease, whereas abscesses on the left side are usually caused by diverticular disease and are seen in an older age group.

Urinary Tract Masses

A **pelvic kidney** may present as a clinically palpable mass. This is readily recognized sonographically by the typical reniform appearance and the absence of a kidney in the normal location. Occasionally, a markedly distended bladder may be mistaken for an ovarian cyst. When a cystic pelvic mass is identified, it is imperative that the bladder be seen separately from the mass. **Bladder diverticula** may also simulate a cystic adnexal mass. The diagnosis can be confirmed by demonstrating communication with the bladder and a changing appearance after voiding. **Dilated distal ureters** may simulate adnexal cysts on transverse scans; however, sagittal scans show their tubular appearance and continuity with the bladder.

POSTPARTUM PELVIC PATHOLOGIC CONDITIONS

Pathologic states in the postpartum period are usually the result of infection and hemorrhage. Specific pathologic conditions occurring in the postpartum period include endometritis, retained products of conception, and ovarian vein thrombophlebitis. **Endometritis** is more frequent following cesarean section than vaginal delivery. It usually occurs in patients who have had prolonged labor or premature rupture of membranes or who have retained products of conception. The most common source of organisms is the normal vaginal flora. Clinically, there is pelvic pain or unexplained fever.

Retained Products of Conception

Retained placental tissue following delivery may cause secondary postpartum hemorrhage or may serve as a nidus for infection. Sonographically, an echogenic mass in the endometrial cavity (Fig. 15-57, *A*) strongly supports this diagnosis.[220,221] A heterogeneous mass may be seen, but it can also be caused by blood clots or infected or necrotic material without the presence of placental tissue.[221] Occasionally, definitive placental tissue may be identified (Fig. 15-57, *B* and *C*).

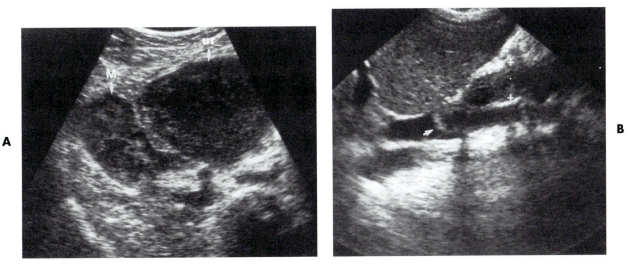

FIG. 15-58. Ovarian vein thrombophlebitis. A, Transverse scan in patient with fever and right lower abdominal pain 4 days following cesarean section shows mass (M) to right of postpartum uterus (UT). B, Sagittal scan of abdomen shows echogenic thrombus in distended right ovarian vein *(between cursors)*. Thrombus is seen extending into inferior vena cava *(arrow)*.

Ovarian Vein Thrombophlebitis

Puerperal ovarian vein thrombosis or thrombophlebitis is an uncommon but potentially life-threatening condition (Fig. 15-58). Patients present with fever, lower abdominal pain, and a palpable mass, usually 48 to 96 hours postpartum. The underlying cause is venous stasis and spread of bacterial infection from endometritis. The right ovarian vein is involved in 90% of cases. Retrograde venous flow occurs in the left ovarian vein during the puerperium, which protects this side from bacterial spread from the uterus.[35] This condition may be diagnosed by sonography, CT, or MRI.[222,223] Sonography may demonstrate an inflammatory mass lateral to the uterus and anterior to the psoas muscle. The ovarian vein may be seen as a tubular, anechoic structure directed cephalad from the mass and containing echogenic thrombus. The thrombus commonly affects the most cephalic portion of the right ovarian vein and can usually be demonstrated sonographically at the junction of the right ovarian vein with the inferior vena cava, sometimes extending into the inferior vena cava.[224] Thrombus in the inferior vena cava may also be seen. Duplex Doppler imaging may demonstrate absence of flow in these veins.[225] Most patients respond to anticoagulant and antibiotic therapy, and follow-up sonography may show resolution of the thrombus and normal flow on duplex Doppler imaging.

Cesarean Section Complications

A lower uterine transverse incision site is commonly used for cesarean section. On sonographic examination, the **incision site** can be identified as an oval, symmetric region of hypoechogenicity relative to the myometrium, located between the posterior wall of

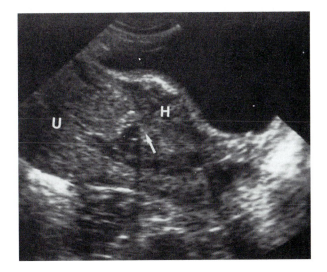

FIG. 15-59. Bladder-flap hematoma. Sagittal scan in patient with fever and lower abdominal pain 8 days following cesarean section shows hematoma (H) between bladder and cesarean section scar *(arrow)*. U, Uterus. (Courtesy of Stephanie R. Wilson, M.D., University of Toronto.)

the bladder and the lower uterine segment.[226] **Sutures** within the incision site may occasionally be recognized as small punctate high-amplitude echoes.

Hematomas may develop from hemorrhage at the incision site (bladder flap hematomas) or within the prevesical space (subfascial hematomas). **Bladder flap hematomas** can be diagnosed sonographically when a complex or anechoic mass greater than 2 cm in diameter is located adjacent to the scar and between the lower uterine segment and the posterior bladder wall (Fig. 15-59). The echogenicity varies depending on the amount of organization within the hematoma.[217] The presence of air within the mass is highly suggestive of an infected hematoma.[227] **Subfascial hematomas** are extraperitoneal in location, contained within the prevesical space, and caused by disruption of the inferior epigastric vessels or their branches during cesarean section[228] or traumatic vaginal delivery.[229] Sonographically, a complex or cystic mass is seen anterior to the bladder. High-frequency, short-focus transducers are frequently necessary to recognize the superficial mass. It is important to identify the rectus muscle in order to distinguish the **superficial wound hematoma,** which is located anterior to the rectus muscle, from the subfascial hematoma located posterior to it.[228] Bladder flap and subfascial hematomas may be seen together in the same patient; however, they have different sources of bleeding and should be treated as separate conditions.

ACKNOWLEDGEMENT

I wish to thank John Lai, R.D.M.S., for his valuable assistance and his contribution to the section on technique and Jocelyne Salem for artwork.

REFERENCES

Normal Pelvic Anatomy

1. Williams PL, Warwick R. *Gray's Anatomy*. 37th ed. Edinburgh: Churchill Livingstone; 1989.
2. Jones HW III, Wentz AC, Burnett LS. *Novak's Textbook of Gynecology*. 11th ed. Baltimore: Williams & Wilkins; 1988.

Technique

3. Cullinan JA, Fleischer AC, Kepple DM et al. Sonohysterography: a technique for endometrial evaluation. *RadioGraphics* 1995;15:501-514.
4. Mendelson EB, Bohm-Velez M, Joseph N et al. Gynecologic imaging: comparison of transabdominal and transvaginal sonography. *Radiology* 1988;166:321-324.
5. Lande IM, Hill MC, Cosco FE et al. Adnexal and cul-de-sac abnormalities: transvaginal sonography. *Radiology* 1988;166:325-332.
6. Leibman AJ, Kruse B, McSweeney MB. Transvaginal sonography: comparison with transabdominal sonography in the diagnosis of pelvic masses. *AJR* 1988;151:89-92.
7. Tessler FN, Schiller VL, Perrella RR et al. Transabdominal versus endovaginal pelvic sonography: prospective study. *Radiology* 1989;170:553-556.
8. Coleman BG, Arger PH, Grumbach K et al. Transvaginal and transabdominal sonography: prospective comparison. *Radiology* 1988;168:639-643.
9. Andolf E, Jörgensen C. A prospective comparison of transabdominal and transvaginal ultrasound with surgical findings in gynecologic disease. *J Ultrasound Med* 1990;9:71-75.
10. DiSantis DJ, Scatarige JC, Kemp G et al. A prospective evaluation of transvaginal sonography for detection of ovarian disease. *AJR* 1993;161:91-94.

Uterus

11. Sample WF, Lippe BM, Gyepes MT. Gray-scale ultrasonography of the normal female pelvis. *Radiology* 1977;125:477-483.
12. Orsini LF, Salardi S, Pilu G et al. Pelvic organs in premenarcheal girls: real-time ultrasonography. *Radiology* 1984;153:113-116.
13. Nussbaum AR, Sanders RC, Jones MD. Neonatal uterine morphology as seen on real-time US. *Radiology* 1986;160:641-643.
14. Siegel MJ. Pediatric gynecologic sonography. *Radiology* 1991;179:593-600.
15. Platt JF, Bree RL, Davidson D. Ultrasound of the normal nongravid uterus: correlation with gross and histopathology. *J Clin Ultrasound* 1990;18:15-19.
16. Miller EI, Thomas RH, Lines P. The atrophic postmenopausal uterus. *J Clin Ultrasound* 1977;5:261-263.
17. Fleischer AC, Kalemeris GC, Machin JE et al. Sonographic depiction of normal and abnormal endometrium with histopathologic correlation. *J Ultrasound Med* 1986;5:445-452.
18. Farrer-Brown G, Beilby JOW, Tarbit MH. The blood supply of the uterus. 2. venous pattern. *Br J Obstet Gynecol Comm* 1970;77:682-689.
19. DuBose TJ, Hill LW, Hennigan HW Jr et al. Sonography of arcuate uterine blood vessels. *J Ultrasound Med* 1985;4:229-233.
20. Occhipinti K, Kutcher R, Rosenblatt R. Sonographic appearance and significance of arcuate artery calcification. *J Ultrasound Med* 1991;10:97-100.
21. Atri M, de Stempel J, Senterman MK et al. Diffuse peripheral uterine calcification (manifestation of Monckeberg's arteriosclerosis) detected by ultrasonography. *J Clin Ultrasound* 1992;20:211-216.
22. Burks DD, Stainken BF, Burkhard TK et al. Uterine inner myometrial echogenic foci: relationship to prior dilatation and curettage and endocervical biopsy. *J Ultrasound Med* 1991;10:487-492.
23. Callen PW, DeMartini WJ, Filly RA. The central uterine cavity echo: a useful anatomic sign in the ultrasonographic evaluation of the female pelvis. *Radiology* 1979;131:187-190.
24. Fleischer AC, Kalemeris GC, Entman SS. Sonographic depiction of the endometrium during normal cycles. *Ultrasound Med Biol* 1986;12:271-277.
25. Forrest TS, Elyaderani MK, Muilenburg MI et al. Cyclic endometrial changes: US assessment with histologic correlation. *Radiology* 1988;167:233-237.
26. Pennes DR, Bowerman RA, Silver TM. Congenital uterine anomalies and associated pregnancies: findings and pitfalls of sonographic diagnosis. *J Ultrasound Med* 1985;4:531-538.
27. Fried AM, Oliff M, Wilson EA et al. Uterine anomalies associated with renal agenesis: role of gray scale ultrasonography. *AJR* 1978;131:973-975.
28. Wiersma AF, Peterson LF, Justema EJ. Uterine anomalies associated with unilateral renal agenesis. *Obstet Gynecol* 1976;47:654-657.
29. Nicolini U, Bellotti M, Bonazzi B et al. Can ultrasound be used to screen uterine malformations? *Fertil Steril* 1987;47:89-93.
30. Yoder IC. Diagnosis of uterine anomalies: relative accuracy of MR imaging, endovaginal sonography, and hysterosalpingography. *Radiology* 1992;185:343.
31. Reuter KL, Daly DC, Cohen SM. Septate versus bicornuate uteri: errors in imaging diagnosis. *Radiology* 1989;172:749-752.
32. Pellerito JS, McCarthy SM, Doyle MB et al. Diagnosis of uterine anomalies: relative accuracy of MR imaging, endovaginal sonography and hysterosalpingography. *Radiology* 1992;183:795-800.
33. Viscomi GN, Gonzalez R, Taylor KJW. Ultrasound detection of uterine abnormalities after diethylstilbestrol (DES) exposure. *Radiology* 1980;136:733-735.

34. Lev-Toaff AS, Toaff ME, Friedman AC. Endovaginal sonographic appearance of a DES uterus. *J Ultrasound Med* 1990;9:661-664.

35. Kurman RJ. *Blaustein's Pathology of the Female Genital Tract.* 4th ed. New York: Springer-Verlag; 1994.

36. Smith JP, Weiser EB, Karnei RF Jr et al. Ultrasonography of rapidly growing uterine leiomyomata associated with anovulatory cycles. *Radiology* 1980;134:713-716.

37. Lev-Toaff AS, Coleman BG, Arger PH et al. Leiomyomas in pregnancy: sonographic study. *Radiology* 1987;164:375-380.

38. Dilts PV Jr, Hopkins MP, Chang AE et al. Rapid growth of leiomyoma in patient receiving tamoxifen. *Am J Obstet Gynecol* 1992;166:167-168.

39. Gross BH, Silver TM, Jaffe MH. Sonographic features of uterine leiomyomas: analysis of 41 proven cases. *J Ultrasound Med* 1983;2:401-406.

40. Kliewer MA, Hertzberg BS, George PY et al. Acoustic shadowing from uterine leiomyomas: sonographic-pathologic correlation. *Radiology* 1995;196:99-102.

41. Baltarowich OH, Kurtz AB, Pennell RG et al. Pitfalls in the sonographic diagnosis of uterine fibroids. *AJR* 1988;151:725-728.

42. Moore L, Wilson S, Rosen B. Giant hydropic uterine leiomyoma in pregnancy: unusual sonographic and Doppler appearance. *J Ultrasound Med* 1994;13:416-418.

43. Fedele L, Bianchi S, Dorta M et al. Transvaginal ultrasonography versus hysteroscopy in the diagnosis of uterine submucous myomas. *Obstet Gynecol* 1991;77:745-748.

44. Karasick S, Lev-Toaff AS, Toaff ME. Imaging of uterine leiomyomas. *AJR* 1992;158:799-805.

45. Dodd GD III, Budzik RF Jr. Lipomatous uterine tumors: diagnosis by ultrasound, CT and MR. *J Comput Assist Tomogr* 1990;14:629-632.

46. Serafini G, Martinoli C, Quadri P et al. Lipomatous tumors of the uterus: ultrasonographic findings in 11 cases. *J Ultrasound Med* 1996;16:195-199.

47. Hertzberg BS, Kliewer MA, George P et al. Lipomatous uterine masses: potential to mimic ovarian dermoids on endovaginal sonography. *J Ultrasound Med* 1995;14:689-692.

48. Siedler D, Laing FC, Jeffrey RB Jr et al. Uterine adenomyosis: a difficult sonographic diagnosis. *J Ultrasound Med* 1987;6:345-349.

49. Bohlman ME, Ensor RE, Sanders RC. Sonographic findings in adenomyosis of the uterus. *AJR* 1987;148:765-766.

50. Fedele L, Bianchi S, Dorta M et al. Transvaginal ultrasonography in the diagnosis of diffuse adenomyosis. *Fertil Steril* 1992;58:94-97.

51. Reinhold C, Atri M, Mehio A et al. Diffuse uterine adenomyosis: morphologic criteria and diagnostic accuracy of endovaginal sonography. *Radiology* 1995;197:609-614.

52. Fedele L, Bianchi S, Dorta M et al. Transvaginal ultrasonography in the differential diagnosis of adenomyosis versus leiomyoma. *Am J Obstet Gynecol* 1992;167:603-606.

53. Togashi K, Ozasa H, Konishi I et al. Enlarged uterus: differentiation between adenomyosis and leiomyoma with MR imaging. *Radiology* 1989;171:531-534.

54. Ascher SM, Arnold LL, Patt RH et al. Adenomyosis: prospective comparison of MR imaging and transvaginal sonography. *Radiology* 1994;190:803-806.

55. Reinhold C, McCarthy S, Bret PM et al. Diffuse adenomyosis: comparison of endovaginal US and MR imaging with histopathologic correlation. *Radiology* 1996;199:151-158.

56. Torres WE, Stones PJ Jr, Thames FM. Ultrasound appearance of pelvic arteriovenous malformation. *J Clin Ultrasound* 1979;7:383-385.

57. Musa AA, Hata T, Hata K et al. Pelvic arteriovenous malformation diagnosed by color flow Doppler imaging. *AJR* 1989; 152:1311-1312.

58. Huang M, Muradali D, Thurston WA et al. Uterine arteriovenous malformations (AVMs): ultrasound and Doppler features with MRI correlation. *Radiology* 1997; in press.

59. Mendelson EB, Bohm-Velez M, Joseph N et al. Endometrial abnormalities: evaluation with transvaginal sonography. *AJR* 1988;150:139-142.

60. Varner RE, Sparks JM, Cameron CD et al. Transvaginal sonography of the endometrium in postmenopausal women. *Obstet Gynecol* 1991;78:195-199.

61. Granberg S, Wickland M, Karlsson B et al. Endometrial thickness as measured by endovaginal ultrasonography for identifying endometrial abnormality. *Am J Obstet Gynecol* 1991;164:47-52.

62. Osmers R, Völkson M, Schauer A. Vaginosonography for early detection of endometrial carcinoma? *Lancet* 1990; 335:1569-1571.

63. Nasri MN, Shepherd JH, Setchell ME et al. The role of vaginal scan in measurement of endometrial thickness in postmenopausal women. *Br J Obstet Gynaecol* 1991;98:470-475.

64. Goldstein SR, Nachtigall M, Snyder JR et al. Endometrial assessment by vaginal ultrasonography before endometrial sampling in patients with postmenopausal bleeding. *Am J Obstet Gynecol* 1990;163:119-123.

65. Karlsson B, Granberg S, Wikland M et al. Transvaginal ultrasonography of the endometrium in women with postmenopausal bleeding: a Nordic multicenter study. *Am J Obstet Gynecol* 1995;172:1488-1494.

66. Shipley CF III, Simmons CL, Nelson GH. Comparison of transvaginal sonography with endometrial biopsy in asymptomatic postmenopausal women. *J Ultrasound Med* 1994; 13:99-104.

67. Lin MC, Gosink BB, Wolf SI et al. Endometrial thickness after menopause: effect of hormone replacement. *Radiology* 1991;180:427-432.

68. Aleem F, Predanic M, Calame R et al. Transvaginal color and pulsed Doppler sonography of the endometrium: a possible role in reducing the number of dilatation and curettage procedures. *J Ultrasound Med* 1995;14:139-145.

69. Levine D, Gosink BB, Johnson LA. Change in endometrial thickness in postmenopausal women undergoing hormone replacement therapy. *Radiology* 1995;197:603-608.

70. Lewit N, Thaler I, Rottem S. The uterus: a new look with transvaginal sonography. *J Clin Ultrasound* 1990;18:331-336.

71. Breckenridge JW, Kurtz AB, Ritchie WGM et al. Postmenopausal uterine fluid collection: indicator of carcinoma. *AJR* 1982;139:529-534.

72. McCarthy KA, Hall DA, Kopans DB et al. Postmenopausal endometrial fluid collections: always an indicator of malignancy? *J Ultrasound Med* 1986;5:647-649.

73. Goldstein SR. Postmenopausal endometrial fluid collections revisited: look at the doughnut rather than the hole. *Obstet Gynecol* 1994;83:738-740.

74. Wilson DA, Stacy TM, Smith EI. Ultrasound diagnosis of hydrocolpos and hydrometrocolpos. *Radiology* 1978;128:451-454.

75. Scott WW Jr, Rosenshein NB, Siegelman SS et al. The obstructed uterus. *Radiology* 1981;141:767-770.

76. Sheth S, Hamper UM, Kurman RJ. Thickened endometrium in the postmenopausal woman: sonographic-pathologic correlation. *Radiology* 1993;187:135-139.

77. Hulka CA, Hall DA, McCarthy K et al. Endometrial polyps, hyperplasia and carcinoma in postmenopausal women: differentiation with endovaginal sonography. *Radiology* 1994; 191:755-758.

78. Atri M, Nazarnia S, Aldis AE et al. Transvaginal US appearance of endometrial abnormalities. *RadioGraphics* 1994;14:483-492.

79. Choo YC, Mak KC, Hsu C et al. Postmenopausal uterine bleeding of nonorganic cause. *Obstet Gynecol* 1985;66:225-228.

80. Kupfer MC, Schiller VL, Hansen GC et al. Transvaginal sonographic evaluation of endometrial polyps. *J Ultrasound Med* 1994;13:535-539.

81. Parsons AK, Lense JJ. Sonohysterography for endometrial abnormalities: preliminary results. *J Clin Ultrasound* 1993; 21:87-95.

82. Gaucherand P, Piacenza JM, Salle B et al. Sonohysterography of the uterine cavity: preliminary investigations. *J Clin Ultrasound* 1995;23:339-348.

83. Dubinsky TJ, Parvey HR, Gormaz G et al. Transvaginal hysterosonography in the evaluation of small endoluminal masses. *J Ultrasound Med* 1995;14:1-6.

84. Karlsson B, Granberg S, Hellberg P et al. Comparative study of transvaginal sonography and hysteroscopy for the detection of pathologic endometrial lesions in women with postmenopausal bleeding. *J Ultrasound Med* 1994;13:757-762.

85. Malfetano JH. Tamoxifen-associated endometrial carcinoma in postmenopausal breast cancer patients. *Gynecol Oncol* 1990;39:82-84.

86. Kedar RP, Bourne TH, Powles TJ et al. Effects of tamoxifen on uterus and ovaries of postmenopausal women in a randomised breast cancer prevention trial. *Lancet* 1994; 343:1318-1321.

87. Lahti E, Blanco G, Kauppila A et al. Endometrial changes in postmenopausal breast cancer patients receiving tamoxifen. *Obstet Gynecol* 1993;81:660-664.

88. Cohen I, Rosen DJD, Tepper R et al. Ultrasonographic evaluation of the endometrium and correlation with endometrial sampling in postmenopausal patients treated with tamoxifen. *J Ultrasound Med* 1993;5:275-280.

89. Hulka CA, Hall DA. Endometrial abnormalities associated with tamoxifen therapy for breast cancer: sonographic and pathologic correlation. *AJR* 1993;160:809-814.

90. Goldstein SR. Unusual ultrasonographic appearance of the uterus in patients receiving tamoxifen. *Am J Obstet Gynecol* 1994;170:447-451.

91. Bourne TH, Campbell S, Steer CV et al. Detection of endometrial cancer by transvaginal ultrasonography with color flow imaging and blood flow analysis: a preliminary report. *Gynecol Oncol* 1991;40:253-259.

92. Weiner Z, Beck D, Rottem S et al. Uterine artery flow velocity waveforms and color flow imaging in women with perimenopausal and postmenopausal bleeding: correlation to endometrial histopathology. *Acta Obstet Gynecol Scand* 1993;72:162-166.

93. Chan FY, Chau MT, Pun TC et al. Limitations of transvaginal sonography and color Doppler imaging in the differentiation of endometrial carcinoma from benign lesions. *J Ultrasound Med* 1994;13:623-628.

94. Carter JR, Lau M, Saltzman AK et al. Gray scale and color flow Doppler characterization of uterine tumors. *J Ultrasound Med* 1994;13:835-840.

95. Sladkevicius P, Valentin L, Marsal K. Endometrial thickness and Doppler velocimetry of the uterine arteries as discriminators of endometrial status in women with postmenopausal bleeding: a comparative study. *Am J Obstet Gynecol* 1994; 171:722-728.

96. Kurjak A, Shalan H, Sosic A et al. Endometrial carcinoma in postmenopausal women: evaluation by transvaginal color Doppler ultrasonography. *Am J Obstet Gynecol* 1993; 169:1597-1603.

97. Sheth S, Hamper UM, McCollum ME et al. Endometrial blood flow analysis in postmenopausal women: can it help differentiate benign from malignant causes of endometrial thickening? *Radiology* 1995;195:661-665.

98. Fleischer AC, Dudley BS, Entman SS et al. Myometrial invasion by endometrial carcinoma: sonographic assessment. *Radiology* 1987;162:307-310.

99. Cacciatore B, Lehtovirta P, Wahlström T et al. Preoperative sonographic evaluation of endometrial cancer. *Am J Obstet Gynecol* 1989;160:133-137.

100. Gordon AN, Fleischer AC, Reed GW. Depth of myometrial invasion in endometrial cancer: preoperative assessment by transvaginal ultrasonography. *Gynecol Oncol* 1990;39:321-327.

101. DelMaschio A, Vanzulli A, Sironi S et al. Estimating the depth of myometrial involvement by endometrial carcinoma: efficacy of transvaginal sonography vs MR imaging. *AJR* 1993;160:533-538.

102. Yamashita Y, Mizutani H, Torashima M et al. Assessment of myometrial invasion by endometrial carcinoma: transvaginal sonography vs contrast-enhanced MR imaging. *AJR* 1993; 161:595-599.

103. Wachsberg RH, Kurtz AB. Gas within the endometrial cavity at postpartum US: a normal finding after spontaneous vaginal delivery. *Radiology* 1992;183:431-433.

104. Fedele L, Bianchi S, Dorta M et al. Intrauterine adhesions: detection with transvaginal US. *Radiology* 1996;199:757-759.

105. Callen PW, Filly RA, Munyer TP. Intrauterine contraceptive devices: evaluation by sonography. *AJR* 1980;135:797-800.

106. Fogel SR, Slasky BS. Sonography of nabothian cysts. *AJR* 1982;138:927-930.

Vagina

107. McCarthy S, Taylor KJW. Sonography of vaginal masses. *AJR* 1983;140:1005-1008.

108. Schoenfeld A, Levavi H, Hirsch M et al. Transvaginal sonography in postmenopausal women. *J Clin Ultrasound* 1990; 18:350-358.

Rectouterine Recess (Posterior Cul-de-sac)

109. Mendelson EB, Bohm-Velez M, Neiman HL et al. Transvaginal sonography in gynecologic imaging. *Semin Ultrasound CT MR* 1988;9:102-121.

110. Davis JA, Gosink BB. Fluid in the female pelvis: cyclic patterns. *J Ultrasound Med* 1986;5:75-79.

111. Koninckx PR, Renaer M, Brosens IA. Origin of peritoneal fluid in women: an ovarian exudation product. *Br J Obstet Gynaecol* 1980;87:177-183.

112. Jeffrey RB, Laing FC. Echogenic clot: a useful sign of pelvic hemoperitoneum. *Radiology* 1982;145:139-141.

113. Nyberg DA, Hughes M, Mack LA et al. Extrauterine findings of ectopic pregnancy at transvaginal US: importance of echogenic fluid. *Radiology* 1991;178:823-826.

Ovary

114. Cohen HL, Shapiro MA, Mandel FS et al. Normal ovaries in neonates and infants: a sonographic study of 77 patients 1 day to 24 months old. *AJR* 1993;160:583-586.

115. Cohen HL, Eisenberg P, Mandel F et al. Ovarian cysts are common in premenarchal girls: a sonographic study of 101 children 2-12 years old. *AJR* 1992;159:89-91.

116. Cohen HL, Tice HM, Mandel FS. Ovarian volumes measured by US: bigger than we think. *Radiology* 1990;177:189-192.

117. van Nagel JR Jr, Higgins RV, Donaldson ES et al. Transvaginal sonography as a screening method for ovarian cancer. *Cancer* 1990;65:573-577.

118. Brandt KR, Thurmond AS, McCarthy JL. Focal calcifications in otherwise ultrasonographically normal ovaries. *Radiology* 1996;198:415-417.

119. Goswamy RK, Campbell S, Royston JP et al. Ovarian size in postmenopausal women. *Br J Obstet Gynaecol* 1988;95:795-801.

120. Granberg S, Wickland M. A comparison between ultrasound and gynecologic examination for detection of enlarged ovaries in a group of women at risk for ovarian carcinoma. *J Ultrasound Med* 1988;7:59-64.

121. Andolf E, Jörgensen C, Svalenius E et al. Ultrasound measurement of the ovarian volume. *Acta Obstet Gynecol Scand* 1987;66:387-389.

122. Hall DA, McCarthy KA, Kopans DB. Sonographic visualization of the normal postmenopausal ovary. *J Ultrasound Med* 1986;5:9-11.

123. Fleischer AC, McKee MS, Gordon AN et al. Transvaginal sonography of postmenopausal ovaries with pathologic correlation. *J Ultrasound Med* 1990;9:637-644.

124. Wolf SI, Gosink BB, Feldesman MR et al. Prevalence of simple adnexal cysts in postmenopausal women. *Radiology* 1991; 180:65-71.

125. Levine D, Gosink BB, Wolf SI et al. Simple adnexal cysts: the natural history in postmenopausal women. *Radiology* 1992; 184:653-659.

126. Hall DA, McCarthy KA. The significance of the postmenopausal simple adnexal cyst. *J Ultrasound Med* 1986; 5:503-505.

127. Rulin MC, Preston AL. Adnexal masses in postmenopausal women. *Obstet Gynecol* 1987;70:578-581.

128. Andolf E, Jörgensen C. Simple adnexal cysts diagnosed by ultrasound in postmenopausal women. *J Clin Ultrasound* 1988;16:301-303.

129. Goldstein SR, Subramanyam B, Snyder JR et al. The postmenopausal cystic adnexal mass: the potential role of ultrasound in conservative management. *Obstet Gynecol* 1989; 73:8-10.

130. Hall DA. Sonographic appearance of the normal ovary, of polycystic ovary disease, and of functional ovarian cysts. *Semin Ultrasound* 1983;4:149-165.

131. Baltarowich OH, Kurtz AB, Pasto ME et al. The spectrum of sonographic findings in hemorrhagic ovarian cysts. *AJR* 1987;148:901-905.

132. Yoffe N, Bronshtein M, Brandes J et al. Hemorrhagic ovarian cyst detection by transvaginal sonography: the great imitator. *Gynecol Endocrinol* 1991;5:123-129.

133. Phillips HE, McGahan JP. Ovarian remnant syndrome. *Radiology* 1982;142:487-488.

134. Athey PA, Cooper NB. Sonographic features of parovarian cysts. *AJR* 1985;144:83-86.

135. Alpern MB, Sandler MA, Madrazo BL. Sonographic features of parovarian cysts and their complications. *AJR* 1984; 143:157-160.

136. Kim JS, Woo SK, Suh SJ et al. Sonographic diagnosis of paraovarian cysts: value of detecting a separate ipsilateral ovary. *AJR* 1995;164:1441-1444.

137. Hoffer FA, Kozakewich H, Colodny A et al. Peritoneal inclusion cysts: ovarian fluid in peritoneal adhesions. *Radiology* 1988;169:189-191.

138. Sohaey R, Gardner TL, Woodward PJ et al. Sonographic diagnosis of peritoneal inclusion cysts. *J Ultrasound Med* 1995;14:913-917.

139. Friedman H, Vogelzang RL, Mendelson EB et al. Endometriosis detection by US with laparoscopic correlation. *Radiology* 1985;157:217-220.

140. Kupfer MC, Schwimmer SR, Lebovic J. Transvaginal sonographic appearance of endometriomata: spectrum of findings. *J Ultrasound Med* 1992;11:129-133.

141. Athey PA, Diment DD. The spectrum of sonographic findings in endometriomas. *J Ultrasound Med* 1989;8:487-491.

142. Yeh HC, Futterweit W, Thornton JC. Polycystic ovarian disease: US features in 104 patients. *Radiology* 1987;163:111-116.

143. Hann LE, Hall DA, McArdle CR et al. Polycystic ovarian disease: sonographic spectrum. *Radiology* 1984;150:531-534.

144. Pache TD, Wladimiroff JW, Hop WCJ et al. How to discriminate between normal and polycystic ovaries: transvaginal US study. *Radiology* 1992;183:421-423.

145. Ardaens Y, Robert Y, Lemaitre L et al. Polycystic ovarian disease: contribution of vaginal endosonography and reassessment of ultrasonic diagnosis. *Fertil Steril* 1991;55:1062-1068.

146. Sommerville M, Grimes DA, Koonings PP et al. Ovarian neoplasms and the risk of adnexal torsion. *Am J Obstet Gynecol* 1991;164:577-578.

147. Graif M, Itzchak Y. Sonographic evaluation of ovarian torsion in childhood and adolescence. *AJR* 1988;150:647-649.

148. Fleischer AC, Stein SM, Cullinan JA et al. Color Doppler sonography of adnexal torsion. *J Ultrasound Med* 1995; 14:523-528.

149. Stark JE, Siegel MJ. Ovarian torsion in prepubertal and pubertal girls: sonographic findings. *AJR* 1994;163:1479-1482.

150. Rosado WM, Trambert MA, Gosink BB et al. Adnexal torsion: diagnosis by using Doppler sonography. *AJR* 1992;159:1251-1253.

151. Kapadia R, Sternhill V, Schwartz E. Massive edema of the ovary. *J Clin Ultrasound* 1982;10:469-471.

152. Lee AR, Kim KH, Lee BH et al. Massive edema of the ovary: imaging findings. *AJR* 1993;161:343-344.

153. Hill LM, Pelekanos M, Kanbour A. Massive edema of an ovary previously fixed to the pelvic side wall. *J Ultrasound Med* 1993;12:629-632.

154. Wingo PA, Tong T, Bolden S. Cancer statistics, 1995. *CA Cancer J Clin* 1995;45:8-30.

155. Kerlikowske K, Brown JS, Grady DG. Should women with familial ovarian cancer undergo prophylactic oophorectomy? *Obstet Gynecol* 1992;80:700-707.

156. Lynch HT, Watson P, Lynch JF et al. Hereditary ovarian cancer: heterogeneity in age at onset. *Cancer* 1993;71:573-581.

157. Einhorn N, Sjövall K, Knapp RC et al. Prospective evaluation of serum CA125 levels for early detection of ovarian cancer. *Obstet Gynecol* 1992;80:14-18.

158. Jacobs I, Davies AP, Bridges J et al. Prevalence screening for ovarian cancer in postmenopausal women by CA 125 measurement and ultrasonography. *BMJ* 1993;306:1030-1034.

159. Campbell S, Bhan V, Royston P et al. Transabdominal ultrasound screening for early ovarian cancer. *BMJ* 1989; 299:1363-1367.

160. DePriest PD, van Nagell JR Jr, Gallion HH et al. Ovarian cancer screening in asymptomatic postmenopausal women. *Gynecol Oncol* 1993;51:205-209.

161. Bast RC Jr, Klug TL, St. John E et al. A radioimmunoassay using a monoclonal antibody to monitor the course of epithelial ovarian cancer. *N Engl J Med* 1983;309:883-887.

162. Jacobs I, Bast RC Jr. The CA 125 tumor-associated antigen: a review of the literature. *Hum Reprod* 1989;4:1-12.

163. Taylor KJW, Schwartz PE. Screening for early ovarian cancer. *Radiology* 1994;192:1-10.

164. Kurjak A, Shalan H, Kupesic S et al. An attempt to screen asymptomatic women for ovarian and endometrial cancer with transvaginal color and pulsed Doppler sonography. *J Ultrasound Med* 1994;13:295-301.

165. Bourne TH, Campbell S, Reynolds KM et al. Screening for early familial ovarian cancer with transvaginal ultrasonography and colour blood flow imaging. *BMJ* 1993;306:1025-1029.

166. Karlan BY, Raffel LJ, Crvenkovic G et al. A multidisciplinary approach to the early detection of ovarian carcinoma: rationale, protocol design, and early results. *Am J Obstet Gynecol* 1993;169:494-501.

167. Weiner Z, Beck D, Shteiner M et al. Screening for ovarian cancer in women with breast cancer with transvaginal sonography and color flow imaging. *J Ultrasound Med* 1993; 12:387-393.

168. Moyle JW, Rochester D, Sider L et al. Sonography of ovarian tumors: predictability of tumor type. *AJR* 1983;141:985-991.

169. Granberg S, Wickland M, Jansson I. Macroscopic characterization of ovarian tumors and the relation to the histologic diagnosis: criteria to be used for ultrasound evaluation. *Gynecol Oncol* 1989;35:139-144.

170. Finkler NJ, Benacerraf B, Lavin PT et al. Comparison of serum CA 125, clinical impression, and ultrasound in the preoperative evaluation of ovarian masses. *Obstet Gynecol* 1988;72:659-664.

171. Sassone AM, Timor-Tritsch IE, Artner A et al. Transvaginal sonographic characterization of ovarian disease: evaluation of a new scoring system to predict ovarian malignancy. *Obstet Gynecol* 1991;78:70-76.

172. DePriest PD, van Nagell JR Jr, Gallion HH et al. Ovarian cancer screening in asymptomatic postmenopausal women. *Gynecol Oncol* 1993;51:205-209.

173. Folkman J, Watson K, Ingber D et al. Induction of angiogenesis during the transition from hyperplasia to neoplasia. *Nature* 1989;339:58-61.

174. Bourne T, Campbell S, Steer C et al. Transvaginal color flow imaging: a possible new screening technique for ovarian cancer. *Br Med J* 1989;399:1367-1370.

175. Kurjak A, Zalud I, Alfirevic Z. Evaluation of adnexal masses with transvaginal color ultrasound. *J Ultrasound Med* 1991;10:295-297.

176. Weiner Z, Thaler I, Beck D et al. Differentiating malignant from benign ovarian tumors with transvaginal color flow imaging. *Obstet Gynecol* 1992;79:159-162.

177. Fleischer AC, Rodgers WH, Rao BK et al. Assessment of ovarian tumor vascularity with transvaginal color Doppler sonography. *J Ultrasound Med* 1991;10:563-568.

178. Hamper UM, Sheth S, Abbas FM et al. Transvaginal color Doppler sonography of adnexal masses: differences in blood flow impedance in benign and malignant lesions. *AJR* 1993;160:1225-1228.

179. Tekay A, Jouppila P. Validity of pulsatility and resistance indices in classification of adnexal tumors with transvaginal color Doppler ultrasound. *Ultrasound Obstet Gynecol* 1992; 2:338-344.

180. Brown DL, Frates MC, Laing FC et al. Ovarian masses: can benign and malignant lesions be differentiated with color and pulsed Doppler US? *Radiology* 1994;190:333-336.

181. Stein SM, Laifer-Narin S, Johnson MB et al. Differentiation of benign and malignant adnexal masses: relative value of grayscale, color Doppler, and spectral Doppler sonography. *AJR* 1995;164:381-386.

182. Jain KA. Prospective evaluation of adnexal masses with endovaginal gray-scale and duplex and color Doppler US: correlation with pathologic findings. *Radiology* 1994;191:63-67.

183. Levine D, Feldstein VA, Babcook CJ et al. Sonography of ovarian masses: poor sensitivity of resistive index for identifying malignant lesions. *AJR* 1994;162:1355-1359.

184. Bromley B, Goodman H, Benacerraf BR. Comparison between sonographic morphology and Doppler waveform for the diagnosis of ovarian malignancy. *Obstet Gynecol* 1994;83:434-437.

185. Salem S, White LM, Lai J. Doppler sonography of adnexal masses: the predictive value of the pulsatility index in benign and malignant disease. *AJR* 1994;163:1147-1150.

186. Carter J, Saltzman A, Hartenbach E et al. Flow characteristics in benign and malignant gynecologic tumors using transvaginal color flow Doppler. *Obstet Gynecol* 1994; 83:125-130.

187. Buy JN, Ghossain MA, Hugol D et al. Characterization of adnexal masses: combination of color Doppler and conventional sonography compared with spectral Doppler analysis alone and conventional sonography alone. *AJR* 1996; 166:385-393.

188. Fleisher AC, Rodgers WH, Kepple DM et al. Color Doppler sonography of ovarian masses: a multiparameter analysis. *J Ultrasound Med* 1993;12:41-48.

189. Fleischer AC, Cullinan JA, Kepple DM et al. Conventional and color Doppler transvaginal sonography of pelvic masses: a comparison of relative histologic specificities. *J Ultrasound Med* 1993;12:705-712.

190. Laing FC. US analysis of adnexal masses: the art of making the correct diagnosis. *Radiology* 1994;191:21-22.

191. Williams AG, Mettler FA, Wicks JD. Cystic and solid ovarian neoplasms. *Semin Ultrasound* 1983;4:166-183.

192. Wagner BJ, Buck JL, Seidman JD et al. Ovarian epithelial neoplasms: radiologic-pathologic correlation. *Radiographics* 1994;14:1351-1374.

193. Athey PA, Siegel MF. Sonographic features of Brenner tumor of the ovary. *J Ultrasound Med* 1987;6:367-372.

194. Brammer HM III, Buck JL, Hayes WS et al. Malignant germ cell tumors of the ovary: radiologic-pathologic correlation. *Radiographics* 1990;10:715-724.

195. Quinn SF, Erickson S, Black WC. Cystic ovarian teratomas: the sonographic appearance of the dermoid plug. *Radiology* 1985;155:477-478.

196. Sheth S, Fishman EK, Buck JL et al. The variable sonographic appearances of ovarian teratomas: correlation with CT. *AJR* 1988;151:331-334.

197. Guttman PH Jr. In search of the elusive benign cystic ovarian teratoma: application of the ultrasound "tip of the iceberg" sign. *J Clin Ultrasound* 1977;5:403-406.

198. Bronshtein M, Yoffe N, Brandes JM et al. Hair as a sonographic marker of ovarian teratomas: improved identification using transvaginal sonography and simulation model. *J Clin Ultrasound* 1991;19:351-355.

199. Malde HM, Kedar RP, Chadha D et al. Dermoid mesh: a sonographic sign of ovarian teratoma. Letter *AJR* 1992;159:1349-1350.

200. O'Malley BP, Richmond H. Struma ovarii. *J Ultrasound Med* 1982;1:177-178.

201. Tanaka YO, Kurosaki Y, Nishida M et al. Ovarian dysgerminoma: MR and CT appearance. *J Comput Assist Tomogr* 1994;18:443-448.

202. Kim SH, Kang SB. Ovarian dysgerminoma: Color Doppler ultrasonographic findings and comparison with CT and MR imaging findings. *J Ultrasound Med* 1995;14:843-848.

203. Stephenson WM, Laing FC. Sonography of ovarian fibromas. *AJR* 1985;144:1239-1240.

204. Athey PA, Malone RS. Sonography of ovarian fibromas/thecomas. *J Ultrasound Med* 1987;6:431-436.

205. Athey PA, Butters HE. Sonographic and CT appearance of Krukenberg tumors. *J Clin Ultrasound* 1984;12:205-210.

206. Shimizu H, Yamasaki M, Ohama K et al. Characteristic ultrasonographic appearance of the Krukenberg tumor. *J Clin Ultrasound* 1990;18:697-703.

Fallopian Tube

207. Timor-Tritsch IE, Rottem S. Transvaginal ultrasonographic study of the fallopian tube. *Obstet Gynecol* 1987;70:424-428.

208. Patten RM, Vincent LM, Wolner-Hanssen P et al. Pelvic inflammatory disease: endovaginal sonography with laparoscopic correlation. *J Ultrasound Med* 1990;9:681-689.

209. Tessler FN, Perrella RR, Fleischer AC et al. Endovaginal sonographic diagnosis of dilated fallopian tubes. *AJR* 1989;153:523-525.

210. Bulas DI, Ahlstrom PA, Sivit CJ et al. Pelvic inflammatory disease in the adolescent: comparison of transabdominal and transvaginal sonographic evaluation. *Radiology* 1992; 183:435-439.

211. vanSonnenberg E, D'Agostino HB, Casola G et al. US-guided transvaginal drainage of pelvic abscesses and fluid collections. *Radiology* 1991;181:53-56.

212. Feld R, Eschelman DJ, Sagerman JE et al. Treatment of pelvic abscesses and other fluid collections: efficacy of transvaginal sonographically guided aspiration and drainage. *AJR* 1994;163:1141-1145.

213. Sherer DM, Liberto L, Abramowicz JS et al. Endovaginal sonographic features associated with isolated torsion of the fallopian tube. *J Ultrasound Med* 1991;10:107-109.

214. Russin LD. Hydrosalpinx and tubal torsion: a late complication of tubal ligation. *Radiology* 1986;159:115-116.

215. Subramanyam BR, Raghavendra BN, Whalen CA et al. Ultrasonic features of fallopian tube carcinoma. *J Ultrasound Med* 1984;3:391-393.

216. Ajjimakorn S, Bhamarapravati Y. Transvaginal ultrasound and the diagnosis of fallopian tube carcinoma. *J Clin Ultrasound* 1991;19:116-119.

Nongynecologic Pelvic Masses

217. Wicks JD, Silver TM, Bree RL. Gray scale features of hematomas: an ultrasonic spectrum. *AJR* 1978;131:977-980.

218. Kurtz AB, Rubin CS, Kramer FL et al. Ultrasound evaluation of the posterior pelvic compartment. *Radiology* 1979; 132:677-682.

219. Salem S, O'Malley BP, Hiltz CW. Ultrasonographic appearance of gastrointestinal masses. *J Can Assoc Radiol* 1980;31:163-167.

Postpartum Pelvic Pathology

220. Lee CY, Madrazo B, Drukker BH. Ultrasonic evaluation of the postpartum uterus in the management of postpartum bleeding. *Obstet Gynecol* 1981;58:227-232.

221. Hertzberg BS, Bowie JD. Ultrasound of the postpartum uterus: prediction of retained placental tissue. *J Ultrasound Med* 1991;10:451-456.

222. Wilson PC, Lerner RM. Diagnosis of ovarian vein thrombophlebitis by ultrasonography. *J Ultrasound Med* 1983; 2:187-190.

223. Savader SJ, Otero RR, Savader BL. Puerperal ovarian vein thrombosis: evaluation with CT, US, and MR imaging. *Radiology* 1988;167:637-639.

224. Grant TH, Schoettle BW, Buchsbaum MS. Postpartum ovarian vein thrombosis: diagnosis by clot protrusion into the inferior vena cava at sonography. *AJR* 1993;160:551-552.

225. Baran GW, Frisch KM. Duplex Doppler evaluation of puerperal ovarian vein thrombosis. *AJR* 1987;149:321-322.

226. Baker ME, Kay H, Mahony BS et al. Sonography of the low transverse incision, cesarean section: a prospective study. *J Ultrasound Med* 1988;7:389-393.

227. Baker ME, Bowie JD, Killam AP. Sonography of post-cesarean-section bladder-flap hematoma. *AJR* 1985;144:757-759.

228. Wiener MD, Bowie JD, Baker ME et al. Sonography of subfascial hematoma after cesarean delivery. *AJR* 1987;148:907-910.

229. Al-Naib S. Sonographic appearance of postpartum retropubic hematoma. *J Clin Ultrasound* 1990;18:520-521.

CHAPTER 16

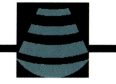

The Thorax

·

William E. Brant, M.D.

Ultrasound is a reliable and efficient imaging method to evaluate a wide range of perplexing clinical problems in the chest and to guide diagnostic and therapeutic invasive procedures.[1] Although the ribs, spine, and air-filled lung act as barriers to ultrasound visualization of intrathoracic diseases, the presence of fluid in the pleural space and tumor, consolidation, or atelectasis in the lung provide ample sonographic windows for evaluation. When film radiography is unable to clarify a chest abnormality, sonography may further characterize the abnormality and limit the differential diagnosis. Sonography can be used to differentiate pleural from parenchymal lesions, to visualize diseased parenchyma hidden by pleural effusion, and to detect pleural septations and other pleural abnormalities not even suspected by other imaging modalities.[2] Ultrasound clearly demonstrates the diaphragm and differentiates subpulmonic effusion from subphrenic abscess. Because ultrasound is portable, it can be readily used at the bedside of critically ill patients to evaluate thoracic disease and to provide safe and accurate guidance for interventional procedures.[3] The patient can be examined in any position, minimizing the need for moving patients on life support devices. Cooperative patients can be maneuvered into a variety of positions to optimize sonographic visualization of the mediastinum and deep thoracic structures. Ultrasound can be effectively used to guide a variety of interventional procedures in the thorax.[4] Most needle placements can be performed under direct and constant visualization, maximizing accuracy and patient safety.

PLEURAL SPACE

The pleural space is superficial and readily examined by ultrasound using either a direct intercostal or an abdominal approach. A high-frequency (5 to 7.5-MHz) linear transducer applied directly to the chest (direct intercostal approach) provides a broad, near field-of-view that allows excellent visualization of the pleural space (Fig. 16-1, *A*). The lower reaches of the pleural space may be effectively examined by use of sector or convex-array (3.5-MHz) transducers directed superiorly from the abdomen (abdominal approach). The liver and spleen provide sonographic windows to the thorax. Sector transducers are frequently unsatisfactory for examination of the pleural space when applied directly to the chest (Fig. 16-1, *B*). The sector scanner has a narrow view in the near field, and the pleural space is frequently obscured by near-field artifacts.

Normal Sonographic Appearance
Direct Intercostal Approach. The normal pleural space is readily recognized when the ribs are

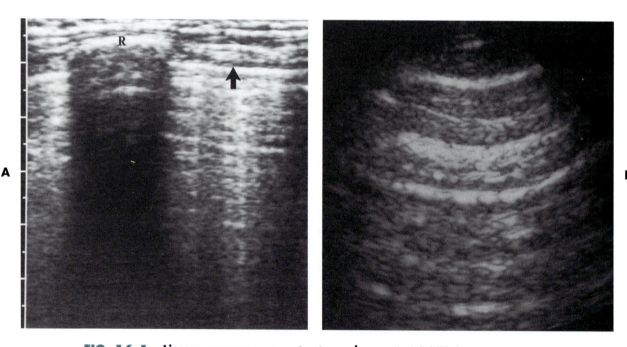

FIG. 16-1. **Linear array versus sector transducer.** **A,** A 5-MHz linear-array transducer applied directly to the chest produces an image of a rib, *R,* and normal visceral pleural-pulmonary interface *(arrow)*. The normal pleural space is the hypoechoic line just superficial to the interface. **B,** A 3.5-MHz sector transducer applied directly to the chest produces a confusing image of reverberation artifacts. No anatomic landmarks can be recognized. The normal pleural space is obscured by artifacts in the narrow field close to the transducer surface.

used as sonographic landmarks (Fig. 16-2). With a linear-array transducer oriented perpendicular to the intercostal spaces, the ribs are displayed as rounded echogenic interfaces with prominent acoustic shadowing. Intercostal muscle is visualized between the rib shadows. The location and depth of the ribs are noted, and the thickness of the subcutaneous tissues and the overlying muscles of the chest wall are determined. The **pleural space** is located within 1 cm of depth from the rib interface. The **air-filled lung,** covered by **visceral pleura,** is a potent reflector of the ultrasound beam, blocking sound penetration deeper into the chest and producing a bright, linear interface that moves with respiration. The normal back-and-forth movement of the lung surface with respiration has been called the **"gliding sign."**[5] The bright, linear interface of the lung surface is the sonographic marker of the visceral pleura. A thin, dark line of **pleural fluid** is normally present, separating the parietal from the visceral pleura. The **parietal pleura** appears as a less distinct, weakly echogenic line, often obscured by reverberation artifact. Its location is inferred by its relationship to the ribs and the visceral pleura.

Abdominal Approach. When imaged from the abdomen, the diaphragm appears as a bright, curving, echogenic line that moves with respiration (Fig. 16-3). The normal diaphragm is approximately 5 mm thick and is covered by parietal pleura on its thoracic side and by peritoneum on its abdominal side. On occasion, the muscle of the diaphragm may

be demonstrated as a thin, dark line just above the much brighter echo of its inferior surface. When the lung above the diaphragm is air-filled, the curved surface of the diaphragm-lung interface acts as a **specular** (mirrorlike) **reflector.**[6] An artifactual, **mirror-image** reflection of the liver or spleen is displayed above the diaphragm. The presence of this mirror image, although easily recognized as an artifact, should also be viewed as definitive evidence of the presence of air-filled lung and absence of pleural fluid above the diaphragm.

Pleural Fluid

Before embarking on a search for pleural fluid by ultrasound, the patient's chest radiograph or chest CT scan should be reviewed. The location of pleural lesions should be noted for correlation with the ultrasound examination. Areas of suspected loculated pleural fluid or pleural thickening can then be carefully examined.

Direct Intercostal Approach. Even minute amounts of pleural fluid can be detected by using a high-resolution linear-array transducer applied directly to the chest. Most pleural fluid is relatively anechoic and is easily recognized as an area of echolucency separating the parietal and visceral pleura (Fig. 16-4).[7-9] The parietal pleura is identified by its position approximately 1 cm deep to the ribs. The visceral pleura is identified by observing motion of the lung as the patient breathes. **Ultrasound signs**

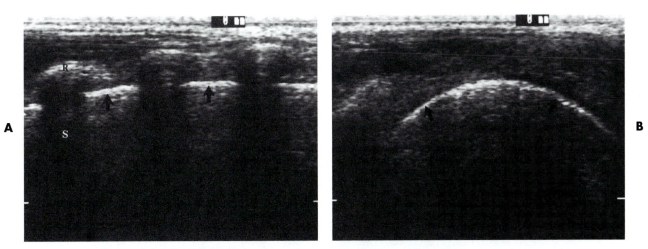

A   **B**

FIG. 16-2. Normal pleural space (direct intercostal approach). A, Longitudinal image from a linear-array transducer applied directly to the chest demonstrates three ribs and the normal pleural space. The ribs produce a bright surface reflection, *R,* and a dense acoustic shadow, *S.* The normal visceral pleura–air-filled lung interface *(arrow)* is localized within 1 cm deep to the rib surface. The pleural space is the thin hypoechoic line just superficial to the interface. Intercostal muscles are seen between the ribs. **B,** A transverse image obtained in an intercostal space with a linear-array transducer demonstrates the curving normal visceral pleura–air-filled lung interface *(arrows).* The location of the visceral pleura is confirmed by observing the motion of the lung interface with respiration, "the gliding sign." Note the pattern of bright echoes, diminishing in intensity with depth, produced by reverberation artifact on both images.

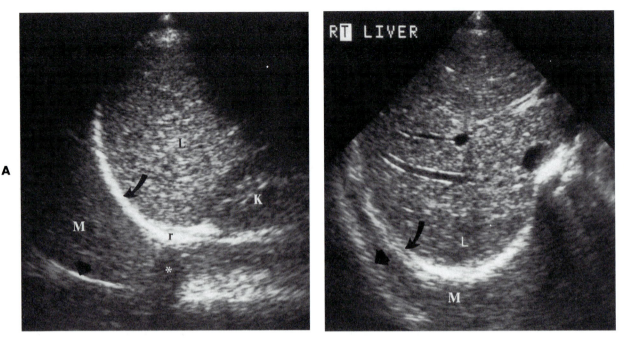

FIG. 16-3. Normal pleural space (abdominal approach). **A,** Longitudinal image obtained through the liver, *L*, and kidney, *K*, with a 3.5-MHz sector transducer directed at the diaphragm. The diaphragm-lung-surface complex produces a bright, curving, linear echo *(curved arrow)*. Mirror-image reflections of the liver, *M*, and the diaphragm *(arrowhead)* are displayed above the diaphragm. The limits of the patient's chest are marked by a rib, *r*, identified by its accompanying shadow, *. The image beyond the level of the rib is entirely artifactual. **B,** Transverse image directed through the liver, *L*, shows mirror-image reflections of the liver, *M*, and diaphragm *(arrowhead)*. The curved arrow shows the true diaphragm. The presence of a mirror-image reflection of the liver above the diaphragm is evidence of the absence of pleural effusion.

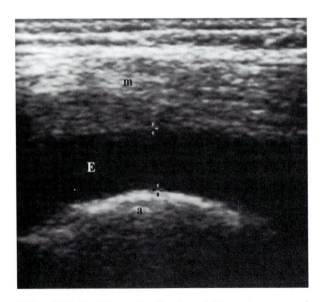

FIG. 16-4. Pleural effusion (direct intercostal approach). Image obtained in an intercostal space using a linear-array transducer demonstrates a small pleural effusion, *E*, as a band of echolucency separating the parietal and visceral pleura *(marked by +)*. *m,* Intercostal muscle; *a,* air-filled lung.

of pleural fluid include hypoechoic fluid separating the visceral and parietal pleura (see Fig. 16-4), floating echogenic particles (Fig. 16-5), moving septations within the pleural space (Fig. 16-6), and moving lung suspended within fluid (see Fig. 16-5). The **quantity** of pleural fluid can be estimated by measuring the maximum perpendicular distance between the lung surface and the chest wall.[10] The scan is performed with the patient in the supine position and holding maximum inspiration. Measurement is made just above the level of the diaphragm. A 20 mm width has a mean volume of 380 ml ± 130 ml. A 40 mm measurement corresponded to a mean volume of 1000 ml ± 330 ml.

SONOGRAPHIC SIGNS OF PLEURAL FLUID

Hypoechoic fluid separating the visceral and parietal pleura
Floating echogenic particles
Moving septations within the pleural space
Moving lung suspended within fluid

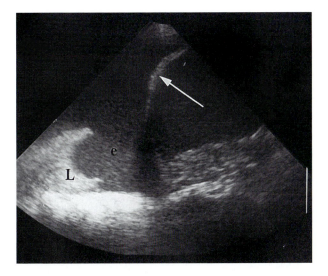

FIG. 16-5. Floating echogenic particles. Floating echogenic particles within the pleural effusion, *e*, confirm the liquid nature of the effusion and are evidence of an exudative effusion. Atelectatic lung, *L*, moved with respiration within the effusion. The diaphragm is seen as a bright curving line *(arrow)* on this image obtained via an abdominal approach.

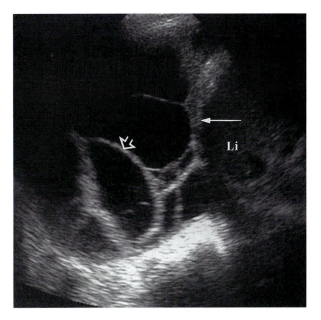

FIG. 16-6. Pleural space septations. Longitudinal image from an abdominal approach demonstrates a complex network of septations *(open arrow)* bridging the pleural space. The diaphragmatic pleura is thickened *(long arrow)*. This exudative effusion was due to tuberculosis. *Li*, Liver.

Abdominal Approach. Pleural effusions are commonly detected during routine sonographic examinations of the abdomen. The **signs of pleural effusion using an abdominal approach** include hypoechoic fluid above the diaphragm (Fig. 16-7), visualization of the inside of the thorax through the fluid collection (see Fig. 16-7), absence of the mirror-image reflection of the liver or spleen above the diaphragm (see Fig. 16-7; Fig. 16-8), and inversion of the diaphragm with large effusions. Because the air-filled lung will block transmission of sound, the ribs and inside of the bony thorax are not normally visualized above the diaphragm when scanning from the abdomen. The presence of pleural fluid allows transmission of sound and visualization of these structures. Artifactual duplication of the diaphragm must not be mistaken for visualization of the inside of the bony thorax. The inside of the bony thorax forms a straight

> ### SONOGRAPHIC SIGNS OF PLEURAL FLUID VIA ABDOMINAL VIEW
>
> Hypoechoic fluid above the diaphragm
> Visualization of the inside of the thorax through the fluid collection
> Absence of the mirror-image reflection of the liver or spleen above the diaphragm
> Inversion of the diaphragm with large effusions

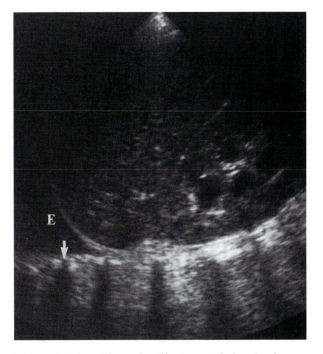

FIG. 16-7. Pleural effusion (abdominal approach). A longitudinal sector scan through the liver shows a pleural effusion, *E*, in the costophrenic angle. The patient's chest wall is marked by the ribs *(arrow)* casting acoustic shadows. The chest wall is visualized above the level of the diaphragm because the pleural effusion allows transmission of ultrasound waves through it. Compare the appearance of the straight true chest wall seen through the effusion on this image with the curving artifactual duplication of the diaphragm seen in a patient without an effusion in Fig. 16-3, *A*.

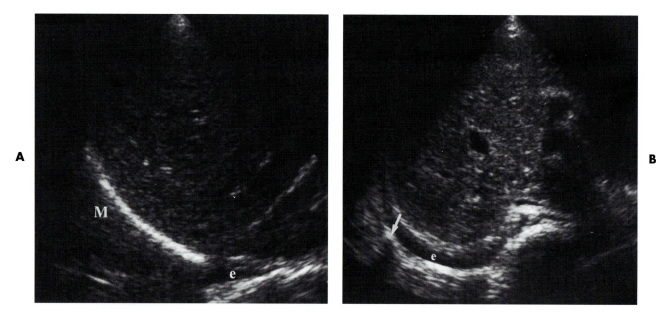

FIG. 16-8. Pleural effusion (abdominal approach). A, Longitudinal scan. A small pleural effusion, *e,* is demonstrated in the extreme costophrenic angle. Air-filled lung above the pleural effusion produces the expected mirror-image reflection, *M,* of the liver. **B,** Transverse image through the liver in the same patient again shows the small pleural effusion, *e.* A rib with its accompanying shadow *(arrow)* marks the limits of the patient's chest wall. Compare with the mirror-image artifacts in Fig. 16-3, *B,* which lack the landmarks of the rib and shadow.

SIGNS OF PLEURAL FLUID

Pleural lesion that changes shape with respiration
Echodensities that float and move with respiration
(within the pleural lesion)
Presence of septations within the pleural lesion (that move with respiration)
"Fluid-color" sign—color Doppler signal within pleural fluid (during respiration with heart motion)

---

line with rib shadows whereas the artifactual reflection of the diaphragm is curved and rib shadows are absent.

Pleural Fluid Versus Pleural Thickening.
Complex pleural fluid may be difficult to differentiate from solid tissue in the pleural space when the fluid is echogenic. Alternatively, pleural thickening or pleural masses may be hypoechoic and difficult to distinguish from pleural fluid.[11] Sonographic features indicating that a pleural lesion is fluid that can be aspirated include[12] a pleural lesion that changes shape with respiration, echodensities that float and move with respiration within the pleural lesion (see Fig. 16-5), presence of septations within the pleural lesion that move with respiration (see Fig. 16-6), and "fluid-color" sign—color Doppler signal within fluid collection in the pleural space during respiration with heart motion.[13] In some

cases sonographic differentiation may not be possible and thoracentesis must be attempted for clarification.

Transudate Versus Exudate. Transudative pleural effusions are essentially ultrafiltrates of plasma and are caused by an imbalance in the homeostatic forces that control the movement of fluid across pleural membranes. They result from an increase in capillary hydrostatic pressure or a decrease in colloid osmotic pressure.[14,15] Pleural membranes are usually normal. Common causes of transudative pleural effusions are listed in a box on page 581. **Exudative pleural effusions** are rich in protein and other constituents of whole blood, implying disease of the pleural membranes and disruption of the integrity of the pleural blood vessels. Most exudates are caused by inflammatory and neoplastic processes. The common causes of exudative pleural effusions are also listed in a box on page 581.

The sonographic appearance of pleural fluid is helpful in differentiating transudates from exudate. Pleural fluid that is anechoic may be either a transudate or an exudate (see Fig. 16-4).[7] Anechoic effusions represent transudative and exudative processes with almost equal frequency.[16] However, fluid that is echogenic, contains floating particulate matter, septations, or fibrin strands, or is associated with pleural nodules or pleural thickening greater than 3 mm is an exudate (see Figs. 16-5 and 16-6)(Table 16-1).[7-9,17] Definitive diagnosis is made by thoracentesis.

Parapneumonic Effusion and Empyema.
Parapneumonic effusion is an exudative pleural effusion associated with pneumonia or lung abscess.[18,19] The visceral pleura is inflamed, and inflammatory cells and fluid leak into the pleural space. Thoracentesis yields fluid with high protein and white blood cell counts but no bacteria. About 40% of bacterial pneumonia have an associated parapneumonic effusion. Gross pus with bacteria or other infectious organisms in the pleural space define an **empyema.** Most empyemas occur by extension of infection from pneumonia. Trauma, surgery, thoracentesis, esophageal rupture, and subdiaphragmatic abscesses are other causes.

Parapneumonic effusions and empyemas may progress to a **fibropurulent stage** characterized by fibrin deposition on the pleura with loculation of fluid and formation of limiting membranes. These fibrin membranes are easily demonstrated by ultrasound.

CAUSES OF TRANSUDATIVE PLEURAL EFFUSIONS

Increased hydrostatic pressure
Congestive heart failure
Superior vena cava obstruction
Constrictive pericarditis

Decreased oncotic pressure
Cirrhosis with ascites
Peritoneal dialysis
Acute glomerulonephritis
Nephrotic syndrome
Urinary tract obstruction
Hypoalbuminemia
Overhydration
Hypothyroidism

Miscellaneous
Misplaced venous catheter

CAUSES OF EXUDATIVE PLEURAL EFFUSIONS

Infections
Parapneumonic effusion
Empyema
Tuberculosis
Fungi (nocardia, actinomycosis)

Neoplasms
Pleural metastases (lung, breast, stomach, ovary)
Pleural mesothelioma
Bronchogenic carcinoma
Lymphoma

Vascular
Pulmonary emboli

Collagen-vascular disease
Systemic lupus erythematosus
Rheumatoid arthritis

Abdominal disease
Subphrenic abscess
Pancreatitis

Trauma
Hydrothorax

Miscellaneous
Drug-induced effusion

TABLE 16-1
TRANSUDATIVE VERSUS EXUDATIVE PLEURAL EFFUSIONS

Transudate	Exudate
Clinical signs	
Pleural fluid protein/serum protein ratio < 0.5	Pleural fluid protein/serum protein ratio > 0.5
Pleural fluid LDH/serum LDH ratio < 0.6	Pleural fluid LDH/serum LDH ratio > 0.6
Pleural fluid LDH < two-thirds upper limit of normal serum LDH	Pleural fluid LDH > two-thirds upper limit of normal serum LDH
Sonographic signs	
Anechoic fluid	Anechoic fluid
	Echogenic fluid
	Floating echodensities
	Septations
	Fibrin strands
	Pleural nodules
	Thickened pleura (> 3 mm)

LDH, Lactate dehydrogenase.

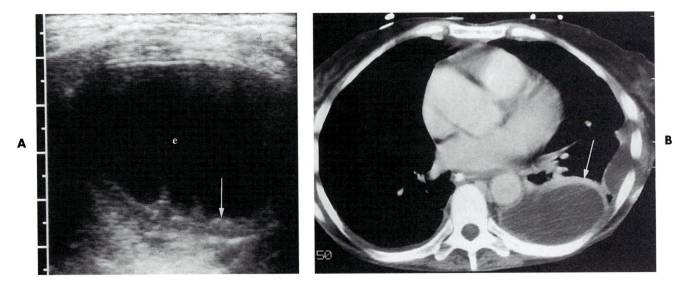

FIG. 16-9. Empyema. A, Transverse ultrasound image through a low left posterior intercostal space demonstrates a located fluid collection, *e,* in the pleural space. Thickened pleura *(arrow)* and septations are evident. The fluid is relatively anechoic, even though gross pus was present on thoracentesis. **B,** Corresponding CT image demonstrates contrast enhancement of the thickened pleura. Perforation of the diaphragm during splenectomy was the cause of the empyema.

The final organization stage produces an inelastic membrane around the lung called a **pleural peel** (Fig. 16-9).[14,19] If untreated, pleurocutaneous or bronchopleural fistulas may further complicate the process. Many of these complicated effusions require catheter drainage for resolution even if bacteria do not actually contaminate the pleural space.

Pleural Thickening

Diffuse Pleural Thickening. Diffuse thickening of the pleura usually indicates pleural fibrosis **(fibrothorax, pleural peel)** or **pleural malignancy.** Diffuse pleural fibrosis most commonly involves the visceral pleura, entrapping the lung and causing restriction of ventilation (Fig. 16-10). It may result from any exudative pleural effusion, asbestos-related effusion, hemothorax, or empyema. Metastatic disease to the pleura may cause diffuse lobulated pleural thickening or multiple discrete pleural masses.[20] Calcification associated with diffuse pleural thickening favors tuberculosis or empyema as the cause.[21] Ultrasound demonstrates solid, smooth, or lobulated pleural tissue that displaces air-filled lung away from the chest wall.[3] Pleural thickening may be more apparent when a pleural effusion is present.

Pleural Plaques. Focal pleural thickening usually indicates fibrosis, which commonly occurs as a result of inflammation. Common causes of pleural plaques include pneumonia, asbestos exposure, pulmonary infarction, trauma, chemical pleurodesis, and drug-related pleural disease. Plaques resulting from asbestos exposure are usually confined to the parietal

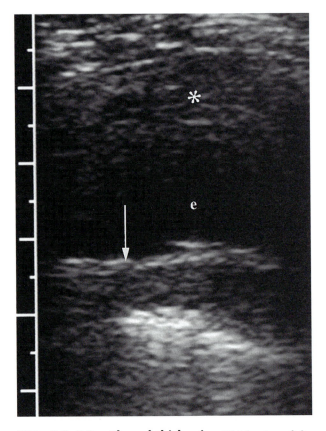

FIG. 16-10. Pleural thickening. Thickening of the visceral pleura *(arrow)* is seen through a pleural effusion, *e,* on this transverse intercostal image. The visceral pleural surface is identified by real-time observation of appropriate movement with respiration. Reverberation artifact, *,* obscures the parietal pleura and near portion of the pleural effusion.

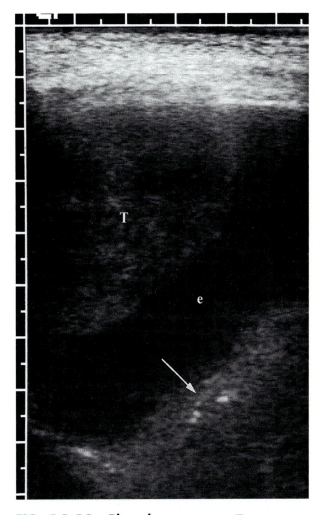

FIG. 16-11. Pleural metastases. Transverse intercostal image demonstrates a large metastatic tumor implant, *T*, on the parietal pleura. A pleural effusion, *e*, is present. The lung *(arrow)* is displaced away from the chest wall. The metastatic deposit was from nonsmall cell lung carcinoma.

pleura. Ultrasound demonstrates pleural plaques as **smooth, elliptical, hypoechoic pleural thickenings.**[22] Visceral pleura plaques are differentiated from parietal pleura plaques by observing the "gliding sign" during respiration. Calcified pleural plaques are irregular, echogenic, and produce acoustic shadowing and comet-tail artifacts.[22]

Pleural Masses

Pleural Metastases. In patients older than 50 years, metastatic disease is second only to congestive heart failure as a cause of pleural effusion.[20] Pleural effusion associated with malignant disease may result from:[20,23]

- Malignant cell implantation on the pleura (common causes: lung, breast, gastrointestinal cancer);
- Obstruction of pleural or pulmonary lymphatics (common causes: lymphoma, breast cancer);
- Obstruction of pulmonary veins (usually by lung cancer);
- Malignant cells shed freely into pleural space (lung and breast cancer); and
- Obstruction of the thoracic duct, resulting in chylous effusion (usually due to lymphoma).

Sonographic findings that favor malignant disease as a cause of pleural effusion are[20,24,25] solid nodules in the pleural space (Fig. 16-11), circumferential pleural thickening, nodular pleural thickening, pleural thickening > 1 cm, and pleural thickening involving the mediastinal parietal pleura.

Pleural Mesothelioma. Malignant mesothelioma is a rare and usually fatal pleural tumor usually (80% of cases) associated with asbestos exposure. Imaging findings are (Fig. 16-12):[24,26]

- Diffuse pleural thickening, often nodular and irregular (86%);
- Calcifications in the pleura (20%);
- Pleural effusion (74%); and
- Focal pleural mass (25%).

Rib destruction occurs with advanced disease. Ultrasound-guided biopsy can be used in most cases to confirm the diagnosis.

Pneumothorax

Pneumothorax is a diagnosis that can be made by ultrasound with careful attention to detail. The visceral pleura–air-filled lung interface produces a bright

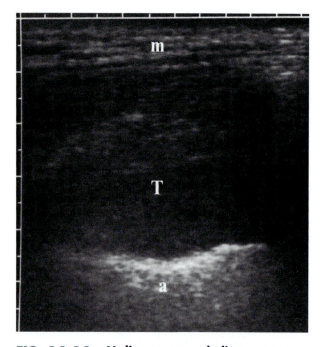

FIG. 16-12. Malignant mesothelioma. A heterogeneous solid mass, *T*, occupies the pleural space, displacing air-filled lung, *a*, and invading intercostal muscle, *m*.

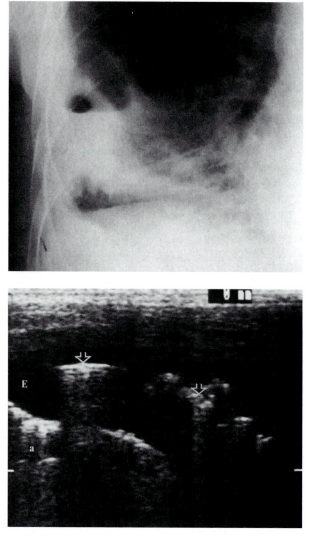

FIG. 16-13. Hydropneumothorax. A, A loculated hydropneumothorax with an air-fluid level is seen in the right lower thorax on this posteroanterior chest radiograph. **B,** A corresponding sonogram obtained in the intercostal space shows the effusion, *E*, containing loculations of air *(arrows)*, which produce bright interfaces with prominent reverberation echoes. The bright linear interface of air in the pleural space does not move with respiration. The surface of displaced air-filled lung, *a*, has a similar appearance, but is observed to move with respiration.

echogenic line of ultrasound reflection that characteristically **moves** with respiratory motion. In contrast, **free air** within the pleural space produces a similar bright echogenic line of sound reflection that **does not move** with respiratory motion.[27-31] Disappearance of a lung or pleural lesion previously visualized during an ultrasound-guided interventional procedure also suggests the development of a pneumothorax.[28] When both air and fluid are present in the pleural space, an air-fluid level can be identified (Fig. 16-13).[29]

Invasive Procedures in the Pleural Space

Ultrasound has become the imaging method of choice for guidance of many procedures in the pleural space.[32]

Diagnostic Thoracentesis.
Sonographic guidance of diagnostic thoracentesis should be done whenever clinically guided thoracentesis is unsuccessful or is judged to be difficult.[32-36] Ultrasound guidance adds accuracy and safety to the procedure.[37] The incidence of pneumothorax is 18% for clinically guided thoracentesis and 3% for sonographically guided thoracentesis.[38] After the physician examines the chest x-ray film, the patient is examined sonographically to identify the largest and most accessible pocket of pleural fluid. The location and depth of the fluid and its relationship to the lung are determined. Vital structures such as the heart and aorta are identified and

avoided. A safe site for thoracentesis is chosen, based on careful diagnostic ultrasound examination that uses the direct approach. Actual puncture of the pleural space can then be performed blindly as long as the patient does not change position. Puncture of the pleural space under continuous ultrasound observation is often not possible because the pleural space is so close to the transducer and the needle is difficult to track from the skin surface. The optimal position for diagnostic thoracentesis is the erect sitting position with the patient's arms resting comfortably on a bedside table. However, if the patient is unable to sit, the procedure may be performed with the patient in the lateral decubitus or supine position.

The puncture site is chosen in the intercostal space so that the needle crosses the top of the rib and avoids the neurovascular bundle coursing along the undersurface of the rib. Puncture of the pleural space should be with the needle perpendicular to the chest wall. The puncture site and surrounding area are cleansed with povidone-iodine solution. A local anesthetic, 1% lidocaine solution, is infiltrated subcutaneously at the puncture site. We use a 22 gauge needle attached to a 12 ml syringe for most diagnostic aspirations. If cytologic examination is planned, at least 100 ml volume of fluid should be obtained. Mild suction is applied while the needle is advanced into the fluid. A characteristic "pop" can usually be felt as the needle punctures the parietal pleura. Care is taken to keep the needle tip well short of the measured depth of the lung surface. The pleural fluid is inspected for color, clarity, and smell, and is sent to the laboratory for Gram stain, bacterial culture, cell count, cytology, chemistries, and any special studies warranted by the patient's clinical condition.

Occasionally the pleural fluid may be too viscous to aspirate through a 22 gauge needle. When the ultrasonographic diagnosis of pleural effusion is secure but fluid cannot be aspirated, the physician must first reexamine the patient to determine the accurate location of the needle within the fluid, then try larger needles (20 or 18 gauge).

Therapeutic Drainage of Symptomatic Effusions.

Large pleural effusions may cause chest pain, dyspnea, or hypoxemia because of impaired gas exchange. These symptoms can be relieved by drainage of most or all of the pleural fluid. Ultrasound can be used to optimize positioning of the drainage catheter and to assess the completeness of fluid removal. To minimize patient discomfort and the risk of infecting the pleural space, complete drainage accomplished as one procedure is preferred to leaving an indwelling catheter. When large pleural effusions are present, the volume of fluid removed at any one setting should not exceed 1 L. Removal of larger amounts may result in complications of acute mediastinal shift, including acute pulmonary edema, shock, and vasovagal syncope.[37] Therapeutic drainage is accomplished as an extension of diagnostic thoracentesis with placement of a flexible catheter into the pleural space to minimize the possibility of trauma to the lung. Short soft and **flexible** catheters, designed for intravenous use, are preferred for this application. The needle-catheter assembly is advanced into the pleural space and the needle is withdrawn, leaving only the catheter within the pleural space. The catheter is connected to a three-way stopcock to which is connected a syringe for aspi-

ration and a bag for fluid collection. This arrangement provides a closed system for repeated aspiration that limits the possibility of contamination of the pleural space. Sonography is used to assess the amount and location of remaining fluid. The patient's position can be altered to access any remaining fluid. Separate loculations of fluid can be removed by additional puncture. When drainage is complete, the catheter is removed. Immediate and 4-hour follow-up chest radiographs should be obtained after all thoracentesis procedures to detect pneumothorax.

Catheter Drainage of Pleural Effusions.

Numerous studies have documented the advantages of image-directed catheter placement over surgically placed catheters for drainage of empyema and complicated parapneumonic effusion.[32,39] Catheter placement with ultrasound guidance is easier, causes fewer complications and less patient discomfort, and has high success rates. Image-guided percutaneous catheter placement is successful in treating empyema in 72% to 92% of cases whereas success rates reported with surgically placed chest tubes are 35% to 80%.[32,39]

Ultrasound is used to identify the largest fluid pocket for catheter placement. Direct puncture of the pleural cavity using the **trocar method** is quicker and easier than using guidewires and catheter exchange techniques. A relatively **stiff** catheter is needed for retention within the pleural space because the continued motion of respiration will place traction on the catheter, resulting in buckling and ineffective drainage. Several catheter systems designed for empyema drainage are commercially available in 10 to 14 French sizes.

To introduce the catheter, the puncture site is infiltrated with local anesthetic and a nick is made in the skin with a no. 11 blade. The catheter-cannula-trocar assembly is advanced directly into the pleural space. The trocar is removed and fluid aspiration attempted. If no fluid is aspirated, the catheter position is adjusted with ultrasound guidance until fluid is easily aspirated. The cannula is directed downward and held firmly in place while the catheter is advanced into the most dependent portion of the pleural space. The cannula is removed and the catheter is attached to a three-way stopcock and drainage bag. Aspiration is performed until ultrasound examination confirms that all fluid has been removed. The pleural cavity is then irrigated several times with sterile saline solution to remove particulate matter. The catheter is sutured to the skin and connected to a standard underwater seal pleural drainage system. The catheter is placed to continuous negative suction (-20 cm water pressure) and the volume of fluid drainage is monitored. When less than 10 ml of fluid drains from the pleural space in 24 hours, the catheter can be removed.

Loculations in the pleural space may prevent complete catheter drainage of pleural fluid. Transcatheter instillation of urokinase or streptokinase has been reported to be useful in lysing fibrin membranes to facilitate drainage.[19,40] Bronchopleural fistula should be suspected in cases that show the presence of both air and fluid in the pleural space, or that are slow to resolve after catheter placement. Propyliodone oil suspension can be injected into the pleural space to perform contrast sinography and demonstrate this complication.[41]

Sclerosis of the Pleural Space.

Malignant pleural effusions are a common cause of progressively disabling dyspnea, cough, and chest pain. Treatment is aimed at relieving symptoms, since most malignant pleural effusions are not curable.[23] Simple thoracentesis and chest tube drainage may provide temporary relief, but nearly all malignant effusions recur within 1 month. Chemical pleurodesis is used to induce adhesions of the visceral and parietal pleural surfaces to prevent accumulation of fluid and air in the pleural space. A variety of agents have been used with success rates in the range of 60% to 70%.[42] Tetracycline has been the most common agent used in the United States, but manufacture of the intravenous suspension used for this application has recently been discontinued.

Ultrasound guidance is used to ensure accurate catheter placement for thoracentesis and instillation of the chemical agents, to assess adequacy of drainage and reaccumulation of fluid, and to identify loculated fluid collections.[43] Therapeutic thoracentesis with a small catheter is performed to remove all pleural fluid. The sclerotherapy agent is injected into the pleural space, and the patient is asked to roll over three or four times to coat the pleural space. The chest catheter is clamped for 24 hours. The patient is instructed to change body position every few minutes to spread the agent over all pleural surfaces. Ultrasound is used to check for reaccumulation of fluid at 24 hours. If no fluid is present, the catheter is removed. If fluid has reaccumulated, sclerotherapy may be repeated.

Current choices of sclerotherapy agents include suspension of sterile talc (2 to 10 g in 50 ml sterile saline), doxycycline in repeated 500 mg doses, and minocycline (300 mg doses).[42,43]

Pleural Biopsy.

Pleural masses and focal areas of pleural thickening are frequently hidden from fluoroscopic view by accompanying pleural fluid. Ultrasound is effective in demonstrating these lesions and guiding needle placement for biopsy. Pleural masses and thickened pleura can frequently be biopsied using standard biopsy needles for histologic or cytologic examination.[44] Normal-thickness pleura in areas of loculated pleural effusion can be biopsied using a reverse-bevel pleural biopsy needle. Mueller et al.[45] provide an excellent description of the technique of pleural biopsy.

Complications of Pleural Invasive Procedures.

Complications of invasive procedures in the pleural space include pneumothorax, hemothorax from laceration of an intercostal artery or vein, vasovagal reaction, infection of the pleural space, and improper placement of needle or catheter into lung, liver, spleen, or kidney. Removal of large amounts of fluid (more than 1 L) may cause reexpansion pulmonary edema.

Pneumothorax is the most frequent complication associated with invasive procedures of the thorax. Pneumothorax rates approach 9% for invasive procedures in the pleural space. Most pneumothoraces are small, self-limiting, and produce minimal symptoms. Some result in progressive loss of lung volume, causing respiratory distress or even respiratory failure in patients with underlying lung disease. The physician performing invasive procedures in the thorax must be familiar with catheter placement for the treatment of pneumothorax.[46]

LUNG PARENCHYMA

Normal Sonographic Appearance

Air-filled lung, covered by visceral pleura, causes a highly reflective interface that blocks transmission of the sound beam into the chest. However, the ultrasound image will display a pattern of bright echoes caused by **acoustic reverberation artifact.**[6] These echoes are usually intense but formless, and diminish in intensity with distance from the transducer (see Figs. 16-1 and 16-2). However, whenever the ultrasound beam is directly perpendicular to the visceral-pleura-lung interface, the bright linear surface of the air-filled lung will be repeatedly duplicated on the image as a series of bright lines at fixed intervals (see Fig. 16-1). The strength of this pattern of reverberation artifacts also diminishes with increasing distance from the transducer. The normal lung surface is identified by its motion, gliding back and forth with inspiration and expiration, the **"gliding sign."** Irregularities of the surface of the lung also cause transient **comet-tail artifacts** that emanate from the lung surface. Although these artifacts may be prominent and confusing on the ultrasound image, they are to be expected and should be recognized as indicators of air-filled lung.

Consolidation

With consolidation, the air spaces of the lung are filled with fluid and inflammatory cells. The highly reflective aerated lung is converted into a firm, dense, solid mass with good sound transmission (Fig. 16-14).

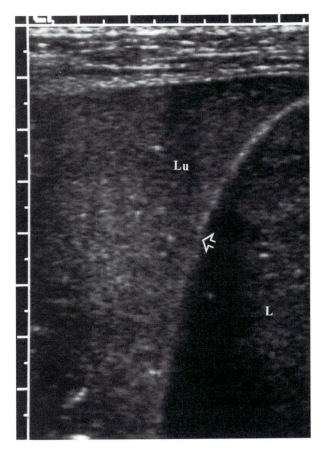

FIG. 16-14. Consolidation. The right lower lobe of lung, *Lu*, is densely consolidated, assuming a level of echogenicity near that of the liver, *L*. The arrow marks the diaphragm.

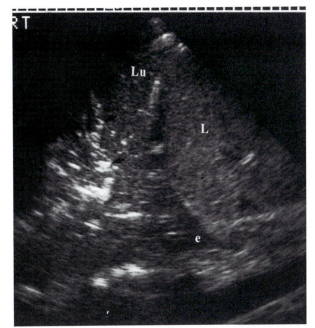

FIG. 16-15. Sonographic air alveolograms. The base of the lung, *Lu*, is densely consolidated, but the more proximal lung has pockets of aerated alveoli *(arrows)*, which produce bright reflections and reverberations. A small pleural effusion, *e*, is also present. Note the poorly defined transition zone between the peripheral consolidated lung and the central air-filled lung. *L*, Liver.

Consolidated lung is hypoechoic as compared with highly reflective aerated lung, and is usually hypoechoic as compared with the liver and spleen because of its high fluid content. The consolidated lung is generally wedge-shaped.[47,48] Air within bronchi surrounded by consolidated lung produces strongly reflective linear branching echoes that can be recognized as **sonographic air bronchograms.**[5,49] Aerated alveoli, surrounded by consolidated lung, produce highly reflective globular echoes that can be recognized as **sonographic air alveolograms** (Fig. 16-15).[5] The high-amplitude echoes produced by trapped air may cause acoustic shadows and reverberation artifacts. Fluid-filled bronchi produce multiple, branching, anechoic tubular structures within the consolidated lung, **sonographic fluid bronchograms.**[5,50] Pulmonary vessels can also be recognized as branching tubular structures. Vessels can be differentiated from bronchi by observing their pulsatility, by tracing their origin to the pulmonary artery, and by the use of Doppler imaging.[50] Identification of sonographic air bronchograms, air alveolograms, fluid bronchograms, and pulmonary vasculature helps to differentiate consolidated lung from parenchymal masses and pleural lesions. Ultrasound also is useful to differentiate pneumonia alone from pneumonia with pleural effusion or empyema. In summary, the **ultrasound findings indicative of lung consolidation** include:

- Solidification of lung tissue, allowing sound transmission (see Fig. 16-14);
- Homogeneous, hypoechoic, wedge-shaped lung;
- Poor definition centrally where consolidation merges with air-filled lung (see Fig. 16-15);
- Sharp definition peripherally, defined by pleural surfaces (see Figs. 16-14 and 16-17);
- Sonographic air bronchograms;
- Sonographic fluid bronchograms;
- Sonographic air alveolograms (see Fig. 16-15);
- Visualization of intraparenchymal pulmonary arteries and veins; and
- Appropriate motion with respiration.

Atelectasis

Atelectasis refers to the absence of air in all or part of the lung with associated collapse of alveoli, resulting in loss of lung volume and crowding of lung blood vessels. Atelectasis is caused by obstruction of supplying bronchi or pressure on the lung due to mass or fluid in the pleural space. Atelectasis frequently accompanies pleural effusion. Atelectatic lung appears as a wedge-shaped density moving through the pleural fluid in time with the patient's respirations (Fig. 16-16). The echogenicity of collapsed lung is usually higher than that of consolidated lung because of lower fluid content (see Fig. 16-5). Crowding of fluid-filled bronchi and blood vessels may be seen within the collapsed portion of the lung. Sonographic air bronchograms are usually not present when bronchial obstruction is the cause of the atelectasis. **Sonographic findings in atelectasis** include[51] wedge-shaped echogenic lung, sharp borders defined by visceral pleura, decreased volume of affected lung, crowding of bronchi and pulmonary blood vessels, sonographic fluid bronchograms, absence of sonographic air bronchograms with bronchial obstruction, and appropriate motion of affected lung with respiration.

SONOGRAPHIC FINDINGS IN ATELECTASIS

Wedge-shaped echogenic lung
Sharp borders defined by visceral pleura
Decreased volume of affected lung
Crowding of bronchi and pulmonary blood vessels
Sonographic fluid bronchograms
Absence of sonographic air bronchograms with
    bronchial obstruction
Appropriate motion of affected lung with respiration

Lung Tumors

Lung tumors that abut the pleural surface appear as masses partially surrounded by highly reflective aerated lung.[47,48,52] The deep margins of the tumor are often well defined, as compared with the poorly defined deep margin seen with consolidation. The tumor stands out in strong relief compared to the surrounding air-filled lung. The linear surface-reflection echo produced by visceral pleura–air-filled lung interface is absent where the tumor abuts the visceral pleura (Fig. 16-17). Echo enhancement is often present deep to the lesion because the tumor is a better sound transmitter than is aerated lung.[48] Lesions smaller than 5 cm are usually hypoechoic compared to aerated lung whereas lesions larger than 5 cm may be isoechoic compared to aerated lung. The increased echogenicity of larger lesions may be caused by internal hemorrhage or necrosis. Cavitary lesions have hyperechoic walls with central echolucent areas (Fig. 16-18). Foci of calcification within lung masses are

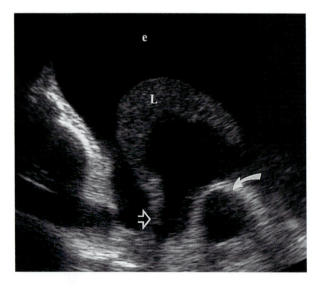

FIG. 16-16. Atelectasis. Compressed and completely collapsed lung, *L*, is suspended in a large, anechoic, transudative, pleural effusion, *e*, in this transverse intercostal image. The lung was observed to move in response to the patient's respiratory efforts. The inferior pulmonary ligament *(open arrow)* and the descending thoracic aorta *(curved arrow)* are well visualized.

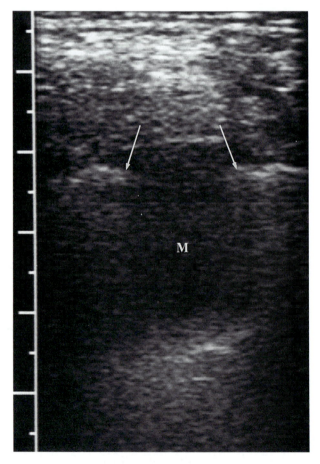

FIG. 16-17. Peripheral lung mass. A hypoechoic mass, *M*, is partially surrounded by brighter aerated lung. The bright, linear, lung-surface echo is interrupted *(arrows)* over the mass. The deep portion of the mass has a relatively well-defined margin with the more central aerated lung. Compare with the image of consolidation in Fig. 16-15.

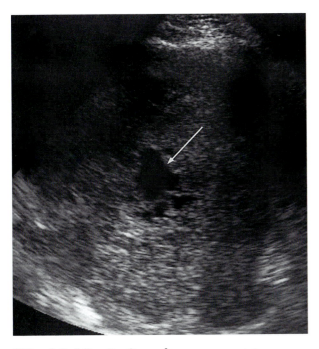

FIG. 16-18. Cavitary lung mass. A large mass replaces most of the right lower lobe of the lung. Cystic areas in the mass correspond to necrosis. Because of severe chronic obstructive pulmonary disease, this patient could not tolerate the supine position for a CT-guided lung biopsy. The biopsy was performed without difficulty using ultrasound guidance, yielding squamous cell carcinoma.

easily demonstrated by ultrasonography.[53] Ultrasound may help define tumor extension to pleura and adjacent structures by observing obliteration of the pleural surface echo and lack of gliding movement of the tumor with respiration.[54,55]

Centrally located lung tumors near the pulmonary hilum may be visualized by ultrasonography when they are associated with peripheral lung consolidation.[47] When the lung tumor causes obstruction to the airways, the tumor is visualized as a mass at the tip of the resulting triangular area of consolidation (Fig. 16-19). Tumors surrounded by consolidated lung appear as a mass within hypoechoic fluid-filled lung.[47] **Sonographic signs of pulmonary tumors** include hypoechoic mass within echogenic aerated lung, absence of linear lung surface reflection echo,[52] relatively well-defined deep margin, absence of tapered edges,[52] absence of sonographic air bronchograms,[4]

SONOGRAPHIC SIGNS OF PULMONARY TUMORS

Hypoechoic mass within echogenic aerated lung
Absence of linear lung surface reflection echo
Relatively well-defined deep margin
Absence of tapered edges
Absence of sonographic air bronchograms
Mass within hypoechoic consolidated lung
Fixation of peripheral tumor during breathing
   (suggesting tumor invasion of the chest wall)

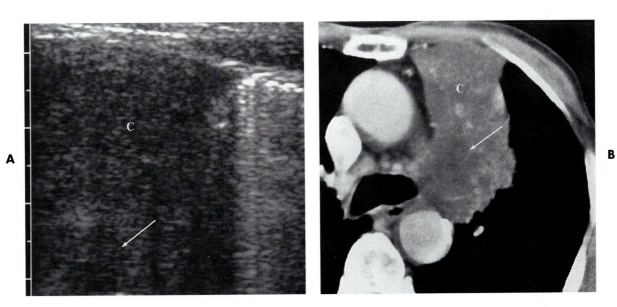

FIG. 16-19. Central lung mass with peripheral consolidation. **A,** Ultrasound and, **B,** corresponding CT image demonstrate a central squamous cell carcinoma *(arrow)* of the lung with peripheral consolidation, *c.* Aerated lung adjacent to the mass produces bright reverberation artifact on the ultrasound.

mass within hypoechoic consolidated lung, and fixation of peripheral tumor during breathing (suggesting tumor invasion of the chest wall).[54,55]

Lung Abscess

A lung abscess is a localized suppurative process characterized by **necrosis** of lung tissue. **Primary lung abscesses** are caused by aspiration, necrotizing pneumonia, septic emboli, or a complication of chronic lung disease. These abscesses are amenable to cure by percutaneously placed drainage catheters.[33,56-58] **Secondary lung abscesses** caused by lung carcinoma, pulmonary sequestration, lung cyst, or bronchoesophageal fistula generally require surgical intervention. Lung abscesses have thick, irregular walls with echogenic debris and air within the internal fluid. Most lung abscesses abut the pleura and can be visualized with ultrasound. **Sonographic findings of lung abscesses** include[56,59] irregular, thick, echogenic walls, hypoechoic central cavity, air echoes within central cavity, and air-fluid level within central cavity. Differentiating lung abscess from empyema is frequently a radiographic challenge. Empyemas are confined within the pleural space and tend to have smooth walls of uniform thickness. Lung parenchyma is compressed and displaced. Lung abscesses destroy lung parenchyma, are associated with surrounding areas of lung consolidation, and have irregular walls of varying thickness. With real-time sonography, a lung abscess will demonstrate expansion of its entire circumference with inspiration.[60] In empyema only the internal wall, the visceral pleura, will show motion with inspiration.

Pulmonary Sequestration

Pulmonary sequestrations are uncommon congenital anomalies that consist of lung tissue that does not communicate with the tracheobronchial tree. Most of these masses occur at the lung bases where they can be evaluated with ultrasound. Diagnosis is made by demonstration of **systemic arterial blood supply** to the sequestered lung tissue (Fig. 16-20).[61] Ultrasound can demonstrate the supplying systemic artery in most cases.[62,63] **Intralobar sequestrations** are contained within visceral pleura and have venous drainage via the pulmonary veins. **Extralobar sequestrations** are covered by their own pleura and have venous drainage via systemic veins. **Ultrasound findings of pulmonary sequestration** include homogeneous solid mass in lower hemithorax (see Fig. 16-20), fluid-filled cysts occasionally present, no bronchi identified, feeding artery identified arising from aorta (key finding) (see Fig. 16-20), draining vein to systemic veins with extralobar sequestration, and draining vein to pulmonary veins with intralobar sequestration.

Invasive Procedures in Lung Parenchyma

Lung Mass Biopsy. Percutaneous transthoracic aspiration biopsy using fluoroscopic guidance is a standard method of obtaining tissue diagnosis of pulmonary parenchymal masses.[64] However, fluoroscopic visualization of lung nodules may be difficult when the nodules are pleural based, at the lung apex, in the axilla, or near the diaphragm or mediastinum.[64-66] In comparison, ultrasonographic visualization of lung masses for guidance of biopsy is best in the areas most difficult to biopsy with fluoroscopic guidance.[48,54,66-68] Ultrasound-guided biopsy is quick, convenient, and safe. Because sonography can visualize aerated lung adjacent to pleural-based nodules better than fluoroscopy, the aerated lung can be avoided more easily.[68] The incidence of pneumothorax for biopsy of pleural-based nodules is 2% with ultrasound guidance, as compared with 11% with fluoroscopic guidance.[65,68] Both ultrasound and fluoroscopic guidance have a reported 90% to 97% sensitivity for the diagnosis of lung cancer.[69-71] Sonography is particularly useful in guiding biopsy of peripheral lung tumors obscured by pleural effusion.

Preliminary inspection of the chest x-ray film is essential in planning the approach to ultrasound-guided biopsy. Most lung lesions may be visualized and biopsied through the intercostal space. Lesions at the lung apex may be approached from either above or below

---

SONOGRAPHIC FINDINGS OF LUNG ABSCESSES

Irregular, thick, echogenic walls
Hypoechoic central cavity
Air echoes within central cavity
Air-fluid level within central cavity

ULTRASOUND FINDINGS OF PULMONARY SEQUESTRATION

Homogeneous solid mass in lower hemithorax
Fluid-filled cysts occasionally present
No bronchi identified
Feeding artery identified arising from aorta (key finding)
Draining vein to systemic veins with extralobar sequestration
Draining vein to pulmonary veins with intralobar sequestration

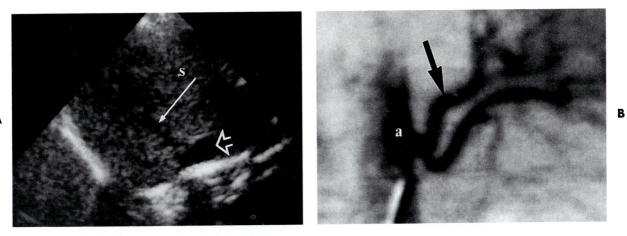

FIG. 16-20. Extralobar pulmonary sequestration. A, Ultrasound image reveals a homogeneous solid mass, *s*, at the left lung base fed by an artery *(long arrow)* arising from the aorta *(open arrow)*. **B,** Image from arteriogram confirms two feeding arteries *(arrow)* originating from the aorta, *a*.

the clavicle.[54] Lesions on the diaphragm may be visualized and biopsied using an upward angle through the liver.[65] Once the lesion is visualized, a safe course for the needle is determined. The needle pass into the lesion is best performed freehand. The patient is asked to suspend respiration while the needle is being advanced into the lesion. The patient may then resume shallow respiration while the needle is allowed to swing freely. The patient is again asked to stop breathing while the biopsy is taken. Fine-needle aspiration (FNA) specimens are given to a cytopathologist for immediate examination for adequacy. Biopsies are repeated until diagnostic tissue is obtained. The presence of a cytopathologist in the biopsy suite is essential to maximize diagnostic yield from FNA while minimizing the number of needle passes.[64] Core biopsy samples for histology can be obtained from large lesions.

Catheter Drainage of Lung Abscess. Most lung abscesses are successfully treated with antibiotics and bronchoscopic internal drainage.[33] Treatment failures are considered candidates for lobectomy. External drainage by catheter was successfully used prior to availability of antibiotics, and has been reaffirmed as a successful treatment method with a low complication rate.[57,58] Ultrasound guidance may be used to accurately direct placement of a large-bore surgical tube or to place a smaller "radiologic" catheter. The technique for catheter placement is similar to that used for empyema drainage.

Complications of Invasive Procedures in the Lung Parenchyma. Pneumothorax and minor bleeding are the most frequent complications of lung biopsy.[64] The significance of pneumothorax is greatest in patients with severely compromised pulmonary function. The risk of bleeding is increased in patients with coagulopathy. Rare complications include major bleeding, air embolism, and neoplastic seeding of the needle tract.

MEDIASTINUM

Because the mediastinum is surrounded by shadowing bone and reflective lung, it offers a challenge to sonographic evaluation. However, with careful attention to technique and patient positioning, most areas of the mediastinum can be effectively examined.[53,71-77] Ultrasound is best for examination of the superior and anterior mediastinum, and is less useful for the posterior mediastinum and paravertebral region.[76,77] When abnormalities are detected, sonographic guidance can be used for biopsy.[78-82] The ability to visualize the needle continually as it courses to the lesion is a significant advantage because this area is so rich with major vascular structures. Detailed knowledge of the three-dimensional anatomy of the mediastinum is critical because the planes of sonographic examination are usually oblique and not readily related to the standard orthogonal planes of computed tomography (CT) and magnetic resonance imaging (MRI).

Normal Sonographic Appearance

The upper mediastinum is accessible to sonographic investigation by use of a **suprasternal approach.**[72] Patients are examined in a supine position with a pillow placed beneath the shoulders and the neck extended. The transducer is placed at the base of the neck and angled caudally behind the manubrium. Oblique sagittal and coronal plane images can be obtained. The innominate veins, common carotid, brachiocephalic, and subclavian arteries are examined (Fig. 16-21). Each vessel is identified by its location and Doppler characteristics. Tortuous vessels, which cause abnormal widening of the mediastinum on chest x-ray films, are easily recognized. Mediastinal masses are precisely localized and characterized as solid, cystic, vascular, or calcified. The relationship of masses to cardiac and vascular structures can be accurately defined.

Parasternal scanning of the mediastinum is aided by placing the patient in the appropriate lateral decubitus position.[73] Gravity enlarges the sonographic window by swinging the mediastinum downward. The ascending aorta, anterior mediastinum, and subcarinal region are best imaged from a **right parasternal** approach with the patient lying with the right side down. The pulmonary trunk and left side of the anterior mediastinum are best imaged with a **left parasternal** approach with the patient in a left lateral decubitus position (Fig. 16-22).

Large posterior masses may be imaged from a **posterior paravertebral approach.** Lesions near the diaphragm are evaluated from the abdomen through the liver or spleen. Large masses displace lung and may

be imaged directly through the intercostal spaces.[53,74]

The **thymus** is a prominent normal anterior mediastinal structure in children up to 8 years of age.[83,84] The thymus has two well-defined, triangle-shaped lobes with homogeneous echogenicity slightly less than the thyroid gland. The normal gland is closely

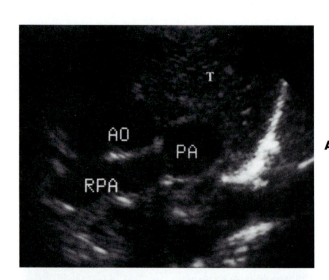

A

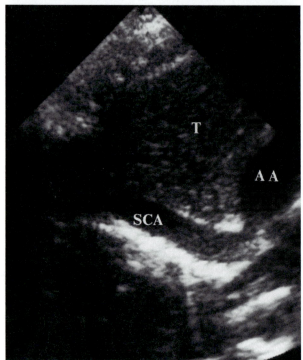

B

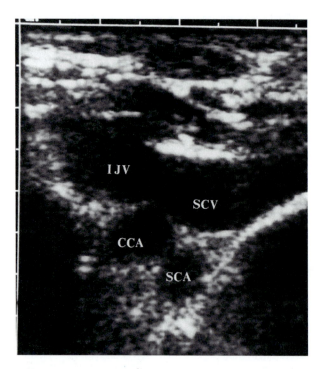

FIG. 16-21. Mediastinum—suprasternal approach. An oblique transverse view into the upper mediastinum is obtained by placing a 5-MHz linear-array transducer at the base of the neck and angling downward behind the manubrium. The junction of the left subclavian vein, *SCV*, with the left internal jugular vein, *IJV*, is demonstrated. The left common carotid artery, *CCA*, and left subclavian artery, *SCA*, are also seen. Vessel identification is confirmed by use of Doppler imaging.

FIG. 16-22. Mediastinum—left parasternal approach. A, Transverse sector scan obtained in an intercostal space from a left parasternal approach demonstrates a prominent thymus, *T*, in a 2-year-old patient. Also clearly seen are the ascending aorta, *AO*, main pulmonary artery, *PA*, at its bifurcation, and the right pulmonary artery, *RPA*. **B,** Sagittal sector scan obtained in the same left parasternal intercostal space as in *A* demonstrates the aortic arch, *AA*, and origin of the left subclavian artery, *SCA*. *T*, Thymus.

applied to mediastinal vessels and may completely encircle the left innominate vein (see Fig. 16-22).[84] In infants less than 2 years old the normal thymus extends from the thoracic inlet to the base of the heart. From age 2 to 8 years the thymus remains a prominent sonographic landmark when scanning the mediastinum, even though it is less obvious on chest radiographs.[83] Progressive fatty replacement makes the thymus blend with mediastinal fat and become sonographically invisible in older children and adults. Sonographic visualization of the thymus in an adult suggests neoplastic disease.[85]

Lymphadenopathy

Since normal mediastinal lymph nodes are generally not seen sonographically, every visualized lymph node should be considered to be abnormally enlarged due to an inflammatory or neoplastic process (Fig. 16-23).[85,86] Most inflammatory nodes are hypoechoic. Neoplastic nodes tend to be hypoechoic when small (< 2 cm), and complex and septated when large. Calcified nodes are echogenic and cast acoustic shadows. **Lymphoma** characteristically causes coalescence of individual nodes into a large, homogeneous, solid mass (Fig. 16-24). With response to therapy, the lymphomatous mass shrinks and becomes more echogenic.[86]

Solid Masses

Accurate sonographic diagnosis of solid mediastinal masses is usually not possible (see box in left column on next page).[85,87] The major role of sonography is to differentiate solid from cystic from vascular masses, and to guide biopsy procedures.[78] However, extension of thyroid tissue into the mediastinum is usually easily demonstrated sonographically by noting continuity with thyroid gland in the neck.

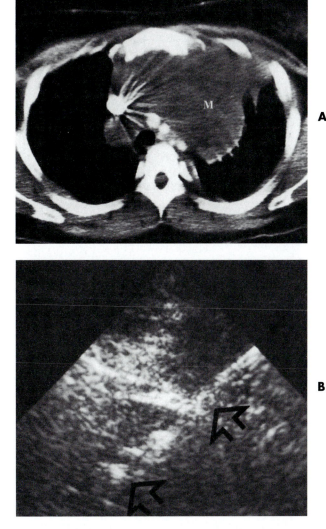

A

B

FIG. 16-24. Biopsy of mediastinal lymphoma. **A,** A CT image of the chest 2 cm above the aortic arch demonstrates a large mass, *M,* in the anterior mediastinum displacing the great vessels posteriorly. **B,** Because the patient was pregnant, acutely ill, and required monitoring in the intensive care unit, biopsy was performed using portable ultrasound guidance at the patient's bedside. Tissue samples for histologic diagnosis of non-Hodgkin's lymphoma were obtained using a 16 gauge core-biopsy needle *(arrows).* Constant observation of needle position by ultrasound safely prevented injury of vascular structures by this large needle. (Courtesy of John P. McGahan, M.D., University of California, Davis Medical Center, Davis, Calif.)

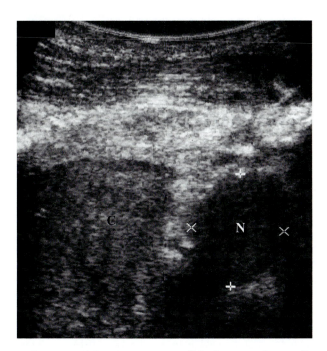

FIG. 16-23. Lung consolidation and mediastinal adenopathy. Transverse intercostal, right-parasternal ultrasound image demonstrates dense consolidation, *C,* of the right upper lobe and an enlarged 2.3 cm hypoechoic node, *N,* in the anterior mediastinum. A large right hilar lung carcinoma caused the consolidation and adenopathy.

CAUSES OF SOLID MEDIASTINAL MASSES

Thymic origin
Normal thymus
Hyperplastic thymus
Thymoma
Thymolipoma
Thymic lymphoma

Lymph nodes
Lymphoma
Metastases
Granulomatous disease
Lymph node hyperplasia

Thyroid origin
Goiter
Thyroid adenoma
Thyroid carcinoma
Thyroiditis

Germ cell tumors
Teratoma
Embryonal cell carcinoma
Choriocarcinoma
Seminoma

Parathyroid origin
Ectopic parathyroid adenoma

Neurogenic origin
Schwannoma
Neurofibroma
Paraganglioma

Primary tumors
Esophageal carcinoma
Tracheal/bronchial tumor
Mesenchymal tumor

CAUSES OF VASCULAR MASSES IN THE MEDIASTINUM

Arterial causes
Tortuous brachiocephalic artery
Aneurysm of the aorta
Aneurysm of the sinus of Valsalva
Right-sided aortic arch
Double aortic arch

Venous causes
Dilated superior vena cava
Esophageal varices
Enlarged azygous vein
Enlarged hemiazygous vein
Congenital anomalies

CAUSES OF CYSTIC MEDIASTINAL MASSES

Thymic mass
Thymoma (cystic degeneration)
Thymic cyst
Thymic lymphoma (cystic degeneration)

Germ cell tumors
Dermoid cyst

Thyroid mass (cystic degeneration)
Adenomatous degeneration
Carcinoma
Adenomatous hyperplasia

Bronchogenic cyst

Pericardial cyst

Vascular Lesions

Ultrasound is an excellent, noninvasive method of diagnosing masses of vascular origin in the mediastinum.[75,85] Many abnormalities seen on chest radiographs and suspected of being of vascular origin can be definitively diagnosed by ultrasound using real-time imaging supplemented by color-flow and spectral Doppler (see top box in the second column).[85,87]

Cystic Masses

Cystic lesions account for about 21% of all primary mediastinal masses.[74,85] Ultrasound is used to characterize wall thickness, septations, vascularity, appearance of internal fluid, location, and relationship to adjacent structures. Differential diagnosis is listed in the bottom box in the second column.

Invasive Procedures in the Mediastinum

Ultrasound is now a fully accepted image-guidance method for percutaneous aspiration or needle biopsy of mediastinal lesions in the anterior and superior mediastinum.[88,89] The simplicity, accuracy, and safety of sonographic guidance are significant advantages for accessible lesions. Large lesions that abut the chest wall are most amenable to ultrasound-directed biopsy (see Fig. 16-17).[90] Ultrasound-guided fine-needle aspiration biopsy is reported to be 77% sensitive for malignancy.[90] Sensitivity is improved to 84% with ultrasound-guided core biopsies for histologic rather than cytologic diagnosis.[78,91,92]

The patient is positioned to optimize ultrasonographic visualization of the lesion and to achieve continuous visualization of the needle path. Adjacent vital structures are visualized and avoided. Pneumothorax, hemoptysis, and hemorrhage are the most common complications reported with mediastinal biopsy procedures.

REFERENCES

1. McLoud TC, Flower CDR. Imaging the pleura: sonography, CT and MR imaging. *AJR* 1991;156:1145-1153.
2. Yu CJ, Yang PC, Wu HD et al. Ultrasound study in unilateral hemithorax opacification. Image comparison with computed tomography. *Am Rev Resp Dis* 1993;147:430-434.
3. Yu C-J, Yang P-C, Chang D-B et al. Diagnostic and therapeutic use of chest sonography: value in critically ill patients. *AJR* 1992;159:695-701.
4. Yang P-C, Kuo S-H, Luh K-T. Ultrasonography and ultrasound-guided needle biopsy of chest diseases: indications, techniques, diagnostic yields and complications. *J Med Ultrasound (Taiwan)* 1993;1:53-63.

Pleural Space

5. Targhetta R, Chavagneux R, Bourgeois JM et al. Sonographic approach to diagnosing pulmonary consolidation. *J Ultrasound Med* 1992;11:667-672.
6. Kremkau FW, Taylor KJW. Artifacts in ultrasound imaging. *J Ultrasound Med* 1986;5:227-237.
7. Yang PC, Luh KT, Chang DB et al. Value of sonography in determining the nature of pleural effusion: analysis of 320 cases. *AJR* 1992;159:29-33.
8. Akhan O, Demirkazik FB, Özmen MN et al. Tuberculous pleural effusions: ultrasonic diagnosis. *J Clin Ultrasound* 1992;20:461-465.
9. Hirsch JH, Rogers JV, Mack LA. Real-time sonography of pleural opacities. *AJR* 1981;136:297-301.
10. Eibenberger KL, Dock WI, Ammann ME et al. Quantification of pleural effusions: sonography versus radiography. *Radiology* 1994;191:681-684.
11. Rosenberg ER. Ultrasound in the assessment of pleural densities. *Chest* 1983;84:283-285.
12. Marks WM, Filly RA, Callen PW. Real-time evaluation of pleural lesions: new observations regarding the probability of obtaining free fluid. *Radiology* 1982;142:163-164.
13. Wu RG, Yang PC, Kuo SH et al. "Fluid color" sign: a useful indicator for discrimination between pleural thickening and pleural effusions. *J Ultrasound Med* 1995;14:767-769.
14. Müller NL. Imaging of the pleura. *Radiology* 1993;186:297-309.
15. Chetty KG. Transudative pleural effusions. *Clin Chest Med* 1985;6:49-54.
16. Hirsch JH, Carter SJ, Chikos PM et al. Ultrasonic evaluation of radiographic opacities of the chest. *AJR* 1978;130:1153-1156.
17. Martinez OC, Serrano BV, Romero RR. Real-time ultrasound evaluation of tuberculous pleural effusions. *J Clin Ultrasound* 1989;17:407-410.
18. Varkey B. Pleural effusions caused by infection. *Postgrad Med* 1986;80:213-223.
19. Light RW. Parapneumonic effusions and empyema. *Clin Chest Med* 1985;6:55-62.
20. Matthay RA, Coppage L, Shaw C et al. Malignancies metastatic to the pleura. *Invest Radiol* 1990;25:601-619.
21. Schmitt WGH, Hubener KH, Rucker HC. Pleural calcification with persistent effusion. *Radiology* 1983;149:633-638.

22. Morgan RA, Pickworth FE, Dubbins PA et al. The ultrasound appearance of asbestos-related pleural plaques. *Clin Radiol* 1991;44:413-6.
23. Olopade OI, Ultmann JE. Malignant effusions. *CA* 1991; 41:166-179.
24. Dynes MC, White EM, Fry WA et al. Imaging manifestations of pleural tumors. *RadioGraphics* 1992;12:1191-1201.
25. Goerg C, Schwerk WB, Goerg K et al. Pleural effusion: an "acoustic window" for sonography of pleural metastases. *J Clin Ultrasound* 1991;19:93-97.
26. Kawashima A, Libshitz HI. Malignant pleural mesothelioma: CT manifestations in 50 cases. *AJR* 1990;155:965-969.
27. Wernecke K, Galanski M, Peters PE et al. Pneumothorax: evaluation by ultrasound—preliminary results. *J Thorac Imag* 1987;2:76-78.
28. Targhetta R, Bourgeois JM, Chavagneux R et al. Ultrasonic signs of pneumothorax: preliminary work. *J Clin Ultrasound* 1993;21:245-250.
29. Targhetta R, Bourgeois JM, Chavagneux R et al. Ultrasonographic approach to diagnosing hydropneumothorax. *Chest* 1992;101:931-934.
30. Lichtenstein DA, Menu Y. A bedside ultrasound sign ruling out pneumothorax in critically ill. Lung sliding. *Chest* 1995;108: 1345-1348.
31. Sistrom CL, Reiheld CT, Gay SB et al. Detection and estimation of the volume of pneumothorax using real-time sonography: efficacy determined by receiver operating characteristic analysis. *AJR* 1996;166:317-321.
32. Klein JS, Schultz S, Heffner JE. Interventional radiology of the chest: image-guided percutaneous drainage of pleural effusions, lung abscesses, and pneumothorax. *AJR* 1995;164:581-588.
33. Illescas FF. Interventional radiology of the pleural space and lung: small diameter catheters. *Radiol Rep* 1989;1:20-31.
34. Weingardt JP, Guico RR, Nemcek AA et al. Ultrasound findings following failed, clinically directed thoracenteses. *J Clin Ultrasound* 1994;22:419-426.
35. Opacic M, Bilac A, Ljubicic N et al. Thoracentesis under ultrasonic control. *Acta Med Iugoslavica* 1991;45:71-75.
36. Mathisen DJ. A surgeon's view of interventional radiology in general thoracic surgery patients. *Semin Intervent Radiol* 1991;8:85-87.
37. Qureshi N, Momin ZA, Brandstetter RD. Thoracentesis in clinical practice. *Heart Lung* 1994;23:376-383.
38. Raptopoulos V, Davis LM, Lee G et al. Factors affecting the development of pneumothorax associated with thoracentesis. *AJR* 1991;156:917-920.
39. Silverman SG, Mueller PR, Saini S et al. Thoracic empyema: management with image-guided catheter drainage. *Radiology* 1988;169:5-9.
40. Moulton JS, Moore PT, Mencini RA. Treatment of loculated pleural effusions with transcatheter intracavitary urokinase. *AJR* 1989;153:941-945.
41. Merriam MA, Cronan JJ, Dorfman GS et al. Radiographically guided percutaneous catheter drainage of pleural fluid collections. *AJR* 1988;151:1113-1116.
42. Seaton KG, Patz EF Jr, Goodman PC. Palliative treatment of malignant pleural effusions: value of small-bore catheter thoracostomy and doxycycline sclerotherapy. *AJR* 1995;164:589-591.
43. Morrison MC, Mueller PR, Lee MJ et al. Sclerotherapy of malignant pleural effusions through sonographically placed small-bore catheters. *AJR* 1992;158:41-43.
44. Chang DB, Yang PC, Luh KT et al. Ultrasound-guided pleural biopsy with Tru-Cut needle. *Chest* 1991;100:1328-1333.

45. Mueller PR, Saini S, Simeone JF et al. Image-guided pleural biopsies: indications, technique, and results in 23 patients. *Radiology* 1988;169:1-4.

46. Conces DJ Jr, Tarver RD, Gray WC et al. Treatment of pneumothoraces utilizing small caliber chest tubes. *Chest* 1988;94:55-57.

Lung Parenchyma

47. Yang P-C, Luh K-T, Wu H-D et al. Lung tumors associated with obstructive pneumonitis: ultrasound studies. *Radiology* 1990;174:717-720.

48. Yang P-C, Luh K-T, Sheu J-C et al. Peripheral pulmonary lesions: ultrasonography and ultrasonically guided aspiration biopsy. *Radiology* 1985;155:451-456.

49. Weinberg B, Diakoumakis EE, Kass EG et al. The air bronchogram: sonographic demonstration. *AJR* 1986;147:593-595.

50. Dorne HL. Differentiation of pulmonary parenchymal consolidation from pleural disease using the sonographic fluid bronchogram. *Radiology* 1986;158:41-42.

51. Ferrari FS, Cozza S, Guazzi G et al. Ultrasound evaluation of chest opacities. *Ultrasound Int* 1995;1:68-74.

52. Targhetta R, Bourgeois JM, Marty-Double C et al. Peripheral pulmonary lesions: ultrasonic features and ultrasonically guided fine needle aspiration biopsy. *J Ultrasound Med* 1993;12:369-374.

53. Rosenberg HK. The complementary roles of ultrasound and plain film radiography in differentiating pediatric chest abnormalities. *RadioGraphics* 1986;6:427-445.

54. Yang P-C, Lee L-N, Luh K-T et al. Ultrasonography of Pancoast tumor. *Chest* 1988;94:124-128.

55. Suzuki N, Saitoh T, Kitamura S. Tumor invasion of the chest wall in lung cancer: diagnosis with US. *Radiology* 1993;187:39-42.

56. Klein JS. Thoracic intervention. *Curr Opinion Radiol* 1992;4:94-103.

57. Yellin A, Yellin EO, Lieberman Y. Percutaneous tube drainage: the treatment of choice for refractory lung abscess. *Ann Thor Surg* 1985;39:266-270.

58. Weissberg D. Percutaneous drainage of lung abscess. *J Thorac Cardiovasc Surg* 1984;87:308-312.

59. Yang PC, Luh KT, Lee YC et al. Lung abscesses: US examination and US-guided transthoracic aspiration. *Radiology* 1991;180:171-175.

60. Simeone JF, Mueller PR, vanSonnenberg E. The uses of diagnostic ultrasound in the thorax. *Clin Chest Med* 1984;5:281-290.

61. Rosado-de-Christenson ML, Frazier AA, Stocker JT et al. From the archives of AFIP. Extralobar sequestration: radiologic-pathologic correlation. *RadioGraphics* 1993;13:425-441.

62. Hernanz-Schulman M, Stein SM, Neblett WW et al. Pulmonary sequestration: diagnosis with color Doppler sonography and a new theory of associated hydrothorax. *Radiology* 1991;180:817-821.

63. West MS, Donaldson JS, Shkolnik A. Pulmonary sequestration: diagnosis by ultrasound. *J Ultrasound Med* 1989;8:125-129.

64. Westcott JL. Percutaneous transthoracic needle biopsy. *Radiology* 1988;169:593-601.

65. Pedersen OM, Aasen TB, Gulsvik A. Fine-needle aspiration biopsy of mediastinal and peripheral pulmonary masses guided by real-time sonography. *Chest* 1986;89:504-508.

66. Ikezoe J, Shusuke S, Higashihara T et al. Sonographically guided needle biopsy for diagnosis of thoracic lesions. *AJR* 1984;143:229-234.

67. Ikezoe J, Morimoto S, Arisawa J et al. Percutaneous biopsy of thoracic lesions: value of sonography for needle guidance. *AJR* 1990;154:1181-1185.

68. Cinti D, Hawkins HB. Aspiration biopsy of peripheral pulmonary masses using real-time sonographic guidance. *AJR* 1984;142:1115-1116.

69. Chen CC, Hsu WH, Huang CM et al. Ultrasound-guided fine-needle aspiration biopsy of solitary pulmonary nodules. *J Clin Ultrasound* 1995;23:531-536.

70. Berquist TH, Bailey PB, Cortese DA et al. Transthoracic needle biopsy accuracy and complications in relation to location and type of lesion. *Mayo Clin Proc* 1980;55:475-481.

71. Das DK, Pant CS, Pant JN et al. Transthoracic (percutaneous) fine needle aspiration cytology diagnosis of pulmonary tuberculosis. *Tubercle Lung Dis* 1995;76:84-89.

Mediastinum

72. Wernecke K, Peters PE, Galanski M. Mediastinal tumors: evaluation with suprasternal sonography. *Radiology* 1986;159:405-409.

73. Wernecke K, Potter R, Peters PE et al. Parasternal mediastinal sonography: sensitivity in the detection of anterior mediastinal and subcarinal tumors. *AJR* 1988;150:1021-1026.

74. Ikezoe J, Morimoto S, Arisawa J et al. Ultrasonography of mediastinal teratoma. *J Clin Ultrasound* 1986;14:513-520.

75. O'Laughlin MP, Huhta JC, Murphy DJ. Ultrasound examination of extracardiac chest masses in children: Doppler diagnosis of a vascular etiology. *J Ultrasound Med* 1987;6:151-157.

76. Wernecke K, Vassallo P, Potter R et al. Mediastinal tumors: sensitivity of detection with sonography compared with CT and radiography. *Radiology* 1990;175:137-143.

77. Betsch B, Berndt R, Knopp MV et al. Comparison of computerized tomography and B-image ultrasound in imaging diagnosis of the mediastinum. Language: German. *Bildebung* 1994;61:295-298.

78. Heilo A. Tumors in the mediastinum: US-guided histologic core-needle biopsy. *Radiology* 1993;189:143-146.

79. Anderson T, Lindgren PG, Elvin A. Ultrasound guided tumour biopsy in the anterior mediastinum. An alternative to thoracotomy and mediastinoscopy. *Acta Radiol* 1992;33:423-426.

80. Yang PC, Chang DB, Yu CJ et al. Ultrasound-guided core biopsy of thoracic tumors. *Am Rev Resp Dis* 1992;146:763-767.

81. Wernecke K, Vassallo P, Peters PE et al. Mediastinal tumors: biopsy under ultrasound guidance. *Radiology* 1989;172:473-476.

82. Tikkakoski T, Lohela P, Leppanen M et al. Ultrasound-guided aspiration biopsy of anterior mediastinal masses. *J Clin Ultrasound* 1991;19:209-214.

83. Adams EJ, Ignotus PI. Sonography of the thymus in healthy children: frequency of visualization, size, appearance. *AJR* 1993;161:153-155.

84. Han BK, Babcock DS, Oestreich AE. Normal thymus in infancy: sonographic characteristics. *Radiology* 1989;170:471-474.

85. Wernecke K, Diederich S. Sonographic features of mediastinal tumors. *AJR* 1994;163:1357-1364.

86. Wernecke K, Vassallo P, Hoffman G et al. Value of sonography in monitoring the therapeutic response of mediastinal lymphoma: comparison with chest radiography and CT. *AJR* 1991;156:265-272.

87. Wernecke K, Vassallo P, Rutsch F et al. Thymic involvement in Hodgkin disease: CT and sonographic findings. *Radiology* 1991;181:375-383.

88. Andersson T, Lindgren PG, Elvin A. Ultrasound guided tumour biopsy in the anterior mediastinum. An alternative to thoracotomy and mediastinoscopy. *Acta Radiol* 1992;33:423-426.

89. Hsu WH, Chiang CD, Hsu JY et al. Ultrasonically guided needle biopsy of anterior mediastinal masses: comparison of carcinomatous and noncarcinomatous masses. *J Clin Ultrasound* 1995;23:349-356.

90. Yu CJ, Chang DB, Wu HD et al. Evaluation of ultrasonically guided biopsies of mediastinal masses. *Chest* 1991;100:399-405.

91. Sawhney S, Jain R, Berry M. Tru-Cut biopsy of mediastinal masses by real-time ultrasound. *Clin Radiol* 1991;44:16-19.

92. Samad SA, Sharifah NA, Zulfiqar MA et al. Ultrasound guided percutaneous biopsies of suspected mediastinal lesions. *Med J Malaysia* 1993;48:421-426.

CHAPTER 17

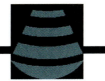

Ultrasound-Guided Biopsy and Drainage of the Abdomen and Pelvis

•

John M. Caspers, M.D.
Carl C. Reading, M.D.
John P. McGahan, M.D.
J. William Charboneau, M.D.

CHAPTER OUTLINE

Ultrasound-guided percutaneous biopsy and abscess drainage have become invaluable diagnostic and therapeutic procedures for the management of patients. Growing experience with ultrasonography and technical advances have significantly broadened the applications of ultrasound as a guidance procedure for interventional techniques. An approach to this topic requires knowledge of the current fundamental methods and applications of these procedures in general and in terms of specific anatomic locations.

ULTRASOUND-GUIDED BIOPSY

Ultrasound-guided needle biopsy is a rapidly growing and important diagnostic technique in radiology practices throughout the world. It has become an accurate, safe, and widely accepted technique for confirmation of suspected malignant masses and characterization of many benign lesions in various intraabdominal locations.[1-6] It also decreases patient costs by obviating the need for an operation, decreasing the duration of hospital stay, and decreasing the number of examinations necessary during a diagnostic evaluation.[7,8]

Traditionally, ultrasound-guided needle biopsy has been used for the biopsy of large, superficial, and cystic masses. Currently, however, because of improvements in instrumentation and biopsy techniques, small, deeply located, and solid masses can also undergo accurate biopsy. Studies have shown that a histologic diagnosis can be made confidently in 90% of cases, even when the mass is 3 cm or smaller.[6,9]

Indications and Contraindications

Most needle biopsies are performed to confirm suspected malignancy before nonsurgical treatment, such as chemotherapy or radiation therapy, is begun. For example, a liver biopsy could be performed to confirm hepatic metastases in a patient with a known primary malignancy. Less often, needle biopsy is performed to determine the nature of an indeterminate lesion, such as a solitary indeterminate solid hepatic mass in a patient with no history of malignancy. Occasionally, needle biopsy is performed on a mass suspected to be benign but in which benignity must be established.[10]

RELATIVE CONTRAINDICATIONS TO NEEDLE BIOPSY

Uncorrectable coagulopathy
Lack of a safe biopsy route
Uncooperative patient

Relative contraindications to needle biopsy include uncorrectable coagulopathy, lack of a safe biopsy route, and an uncooperative patient.

To assess for **coagulopathy**, the primary information comes from the patient's medical history.[11] If the bleeding history is unremarkable, most procedures can be performed without additional laboratory testing. However, if the history suggests a bleeding disorder, prothrombin time, partial thromboplastin time, and platelet count should be assessed.[12] This selective, individually tailored, preprocedural testing, in contrast to pretesting every patient, has been estimated to result in a yearly savings of $20 to $30 million in health care costs.[13] Mild coagulopathies may occur secondary to the use of aspirin and some antibiotics. If present, the procedure may be delayed and the drug discontinued until coagulation measurements become normal.[14] Most coagulopathies can be sufficiently improved by the administration of the appropriate blood products to allow biopsy to be performed. Postbiopsy embolization of the needle tract has been reported to control hemorrhage in patients whose coagulopathy is uncorrectable and in whom the need for biopsy outweighs any risks.[15,16]

The second relative contraindication is the **lack of a safe biopsy route.** A biopsy path extending through large vessels such as the portal vein or inferior vena cava potentially increases the risk of hemorrhage. Also, a biopsy path free of overlying stomach or bowel is a preferable route, although puncture of an overlying loop of bowel is not an absolute contraindication if a small-caliber (21 gauge) needle is used.[17] A biopsy done through ascites has also proved to be safe.[18,19]

The third relative contraindication to needle biopsy is an **uncooperative patient** in whom uncontrolled motion during needle placement increases the risk of tissue laceration and hemorrhage. This is a common problem in pediatric patients and, to overcome it, occasionally it is necessary to administer sedatives.

Imaging Method

Both ultrasonography and computed tomography (CT) can be used as guidance methods for percutaneous needle insertion. The choice of method depends on multiple factors, including lesion size and location, relative visibility of the lesion by the two imaging methods, and equipment availability. Biopsy of many masses can be done with ease under either ultrasound or CT guidance. In these cases the choice of which modality is used is determined mainly by the **personal preference** and experience of the radiologist performing the biopsy.

Ultrasonography. Ultrasonography has several strengths as a biopsy guidance system. It is readily available, relatively inexpensive, and portable; uses no ionizing radiation; and can provide guidance in multiple transverse, longitudinal, or oblique planes. The greatest advantage, however, is that it allows the **real-time visualization** of the needle tip as it passes through tissue planes into the target area in a manner similar to fluoroscopy. This allows precise needle placement and avoidance of important intervening structures. Angled approaches are also easily performed with ultrasound guidance. In addition, **color flow Doppler** imaging can help prevent complications of needle placement by identifying the vascular nature of a mass and by allowing the clinician to avoid vascular structures lying within the needle path.[20,21]

Ultrasound guidance can be used for the biopsy of many organs and regions of the body. The technique is optimal for lesions located superficially or at moderate depth in a thin to average-size person. Biopsy of deep masses and masses in obese patients can be difficult with ultrasonography because of the difficulty in lesion visualization resulting from sound attenuation in the soft tissues. Similarly, lesions located within or behind bone or gas-filled bowel cannot be visualized because of nearly complete reflection of sound from the bone or air interface.

Theoretically, any mass that is well visualized on a sonogram is amenable to ultrasound-guided needle biopsy. In our practice, most liver and kidney biopsies are performed with ultrasound guidance, as are most neck biopsies for thyroid, parathyroid, and cervical nodes. Sometimes the pancreas and other sites in the abdomen and pelvis undergo biopsy with ultrasound guidance if lesion visualization is adequate.[5,17]

Computed Tomography. CT is well established as an accurate guidance method for percutaneous biopsy of most regions in the body. It provides excellent spatial resolution of all structures between the skin and the lesion, and it provides an accurate image of the needle tip. In addition, lesions located deep in the abdomen, retroperitoneum, or within bone are all better seen with CT than with ultrasound. In our practice, many pelvic, adrenal, pancreatic, retroperitoneal, and musculoskeletal biopsies are performed with CT guidance because these structures are often best seen with this imaging method.[5,22]

CT is limited, however, by its lack of continuous visualization of the needle during insertion and biopsy. In most cases, the direction and depth of the needle can be established reliably with minimal need for needle repositioning.

Needle Selection

A variety of needles with a broad spectrum of calibers, lengths, and tip designs are commercially available for use in percutaneous biopsy.[22-28] Conceptually, needles can be grouped into small-caliber (20 to 25 gauge) and large-caliber (14 to 19 gauge) sizes. **Small-caliber needles** are used primarily to obtain specimens for **cytologic analysis.** However, small pieces of tissue may be obtained for histologic examination as well. With these needles, masses behind loops of bowel can be punctured with minimal likelihood of infection. Small-caliber needles are often used to confirm tumor recurrence or metastasis in a patient known to have a previous primary malignancy. Even if the sample is small, the pathologist is usually able to make an accurate diagnosis by comparing the biopsy specimen with the previously obtained tissue.

Large-caliber needles can be used to obtain greater amounts of material for **histologic** as well as cytologic analysis.[25,28] Their use may be necessary to obtain an adequate histologic specimen to confidently diagnose some types of malignancies (such as lymphoma), many benign lesions, and most chronic diffuse parenchymal disease processes (such as hepatic cirrhosis, renal glomerulonephritis, or renal allograft rejection).[29,30]

Needles may also be categorized according to the configuration of the **needle tip.** Most needles have either a noncutting beveled tip (as in conventional injection and spinal needles) or a **tissue-cutting tip** (as in Menghini needles).[25] Noncutting beveled-tip needles easily penetrate soft tissue planes. They are usually used to aspirate fluid and to obtain cytologic specimens. These sharply beveled needles are useful in the biopsy of small masses, such as superficial lymph nodes in the groin or neck, without displacing or deflecting these mobile structures. Needles with a cutting tip are used to obtain a **core of tissue** when histologic analysis is needed. A variation of the cutting tip needle is the side-cutting (Tru-Cut) needle. This type of needle can be used in conjunction with an **automated, spring-loaded biopsy gun.**[31,32] The automated gun offers several advantages over conventional biopsy needles and techniques. A larger core of tissue is obtained consistently. A single pass rather than multiple passes is all that is required in most patients. This often decreases discomfort and theoretically makes the procedure safer. This biopsy device is easy to learn to operate and can be fired with one hand, allowing the other hand to be used for scanning to monitor needle location. There have been no re-

---

ADVANTAGES OF AUTOMATED, SPRING-LOADED BIOPSY GUN

Larger core of tissue consistently obtained
Single pass rather than multiple passes
Easy to learn to operate
Can be fired with one hand, allowing the other hand to be used for scanning to monitor needle location
No increased risk of complications

ports to date of any increased risk of complications from the use of this automated biopsy gun compared with conventional techniques.[33-37]

The preference and level of expertise of the pathologist involved in the interpretation of biopsy specimens are considerations in the selection of needle size and type. **Cytopathologists** deal with small specimens and are trained to diagnose on the basis of only a few cells. Unfortunately, some institutions do not offer cytopathologic interpretation. **Histopathologists**, in contrast, often prefer a large biopsy specimen for interpretation. For example, a large biopsy specimen from a metastatic lesion often allows a more reliable prediction of the likely primary site of the malignancy than does either a tiny sample or a cytologic aspirate. Determination of the probable site of primary malignancy is important in that it allows the oncologist to tailor subsequent treatment optimally.

Biopsy Procedure

Before percutaneous abdominal biopsy is performed, the procedure, risks, alternatives, and benefits should be explained in terms the patient can understand, and **informed consent** should be received. Most patients undergoing abdominal biopsy have a known or suspected malignancy and are concerned about the possible pathologic results. The patients are also apprehensive about the pain and possible complications of abdominal biopsy. Consequently, physicians should be especially sensitive to the psychologic needs of patients undergoing abdominal biopsy. After the procedure is discussed with the patient, any questions the patient might have should be answered fully.

Biopsies are frequently performed on an **outpatient** basis. Discomfort from the procedure is rarely severe and usually is controlled by local anesthesia at the biopsy site after the skin is cleaned and draped. Premedication is usually not necessary. Sedatives and analgesics such as midazolam hydrochloride (Versed) or fentanyl citrate (Sublimaze) can be administered parenterally during the procedure, if necessary.[38,39] An intravenous access may be established before the biopsy is begun in the event that parenteral administration of sedatives, analgesics, or other medications or fluids is required during or after the biopsy procedure. If the patient's history suggests a bleeding disorder, coagulation studies should be reviewed before biopsy.

For sterility, the transducer can be covered with a sterile plastic sheath, but this may degrade image quality and make the transducer more difficult to handle. We prefer to clean the transducer with povidone-iodine (Betadine) and place it directly on the skin.[6] Sterile gel is used as an acoustic coupling agent. After the biopsy procedure, the transducer is soaked for 10 minutes in a bactericidal dialdehyde solution. Caturelli et al.[40] reviewed their 3-year experience using a freehand technique and a similar degree of antisepsis and found no increase in postbiopsy infection.

Most ultrasound-guided biopsies are performed under continuous real-time visualization. Several **needle-guidance systems** designed to facilitate proper needle advancement are commercially available. These guides direct the needle to various depths from the transducer surface, depending on the preselected angle of the guide relative to the transducer (Fig. 17-1).[41-43] Many radiologists prefer

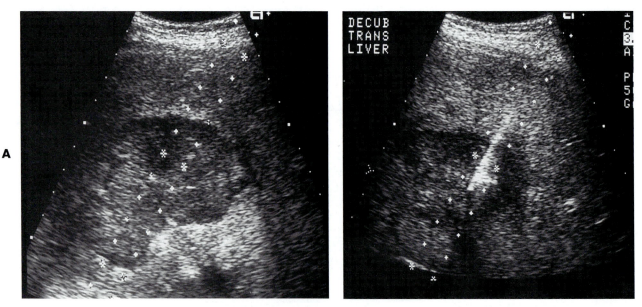

FIG. 17-1. Ultrasound-guided biopsy with a needle guide. A, Sonogram of the liver shows a mass in the right lobe of the liver. **B,** The needle is seen within the preselected angle boundaries with the tip within the mass.

a **"freehand"** approach in which the needle is freely inserted through the skin directly into the view of the transducer without the use of a guide.[4,6] This approach provides great flexibility to the radiologist and allows subtle adjustments to be made during the course of the biopsy, thereby compensating for improper trajectory or patient movement.

When the tip is visualized within the lesion of interest, the biopsy specimen is obtained. If an automated, spring-loaded biopsy device (biopsy gun) that fires both the central stylet and cutting sheath in a rapid forward motion is used, careful attention should be paid to the expected excursion length of the biopsy device. Often the needle tip can be placed at the near edge of the target lesion to avoid the needle passing through the deep margin of the mass into an adjacent critical structure (Fig. 17-2). Some biopsy guns fire only the cutting sheath and not the central stylet. When this type of gun is used, the stylet is advanced to the desired depth within the mass. When the gun is fired, the cutting sheath advances over the stylet, but there is no additional forward motion of the stylet.

Most biopsies are performed by making one or more passes into a mass with a single needle. Occasionally, two needles are used in a **coaxial** manner whereby a large needle is placed into the mass, the stylet removed, and a longer, smaller-caliber needle is placed through the lumen of the first needle, which serves as a guide. Multiple samples can then be obtained with the smaller needle without the need to reposition the larger needle. This technique allows a large amount of tissue to be obtained with only one puncture of the capsule of an organ, which may decrease the risk of hemorrhage. In addition, precise needle placement is performed only once, which saves time in the biopsy of lesions in deep or difficult locations.[44] In our practice, this coaxial technique is frequently used with CT-guided biopsies in deep locations and less often with ultrasound-guided biopsies.

After the biopsy is performed, the patient is observed in the radiology department for 1 to 2 hours, with vital signs checked frequently. In many medical centers, initial cytologic results are available within this time. If the results of the initial cytologic analysis are not conclusive, then a repeat biopsy is usually performed immediately. When core biopsy samples are obtained with needles such as biopsy guns, immediate interpretation of the core biopsy sample can be performed by traditional frozen-section diagnosis. Additional tissue samples are necessary if permanent fixation is needed. Alternatively, "touch" preparation cytology offers rapid diagnosis from one core biopsy sample and preserves the core material for subsequent permanent fixation for histologic diagnosis.[45,46]

Needle Visualization

One of ultrasound's greatest strengths as a biopsy-guidance method is its ability to continuously monitor needle tip advancement under **real-time visualization**. However, this is frequently the most technically difficult aspect of ultrasound-guided biopsy for many radiologists. Beginners may wish to

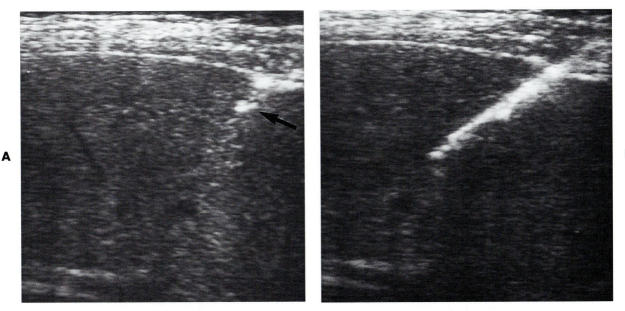

FIG. 17-2. **Ultrasound-guided liver parenchymal biopsy using an automated spring-loaded biopsy device.** **A,** Longitudinal sonogram of the liver shows the needle tip *(arrow)* 1 cm into the liver parenchyma. **B,** Real-time image shows forward excursion of the needle tip during biopsy.

practice on a homemade ultrasound biopsy phantom to develop the coordination necessary for ultrasound-guided procedures.[47-49]

On an ultrasonogram, the needle usually appears as a hyperechoic dot representing the needle tip and less often as a hyperechoic line representing the needle shaft. The most common reason for nonvisualization of the needle tip is **improper alignment** of the needle tip and transducer.[5] To visualize the entire needle, the needle and the central ultrasound beam of the transducer must be in the same plane. When a mechanical needle guide is used, the needle is usually maintained within this central plane. If the "freehand" method of guidance is used, the radiologist must frequently look at the alignment of the needle with the transducer.

When the needle is not visualized, it is usually because the needle is misaligned (either initially aligned off-center relative to the central beam of the transducer or angled away from the central beam of the transducer) (Fig. 17-3). A "bobbing" or in-and-out **jiggling movement** of the biopsy needle during insertion improves needle visualization. This bobbing motion causes deflection of the soft tissues adjacent to the needle and makes the trajectory of the needle much more discernible within the otherwise stationary field.

Needle visualization can also improve by increasing the **reflectivity of the biopsy needle**. Large-caliber needles are more readily visualized than small-caliber needles. Various modifications in needle-tip design have been tried to enhance needle visualization, including scoring the needle tip and using a screw stylet.[50-52] Extra-reflective needles specifically designed for ultrasound guidance are commercially available. Most needles, however, are sufficiently visible sonographically as long as the needle and transducer are aligned.

The **echogenicity of the parenchyma** of the organ undergoing biopsy also affects the visibility of the biopsy needle. If the parenchyma is relatively hypoechoic, such as liver, kidney, or spleen, an echogenic needle can usually be identified easily. Conversely, if the organ is relatively hyperechoic, it is usually difficult to visualize the echogenic needle tip in this background. This factor is responsible for poor needle visualization in biopsies of retroperitoneal structures or in obese patients.

Linear or curved-array transducers are frequently used for guiding procedures because of their good near-field resolution, which allows visualization of the needle after relatively little tissue penetration. The focal zone of the ultrasound beam should also be placed in the near field for better needle visualization. Sector transducers are often used if there is a small acoustic window or if there is a deep lesion situated at steep angles. Some authors have found **color flow Doppler** imaging helpful to visualize needle motion.[53,54] In our experience, however, color flow Doppler imaging has not been helpful in needle-tip localization.

Clear visualization of the biopsy needle is an important element in the success of ultrasound-guided needle biopsies. The various techniques that have been described can be used to enhance needle visualization. However, considerable real-time scanning experience remains the key factor to the successful performance of ultrasound-guided biopsies.

Specific Anatomic Applications

Liver. The liver is the abdominal organ for which percutaneous biopsy is most frequently used. Common indications for biopsy include nonsurgical confirmation of metastatic disease, characterization of focal liver mass(es) with inconclusive imaging, and diagnosis of progression of diffuse parenchymal abnormality. In our practice, liver biopsy is usually performed under ultrasound guidance because of the real-time needle visualization.[5,37,55] The advantage of real-time needle guidance becomes especially obvious when there is significant movement of the organ from respiratory variation. Biopsy of large or superficial lesions is easiest. With experience, deep lesions and lesions as small as 0.5 cm can undergo biopsy with high accuracies (Fig. 17-4).[6,9] In a retrospective study of 2091 ultrasound-guided hepatic biopsies, Buscarini et al.[56] reported an overall accuracy of 95.1% for core hepatic biopsies.

Lesions in the left lobe and in the inferior portion of the right lobe can usually undergo biopsy through a **subcostal approach**. Lesions located superiorly in the dome of the liver present a technical challenge for CT-guided biopsy, but biopsy can be done safely with ultrasound guidance by angling the needle from inferior to superior, usually using an intercostal approach (Fig. 17-5). Although the intercostal approach may enter the pleural space, aerated lung is rarely violated because it is well visualized sonographically and can be avoided (Fig. 17-6). We usually place the patient in the left posterior oblique rather than the supine position when an intercostal approach is used to improve visibility of the liver through the intercostal spaces.

Hepatic biopsies have proved to be safe. Of the rare complications, hemorrhage is the most common.[22,37,56] Previously, most authors concurred that biopsy of vascular lesions should be avoided because of the risk of hemorrhage.[3] However, **vascular hepatic masses** have successfully undergone biopsy with only rare complications.[57-61]

Benign hepatic lesions such as atypical cavernous hemangiomas, focal fatty infiltration, and focal areas of normal liver within a fatty infiltrated liver can occasionally mimic the appearance of malignancy on imaging studies. Biopsy of these processes can be done

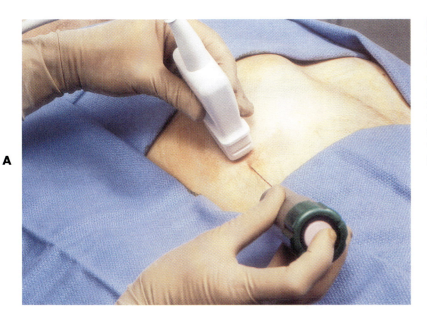

A

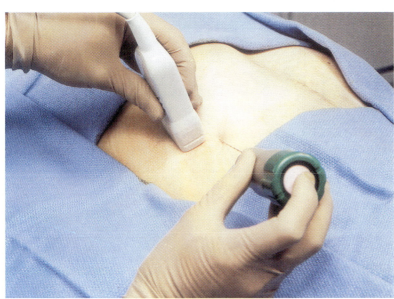

B

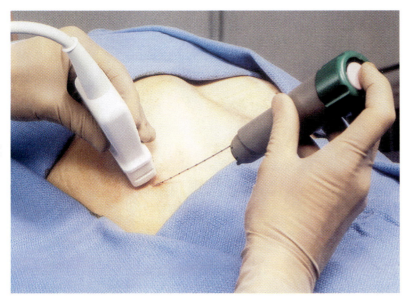

C

FIG. 17-3. **Freehand alignment of biopsy needle with the ultrasound transducer.** **A,** Correct alignment for optimal sonographic visualization. Biopsy needle is aligned precisely within the central plane of the transducer. **B,** Incorrect alignment. Biopsy needle is aligned off-center relative to the transducer. **C,** Incorrect alignment. Biopsy needle is aligned correctly with the center of the transducer but is angled away from the central plane.

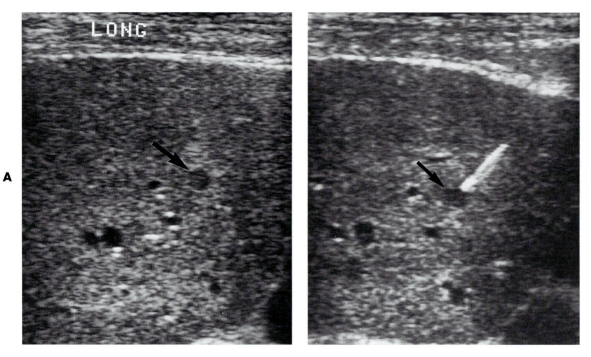

FIG. 17-4. **Ultrasound-guided biopsy of a small, metastatic lesion in the liver from transitional cell carcinoma of bladder.** **A,** Longitudinal image of the right lobe of liver shows 0.5 cm mass in midportion *(arrow)*. **B,** Ultrasound-guided biopsy with an 18-gauge biopsy needle *(arrow)*. (From Charboneau JW, Reading CC, Welch TJ. CT and sonographically guided needle biopsy: current techniques and new innovations. *AJR* 1990;154:1-10.)

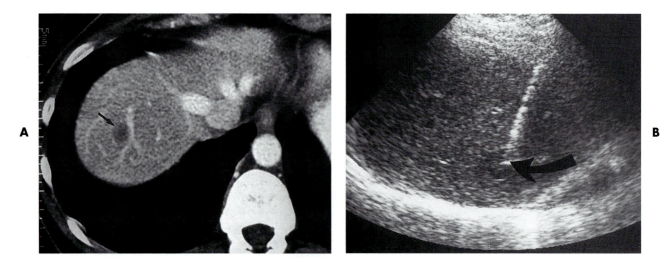

FIG. 17-5. **Ultrasound-guided biopsy of a metastatic lesion located in the dome of the liver from breast carcinoma.** **A,** Contrast-enhanced computed tomogram shows a 1 cm mass near the dome of the liver *(arrow)*. **B,** Ultrasound-guided biopsy needle angled superiorly from a subcostal approach shows the needle tip *(arrow)* in the 1 cm mass.

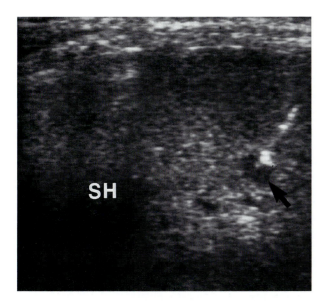

FIG. 17-6. Avoidance of lung. Oblique ultrasonogram of right lobe of liver shows biopsy needle with 1 cm metastatic lesion *(arrow)*. The aerated lung causes posterior acoustic shadowing, *SH*.

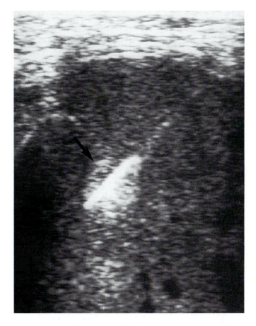

FIG. 17-7. Biopsy of 2 cm cavernous hemangioma. Longitudinal ultrasonogram of the liver shows a 21 gauge needle within a 2 cm hyperechoic mass *(arrow)*.

with ultrasound guidance to exclude malignancy and to confirm their benign nature (Fig. 17-7).[10] Although cavernous hemangiomas are vascular lesions, there have been several reported series in which these masses have undergone successful percutaneous biopsy without significant complications.[55-62] However, there is a case report of a death due to hemorrhage after percutaneous biopsy of a large, subcapsular, hepatic hemangioma with a 21 gauge needle under CT guidance. In this particular case the needle was inserted directly into the mass through the liver capsule without any interposed normal hepatic parenchyma. If normal liver can be interposed between the mass and liver capsule, this may provide a potential tamponade effect if bleeding occurs.[57]

Percutaneous ultrasound-guided biopsy of **portal vein thrombus** has also proved to be a safe and an accurate diagnostic procedure for the staging of **hepatocellular carcinoma.**[63,64] Accurate staging of hepatocellular carcinoma is necessary to determine appropriate treatment. In particular, neoplastic invasion of the main portal vein is a contraindication for hepatic resection or transplantation. Establishing the benign or malignant nature of portal vein thrombosis is therefore critical to patient management.

Pancreas. Most pancreatic biopsies are performed in patients with **ductal adenocarcinoma** when it is considered to be unresectable because of tumor encasement of adjacent major vascular structures such as the celiac axis or superior mesenteric artery. Occasionally, a pancreatic biopsy is performed

to distinguish benign disease, such as chronic pancreatitis, from malignancy. At our institution, most pancreatic biopsies are done with CT guidance because the depth of the pancreas plus the presence of overlying bowel gas and hyperechoic abdominal fat can render ultrasound visualization of the needle difficult. However, biopsy of pancreatic masses in normal-size and slender patients can be done accurately under ultrasound guidance (Fig. 17-8). In general, if the mass is well seen under ultrasound, biopsy can be done readily with ultrasound guidance. A review of 211 CT-guided and 58 ultrasound-guided biopsies of pancreatic lesions demonstrated a CT-guided accuracy of 86% and an ultrasound-guided accuracy of 95%.[17]

In some reported series, the biopsy **success rate** for the diagnosis of pancreatic carcinoma has been lower than the success rate for the diagnosis of malignant lesions in other organs of the abdomen.[17,65,66] However, an increased success rate can be expected when ultrasound guidance is used if the needle is placed into the central hypoechoic portion of the pancreatic mass, which should represent tumor, rather than the adjacent echogenic regions, which are more likely to be nonmalignant pancreatic parenchyma or desmoplastic inflammatory change. In addition, carcinoma of the pancreas is often well-differentiated adenocarcinoma that is difficult to distinguish from normal pancreatic cells on cytologic sample alone.[31,67] Therefore, histologic specimens obtained with cutting needles are helpful.

Cystic pancreatic malignancies are difficult to diagnose accurately by percutaneous biopsy.

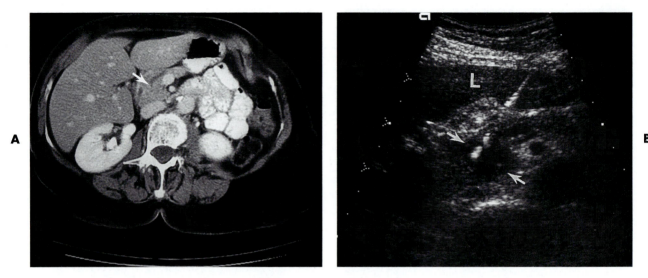

FIG. 17-8. Ultrasound-guided pancreatic biopsy. A, Contrast-enhanced CT scan shows a mildly dilated pancreatic duct with abrupt termination in the head of the pancreas *(arrow)*. No definite mass is identified on CT scan. **B,** Ultrasonogram for guided biopsy shows a 19 gauge needle passing through the left lobe of the liver, *L*, with needle tip within a 2 cm hypoechoic mass in the head of the pancreas *(arrows)*. The biopsy was positive for adenocarcinoma.

Previously, surgical exploration rather than biopsy was recommended for these masses.[3] More recently, analysis of percutaneous fluid aspirates from cystic lesions has been proposed as an aid to distinguishing cystic neoplasms from pseudocysts.[68-70] A high amylase is consistent with a pseudocyst. Columnar cells are suggestive of a neoplastic origin, and a positive stain for mucin is found with mucinous tumors.

The **safety** of percutaneous biopsy of the pancreas has been well established. Although complications are rare, with cited rates from 1.1% to 6.7%, six deaths have been reported.[17,71] Five of these deaths were attributed to pancreatitis and one to sepsis. No pancreatic cancer was found in either the biopsy specimen or postmortem examination of these patients, suggesting an increased risk for developing pancreatitis after biopsy of normal pancreas.[72] The review by Brandt et al.[17] of 269 pancreatic biopsies showed a major complication rate of 1.1% of biopsies and no related deaths. Two patients with major complications had acute pancreatitis, and both of these patients had percutaneous biopsy-proven ductal adenocarcinoma. The potential risk of tumor seeding along the needle track has caused some authorities to recommend that the procedure not be performed in patients who are considered potential surgical candidates.[73] Of 23 reported instances of needle-track seeding, 10 have occurred after biopsy of pancreatic malignancies.[71]

Kidney. Renal masses or parenchyma can undergo biopsy accurately and safely by using sono-graphic guidance.[74] The vast majority of solitary solid renal masses represent renal cell carcinoma. Therefore when a solitary mass is discovered, it is usually removed without prior biopsy. However, if the patient is not a surgical candidate, a biopsy of the mass can provide tissue confirmation of the presumed malignancy. The rare patient with **multiple solid renal masses** often undergoes biopsy to distinguish the potential causes of multiple masses: metastases, lymphoma, or multiple renal cell carcinomas (Fig. 17-9). Although these lesions can be similar in appearance, their treatments differ widely. Thus accurate diagnosis is necessary.

An **atypical cystic renal mass** that has internal debris, solid components, or a thick irregular wall can be aspirated and a biopsy of the solid elements can be done under ultrasound guidance in an attempt to distinguish a complicated benign cyst from renal cell carcinoma. The aspiration of grossly bloody fluid raises the suspicion of malignancy, and the recovery of malignant cells is confirmatory. Alternatively, the aspiration of clear, straw-colored fluid and recovery of benign solid tissue from the wall of the mass support the diagnosis of benign atypical cysts.[75,76]

Sonographic guidance can also be used in the biopsy of kidneys with **diffuse parenchymal disease.** Insertion of the needle into the cortex of the lower-pole renal parenchyma under continuous real-time guidance results in few complications and produces a tissue sample of excellent quality for microscopic analysis.[77,78] Ultrasound-guided biopsy of renal transplants with an 18 gauge automated cutting needle provides a biopsy specimen that is equivalent

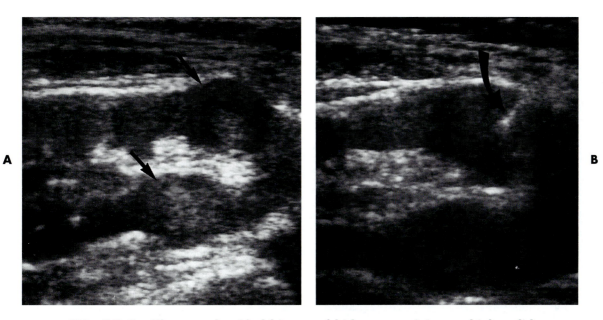

FIG. 17-9. Ultrasound-guided biopsy of kidney containing multiple solid masses—metastases from lung carcinoma. A, Longitudinal ultrasonogram of the right kidney shows two round isoechoic masses *(arrows)* in the lower pole of the kidney. **B,** An 18 gauge biopsy needle *(arrow)* is seen within the anterior mass.

in diagnostic quality to the biopsy specimen obtained by the traditional 14 gauge cutting needle.[79] In addition, there were substantially fewer complications with the 18 gauge biopsy gun than with the 14 gauge needle in these series.

Adrenal Gland. The most common indication for adrenal biopsy is to **confirm metastatic disease** in a patient with an adrenal mass and a known primary malignancy elsewhere.[80] The right adrenal gland is more accessible to ultrasound-guided biopsy than the left adrenal gland because of the sonographic window of the right lobe of the liver (Fig. 17-10). For practical purposes most right adrenal masses need to be at least 2 to 3 cm in diameter to allow adequate visualization and biopsy under ultrasound guidance; most left adrenal masses need to be several centimeters larger. Guidance by CT is often preferable for the biopsy of small adrenal masses. Brightly echogenic fat containing adrenal masses and homogeneous, thin-walled, fluid-filled adrenal masses do not undergo biopsy because these should represent benign adrenal myelolipomas and cysts, respectively. A small (less than 3 cm), homogeneous, smoothly marginated, solid adrenal mass that is discovered incidentally in a patient with no primary malignancy or endocrine abnormalities is likely a benign, nonfunctioning, adrenal adenoma, and no biopsy is done.[81] Follow-up examination in 6 months to 1 year can be performed to confirm lack of change in size or appearance of the mass. Although benign adenomas can be larger than 3 cm, the likelihood of silent adrenal carcinoma increases significantly if an incidentally discovered mass is

larger than 5 cm.[82] However, needle biopsy may not be accurate in these patients because the histologic diagnosis of carcinoma requires the demonstration of adrenal capsular breakthrough and invasion of vascular structures by tumor. Therefore surgical exploration rather than biopsy is often warranted for asymptomatic adrenal masses larger than 5 cm.[83]

Radiologists performing adrenal biopsies should be familiar with the management of a hypertensive crisis from the inadvertent biopsy of a pheochromocytoma.[84,85] If the clinical history suggests pheochromocytoma, further laboratory tests should establish the diagnosis rather than biopsy.

Spleen. The spleen is the abdominal organ that undergoes biopsy least often. Percutaneous splenic biopsy is usually not performed for two reasons. First, it is rare for the spleen to be the only organ in the abdomen involved with the pathologic process such as metastasis (Fig. 17-11). In most cases, when the splenic lesion is visualized, there is also concomitant disease in other abdominal organs, such as the liver or lymph nodes, in which a biopsy can be done. Second, the spleen is a highly vascular organ and the risk of hemorrhage from needle biopsy seems to be high. However, the reported rate of hemorrhage from spleen biopsy is low.[86-88] In one of these series there were no significant complications in more than 1000 splenic biopsies.[86]

The main clinical reason for performing percutaneous biopsy of the spleen at present is to distinguish a metastasis from recurrent lymphoma in a patient who has a new splenic mass but no disease elsewhere in the abdomen. Recurrent lymphoma can often be

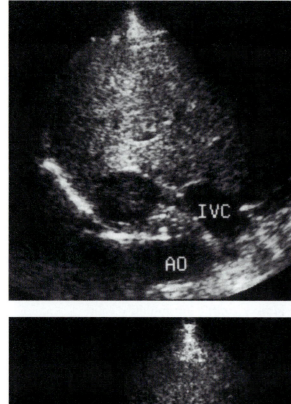

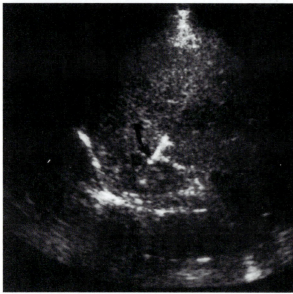

FIG. 17-10. Ultrasound-guided biopsy of right adrenal mass—metastasis from lung carcinoma. **A,** Transverse sonogram through intercostal space and right lobe of liver with patient in the left lateral decubitus position shows a 3 cm solid right adrenal mass. *IVC,* Inferior vena cava; *AO,* aorta. **B,** Transhepatic biopsy with 18 gauge needle *(arrow).*

diagnosed by comparison of the percutaneous biopsy specimen with tissue previously obtained from the patient. In contrast, needle biopsy of the spleen is usually not performed for initial nonoperative diagnosis of lymphoma because of the great difficulty in obtaining an adequate amount of tissue for the complete histopathologic subclassification of lymphoma that is necessary before treatment begins.

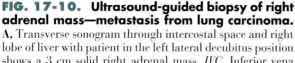

MAJOR COMPLICATIONS OF BIOPSY

Hemorrhage
Pneumothorax
Pancreatitis
Bile leakage
Peritonitis
Needle-track seeding

Accuracy

The accuracy of ultrasound-guided biopsy has been reported as 66% to 97%, depending on the location, size, and histologic type of the lesion.[*] Differences in patient population, technique, and numbers of patients make comparison of these studies difficult. In our series of sonographically guided biopsies of 126 consecutive small ($\leq$ 3 cm), solid masses in various anatomic locations and various histologic types, the accuracy of biopsy was 91%.[6] Biopsy results improved with increasing size of the mass in this group of small lesions; accuracy ranged from 79% in masses of 1 cm or less in diameter to 98% in masses 2 to 3 cm. The accuracy in the liver, where most biopsies were performed, was 96%. Others have also shown accuracies as high as 91% for ultrasound-guided biopsy of small ($<$ 2.5 cm) abdominal masses.[9] Two organ-specific reviews showed accuracies for ultrasound-guided liver biopsy of 94% and ultrasound-guided pancreatic biopsy of 95%.[17,56]

Complications

Radiologically guided percutaneous needle biopsy has widely expanded, in part because of its well-documented safety, with rare and usually minor complications. Several large reviews obtained by multi-institutional questionnaires have reported mortality rates of 0.008% to 0.031% and major complication rates of 0.05% to 0.18%.[71,89,90] A review by Nolsoe et al.[91] of 8000 ultrasound-guided needle punctures at a single institution, including the use of both large-caliber and small-caliber needles, found a slightly higher mortality rate, 0.038%, and a major complication rate of 0.187% (see box above).

A prospective analysis of 3393 biopsies (1825 ultrasound guided and 1568 CT guided) from our institution demonstrated similar results.[37] This study showed a mortality rate of 0.06%, a major complication rate of 0.34% (0.3% ultrasound, 0.5% CT), and a minor complication rate of 2.9% (2.4% ultrasound, 3.3% CT).

Although rare, **hemorrhage** is the most common major complication of solid-organ biopsy and accounts for most deaths in these series. An interesting note from the review by Nelson et al.[37] is that five of the

---

[*]References 2, 5, 6, 17, 31, 41, 55, 56.

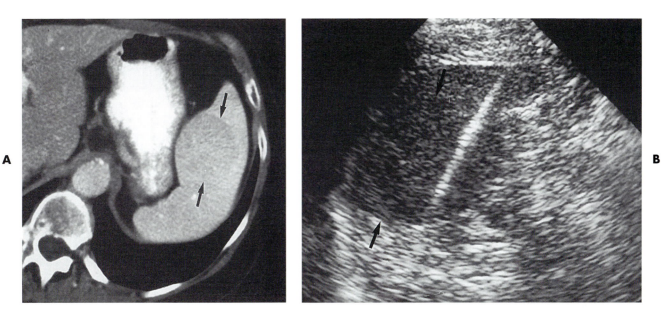

FIG. 17-11. Ultrasound-guided biopsy of melanoma metastasis to the spleen. A, Contrast-enhanced CT scan shows a 5 cm, low-attenuating mass in the spleen *(arrows)*. **B,** Longitudinal ultrasonogram shows biopsy needle in the mass *(arrows)*.

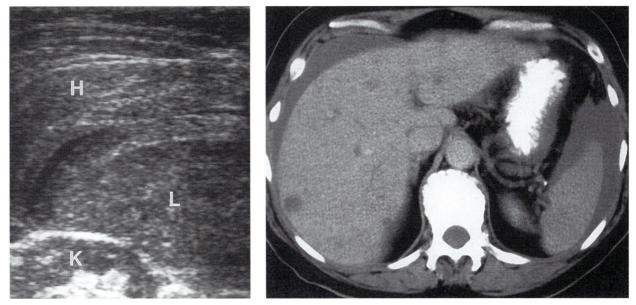

FIG. 17-12. Hemorrhage as a complication of liver biopsy. A, Transverse ultrasonogram shows echogenic material, *H*, surrounding right lobe of liver, *L*. This echogenic material represents fresh hemorrhage and is difficult to distinguish from the adjacent liver because of similarity in echogenicities of hemorrhage and liver. *K*, Kidney. **B,** Computed tomogram with intravenous injection of contrast material clearly shows the fresh intraperitoneal hemorrhage as a crescent of fluid of decreased attenuation that is different from the attenuation of the adjacent spleen and liver, which contain metastases.

eight patients who had significant hemorrhage post-biopsy had normal results of coagulation studies and often did not present until several hours after the biopsy. If hemorrhage is suspected after biopsy and the patient is hemodynamically stable, the patient should be scanned to evaluate for this complication. CT is more accurate than ultrasound to evaluate for acute hemorrhage. On ultrasound, fresh blood has an echogenicity similar to that of surrounding organs and can be overlooked (Fig. 17-12).

Other **major complications** reported secondary to biopsy include pneumothorax, pancreatitis, bile leakage, peritonitis, and needle-track seeding. In the review by Nelson et al.,[37] hemorrhage and significant pneumothorax were the only major complications. **Needle-track seeding** is a rare complication, with only 23 reported cases in the literature and an estimated frequency of 0.005%.[71,92] Although most reports of needle-track seeding have been from biopsy of carcinoma of the pancreas and carcinoma of the prostate, single cases have been reported from biopsies of the liver, kidney, pleura, breast, eye, and retroperitoneum.[93-102] Because seeding is such a rare complication, it should not affect the decision to perform percutaneous biopsy. Vasovagal reactions, pain, fever, transient hematuria, and tiny pneumothoraces not requiring treatment except analgesics or observation were considered minor complications in these studies.

The **differences** in the **complication rates** associated with the use of **larger-caliber cutting needles** and **small-caliber needles** may be overestimated. An early comparative study found complication rates of 0.8% with small-caliber (22 gauge) and 1.4% with large-caliber cutting needles (18 gauge and 19 gauge); this difference was not statistically significant.[103] Welch et al.[22] found equal rates of complications from the use of 18 gauge and 21 gauge biopsy needles (0.3%). The review by Nelson et al.[37] supported this finding (15 to 19 gauge: 3.8%; 20 to 22 gauge: 5.0%). In addition, there was no higher incidence of complications from biopsies performed with automated biopsy cutting needles (0.7%) compared with those done with conventional cutting needles (0.9%).[37]

Percutaneous Tumor Ablation

It is likely that in the future the emphasis of image-guided percutaneous needle biopsy may switch from that of diagnostic biopsy of a suspected abdominal mass to therapeutic ablation of the mass as well. For example, during the last 10 years percutaneously injected alcohol has been used for the ablation of primary hepatic neoplasms with a high degree of success (Fig. 17-13). Unfortunately, results have been less en-

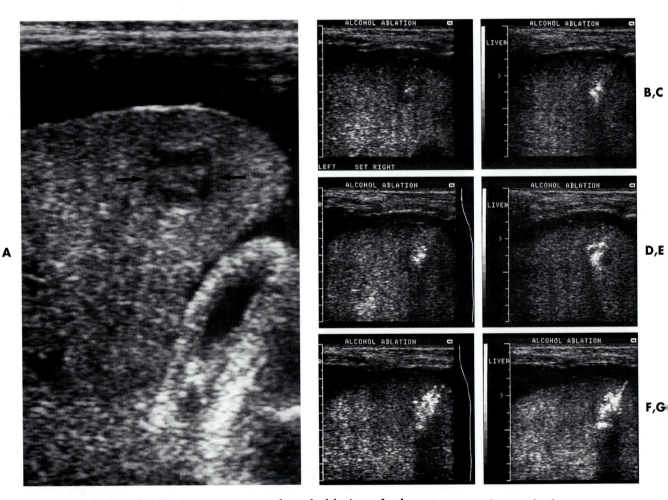

FIG. 17-13. Percutaneous ethanol ablation of a hepatoma. A, Longitudinal ultrasonogram of right lobe of liver shows ascites and a 1.5 cm hypoechoic solid mass *(arrows)*, which proved to be a hepatoma on subsequent needle biopsy. **B** to **G,** Multiple injections of ethanol injection through a 21 gauge needle caused the mass to become hyperechoic because of microbubbles.

couraging for the treatment of hepatic metastases with alcohol.[104-108] It may be that additional newer thermal ablation methods, including radiofrequency electrocautery and laser photocoagulation, which can be administered via a percutaneously placed needle, will be useful in the treatment of metastatic disease.[108-110] These new percutaneous treatment methods are the natural extension of the percutaneous biopsy techniques that have been discussed in this chapter and hold promise for the treatment of metastatic malignancies in the future.

ULTRASOUND-GUIDED DRAINAGE

Like needle biopsy, percutaneous aspiration and drainage procedures have gained wide acceptance in clinical practice because of their safety, simplicity, and effectiveness. Although needle puncture and aspiration were first described in 1930,[111] only more recently have percutaneous abdominal aspiration and drainage become popular techniques. The development of newer guidance methods and refinement of catheters have been responsible for this increase.[112,113] Modalities such as sonography and CT allow for precise needle placement for superficial and deep abdominal fluid collections or abscesses.[114]

Indications and Contraindications

The indications for image-guided percutaneous abscess drainage continue to expand. Initial criteria specified that the fluid collection be unilocular with no communications, and surgical backup was considered essential.[113,115] Currently, percutaneous abscess drainage is performed safely for solitary, multilocular, and multifocal fluid collections with or without communication to the gastrointestinal tract.[115,116] More recently, indications include complex solid organ abscesses, enteric-related abdominal abscesses, even with underlying bowel pathology (i.e., appendicitis and diverticulitis), tuboovarian abscesses, and percutaneous cholecystostomy for an inflamed gallbladder.

Most percutaneous abscess drainage is performed **to facilitate a cure** and thus obviates the risks and morbidity of general anesthesia and operation. Other times it is a **temporizing procedure** that either postpones the definitive operation until the patient is stable (such as periappendiceal abscess drainage) or permits a single-stage surgery rather than a multistage surgery (such as peridiverticular abscess drainage). This is particularly desirable in elderly, high-risk patients who present with sepsis. Poorly defined fluid in the peritoneum with an underlying surgically correctable abnormality (such as perforated colon with generalized peritonitis) should not be drained percutaneously and is best treated with an operation.

Contraindications to image-guided percutaneous catheter drainage are all relative contraindications and are similar to those of percutaneous biopsy discussed earlier in this chapter. Lack of a safe route for percutaneous drainage precludes the procedure; however, this is uncommon. Unlike percutaneous biopsy where bowel may be traversed without complications, fluid aspiration and percutaneous abscess drainage through bowel should be avoided. Bleeding diathesis should be maximally corrected, and appropriate sedation (local and systemic) should be given to the uncooperative patient.

Imaging Method

Selection of an imaging modality, whether ultrasonography, CT, or fluoroscopy, for guidance of aspiration and drainage is influenced by several factors, including the location of the fluid collection as well as the strengths and weaknesses of each imaging modality as discussed earlier in this chapter. For instance, a simple paracentesis is best performed under ultrasound guidance (Fig. 17-14). More complicated drainage procedures in the retroperitoneum or pelvis are best performed with CT guidance. More superficial abdominal fluid collections may be performed easily with ultrasound guidance; however, obtaining a CT scan before the procedure provides an anatomic map for planning a safe access route.

In certain anatomic areas such as the gallbladder, biliary tract, and kidneys, combined ultrasound-fluoroscopic guidance of catheter placement may be preferred. The combined use of ultrasound for initial

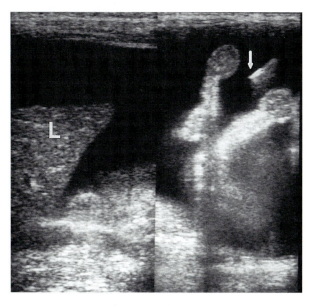

FIG. 17-14. Ultrasound-guided paracentesis. Longitudinal dual ultrasound image shows aspiration needle tip *(arrow)* in ascites, which surrounds the liver, *L*, and loops of bowel.

needle placement and fluoroscopy for catheter placement, via the guidewire exchange technique, optimizes the strengths of both guidance systems. Fluoroscopy may then be used to opacify the area drained and to confirm final catheter placement and the adequacy of drainage.[117,118]

No single method of guidance for percutaneous guidance is appropriate for all abdominal fluid collections or abscesses. Part of the intrigue in implementing abdominal interventional procedures is that each case is different. The approach to any fluid collection or potential abscess must be tailored to the patient, procedure, and specific circumstances.

Catheter Selection

Various catheters and introducing systems are available for percutaneous abscess drainage.[119] The catheter and introducing system chosen depend most on personal preference. As with most interventional procedures, it is important for the radiologist to be familiar and comfortable with the system (Fig. 17-15). In general, thicker fluid is best drained with larger-caliber catheters. A 10 to 14 French catheter provides adequate drainage for virtually all abscesses. A sump catheter (double lumen) may also aid in the drainage of thick fluid collections in the abdomen. Smaller (6 to 8 French) catheters are adequate for less viscous collections. Catheters with retention devices, such as locking Cope loop catheters, are being used more frequently to prevent catheter dislodgment.

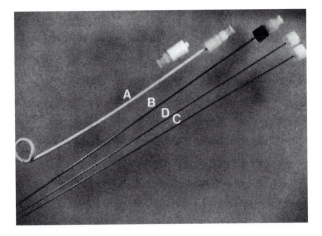

FIG. 17-15. **McGahan drainage catheter is composed of four components, including a 25 cm long pigtail catheter with** **A,** a locking Cope loop, **B,** a cannula, and **C,** an inner blunted obturator used to straighten the catheter. Once the catheter and cannula are assembled, the inner blunted obturator is removed and can be replaced with a sharp inner stylet, **D,** so the catheter may be inserted via the trocar method. (From McGahan JP. A new catheter design for percutaneous cholecystostomy. *Radiology* 1988;166:49-52.)

Drainage Procedure

Patient Preparation. The procedure and risks should be explained to the patient and **informed consent** should be received. The patient's hemostatic status should be assessed through clinical history and, if necessary, coagulation studies should be done. **Intravenous access** is obtained in all patients for the administration of medications and for emergency access in case the patient develops complications from the procedure, such as hemorrhage. Patients often receive **broad-spectrum antibiotics intravenously** to decrease the possibility of sepsis. Satisfactory **analgesia** is necessary throughout the procedure to provide optimal patient comfort and cooperation. Local anesthesia is usually sufficient for needle aspiration; however, intravenous administration of sedatives and analgesics such as midazolam hydrochloride (Versed) or fentanyl citrate (Sublimaze) is beneficial for percutaneous catheter insertion.

Diagnostic Aspiration. Because fluid collections often have a nonspecific appearance, diagnostic aspiration is the first step. A fine needle is guided into the fluid collection by the selected imaging modality. This needle insertion defines a precise and safe route to the fluid collection. A small amount of fluid is aspirated and sent for appropriate microbiologic evaluation. The resulting culture and sensitivity data are used to modify the antibiotic therapy. If the fluid does not appear infected (i.e., clear, colorless, and odorless), the clinician may elect to completely aspirate the cavity and not perform the drainage procedure. If pus is aspirated, care should be taken to aspirate only a small amount of fluid because any decrease in the cavity size may make subsequent catheter placement more difficult.

Catheter Placement. Catheter insertion can be performed using the trocar or Seldinger technique, and the decision to use one or the other usually depends on the preference of the operator. In the **trocar technique** (Fig. 17-16) the fine needle is used as a tandem localizer. The catheter fits over a stiffening cannula, and a sharp inner stylet is placed within the cannula for insertion. The catheter assembly is advanced into the fluid collection. The catheter is then pushed from the cannula, and the distal loop is formed and tightened to secure the catheter within the fluid collection. This method works best for large and superficial fluid collections.

With the **Seldinger technique** (guidewire exchange technique) (Fig. 17-17), a guidewire is advanced through the aspiration needle and coiled within the fluid collection. The needle is then removed and the guidewire is used as an anchor for passage of a dilator to widen the catheter track. The catheter-cannula assembly is placed over the guidewire into the fluid collection. The guidewire and inner cannula are

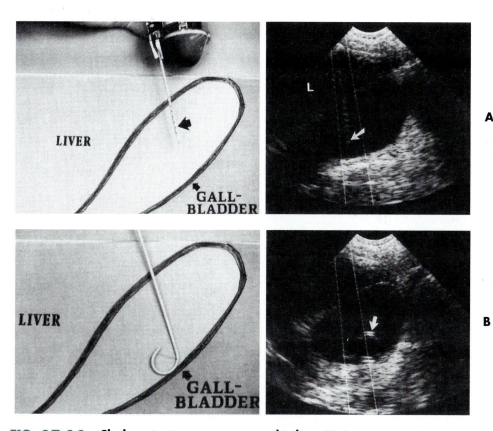

FIG. 17-16. Cholecystostomy—trocar method. A, With ultrasound guidance and use of a needle guide, a cholecystostomy catheter *(arrow)* is placed transhepatically via the trocar method into the gallbladder. *L,* Liver. **B,** Once in the gallbladder, the stylet and the cannula are removed while the catheter is simultaneously advanced into the gallbladder and the distal loop in the catheter *(arrow)* is reformed. (From McGahan JP. Gallbladder. In: McGahan JP, ed. *Interventional Ultrasound.* Baltimore: Williams & Wilkins; 1990.)

removed while the catheter is simultaneously advanced. The distal Cope loop of the catheter is reformed to prevent catheter dislodgment. If catheter visualization is difficult, the use of color flow Doppler imaging may improve ultrasound visualization. During aspiration or irrigation, Doppler shifts improve catheter visualization (Fig. 17-18).

Drainage. After the drainage catheter is placed, the cavity is completely aspirated and gently irrigated. Care should be taken to not distend the cavity during the irrigation because this may increase the risk of bacteremia. Repeat images are obtained to determine the size of the residual cavity, the position of the drainage tube, and whether all the abscess communicates with the drainage tube. If the abscess cavity has not completely resolved, the drainage catheter may need to be repositioned or a second drain may need to be placed. Correct catheter position and adequate catheter size are the most important factors for successful drainage.[120]

Follow-Up Care. All drains must be **irrigated regularly.** Injection of 10 ml isotonic saline three or four times a day is usually sufficient. If drainage is especially tenacious, more frequent irrigations with greater vol-

umes of saline may be necessary. The fluid collection can be drained either dependently or by low intermittent suction. The character and volume of the output should be recorded each nursing shift and checked daily on rounds by the radiology service.[121] If the drainage changes significantly in volume or character or if fever recurs, the patient should be reexamined to check for fistulas, catheter blockage, reaccumulation of the abscess, or a previously undiagnosed collection.

Twenty-four to 48 hours after tube placement, a **sinogram** should be performed to look at the abscess cavity size, completeness of drainage, and catheter position, and to look for fistulas. Simple abscess cavities may drain for 5 to 10 days. Abscesses secondary to fistulas from bowel or biliary or urinary tracts may drain for 6 weeks or longer. As long as drainage persists, sinograms are performed every 3 to 4 days and the drains are left in place. Outpatient care is possible for selected patients.

Catheter Removal. There are **three criteria** for catheter removal:
• **Negligible drainage in 24 hours;**
• **Patient afebrile;**
• **Minimal residual cavity.**

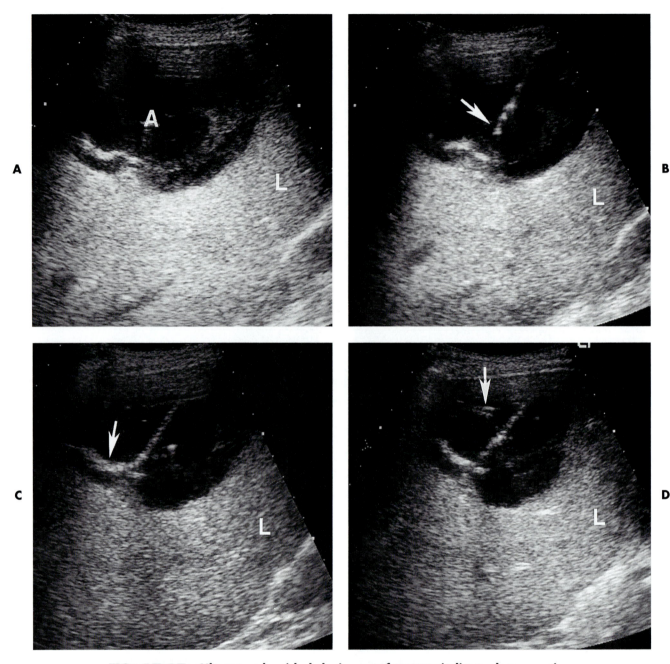

FIG. 17-17. **Ultrasound-guided drainage of pyogenic liver abscess using the Seldinger technique.** **A,** Longitudinal ultrasonogram shows an 8 cm abscess, *A,* in the liver, *L.* **B,** Aspiration needle *(arrow)* insertion into the abscess. **C,** A guidewire is inserted and a dilator *(arrow)* is placed over the guidewire. **D,** Once the catheter-cannula is within the abscess, the guidewire and inner cannula are removed while the catheter is advanced and the pigtail is formed *(arrow).*

Drains in small, superficial abscess cavities can be pulled all at once whereas drains in large, deeper cavities may be gradually removed over a few days, which promotes healing by secondary intention.

Specific Anatomic Applications

Liver. Percutaneous catheter drainage is considered the initial treatment of choice for **pyogenic liver abscesses** (see Fig. 17-17). Pyogenic liver abscesses are most often a secondary development of seeding from intestinal sources, such as appendicitis or diverticulitis; as a direct extension from cholecystitis or cholangitis; or secondary to operation or trauma. Like abscesses elsewhere in the body, the sonographic appearance of hepatic abscesses is usually one of a complex fluid collection. Both ultrasonography and CT pro-

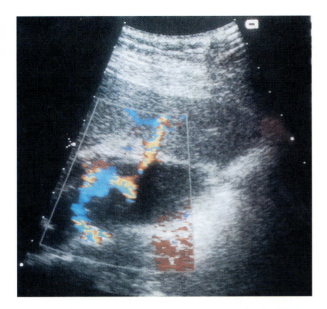

FIG. 17-18. Catheter visualization aided by color flow Doppler imaging. Transverse color Doppler image of percutaneous cholecystotomy tube demonstrates flow in catheter during aspiration that improves catheter visualization.

vide excellent guidance for percutaneous drainage of hepatic abscesses. The cure rate ranges from 67% to 90%.[122-124] Complications of percutaneous hepatic abscess drainage include sepsis, hemorrhage, and catheter transgression of the pleura. Because of these complications, some authors have recently suggested treating pyogenic liver abscesses with antibiotics and percutaneous needle aspiration, without catheter drainage.[125]

Most intrahepatic **amebic** abscesses are treated with metronidazole with 85% to 90% success.[126] However, percutaneous abscess drainage of amebic abscesses is indicated if the diagnosis is uncertain, the patient is not responding to medical treatment, or there are signs of abscess cavity rupture.[125] Catheter drainage in these situations is safe and generally provides a rapid cure; the catheter can often be removed within a few days.[115,126,127]

Previously, hepatic abscesses infected with **Echinococcus** organisms were considered a contraindication to percutaneous abscess drainage because of the concern about anaphylaxis. More recently, these abscesses have not only been percutaneously drained safely but have also been successfully treated with transcatheter sclerotherapy.[128,129]

Abdominal and Pelvic Abscesses. Most abdominal and pelvic abscesses are secondary to operation or related to underlying bowel abnormality. Percutaneous abscess drainage for postoperative abdominal abscesses has become the accepted primary treatment of choice, with cure being the procedural

goal.[115] More recently, percutaneous abscess drainage has played a principal role in the treatment of **diverticular, appendiceal,** and **Crohn's** related abscesses.[130-136] Drainage of abscesses in these acutely ill patients can help alleviate sepsis and permit the necessary curative surgical treatment on an elective basis.

Drainage of abdominal abscesses is often best performed with CT guidance, which allows for the best visualization of adjacent bowel loops, thereby avoiding traversing bowel. CT also provides an overview of the entire abdomen, which is essential to be certain that all collections are drained. Ultrasonography can also provide excellent guidance for percutaneous abscess drainage; however, careful review of CT scans assists in planning an approach free of intervening bowel. Ultrasonography is especially valuable in the treatment of critically ill patients who are not able to be transported to the radiology department.[137]

Pelvic abscesses are of variable origin and have been notoriously difficult to access because of their deep location, overlying bowel, blood vessels, bony pelvis, and bladder. Traditional approaches include an anterior transperineal approach or a posterior transgluteal approach. The transgluteal approach is relatively painful, and care must be taken to avoid the sciatic nerve. Small, deep, pelvic abscesses may be difficult to access safely via traditional approaches.

Experience with **ultrasound-guided transrectal and transvaginal drainage** is growing, and these techniques appear to be effective and well-tolerated procedures in appropriate patients[138-144] (Fig. 17-19). Needle guides are available for endovaginal probes that help guide the needle into the fluid collection. The use of the Seldinger technique (as opposed to the trocar method) and the combination of ultrasound and fluoroscopic guidance have been found by some authors to improve the technical ease of transvaginal and transrectal ultrasound drainage.[141,143,145] For nonpurulent collections, immediate catheter drainage is not necessarily indicated; most of these patients respond to a one-step aspiration, lavage, and antibiotic therapy based on results of cultures of the aspirates.[143,144] In regard to **tuboovarian abscesses,** ultrasound-guided transvaginal drainage has also been shown to be a successful alternative to operation in patients who fail standard initial antibiotic treatment.[141,146]

Enteric abscesses often have **communication** with the gastrointestinal tract. For these abscesses to be drained successfully, one must first recognize that a communication exists, and the communication must be allowed to close before removal of the catheter.[115] Fistulas will not close if there is distal obstruction, tumor, or persistent infection. Unfortunately, even with the most aggressive techniques, success in treating abscesses with communication is lower than for noncommunicating abscesses.[122,147]

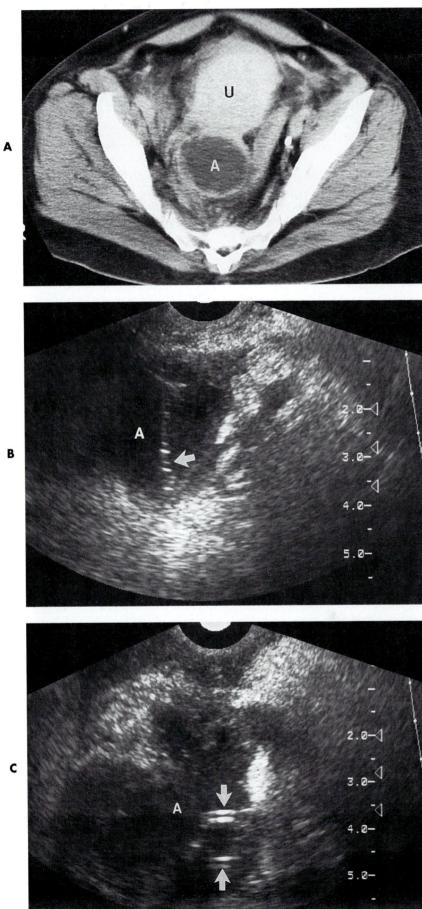

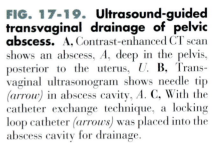

FIG. 17-19. Ultrasound-guided transvaginal drainage of pelvic abscess. A, Contrast-enhanced CT scan shows an abscess, *A,* deep in the pelvis, posterior to the uterus, *U.* **B,** Transvaginal ultrasonogram shows needle tip *(arrow)* in abscess cavity, *A.* **C,** With the catheter exchange technique, a locking loop catheter *(arrows)* was placed into the abscess cavity for drainage.

Gallbladder

Gallbladder Aspirate. Gallbladder aspiration is used as a method of diagnosis of acute cholecystitis in the hospitalized patient. With ultrasound guidance, a 22 gauge needle is placed transhepatically into the gallbladder (Fig. 17-20). A small amount of bile is aspirated and an immediate Gram stain is performed; the remaining bile is sent for culture. The needle is then removed. If the Gram stain demonstrates bacteria or leukocytes or bile culture reveals bacteriologic growth, this is thought to indicate gallbladder inflammation associated with acute cholecystitis.[148] Subsequently, it was shown that a positive result of gallbladder aspiration indicates acute cholecystitis with a specificity of 87%, but there is a low sensitivity (< 50%) of a gallbladder aspirate in predicting acute cholecystitis in the hospitalized patient.[149] Therefore a negative aspirate result does not exclude the diagnosis of acute cholecystitis. It is reasoned that a sterile aspirate occurs in patients with acute cholecystitis because the patients, while septic, are receiving concomitant, multiple, intravenous antibiotic administration, rendering the bile sterile. These early studies demonstrated the safety of percutaneous gallbladder aspiration.

More recently, Swobodnik et al.[150] reported that gallbladder aspiration has been used to classify gallstones as either pigmented or cholesterol stones. Fine-needle puncture of the gallbladder with ultrasound guidance was performed in 118 symptomatic patients with gallstones. Gallbladder puncture was success-

fully performed at the first attempt using a 22 gauge needle and continuous ultrasound guidance in all patients. Aspirate volume varied between 3 and 88 ml. Biliary analysis found an increase of the cholesterol saturation index in patients with cholesterol gallstones relative to that of patients with pigmented gallstones. Also, nucleation time was prolonged in patients with pigmented stones to 19.3 days compared with 1.8 days for patients with cholesterol stones. These values were statistically significant. These authors think that diagnostic percutaneous gallbladder aspiration is a safe and valuable technique in the diagnostic work-up of gallstone patients to determine their suitability for nonoperative treatment.

Tudyka et al.[151] also performed bile sampling of the gallbladder fluid in 207 patients with gallstones. Again, a 22 gauge needle was inserted into the gallbladder using continuous real-time guidance. There were no major complications such as bleeding, bile leak, or inflammation in any of the patients. They performed bacteriologic tests and culture and sensitivity tests and analyzed bile lipids, cholesterol saturation index, and total lipid concentration in all these patients. They also thought that fine-needle puncture of the gallbladder represented an important diagnostic procedure in evaluation of cholelithiasis that is easily performed without major side effects by an experienced physician.

Percutaneous Cholecystostomy. Cholecystectomy is the accepted method of treatment of both acute and chronic **cholecystitis**. Although elective cholecystectomy for chronic cholecystitis is associated with a low mortality, there are conflicting reports concerning the management of patients with acute cholecystitis, especially with reference to optimal time for intervention. Some surgeons prefer emergency cholecystectomy, but others advocate delaying cholecystectomy until the patient is in a less toxic condition. Emergency cholecystectomy has been shown to have a mortality rate as high as 19% in the elderly.[152] This high mortality is most certainly a reflection of not only the cholecystitis but also the poor overall medical condition of these patients. Emergency surgical cholecystostomy has been championed as a lifesaving, although temporizing, procedure in the elderly, debilitated, or critically ill patient who presents too great a surgical or anesthetic risk for formal cholecystectomy. Surgical cholecystostomy is a simpler procedure than cholecystectomy, yet it too may be associated with high mortality because of the underlying medical problems in this group of patients.[153] A major advantage of ultrasound-guided cholecystostomy is that the procedure may be performed at the patient's bedside. Thus critically ill patients need not be moved to surgery or the radiology department, which offers an alternative to surgical cholecystectomy in critically ill patients.

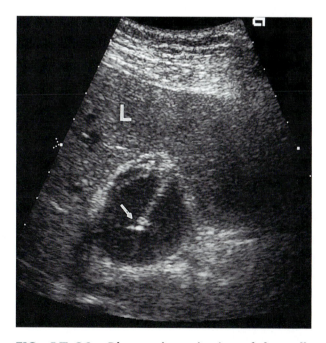

FIG. 17-20. Diagnostic aspiration of the gallbladder. By using the freehand technique, a 22 gauge needle *(arrow)* is passed transhepatically into the gallbladder. The stylet is removed and the bile is aspirated under ultrasound guidance. *L,* Liver.

A review of 182 percutaneous ultrasound-guided cholecystostomies indicates that **complications** are few; there were 14 technical problems or complications (7%) and 1 reported death.[154] Many of the technical problems were due to dislodgment of early catheters designed without a securing device. Newer catheters include some type of securing device. The Hawkins accordion catheter, a self-retaining catheter, may be placed using a coaxial technique after initial puncture with a 22 gauge needle.[155,156] The McGahan drainage catheter set has a distal Cope loop to prevent catheter dislodgment (see Fig. 17-15).[156,157] The catheter is easily placed with ultrasound guidance using a transhepatic route by either the trocar method or guidewire exchange technique (see Fig. 17-16).

More recently, reports have validated the safety and effectiveness of percutaneous cholecystostomy for the treatment of **acute acalculus cholecystitis.** Browning et al.[158] published a report of percutaneous cholecystostomy attempted on 50 occasions in 49 patients. Percutaneous cholecystostomy was successful in 49 of 50 catheter placements (98%), and 40 of the 50 cholecystostomies (80%) were performed at the patients' bedside. There was clinical improvement in 63% of the patients based on a 72-hour decrease in temperature to less than 37.3°C, normalization of leukocyte count, and a resolution of abdominal pain. Similarly, Boland et al.[159] reviewed their experience of percutaneous cholecystostomy in 82 critically ill patients. They also found that this was a successful technique, and there was dramatic improvement in 48 patients (59%) within 48 hours. Browning et al.[158] and Boland et al.[159] felt that acute cholecystitis is difficult to diagnose in hospitalized patients and that percutaneous cholecystostomy serves as a diagnostic and a therapeutic maneuver in these patients. It is a safe and effective method to clear the gallbladder as a potential source of sepsis in these patients.[159]

There are several other applications for percutaneous cholecystostomy, including drainage of the biliary system in patients with failed transhepatic biliary drainage. The cystic duct must be patent to provide a route of drainage for the rest of the biliary system.[156] Percutaneous cholecystostomy may be used as an alternative; it is a less invasive procedure than transhepatic cholangiography or drainage in patients in whom transhepatic cholangiography or drainage is difficult or unsuccessful. Creasy et al.[160] performed percutaneous transperitoneal cholecystostomy in 44 patients. In those patients in whom there was not cystic duct obstruction, **antegrade cholecystography** was successful in visualizing the common bile duct in all but 2 patients (Fig. 17-21). This technique was successful in visualizing common duct calculi in 8 of 9 patients. They felt that antegrade cholecystography is an easy and safe method for not only visual-

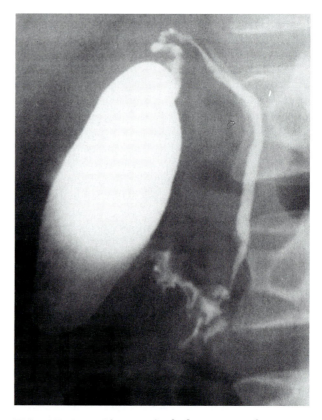

FIG. 17-21. Diagnostic cholecystography. Cholangiogram performed after gallbladder puncture demonstrates preferential flow of contrast medium into the common duct rather than intrahepatic ducts in this nonobstructed system. (From McGahan JP. Gallbladder. In: McGahan JP, ed. *Interventional Ultrasound.* Baltimore: Williams & Wilkins; 1990.)

izing the gallbladder anatomy but also evaluating the common duct for associated biliary ductal problems or common duct calculi.

Previously, percutaneous cholecystostomy was used as a method to access the gallbladder for treatment of cholelithiasis by **contact stone dissolution, basket removal,** or **percutaneous fragmentation** of stones.[161-165] However, these methods are less frequently used,[164] but in situations in which they are used, ultrasound may serve as a guidance method for gallbladder access.

Biliary Tract

Percutaneous Transhepatic Drainage. Percutaneous transhepatic cholangiography and drainage is traditionally performed using "blind" cholangiography with fluoroscopy for initial needle placement. However, the combined use of sonography for the initial needle puncture and fluoroscopy for final catheter placement via the guidewire exchange technique optimizes the advantages of both guidance systems for performance of percutaneous transhepatic cholangiography, biliary drainage, and other invasive procedures.[117] Selected ducts may be punctured under ultrasound guidance for percutaneous transhepatic cholangiography or as the site of definitive catheter placement. In patients with segmental biliary obstruction, a "blind" technique allows initial opacification of the biliary system only by chance. However, sonography may allow direct puncture of the appropriate biliary duct. Some authors have advocated the use of ultrasound alone for percutaneous transhepatic biliary drainage.[166] These authors used complete ultrasound guidance for percutaneous transhepatic cholangiography and drainage in patients with hilar cholangiocarcinoma. Ultrasound guidance was successful for percutaneous puncture and drainage in these patients. There was only one major complication in this group in which one patient with ascites and severe cholangitis had bacterial peritonitis.[166]

Pancreas

Pancreatic Fluid. There are several different terms for pancreatic inflammatory fluid collections or masses.[117] **Peripancreatic fluid collections** without mature walls may develop during an episode of acute pancreatitis. Many of these disappear spontaneously. Ultrasound-guided needle aspiration may be used to determine if these fluid collections are infected. After an episode of acute pancreatitis, a mature fibrous wall develops around a fluid collection; this is best termed a **"pancreatic pseudocyst."** Needle aspiration may be used to determine if it is sterile or infected. There is a high rate of recurrence of pancreatic pseudocysts with simple aspiration.

However, vanSonnenberg et al.[167] published their experience with percutaneous drainage of pseudocysts with excellent results. The overall cure rate by catheter drainage alone was 90.1%; this includes 48 of 51 infected pseudocysts (94%) and 43 of 50 noninfected pseudocysts (86%). In most of these patients, CT rather than sonography was the primary method of guidance, although sonography may be used for guidance of drainage (Fig. 17-22). While vanSonnenberg et al.[167] most commonly used the transperitoneal or retroperitoneal route for drainage, others[168] have advocated use of transgastric drainage of pseudocysts.

Kumar et al.[169] published their work with 57 patients, comparing CT to ultrasonography in evaluation and percutaneous intervention in patients with acute pancreatitis. Although CT was thought to be superior to ultrasonography in evaluation of acute pancreatitis, ultrasonography was thought to provide easy guidance for percutaneous interventional procedures, such as fluid aspiration, in these patients.

Pancreatic necrosis deserves special consideration. Large areas of pancreatic necrosis with surrounding fluid collections require surgical debridement. Percutaneous drainage may be temporizing in drainage of the surrounding fluid collections but is not curative. Pancreatic phlegmons develop after pancreatic necrosis and inflammation of the pancreatic tissues and are also not amenable to catheter drainage. Ultrasound may be used to guide needle aspiration of fluid in these situations to check if the fluid is infected. **Pancreatic abscesses** may be treated with percutaneous drainage.[167,168]

Pancreatography. Ultrasound may be used to guide percutaneous aspiration and opacification of the pancreatic ductal system. Chong et al.[170] reviewed their experience with ultrasound-guided percutaneous pancreatography. Percutaneous pancreatography was attempted in 63 patients with chronic pancreatitis. In 52 of these patients, endoscopic retrograde pancreatography was unsuccessful or did not completely visualize all of the pancreatic duct. Therefore percutaneous pancreatography under ultrasound guidance was attempted. Percutaneous ultrasound-guided pancreatography was successful in 54 of 63 patients (86%). The percutaneous procedure clearly mapped the full ductal anatomy, depicted the relationship of the ducts with peripancreatic fluid collections that were noted on CT or ultrasonography, and allowed ease of duct drainage after injection of contrast medium. These authors felt that this technique was safe and provided additional imaging information in patients with chronic pancreatitis.

Kidney

Renal Cyst Sclerosis. There have been a small number of publications regarding ultrasound-guided renal cyst puncture with cyst sclerosis. Zama[171] (26 renal cysts) and Nishimura et al.[172] (69 renal cyst punctures) used absolute alcohol as a sclerosing agent after a cyst puncture under ultrasound guidance.

Perinephric Abscess or Fluid Collections. Fluid collections that occur in the retroperitoneal space include abscesses, urinomas, lymphoceles, and hematomas. CT is usually performed to identify the fluid collection and its extent. Either ultrasonography or CT may be used for aspiration or drainage of these fluid collections. Perinephric fluid aspirations are performed in a fashion similar to renal cyst aspiration. If drainage is needed, the Seldinger technique may be used with sonography for initial needle placement and fluoroscopy for catheter placement (Fig. 17-23).

Text continued on p. 624

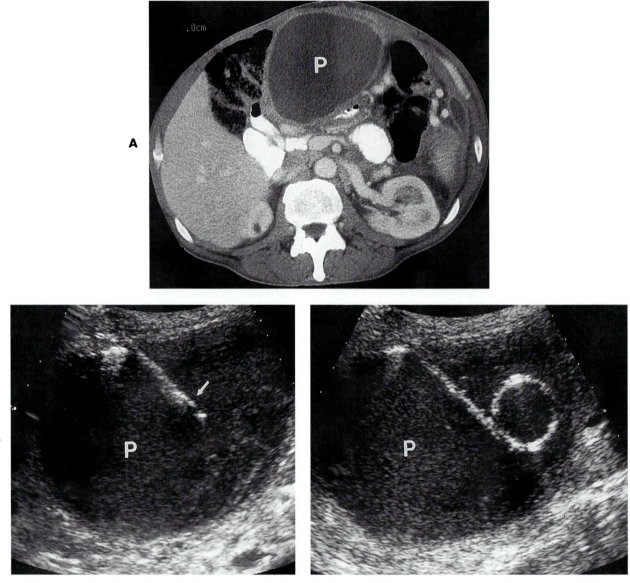

FIG. 17-22. Ultrasound-guided pancreatic pseudocyst drainage. A, Contrast-enhanced CT scan shows a large fluid collection (*P,* pseudocyst) anterior and superior to the pancreas. **B,** Sonogram shows aspiration needle *(arrow)* in the pseudocyst, which contains echogenic debris. **C,** With the catheter exchange technique, a locking loop catheter was placed into pancreatic pseudocyst for drainage.

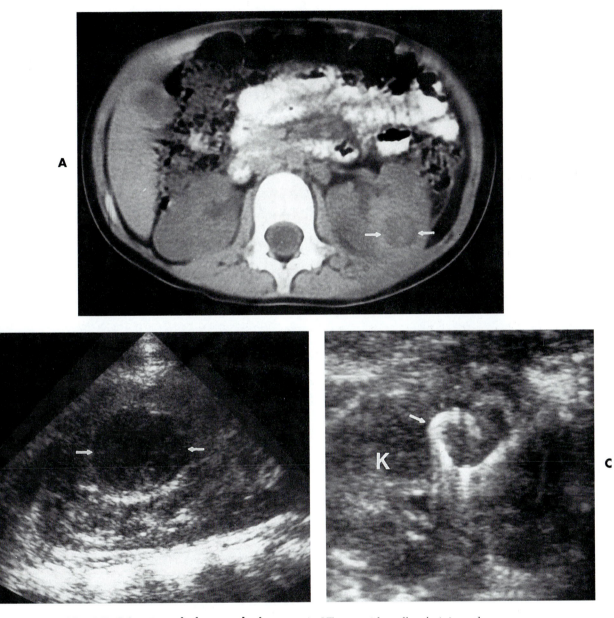

FIG. 17-23. **Renal abscess drainage.** **A,** CT scan with orally administered contrast material shows only a small 2.5 cm, low-attenuating mass *(arrows)* in the midleft kidney. **B,** Longitudinal ultrasonogram of the left kidney shows a 2.5 cm cystic mass with internal debris *(arrows)*. **C,** Transverse image of the kidney, *K.* With the Seldinger technique, a locking loop catheter *(arrow)* was placed into the renal abscess.

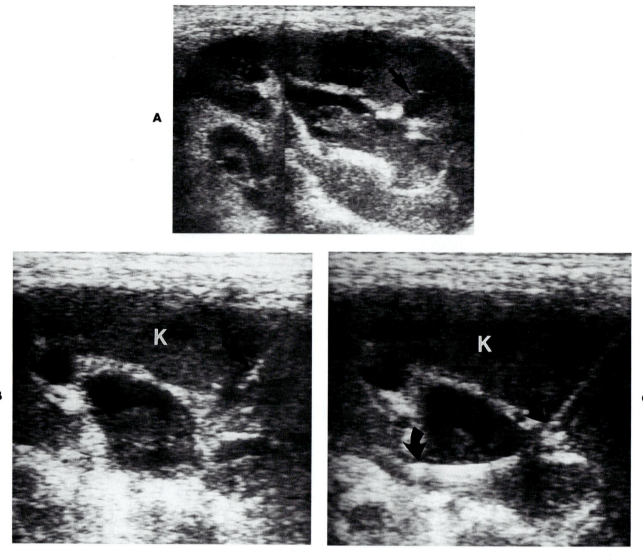

FIG. 17-24. **Ultrasound-guided percutaneous nephrostomy.** **A,** Longitudinal sonogram shows pyelocaliectasis with debris in renal collecting system. The dilated calyx in the lower pole *(arrow)* would be optimal for nephrostomy access. **B,** Longitudinal sonogram shows the needle tip *(arrow)* in the dilated lower pole calyx. *K*, Kidney. **C,** After a guidewire is advanced into the renal collecting system, the catheter *(arrows)* is placed in the renal pelvis by the Seldinger technique.

Percutaneous nephrostomy. Recently, sonography has gained wide acceptance as the imaging modality for initial needle placement for percutaneous nephrostomy (Fig. 17-24). After the dilated collecting system is accessed, a catheter is placed via the Seldinger technique using fluoroscopic control.[173] Saitoh[174] demonstrated that color flow Doppler imaging is useful in supplementing ultrasound guidance in renal biopsies, nephrostomies, and renal cyst punctures. Puncture of intrarenal vessels could be avoided by using color flow Doppler imaging in performance of interventional procedures.

REFERENCES
Ultrasound-Guided Biopsy

1. Bernardino ME. Percutaneous biopsy. *AJR* 1984;142:41-45.
2. Grant EG, Richardson JD, Smirniotopoulos JG et al. Fine-needle biopsy directed by real-time sonography: technique and accuracy. *AJR* 1983;141:29-32.
3. Gazelle GS, Haaga JR. Guided percutaneous biopsy of intraabdominal lesions. *AJR* 1989;153:929-935.
4. Matalon TA, Silver B. US guidance of interventional procedures. *Radiology* 1990;174:43-47.
5. Charboneau JW, Reading CC, Welsh TJ. CT and sonographically guided needle biopsy: current techniques and new innovations. *AJR* 1990;154:1-10.

6. Reading CC, Charboneau JW, James EM et al. Sonographically guided percutaneous biopsy of small (3 cm or less) masses. *AJR* 1988;151:189-192.

7. Mitty HA, Efremidis SC, Yeh HC. Impact of fine-needle biopsy on management of patients with carcinoma of the pancreas. *AJR* 1981;137:1119-1121.

8. Bret PM, Fond A, Casola G et al. Abdominal lesions: a prospective study of clinical efficacy of percutaneous fine-needle biopsy. *Radiology* 1986;159:345-346.

9. Downey DB, Wilson SR. Ultrasonographically guided biopsy of small intra-abdominal masses. *Can Assoc Radiol J* 1993;44:350-353.

10. Spamer C, Brambs HJ, Koch HK et al. Benign circumscribed lesions of the liver diagnosed by ultrasonically guided fine-needle biopsy. *J Clin Ultrasound* 1986;14:83-88.

11. Rapaport SI. Preoperative hemostatic evaluation: which tests, if any? *Blood* 1983;61:229-231.

12. Silverman SG, Mueller PR, Pfister RC. Hemostatic evaluation before abdominal interventions: an overview and proposal. *AJR* 1990;154:233-238.

13. Murphy TP, Dorfman GS, Becker J. Use of preprocedural tests by interventional radiologists. *Radiology* 1993;186:213-220.

14. Rapaport SI. Assessing hemostatic function before abdominal interventions. *AJR* 1990;154:239-240.

15. Zins M, Vilgrain V, Gayno S et al. US-guided percutaneous liver biopsy with plugging of the needle track: a prospective study in 72 high-risk patients. *Radiology* 1992;184:841-843.

16. Crummy AB, McDermott JC, Wojtowycz M. A technique for embolization of biopsy tracts. *AJR* 1989;153:67-68.

17. Brandt KR, Charboneau JW, Stephens DH et al. CT- and US-guided biopsy of the pancreas. *Radiology* 1993;187:99-104.

18. Murphy FB, Barefield KP, Steinberg HV et al. CT- or sonography-guided biopsy of the liver in the presence of ascites: frequency of complications. *AJR* 1988;151:485-486.

19. Little AF, Ferris JV, Dodd GD III et al. Image-guided percutaneous hepatic biopsy: effect of ascites on the complication rate. *Radiology* 1996;199:79-83.

20. McGahan JP, Anderson MW. Pulsed Doppler sonography as an aid in ultrasound-guided aspiration biopsy. *Gastrointest Radiol* 1987;12:279-284.

21. Longo JM, Bilbao JI, Barettino MD et al. Percutaneous vascular and nonvascular puncture under US guidance: role of color Doppler imaging. *RadioGraphics* 1994;14:959-972.

22. Welch TJ, Sheedy PF II, Johnson CD et al. CT-guided biopsy: prospective analysis of 1,000 procedures. *Radiology* 1989;171:493-496.

23. Isler RJ, Ferrucci JT Jr, Wittenberg J et al. Tissue core biopsy of abdominal tumors with a 22 gauge cutting needle. *AJR* 1981;136:725-728.

24. Wittenberg J, Mueller PR, Ferrucci JT Jr et al. Percutaneous core biopsy of abdominal tumors using 22 gauge needles: further observations. *AJR* 1982;139:75-80.

25. Andriole JG, Haaga JR, Adams RB et al. Biopsy needle characteristics assessed in the laboratory. *Radiology* 1983;148:659-662.

26. Lieberman RP, Hafez GR, Crummy AB. Histology from aspiration biopsy: Turner needle experience. *AJR* 1982;138:561-564.

27. Pagani JJ. Biopsy of focal hepatic lesions. Comparison of 18 and 22 gauge needles. *Radiology* 1983;147:673-675.

28. Haaga JR, LiPuma JP, Bryan PJ et al. Clinical comparison of small- and large-caliber cutting needles for biopsy. *Radiology* 1983;146:665-667.

29. Ubhi CS, Irving HC, Guillou PJ et al. A new technique for renal allograft biopsy. *Br J Radiol* 1987;60:599-600.

30. Erwin BC, Brynes RK, Chan WC et al. Percutaneous needle biopsy in the diagnosis and classification of lymphoma. *Cancer* 1986;57:1074-1078.

31. Jennings PE, Donald JJ, Coral A et al. Ultrasound-guided core biopsy. *Lancet* 1989;1:1369-1371.

32. Parker SH, Hopper KD, Yakes WF et al. Image-directed percutaneous biopsies with a biopsy gun. *Radiology* 1989;171:663-669.

33. Hopper KD, Baird DE, Reddy VV et al. Efficacy of automated biopsy guns versus conventional biopsy needles in the pygmy pig. *Radiology* 1990;176:671-676.

34. Poster RB, Jones DB, Spirt BA. Percutaneous pediatric renal biopsy: use of the biopsy gun. *Radiology* 1990;176:725-727.

35. Elvin A, Andersson T, Scheibenpflug L et al. Biopsy of the pancreas with a biopsy gun. *Radiology* 1990;176:677-679.

36. Parker SH, Lovin JD, Jobe WE et al. Sterotactic breast biopsy with a biopsy gun. *Radiology* 1990;176:741-747.

37. Nelson DL, Reading CC, Welch TJ et al. Complications of percutaneous needle biopsy: a prospective study employing both large- and fine-needle techniques. (In preparation).

38. Miller DL, Wall RT. Fentanyl and diazepam for analgesia and sedation during radiologic special procedures. *Radiology* 1987;162:195-198.

39. Hurlbert BJ, Landers DF. Sedation and analgesia for interventional radiologic procedures in adults. *Semin Interven Radiol* 1987;4:151-160.

40. Caturelli E, Giacobbe A, Facciorusso D et al. Free-hand technique with ordinary antisepsis in abdominal US-guided fine-needle punctures: three-year experience. *Radiology* 1996;199:721-723.

41. Rizzatto G, Solbiati L, Croce F et al. Aspiration biopsy of superficial lesions: ultrasonic guidance with a linear-array probe. *AJR* 1987;148:623-625.

42. Buonocore E, Skipper GJ. Steerable real-time sonographically guided needle biopsy. *AJR* 1981;136:387-392.

43. Reid MH. Real-time sonographic needle biopsy guide. *AJR* 1983;140:162-163.

44. Moulton JS, Moore PT. Coaxial percutaneous biopsy technique with automated biopsy devices: value in improving accuracy and negative predictive value. *Radiology* 1993;186:515-522.

45. Hahn PF, Eisenberg PJ, Pitman MB et al. Cytopathologic touch preparations (imprints) from core needle biopsies: accuracy compared with that of fine-needle aspirates. *AJR* 1995;165:1277-1279.

46. Miller DA, Carrasco CH, Katz RL et al. Fine needle aspiration biopsy: the role of immediate cytologic assessment. *AJR* 1986;147:155-158.

47. McNamara MP Jr, McNamara ME. Preparation of a home-made ultrasound biopsy phantom. *J Clin Ultrasound* 1989;17:456-458.

48. Fornage BD. A simple phantom for training in ultrasound-guided needle biopsy using the freehand technique. *J Ultrasound Med* 1989;8:701-703.

49. Georgian-Smith D, Shiels WE II. Freehand interventional sonography in the breast: basic principles and clinical applications. *RadioGraphics* 1996;16:149-161.

50. Heckemann R, Seidel KJ. The sonographic appearance and contrast enhancement of puncture needles. *J Clin Ultrasound* 1983;11:265-268.

51. McGahan JP. Laboratory assessment of ultrasonic needle and catheter visualization. *J Ultrasound Med* 1986;5:373-377.

52. Reading CC, Charboneau JW, Felmlee JP et al. US-guided percutaneous biopsy: use of a screw biopsy stylet to aid needle detection. *Radiology* 1987;163:280-281.

53. Hamper UM, Savader BL, Sheth S. Improved needle-tip visualization by color Doppler sonography. *AJR* 1991;156:401-402.

54. Cockburn JF, Cosgrove DO. Device to enhance visibility of needle or catheter tip at color Doppler US. *Radiology* 1995;195:570-572.

55. Bret PM, Sente JM, Bretagnolle M et al. Ultrasonically guided fine-needle biopsy in focal intrahepatic lesions: six years' experience. *Can Assoc Radiol J* 1986;37:5-8.

56. Buscarini L, Fornari F, Bolondi L et al. Ultrasound-guided fine-needle biopsy of focal liver lesions: techniques, diagnostic accuracy and complications: a retrospective study on 2091 biopsies. *J Hepatol* 1990;11:344-348.

57. Terriff BA, Gibney RG, Scudamore CH. Fatality from fine-needle aspiration biopsy of a hepatic hemangioma (letter to the editor). *AJR* 1990;154:203-204.

58. Solbiati L, Livraghi T, De Pra L et al. Fine-needle biopsy of hepatic hemangioma with sonographic guidance. *AJR* 1985;144:471-474.

59. Nakaizumi A, Iishi H, Yamamoto R et al. Diagnosis of hepatic cavernous hemangioma by fine needle aspiration biopsy under ultrasonic guidance. *Gastrointest Radiol* 1990;15:39-42.

60. Cronan JJ, Esparza AR, Dorfman GS et al. Cavernous hemangioma of the liver: role of percutaneous biopsy. *Radiology* 1988;166:135-138.

61. Caturelli E, Rapaccini GL, Sabelli C et al. Ultrasound-guided fine-needle aspiration biopsy in the diagnosis of hepatic hemangioma. *Liver* 1986;6:326-330.

62. Tung GA, Cronan JJ. Percutaneous needle biopsy of hepatic cavernous hemangioma. *J Clin Gastroenterol* 1993;16:117-122.

63. Dodd GD III, Carr BI. Percutaneous biopsy of portal vein thrombus: a new staging technique for hepatocellular carcinoma. *AJR* 1993;161:229-233.

64. Vilana R, Bru C, Bruix J et al. Fine-needle aspiration biopsy of portal vein thrombus: value in detecting malignant thrombosis. *AJR* 1993;160:1285-1287.

65. Lees WR, Hall-Craggs MA, Manhire A. Five years' experience of fine-needle aspiration biopsy: 454 consecutive cases. *Clin Radiol* 1985;36:517-520.

66. Hall-Craggs MA, Lees WR. Fine-needle aspiration biopsy: pancreatic and biliary tumors. *AJR* 1986;147:399-403.

67. Mitchell ML, Carney CN. Cytologic criteria for the diagnosis of pancreatic carcinoma. *Am J Clin Pathol* 1985;83:171-176.

68. Lewandrowski K, Lee J, Southern J et al. Cyst fluid analysis in the differential diagnosis of pancreatic cysts: a new approach to the preoperative assessment of pancreatic cystic lesions. *AJR* 1995;164:815-819.

69. Yong WH, Southern JF, Pins MR et al. Cyst fluid NB/70K concentration and leukocyte esterase: two new markers for differentiating pancreatic serous tumors from pseudocysts. *Pancreas* 1995;10:342-346.

70. Carlson S, Johnson CD. Biopsy of cystic pancreatic neoplasms. (In press).

71. Smith EH. Complications of percutaneous abdominal fine-needle biopsy. *Radiology* 1991;178:253-258.

72. Mueller PR, Miketic LM, Simeone JF et al. Severe acute pancreatitis after percutaneous biopsy of the pancreas. *AJR* 1988;151:493-494.

73. Warshaw AL, Fernandez-del Castillo C. Pancreatic carcinoma. *N Engl J Med* 1992;326:455-465.

74. Nadel L, Baumgartner BR, Bernardino ME. Percutaneous renal biopsies: accuracy, safety, and indications. *Urol Radiol* 1986;8:67-71.

75. Lindsay DJ, Lyons EA, Levi CS. Urinary tract. In: McGahan JP, ed. *Interventional Ultrasound*. Baltimore: Williams & Wilkins; 1990:199-210.

76. Clayman RV, Williams RD, Fraley EE. The pursuit of the renal mass. *N Engl J Med* 1979;300:72-74.

77. Yoshimoto M, Fujisawa S, Sudo M. Percutaneous renal biopsy well-visualized by orthogonal ultrasound application using linear scanning. *Clin Nephrol* 1988;30:106-110.

78. Rapaccini GL, Pompili M, Caturelli E et al. Real-time ultrasound guided renal biopsy in diffuse renal disease: 114 consecutive cases. *Surg Endosc* 1989;3:42-45.

79. Bogan ML, Kopecky KK, Kraft JL et al. Needle biopsy of renal allografts: comparison of two techniques. *Radiology* 1990;174:273-275.

80. Welch TJ, Sheedy PF II, Stephens DH et al. Percutaneous adrenal biopsy: review of a 10-year experience. *Radiology* 1994;193:341-344.

81. Dunnick NR. Hanson lecture. Adrenal imaging: current status. *AJR* 1990;154:927-936.

82. Dunnick NR, Heaston D, Halvorsen R et al. CT appearance of adrenal cortical carcinoma. *J Comput Assist Tomogr* 1982;6:978-982.

83. Bernardino ME. Management of the asymptomatic patient with a unilateral adrenal mass. *Radiology* 1988;166:121-123.

84. Casola G, Nicolet V, vanSonnenberg E et al. Unsuspected pheochromocytoma: risk of blood-pressure alterations during percutaneous adrenal biopsy. *Radiology* 1986;159:733-735.

85. McCorkell SJ, Niles NL. Fine-needle aspiration of catecholamine-producing adrenal masses: a possibly fatal mistake. *AJR* 1985;145:113-114.

86. Soderstrom N. How to use cytodiagnostic spleen puncture. *Acta Med Scand* 1976;199:1-5.

87. Jansson SE, Bondestam S, Heinonen E et al. Value of liver and spleen aspiration biopsy in malignant diseases when these organs show no signs of involvement in sonography. *Acta Med Scand* 1983;213:279-281.

88. Solbiati L, Bossi MC, Bellotti E et al. Focal lesions in the spleen: sonographic patterns and guided biopsy. *AJR* 1983;140:59-65.

89. Livraghi T, Damascelli B, Lombardi C et al. Risk in fine-needle abdominal biopsy. *J Clin Ultrasound* 1983;11:77-81.

90. Fornari F, Civardi G, Cavanna L et al. Complications of ultrasonically guided fine-needle abdominal biopsy. Results of a multicenter Italian study and review of the literature. The Cooperative Italian Study Group. *Scand J Gastroenterol* 1989;24:949-955.

91. Nolsoe C, Nielsen L, Torp-Pedersen S et al. Major complications and deaths due to interventional ultrasonography: a review of 8000 cases. *J Clin Ultrasound* 1990;18:179-184.

92. Ryd W, Hagmar B, Eriksson O. Local tumour cell seeding by fine-needle aspiration biopsy. A semiquantitative study. *Acta Pathol Microbiol Immunol Scand [A]* 1983;91:17-21.

93. Bergenfeldt M, Genell S, Lindholm K et al. Needle-tract seeding after percutaneous fine-needle biopsy of pancreatic carcinoma. Case report. *Acta Chir Scand* 1988;154:77-79.

94. Caturelli E, Rapaccini GL, Anti M et al. Malignant seeding after fine-needle aspiration biopsy of the pancreas. *Diagn Imag Clin Med* 1985;54:88-91.

95. Haddad FS, Somsin AA. Seeding and perineal implantation of prostatic cancer in the track of the biopsy needle: three case reports and a review of the literature. *J Surg Oncol* 1987;35:184-191.

96. Greenstein A, Merimsky E, Baratz M et al. Late appearance of perineal implantation of prostatic carcinoma after perineal needle biopsy. *Urology* 1989;33:59-60.

97. Onodera H, Oikawa M, Abe M et al. Cutaneous seeding of hepatocellular carcinoma after fine-needle aspiration biopsy. *J Ultrasound Med* 1987;6:273-275.

98. Kiser GC, Totonchy M, Barry JM. Needle tract seeding after percutaneous renal adenocarcinoma aspiration. *J Urol* 1986;136:1292-1293.

99. Muller NL, Bergin CJ, Miller RR et al. Seeding of malignant cells into the needle track after lung and pleural biopsy. *J Can Assoc Radiol* 1986;37:192-194.

100. Fajardo LL. Breast tumor seeding along localization guide wire tracks (letter to the editor). *Radiology* 1988;169:580-581.

101. Glasgow BJ, Brown HH, Zargoza AM et al. Quantitation of tumor seeding from fine needle aspiration of ocular melanomas. *Am J Ophthalmol* 1988;105:538-546.

102. Hidai H, Sakuramoto T, Miura T et al. Needle tract seeding following puncture of retroperitoneal liposarcoma. *Eur Urol* 1983;9:368-369.

103. Martino CR, Haaga JR, Bryan PJ et al. CT-guided liver biopsies: eight years' experience. Work in progress. *Radiology* 1984;152:755-757.

104. Reading CC. Ultrasound-guided percutaneous ethanol ablation of solid and cystic masses of the liver, kidney, thyroid, and parathyroid. *Ultrasound Quart* 1994;12:67-88.

105. Livraghi T, Vettori C. Percutaneous ethanol injection therapy of hepatoma. *Cardiovasc Intervent Radiol* 1990;13:146-152.

106. Shiina S, Tagawa K, Niwa Y et al. Percutaneous ethanol injection therapy for hepatocellular carcinoma: results in 146 patients. *AJR* 1993;160:1023-1028.

107. Livraghi T, Solbiati L. Percutaneous ethanol injection in liver cancer: method and results. *Semin Interven Radiol* 1993; 10:69-77.

108. McGahan JP, Schneider P, Brock JM et al. Treatment of liver tumors by percutaneous radiofrequency electrocautery. *Semin Interven Radiol* 1993;10:143-149.

109. Amin Z, Donald JJ, Masters A et al. Hepatic metastases: interstitial laser photocoagulation with real-time US monitoring and dynamic CT evaluation of treatment. *Radiology* 1993;187:339-347.

110. Nolsoe CP, Torp-Pedersen S, Burcharth F et al. Interstitial hyperthermia of colorectal liver metastases with a US-guided Nd-YAG laser with a diffuser tip: a pilot clinical study. *Radiology* 1993;187:333-337.

Ultrasound-Guided Drainage

111. Blady JV. Aspiration biopsy of tumors in obscure or difficult locations under roentgenoscopic guidance. *AJR* 1939;42:515-524.

112. Gronvall S, Gammelgaard J, Haubek A et al. Drainage of abdominal abscesses guided by sonography. *AJR* 1982;138:527-529.

113. Haaga JR, Alfidi RJ, Havrilla TR et al. CT detection and aspiration of abdominal abscesses. *AJR* 1977;128:465-474.

114. McGahan JP, Hanson F. Ultrasonographic aspiration and biopsy techniques. In: Dublin AB, ed. *Outpatient Invasive Radiologic Procedures: Diagnostic and Therapeutic.* Philadelphia: WB Saunders Co; 1989:79-113.

115. vanSonnenberg E, D'Agostino HB, Casola G et al. Percutaneous abscess drainage: current concepts. *Radiology* 1991;181:617-626.

116. Gazelle GS, Mueller PR. Abdominal abscess. Imaging and intervention. *Radiol Clin North Am* 1994;32:913-932.

117. McGahan JP, Raduns K. Biliary drainage using combined ultrasound fluoroscopic guidance. *J Intervent Radiol* 1990; 5:33-37.

118. McGahan JP. Aspiration and biopsy—advantages of sonographic guidance. In: McGahan JP, ed. *Controversies in Ultrasound: Clinics in Diagnostic Ultrasound.* New York: Churchill Livingstone; 1987;20:249-270.

119. McGahan JP, Brant WE. Principles, instrumentation, and guidance systems. In: McGahan JP, ed. *Interventional Ultrasound* Baltimore: Williams & Wilkins; 1990:1-20.

120. Deveney CW, Lurie K, Deveney KE. Improved treatment of intra-abdominal abscess. A result of improved localization, drainage, and patient care, not technique. *Arch Surg* 1988; 123:1126-1130.

121. Goldberg MA, Mueller PR, Saini S et al. Importance of daily rounds by the radiologist after interventional procedures of the abdomen and chest. *Radiology* 1991;180:767-770.

122. Lambiase RE, Deyoe L, Cronan JJ et al. Percutaneous drainage of 335 consecutive abscesses: results of primary drainage with 1-year follow-up. *Radiology* 1992;184:167-179.

123. Johnson RD, Mueller PR, Ferrucci JT Jr. et al. Percutaneous drainage of pyogenic liver abscesses. *AJR* 1985;144:463-467.

124. vanSonnenberg E, Mueller PR, Ferrucci JT Jr. Percutaneous drainage of 250 abdominal abscesses and fluid collections. Pt I. Results, failures, and complications. *Radiology* 1984; 151:337-341.

125. Giorgio A, Tarantino L, Mariniello N et al. Pyogenic liver abscesses: 13 years of experience in percutaneous needle aspiration with US guidance. *Radiology* 1995;195:122-124.

126. vanSonnenberg E, Mueller PR, Schiffman HR. Intrahepatic amebic abscesses: indications and results of percutaneous catheter drainage. *Radiology* 1985;156:631-635.

127. Van Allan RJ, Katz MD, Johnson MB et al. Uncomplicated amebic liver abscess: prospective evaluation of percutaneous therapeutic aspiration. *Radiology* 1992;183:827-830.

128. Filice C, Pirola F, Brunetti E et al. A new therapeutic approach for hydatid liver cysts. Aspiration and alcohol injection under sonographic guidance. *Gastroenterology* 1990; 98:1366-1368.

129. Khuroo MS, Zargar SA, Mahajan R. *Echinococcus granulosus* cysts in the liver: management with percutaneous drainage. *Radiology* 1991;180:141-145.

130. Casola G, vanSonnenberg E, Neff CC et al. Abscesses in Crohn disease: percutaneous drainage. *Radiology* 1987; 163:19-22.

131. Safrit HD, Mauro MA, Jaques PF. Percutaneous abscess drainage in Crohn's disease. *AJR* 1987;148:859-862.

132. Mueller PR, Saini S, Wittenburg J et al. Sigmoid diverticular abscesses: percutaneous drainage as an adjunct to surgical resection in 24 cases. *Radiology* 1987;164:321-325.

133. Stabile BE, Puccio E, vanSonnenberg E et al. Preoperative percutaneous drainage of diverticular abscesses. *Am J Surg* 1990;159:99-104.

134. Neff CC, vanSonnenberg E, Casola G et al. Diverticular abscesses: percutaneous drainage. *Radiology* 1987;163:15-18.

135. vanSonnenberg E, Wittich GR, Casola G et al. Periappendiceal abscesses: percutaneous drainage. *Radiology* 1987;163:23-26.

136. Jeffrey RB Jr, Tolentino CS, Federle MP et al. Percutaneous drainage of periappendiceal abscesses: review of 20 patients. *AJR* 1987;149:59-62.

137. McGahan JP, Anderson MW, Walter JP. Portable real-time sonographic and needle guidance systems for aspiration and drainage. *AJR* 1986;147:1241-1246.

138. Nosher JL, Needell GS, Amorosa JK et al. Transrectal pelvic abscess drainage with sonographic guidance. *AJR* 1986; 146:1047-1048.

139. Nosher JL, Winchman HK, Needell GS. Transvaginal pelvic abscess drainage with US guidance. *Radiology* 1987;165: 872-873.

140. Abbitt PL, Goldwag S, Urbanski S. Endovaginal sonography for guidance in draining pelvic fluid collections. *AJR* 1990;154:849-850.

141. vanSonnenberg E, D'Agostino HB, Casola G et al. US-guided transvaginal drainage of pelvic abscesses and fluid collections. *Radiology* 1991;181:53-56.

142. Alexander AA, Eschelman DJ, Nazarian LN et al. Transrectal sonographically guided drainage of deep pelvic abscesses. *AJR* 1994;162:1227-1230.

143. Feld R, Eschelman DJ, Sagerman JE et al. Treatment of pelvic abscesses and other fluid collections: efficacy of transvaginal sonographically guided aspiration and drainage. *AJR* 1994;163:1141-1145.

144. Kuligowska E, Keller E, Ferrucci JT. Treatment of pelvic abscesses: value of one-step sonographically guided transrectal needle aspiration and lavage. *AJR* 1995;164:201-206.

145. Kastan DJ, Nelsen KM, Shetty PC et al. Combined transrectal sonographic and fluoroscopic guidance for deep pelvic abscess drainage. *J Ultrasound Med* 1996;15:235-239.

146. Nelson AL, Sinow RM, Renslo R et al. Endovaginal ultrasonographically guided transvaginal drainage for treatment of pelvic abscesses. *Am J Obstet Gynecol* 1995;172:1926-1932.

147. Schuster MR, Crummy AB, Wojtowycz MM et al. Abdominal abscesses associated with enteric fistulas: percutaneous management. *J Vasc Intervent Radiol* 1992;3:359-363.

148. McGahan JP, Walter JP. Diagnostic percutaneous aspiration of the gallbladder. *Radiology* 1985;155:619-622.

149. McGahan JP, Lindfors KK. Acute cholecystitis: diagnostic accuracy of percutaneous aspiration of the gallbladder. *Radiology* 1988;167:669-671.

150. Swobodnik W, Hagert N, Janowitz P et al. Diagnostic fine-needle puncture of the gallbladder with US guidance. *Radiology* 1991;178:755-758.

151. Tudyka J, Kratzer W, Kuhn K et al. Diagnostic value of fine-needle puncture of the gallbladder: side effects, safety, and prognostic value. *Hepatology* 1995;21:1303-1307.

152. Houghton PW, Jenkinson LR, Donaldson LA. Cholecystectomy in the elderly: a prospective study. *Br J Surg* 1985;72:220-222.

153. Jurkovich GJ, Dyess DL, Ferrara JJ. Cholecystostomy. Expected outcome in primary and secondary biliary disorders. *Am Surg* 1988;54:40-44.

154. McGahan JP, Lindfors KK. Percutaneous cholecystostomy: an alternative to surgical cholecystostomy for acute cholecystitis? *Radiology* 1989;173:481-485.

155. Hawkins IF Jr. Percutaneous cholecystostomy. *Semin Intervent Radiol* 1985;2:97-103.

156. McGahan JP. Gallbladder. In: McGahan JP, ed. *Interventional Ultrasound*. Baltimore: Williams & Wilkins; 1990:159-170.

157. McGahan JP. A new catheter design for percutaneous cholecystostomy. *Radiology* 1988;166:49-52.

158. Browning PD, McGahan JP, Gerscovich EO. Percutaneous cholecystostomy for suspected acute cholecystitis in the hospitalized patient. *J Vasc Intervent Radiol* 1993;4:531-538.

159. Boland GW, Lee MJ, Leung J et al. Percutaneous cholecystostomy in critically ill patients: early response and final outcome in 82 patients. *AJR* 1994;163:339-342.

160. Creasy TS, Gronvall S, Stage JG. Assessment of the biliary tract by antegrade cholecystography after percutaneous cholecystostomy in patients with acute cholecystitis. *Br J Radiol* 1993;66:662-666.

161. Donald JJ, Cheslyn-Curtis S, Gillams AR et al. Percutaneous cholecystolithotomy: is gall stone recurrence inevitable? *Gut* 1994;35:692-695.

162. Lux G, Ell C, Hochberger J et al. The first successful endoscopic retrograde laser lithotripsy of common bile duct stones in man using a pulsed neodymium-YAG laser. *Endoscopy* 1986;18:144-145.

163. Martin EC, Wolff M, Neff RA et al. Use of the electrohydraulic lithotriptor in the biliary tree in dogs. *Radiology* 1981;139:215-217.

164. May GR, Thistle JL. Percutaneous cholecystostomy for gallstone dissolution by methyl tert-butyl ether (scientific program). *Radiology* 1986;161(P):90.

165. Gillams A, Donald JJ, Russell RC et al. The percutaneous rotary lithotrite: a new approach to the treatment of symptomatic cholecystolithiasis. *Gut* 1993;34:837-842.

166. Lameris JS, Hesselink EJ, Van Leeuwen PA et al. Ultrasound-guided percutaneous transhepatic cholangiography and drainage in patients with hilar cholangiocarcinoma. *Semin Liver Dis* 1990;10:121-125.

167. vanSonnenberg E, Wittich GR, Casola G et al. Percutaneous drainage of infected and noninfected pancreatic pseudocysts: experience in 101 cases. *Radiology* 1989;170:757-761.

168. Bret PM. Pancreas. In: McGahan JP, ed. *Interventional Ultrasound*. Baltimore: Williams & Wilkins; 1990:171-192.

169. Kumar P, Mukhopadhyay S, Sandhu M et al. Ultrasonography, computed tomography and percutaneous intervention in acute pancreatitis: a serial study. *Australas Radiol* 1995;39:145-152.

170. Chong WK, Theis B, Russell RC et al. US-guided percutaneous pancreatography: an essential tool for imaging pancratitis. *RadioGraphics* 1992;12:79-90.

171. Zama S. Percutaneous renal cyst puncture and ethanol instillation. *Hinyokika Kiyo* 1994;40:9-13.

172. Nishimura K, Tsujimura A, Matsumiya K et al. Clinical experience of percutaneous renal cyst puncture in recent six years. *Hinyokika Kiyo* 1993;39:121-125.

173. Pedersen H, Juul N. Ultrasound-guided percutaneous nephrostomy in the treatment of advanced gynecologic malignancy. *Acta Obstet Gynecol Scand* 1988;67:199-201.

174. Saitoh M. Color Doppler flow imaging in interventional ultrasound of the kidney. *Scand J Urol Nephrol Suppl* 1991;137:59-64.

PART III

Intraoperative Sonography

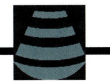

CHAPTER 18

Intraoperative Sonography of the Brain

•

Jonathan M. Rubin, M.D., Ph.D.
William F. Chandler, M.D.

TECHNIQUE

Orientation

The most difficult aspect of using intraoperative sonography is becoming oriented to the slices generated during surgery. Because ultrasound sections are generated at the surgical site, the orientation of the images almost never corresponds to standard anatomic sections. For example, a near-true coronal section of the brain is imaged through the anterior fontanelle of the neonate. From this midline acoustic window, the hemispheres are symmetrically imaged on both sides of the interhemispheric fissure/falx, which is positioned along the central ray of each scanned section. However, neurosurgeons rarely operate directly over the midline because this would necessitate dissecting through the superior sagittal sinus. Instead, they usually try to enter the cranium directly over the area of interest. Images made from such sites produce slices with unusual perspectives (Fig. 18-1). For instance, when scanning over the convexities, the falx does not appear as a line projecting along the midline in coronal sections, but is tipped slightly from the vertical; for parietal craniotomies, this is a slight obliquity, but approaches an angle of 90 degrees from vertical when scanning on the temporal lobe. Such changes in perspective can be disorienting for a surgeon with limited experience. The inability to recognize the normal anatomy because of these strange perspectives can cause significant consternation and frustration in an environment as tense as an operating room.

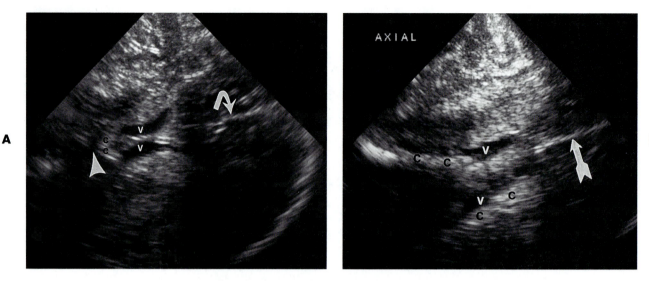

A

B

FIG. 18-1. **Intraoperative sonogram demonstrates tipped field of view.**
A, Angled coronal sonogram on the temporal lobe. Interhemispheric fissure/falx *(curved arrow)* projects down in the 3 o'clock position. Lateral ventricles, *v,* with echogenic choroid plexus, *c,* converging through foramina of Monro into a small third ventricle *(arrowhead)* are shown. **B,** Axial intraoperative scan made on surface of the temporal lobe. Choroid plexus, *c,* lateral ventricles, *v,* interhemispheric fissure/falx *(arrow)* are marked.

INTRAOPERATIVE BRAIN SCANNING

Begin with 3 or 5 MHz for whole brain slices.
Find choroid plexus, lateral ventricles, falx, and tentorium.
Place transducer in center of surgical field.
Rotate transducer to obtain standard anatomic sections.
Slide across the craniotomy in that plane.
Rotate transducer 90 degrees to study normal anatomy.
Avoid random scanning.
Find lesion relationship to normal anatomy.
Use 5-MHz or higher transducer for surgical guidance.

To avoid these problems, the radiologist should follow a few basic rules (see box above). First, begin scanning at a frequency low enough for the sound to traverse the entire brain, generally **about 3 MHz**. Although the spatial resolution of scans at these frequencies is not optimal for performing surgical guidance, these images are very useful for orientation. These **"whole brain" slices** should make it possible to distinguish the anatomy on the abnormal and normal sides of the brain. The **choroid plexus, lateral ventricles, falx,** and **tentorium** are easy to recognize (see Fig. 18-1). By identifying these structures,

the operator can produce a slice that corresponds to a standard anatomic section. This can be done as follows: after placing the transducer in the center of the surgical field, the operator should rotate, not slide, the scan head until it is possible to see a recognizable relationship between the above structures. There are **at least two standard orientations** that can be produced from any craniotomy. For example, a sagittal or coronal slice can be produced from a parietal craniotomy, a transaxial or coronal slice from a temporal craniotomy, and a transaxial or sagittal slice from a frontal craniotomy. Once a recognizable section has been produced, the operator should slide the transducer, maintaining the same orientation, from one edge of the craniotomy to the other. By scanning the entire brain in that one orientation, both lateral ventricles, the choroid plexus, the falx, and the tentorium should be visible in standard, well-known relationships. After completing this series of scans, the operator should rotate the transducer 90 degrees and scan the brain in the orthogonal orientation, again identifying the normal structures. Only after a complete familiarity with the field and its relationship to the craniotomy has been obtained should the search for the lesion begin. The lesion should basically be ignored until all of the intracranial relationships relative to the particular craniotomy are understood. The maxim here is be systematic and avoid random scanning.

Once the orientation is understood, the transducer should be changed to a higher frequency, **5 MHz or**

BASIC BRAIN INTRAOPERATIVE TECHNIQUE

Sterile gel between drape and transducer
Sterile transducer drapes with two layers
Saline drip onto brain instead of gel

higher, to interrogate the lesion. Unless a major error has been made, the lesion of interest will be on the same side of the head as the craniotomy. There is little reason for scanning across the falx once the orientation sequence has been completed. A correctly positioned craniotomy almost always places the area of interest in the near field of the transducer, usually within 6 cm of the scan head. There is rarely any reason to scan such lesions at frequencies of less than 5 MHz. Therefore the typical case will require a low-frequency transducer (3–5 MHz) for orientation and a higher-frequency transducer (5 MHz or more) for surgical guidance.

Draping the Transducer

Although sterilizable transducers are now available, many scan heads cannot be sterilized and must be draped for sterility. There are many different draping schemes, and we have covered scan heads with various objects, including sterile latex surgical gloves or transparent microscope drapes.[1-4] Each of these works well; the reader could probably devise a draping method that would perform as well. The problem with many of these "home-grown" techniques is that usually they cover the transducer with any thin material that happens to be handy in the operating room at the time. In these cases the potential for tearing the drape on the rough bony margin of a craniotomy is great. To avoid this hazard the scan head should ideally be draped with at least two layers of protective material. Alternatively, a commercially marketed draping system can be used (Fig. 18-2). Besides being convenient to use, some commercial draping kits have the additional benefit of a hard, tightly fitting cap that covers both the drape and the scan head. This cap negates the possibility of contamination of the field.

Some machines have sterilizable transducers. These seem to be in the minority, since gas sterilization can corrupt the plastic casing of the scan head in some circumstances.

Once draped, the scan head can be touched gently to the dura or directly to the cortex. Experience has shown little difference in image quality whether scanning on the dura mater or the cortex.[4] Saline, dripped onto the surface of the brain, acts as the coupling

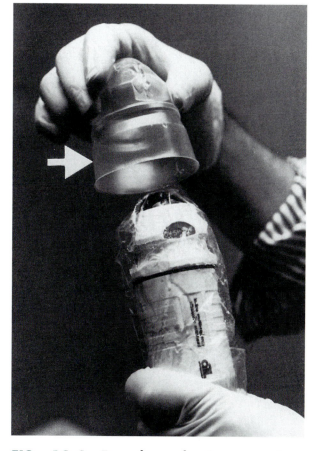

FIG. 18-2. Transducer draping procedure. Photograph shows the application of a protective plastic cap *(arrow)* to a draped scan head and cable using a commercially available draping system. (CIVCO Medical Instruments Co, Kalona, Iowa.)

agent. If necessary, the wound itself can be filled with saline, creating a natural fluid path for scanning.[5]

Time Requirements

One major disadvantage of intraoperative scanning has been the time the radiologist must commit to these procedures. Quencer and Montalvo[6] determined that they spent an average of 52 minutes in the operating room for craniotomies. However, complex cases could last as long as an hour and a half, which is a significant commitment of time. Yet, in our experience, Quencer and Montalvo's numbers are very liberal, and the radiologist's involvement need be nowhere near this great. First, in 18% of their cases, Quencer and Montalvo noted that the radiologist was able to leave the operating room for long periods of time, an average of 48 minutes. Second, we have found that as surgeons become more and more adept at the technique, the radiologist is needed less for the mundane techniques of scanning basics, draping the scan head, and guidance; he or she assumes the role of a consul-

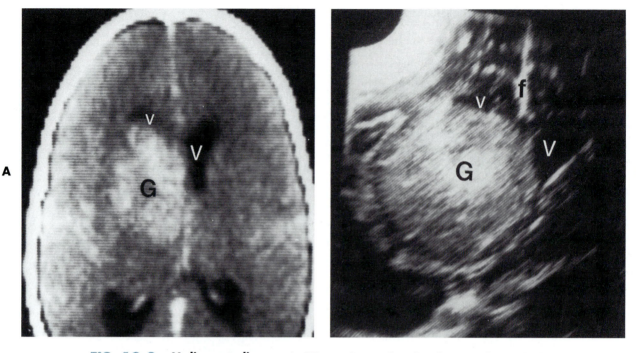

FIG. 18-3. **Malignant glioma.** **A,** CT scan shows a densely enhancing glioma, *G,* that is distorting the lateral ventricles, *V.* **B,** Coronal sonogram of the highly echogenic glioma, *G,* again shows the compressed ventricles, *V,* and the abutting falx, *f.* (From Chandler WF. Use of ultrasound imaging during intracranial operations. In: Rubin JM, Chandler WF, eds. *Ultrasound in Neurosurgery.* New York: Raven Press; 1990.)

tant. In fact, we have frequently found that it often takes more time to change into operating room attire than it does to monitor a case.

Yet there is often no way the radiologist can expedite a complex case. A significant time commitment is sometimes necessary for a favorable surgical result.[6] The realization that the radiologist's imaging skills improved the outcome of surgery and the quality of care the patient received is a valuable reward.[7]

TUMORS

High-Grade Gliomas

Tumors in general and high-grade gliomas in particular have very characteristic sonographic appearances. These **tumors are almost always more echogenic** than the background brain substance (Fig. 18-3).[3,7,8-14] Only **cysts**, which frequently arise in these tumors, are hypoechoic and have the typical properties of increased through-transmission and sharp margins (Fig. 18-4). At times it is possible to identify either a tumor nodule within a cyst or a cyst with a hyperechoic ring corresponding to tumor around its edge.

It is clear that ultrasound is the primary imaging modality for cysts.[12,14-16] Computed tomography (CT) and, less often, magnetic resonance imaging (MRI) can have difficulty in distinguishing solid from cystic

lesions.[7,12,17-19] Identification of these cysts is crucial because the neurosurgeon may need to drain them in order to decompress the brain before opening the dura mater (Fig. 18-5).[20,21]

Tumor Versus Edema and Necrosis

The distinction between degrees of echogenicity in high-grade gliomas is an interesting one. When performing a biopsy, those portions of a lesion containing viable tumor should be sampled and areas of necrosis or edema should be avoided. McGahan et al.[21] showed that the **areas of highest echogenicity in high-grade gliomas usually correspond to areas of necrosis** whereas the relatively lower echogenicity ring immediately around the necrotic area generally represents tumor. Although there is some debate,[3,16] and one group[22] has suggested that vasogenic edema is hypoechoic whereas cytotoxic edema is echogenic, edema is now generally thought to be echogenic in the brain and spinal cord (Fig. 18-6).[23,24] This echogenicity is problematic when trying to discriminate tumor margins from edema.[11,22,23,25-27] In fact, **edema can obscure the margins of lesions** on sonography relative to CT and MRI (see Fig. 18-6). Yet edema is more of a problem in identifying and delineating low-grade astrocytomas whose lesions are often more homogeneous than those of high-grade malignancies.[22]

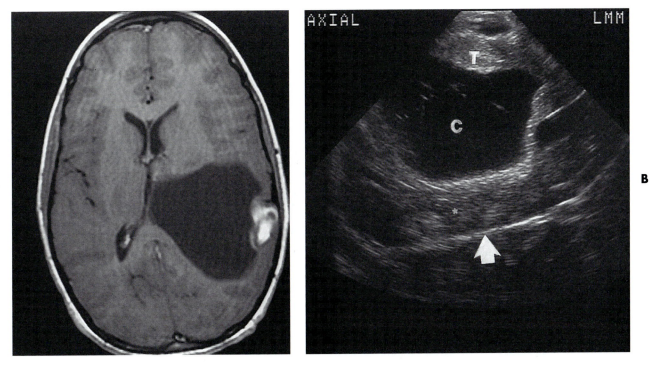

FIG. 18-4. **Ganglioglioma.** **A,** Postgadolinium T1-weighted axial scan (TR = 550, TE = 16) demonstrates a large left parietal cystic mass with an enhancing mural nodule. **B,** Axial intraoperative sonogram performed on the left parietal dura demonstrates the mural tumor nodule, *T,* just under the calvarial defect and the cystic component of the mass, *C,* of the mass deep to the nodule. There is increased through-transmission, *, noted in the brain substance behind the cyst. The interhemispheric fissure/falx *(arrow)* is marked. (Courtesy of Lori L. Barr, M.D., Children's Hospital Medical Center, Cincinnati, Ohio.)

BRAIN LESION CHARACTERISTICS

Echogenic lesions
Necrotic tumor
Tumors
Tumor nodules in cysts
Edema around tumor
Postoperative gliosis

Echogenicity like brain or like edema
Low-grade tumors

Anechoic
Cysts
Center of echogenic abscess

Tumor Margins and Tumor Size on Sonography

Although tumor margins are often better seen on ultrasound than CT, comparison of tumor size between modalities seems to vary greatly. Enzmann et al.[22] reported that nonenhancing masses on CT scans could appear larger, equal, or smaller on ultrasound. However, lesions enhancing with contrast on CT scans were always less than or equal to the size on the corresponding sonogram. Hypodense or isodense mass margins were seen more clearly on ultrasound than CT; ultrasound more accurately defined tumor extension if there had been no breakdown of the blood-brain barrier.[22] Another group found that CT consistently overestimated tumor size.[16]

An elegant comparative study between ultrasound and CT where CT was the gold standard was performed by LeRoux et al.[28] Twenty-two patients with primary and metastatic brain tumors were evaluated. In patients undergoing surgery for the first time, ultrasound tumor volumes closely matched CT findings: 101.69% ± 24.7%. Preoperative sonography was more likely to improve the delineation of tumor margins relative to CT. However, in patients undergoing subsequent surgery, ultrasound overestimated the tumor volumes by about 40%. **Postoperative gliosis** appeared similar to tumor on sonography, thus enlarging the apparent masses.

More recent studies have confirmed that sonography improves the ability to depict the **internal structure of gliomas** relative to CT and MRI.[25,26] However, this same group commented that since edema is generally echogenic on ultrasound, the **margins of lesions** are often better seen with CT and MRI.

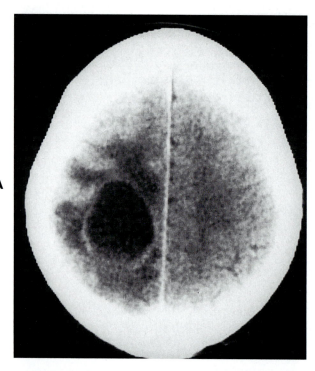

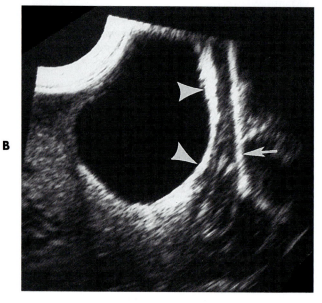

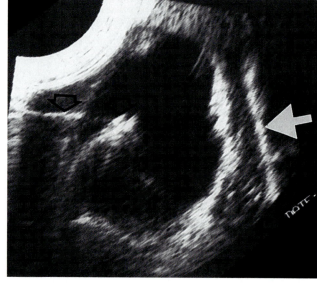

FIG. 18-5. Cystic astrocytoma. A, CT scan of posterior right frontal lobe cystic astrocytoma. **B,** Coronal intraoperative sonogram shows a medial echogenic ring of tumor *(arrowheads)*. Obvious increased through-transmission is seen behind the cyst. Falx is identified *(arrow)*. **C,** Coronal scan showing a needle *(open black arrows)* entering the cyst. The falx *(solid white arrow)* is again marked.

In general, high-grade astrocytomas, which are large when discovered, do not present localization problems for neurosurgeons.[15] The value of sonography in these cases lies in **determining the borders of lesions** or in **defining a safe access to a deep tumor**. This localization often can be more accurate and precise than on preoperative imaging examinations such as CT.[22] Sonography can also be useful in **identifying residual tumor** when a total removal has been attempted.[11,12,15] Some investigators have found the efficacy of postoperative evaluation for residual tumor to be limited, however.[26] Many of these masses are only biopsied, and although ultrasound certainly can be used to guide biopsies of these lesions, biopsies are often done under CT or MRI guidance.

Pitfalls in Tumor Localization

When scanning across a sulcus, the **sulcus can look like a solid mass** if the sound beam is parallel to it (Fig. 18-7).[11,29] This fact, which is well recognized in scans of neonatal heads, can lead to biopsies of normal brain if unrecognized in the operating room. To avoid this pitfall, every suspected mass must be scanned in two orthogonal planes. **A mass will look solid in both planes,** but a sulcus will look like a line in one of the orientations (see Fig. 18-7).

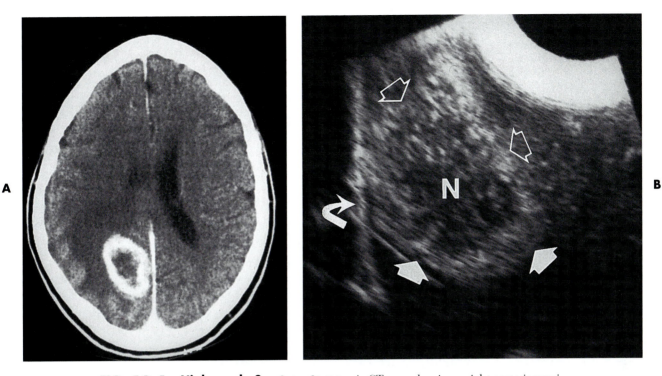

FIG. 18-6. High grade 3 astrocytoma. A, CT scan showing a right posterior pari-etal tumor with a necrotic center and surrounding edema. **B,** Coronal ultrasound image showing the tumor mass *(arrows)*. The more superior and medial margins *(open arrows)* are less well defined compared with the deeper boundaries *(solid arrows)* because of more echogenic, edematous brain in those regions creating decreased relative contrast. The necrotic center of the mass, *N,* and the falx *(curved arrow)* are marked.

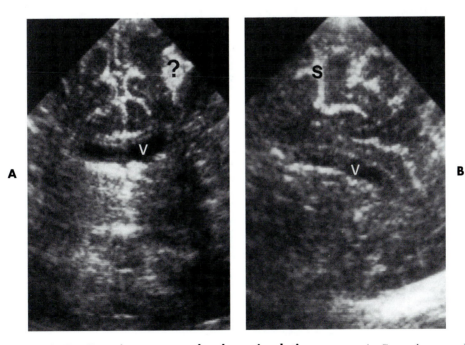

FIG. 18-7. Prominent normal sulcus simulating mass. A, Coronal neonatal brain ultrasound scan shows an apparent parietal mass (?). *V,* Lateral ventricle. **B,** 90 degree rotation of the transducer over the presumed mass produces a line, *S,* proving it is a sulcus. *V,* Ventricle. (From Bowerman RA. Tangential sulcal echoes: potential pitfall in the diagnosis of parenchymal lesions on cranial sonography. *J Ultrasound Med* 1987;6:685-689.)

Low-Grade Astrocytomas

Determining the precise location of these slow-growing, infiltrating lesions can be difficult. Even though they may be obvious on CT or MRI, in surgery they may appear very much like normal brain on gross

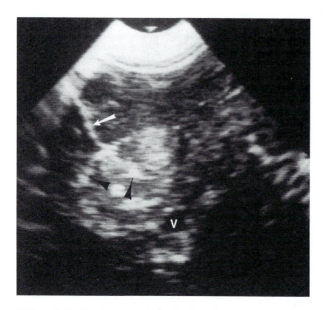

FIG. 18-8. Low-grade astrocytoma crossing midline. Coronal scan shows hyperechoic tumor invading the falx *(arrow)* and crossing the midline. Destroyed sulci *(arrowheads)* are within the mass. *v,* Lateral ventricle.

inspection or even on pathologic frozen section.[14,30] Although low-grade astrocytomas may be difficult to visualize sonographically, lesions difficult or impossible to identify on CT scans often are easily seen on ultrasound (Fig. 18-8).[31] Low-grade gliomas are invariably **more echogenic than normal brain**.[22,31,32] However, the degree of echogenicity in low-grade malignancies is less than for higher-grade malignancies. Tumoral echogenicity can be similar to that of edematous brain,[23,32] making the boundary between edema and tumor difficult to identify. The poorly defined margin may also be due to infiltrating tumor.

Tumor Versus Edema

A helpful clue for distinguishing tumor from edema is that **tumors invade** whereas edema does not. Therefore tumors usually disrupt or destroy sulcal morphology whereas edema spreads around sulci, sparing them (see Fig. 18-8; Figs. 18-9 and 18-10). This sign, although generally useful, has been known

PITFALLS IN TUMOR LOCALIZATION

Sulcus looks like a solid mass in one plane
Edema obscures tumor margins
Tumor infiltration may obscure margins

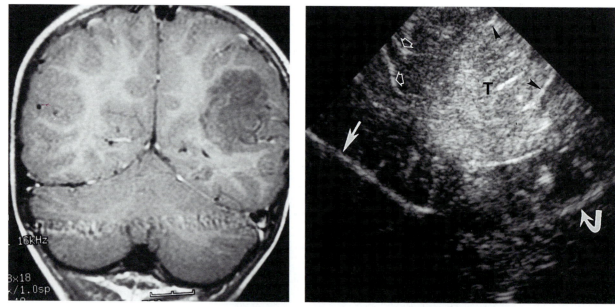

FIG. 18-9. Oligodendroglioma. A, Coronal T1-weighted MRI scan showing left parietal mass. **B,** Tipped coronal intraoperative ultrasound scan showing the highly echogenic tumor, *T.* Note the irregular margins. Several invaded sulci *(arrowheads)* are seen within the mass. The interhemispheric fissure/falx *(arrow)* is projecting in obliquely from about the 9 o'clock position. A portion of the tentorium is seen under the mass *(curved arrow)*. Normal sulci *(open arrows)* are noted projecting into mildly echogenic, edematous brain above the tumor.

to fail.[11] In addition, unlike high-grade tumors, focal areas of increased echogenicity are more likely to correspond to areas of viable tumor in low-grade gliomas[32] (see Fig. 18-9). Hence areas of local increased echogenicity can be used to identify viable tumor and often represent prime sites for biopsy.[32]

Unusual Approaches

Before sonography, surgeons had to approach masses from the most direct and often shortest path. If this path transgressed an inviolable portion of the brain such as the motor strip or the primary speech area, an otherwise resectable lesion was considered inoper-

able. However, using sonography, surgeons can **approach lesions from any number of oblique directions.** Mapping the motor strip or speech area can be done before a resection while the patient is awake; a surgical path can be designed through a silent area to avoid these essential areas and still intersect the lesion, making an otherwise nonresectable lesion resectable (Fig. 18-11). Patients should not have deficits after such operations. Because of increased flexibility, rapid localization of tumors, and increased precision in tumor removal, sonography has led to major decreases in the morbidity and mortality rates associated with brain tumor resections.[27]

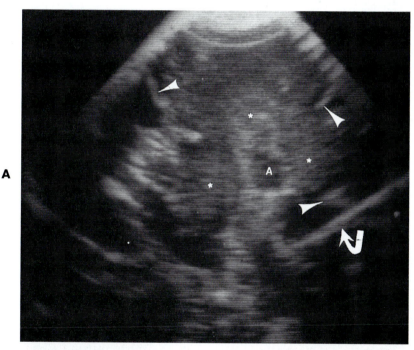

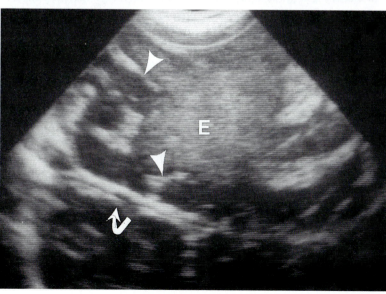

FIG. 18-10. A, Deep frontal abscess cavity, **A,** with surrounding echogenic edematous brain,*. Several preserved sulci *(arrowheads)* and falx projecting down from the right-hand side of the image *(curved arrow)* are marked. **B, After aspiration of the abscess,** echogenic edematous brain, *E,* remains visible. Normal sulci *(arrowheads)* and interhemispheric fissure/falx, now projecting down from the 9 o'clock position *(curved arrow),* are again marked.

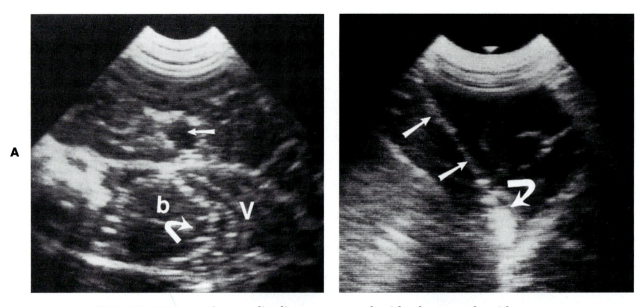

FIG. 18-11. **Cystic ganglioglioma removed with ultrasound guidance.** A. Transaxial sonogram shows the cystic mass *(arrow)* lying underneath the primary speech center against the midbrain, *b*, and cerebellar vermis, *V* (multiple curved folia). Aqueduct of Sylvius *(curved arrow)*. **B,** Needle *(straight arrows)* passing through a silent area into the lesion *(curved arrow)*. The needle tip has concentric rings etched into it, making it extremely echogenic.

Other Tumors

The entire gamut of brain tumors has been imaged by sonography. These lesions have been uniformly more echogenic than the surrounding brain. **Meningiomas** can be detected deep on the falx, at the base of the skull, within the ventricular system, or simply on the convexity.[2] They can be highly attenuating and are very echogenic.

Metastases to the brain can easily be identified.[7,10-14,22,33] Solitary metastases are often resected; typically, they have well-defined margins with surrounding edema. In addition, associated masses such as hematomas occurring with vascular metastases such as melanomas or renal cell carcinomas can be readily separated from the tumor (Fig. 18-12). Superficial metastases present few problems, but deep lesions can be difficult to locate. Sonography can also be valuable for certain superficial metastases by making resection possible. With a lesion near the motor strip, the surgeon can locate a silent area for an approach. With sonographic guidance through the silent area, the lesion becomes resectable.

Posterior fossa tumors such as hemangioblastomas, dermoids, epidermoids, ependymomas, and medulloblastomas can easily be seen with sonography, and the solid or cystic nature of a lesion may be accurately determined where CT is not reliable (Fig. 18-13).[30]

Multiple, closely spaced folia make the cerebellum echogenic. The important relationship of a mass to the fourth ventricle can also be made with sonography (see Fig. 18-13).

Biopsy

Sonographically guided intraoperative biopsies can be performed with standard biopsy guides or free-hand approaches.[34-39] The choice largely depends on the surgeon's tastes. However, it is often helpful to alter a biopsy needle's surface to improve identification of the needle tip. Because the length of the surface of the needle is much larger than a wavelength, it constitutes a specular reflector. Because of this, the angle of reflection is highly dependent on the angle of incidence.[40,41] If the needle is inserted at an oblique angle to the transducer, most of the sound that strikes the needle will scatter away from the surface of the transducer, decreasing the backscattered energy, which makes the needle and its tip harder to see. One way to prevent this is to roughen or etch the surface of the needle or catheter tip.[42-44] If the roughened surface has irregularities that approximate the size of one wavelength, the backscatter is no longer directionally dependent. Significantly more sound is scattered in the direction of the transducer, which makes it easier to see the needle (see Fig. 18-11).

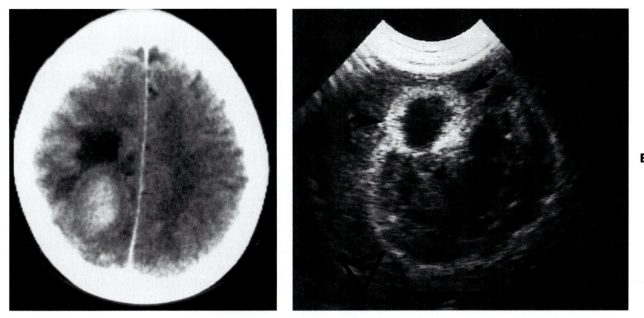

FIG. 18-12. Renal cell carcinoma metastasis. A, CT scan demonstrates right anterior parietal tumor with a high-density hematoma in it. **B,** Ultrasound scan showing a small tumor nodule with a highly echogenic rim *(solid arrows)*. Deep to the tumor is a larger mass with less echogenic walls, which is the hematoma *(open arrows)*.

INFECTION

Abscesses of various sizes and in various stages of development can be seen sonographically.[14,15,45] The margins of an abscess are almost always hyperechoic whereas the central echogenicity varies, depending on the degree of liquefaction. The hyperechoic margins in the early stages of an abscess are caused by marked cellular infiltration whereas collagen deposition causes the increased echogenicity later on.[45] Surrounding edema or cerebritis is nearly always echogenic, and distinguishing between the two by ultrasound is difficult if not impossible. Clearly it is possible to aspirate such lesions under ultrasonic guidance (see Fig. 18-10).

TRAUMA

Sonography has proven to be a useful modality for localizing foreign bodies in the extremities, and it can be useful in identifying bone fragments or foreign bodies in the brain (Fig. 18-14).[46-50] The acoustic impedances of the standard materials searched for, such as **metal, bone, wood fragments,** and **glass,** are different enough from soft tissue to make them readily distinguishable. In general, they all produce bright reflections with or without associated acoustic shadows that help pinpoint their locations. Foreign materials will have backscatter differences—the reflections from wood are less than those from bone or metal.[47] Except for **metal,** which produces a characteristic **"comet-tail"** artifact (see Fig. 18-14; Fig. 18-15 on p. 644),[47,51,52] the nature of the shadows does not distinguish one material from another.[53] This creates a problem because one pitfall is **air,** which is often present in these wounds along with the foreign bodies. In fact, air can be incorporated directly into wood fragments.[47] Because air also casts shadows, the operator may have difficulty deciding whether a shadow arises from a foreign body or from air in the wound. If the search does not involve finding a large number of fragments, a preoperative CT scan pinpointing the fragment locations can limit the search and distinguish air from solid, shadowing materials.

The ultrasound appearance of **intracranial hematomas** is well known from the literature on intraoperative and neonatal neurosonography.[14,15,47,54] Hematomas initially start out as hypoechoic masses during active bleeding, but within a minute after clot formation, the mass becomes echogenic with the increased echogenicity caused by red cell aggregation.[55-57] The central echogenicity begins to decrease after a period of 3 to 4 days until the hematoma becomes centrally hypoechoic with an echogenic rim.

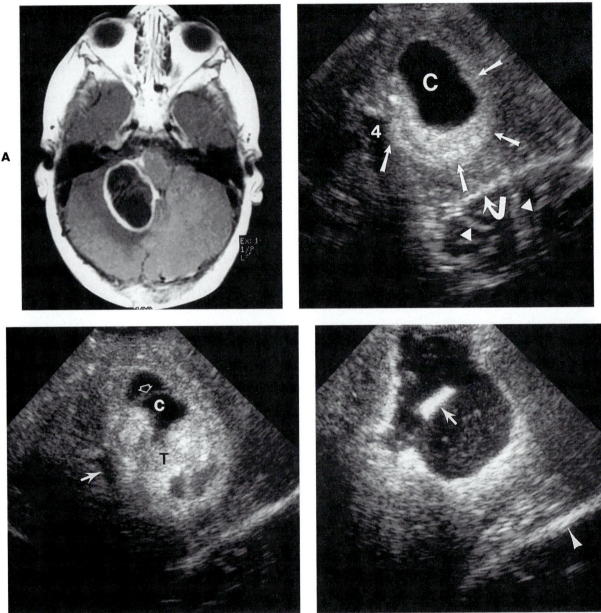

FIG. 18-13. Ependymoma—preresection and postresection. A, MRI scan postgadolinium demonstrating partly cystic mass in the posterior fossa. **B,** Axial sonogram with posterior at top of the image reflecting the way the surgeon would view the anatomy. The image shows the fourth ventricle, *4*, partially compressed posteriorly by the tumor. The cystic center, *c*, and echogenic tumor margin *(arrows)* are easily seen. Anterior to the tumor, the tentorium can be seen *(curved arrow)*, at least on the right side, with supratentorial brain deep to it. Several supratentorial sulci are also marked *(arrowheads)*. **C,** Another axial scan taken at 7 MHz showing the huge echogenic tumor mass, *T*, compressing and displacing the fourth ventricle *(arrow)* laterally. A septum *(open arrow)* is seen in the tumor cyst. **D,** Postresection axial scan showing the saline-filled wound with a gelfoam bar *(arrow)* in it. The tentorium is visible anteriorly *(arrowhead)*.

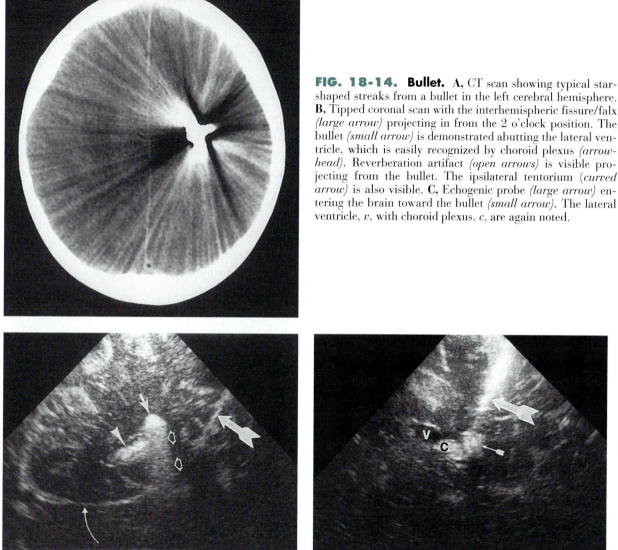

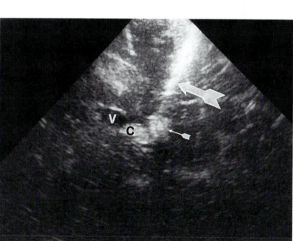

FIG. 18-14. Bullet. **A,** CT scan showing typical star-shaped streaks from a bullet in the left cerebral hemisphere. **B,** Tipped coronal scan with the interhemispheric fissure/falx *(large arrow)* projecting in from the 2 o'clock position. The bullet *(small arrow)* is demonstrated abutting the lateral ventricle, which is easily recognized by choroid plexus *(arrowhead)*. Reverberation artifact *(open arrows)* is visible projecting from the bullet. The ipsilateral tentorium *(curved arrow)* is also visible. **C,** Echogenic probe *(large arrow)* entering the brain toward the bullet *(small arrow)*. The lateral ventricle, *v*, with choroid plexus, *c*, are again noted.

The echogenic rim initially is caused by red cell aggregation, but the rim is eventually collagenized. Histologically, the area of decreased echogenicity corresponds to the breakdown of red blood cells.[58] This decrease in echogenicity continues for about 2 weeks, when the clot starts looking primarily hypoechoic.[58] The upshot of this transition is that hematomas can look different sonographically, depending on their time of formation relative to the time of scanning. Thus it is theoretically possible for a hematoma to be isoechoic with the brain, but this does not usually happen in actual practice.

The diagnosis of a hematoma is rarely based on the sonogram alone. A recent history of trauma, a high-density lesion on a CT scan, and a lesion with slight hyperintensity relative to surrounding brain on T1-weighted MRI scans will all help in making the diagnosis. The usefulness of sonography is in localizing the hematoma and monitoring its drainage. These lesions are easy to locate and, since the diameters of "brain needles" are often several millimeters, it is usually possible to clearly visualize a needle while decompressing these lesions transdurally (Fig. 18-16). Sonography can also be used for confirming that the hematoma has been totally aspirated without opening the dura.

The development of a hematoma as a surgical complication is a corollary of ultrasound's application in trauma.[8,15,59] Because acute brain swelling during

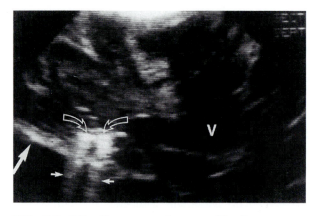

FIG. 18-15. Postoperative metallic clips. Transaxial scan shows two highly echogenic clips *(curved arrows)* with comet-tail artifacts behind them *(small arrows)* on feeding vessels of arteriovenous malformation. Falx *(large arrow)*. *V,* Ipsilateral lateral ventricle. (From Rubin JM, Carson PL. Physics and techniques. In: Rubin JM, Chandler WF, eds. *Ultrasound in Neurosurgery.* New York: Raven Press; 1990.)

surgery is a potential catastrophe, immediate localization of a developing hematoma is essential. In these circumstances the surgeon is totally blind without sonography. Ultrasound can immediately locate a developing hematoma, and the lesion can be resected or drained under directed guidance if necessary (Fig. 18-17). If the hemorrhage is entirely intraventricular (see Fig. 18-17), only a ventricular catheter is needed for drainage after surgery.

SHUNTS

It has never been difficult to introduce catheters into enlarged ventricles; neurosurgeons have been doing so for years. Yet problems can arise even in the most routine cases. For instance, the tip of the catheter can pass through the foramen of Monro and enter the third ventricle (Fig. 18-18). Sometimes the tip can actually become embedded in the thalamus or caudate nucleus, or postshunt bleeding can occur.[59,60] A common problem is the proximity of the catheter tip to the choroid plexus. It is believed that **80% of proximal shunt obstructions are caused by entanglement of the shunt tip with the choroid plexus.**[61] Theoretically, the longevity of shunts would improve if shunt tips could be positioned away from the choroid plexus in the frontal horn of a lateral ventricle.* Because of the high echogenicity of the choroid plexus

*References 3, 10, 20, 59, 62.

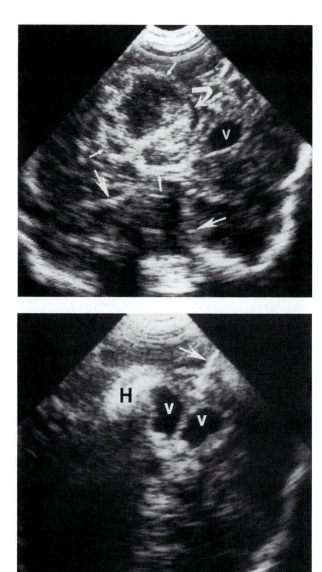

FIG. 18-16. Hematoma. A, Coronal scan shows a large, complex mass *(small arrows)* in the right cerebral hemisphere that compresses the right lateral ventricle *(curved arrow)*. Left lateral ventricle, *v,* falx *(open arrow),* and two leaves of the tentorium *(large arrows).* **B,** Postdrainage coronal scan shows a small residual hematoma, *H,* after drainage. Lateral ventricles, *v,* are both expanded. Falx *(arrow)*.

on sonography, it is easy to place the tips of catheters in portions of the ventricles away from the choroid plexus (see Fig. 18-18).* Furthermore, it is simple to confirm the position of the shunt tip and shunt patency by merely pumping the shunt or injecting small amounts of saline.[3,20,62,63] This maneuver introduces microbubbles that are highly echogenic and easily visible.[63,64] In at least one early series, the longevity of shunts placed under ultrasound guidance was about twice that of nonultrasound-guided shunts.[59]

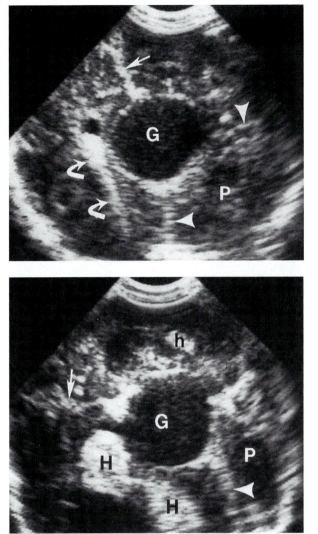

A

B

FIG. 18-17. Vein of Galen aneurysm. A, Prehemorrage coronal sonogram shows a hypoechoic vein of Galen, *G*. **B,** Coronal sonogram more tipped to the right shows two intraventricular hematomas, *H* and *h*, that occurred at surgery. Falx *(straight arrow)*. Echogenic choroid plexus in the contralateral ventricle *(curved arrows)*. Leaves of the tentorium *(arrowheads)*. *P*, Posterior fossa.

Although large ventricles are easy to hit, placing catheters into small ventricles for pressure monitoring or for chemotherapy can be difficult.[3,20] In such cases, sonography can be useful in localizing the ventricle and confirming the position of the catheter.[65]

Two main approaches have been used. In young children with an anterior fontanelle, catheters can be introduced through posterior parieto-occipital trephines or craniotomies while simultaneously **monitoring the catheter's progress from the infant's**

fontanelle.[3,59,62,65] Because the site of scanning is almost perpendicular to the catheter, the catheter is extremely well seen (Fig. 18-19).[65]

Another approach that has been used **in adults** is to produce a **keyhole-shaped craniotomy near the coronal suture.**[35] The large portion of the keyhole, generally a small trephine, is for positioning the scan head. A small extension off the trephine is used as a site for introduction of the shunt catheter. The catheter is passed through the smaller hole and monitored under ultrasound guidance. Once the catheter tip has entered the ventricle, the extruding catheter can be attached conveniently to a reservoir positioned over the smaller hole. The reservoir rests on the bone surrounding the smaller hole and stabilizes the position of the catheter.

VASCULAR LESIONS

Arteriovenous Malformation

Despite the success of gray-scale ultrasonography for most neurosurgical applications, its utility for arteriovenous malformations (**AVMs**) has been limited because the **gray-scale contrast between large portions of these lesions and the rest of the brain is low.**[14,15,59] This is particularly true for the hypoechoic, large, feeding arteries and draining veins, which must be identified for any localizing procedure to have full utility in these instances.[14,15,59]

It is clear that even though portions of AVMs can be imaged in gray-scale,[15,59,66,67] the surgeon cannot be certain that the entire lesion with its associated vasculature has been seen (Fig. 18-20).[15,59] In one report, two AVMs were studied; one was seen and the other was termed "subtle," although the associated arteries and veins were seen in both.[59] In another study, a group of 11 AVMs was studied by intraoperative gray-scale imaging alone; only about one half of the lesions could be visualized at all.[15] The identification of draining veins and feeding arteries was at best incomplete; however, the ability to distinguish these vessels intraoperatively would be useful.[66] In particular, the clipping of draining veins too early during surgery can cause a disastrous venous infarction.

Pulsed Doppler imaging seems to have a natural role in these cases.[66,67] It would appear at first glance that the problems of localizing subcortical AVMs and discriminating between feeding arteries and draining veins would be easy by this modality. Yet, considering the complexity of these lesions, the mere mapping of a complex, three-dimensional tangle of vessels with a point sample volume is daunting if not impossible. Furthermore, the velocity waveforms within these vessels can be misleading. It is a well-known property of vascular malformations that veins can be "arterial-

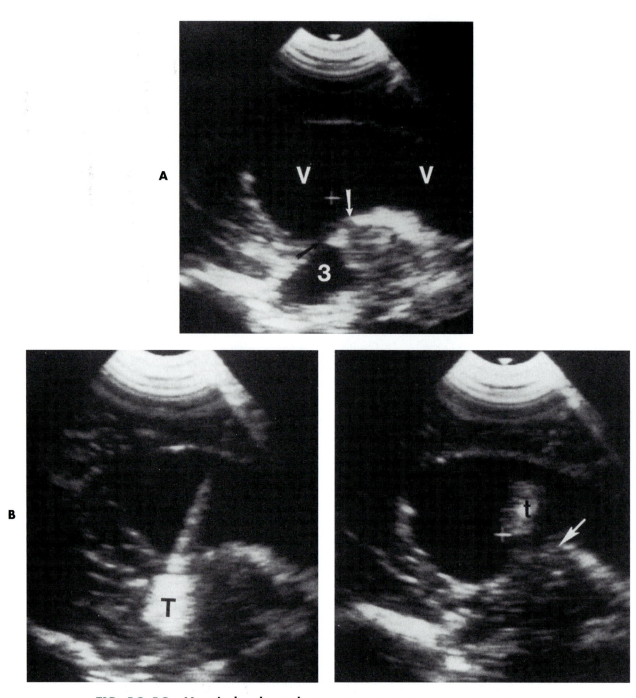

FIG. 18-18. Ventricular shunt placement. A, Sagittal sonogram shows the anterior margin of the choroid plexus *(white arrow)*. B, Repeat scan shows the catheter tip, *T*, had migrated through the foramen of Monro into the third ventricle. C, Follow-up scan shows catheter tip, *t*, pulled back into the lateral ventricle. Body of the lateral ventricle, *V*. Foramen of Monro *(black arrow)*. Third ventricle, *3*. The + in the lateral ventricle marks the target for the catheter.

ized."[68] Thus arterial signals can be detected in what are known to be draining veins, although some veins definitely will have venous signals. As a result, the Doppler signals themselves can be misleading, and because these vessels often are barely visible if not invisible on gray-scale imaging the addition of pulsed

Doppler imaging offers little to the surgical resection of these lesions.

In contrast, color flow Doppler sonography can be an accurate technique to detect and determine the extent of **AVMs**. The mapping of the lesions themselves is greatly **enhanced by the color con-**

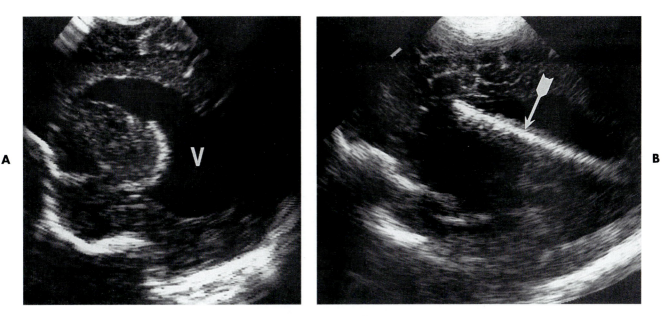

FIG. 18-19. Pediatric ventricular shunt placement. A, Sagittal sonogram made through the anterior fontanelle demonstrating a dilated lateral ventricle, *V*. **B,** Sagittal scan performed after positioning a shunt catheter *(arrow)* through a posterior craniectomy. The tip of the shunt is in the frontal horn. (From Babcock DS, Barr LL, Crone KR. Intraoperative uses of ultrasound in the pediatric neurosurgical patient. *Pediatr Neurosurg* 1992;18:34-91.)

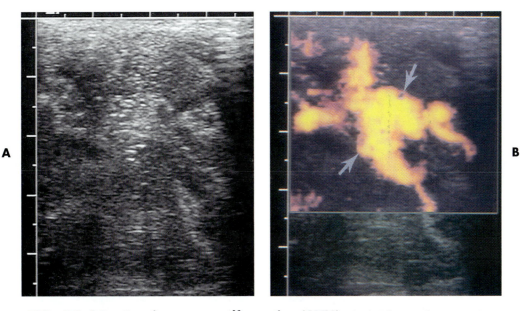

FIG. 18-20. Arteriovenous malformation (AVM). A, Axial scan demonstrating ill-defined coarsening of the echo texture and increased echogenicity representing an AVM of the left temporal lobe. **B,** Power Doppler scan clearly delineating the margins of the mass *(arrows)* as well as feeding arteries and draining veins. (Courtesy of Lori L. Barr, M.D., Children's Hospital Medical Center, Cincinnati, Ohio.)

trast generated by the high velocity of the blood flowing through them (Figs. 18-21 to 18-23). In particular, high-velocity, multidirectional flows in AVMs are displayed as areas with multiple colors lying side by side in an apparently random fashion. The multiple flow directions and aliasing intro-

duced by the high velocities are responsible for this appearance.

This **localized, chaotic, turbulent flow is the sine qua non of AVMs**; it must be present to identify lesions definitively. Vascular lesions can be difficult or impossible to image in cases where there is slow

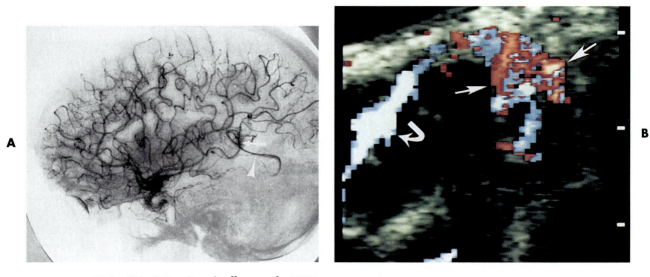

FIG. 18-21. Surgically occult AVM. A, Preoperative cerebral angiogram with subtraction technique of an AVM *(arrow)* at the posterior aspect of the sylvian fissure that was incompletely resected. Large early draining vein *(arrowhead)*. **B,** Color flow Doppler scan shows small subcortical AVM *(arrows)* with a presumed feeding artery *(curved arrow)*.

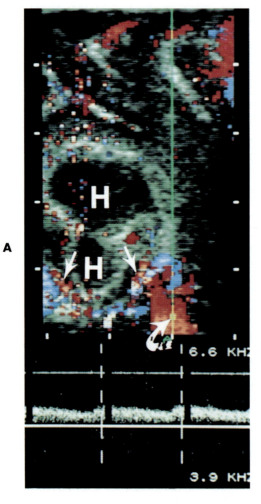

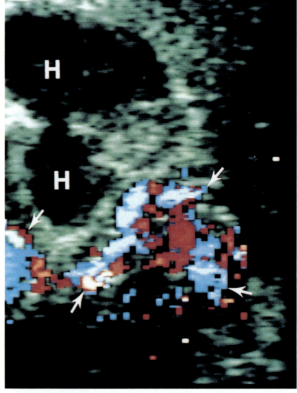

FIG. 18-22. Hematoma and associated AVM.
A, Color flow Doppler scan shows a hypoechoic hematoma, *H,* superficial to the AVM *(arrows)*. Sample volume *(curved arrow)* within a large draining vein containing a venous signal. **B,** Magnified image shows the hematoma, *H,* and the AVM *(arrows)*.

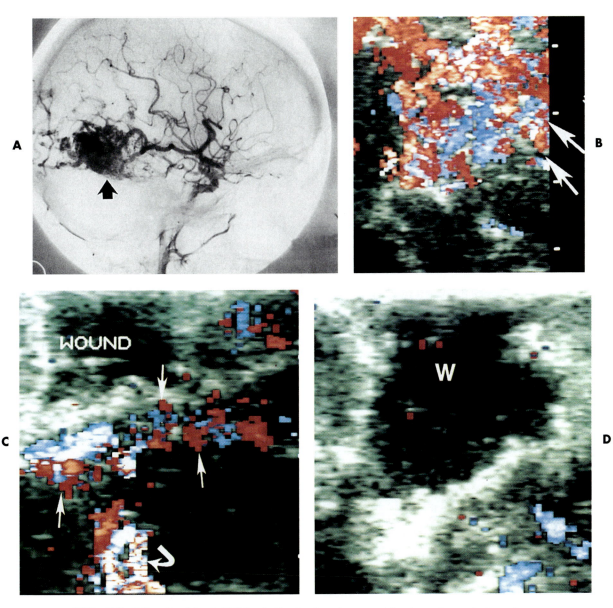

FIG. 18-23. Residual AVM. A, Cerebral angiogram with subtraction technique shows a large, posterior, temporal AVM *(arrows)*. **B,** Color flow Doppler image shows classic turbulent flow of the AVM *(arrows)*. **C,** Initial postresection scan (presumed totally resected) shows at the base of the saline-filled wound a residual AVM with multiple vessels of varied colors *(arrows)* with a high velocity, aliasing vessel *(curved arrow)* deep to the lesion. **D,** Second postresection scan shows no abnormal vessels in the base of the wound, *W.*

flow, such as **venous angiomas,** or where there has been an intervention prior to surgery that decreases flow, such as endovascular embolization. Improvements in slow-flow imaging techniques may eventually help in these cases, but any improvement still will require a knowledge of the lesion's approximate position because any slow-flow technique will produce aliasing and complex signal patterns in neighboring normal vessels, making them look abnormal. These normal vessels could then be mistaken for the lesion itself.

A knowledge of a lesion's approximate position is also necessary when identifying feeding arteries and draining veins. Although in theory the arteries should be able to be distinguished from veins by their flow directions relative to the AVM, in practice, because of the complex tangle of vessels, this determination becomes almost impossible to evaluate, even with the use of color. Furthermore, the waveforms themselves can be misleading. However, it should be noted that although an arterial pattern can occur in either arteries or veins, a venous pattern is likely to occur only in veins.

Despite these limitations, color flow Doppler imaging is still a useful imaging technique for surgery on AVMs.[69,70] In one report, color flow Doppler imaging was determined to be useful in 8 of 12 intracerebral AVMs.[70] In 3 of the 4 cases in which it was not useful, the cause was either equipment or procedure related, and was unrelated to the technique itself. The benefits of the method include identification of deep or hard to find lesions (see Fig. 18-21), localization of AVMs relative to adjacent hematomas (see Fig. 18-22), and confirmation of complete resection of lesions that are presumed to have been totally removed (see Fig. 18-23).

The latter two advantages are particularly interesting. By removing an AVM-associated hematoma, the surgeon can reduce the intracerebral volume and more easily gain access to the AVM itself. In one case the intracerebral pressure produced by a hematoma was so high that the AVM only became visible as the hematoma was aspirated.

Color flow Doppler sonography has proven extremely useful in localizing residual AVMs in certain cases where a total resection had been attempted but not accomplished (see Fig. 18-23). A finding of no residual AVM on a postresection scan is conclusive evidence that total removal has been achieved. Without intraoperative confirmation, follow-up surgery may be necessary to remove the portions of an AVM that were missed the first time.[69,70]

Aneurysm

Cerebral aneurysms can also be seen with remarkable clarity using intraoperative ultrasound.[27,71] However, except in certain cases, localization of these lesions is rarely a problem because aneurysms usually occur at well-defined, easily localized vascular bifurcations. There are, however, specific examples, such as mycotic aneurysms, where rapid localization of lesions is difficult without sonography.[14]

In certain circumstances, pulsed Doppler sonography has proven to be useful in aneurysm surgery.[72] In particular, spectral Doppler waveforms can be used to

> **COLOR FLOW DOPPLER IMAGING BENEFITS FOR AVMs**
>
> Identification of deep or hard to find lesions
> Localization of AVMs relative to adjacent hematomas
> Confirmation of complete resection of lesions presumed to have been totally removed

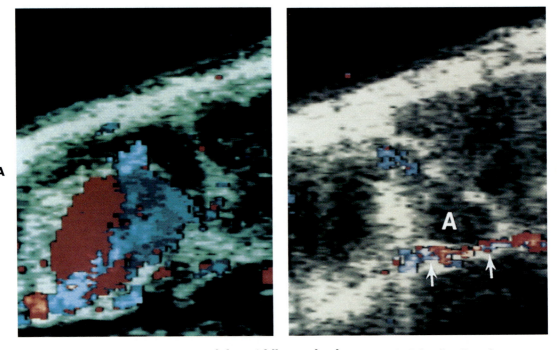

FIG. 18-24. Aneurysm of the middle cerebral artery. A, Color flow Doppler image of giant aneurysm with swirling blood demonstrated by the red-blue color separation. **B,** Postclipping scan demonstrating no flow in the aneurysm, *A.* Interestingly, there is probably spasm in the source artery *(arrows)*, which contains multiple and varied colors. These represent either multiple flow speeds or flow directions or both. Such a finding would occur with spasm and/or turbulence. (See references 7, 8, 10, 12, 14, 15.)

evaluate changes in blood flow in the parent artery as the neck of the aneurysm is occluded. A rapidly increasing velocity can herald the onset of spasm in the native vessel. Color flow Doppler sonography can also be used to evaluate flow in an aneurysm while the neck is being surgically occluded (Fig. 18-24).[69] It can be particularly useful in cases of giant aneurysms where the neck may be wide and difficult to occlude. Although there are only a few such cases, it seems likely that arterial spasm in the parent vessel could be determined with color flow Doppler sonography as well.

REFERENCES
Technique

1. Rubin JM, Mirfakhraee M, Duda E et al. Intraoperative ultrasound examination of the brain. *Radiology* 1980;137:831-832.
2. Rubin JM, Dohrmann GJ, Greenberg M et al. Intraoperative sonography of meningiomas. *Am J Neuroradiol* 1982;3:305-308.
3. Chandler WF, Knake JE, McGillicuddy JE et al. Intraoperative use of real-time ultrasonography in neurosurgery. *J Neurosurg* 1982;57:157-163.
4. Gooding GAW, Edwards MSB, Rabkin AE et al. Intraoperative real-time ultrasound in the localization of intracranial neoplasms. *Radiology* 1983;146:459-462.
5. DiPietro MA, Venes JL. Intraoperative sonography of the Arnold-Chiari malformations. In: Rubin JM, Chandler WF, eds. *Ultrasound in Neurosurgery.* New York: Raven Press; 1990:183-199.
6. Quencer RM, Montalvo BM. Time requirements for intraoperative neurosonography. *AJR* 1986;146:815-818.
7. Rubin JM, Dohrmann GJ. Intraoperative neurosurgical ultrasound in the localization and characterization of intracranial masses. *Radiology* 1983;148:519-524.

Tumors

8. Masuzawa H, Kamitani H, Sato J et al. Intraoperative application of sector scanning electronic ultrasound in neurosurgery. *Neurol Med Chir* 1981;21:277-285.
9. Shkolnick A, Tomita T, Raimondi AJ et al. Work in progress. Intraoperative neurosurgical ultrasound: localization of brain tumors in infants and children. *Radiology* 1983;148:525-527.
10. Knake JE, Chandler WF, McGillicuddy JE et al. Intraoperative sonography for brain tumor localization and ventricular shunt placement. *AJR* 1982;139:733-738.
11. Pasto ME, Rifkin MD. Intraoperative ultrasound examination of the brain: possible pitfalls in diagnosis and biopsy guidance. *J Ultrasound Med* 1984;3:245-249.
12. Gooding GAW, Boggan JE, Weinstein PR. Characterization of intracranial neoplasms by computed tomography and intraoperative sonography. *Am J Neuroradiol* 1984;5:517-520.
13. Smith WL, Menezes A, Franken EA. Cranial ultrasound in the diagnosis of malignant brain tumors. *J Clin Ultrasound* 1983;11:97-100.
14. Chandler WF, Rubin JM. The application of ultrasound during brain surgery. *World J Surg* 1987;11:558-569.
15. Rubin JM, Dohrmann GJ. Efficacy of intraoperative ultrasound for evaluating intracranial masses. *Radiology* 1985;157:509-511.
16. Machi J, Sigel B, Jafar JJ et al. Criteria for using imaging ultrasound during brain and spinal cord surgery. *J Ultrasound Med* 1984;3:155-161.

17. Latchaw RE, Gold LHA, Moore JS Jr et al. The nonspecificity of absorption coefficients in the differentiation of solid tumors and cystic lesions. *Radiology* 1977;125:141-144.
18. Handa J, Nakano Y, Handa H. Computed tomography in the differential diagnosis of low-density intracranial lesions. *Surg Neurol* 1978;10:179-185.
19. Kjos BO, Brant-Zawadzki M, Kucharczyk W et al. Cystic intracranial lesions: magnetic resonance imaging. *Radiology* 1985;155:363-369.
20. Rubin JM, Dohrmann GJ. Use of ultrasonically guided probes and catheters in neurosurgery. *Surg Neurol* 1982;18:143-148.
21. McGahan JP, Ellis WG, Budenz RW et al. Brain gliomas: sonographic characterization. *Radiology* 1986;159:485-492.
22. Enzmann DR, Wheat R, Marshall WH et al. Tumors of the central nervous system studied by computed tomography and ultrasound. *Radiology* 1985;154:393-399.
23. Smith SJ, Vogelzang RL, Marzano MI et al. Brain edema: ultrasound examination. *Radiology* 1985;155:379-382.
24. Platt JF, Rubin JM, Chandler WF et al. Intraoperative spinal sonography in the evaluation of intramedullary tumors. *J Ultrasound Med* 1988;7:317-325.
25. Auer LM, van Velthoven V. Intraoperative ultrasound (US) imaging. Comparison of pathomorphological findings in US and CT. *Acta Neurochir (Wien)* 1990;104:84-95.
26. van Velthoven V, Auer LM. Practical application of intraoperative ultrasound imaging. *Acta Neurochir (Wien)* 1990;105:5-13.
27. Roselli R, Iacoangeli M, Pentimalli L et al. Intraoperative real-time ultrasonography in the microsurgical removal of subcortical or deep-seated brain tumors. *Acta Chir Beig* 1993;93:185-187.
28. LeRoux PD, Berger MS, Ojemann GA et al. Correlation of intraoperative ultrasound tumor volumes and margins with preoperative computerized tomography scans: an intraoperative method to enhance tumor resection. *J Neurosurg* 1989;71:691-698.
29. Bowerman RA. Tangential sulcal echoes: potential pitfall in the diagnosis of parenchymal lesions on cranial sonography. *J Ultrasound Med* 1987;6:685-689.
30. Chandler WF. Use of ultrasound imaging during intracranial operations. In: Rubin JM, Chandler WF, eds. *Ultrasound in Neurosurgery.* New York: Raven Press; 1990:67-106.
31. Knake JE, Chandler WF, Gabrielsen TO et al. Intraoperative sonographic delineation of low-grade brain neoplasms defined poorly by computed tomography. *Radiology* 1984;151:735-739.
32. Hatfield MK, Rubin JM, Gebarski SS et al. Intraoperative sonography in low-grade gliomas. *J Ultrasound Med* 1989;8:131-134.
33. Lange SC, Howe JF, Shuman WP et al. Intraoperative ultrasound detection of metastatic tumors in the central cortex. *Neurosurgery* 1982;11:219-222.
34. Tsutsumi Y, Andoh Y, Inoue N. Ultrasound-guided biopsy for deep-seated brain tumors. *J Neurosurg* 1982;57:164-167.
35. Tsutsumi Y, Andoh Y, Sakaguchi J. A new ultrasound-guided brain biopsy technique through a burr hole. *Acta Neurochir (Wien)* 1989;96:72-75.
36. Enzmann DR, Irwin KM, Fine IM et al. Intraoperative and outpatient echoencephalography through a burr hole. *Neuroradiology* 1984;26:57-59.
37. Enzmann DR, Irwin KM, Marshall WH et al. Intraoperative sonography through a burr hole: guide for brain biopsy. *Am J Neuroradiol* 1984;5:243-246.
38. Berger MS. Ultrasound guided stereotactic biopsy using the Diasonics neuro-biopsy device for deep-seated intracranial lesions. Presented at the Annual Meeting of the American Association of Neurological Surgeons; April 21-25, 1985; Atlanta, Ga.

39. Sutcliffe JC, Battersby RDE. Intraoperative ultrasound-guided biopsy of intracranial lesions: comparison with freehand biopsy. *Brit J Neurosurg* 1991;5:163-168.

40. Rubin JM, Carson PL. Physics and techniques. In: Rubin JM, Chandler WF, eds. *Ultrasound in Neurosurgery*. New York: Raven Press; 1990:1-67.

41. McDicken WW. *Diagnostic Ultrasonics: Principles and Use of Instruments*. New York: John Wiley & Sons; 1976.

42. Rubin JM, Dohrmann GJ. A cannula for use in ultrasonically-guided biopsies of the brain. *J Neurosurg* 1983;59:905-907.

43. Heckermann R, Seidel KJ. The sonographic appearance and contrast of puncture needles. *J Clin Ultrasound* 1983;11:265-268.

44. McGahan JP. Laboratory assessment of ultrasonic needle and catheter visualization. *J Ultrasound Med* 1986;5:373-377.

Infection

45. Enzmann DR, Britt RH, Lyons B et al. High-resolution ultrasound evaluation of experimental brain abscess evolution: comparison with computed tomography and neuropathology. *Radiology* 1982;142:95-102.

46. Wood JH, Parver M, Doppman JL et al. Experimental intraoperative localization of retained intracerebral bone fragments using transdural ultrasound. *J Neurosurg* 1977;46:65-71.

47. Enzmann DR, Britt RH, Lyons B et al. Experimental study of high-resolution ultrasound imaging of hemorrhage, bone fragments, and foreign bodies in head trauma. *J Neurosurg* 1981;54:304-309.

48. Fornage BD, Schernberg FL. Sonographic diagnosis of foreign bodies of the distal extremities. *AJR* 1986;147:567-569.

49. Fornage BD, Schernberg FL. Sonographic pre-operative localization of a foreign body in the hand. *J Ultrasound Med* 1987;6:217-219.

50. Gooding GAW, Gardiman T, Sumers M et al. Sonography of the hand and foot in foreign body detection. *J Ultrasound Med* 1987;6:441-447.

51. Wendell BA, Athey A. Ultrasonic appearance of metallic foreign bodies in parenchymal organs. *J Clin Ultrasound* 1981;9:133-135.

52. Ziskin MC, Thickman DI, Goldenberg WJ et al. The comet tail artifact. *J Ultrasound Med* 1982;1:1-7.

53. Rubin JM, Adler RS, Bude RO et al. Clean and dirty shadowing: a reappraisal. *Radiology* 1991;181:231-236.

54. Grode ML, Komaiko MS. The role of intraoperative ultrasound in neurosurgery. *Neurosurgery* 1983;12:624-628.

55. Lillehei KO, Chandler WF, Knake JF. Real time ultrasound characteristics of the acute intracerebral hemorrhage as studied in the canine model. *Neurosurgery* 1984;14:48-51.

56. Sigel B, Machi J, Beitler JC et al. Red cell aggregation as a cause of blood-flow echogenicity. *Radiology* 1983;148:799-802.

57. Sigel B, Coelho JC, Spigos DG et al. Ultrasonography of blood during stasis and coagulation. *Invest Radiol* 1981;16:71-76.

58. Enzmann DR, Britt RH, Lyons BE et al. Natural history of experimental intracerebral hemorrhage: sonography, computed tomography and neuropathology. *Am J Neuroradiol* 1981;2:517-526.

59. Merritt CRB, Coulon R, Connolly E. Intraoperative neurosurgical ultrasound: transdural and transfontanelle applications. *Radiology* 1983;148:513-517.

Shunts

60. Mahony BS, Gross BH, Callen PW et al. Intraventricular hemorrhage following ventriculoperitoneal shunt placement: real-time ultrasonographic demonstration. *J Ultrasound Med* 1983;2:143-145.

61. Sekhar LN, Moossy J, Guthkelch AN. Malfunctioning ventriculoperitoneal shunts: clinical and pathological features. *J Neurosurg* 1982;56:411-416.

62. Shkolnik A, McLone DG. Intraoperative real-time ultrasonic guidance of ventricular shunt placement in infants. *Radiology* 1981;141:515-517.

63. Widder DJ, Davis KR, Taveras JM. Assessment of ventricular shunt patency by sonography: a new noninvasive test. *AJR* 1986;147:353-356.

64. Widder DJ, Simeone JF. Microbubbles as a contrast agent for neurosonography and ultrasound-guided catheter manipulation: in vitro studies. *AJR* 1986;147:347-352.

65. Babcock DS, Barr LL, Crone KR. Intraoperative uses of ultrasound in the pediatric neurosurgical patient. *Pediatr Neurosurg* 1992;18:84-91.

Vascular Lesions

66. Nornes H, Grip A, Wikeby P. Intraoperative evaluation of cerebral hemodynamics using directional Doppler technique. Pt 1. Arteriovenous malformations. *J Neurosurg* 1979;50:145-151.

67. Fasano VA, Ponzio RM, Liboni W et al. Preliminary experiences with "real-time" intraoperative ultrasonography associated to the laser and ultrasonic aspirator in neurosurgery. *Surg Neurol* 1983;19:318-323.

68. Helvie MA, Rubin JM. Evaluation of traumatic groin arteriovenous fistulas with duplex Doppler sonography. *J Ultrasound Med* 1989;8:21-24.

69. Black KL, Rubin JM, Chandler WF et al. Intraoperative color flow Doppler imaging of AVMs and aneurysms. *J Neurosurg* 1988;68:635-639.

70. Rubin JM, Hatfield MK, Chandler WF et al. Intracerebral arteriovenous malformations: intraoperative color Doppler flow imaging. *Radiology* 1989;170:219-222.

71. Hyodo A, Mizukami M, Tazawa T et al. Intraoperative use of real-time ultrasonography applied to aneurysm surgery. *Neurosurgery* 1983;13:642-645.

72. Nornes H, Grip A, Wikeby P. Intraoperative evaluation of cerebral hemodynamics using directional Doppler technique. Pt 2. Saccular aneurysms. *J Neurosurg* 1979;50:570-577.

CHAPTER 19

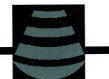

Intraoperative Sonography of the Spine

•

Berta Maria Montalvo, M. D.
Steven Falcone, M. D.

SPINAL SONOGRAPHIC INDICATIONS

Herniated disks
Canal stenosis
Spine fractures
Tumors and cysts
Inflammatory masses
Congenital anomalies

retracting delicate neural tissues. The dynamic nature of real-time sonography also affords the surgeon the opportunity to continually monitor the progress and adequacy of the surgical process.

INDICATIONS

Since its introduction in 1982,[1] intraoperative spinal sonography has been used for the intraoperative management of lesions that compress or fix neural elements. These include herniated disks, canal stenosis, spine fractures, tumors and cysts, inflammatory masses, and congenital anomalies.

Sonography has also been used to locate foreign bodies and to guide procedures like biopsies, drainages, and shunt placements. Sonography has significantly improved the effectiveness and precision of each of these applications, and its use should be universal.

Clinical outcome of spinal surgery depends not only on accurate preoperative diagnosis but also on the proper identification and localization of lesions during surgery and their adequate correction. The use of high-resolution sonography in the operating room has provided the spinal surgeon with a new vision. Without sonography the surgeon had a limited field of view and often had to rely on indirect signs, such as transmitted pulsations, to assess completeness of decompression. With sonography the contents of the thecal sac are precisely depicted, and a view of the ventral canal is obtained without incurring the risk of

TECHNIQUE

We use a portable sonographic machine appropriate for the operating room equipped with preset parameters, high-resolution (7 to 10 MHz) sector, curved array, or linear transducers on a long cord, a camera, and a video tape recorder. In the operating room the transducer and cord are draped in a long, sterile sheath; sterile gel serves as an acoustic couplet between the transducer and sterile sheath.

The radiologist and the surgeon review the preoperative examinations to establish the surgical approach to the case, specifically the level and extent of the surgical exposure. Most patients undergo surgery in the prone position and therefore are examined from a posterior approach. The paraspinal muscles are retracted, the initial laminectomy is performed, and sterile fluid is poured into the wound to serve as an acoustic water path. The tip of the draped transducer is then introduced into the water bath, and the surgeon scans the spinal canal and its contents in the transverse and longitudinal planes. Longitudinal scans are oriented so that the cephalad direction will lie to the left of the image; transverse scans are oriented with the left side of the patient on the left (the reverse of usual anatomic displays) because the patient is prone.

The radiologist and the surgeon review the pertinent findings in the initial scan that may influence the surgical approach. The progress of surgery is monitored with sonography, and the final sonogram documents the results of the surgery.

Limitations

The diagnostic capabilities of intraoperative spinal sonography are limited by the field of view, which is determined by the extent of the laminectomy performed because bone interferes with the transmission of the ultrasound beam. Structures that lie under unresected bone will not be visualized because of acoustic shadowing. **A laminectomy that measures at least 1.5 cm by 1 cm is necessary for adequate visualization of the canal and its contents.** A laminectomy of this size does not affect spinal stability and in most cases does not require added resection. Sonography cannot be used in microsurgery for disk disease because of the small size of the laminectomy.

Substances other than bone may also interfere with the transmission of sound and will obscure visualization of deeper structures. Specifically, dura mater that is calcified dorsally will interfere with visualization of the thecal sac contents and all other structures that lie ventral to the calcification. Gelfoam, used routinely for hemostasis during surgery, has a characteristic appearance, exhibiting a bright interface and a shadowing artifact of reverberations. In large amounts Gelfoam obscures adjacent structures; in small amounts it may be confused with a pathologic process. Therefore prior to scanning **it is desirable to remove all Gelfoam from the operative field.**

SONOGRAPHIC ANATOMY

The **spinal cord** and **cauda equina** are contained within the thecal sac surrounded by anechoic cerebrospinal fluid.[2,3] On transverse views, the cord is oval in shape in the cervical region and round in the thoracic area. The distal cord tapers to the conus medullaris, a characteristic best appreciated on sagittal views. The surface of the cord is brightly reflective, presumably secondary to the pial covering. The parenchyma of the cord is homogeneous and hypoechoic, and the gray and white matter are not individually visualized.[2,3] A midline, echogenic structure is seen within the ventral half of the cord. This central echo has a punctate appearance on transverse views and a linear interface on longitudinal sections. The central echo has been shown to represent the central aspect of the **anterior median** fissure.[4-6] **Denticulate ligaments** tether the cord laterally and are seen as bright, linear interfaces on transverse views. Dorsal arachnoid septations course from the posterior surface of the cord to the dorsal arachnoid and are seen as bright interfaces within the dorsal cerebrospinal fluid (Fig. 19-1).

Dorsal and ventral **nerve roots** are only rarely seen at the cervical, upper, and midthoracic region. They are routinely seen clustering around the conus medullaris as they descend to form the cauda equina. Individual nerve roots typically appear as two parallel, bright, linear echoes, short on transverse views and long and tubular on longitudinal sections. They are most numerous in the upper lumbar canal where the cauda equina can look like a tangle of spaghetti; at this level it may be difficult to resolve individual nerve roots. The number of spinal nerve roots decreases as the roots exit segmentally, so fewer roots are seen in the distal lumbar region (Fig. 19-2).

The shape of the spinal canal varies at different levels. On transverse images following laminectomy the canal at the cervical and lumbar regions resembles an open rectangle whereas in the thoracic region it approximates the shape of a semicircle. On longitudinal examination the dorsal aspect of the vertebral body, a characteristically bright interface, is interrupted by the intervertebral space, a structure of medium echogenicity that exhibits acoustic transmission. In the lumbar region, ventral epidural fat is abundant, usually hyperechoic, and symmetrically distributed in the epidural space.

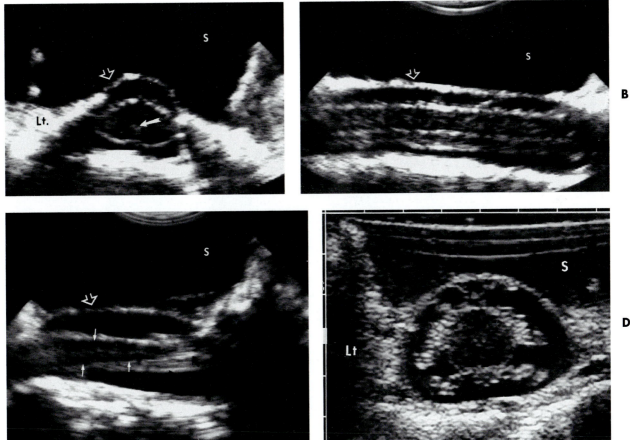

FIG. 19-1. Normal spinal cord. A, Transverse and, **B,** longitudinal scans of the cervical cord show an echogenic line *(open arrowhead)* that represents the dorsal dura-arachnoid layer. Spinal fluid surrounds the cord, which is seen as a hypoechoic structure with echogenic boundaries. The central echo of the cord *(straight arrow)* represents the central aspect of the anterior median fissure. **C,** Longitudinal image of the lower thoracic cord shows the conus medullaris, which is the tapering end of the cord *(white arrows)*. The exiting nerve roots *(black arrows)* are hyperechoic. **D,** Transverse view of the distal spinal cord/proximal cauda equina. Except for the central echo complex, the spinal cord parenchyma is fairly homogeneous and hypoechoic. Surrounding the spinal cord are multiple echogenic foci representing the nerve roots of the proximal cauda equina. *S,* Saline, *Lt,* left. (**A** and **B** from Quencer RM, Montalvo BM. Normal intraoperative spinal sonography. *Am J Neuroradiol* 1984;5:501-505; *AJR* 1984;143:1301-1305. **C** from Montalvo BM, Quencer RM. Intraoperative sonography in spinal surgery: current state of the art. *Neuroradiology* 1986;28:551-590. **D** courtesy of J. William Charboneau, M.D., Mayo Clinic, Rochester, Minn.)

CORD COMPRESSION

Sonographic Criteria for Decompression

Sonography is commonly used to evaluate spinal lesions that compress the spinal cord, thecal sac, or cauda equina. To determine the adequacy of surgical decompression, several criteria have been established.[7-10] Lack of displacement of neural elements is shown by normal or near normal shape of the spinal cord, rounded thecal sac in the lumbar spine, normal course of the cauda equina, absence of initially identified soft tissue or bony mass, normal or near normal shape of the spinal canal, open rectangle in the lumbar region, space visualized between the thecal sac and the bony canal laterally, and no displacement of the spinal cord or cauda equina.

ULTRASOUND CRITERIA OF DECOMPRESSION

Normal or near normal shape of the spinal cord
Rounded thecal sac in the lumbar spine
Normal course of the cauda equina
Absence of initially identified soft tissue or bony mass
Normal or near normal shape of the spinal canal
Open rectangle in the lumbar region
Space visualized between the thecal sac and the bony canal laterally
No displacement of spinal cord or cauda equina

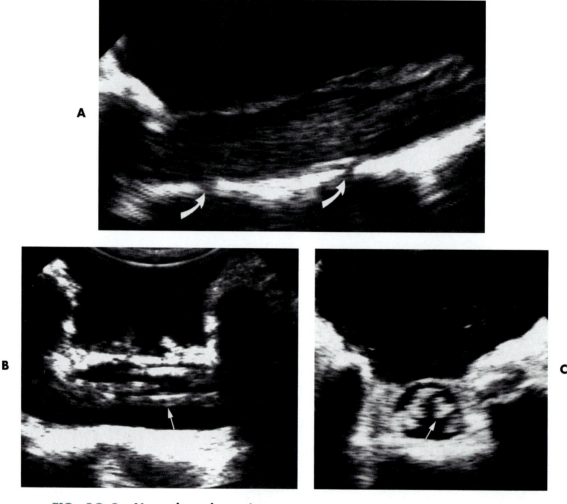

FIG. 19-2. Normal cauda equina. A, Superior (proximal) cauda equina, longitudinal scan. The nerve roots of the cauda equina are small tubular structures that are difficult to resolve individually in the superior lumbar canal. The dorsal surface of the vertebral bodies is delineated by the highly echogenic lines, which are interrupted by intervertebral disk spaces *(curved arrows).* **B** and **C,** Inferior (distal) cauda equina. Longitudinal, *B,* and transverse, *C,* images at this level show the individual nerve roots *(arrows)* within the subarachnoid space.

Of these, the single most important criterion is the lack of displacement of either the spinal cord or the cauda equina.[7-9]

Herniated Disks

Herniated disks within the spinal canal can be differentiated from surrounding normal and abnormal structures by their typical sonographic appearance. **Disks** are sharply marginated, exhibit medium echogenicity, can be clearly seen in two views, and are located immediately adjacent to the intervertebral disk space where they compress neural structures (Fig. 19-3). In **spondylolisthesis**, longitudinal sonograms can establish the presence of a herniated disk when the characteristic soft tissue mass is seen protruding into the canal between the edges of the subluxed vertebrae. Spondylolisthesis without associated disk herniation is seen as a displacement of the normal dorsal vertebral surface (Fig. 19-4). **Ventral epidural fat** should not be confused with a disk as it appears homogeneously hyperechoic, does not displace neural elements, and is symmetrical in distribution. **Scar**, on the other hand, may be heterogeneous, brightly echogenic, and mimic fat, or it may be of medium echogenicity and mimic disk. The identifying characteristic of scar is the absence of a well-defined interface with surrounding tissues (Fig. 19-5). **Swollen roots** are round and well defined on transverse views, but unlike herniated disks, they are poorly defined on longitudinal views.

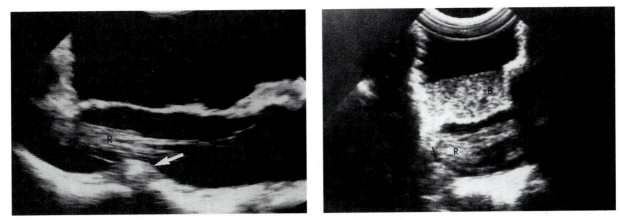

A **B**

FIG. 19-3. Herniated disk, longitudinal scans. A, Herniated disk *(white arrow)* is located at the intervertebral interspace. It appears as a sharply marginated soft tissue mass that touches the nerve roots, *R*, in the lumbar region. **B,** When the herniated disk *(black arrow)* is located at the edge of the laminectomy, it may be missed, but compression of the adjacent nerve roots, *R*, helps define the soft-tissue mass. *B*, Fresh blood in the saline dorsal to the dura.

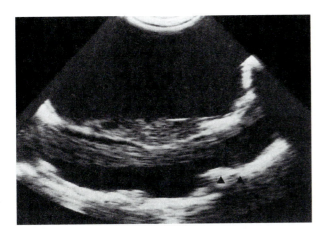

FIG. 19-4. Spondylolisthesis. In contrast to a disk, spondylolisthesis is seen as displacement of the normal dorsal surface of the vertebral body *(arrowheads)*, which does not compress neural elements.

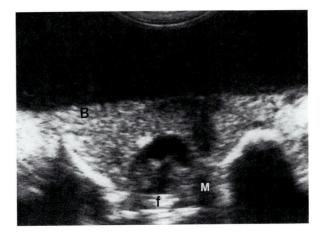

FIG. 19-5. Scar. Transverse image shows a poorly marginated mass, *M*, adjacent to the right side of the thecal sac. This poor margination is characteristic of a scar rather than a herniated disk. Note the bright echogenicity of epidural fat, *f*. *B*, Blood saline layer.

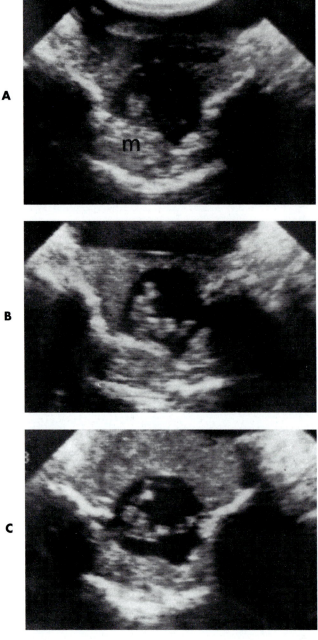

FIG. 19-6. Occult residual herniated disk.
Transverse images. **A,** After posterior and lateral bone decompression a soft-tissue mass, *M,* with well-defined edges is seen, which deforms the ventrolateral aspect of the thecal sac. This appearance is typical of a disk. **B,** Following diskectomy, residual disk material, which was surgically occult, is visible sonographically, and the thecal sac continues to be deformed. **C,** After the residual occult fragment was removed, no soft-tissue mass remains and the thecal sac is nearly normal in shape. The diskectomy is now judged to be complete.

The ability of sonography to discriminate a disk from other structures has important implications in the surgical management of disk herniation. Because a common cause of failed back surgery is residual disk material,[11] the removal of as much abnormal disk as possible from the spinal canal is a crucial goal of surgery. In our series, **40% of patients examined after routine diskectomy were found to have unsuspected residual fragments**, which were then removed (Fig. 19-6).[9]

Canal Stenosis

Failure to recognize and adequately treat lateral stenosis is the most common cause of failed back surgery.[11] Sonography provides an immediate evaluation of the effect of bone on adjacent neural tissue during decompression surgery of the lumbar canal for stenosis. Sonography shows when sufficient bone has been removed to result in a decompressed canal. The sac will assume a normal rounded configuration, and space will be visualized between the sac and the remaining lateral facet. When sonography shows that the thecal sac is encroached laterally by facets at a symptomatic level, the surgeon will extend the facetectomies (Fig. 19-7). Similarly, if sonography shows that the sac is compressed by a ventral spur, spur resection may be attempted. About 20% of patients examined with sonography after posterolateral decompression for canal stenosis had persistent encroachment of the neural elements by bone and had to undergo further bony removal to achieve optimal decompression.[9]

Fractures

Open reduction and stabilization with fusion and metallic rod instruments is the accepted management of patients with unstable thoracic and lumbar fractures because they experience less pain and are mobilized and rehabilitated earlier than when treated with postural reduction alone. The degree of neurologic improvement in patients with incomplete neurologic deficits and bone in the canal may be related to the adequacy of neural element decompression. The bone that compresses the neural elements is usually hidden from view by the spinal cord and thecal sac. "Blind" placement of metallic rods results in inadequate reduction and distraction in a high percentage of cases.[12,13] Mobilizing the spinal cord or thecal sac is risky. Sonography safely provides an accurate view of the ventral canal and evaluates the shape of the spinal canal, the presence of bone in the canal, and the degree of compression of spinal cord or cauda equina (Figs. 19-8 and 19-9). In addition, the extent of intramedullary injuries and the location of the conus medullaris may be assessed.[14-16]

Decompression was inadequate in about half of the 41 unstable spine fracture patients we studied sonographically who had metallic rod fixation.[16] In this setting the surgeon may elect to reposition the rods or to resect or reduce the bone fragment; repeat sonography can document the successful decompression.

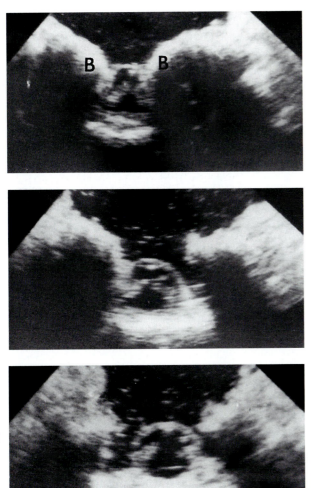

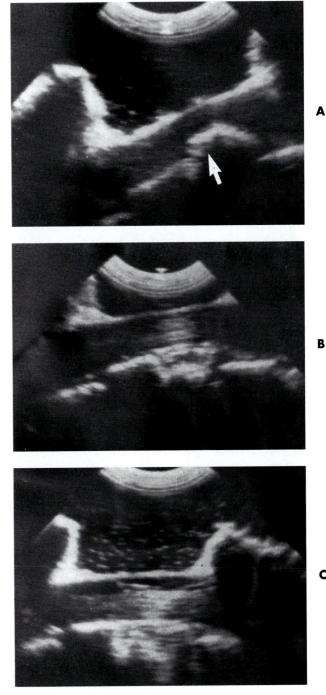

FIG. 19-7. Decompression of spinal canal stenosis. **A,** Transverse image shows inadequate lateral bone decompression following bilateral facetectomies. Residual bony masses, *B,* deform the thecal sac, which is triangular and narrowed. **B,** Extended right facetectomy. The right side of the thecal sac is rounded and there is space between the residual facet and the sac, but bony compression persists on the left. **C,** Extended left facetectomy. The left side of the thecal sac is now rounded and there is a wide space between the sac and residual bone.

The use of sonography during metallic rod instrumentation for unstable thoracic and lumbar fractures **improves the rate of adequate decompression from about 50% to 80%.**

Fragments

Patients who have intracanalicular metallic or bony fragments as a result of recent gunshot wounds undergo surgery to remove these fragments to relieve pain or prevent its development and with the goal of partially reversing any incomplete neurologic deficit that may exist. Sonography has proved to be an effective and fast-localizing tool in these cases and is useful

FIG. 19-8. Decompression of upper lumbar fracture. Longitudinal images. **A,** Displaced bone fragment *(arrow)* protrudes into the canal, significantly compressing the cauda equina. **B,** Metallic rods were inserted and distracted, and neural compression reduced, but still present. **C,** The bone fragment was removed after posterolateral decompression; vertebral alignment is nearly normal, and the cauda equina follows a normal course. (From Montalvo BM, Quencer RM, Green BA et al. Intraoperative sonography in spinal trauma. *Radiology* 1984;153:125-134.)

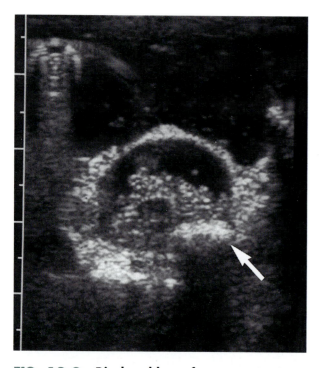

FIG. 19-9. Displaced bone fragment. Axial scan at the distal spinal cord shows a linear echogenic structure *(arrow)* with shadowing compatible with a bone fragment. This piece of fractured bone compresses the right ventral spinal cord and thecal sac. Intraoperative ultrasound is useful in assessing for adequate decompression. (Courtesy of J. William Charboneau, M.D., Mayo Clinic, Rochester, Minn.)

in the evaluation and management of associated lesions, such as intramedullary or subarachnoid cysts (Fig. 19-10).[17]

POSTTRAUMATIC MYELOPATHY

Posttraumatic cystic myelopathy is a frequent complication of spinal trauma, and it is currently best diagnosed with magnetic resonance imaging (MRI). The syndrome presents with pain, spasticity, hyperhidrosis, and ascending motor and sensory loss. The cord lesion is a round or oval cyst that may be lobulated and contain fibroglial scars. It is often associated with myelomalacia of the adjacent cord, cord compression by bone, adhesions that tether the cord, and subarachnoid cysts.[18,19]

MRI reliably diagnoses posttraumatic cysts. Sonography is excellent in distinguishing intramedullary from subarachnoid cysts and from surrounding myelomalacia. **Posttraumatic intramedullary cysts** have the typical anechoic appearance of cysts on sonography, occur in small, normal-size, or enlarged cords, and may be septated (Fig. 19-11). Surgical management of intramedullary cysts consists of shunting the cyst into the pleural or peritoneal space and lysing the associated adhesions that tether the cord as well as removing other causes of extrinsic cord

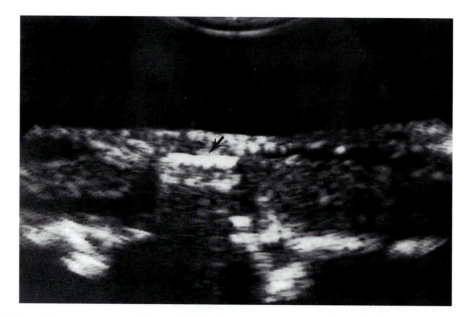

FIG. 19-10. Surgically occult bullet fragment in thoracic cord. Intrathecal bullet fragment *(arrow)* was not palpable because of abundant scar (between cord, bullet, and dura) but was easily identified with sonography by its typical, very bright interface with reverberative shadowing. The spinal cord has lost its normal architecture and is uniformly hyperechoic with loss of the normal central echo. These findings are typical of myelomalacia. (From Montalvo BM, Quencer RM, Green BA et al. Intraoperative sonography in spinal trauma. *Radiology* 1984;153:125-134.)

compression. Surgery prevents further cyst enlargement and frequently reverses recently developed symptoms. Sonography locates the cyst prior to the opening up of the dura; it helps the surgeon choose the optimal place to enter the cyst with least damage to the intact spinal cord. Intracystic fibroglial scars that may compartmentalize the cyst into separate locules are identified as thin septa and lysed by the surgeon (see Fig. 19-10). Sonography is used after shunting to evaluate adequacy of cyst decompression.[20,21] If collapse of the cyst is incomplete, the catheter may be repositioned, intracystic scars may be lysed, or a second catheter may be inserted, depending on the cause for the lack of decompression. Persistent cord tethering caused by adhesions can also be seen and the adhesions lysed.

Myelomalacia may precede the development of a posttraumatic spinal cord cyst[19,22-26] and may result in a posttraumatic myelopathy.[2,18,23,27-29] As in cystic posttraumatic myelopathy, the syndrome of the posttraumatic noncystic myelopathy is associated with ascending motor and sensory loss, progressive spasticity, autonomic dysreflexia, worsening bowel and/or bladder function, and local or radicular pain.* Surgical and intraoperative sonographic evaluation has consistently demonstrated associated arachnoid adhesions and cord tethering (Fig. 19-12).

Although there are certain characteristics on MRI scan that may suggest the presence of myeloma-

*References 22, 23, 27, 30, 31.

lacia, it may be difficult to distinguish from an intramedullary cyst. Intraoperative sonography is superior in this distinction. On sonography, **myelomalacia appears as an area of abnormal spinal cord echotexture with loss of the central echo** (see Fig. 19-12; Figs. 19-13 and 19-14). Compared to the normal spinal cord, the parenchyma may be hypoechoic, hyperechoic, or contain microcysts.[27] Spinal cord expansion may be seen. The spinal cord is invariably **tethered by fibrous intradural adhesions.** Dorsal tethering of the spinal cord is most common.

Distinction between a confluent intramedullary cyst from myelomalacia is more than an academic exercise if surgical intervention is contemplated. In patients with a progressive posttraumatic myelomalacic myelopathy, **lysis of surrounding spinal cord adhesions** and untethering of the cord resulted in clinical improvement.[27] Recreation of a subarachnoid space with a dural allograft is important to help prevent retethering of the spinal cord. Intraoperative sonography can assist in assessing for adequate untethering of the spinal cord.

Subarachnoid cysts are seen as anechoic extramedullary collections that displace the cord and may have fibrous septations. Their shunting can be monitored with sonography (see Fig. 19-13).[15-21,30]

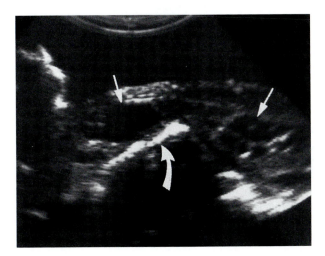

FIG. 19-11. Posttraumatic cystic myelopathy. Longitudinal scan shows a large, angulated, bony fragment *(curved arrow)* that compresses the cord. Multiloculated intramedullary cysts *(arrows)* are observed cranial and caudal to the compression. The compressing bone was removed, and by sonographic guidance, a catheter was inserted to lyse the septations and collapse the cysts.

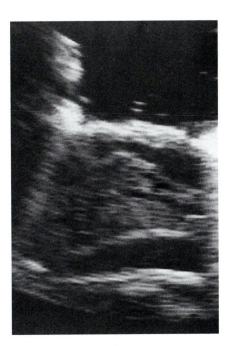

FIG. 19-12. Spinal cord tethering. Longitudinal scan of the cervical cord was performed through a small window and anterior approach. The spinal cord echo texture is inhomogeneous with loss of the central echo. The cord is deviated or "pulled" anteriorly by arachnoid adhesions. After confirming the position of the spinal cord the surgeon opened the dura and lysed the adhesions.

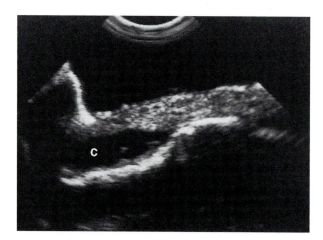

FIG. 19-13. Subarachnoid cyst, bone fragment, and myelomalacia. Echogenic, myelomalacic cord is tethered and inseparable from the dorsal dura and is compressed by a posteriorly displaced bone fragment. A large, subarachnoid cyst, C, displaces the cord cephalad to the site of bone compression. Small, intracystic scars are evident as tiny, echogenic foci. (From Quencer RM, Montalvo BM, Green BA et al. Intraoperative spinal sonography of soft tissue masses of the spinal cord and spinal canal. *Am J Neuroradiol* 1984;5:507-515; *AJR* 1984;143:1307-1315.)

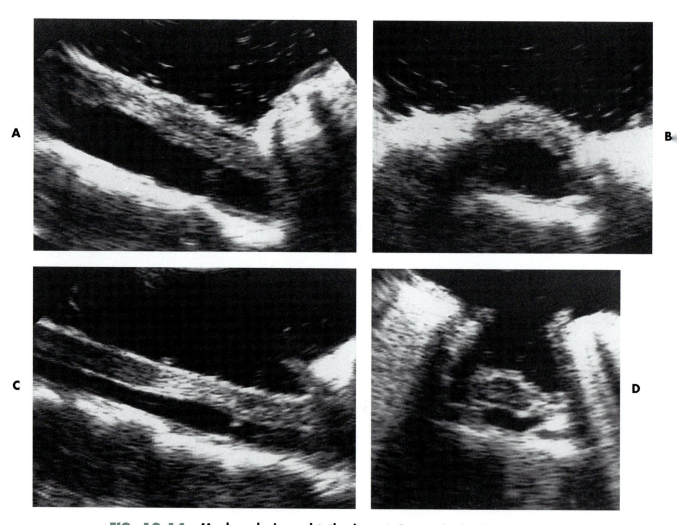

FIG. 19-14. Myelomalacia and tethering. A, Longitudinal and, B, axial scan of the cervical cord demonstrates dorsal tethering against a thickened dura. Abnormal increased echogenicity is present in the spinal cord. Scans performed after untethering, C and D, with the spinal cord in a more normal position in the spinal canal. Note decrease in size of the ventral subarachnoid space. (From reference 27.)

TUMORS

The sonographic characteristics of intramedullary tumors are nonspecific.[7,32-39] Most tumors enlarge the cord, efface the central echo, and are either isoechoic or hyperechoic compared to normal cord tissue (Figs. 19-15 to 19-18). **Ependymomas, metastases,** and **dermoids** are typically well-demarcated hyperechoic lesions. **Astrocytomas** and **ependymomas** may also undergo cystic degeneration, which is seen as a cystic region within the tumor. Cord enlargement caused by syringomyelia can be easily differentiated from neoplasm in most cases.[36] Calcification is a nonspecific finding and may be seen with ependymoma, astrocytoma, and dermoid. Color flow Doppler ultrasound has been shown to be of great value in detection of **hemangioblastomas,** which are characteristically hypervascular.[40]

For purposes of biopsy, surgeons have traditionally chosen an area of gross cord enlargement; however, the cord may be enlarged secondary to syringohydromyelia, cord edema, or cystic degeneration, and biopsies directed at these areas will be nondiagnostic (see Fig. 19-15). Sonography determines the optimal site for biopsy by identifying the region of solid cord enlargement where the central echo is absent. Sonography is especially valuable to guide a biopsy of the solid component of a tumor that has associated cystic changes. With the use of sonography, fewer passes are needed for a diagnostic biopsy, unnecessary damage to the cord is avoided, and repeat surgery because of nondiagnostic biopsies is obviated.[33]

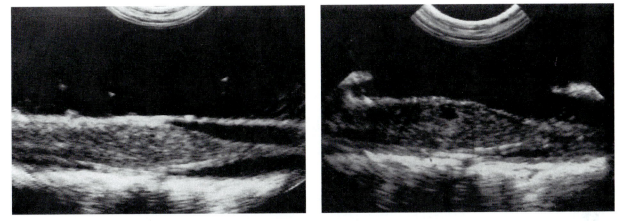

FIG. 19-15. Biopsy of intramedullary tumor. A, Intramedullary metastatic disease enlarges the conus medullaris and effaces the central echo. The exact site of the biopsy can be chosen prior to opening the dura. **B,** A small cystic space confirms that the biopsy was performed in the area of abnormal cord. Notice that the posterior dura is now open.

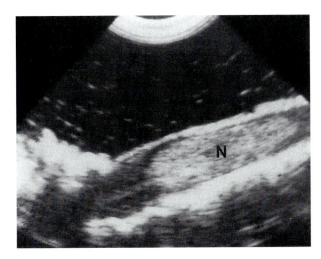

FIG. 19-16. Diffuse thoracic cord enlargement with focal astrocytoma. Sonography clearly distinguishes the area of cord enlargement caused by neoplasm (*N,* oval echogenic area) from nonneoplastic enlargement seen superiorly. Note the presence of the central echo in the region of the cord free of tumor and the absence of the central echo in the neoplastic region. Areas of cord enlargement do not necessarily represent tumor, as in this case in which a prior nondiagnostic biopsy was performed without the use of sonography. The tumor is echogenic, well defined, and effaces the central echo.

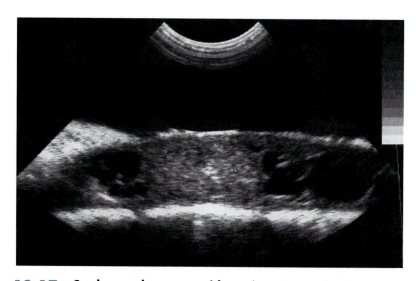

FIG. 19-17. Cord ependymoma with syrinx. Longitudinal scan shows focal spinal cord enlargement by a heterogeneous mass. Rostral and caudal to the mass are reactive cord cysts. (Courtesy of J. William Charboneau, M.D., Mayo Clinic, Rochester, Minn.)

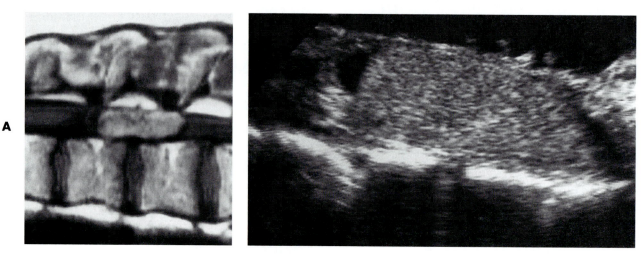

A   B

FIG. 19-18. Filar ependymoma. **A,** T1-weighted gadolinium-enhanced sagittal MRI scan oriented in prone position. An enhancing intradural mass is present at the L1-L2 level. Note small superior cystic collection. Is this cystic collection part of the mass or loculated cerebrospinal fluid? **B,** Intraoperative longitudinal ultrasound confirms the cystic component of the mass in its superior aspect.

Extramedullary masses, such as **metastases, meningiomas, neurinomas, neurofibromas, lipomas,** and **dermoids,** are round or oval in shape, have well-demarcated borders, are hyperechoic, and compress the cord or nerve roots in proportion to their size (Figs. 19-19 to 19-21).[7,33,37] Sonography is valuable in planning surgical resection of these masses. It is used to localize the mass prior to opening the dura, define its craniocaudal and anteroposterior extent, which may not be appreciated visually, and to demonstrate its relationship to normal spinal cord or nerve roots. Sonography can also detect surgically occult residual tumor, which can then be excised, ensuring an optimal result (see Fig. 19-19).[38] When tumors are unresectable, sonography guides the debulking procedures to ensure optimal decompression of the spinal cord or cauda equina.

INFECTION

The use of intraoperative sonography is critical in the surgical management of epidural abscesses.[33,41,42]

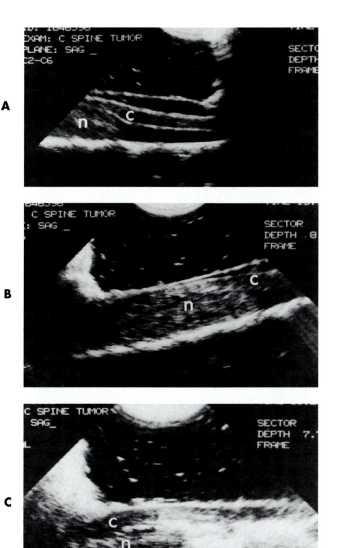

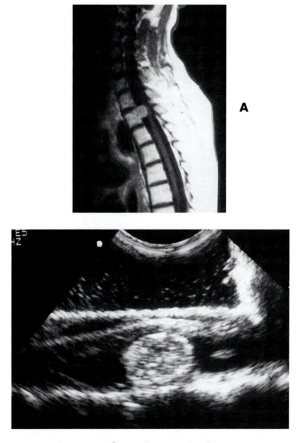

FIG. 19-20. Thoracic meningioma. A, Sagittal postcontrast T1-weighted MRI scan reveals a well-defined, round, homogeneously enhancing intradural mass ventral to the upper thoracic spinal cord. There is associated cord compression. **B,** Intraoperative longitudinal scan helps the surgeon localize the round mass ventral to the cord. (Courtesy of Tom Winter, M.D.)

FIG. 19-19. Partial resection of neurinoma ventral to cervical cord. Longitudinal scans. **A** and **B,** Prior to resection, sonography defines the ventral location and craniocaudal extent of the neurinoma. **C,** Scan after resection shows residual neurinoma, *n,* in the cranial aspect of the canal. The more caudal region of the canal is partially obscured by acoustic shadow from Gelfoam. *c,* Cervical cord. (From Quencer RM, Montalvo BM, Naidich TP et al. Intraoperative sonography in spinal dysraphism and syringohydromyelia. *Am J Neuroradiol* 1987;8:329-337; *AJR* 1987; 148:1005-1013.)

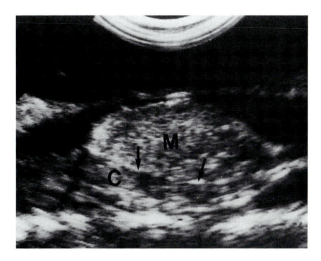

FIG. 19-21. Lipoma from conus medullaris. Sonogram prior to opening the dura shows a well-defined, oval, hyperechoic mass, *M,* posterior to the conus, *C,* in a subpial location. The preoperative imaging studies suggested that the mass was within the conus rather than adjacent to it. Note the well-defined interface *(arrows)* between the mass and conus medullaris.

Epidural abscesses appear as localized echogenic masses compressing the dural sac (Figs. 19-22 and 19-23). With ultrasound, extradural location, extent in the spinal canal, and their relationship to the spinal cord are clear. Sonography is particularly valuable in the localization of ventral abscesses that are difficult to

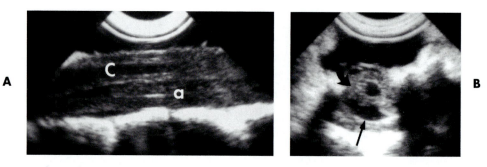

FIG. 19-22. Ventral epidural abscess and meningitis. A, Longitudinal view at the level of the conus, *C*, shows an extensive hyperechoic abscess, *a*, elevating the ventral dura and posteriorly displacing the thecal sac, which contains the conus medullaris and cauda equina. **B,** Transverse scan after evacuation. The ventral dura *(straight arrow)* has returned to a normal position, confirming adequate drainage. An abundance of diffuse hyperechoic material *(curved arrow)* surrounds the conus and distends the sac. This appearance is typical of meningitis.

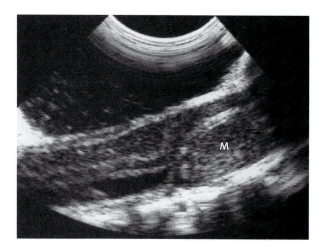

FIG. 19-23. Tuberculous abscess. Longitudinal view shows a well-circumscribed ventral mass, *M*, isoechoic to the cord, displacing the dura dorsally and compressing the spinal cord. The mass represents a tuberculous abscess. (Courtesy of J. William Charboneau, M.D., Mayo Clinic, Rochester, Minn.)

visualize surgically (see Fig. 19-22). Associated **meningitis** can be distinguished from abscess, and appears as diffuse echogenic material that distends the subarachnoid space and replaces the normal anechoic cerebrospinal fluid (see Fig. 19-22). Sonography helps the surgeon plan the evacuation of epidural abscesses, monitors this process to ensure optimal decompression, and prevents unnecessary manipulation of the spinal cord.[41]

CONGENITAL LESIONS

Spinal dysraphism represents a failure of normal midline fusion and may be associated with multiple lesions, including **congenital tumors, diastematomyelia, syringohydromyelia, meningocele, myelomeningocele,** and **tethered cord.** Each of these anomalies may occur in isolation or in combination with other dysraphic states. Surgery in these cases is performed primarily to free the spinal cord from tethering and to effectively decompress neural tissue. Sonography has proven to be useful in many of these conditions.

As with acquired spinal masses, sonography of congenital tumors defines their extent and their relationship to normal neural tissue. **Lipomas** appear as highly echogenic masses that may be found in the filum terminale (see Fig. 19-21; Fig. 19-24). The location and extent of tumor may alter the surgical approach. If sonography demonstrates that the cord is surrounded by tumor and the patient is neurologically normal, the surgeon may take a less aggressive approach and may not completely resect the tumor, particularly if it would require extensive cord retraction.

In diastematomyelia, sonography can display the cleft of the cord, the site and length of associated bone spurs or fibrous septa, and the nature of any adhesions present, as well as any associated tumors and/or hydromyelic cavities (Fig. 19-25).

Syringohydromyelic cavities are easily detected sonographically and usually managed by shunting to the subarachnoid space or, if small, by fenestration of the cavity (Figs. 19-26 and 19-27). The distal end of the syrinx cavity is identified so that a shunt can be passed into the cavity through the lowest possible portion of the spinal cord, minimizing the risk of neurologic deficit. Any septa that may compartmentalize the syrinx into separate lobules can also be identified with sonography. Successful decompression of the syrinx by a shunt or fenestration can be documented prior to finalizing surgery.[43]

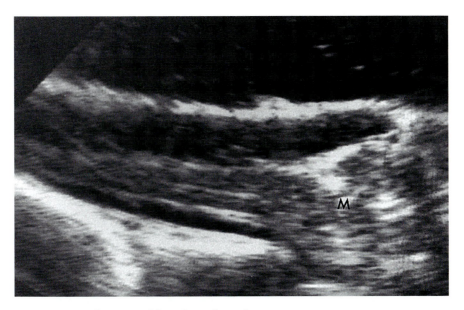

FIG. 19-24. Lipoma with tethered cord. Longitudinal scan in the lower lumbar region demonstrates an abnormally low position of the spinal cord. The central echo is obscured by an expansile mass, *M*. This intradural pial lipoma infiltrates the spinal cord parenchyma.

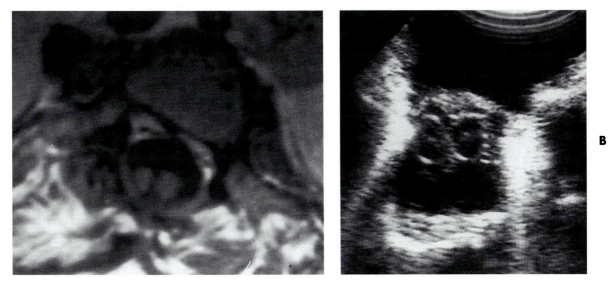

FIG. 19-25. Diastematomyelia. **A,** T1-weighted axial MRI scan at a lower lumbar segment reveals two hemicords in a single dural sac. The posterior elements are malformed and unfused. **B,** Transverse prone sonographic view at the same level as **A** shows the two hemicords each with their own central echo. Focal thickening of the dura is seen dorsally in both **A** and **B.**

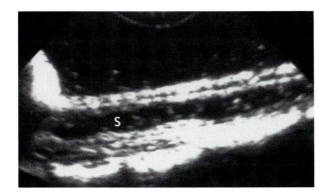

FIG. 19-26. Syrinx. Longitudinal image of the cervical cord through an intact dura mater. A long, mostly anechoic, cystic space, *s*, is seen within the cord. Note the small echogenic foci, which are most likely scar and are commonly seen in these congenital lesions.

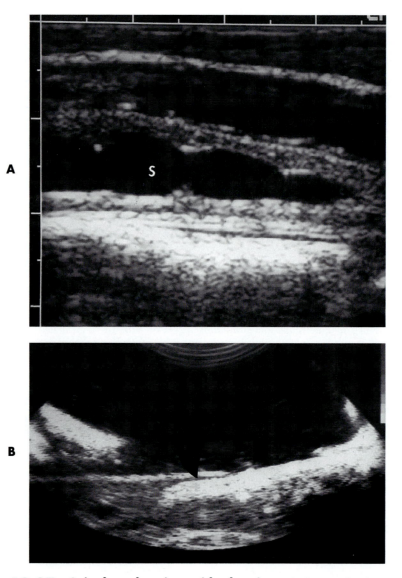

FIG. 19-27. Spinal cord syrinx with shunting. A, Longitudinal scan demonstrates a typical cord syrinx, *s,* of the thoracic cord. A shunt catheter was placed within the cyst with intraoperative sonographic monitoring. **B,** Longitudinal scan confirms intramedullary location of the shunt. The catheter is highly echogenic *(curved arrow).* The cyst is nearly completely collapsed with a small residual cyst in the cephalad aspect of the cord.

REFERENCES
Indications
1. Dohrmann GJ, Rubin JM. Intraoperative ultrasound imaging of the spinal cord: syringomyelia, cysts and tumors—a preliminary report. *Surg Neurol* 1982;18(6):395-399.

Sonographic Anatomy
2. Quencer RM, Montalvo BM. Normal intraoperative spinal sonography. *Am J Neuroradiol* 1984;5:501-505; *AJR* 1984;143:1301-1305.
3. Montalvo BM, Quencer RM. Intraoperative sonography. In: Schnitzlein HN, Murtagh FR, eds. *Imaging Anatomy of the Head and Spine.* 2nd ed. Baltimore, Md: Urban and Schwarzenberg; 1990:443-451.
4. Skaggs PH, Montalvo BM. Sonographic anatomic correlation in the spine. *Radiology* 1984;153(P):326.

5. Montalvo BM, Skaggs PH. The central canal of the spinal cord: ultrasonic identification. (Letter to the editor.) *Radiology* 1985;155:535.
6. Nelson MD Jr, Sedler JA, Gilles FH. Spinal cord central echo complex: histoanatomic correlation. *Radiology* 1989;170:479-481.

Cord Compression
7. Montalvo BM, Quencer RM. Intraoperative sonography in spinal surgery: current state of the art. *Neuroradiology* 1986;28:551-590.
8. Montalvo BM. The role of intraoperative ultrasonography in the management of spinal lesions. In: Rifkin MD, ed. *Clinics in Diagnostic Ultrasound 22: Intraoperative and Endoscopic Ultrasonography.* New York: Churchill Livingstone; 1987:33-63.

9. Montalvo BM, Quencer RM, Brown MD et al. Lumbar disk herniation and canal stenosis: value of intraoperative sonography in diagnosis and surgical management. *Am J Neuroradiol* 1990;11:31-40; *AJR* 1990;154:821-830.

10. Imamura H, Iwasaki Y, Hida K et al. Intraoperative spinal sonography in the cervical anterior approach. *Neurol Med Chir* 1995;34(3):144-147.

11. Burton CV, Kirkaldy-Willis WH, Yong-Hing K. Causes of failure of surgery on the lumbar spine. *Clin Orthop* 1981;157:191-199.

12. Montalvo BM, Quencer RM, Green BA et al. Intraoperative sonography in spinal trauma. *Radiology* 1984;153:125-134.

13. Eismont FJ, Green BA, Berkowitz BM et al. The role of intraoperative ultrasonography in the treatment of thoracic and lumbar spine fractures. *Spine* 1984;9(8):782-787.

14. Quencer RM, Montalvo BM, Eismont FJ et al. Intraoperative spinal sonography in thoracic and lumbar fractures: evaluation of Harrington rod instrumentation. *Am J Neuroradiol* 1985;6:353-359; *AJR* 1985;145:343-349.

15. Flesch JR, Leider LL, Erickson DL et al. Harrington instrumentation and spinal fusion for unstable fractures and fracture/dislocations of the thoracic and lumbar spine. *J Bone Joint Surg* 1977;59:143-153.

16. Yosipovitch Z, Robin GC, Makin M. Open reduction of unstable thoracolumbar spinal injuries and fixation with Harrington rods. *J Bone Joint Surg* 1977;59:1003-1015.

17. Montalvo BM, Quencer RM, Green BA et al. Intraoperative spinal sonography in gunshot wounds to the spine. *Radiology* 1984;153(P):260.

Posttraumatic Myelopathy

18. Osborne DRS, Vavoulis G, Nashold BS et al. Late sequelae of spinal cord trauma. *J Neurosurg* 1982;57:18-23.

19. Quencer RM, Green BA, Eismont FJ. Posttraumatic spinal cord cysts: clinical features and characterization with metrizamide computed tomography. *Radiology* 1983;146:415-423.

20. Quencer RM, Morse BMM, Green BA. Intraoperative spinal sonography: adjunct to metrizamide computed tomography in the assessment and surgical decompression of posttraumatic spinal cord cysts. *Am J Neuroradiol* 1984;5:71-79; *AJR* 1984;142:593-601.

21. Sklar E, Quencer RM, Green BA et al. Acquired spinal subarachnoid cysts: evaluation with MR, CT myelography, and intraoperative sonography. *Am J Neuroradiol* 1989;10:1097-1104; *AJR* 153:1057-1064.

22. MacDonald RL, Findlay JM, Tator CH. Microcystic spinal cord degeneration causing post-traumatic myelopathy. Report of two cases. *J Neurosurg* 1988;68:466-471.

23. Fox JL, Wener L, Drennan DC et al. Central spinal cord injury: magnetic resonance imaging confirmation and operative considerations. *Neurosurgery* 1988;22:340-347.

24. Umbach I, Heilporn A. Review article: post-spinal cord injury syringomyelia. *Paraplegia* 1991;29:219-221.

25. McLean DR, Miller JDR, Allen PBR et al. Post-traumatic syringomyelia. *J Neurosurg* 1973;39:485-492.

26. Seibert CE, Dreizbach JN, Swanson WB et al. Progressive post-traumatic cystic myelopathy. *Am J Neuroradiol* 1981;2:115-119.

27. Falcone S, Quencer RM, Green BA et al. Progressive post-traumatic myelomacic myelopathy: imaging and clinical features. *Am J Neuroradiol* 1994;15:747-754.

28. Kawakami N, Mimatsu K, Kato F et al. Intraoperative ultrasonographic evaluation of the spinal cord in cervical myelopathy. *Spine* 1994;19(1):34-41.

29. Ragnarsson TS, Durwood QJ, Nordgren RE. Spinal cord tethering after traumatic paraplegia with late neurologic deterioration. *J Neurosurg* 1986;64:397-401.

30. Gebarski SS, Maynard FW, Gabrielsen TO et al. Posttraumatic progressive myelopathy. *Radiology* 1985;157:379-385.

31. Stevens JM, Olney JS, Kendall BE. Post-traumatic cystic and non-cystic myelopathy. *Neuroradiology* 1985;27:48-56.

Tumors

32. Knake JE, Chandler WF, McGillicuddy JE et al. Intraoperative spinal sonography of intraspinal tumors: initial experience. *Am J Neuroradiol* 1983;4:1199-1201.

33. Quencer RM, Montalvo BM, Green BA et al. Intraoperative spinal sonography of soft-tissue masses of the spinal cord and spinal canal. *Am J Neuroradiol* 1984;5:507-515; *AJR* 1984;143:1307-1315.

34. Platt JF, Rubin JM, Chandler WF et al. Intraoperative spinal sonography in the evaluation of intramedullary tumors. *J Ultrasound Med* 1988;7:317-325.

35. Post MJD, Quencer RM, Green BA et al. Intramedullary spinal cord metastases, mainly of nonneurogenic origin. *Am J Neuroradiol* 1987;8:339-346; *AJR* 1987;148:1015-1022.

36. Hutchins WW, Volgelzang RL, Neiman HL et al. Differentiation of tumor from syringohydromyelia: intraoperative neurosonography of the spinal cord. *Radiology* 1984;151:171-174.

37. Mimatsu K, Kawakami N, Kato F et al. Intraoperative ultrasonography of extramedullary spinal tumours. *Neuroradiology* 1992;34(5):440-443.

38. Matsuzaki H, Tokuhashi Y, Wakabayashi K et al. Clinical values of intraoperative ultrasonography for spinal tumors. *Spine* 1992;17(11):1392-1399.

39. Kawakami N, Mimatsu K, Kato F. Intraoperative sonography of intramedullary spinal cord tumours. *Neuroradiology* 1992;34(5):436-439.

40. Avila NA, Shawker TH, Choyke PL et al. Cerebellar and spinal hemangioblastomas: evaluation with intraoperative gray-scale and color Doppler flow US. *Radiology* 1993;188(1):143-147.

Infection

41. Post MJD, Quencer RM, Montalvo BM et al. Spinal infection: evaluation with MR imaging and intraoperative US. *Radiology* 1988;169:765-771.

42. Mak KH, Au KK, Fung KY et al. Spinal epidural abscess: a report of nine cases and the use of intra-operative ultrasonography. *Austral NZ J Surg* 1996;66(5):287-290.

Congenital Lesions

43. Quencer RM, Montalvo BM, Naidich TP et al. Intraoperative sonography in spinal dysraphism and syringohydromyelia. *Am J Neuroradiol* 1987;8:329-337; *AJR* 1987;148:1005-1013.

CHAPTER 20

Intraoperative and Laparoscopic Sonography of the Abdomen

•

Robert A. Lee, M.D.

Robert A. Kane, M.D., F.A.C.R.

Eric J. Lantz, M.D.

J. William Charboneau, M.D.

Intraoperative ultrasonography (IOUS) is a dynamic and rapidly growing imaging technique providing important real-time information to the radiologist and the surgeon. It identifies and characterizes lesions seen on preoperative imaging and discovers new lesions not detected by preoperative imaging or surgical inspection and palpation. IOUS is usually the final imaging procedure, and it requires clear communication between the radiologist and the surgeon. The ultimate goal is to correlate preoperative images, surgical inspection and palpation, and IOUS findings to determine the most appropriate surgical procedure.[1,2] Continued growth of IOUS is expected as more surgeons become aware of its usefulness and as laparoscopic ultrasound techniques and intraoperative ultrasound-guided tumor ablation techniques are improved.

A-mode IOUS was first used in the early 1960s for evaluating the biliary system for calculi.[3,4] Image quality was not ideal, and interpretation was difficult. However, a number of technical advances have made IOUS both practical and useful. Over the past 15 years there has been a resurgence in the use of IOUS because equipment advances have allowed real-time images of high quality to be produced in the operating room. Smaller, dedicated IOUS probes have also been developed, which make the routine use of ultrasonography in the operating room easier. Although IOUS accounts for a small percentage (fewer than 1%) of ultrasound examinations in our practices, its rate of growth has been rapid, and the number of IOUS examinations has increased by more than 200% during the past 5 years.[5] In 1996 we performed approximately 500 IOUS examinations.

Many of the technical problems and limitations in routine abdominal ultrasonography are not present in the operating room after laparotomy. Shadowing from bony structures, such as the ribs, and sound attenuation in the body wall are no longer present. All bowel can easily be moved out of the way to scan a particular solid organ or vascular structure. This allows high-frequency, high-resolution ultrasound probes to be used directly on the surface of the organ being examined. When these technical problems affecting image quality have been removed or minimized in the operating room, high-resolution images of high quality are routinely obtained, allowing superb lesion detection, localization, and characterization.

For the radiologist, the most important and significant drawback of IOUS is the time away from the radiology department. Because of this requirement, many radiologists have been reluctant to become involved with IOUS. Depending on the complexity of the case, the radiologists and the ultrasound equipment can be out of the department for 30 min to 1 hr or longer. Therefore IOUS cases should be prescheduled the day before surgery so that an experienced radiologist and the proper equipment are available. The surgeon should notify the radiologist 20 to 30 min before the actual scanning is to be done to allow sufficient time for equipment transportation and preparation and for the radiologist to scrub in. Time invested in the operating room is well spent if the radiologist has a high level of scanning skills and experience so that patient care is significantly improved.

EQUIPMENT

Standard ultrasound equipment used for general ultrasonography can be used in the operating room. Standard curvilinear and linear array transducers of various frequencies are widely available. The curved array transducers have a large field of view that can detect masses and easily display their orientation and relationships to important vessels. The entire organ can be rapidly surveyed with the large field of view of curved array transducers. However, because of the larger size of this transducer, some small peritoneal spaces are inaccessible. In addition, the near field of view and resolution are inferior to those of the dedicated intraoperative transducers.

Dedicated intraoperative transducers are small and of a high frequency. Their small size allows the transducer to be cradled in the examiner's hand and easily maneuvered into small peritoneal spaces.[6-8] Linear array 7-MHz and 5-MHz intraoperative transducers have a clear near field of view and can be used on all intraabdominal organs. They provide penetration up to approximately 8 cm and have excellent spatial and contrast resolution. A disadvantage of these dedicated intraoperative linear array transducers is the small rectangular field of view, which can make orientation difficult, particularly during scanning of a large organ, such as the liver. The combination of curvilinear transducer and dedicated IOUS probes may be used when a large organ such as the liver is scanned (Fig. 20-1). The curvilinear transducer demonstrates a global perspective of relationships of large tumors

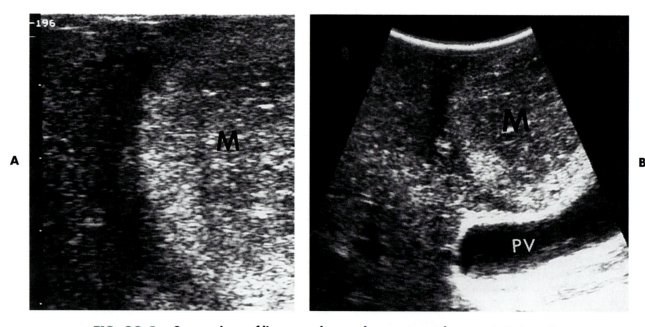

FIG. 20-1. Comparison of linear and curved array transducers. A, Dedicated, linear array IOUS transducer has a relatively small field of view, which demonstrates only a portion of a large hepatic metastasis, *M.* B, Larger, standard curvilinear transducer better demonstrates the relationship of the large metastasis, *M,* to the portal vein, *pv.*

and key structures.[8] The dedicated IOUS transducer can then be used to detect small, occult masses. With experience, the familiar vascular landmarks within the liver are easily recognized.[8] Knowledge of portal and hepatic venous anatomy allows the radiologist to assist in a complete and safe surgical resection.

The ultrasound transducers used in the operating room must have sterile surfaces. Some ultrasound transducers can be **gas sterilized** (ethylene oxide). However, the high temperatures used can potentially damage the transducer; therefore some manufacturers do not recommend this technique. The manufacturers that allow gas sterilization are usually very specific in their recommendations. Sterilization with low-concentration ethylene oxide typically requires 4 hrs and is followed by 18 hrs of rest and aeration. Consequently, the transducer can be used only once a day.[5,8] Transducers can also be **sterilized by immersion in liquid** (glutaraldehyde), which also requires a significant delay before the ultrasound transducer can be used again.[8] In addition, some surgeons do not allow any glutaraldehyde to come in contact with visceral surfaces or in the peritoneal cavity. Therefore the sterilization method must be chosen in consultation with the surgeon.[8] This can become a problem if the transducer must be used in consecutive intraoperative cases. In many practices the ultrasound transducer is **covered by a sterile latex or plastic sleeve**. Gel must be applied into the sleeve to couple the transducer to the sleeve. Great care must be taken to be certain no air bubbles are present between the head of the transducer and the sterile sleeve covering it.[5] This method allows several uses of the same intraoperative probe on the same day. However, the sleeve-draped transducer is slightly more cumbersome to use than is the nondraped sterile transducer.

TECHNIQUE

IOUS often provides important clinical information that cannot be obtained by any other means. For the technique to be most effective, there should be clear communication and cooperation between the radiologist and the surgeon. Intraoperative cases should be prescheduled to allow the proper equipment and personnel to be available. Ideally, the radiologist reviews preoperative images before surgery. This is sometimes not possible, but the images are invariably available in the operating room and can be reviewed before the radiologist scrubs in. After the review, the radiologist knows the location of the suspected malignant masses and indeterminate lesions that need further characterization. In our practice, a radiologist experienced in IOUS scrubs in and scans the organ of interest. To avoid confusion, we always try to scan from the patient's right side as if we were performing a routine ul-

trasound examination. The normal moisture on the surface of the organ to be evaluated can provide acoustic coupling. Warm saline is frequently poured into the peritoneal cavity to enhance acoustic coupling. The saline can also be used as a standoff agent during a search for surface lesions. Surface lesions can be difficult to detect if the transducer is directly in contact with the mass. The contrast between the surface lesion and the normal organ parenchyma often becomes much more apparent if a standoff agent such as sterile saline is used. In most cases, the organ to be evaluated has been exposed and mobilized before scanning. The entire organ should be scanned along with the adjacent structures, such as regional lymph nodes. When a mass is localized, it should be characterized and its relationship to vascular structures carefully delineated.

HEPATOBILIARY SYSTEM

Liver

Indications and Applications. Examination of the liver is the most common IOUS procedure performed in our practice and is usually done to evaluate for colorectal metastasis.[5] The presence and extent of colorectal liver metastasis are important factors for long-term survival. Liver failure due to extensive hepatic metastatic disease accounts for 60% to 70% of the deaths in patients with colorectal cancer.[9] The 5-year survival rate for patients undergoing surgical resection for hepatic colorectal metastasis is 20% to 30%.[10] In contrast, the average survival rate in patients with liver metastasis without surgery is approximately 8 to 9 months, with no patients surviving longer than 5 years.[11] Therefore the surgical resectability of hepatic colorectal metastasis has a major impact on long-term survival. In addition to its use for hepatic metastasis, IOUS can be used for evaluation of primary hepatic malignant lesions such as hepatocellular carcinoma and cholangiocarcinoma.

Detection of Occult Masses. Detection of occult hepatic masses is an important application for IOUS (Fig. 20-2). Malignant lesions in patients with

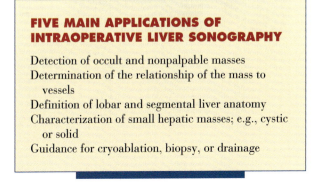

FIVE MAIN APPLICATIONS OF INTRAOPERATIVE LIVER SONOGRAPHY

Detection of occult and nonpalpable masses
Determination of the relationship of the mass to vessels
Definition of lobar and segmental liver anatomy
Characterization of small hepatic masses; e.g., cystic or solid
Guidance for cryoablation, biopsy, or drainage

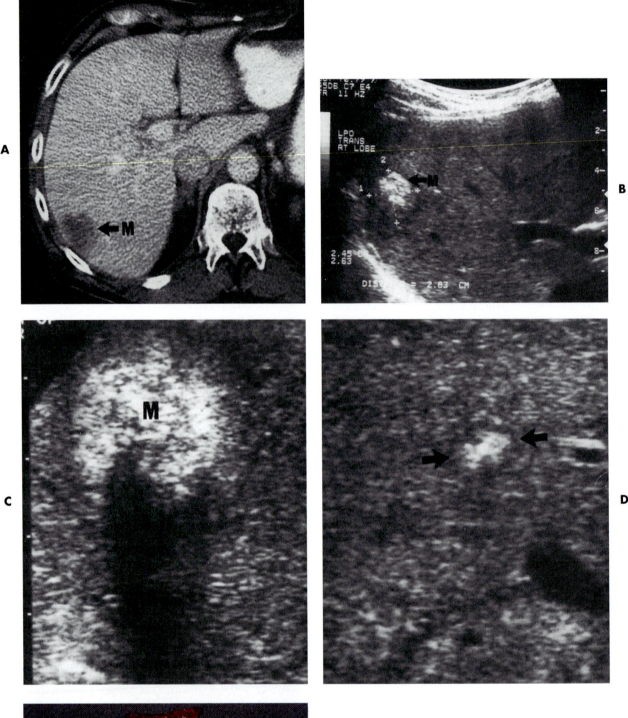

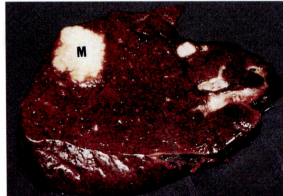

FIG. 20-2. Hepatic metastases from adenocarcinoma of colon. A, Contrast-enhanced CT scan shows solitary metastasis, *M*. B, Transverse preoperative sonogram shows solitary hyperechoic hepatic mass, *M*. C and D, Intraoperative sonograms show mass previously identified, *M*. Additional small metastasis *(arrows)* was identified. Microcalcification within larger mass is causing acoustic shadowing. E, Photograph of gross specimen shows both metastases, *M* and *arrow*.

otherwise normal hepatic parenchyma can be nonpalpable if they are small or located deep in the hepatic parenchyma.[12] The detection rate of hepatic lesions with preoperative imaging depends on the type and quality of imaging technique. Preoperative computed tomography (CT), magnetic resonance imaging (MRI), or ultrasonography typically detect only 60% to 80% of hepatic masses.[12-15] With IOUS, it has been estimated that 93% to 98% of the hepatic lesions are detected.[16-18] In a study by Kane et al., preoperative imaging detected 67% of the hepatic lesions; 78% of the hepatic lesions were detected when preoperative imaging was combined with surgical inspection and palpation. However, 97% of the hepatic masses were identified with IOUS.[1] If additional hepatic malignant lesions are detected with IOUS and then surgically removed, the 5-year survival rate in this subgroup of patients theoretically could improve. Lesions as small as 3 to 5 mm can be detected at the time of IOUS.

IOUS is of value in the detection of occult, nonpalpable **hepatocellular carcinoma** in a cirrhotic liver. In a series reported by Sheu et al.,[19] 49% of hepatocellular carcinomas less than 3 cm in diameter could not be localized with inspection or palpation. In a series reported by Jin-Chuan et al.,[20] 46% of hepatocellular carcinomas could not be localized by palpation or visual inspection. In these patients IOUS is of great value in localizing the mass so that it can be resected with adequate surgical margins (Fig. 20-3).

Determination of Relationships. IOUS also has a role in surgical planning in known, palpable hepatic masses. IOUS is uniquely suited to **demonstrate the relationship** of known hepatic masses to the hepatic vascularity and the biliary system (Figs. 20-4 to 20-6). Additional information obtained by IOUS sometimes changes the planned surgical procedure. At the Mayo Clinic, we reviewed 150 operations for hepatic malignant disease (103 metastatic and 47 primary hepatic tumors). Fourteen percent of the operations were either extended (11%) or aborted (3%) on the basis of information provided only by IOUS.[5] Several other studies have shown a significantly greater effect on operative decision making. For example, in a study by Parker et al.,[13] IOUS of the liver was 98% sensitive for lesion detection, compared with 77% for preoperative CT. IOUS affected operative management in 49% of the patients either by allowing a lesser procedure than expected or by facilitating a more extensive resection. In another study, Kane et al.[1] found that in 19 of 46 patients (41%), the surgical procedures were altered because of IOUS. In some cases, IOUS demonstrates that the lesion is unresectable because of invasion into the main bile duct or into vessels.

Characterization of Masses. IOUS is also invaluable in **characterizing** small, indeterminate hepatic lesions seen on preoperative radiologic studies or detected by surgical palpation. Small cysts can be dif-

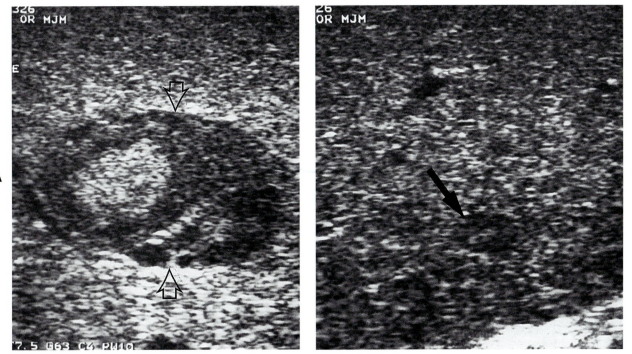

FIG. 20-3. Nonpalpable hepatoma. A, IOUS localizes a nonpalpable hematoma *(open arrows).* B, Second, small, nonpalpable hematoma *(arrow)* was also localized with IOUS.

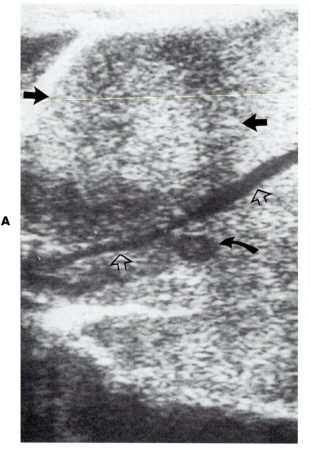

A

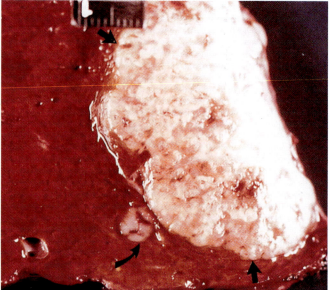

B

FIG. 20-4. Extent of hepatic metastasis provided by operative sonography. **A,** Oblique longitudinal intraoperative scan in patient with metastatic adenocarcinoma of colon shows large metastasis *(black arrows)* adjacent to left hepatic vein *(open arrows)*. This mass was identified on preoperative imaging. Second satellite metastasis *(curved arrow)* is identified posterior to hepatic vein. Because of tumor spread beyond left hepatic vein, a more extensive hepatic resection was required. **B,** Photograph of gross specimen demonstrating both metastases. *Straight arrow,* Large metastases; *curved arrow,* satellite metastases.

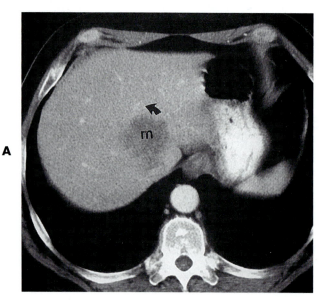

A

FIG. 20-5. Metastasis encasing hepatic vein. A, Contrast-enhanced CT demonstrates a metastasis, *m,* near the middle hepatic vein *(curved arrow)*.

Continued.

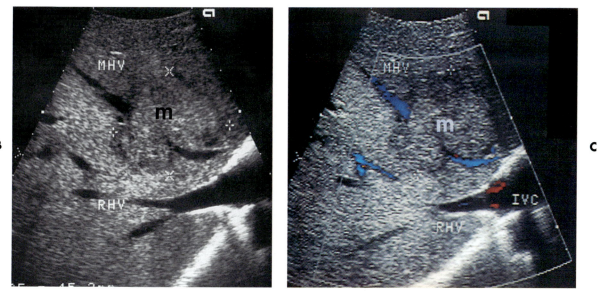

FIG. 20-5, cont'd. B and C, IOUS shows the metastasis, *m*, encasing the middle hepatic vein, *MHV. RHV,* Right hepatic vein.

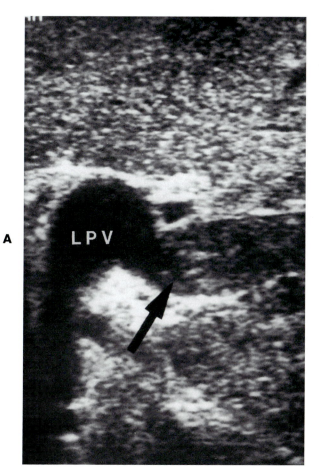

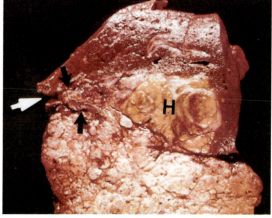

FIG. 20-6. Tumor thrombus of left portal vein. A, Intraoperative sonogram shows tumor thrombus *(arrow)* in left portal vein, *LPV.* B, Photograph of gross specimen shows collapsed portal vein proximally *(white arrow)* with tumor thrombus distally *(black arrows). H,* Hepatocellular carcinoma.

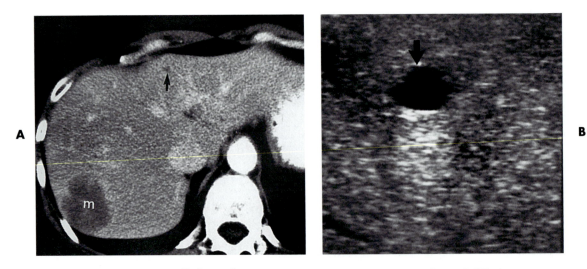

FIG. 20-7. Small hepatic cysts. A, Preoperative contrast-enhanced CT shows a metastasis, *m*, in the right lobe and a small indeterminate lesion in the left lobe *(arrow)*. B, Intraoperative sonogram shows a 0.6 cm hepatic cyst *(arrow)* in the left lobe.

INDICATIONS FOR INTRAOPERATIVE BILIARY SONOGRAPHY

Identification of biliary calculi
Identification of biliary neoplasms
Localization of the common bile duct and its
   relationship to other structures

ficult to differentiate from small metastatic lesions with CT because of partial volume-averaging effects. With IOUS, however, small **cysts** can be easily identified and characterized as benign (Fig. 20-7). Likewise, small **hemangiomas** typically appear as small, uniformly hyperechoic nodules without a peripheral halo (Fig. 20-8).

Guidance for Intervention. Some hepatic lesions are indeterminate by ultrasound criteria and may require **biopsy** for accurate diagnosis. This can be safely and easily accomplished in the operating room with ultrasound guidance (Fig. 20-9). The technique of intraoperative biopsy using ultrasound guidance is described in Chapter 17.

Gallbladder and Bile Ducts

The gallbladder and bile ducts can be evaluated for **calculi** with IOUS.[21-25] Although gallstones are usually detected by preoperative ultrasonography, they are occasionally noted incidentally at the time of IOUS of the liver (Fig. 20-10). IOUS is also used to screen the common bile duct for stones during cholecystectomy. In a series of 449 patients who underwent both intra-

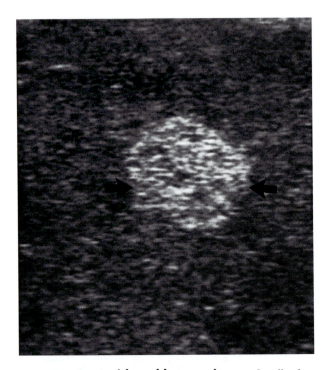

FIG. 20-8. Incidental hemangioma. Small echogenic hemangioma *(arrows)* with a scalloped margin and tiny cystic spaces. Note there is no peripheral halo around the hemangioma.

operative cholangiography and IOUS, the accuracy was 98% for IOUS and 94% for cholangiography.[21]

Primary and secondary neoplasms of the gallbladder and bile ducts may cause a focal mass or wall thickening (Fig. 20-11). IOUS can localize the mass and define its extent. Adjacent normal structures and lymph nodes can also be surveyed with IOUS.

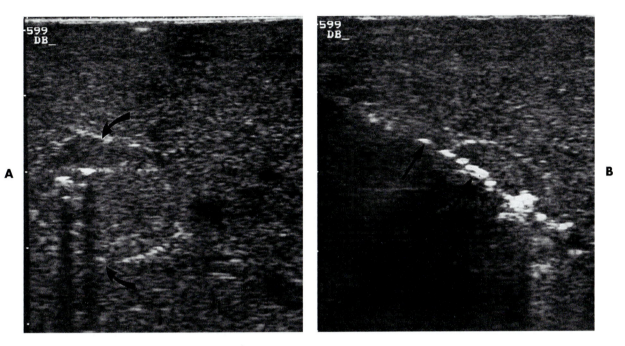

FIG. 20-9. IOUS-guided liver biopsy. **A,** Nearly isoechoic mass *(arrows)* with tiny calcifications. **B,** IOUS-guided biopsy needle *(straight arrows)* within the mass, which was an atypical hemangioma.

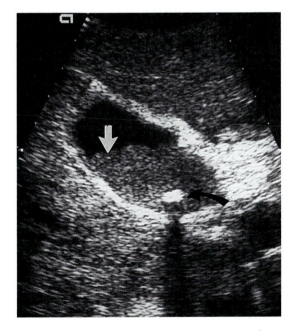

FIG. 20-10. Incidental gallstone *(curved arrow)* and biliary sludge *(straight arrow)*.

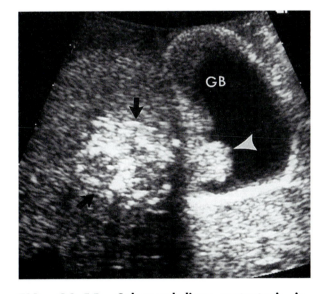

FIG. 20-11. Colorectal liver metastasis invading gallbladder. IOUS shows a colorectal metastasis *(arrows)* with microcalcifications invading *(arrowhead)* the gallbladder, *GB.*

Localizing a normal common bile duct (CBD) can also be important if it is to be preserved during surgery. IOUS accurately localizes the CBD and demonstrates its relationship to adjacent masses and fluid collection. This helps plan surgery and hopefully avoid damage to the CBD (Fig. 20-12).

PANCREAS

Carcinoma

The most common pancreatic malignant lesion is **ductal adenocarcinoma,** and few patients with this tumor are surgical candidates at presentation

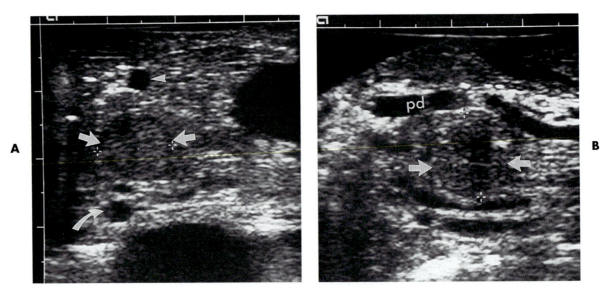

FIG. 20-12. **Insulinoma near common bile duct.** **A,** Transverse and, **B,** longitudinal images demonstrate a small, discrete, hypoechoic insulinoma *(white arrows)*. Pancreatic duct, *pd* (**B**) and *white arrowhead* (**A**), and common bile duct *(curved arrow)* are in close proximity to the insulinoma.

because of either metastatic or unresectable disease. Patients with small tumors (less than 2 cm) that have no vascular invasion or lymph node metastasis have the best prognosis.[26-29] The 5-year survival rate after pancreatoduodenectomy is between 18% and 33%.[26-30]

Multiple preoperative imaging studies can be obtained to diagnose pancreatic ductal adenocarcinoma; they include CT, ultrasonography, endoscopic retrograde cholangiopancreatography (ERCP), MRI, and endoscopic ultrasonography. IOUS is rarely used at our institution in patients with pancreatic ductal adenocarcinoma because most of these cancers are easily palpable and the lack of resectability is apparent by inspection and palpation. IOUS can be used to detect and determine the extent of a small, nonpalpable pancreatic mass.[31-33] Pancreatic ductal adenocarcinoma is usually a hypoechoic, solid mass with irregular margins (Fig. 20-13). It frequently obstructs the pancreatic duct and common bile duct and causes dilatation up to the level of the mass. IOUS can also be used to detect abnormal regional lymph nodes, vascular encasement by neoplasm, and liver metastatic lesions.[33] Demonstrating occult liver metastatic lesions with IOUS can prevent an unnecessary attempt at surgical resection.[33]

Pancreatitis

IOUS may be used to evaluate the multiple complications associated with chronic pancreatitis, including pseudocyst, abscesses, and secondary involvement of the gastrointestinal tract, biliary tract, or abdominal vessels by the inflammatory process. Although most

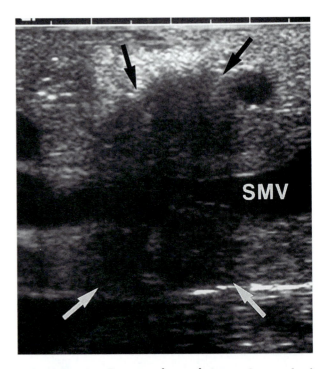

FIG. 20-13. **Pancreatic carcinoma.** Longitudinal IOUS demonstrates a small, hypoechoic, ductal adenocarcinoma *(arrows)* surrounding the superior mesenteric vein, *SMV.* (Courtesy of Sharlene Teefey, M.D.)

pseudocysts and abscesses can be readily identified with preoperative imaging, IOUS can help localize and drain these fluid collections and their extensions (Fig. 20-14). Occasionally, previously unrecognized fluid collections can be identified with IOUS.[32,34,35]

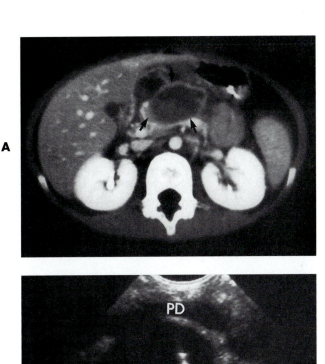

The pancreatic duct and intraductal calcifications are easily identified with IOUS (Fig. 20-15). Also, IOUS can differentiate inflamed pancreatic parenchyma from the pseudocyst and thus save the parenchyma from unnecessary surgical removal.

In some patients, distinguishing between **chronic pancreatitis** and **pancreatic cancer** is difficult with imaging studies and clinical history.[33] In addition, small ductal adenocarcinomas can obstruct the pancreatic duct and cause secondary pancreatitis that may obscure the primary neoplasm. Ultrasound guidance may be used for biopsy of indeterminate masses within the pancreas to determine whether they are inflammatory or malignant.[33] This may be done percutaneously or in the operating room after laparotomy.

Islet Cell Neoplasm

Insulinoma. A highly valuable application for IOUS is the localization of an islet cell neoplasm, such as insulinoma. Imaging and attempted localization of islet cell neoplasms can be frustrating to the radiologist, clinician, surgeon, and patient. Islet cell neoplasms often produce excessive hormone so that the clinician can make a firm clinical diagnosis. Afterward, the patient is often referred to the radiologist for localization of the neoplasm producing the excessive hormone. Various preoperative imaging studies, including ultrasonography, CT, MRI, angiography, venous sampling, and radionuclide scanning, are used to localize islet cell neoplasms with variable results. However, islet cell neoplasms are frequently small and difficult to localize preoperatively.

At our institution, the most common pancreatic application for IOUS is to localize a small insulinoma. Insulinomas are usually small, solitary, and benign.[36,37] The insulinoma produces excessive insulin, which

FIG. 20-14. Drainage of pseudocyst. A, Preoperative contrast-enhanced CT shows pseudocyst *(arrows)* with dependent debris. **B,** Intraoperative sonogram shows pseudocyst *(arrows)* communicating with pancreatic duct, *PD*. Under ultrasound guidance, needle was placed *(bright linear echoes)* into pancreatic pseudocyst.

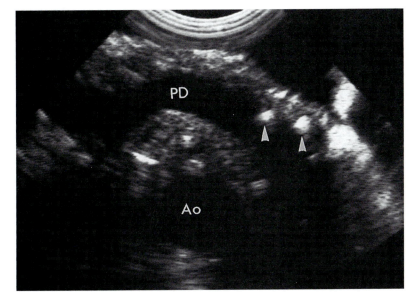

FIG. 20-15. Chronic pancreatitis. Transverse IOUS shows a dilated pancreatic duct, *PD*, with ductal calcifications *(arrowheads). Ao,* Aorta.

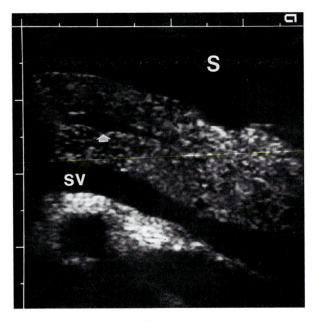

FIG. 20-16. Normal pancreas. Saline, *S*, anterior to the pancreas improves visualization of the anterior surface of the pancreas. Pancreatic duct *(arrow). SV*, Splenic vein.

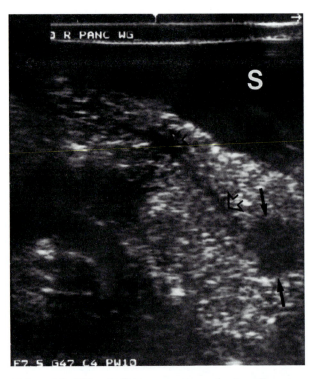

FIG. 20-17. Solitary pancreatic insulinoma. Transverse IOUS shows 0.8 cm hypoechoic mass *(black arrows)* in pancreatic tail adjacent to pancreatic duct *(open arrows)*. *S*, Saline.

causes hypoglycemia. Once the laboratory evidence establishes that the patient has an insulinoma, surgical intervention is needed to prevent a neurologic catastrophe caused by severe hypoglycemia. Experienced pancreatic surgeons working with experienced radiologists can localize nearly all insulinomas during surgery by using a combination of inspection, palpation, and IOUS.[36-41] Because of this capability, we usually perform a minimal number of preoperative examinations for localization.

High-frequency (7-MHz) transducers are essential in searching for an insulinoma. Warm saline is poured into the abdomen to provide acoustic coupling and a standoff medium. Identifying small insulinomas on the surface of the pancreas can be difficult if the transducer is placed directly on them. Scanning slightly off the surface with saline as a standoff medium makes detection of surface lesions easier. The normal pancreas has a uniform, coarse, hyperechoic echotexture (Fig. 20-16). Ninety percent of insulinomas are discrete, small, well-defined hypoechoic nodules (Fig. 20-17).[41] In addition to detecting the tumor, IOUS should demonstrate the relationship of the insulinoma to the pancreatic ducts. If the insulinoma is located a safe distance away from and superficial to the pancreatic duct, enucleation is performed. However, if the insulinoma is deeply situated or very near the pancreatic duct, safe enucleation is not possible without transecting the pancreatic duct (see Fig. 20-12). Instead, pan-

creatic resection is performed. If the insulinoma is nonpalpable, a localizing needle can be placed near it (Fig. 20-18).

Ten percent of insulinomas are hyperechoic or isoechoic relative to the pancreas.[41] Insulinomas in young patients are more difficult to detect probably because the pancreatic parenchyma is less echogenic and can be isoechoic with the insulinoma. In these cases, the insulinoma can be detected if the edge effect from its smooth margin is detected or the fine echotexture of the insulinoma is detected in contrast to the coarse echotexture of the pancreatic parenchyma.[41]

Gastrinoma. Gastrinoma is the second most common functioning neuroendocrine tumor. Gastrinomas produce gastrin, which causes excess secretion of gastric acid and leads to severe diarrhea and gastric ulcers (i.e., Zollinger-Ellison syndrome). Gastrinomas are often difficult to localize. Twenty to forty percent of gastrinomas are multiple, and 60% to 90% are malignant.[42] Gastrinomas are extrapancreatic in 20% to 40% of patients[42] and are often located in the wall of the duodenum (Fig. 20-19). Ninety percent of gastrinomas lie in a region known as the "gastrinoma triangle."[36,43] The boundaries of the gastrinoma triangle are the second and third portions of the duodenum inferiorly, the junction of the cystic and

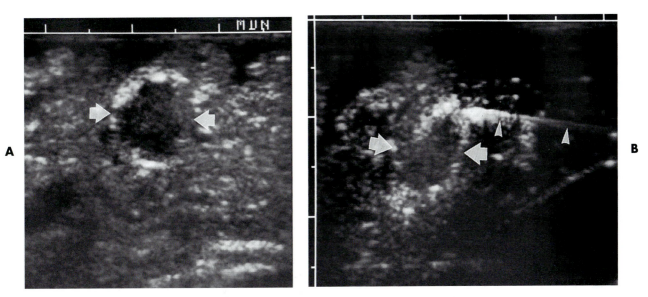

FIG. 20-18. Nonpalpable insulinoma. A, Nonpalpable, 1 cm insulinoma *(arrows)* identified with IOUS. **B,** Under IOUS guidance, a localizing needle *(arrowheads)* was placed next to the insulinoma *(arrows).*

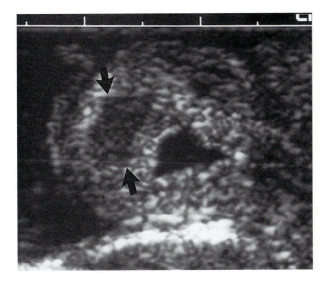

FIG. 20-19. Gastrinoma *(arrows)* located in the wall of the duodenum.

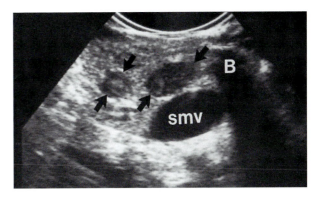

FIG. 20-20. MEN syndrome—multiple pancreatic insulinomas. Transverse scan in patient with multiple endocrine neoplasia syndrome, type I, shows two hypoechoic insulinomas *(arrows)* within pancreatic head. *smv,* Superior mesenteric vein. *B,* bowel.

common bile ducts superiorly, and the junction of the head and neck of the pancreas medially.[36,43] This area should be carefully scanned during IOUS. Unfortunately, many gastrinomas cannot be found despite careful preoperative imaging, laparotomy, careful surgical inspection and palpation, and IOUS.

Multiple Endocrine Neoplasia. Multiple endocrine neoplasia, type I (MEN I) is associated with tumors of the pancreas, parathyroid glands, pituitary gland, adrenal cortex, and thyroid. MEN I is an autosomal-dominant trait with high penetrance. Pancreatic tumors are usually multifocal and account for most of the morbidity and mortality in patients with MEN I. Patients with MEN I often have several adenomas less than 1 cm in diameter and require near-total pancreatectomy for cure (Fig. 20-20).[41,44] The head of the pancreas must be carefully scanned and palpated because residual adenomas may cause the patient's symptoms to persist postoperatively.

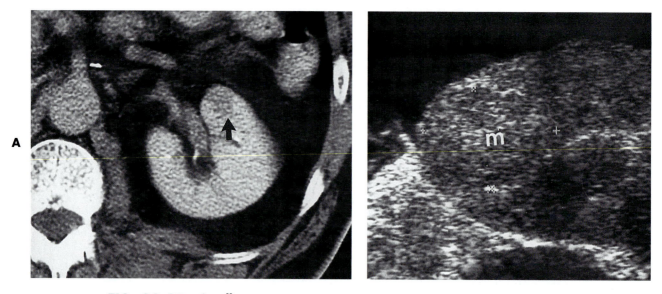

FIG. 20-21. Small oncocytoma. A, Contrast-enhanced CT shows a small, indeterminate, left renal mass *(arrow)*. **B,** IOUS demonstrates small, solid, renal mass, *m*, which is nearly isoechoic with adjacent renal parenchyma. This mass was not palpable.

RENAL

Masses

IOUS can be of value in kidney-sparing surgery. Partial nephrectomy for renal malignant disease should be considered in patients with bilateral renal malignant lesions, a mass in a solitary kidney, renal insufficiency, or significant abnormalities in the contralateral kidney.[45-49] The goal is to preserve renal parenchyma to avoid dialysis. Some authors have recommended partial nephrectomy for small, localized renal cell carcinomas in patients with a normal contralateral kidney.[47-49] Local recurrence affects 3% to 13% of patients after partial nephrectomy.[50-55] To prevent recurrence, the entire malignant tumor must be removed with adequate surgical margins. Simple enucleation of renal cell carcinomas frequently results in incomplete tumor excision.[56,57] Mukamel et al. reported that 20% of kidneys with a dominant renal cell carcinoma also had separate adenocarcinomas in another area of the renal parenchyma.[58] Gilbert et al. were the first group to use IOUS in patients who were candidates for partial nephrectomy.[59] Since then, several groups have shown that IOUS is useful in surgical procedures that spare the renal parenchyma.[40,41,53-56] Sonography is useful to **locate occult, nonpalpable tumors,** to **delineate the boundaries of the renal mass,** and to **guide partial nephrectomy** (Fig. 20-21). IOUS is especially valuable if a lesion is deeply located and therefore difficult to palpate.

IOUS can also be useful in **characterizing indeterminate renal masses** (Figs. 20-22 to 20-24).

Depending on CT slice thickness and the size of the renal lesion, it may be difficult to determine whether a small renal lesion is cystic or solid. IOUS can readily characterize small cystic lesions and thus prevent unnecessary resection. IOUS can also be used to guide biopsy of an indeterminate renal mass. For example, a small renal cell carcinoma may appear hyperechoic and indistinguishable from a small angiolipoma (Fig. 20-25).

Vascular

Technical problems encountered by the surgeon during renal revascularization procedures have traditionally been difficult to accurately assess. A variety of methods have been used, including palpation, continuous wave Doppler analysis, and arteriography, but each has limitations. In recent years sonography has been increasingly used intraoperatively to evaluate the main renal arteries occasionally before, but more often following the surgical procedure. Most patients evaluated are undergoing transaortic **renal artery endarterectomy** or **renal artery bypass grafting** to treat renal artery stenosis that has led to hypertension and/or renal insufficiency. Gray-scale, spectral, and color flow Doppler sonography allow detection of abnormalities at the time of the operation, thereby improving the chance for a successful outcome. In our experience, abnormalities requiring surgical revision have been detected in 9% to 11% of reconstructed main renal arteries scanned intraoperatively.[63,64] Data suggest that clinical outcomes of patients requiring intraoperative revision are favorable and similar to those with normal IOUS studies.

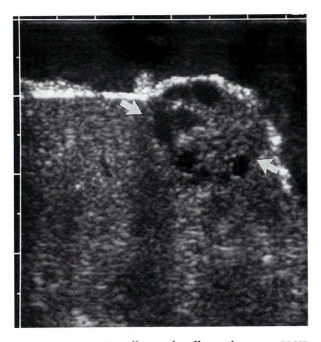

FIG. 20-22. Small renal cell carcinoma. IOUS demonstrates a 1.5 cm, mixed solid and cystic mass *(arrows)* in the cortex of the kidney.

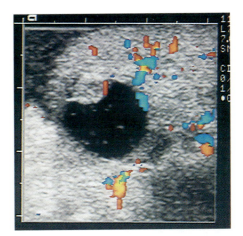

FIG. 20-23. Small renal cell carcinoma in wall of cyst. Transverse image demonstrates a 1.5 cm cyst with a 0.5 cm mural nodule, which was a low-grade, non-palpable, renal cell carcinoma in a patient with Hippel-Lindau syndrome.

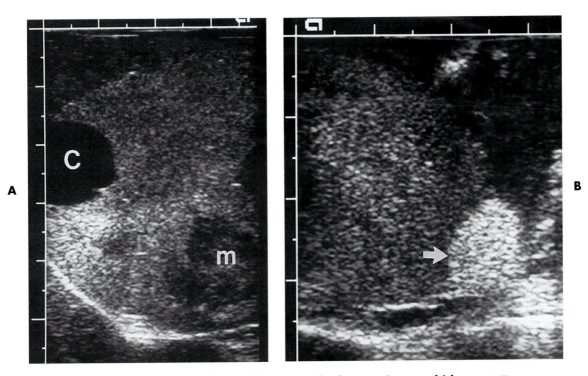

FIG. 20-24. Cyst, angiomyolipoma, and adenoma in same kidney. A, Transverse IOUS image of kidney shows a benign cyst, *C*, and a hypoechoic solid mass, *M*, which proved to be an adenoma. **B,** At a different level a small, hyperechoic angiomyolipoma *(arrow)* was seen.

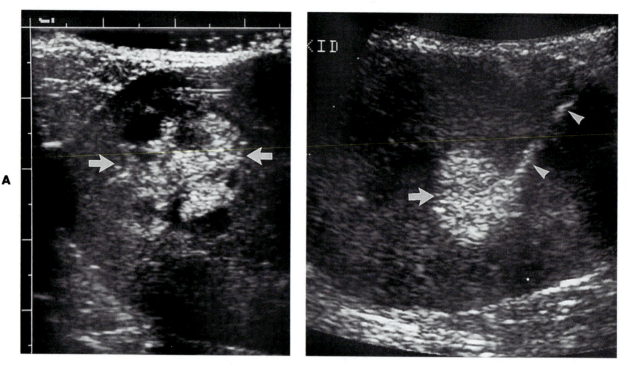

FIG. 20-25. Incidentally detected low-grade renal cell carcinoma. A, IOUS of the liver in a patient with a hepatoma discovered an incidental, echogenic, right renal mass *(arrows)*. **B,** Under IOUS guidance, a biopsy needle *(arrowheads)* was placed into the mass *(arrow)*, which proved to be a low-grade renal cell carcinoma.

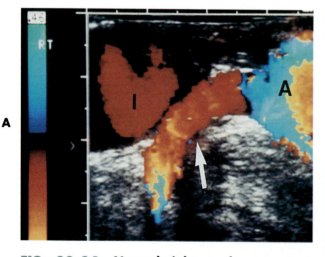

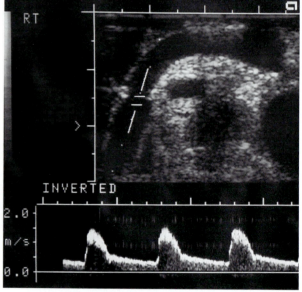

FIG. 20-26. Normal right renal artery post-endarterectomy. A, Transverse scan shows right renal artery *(arrow)* arising from the aorta, *A*, and passing behind the IVC, *I*. **B,** Right renal artery bypass graft. Spectral Doppler scan shows a normal, low-resistance waveform.

Scanning is performed through the operative incision using a high-frequency transducer covered with a sterile plastic sheath. The surgeon provides exposure as needed, and the wound is filled with saline or water, which provides the acoustic window. Gray-scale, spec-tral, and color wave Doppler analysis complement each other in evaluation of the renal arteries. A smooth lumen and uniform flow with prompt systolic upstroke and a low resistance pattern are typical of normal renal arteries (Fig. 20-26).

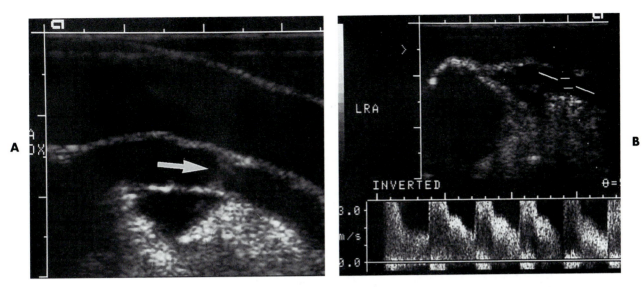

FIG. 20-27. **Residual stenosis after endarterectomy.** **A,** Longitudinal image of the left renal artery shows residual plaque *(arrow).* **B,** Spectral Doppler exam shows elevated flow velocities and turbulence, indicating significant stenosis. This was surgically revised.

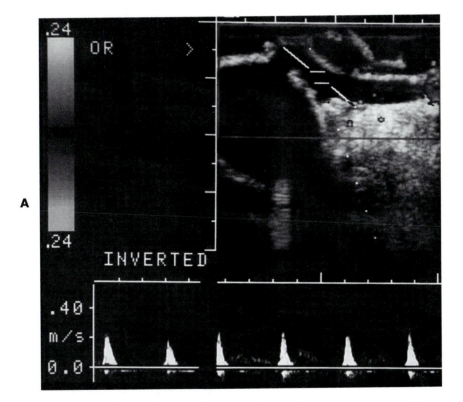

FIG. 20-28. **Left renal artery thrombosis.** **A,** Transverse duplex scan following left renal artery bypass using saphenous vein graft shows low-velocity, high-resistance waveform in proximal left renal artery, suggesting obstruction distally. *Continued.*

RENOVASCULAR ABNORMALITIES THAT MAY BE DETECTED SONOGRAPHICALLY

Residual renal artery or anastomotic stenosis (Fig. 20-27)

Thrombosis/occlusion of the graft or renal artery (Fig. 20-28)

Intimal flap or dissection (Figs. 20-29 and 20-30)

Extrinsic compression or kinking of the graft or renal artery

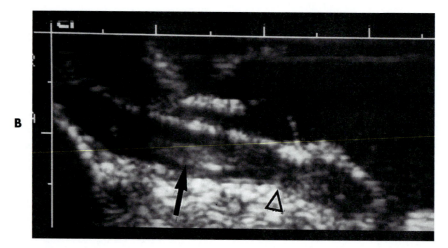

FIG. 20-28, cont'd. **B,** Gray-scale image more distally demonstrates mild narrowing at distal anastomosis *(arrowhead)* with partial thrombosis of renal artery lumen *(arrow)*. (From Lantz EJ, Charboneau JW, Hallett JW et al. Intraoperative color Doppler sonography during renal artery revascularization. *AJR* 1994;162:859-863.)

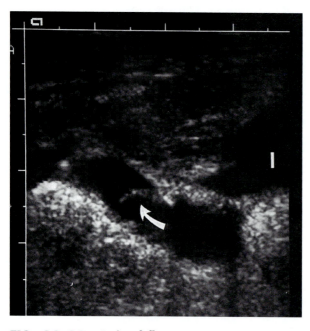

FIG. 20-29. **Intimal flap.** Transverse scan of right renal artery following endarterectomy shows intimal flap *(arrows)* in vessel lumen, *I*–IVC. Vessel was opened and flap was repaired.

LAPAROSCOPIC SONOGRAPHY

The latest development in IOUS has been the application of specially designed probes that can be inserted through standard laparoscopic ports that are typically no more than 10 to 11 mm in size. Because these laparoscopy ports are at some distance from the intraabdominal organs, the laparoscopic ultrasound (LUS) probes must be mounted on a long,

> ### LAPAROSCOPIC ULTRASOUND PROBE FEATURES
>
> **Center frequency ranging from 5 to 7.5 MHz**
> **Long, rigid shaft of at least 15 to 20 cm in length**
> **Real-time gray-scale**
>   As well as Doppler and color flow capability
> **Linear array or curvilinear array**
>   Transducers with crystal length ranging from approximately 1 to 3 cm
> **Sterile sheaths specifically designed for each individual probe**

thin shaft. The earliest reports of laparoscopic ultrasound used A-mode ultrasonography for diagnosis of intraabdominal pathology, although this was of limited usefulness.[65,66] Miniaturization techniques were then applied to conventional gray-scale scanners, both mechanical and electronic types, allowing for a substantial decrease in probe size, thus making laparoscopic real-time ultrasound feasible.[67-69] The ultimate in miniaturization has been the catheter-based transducers, which were originally developed for intravascular ultrasound, but which have also been used laparoscopically.[70] The extremely small size of catheter-mounted transducers makes the field of view so small as to limit practical usefulness in the abdomen.

Currently, a number of commercial ultrasound manufacturers produce laparoscopic ultrasound probes, most of which share the following features in common: center frequency ranging from 5 to 7.5 MHz; long, rigid shaft of at least 15 to 20 cm in length;

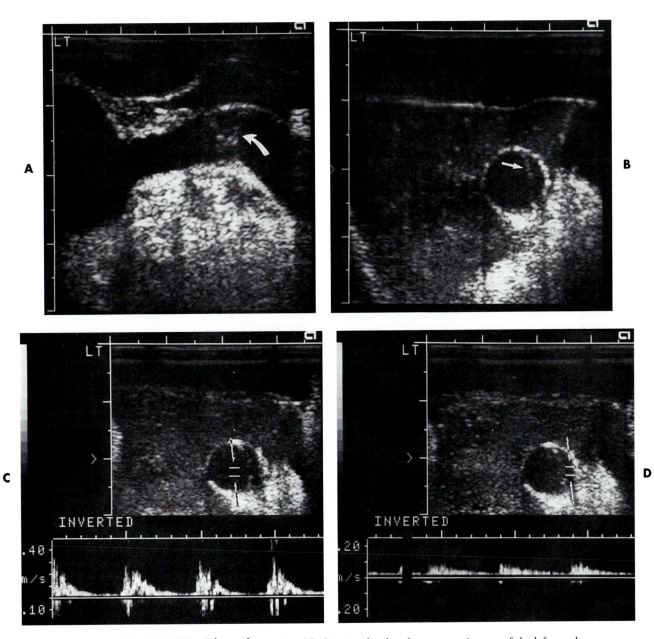

FIG. 20-30. **Dissection.** A and B, Longitudinal and transverse images of the left renal artery following endarterectomy show an intimal dissection *(arrow)*. C and D, Spectral Doppler scan shows the two lumens have different waveforms. (From Lantz EJ, Charboneau JW, Hallett JW et al. Intraoperative color Doppler sonography during renal artery revascularization. *AJR* 1994;162:859-863.)

real-time gray-scale as well as Doppler and color flow capability; linear array or curvilinear array transducers with crystal length ranging from approximately 1 to 3 cm; and sterile sheaths specifically designed for each individual probe.

Technique

Most of the available equipment also will feature a flexible tip including the imaging crystal some distance up the shaft. Some systems will flex and extend in one plane while other systems can steer to the right and left

as well as offer flexion and extension capability. Movement of the flexible portion of the probe is controlled by the operator using mechanisms that are similar to controls for flexible endoscopes. The ability to flex or extend the probe is of critical importance in maintaining contact with organs having curved surfaces such as the liver. A strictly rigid system often loses acoustic coupling because of its inability to maintain direct contact with the organ surface. An alternative approach for a nonflexing system is to fill the abdominal cavity with fluid and scan through the fluid as an acoustic medium. This may work reasonably well for assessing the pancreas but is extremely awkward, since the abdomen is already markedly distended with CO_2 to facilitate the laparoscopy.

There is usually sufficient moisture naturally to allow good acoustic contrast with the target organs, but sterile saline may be used to moisten surfaces, if necessary. Acoustic coupling must be maintained within the sterile probe cover as well, either by using sterile gel on or sterile water inside the sheath to provide an acoustic coupling medium for the imaging array. In addition to the sterile sheath covering the probe and shaft, a larger sterile cover is also used to cover the handle of the probe, its control mechanisms, and the electrical cord.

It is important that the probe frequency be sufficient to image the entire organ being studied. While a frequency of 7 MHz may be entirely adequate for assessment of the pancreas, bile duct, and gallbladder, the attenuation of a 7-MHz beam in the liver would allow for only 6 to 7 cm penetration. Consequently, 5-MHz frequency is preferred for the liver, which would allow penetration to a depth of 10 to 12 cm. Most livers therefore could be scanned from the anterior surface, which is smooth and well suited for laparoscopic scanning. Attempts to scan the undersurface of the liver are fraught with difficulty because of the uneven surfaces as well as ligamentous attachments, intervening organs such as the gallbladder and duodenum, and other impediments to effective scanning.

Because the probe sizes are necessarily small, the amount of time required to completely image an organ is substantially longer than imaging with standard IOUS probes. A complete scan requires overlapping images throughout the entire organ. IOUS probes are two to four times as large as laparoscopic probes and consequently the time of examination is substantially longer using the laparoscopic approach. For instance, complete assessment of the liver might take less than 5 min using intraoperative probes, but would take 15 to 20 min with an LUS examination.

Another limitation of LUS is the fact that the probe is pivoting on a single point in space (i.e., the entry laparoscopic port). This limits the freedom of motion of the scan head such that it is impossible to maintain the probe in standard transverse or longitudinal orientations. Because the probe is pivoting, the resultant image planes are most often at some obliquity to either a transverse or longitudinal image plane. This can cause disorientation and also some difficulty in ensuring that the image planes overlap one another. In liver imaging, while the right subcostal port may be sufficient for imaging the right lobe, and at times the left lobe, the lateral segment of the left lobe and caudate lobes cannot be adequately imaged from this site. If this is the case, the probe must be moved to another port, usually in the periumbilical, left subcostal, or epigastric region, to complete the assessment of the left lobe.

It is important to observe the insertion of the LUS probe under direct visualization using the fiberoptic laparoscope. There is little, if any, sense of feel as to where the probe tip is located and, to avoid inadvertent injury to tissues and vessels, the probe placement should be observed continuously on the TV monitor. Split-screen presentation of both the laparoscopic and real-time ultrasound images on the same monitor is convenient and requires only an inexpensive beam-splitter.

Liver

An organized, systematic approach to LUS of the liver is of paramount importance, keeping in mind that the imaging fields should overlap one another for complete assessment of the liver parenchyma. We prefer to begin at the dome of the liver, scanning across the dome, and then repositioning the probe slightly more caudal in position but no more than the length of the imaging crystal. After repositioning, a second sweep across the liver is performed, the probe is then moved further caudally and another sweep obtained, and so on. It is important to remember that the fields must overlap to avoid the potential for missing lesions in unscanned areas of the liver. Some laparoscopic systems present a sector format image, and this can be misleading in giving the false assurance that a large portion of the liver is imaged with each sweep. Although this is true in the far field, the extreme near field is only as wide as the length of the imaging crystal.

If the falciform ligament is well developed and obstructs access to the left, the probe is repositioned in a different port and more scans are obtained from the dome to the free edge of the left lateral segment and caudate lobe.

It is well known that many primary or metastatic hepatic tumors are found to be unresectable at the time of laparotomy, despite multiple preoperative

---

GOALS OF LAPAROSCOPIC ULTRASOUND

To detect and characterize all possible liver lesions

To accurately localize these lesions to lobes and segments

To assess the relationship of tumors to vascular and biliary structures

To assess for invasion

To guide biopsy and aspirations under real-time visualization

To guide minimally invasive ablative techniques

imaging studies. This may be due to the presence of tumor in lymph nodes or tumor deposits in the mesentery and on the peritoneal surfaces. In one prospective study of 29 patients with hepatic malignancy, all tumors judged resectable by preoperative imaging studies, 48% of the tumors were deemed unresectable because of laparoscopic findings that included peritoneal seeding, satellite liver lesions, and unsuspected cirrhosis.[71] However, another 20% of the tumors had unresectable disease not identified at laparoscopy. This is where LUS may play a key role.

IOUS consistently detects 20% to 30% more liver lesions than are shown on preoperative imaging studies.[72] LUS shares this same enhanced capacity for detection of tiny liver lesions (Fig. 20-31). In one small series of 11 patients, significant additional findings were obtained at LUS, including additional masses, metastatic lymphadenopathy, or vascular involvement, thereby influencing surgical decision-making. In 5 cases, LUS-guided biopsies were successfully performed.[73] In another larger study of 50 patients, 43 of whom had successful LUS, 33% more liver lesions were depicted with LUS than were visible through the laparoscope, and LUS added additional staging information in 42%. This resulted in a resectability rate of 93% among patients having laparoscopy and LUS performed as compared with only 48% successful resections in patients without laparoscopy.[74]

The majority of additional liver lesions detected are very small, typically 1 cm or less in size, and therefore are below resolution limits for conventional imaging (Fig. 20-32). This is identical to the experience with open IOUS. Not all nodules detected proved to be cancer, however, and biopsy may be important to assess unsuspected lesions demonstrated only by LUS (Fig. 20-33). Biopsy of large or fairly superficial lesions can be accomplished readily by use of extra-long biopsy needles puncturing through the anterior abdominal wall and entering the liver immediately adjacent to the laparoscopic probe, which is positioned directly over the lesion. However, small and deeply seated lesions are more difficult to biopsy, and some type of real-time biopsy guide similar to those available on conventional ultrasound probes would prove useful. Unfortunately, at present there is no commercially available system with adequate real-time biopsy guidance.

Invasion or obstruction of bile ducts can be readily demonstrated as well as vascular invasion into the portal or hepatic veins, which is seen most often in hepatocellular carcinoma. Assessment of aberrant vascular supply to the liver may also be important in influencing the type of resection performed, particularly in patients with replaced or accessory left hepatic or right hepatic arteries (Fig. 20-34). Accessory hepatic venous drainage, particularly in the inferior right

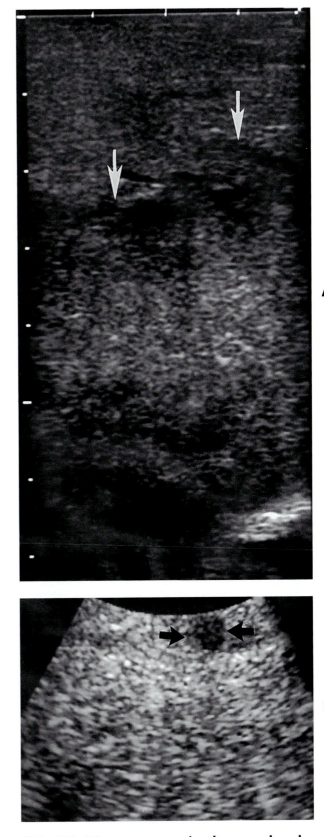

FIG. 20-31. Laparoscopic ultrasound—colorectal metastases. A. Large left lobe metastasis *(white arrows)*. **B.** Superficial 5 mm right lobe metastasis not visible via the laparoscope and not seen on preoperative imaging studies *(black arrows)*.

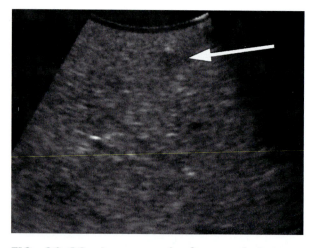

FIG. 20-32. **Laparoscopic ultrasound—hepato-cellular** carcinoma; 4 mm tumor deposit *(arrow)* only detectable by LUS.

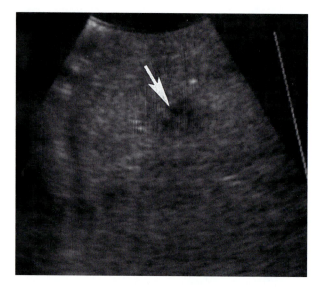

FIG. 20-33. **Laparoscopic ultrasound demonstrates a small area of focal nodular hyperplasia *(arrows)*, which simulates a metastasis.**

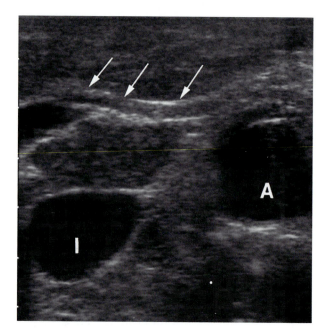

FIG. 20-34. **Laparoscopic ultrasound demonstrates a replaced left hepatic artery** *(arrows)* arising from the left gastric artery. *A,* Aorta; *I,* IVC.

lobe, is frequently seen, and an awareness of this is important for the surgeon in order to avoid unnecessary traction and trauma to this accessory vein, which could lead to substantial and even life-threatening hemorrhage.

Gallbladder and Bile Ducts

Initially, there was great expectation for the use of LUS techniques in assessing patients undergoing laparoscopic cholecystectomy. In particular, LUS was believed to be at least equivalent, if not superior, to laparoscopic intraoperative cholangiography, which can be a difficult and technically challenging study to per-

form. In a study by Liu et al., 1 of 7 patients undergoing laparoscopic cholecystectomy had **common duct stones** identified by LUS leading to an open surgical approach with removal of multiple intrahepatic and common bile duct stones.[9] However, in a larger study of 150 patients in whom 129 successful LUS examinations were obtained, although visualization of the common bile duct was good in most cases, unexpected common bile duct pathology was only detected in 5 cases (approximately 3%).[75] In our experience, if there are any clinical, laboratory, or imaging findings suspicious for common bile duct pathology during the preoperative work-up of patients with gallstones, these patients are referred immediately for ERCP prior to laparoscopic cholecystectomy. If stones are demonstrated on the ERCP study, sphincterotomy and stone extraction techniques are performed, and in most cases the patient may still undergo successful laparoscopic cholecystectomy.

LUS may play a role in other types of biliary pathology. Certainly in patients with **gallbladder carcinoma,** since the long-term survival is so poor, it would be appropriate to perform laparoscopic assessment for metastatic disease in the liver, adjacent lymph nodes, or peritoneal surfaces to avoid unnecessary and unsuccessful laparotomy (Fig. 20-35). Tumors of the biliary tract such as **cholangiocarcinoma** and inflammatory conditions such as **sclerosing cholangitis** (Fig. 20-36) and **oriental cholangiohepatitis** may also benefit from LUS evaluation. The goal is to assess for extent of tumor; site of intrahepatic bile duct di-

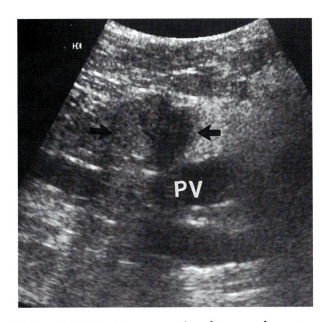

FIG. 20-35. Laparoscopic ultrasound—metastatic gallbladder carcinoma. Scan of the porta hepatis demonstrates metastatic lymphadenopathy *(arrows)* anterior to the portal vein, *PV.*

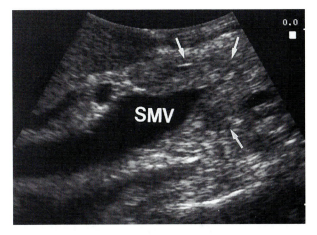

FIG. 20-37. Laparoscopic ultrasound—pancreatic carcinoma. Longitudinal scan shows a mass *(arrows)* encasing the superior mesenteric vein, *SMV,* just distal to the confluence, indicating unresectability.

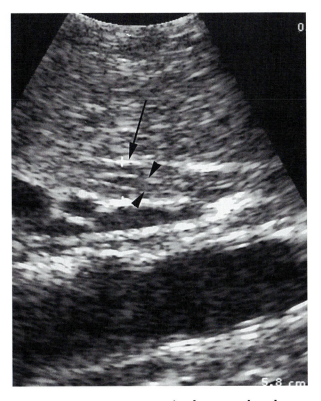

FIG. 20-36. Laparoscopic ultrasound—sclerosing cholangitis. Longitudinal image demonstrates diffuse wall thickening of the common bile duct *(arrow)* with a barely visible narrowed lumen *(arrowheads).*

latation; potential for surgical bypass procedures; and location of obstructed ducts, stones, and periductal infected collections for drainage.

Pancreas

LUS has been advocated for evaluation and staging of **carcinoma** of the pancreas and periampullary region. In one series of 70 patients with presumed stage 1 carcinoma of the head of the pancreas, 21 of this group proved to have distant metastases, and 16 of the 21 were detected by laparoscopy and LUS.[76] Of this group, 3 patients had liver metastases missed at the dome of the liver, all of which were less than 5 mm in size, and 2 further patients had lymph node metastases at the celiac axis, which were missed by LUS. The authors also noted a 93% positive predictive value for vascular invasion by LUS, but a sensitivity of only 59%. In this series, the preoperative stage was upgraded in 41% and laparotomy was avoided in 19%. A second study of 40 patients with carcinoma of the pancreatic head or periampullary region showed similar findings in which laparoscopy with LUS demonstrated occult metastatic disease in 35%. The addition of LUS to laparoscopy increased specificity for predicting tumor resectability.[77]

Possible LUS findings that indicate unresectability include liver metastases, lymph node metastases, and direct vascular invasion of the portal vein or the superior mesenteric vein (Fig. 20-37). While these findings can be assessed by preoperative ultrasound and other imaging studies, the increased resolution available by LUS techniques can undoubtedly increase the detection rate for small liver metastases. Whether the accuracy for detection of lymphadenopathy is increased remains a subject of dispute as there are no conclusive studies documenting this. Similarly, there has been no prospective study to compare the preoperative definition of vascular invasion to LUS findings, but both **lymphadenopathy** and **vascular invasion** can be well demonstrated by LUS. Further studies will hopefully better define the precise role of laparoscopy and LUS in evaluation of patients with carcinoma of the pancreas.

Thus far there has been little, if any, experience with the use of LUS in patients with nonmalignant pancreatic disease. But LUS guidance for minimally invasive approaches to pseudocyst drainage might prove useful.

Other Applications

There are some reports in the literature of LUS used for **staging of hollow viscous tumors**. In one report, 56 patients with carcinoma of the esophagus and cardia were undergoing laparoscopy for assessment of peritoneal metastases; they also had LUS of the liver and celiac lymph nodes. In 5% of patients, the laparotomy was canceled secondary to metastatic disease, and an additional 5% metastases were suspected but required laparotomy to confirm with biopsy. In 1 patient, LUS missed a liver metastasis in segment 7. Out of this combined group, the preoperative stage was changed and metastases detected primarily in patients with cancer of the stomach and rarely in patients with esophageal cancer.[78] In another report of a mixed group of 40 patients with upper gastrointestinal tumors, laparoscopy added information in 40%, including finding peritoneal, liver, and nodal metastases.[79] In a subgroup of 20 of these patients, LUS led to a stage change in 7 (35%) by detecting liver metastases in 3 and lymph node metastases in 4.

A report was also published on the use of LUS to localize **renal stones** in a patient undergoing laparoscopic nephrolithotomy. Color flow Doppler via the laparoscopic ultrasound device was also useful for identifying an area of minimal vascularity to select for the cortical incision site, thereby hopefully minimizing renal cortical tissue damage.[80] LUS has also been described for use in gynecologic surgical procedures, particularly in evaluation of **hydrosalpinx**.[73]

CRYOSURGERY OF THE LIVER

Cryoablation of liver tumors using liquid nitrogen at $-196°C$ circulating through an enclosed cryoprobe has proved to be a successful alternative to surgical resection. It is used when resection is unfeasible for technical reasons such as tumor location, multiplicity of tumor sites, lack of sufficient liver reserve, or other comorbid diseases. Cryosurgery may also be used in conjunction with surgical resection, either to treat other sites of tumor within the liver or to freeze positive or close resection margins.

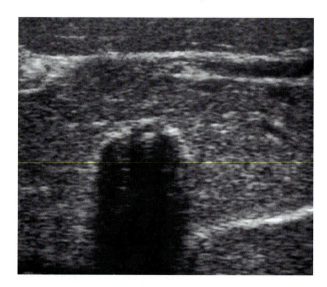

FIG. 20-38. Cryolesion. The "freeze front" appears as a hyperechoic, hemispherical rim with complete acoustic shadowing posteriorly.

> ### ADVANTAGES OF IOUS IN THE PERFORMANCE OF HEPATIC CRYOSURGERY
>
> Detection of occult tumor within the liver
> Evaluation of the relationship of tumor to the surrounding hepatic vasculature and biliary system
> Guidance for tumor biopsy
> Real-time guidance for accurate placement of the cryoprobe(s)
> Continuous real-time monitoring of the developing cryolesion in multiple planes to assure complete cryoablation of the tumor

tive or close resection margins. Monitoring the cryolesion visually or by palpation is not adequate to ensure appropriate tumor ablation. Needle-mounted thermocouples offer some improvement in monitoring the cryoablation. This is impractical because innumerable thermocouples would be required for precise monitoring of irregular tumor margins, since each thermocouple reads accurately only at its precise location and a change in position of 1 to 2 mm may alter the temperature recording by as much as 10°C to 15°C.[81]

The in vitro demonstration by Onik et al. that a cryolesion can be accurately visualized by sonography has allowed for an efficient and effective means of monitoring cryoablation in the liver.[82] The "freeze front" is visualized as a curvilinear hyperechoic rim, deep to which there is virtually complete acoustic shadowing (Fig. 20-38). Using this approach, a sono-

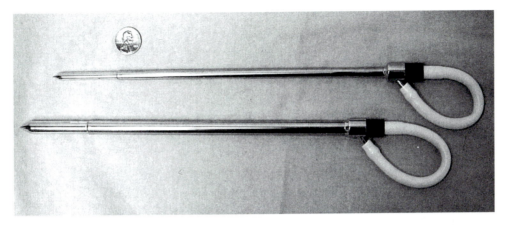

FIG. 20-39. Cryoprobes 5 mm and 10 mm diameter. Note the conical tips, which are suitable for direct penetration into liver tumors.

graphic-pathologic correlation study was performed on patients during surgery for liver tumors. There was a precise correlation between the echogenic delineation of the cryolesion on ultrasound and the gross and microscopic pathologic definition of the boundaries of cryonecrosis. The boundary between normal healthy tissue and the frozen cryolesion is sharp, with the frozen tissue showing clear evidence of coagulation necrosis.[83]

Technique

The IOUS studies are performed using linear array or curvilinear probes, preferably with a center frequency at approximately 5 MHz. It is essential to use a probe capable of imaging 10 to 12 cm of liver tissue without adverse effects on image quality because of attenuation. The lesions found within the liver are assessed for size, location, and proximity to major hepatic and portal vasculature. Lesions that abut major vessels present a particular problem because the flowing blood may interfere with successful cryoablation of that portion of the tumor that abuts the large vessel. Freezing temperature must range down to $-25°C$ to $-30°C$ to ensure a lethal freeze. Consequently, if the tumor is seen to be contiguous to a large vessel and cryosurgery is still the treatment of choice, steps may be taken to temporarily interrupt blood flow. These include a Pringle maneuver (temporarily cross-clamping the vessels at the porta hepatis) or cinching a hepatic vein temporarily to prevent reflux during the time of freezing.[85]

Ultrasound is also important in assessing the proximity of tumors to the major right and left bile ducts and gallbladder. The biliary epithelium is exquisitely sensitive to freezing and will undergo necrosis if frozen, resulting in major bile leaks. Consequently, a tumor in close proximity to the gallbladder would require a cholecystectomy prior to freezing. Tumors in the central portion of the liver abutting the main right and left bile ducts present a more difficult problem, as there is no method to protect the biliary epithelium. This may be a relative contraindication to cryoablation of tumors in that location.

Guidance for cryoprobe placement can be performed in several ways. We use cryoprobes with conical pointed tips (Fig. 20-39). These can often be placed by hand directly into the liver tumor using real-time ultrasound guidance for direction and assessment of accurate placement. A single cryoprobe should bisect the lesion and extend all the way through the lesion such that the tip of the probe is at the deep margin of tumor. The freezing extends primarily perpendicular to the cryoprobe with very little forward propagation of ice. Consequently, if the probe is not placed through the entire lesion, the deep margin may not be adequately frozen. Larger lesions may require more than one probe placement, and the spacing of multiple cryoprobes can be precisely controlled using IOUS guidance.

If a lesion is not palpable, direct insertion of the cryoprobe may be difficult. There are two methods to deal with this problem. An 18-gauge biopsy needle may be initially placed with ultrasound guidance. When satisfactory positioning is accomplished, a tandem placement of the cryoprobe may be successful. Another method involves the placement of a needle into the lesion followed by a guidewire that is stiff enough to allow passage of dilators and, subsequently, a sheath through which the cryoprobe can be placed in the desired position.[86]

Freezing is monitored in real time in multiple planes to assess growth of the cryolesion through and beyond the tumor into the adjacent normal liver (Fig. 20-40). The goal is to extend the cryolesion for approximately 1 cm beyond the tumor into normal liver to ensure adequate treatment margins. The visible

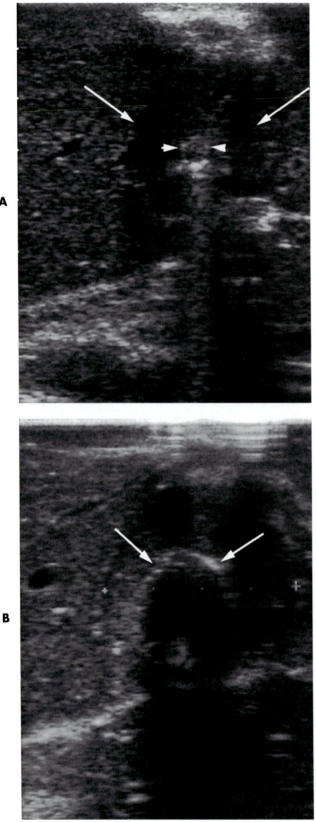

A

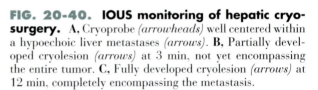

FIG. 20-40. IOUS monitoring of hepatic cryosurgery. A, Cryoprobe *(arrowheads)* well centered within a hypoechoic liver metastases *(arrows)*. **B,** Partially developed cryolesion *(arrows)* at 3 min, not yet encompassing the entire tumor. **C,** Fully developed cryolesion *(arrows)* at 12 min, completely encompassing the metastasis.

B

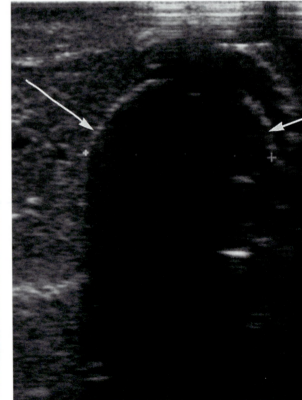

C

freeze front corresponds to 0°C, where ice formation begins, but the lethal temperatures of $-25°$ or colder are reached only 2 to 3 mm inside the visible ice edge. Experimental in vitro and *in vivo* data suggest that more than one freeze-thaw cycle is necessary for complete tumor destruction.[87] Consequently, after reaching maximal desired size, the cryolesion is allowed to thaw spontaneously until the periphery of the tumor is again visualized. At this point a second freeze cycle is undertaken, again with continuous real-time monitoring. The importance of excellent IOUS cannot be overstated to assure effective cryosurgical treatment of liver tumors.

Results

Although surgical resection of hepatic metastases remains the standard of care, only a small percentage of patients (less than 20%) are candidates for surgical resection because of multiple sites of tumor in both right and left lobes or because of comorbid disease processes that make surgical resection impossible. Some of these patients are amenable to cryosurgical ablation, which has the advantage of preserving more functional liver tissue as well as having less morbidity and shorter recuperative time. Actuarial analysis using the Kaplan-Meier method projects a 30% to 40% 5-year survival rate in patients undergoing cryosurgical ablation of colorectal metastases. Not all of these patients are cured, and recurrence after 5 years can occur, but the actuarial survival curve is similar to the survival curve for surgical resection.[86,87] Consequently, the cryosurgical option may provide potential curative treatment to a group of patients in whom no other curative options are available. It is a safe and effective alternative to surgical resection or may indeed be used in combination with surgical resection, treating several sites of tumor simultaneously. Further study with more prolonged survival data is necessary to ascertain the precise role of hepatic cryosurgery in the treatment of liver cancer.

REFERENCES

Hepatobiliary System

1. Kane, RA, Hughes LA, Cua EJ et al. The impact of intraoperative ultrasonography on surgery for liver neoplasms. *J Ultrasound Med* 1994;13:1-6.
2. Boldrini G, deGaetano AM, Giovanni I et al. The systematic use of operative ultrasound for detection of liver metastasis during colorectal surgery. *World J Surg* 1987;11:622-627.
3. Eiseman B, Greenlaw RH, Gallagher JQ. Localization of common duct stones by ultrasound. *Arch Surg* 1965;91:195-199.
4. Knight PR, Newell JA. Operative use of ultrasonics in cholelithiasis. *Lancet* 1963;1:1023-1025.
5. Reading CC. Intraoperative ultrasonography. *Abdom Imaging* 1996;21:21-29.
6. Mack LA, Lee RA, Nyberg DA. Intraoperative sonography of the abdomen. In: Rumack CM, Wilson SR, Charboneau JW, eds. *Diagnostic Ultrasound*, St Louis: Mosby-Year Book; 1991:492-504.
7. Kane RA. Intraoperative ultrasound. In: Wilson SR, Charboneau JW, Leopold GR, eds. *Ultrasound: Categorical Course Syllabus*. Presented at the American Roentgen Ray Society 93rd Annual Meeting; 1993; San Francisco.
8. Kraskal JB, Kane RA. Intraoperative ultrasonography of the liver. *Crit Rev Diagn Imag* 1995;36(3):175-226.
9. Foster JH, Ensminger WF. Treatment of metastatic cancer to liver. In: De Vita et al., eds. *Cancer: Principles and Practice of Oncology*. Lippincott: Philadelphia; 1985:2117.
10. Hughes K, Scheele J, Sugarbaker PH. Surgery for colorectal cancer metastatic to the liver: optimizing the results of treatment. *Surg Clin North Am* 1989;69:339-359.
11. Bengmark S, Hafstrom L. The natural course of liver cancer. *Prog Clin Cancer* 1978;7:195-200.
12. Clarke MP, Kane RA, Steele GD et al. Prospective comparison of preoperative imaging and intraoperative ultrasonography in the detection of liver tumors. *Surgery* 1989;106:849-855.
13. Parker GA, Lawrence W, Horsley JS et al. Intraoperative ultrasound of the liver affects operative decision making. *Ann Surg* 1989;209:569-588.
14. Wernecke K, Rummeny E, Bongartz G et al. Detection of hepatic masses in patients with carcinoma: comparative sensitivities of sonography, CT, and MR imaging. *AJR* 1991;157:731-739.
15. Sitzmann JV, Coleman J, Pitt HA et al. Preoperative assessment of malignant hepatic tumors. *Am J Surg* 1990;159:137-143.
16. Machi J, Isomoto H, Kurohiji T et al. Accuracy of intraoperative ultrasonography in diagnosing liver metastasis from colorectal cancer: evaluation with postoperative follow-up results. *World J Surg* 1991;15:551-557.
17. Igawa S, Sakai K, Kinoshita H et al. Intraoperative sonography: clinical usefulness in liver surgery. *Radiology* 1985;156:473.
18. Gozzetti G, Mazziotti A, Bolondi L et al. Intraoperative ultrasonography in surgery for liver tumors. *Surgery* 1986;99:523.
19. Sheu JC, Lee CS, Sung JL et al. Intraoperative hepatic ultrasonography: an indispensable procedure in resection of small hepatocellular carcinoma. *Surgery* 1985;97:97-193.
20. Jin-Chuan, Chue-Shue L, Jeui-Low S et al. Hepatic ultrasonography: an indispensable procedure in resection of small hepatocellular carcinomas. *Surgery* 1987;97-103.
21. Jakimowicz JJ, Rutten H, Jurgens PJ et al. Comparison of operative ultrasonography and radiography in screening of the common bile duct for calculi. *World J Surg* 1987;11:628-634.
22. Dunnington GL. Intraoperative ultrasonography in abdominal surgery. *Surg Ann* 1993;24:101-125.
23. Sigel B, Machi J, Anderson KW et al. Operative sonography of the biliary tree and pancreas. *Semin Ultrasound CT MRI* 1985;6:2-4.
24. Mack LA, Nyberg DA. Intraoperative ultrasonography of the gallbladder and biliary tract. In: Rifkin MD, ed. *Intraoperative and Endoscopic Ultrasonography*. New York: Churchill Livingstone; 1987:105-120.
25. Herbst CA, Mittlestaedt CA, Staab EV et al. Intraoperative ultrasonography evaluation of the gallbladder in morbidly obese patients. *Ann Surg* 1984;200:691-692.

Pancreas

26. Charnsangavej C. Pancreatic duct adenocarcinoma: diagnosis and staging by CT and MR imaging. In: Freeny PC et al., eds. *Radiology of the liver, biliary tract, and pancreas. Categorical course syllabus. American Roentgen Ray Society* 1996:165-171.

27. Trede M, Schwall G, Saeger HD. Survival after pancreatoduodenectomy. *Ann Surg* 1990;211:447-458.

28. Cameron JL, Crist DW, Sitzman, JV et al. Factors influencing survival after pancreatoduodenectomy for pancreatic cancer. *Am J Surg* 1991;165:68-73.

29. Geer RJ, Brennan MF. Prognostic indicators for survival after resection of pancreatic adenocarcinoma. *Am J Surg* 1993; 165:68-73.

30. Douglass HO Jr, Tepper J, Leichman L. Neoplasms of the exocrine pancreas. In: Holland JF, Frei E III, Bast RC Jr et al., eds. *Cancer Medicine*. Philadelphia: Lea & Febiger; 1993: 1466-1484.

31. Rifkin MD, Weiss SM. Intraoperative sonographic identification of nonpalpable pancreatic masses. *J Ultrasound Med* 1984;3:409-411.

32. Sigel B, Machi J, Ramos JR et al. The role of imaging ultrasound during pancreatic surgery. *Ann Surg* 1984;200(4): 486-493.

33. Serio G, Fugazzola C, Iacono C et al. Intraoperative ultrasonography in pancreatic cancer. *Int J Pancreatol* 1992; 11(1):31-41.

34. Freeny P. Radiologic imaging of chronic pancreatitis. In: Freeny PC et al., eds. Radiology of the liver, biliary tract, and pancreas. Categorical course syllabus. *American Roentgen Ray Society* 1996;157-163.

35. Printz H, Klotter JH, Nies C et al. Intraoperative ultrasonography in surgery for chronic pancreatitis. *Int J Pancreatol* 1992;12(3):233-237.

36. Gorman B, Reading C. Imaging of gastrointestinal neuroendocrine tumors. In: Freeny PC et al., eds. Radiology of the liver, biliary tract, and pancreas. Categorical course syllabus. *American Roentgen Ray Society* 1996:191-198.

37. Gorman B, Charboneau JW, James EM et al. Benign pancreatic insulinomas: preoperative and intraoperative sonographic localization. *AJR* 1986;147:929-934.

38. Zeiger MA, Shawker TH, Norton JA. Use of intraoperative ultrasonography to localize islet cell tumors. *World J Surg* 1993;174:448-454.

39. Bottger TC, Junginger T. Is preoperative radiographic localization of islet cell tumors in patients with insulinoma necessary? *World J Surg* 1993;17:427-432.

40. vanHeerden JA, Grant CS, Czako PF et al. Occult functioning insulinomas: which localizing studies are indicated? *Surgery* 1992;112(6):1010-1014.

41. Charboneau JW, Gorman B, Reading CC et al. Intraoperative ultrasonography of pancreatic endocrine tumors. In: Rifkin MD, ed. *Clinics in Diagnostic Ultrasound—Intraoperative and Endoscopic Ultrasound.* 7(22):123-134, 1987.

42. Sugg SL, Norton SL, Fraker DL et al. A prospective study of intraoperative methods to diagnose and resect duodenal gastrinomas. *Ann Surg* 1993;218(2):138-144.

43. Stabile BE, Morrow DJ, Passaro E Jr. The gastrinoma triangle: operative implications. *Am J Surg* 1984;147:25-31.

44. Davies PF, Shevland JE, Shepherd JJ. Ultrasonography of the pancreas in patients with MEN I. *J Ultrasound Med* 1993;12(2):67-72.

Renal

45. Polascik TJ, Meng MV, Epstein JI et al. Intraoperative sonography for the evaluation and management of renal tumors: experience with 100 patients. *J Urol* 1995;154:1676-1680.

46. Walther MM, Choyke PL, Hayes W et al. Evaluation of color Doppler intraoperative ultrasound in parenchymal sparing renal surgery. *J Urol* 1994;152:1984-1987.

47. Morgan WR, Zincke H. Progression and survival after renalconserving surgery for renal cell carcinoma: experience in 104 patients and extended followup. *J Urol* 1990;144:852-858.

48. Steinbach F, Stöckle M, Müller SC et al. Conservative surgery of renal cell tumors in 140 patients: 21 years of experience. *J Urol* 1992;148:24-30.

49. Campbell SC, Novick AC, Streem SB et al. Complications of nephron sparing surgery for renal tumors. *J Urol* 1994; 151:1177.

50. Carini M, Selli C, Barbanti G et al. Conservative surgical treatment of renal cell carcinoma: clinical experience and reappraisal of indications. *J Urol* 1988;140:725-731.

51. Novick AC, Streem S, Montie JE et al. Conservative surgery for renal cell carcinoma: a single-center experience with 100 patients. *J Urol* 1989;141:835-839.

52. Zincke H, Engen DE, Henning KM et al. Treatment of renal cell carcinoma by in situ partial nephrectomy and extracorporeal operation with autotransplantation. *Mayo Clin Proc* 1985;60:651-662.

53. Novick AC, Zincke H, Neves RJ et al. Surgical enucleation for renal cell carcinoma. *J Urol* 1986;135:235-238.

54. Smith RB, deKernian JB, Ehrlich RM et al. Bilateral renal cell carcinoma and renal cell carcinoma in the solitary kidney. *J Urol* 1984;132:450-454.

55. Topley M, Novick AC, Montie JE. Long-term results following partial nephrectomy for localized renal adenocarcinoma. *J Urol* 1984;131:1050-1052.

56. Blackley SK, Ladaga L, Woolfitt RA et al. Ex situ study of the effectiveness of enucleation in patients with renal cell carcinoma. *J Urol* 1988;140:6-10.

57. Marshall FF, Taxy JB, Fishman EK et al. The feasibility of surgical enucleation for renal cell carcinoma. *J Urol* 1986; 135:231-234.

58. Mukamel E, Konichezky M, Engelstein D et al. Incidental small renal tumors accompanying clinically overt renal cell carcinoma. *J Urol* 1988;140:22-24.

59. Gilbert BR, Russo P, Zirinsky K et al. Intraoperative sonography: application in renal cell carcinoma. *J Urol* 1988; 139:582-584.

60. Assimos DG, Hanson KJ. Role of intraoperative ultrasonography in urology. *Semin Urol* 1994;12(4):283-291.

61. Marshall FF, Holdford SS, Hamper UM. Intraoperative sonography of renal tumors. *J Urol* 1992;148:1393-1396.

62. Campbell SC, Novick AC, Streem SB et al. Complication of nephron sparing surgery for renal tumors. *J Urol* 1994; 151:1177-1180.

63. Dougherty MJ, Hallett JW, Naessens JM et al. Optimizing technical success of renal revascularization: the impact of intraoperative color flow duplex ultrasonography. *J Vasc Surg* 1993;7:849-857.

64. Lantz EJ, Charboneau JW, Hallett JW et al. Intraoperative color Doppler sonography during renal artery revascularization. *AJR* 1994;162:859-863.

Laparoscopic Sonography

65. Yamakawa K, Naito S, Azuma K et al. Laparoscopic diagnosis of the intra-abdominal organs. *Jpn J Gastroenterol* 1958;55: 741-747.

66. Yamakawa K, Yoshioka A, Shimizu K et al. Laparoechography: an ultrasonic diagnosis under laparoscopic observation. *Jpn Med Ultrasonics* 1964;2:26.

67. Fukuda M, Mima S, Tanabe T et al. Endoscopic sonography of the liver: diagnostic application of the echolaparoscope to localize intrahepatic lesions. *Scand J Gastroenterol* 1984;19 (suppl 94):24-38.

68. Frank K, Bliesze H, Honhof JA et al. Laparoscopic sonography: a new approach to intra-abdominal disease. *J Clin Ultrasound* 1985;13:60-65.

69. Fornari F, Civardi G, Cavanna L et al. Laparoscopic ultrasonography in the study of liver diseases. *Surg Endosc* 1989;3:33-37.

70. Goldberg BB, Liu JB, Merton DA et al. Sonographically guided laparoscopy and mediastinoscopy using miniature catheter-based transducers. *J Ultrasound Med* 1993;12:49-54.

71. Babineau TJ, Lewis WD, Jenkins RJ et al. Role of staging laparoscopy in the treatment of hepatic malignancy. *Am J Surg* 1994;167:151-155.

72. Kane RA, Hughes LA, Cua EJ et al. The impact of intraoperative ultrasonography on surgery for liver neoplasms. *J Ultrasound Med* 1994;13:1-6.

73. Liu JB, Feld RI, Goldberg BB et al. Laparoscopic gray-scale and color Doppler US: preliminary animal and clinical studies. *Radiology* 1995;194:851-857.

74. John TG, Greig JD, Crosbie JL et al. Superior staging of liver tumors with laparoscopy and laparoscopic ultrasound. *Ann Surg* 1994;220(6):711-719.

75. Jakimowicz J. Laparoscopic intraoperative ultrasonography, equipment, and technique. *Semin Laparoscopic Surg* 1994; 1(1):52-61.

76. Bemelman WA, DeWit LT, van Delden OM et al. Diagnostic laparoscopy combined with laparoscopic ultrasonography in staging of cancer of the pancreatic head region. *Br J Surg* 1995;82:820-824.

77. John TG, Greig JD, Carter DC et al. Carcinoma of the pancreatic head and periampullary region: tumor staging with laparoscopy and laparoscopic ultrasonography. *Ann Surg* 1995;221(2):156-164.

78. Bemelman WA, van Delden OM, van Lanschot JJB et al. Laparoscopy and laparoscopic ultrasonography in staging of carcinoma of the esophagus and gastric cardia. *J Am Coll Surg* 1995;181:421-425.

79. Hünerbein M, Rau B, Schlag PM. Laparoscopy and laparoscopic ultrasound for staging of upper gastrointestinal tumours. *Eur J Surg Oncol* 1995;21:50-55.

80. van Cangh P, Abi Aad AS, Lorge F et al. Laparoscopic nephrolithotomy: the value of intracorporeal sonography and color Doppler. *Urology* 1995;45(3):516-519.

81. Cooper IS. Cryogenic surgery. *N Engl J Med* 1963;268:743-749.

Cryosurgery

82. Onik G, Cooper C, Goldberg HI et al. Ultrasonic characteristics of frozen liver. *Cryobiology* 1984;21:321-328.

83. Onik G, Kane R, Steele G et al. Monitoring hepatic cryosurgery with sonography. *AJR* 1986;147:665-669.

84. Ravikumar TS, Kane R, Cady B et al. A 5-year study of cryosurgery in the treatment of liver tumors. *Arch Surg* 1991;126:1520-1524.

85. Kane RA. Ultrasound-guided hepatic cryosurgery for tumor ablation. *Semin Interven Rad* 1993;10(2):132-142.

86. Onik G, Rubinsky B, Zemel R et al. Ultrasound-guided hepatic cryosurgery in the treatment of metastatic colon carcinoma: preliminary results. *Cancer* 1991;67:901-907.

87. Ravikumar TS, Steele G Jr, Kane R et al. Experimental and clinical observations on hepatic cryosurgery for colorectal metastases. *Cancer Res* 1991;51:6323-6327.

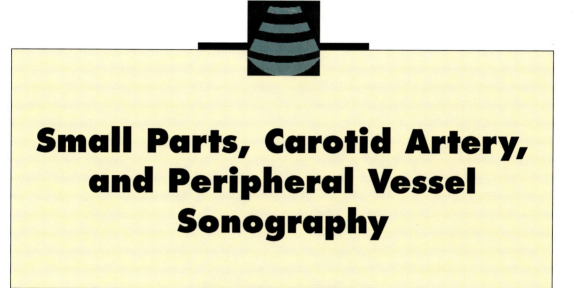

PART IV

Small Parts, Carotid Artery, and Peripheral Vessel Sonography

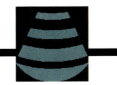

The Thyroid Gland

•

Luigi Solbiati, M.D.
J. William Charboneau, M.D.
E. Meredith James, M.D., F.A.C.R.
Ian D. Hay, M.B., Ph.D., F.A.C.E., F.A.C.P., F.R.C.P.

Because of the superficial location of the thyroid gland, high-resolution real-time gray scale and color Doppler sonography can demonstrate normal thyroid anatomy and pathologic conditions with remarkable clarity. As a result, this technique has come to play an increasingly important role in the diagnostic evaluation of thyroid diseases. Sonography, however, is only one of several diagnostic methods currently available for use in evaluation of the thyroid. In order to use it effectively and economically, it is important to understand its current capabilities and limitations.

INSTRUMENTATION AND TECHNIQUE

High-frequency transducers (7.5-15.0 MHz) currently provide both deep ultrasound penetration—up to 5 cm—and high-definition images, with a resolution of 0.7 to 1.0 mm. No other imaging method can achieve this degree of spatial resolution. Linear-array transducers are preferred to sector transducers because of the wider near field of view and the capability to combine high-frequency gray scale and color Doppler images. The thyroid gland is one of the most vascular organs of the body. As a result, Doppler examination may provide useful diagnostic information in some thyroid diseases.

The patient is typically examined in the supine position, with the neck extended. A small pad may be placed under the shoulders to provide better exposure of the neck, particularly in patients with a short, stocky habitus. The thyroid gland must be examined thoroughly in both transverse and longitudinal planes. Imaging of the lower poles can be enhanced by asking the patient to swallow, which momentarily raises the thyroid gland in the neck. The entire gland, including the isthmus, must be examined. The examination should also be extended laterally to include the region of the carotid artery and jugular vein in order to identify enlarged jugular chain lymph nodes, superiorly to visualize submandibular adenopathy, and inferiorly to define any pathologic supraclavicular lymph nodes.

In addition to the images recorded during the examination, some examiners include in the permanent record a diagrammatic representation of the neck showing the location(s) of any abnormal findings (Fig. 21-1). This cervical "map" helps to communicate the anatomic relationships of the pathology more clearly to the referring clinician and his/her patient. It also serves as a useful reference for the radiologist and sonographer for follow-up examinations.

ANATOMY

The thyroid gland is located in the anteroinferior part of the neck (infrahyoid compartment) in a space outlined by muscle, trachea, esophagus, carotid arteries, and jugular veins (Fig. 21-2). The thyroid gland is made up of two lobes located along either side of the trachea and connected across the midline by the isthmus, a thin structure draping over the anterior tracheal wall at the level of the junction of the middle and lower thirds of the thyroid gland. From 10% to 40% of normal patients have a small thyroid (pyramidal) lobe arising superiorly from the isthmus and lying in front of the thyroid cartilage.[1] It can be regularly visualized in younger patients, but it undergoes progressive atrophy in adulthood and becomes invisible. The size and shape of the thyroid lobes vary widely in normal patients. In tall individuals, the lateral lobes have a longitudinally elongated shape on the sagittal scans, while in shorter individuals the gland is more oval. As a result, the normal dimensions of the lobes have a wide range of variability. In the newborn, the gland is 18 to 20 mm long, with an anteroposterior (AP) diameter of 8 to 9 mm. By one year of age, the mean length is 25 mm and the anteroposterior diameter is 12 to 15 mm.[2] In adults, the mean length is approximately 40 to 60 mm and the mean anteroposterior diameter is 13 to 18 mm. The mean thickness of the isthmus is 4 to 6 mm.[3]

Sonography is an accurate method to use in calculating **thyroid volume**. In approximately one-third of cases, the sonographic measurement of volume differs from the physical size estimate derived from examination.[4] Thyroid volume measurements may be useful for goiter size determination in order to assess the need for surgery, to permit calculation of the dose of I[131] needed for treating thyrotoxicosis, and to evaluate the response to suppression treatments.[5] Thyroid volume can be calculated with linear parameters or more precisely with mathematical formulas. Among the linear parameters, the anteroposterior diameter is the most precise, since it is relatively independent of possible dimensional asymmetry between the two lobes. When the AP diameter is more than 2 cm, the thyroid gland may be considered enlarged. The most precise method of calculating thyroid volume is an integration of formulas of serial areas obtained from contiguous ultra-

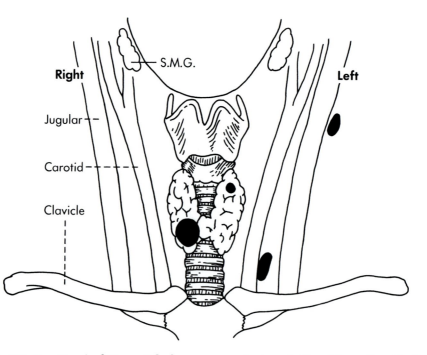

FIG. 21-1. Cervical "map" helps communicate relationships of pathology to clinicians and serves as a reference for follow-up examinations. SMG, submandibular gland.

sound scans.[6] In neonates, thyroid volume ranges from 0.40 to 1.40 ml, increasing by approximately 1.0 to 1.3 ml for each 10 kg of weight up to a normal volume in adults of 10 to 11 ± 3 ml.[6] Thyroid volume is generally larger in patients living in regions with iodine deficiency and in patients who have acute hepatitis or chronic renal failure; it is smaller in patients who have chronic hepatitis or have been treated with thyroxine or radioactive iodine.[5,6]

Normal **thyroid parenchyma** has a homogeneous medium- to high-level echogenicity which makes detection of focal cystic or hypoechoic thyroid lesions relatively easy in most cases (Fig. 21-2). The thin hyperechoic line that bounds the thyroid lobes is the capsule, which is often identifiable by ultrasound. It may become calcified in patients who have uremia or disorders of calcium metabolism. With currently available high-sensitivity Doppler instruments, the rich vascularity of the gland can be seen and is most pronounced at the superior and inferior poles (Fig. 21-3). The **superior thyroid artery and vein** are found at the upper pole of each lobe. The **inferior thyroid vein** is found at the lower pole and the **inferior thyroid artery** is located posterior to the lower third of each lobe (Fig. 21-4). The mean diameter of the arteries is 1 to 2 mm, while the lower veins can be up to

8 mm in diameter. Normally, peak systolic velocities reach 20 to 40 cm/sec in the major thyroid arteries and 15 to 30 cm/sec in intraparenchymal arteries. It should be noted that these are the highest velocities found in vessels supplying superficial organs.

The **sternohyoid** and **omohyoid muscles** are seen as thin, hypoechoic bands anterior to the thyroid gland (Fig. 21-2). The **sternocleidomastoid muscle** is seen as a larger oval band that lies lateral to the thyroid gland. An important anatomic landmark is the **longus colli muscle** which is located posterior to each thyroid lobe, in close contact with the prevertebral space.

The recurrent laryngeal nerve and the inferior thyroid artery pass in the angle between the trachea, esophagus, and thyroid lobe. By careful scanning with gray scale and color Doppler, these structures can be located. On longitudinal scans, the recurrent laryngeal nerve and inferior thyroid artery may be seen as a thin hypoechoic band located between the thyroid lobe and esophagus on the left, and the thyroid lobe and longus colli muscle on the right. The esophagus, primarily a midline structure, may be found laterally and is usually on the left side. It is clearly identified by the target appearance of bowel in the transverse plane and by its peristaltic movements when the patient swallows.

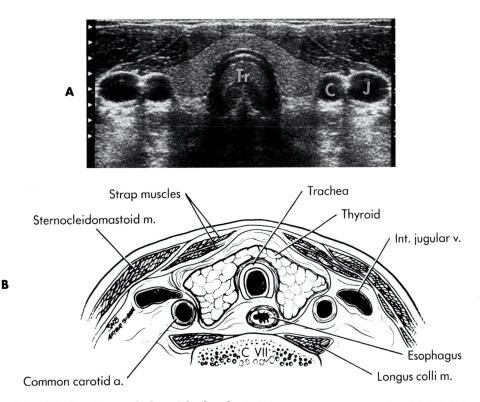

FIG. 21-2. Normal thyroid gland. A, Transverse sonogram made with 7.5 MHz linear array transducer. **B,** Corresponding anatomic drawing. Tr, Tracheal air shadow. C, common carotid artery. J, jugular vein. (From James EM, Charboneau JW. High-frequency (10 MHz) thyroid ultrasonography. *Semin Ultrasound, CT, MR* 1985;6:294-309.)

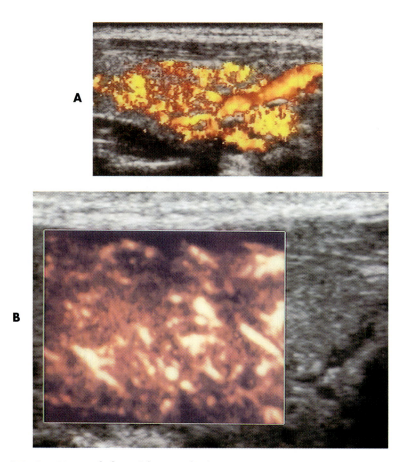

FIG. 21-3. Normal thyroid vascularity. A and B, New, highly sensitive color and power Doppler instruments demonstrate the rich vascular network of the normal gland on these longitudinal images.

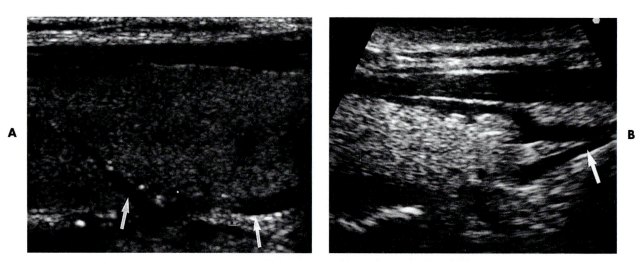

FIG. 21-4. Major blood vessels of the thyroid gland on longitudinal scans.
A, Inferior thyroid artery *(arrows)* along the posterior surface. B, Inferior thyroid vein *(arrow)* branches at the inferior pole of the thyroid.

CONGENITAL THYROID ABNORMALITIES

Congenital conditions of the thyroid gland include **agenesis** of one lobe or the whole gland, varying degrees of **hypoplasia**, and **ectopia**. Ultrasonography can be used to help establish the diagnosis of **hypoplasia** by demonstrating a diminutively sized gland. High-frequency ultrasound can also be used in the study of **congenital hypothyroidism**.[7] Measurement of thyroid lobes can be used to differentiate agenesis (absent gland) from goitrous hypothyroidism (gland enlargement). Radionuclide scans are more commonly used to detect ectopic thyroid tissue, e.g., in a lingual or suprahyoid position.

NODULAR THYROID DISEASE

Many thyroid diseases can present clinically with one or more thyroid nodules. Such nodules represent common and controversial clinical problems. Epidemiologic studies estimate that between 4% and 7% of the adult population in the United States have palpable thyroid nodules, with women being more frequently affected than men.[8,9] Exposure to ionizing radiation increases the incidence of benign and malignant nodules, with 20% to 30% of a radiation-exposed population having palpable thyroid disease.[10,11]

Although nodular thyroid disease is relatively common, thyroid cancer is rare and accounts for less than 1% of all malignant neoplasms.[12] In fact, the overwhelming majority of thyroid nodules are benign. The clinical challenge is to distinguish the few clinically significant malignant nodules from the many benign ones and, thus, to identify those patients for whom surgical excision is genuinely indicated. This task is complicated by the fact that much of the nodular disease of the thyroid gland is clinically occult (less than 1.5 cm) but can be readily detected by high-resolution sonography. The question of how to manage these small nodules discovered incidentally by sonography is an important one and it will be addressed later in this chapter.

Pathologic Features and Sonographic Correlates

Hyperplasia and Goiter.
Approximately 80% of nodular thyroid disease is due to **hyperplasia** of the gland, and it occurs in up to 5% of any population.[13] Its etiology includes **iodine deficiency** (endemic), **disorders of hormonogenesis** (hereditary familial forms), and **poor utilization of iodine** as a result of medication. When hyperplasia leads to an overall increase in size or volume of the gland, the term **"goiter"** is used. The peak age of patients with goiter is between 35 and 50 years, and females are three times more likely than males to have the disease.

Histologically, the initial stage is cellular hyperplasia of the thyroid acini, which is followed by micronodule and macronodule formation. Hyperplastic nodules often undergo liquefactive degeneration with the accumulation of blood, serous fluid, and colloid substance. Pathologically, they are often referred to as **hyperplastic, adenomatous, or colloid nodules**. Many cystic thyroid lesions are hyperplastic nodules that have undergone extensive liquefactive degeneration. Pathologically, true epithelial-lined cysts of the thyroid gland are rare. In the course of this cystic degenerative process, calcification, which is often coarse and perinodular, may occur.[5,14] Hyperplastic nodule function may have decreased, may have remained normal, or may have increased (toxic nodules).

Sonographically, most hyperplastic or adenomatous nodules are isoechoic compared to normal thyroid tissue (Fig. 21-5). As the size of the mass increases, it may become hyperechoic due to the numerous interfaces between cells and colloid substance.[5,15] Less frequently, a

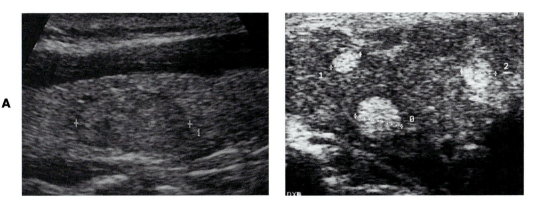

FIG. 21-5. Hyperplastic (adenomatous) nodules. A, Oval homogeneous isoechoic nodule *(calipers)* with thin and regular peripheral halo. **B,** Multiple hyperechoic nodules *(calipers)*.

hypoechoic sponge-like pattern is seen. When the nodule is isoechoic or hyperechoic, a thin peripheral hypoechoic halo is commonly seen (Fig. 21-5); it is most likely due to perinodular blood vessels and mild edema or compression of the adjacent normal parenchyma. Perinodular blood vessels are easily detected with the use of color Doppler sonography.[5,16,17] Hyperfunctioning (autonomous) nodules usually exhibit an abundant perinodular and intranodular vascularity.[16,17]

The degenerative changes of goitrous nodules correspond to their sonographic appearances: purely anechoic areas are due to serous or colloid fluid (Fig. 21-6, A, B); echogenic fluid or moving fluid-fluid levels correspond to hemorrhage (Fig. 21-6, C, D);[18] bright echogenic foci with comet-tail artifacts are likely to be due to the presence of dense colloid material (Fig. 21-6, E, F);[19] intracystic, thin septations probably correspond to attenuated strands of thyroid tissue (Fig. 21-6, G, H). On color Doppler these septations are avascular. Intracystic solid projections, or papillae, with or without color Doppler signals, are common, and this appearance can be similar to the rare cystic papillary thyroid carcinoma.[16,17]

Adenoma. Adenomas represent only 5% to 10% of all nodular disease of the thyroid and are seven times more common in females than in males.[5] Most result in no thyroid dysfunction; a minority (probably <10%) hyperfunction, develop autonomy and may cause thyrotoxicosis. Most adenomas are solitary but they may also develop as part of a multinodular process.

The **benign follicular adenoma** is a true thyroid neoplasm that is characterized by compression of adjacent tissues and fibrous encapsulation. Various subtypes of follicular adenoma include the fetal adenoma, Hurthle cell adenoma, and embryonal adenoma, each distinguished according to the character and pattern of cell proliferation. The cytologic features of follicular adenomas are generally indistinguishable from those of follicular carcinoma. Vascular and capsular invasion are the hallmarks of follicular carcinoma, and these features are identified by histologic, rather than cytologic, analysis. Needle biopsy is therefore not a reliable method to distinguish between follicular carcinoma and cellular adenoma. Therefore, such tumors are usually surgically removed.

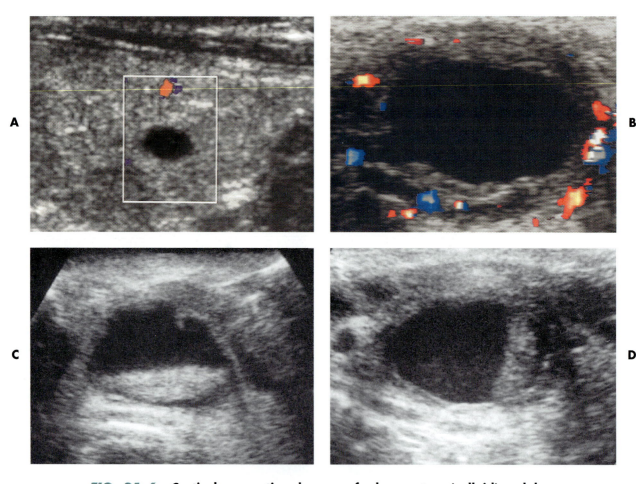

FIG. 21-6. Cystic degenerative changes of adenomatous (colloid) nodules. **A,** Small, discrete, purely cystic lesion. **B,** Cystic change in solid hypoechoic nodule. **C** and **D,** Hemorrhage in cystic nodule; the flat debris layer is horizontal in supine position (C) and vertical in upright position (D).   *Continued.*

Sonographically, adenomas are usually solid masses that may be hyperechoic, isoechoic, or hypoechoic. They often have a peripheral hypoechoic halo that is thick and smooth (Fig. 21-7, *A*). This halo is due to the fibrous capsule and blood vessels, which can be readily seen by color Doppler. Often, vessels pass from the periphery to the central regions of the nodule, creating a "spoke-and-wheel–like" appearance (Fig. 21-7, *B*). Hyperfunctioning (autonomous) adenomas sometimes exhibit abundant blood flow which may be peripheral and/or internally located (Fig. 21-8).[20]

Carcinoma. In most patients with primary thyroid cancer, the tumors are of epithelial origin and are derived from either the follicular or the parafollicular cells.[12] Malignant thyroid tumors of mesenchymal origin are exceedingly rare, as are metastases to the thyroid. Most thyroid cancers are well differentiated, and papillary carcinoma (including so-called mixed papillary and follicular carcinoma) now accounts for 75% to 90% of all cases.[12,21] In contrast, medullary, follicular, and anaplastic carcinoma, combined, represent only 10% to 25% of all thyroid carcinomas currently diagnosed in North America.

Although it can occur in patients of any age, **papillary cancer** is especially prevalent in younger patients.[12] Females are affected more often than males. On microscopic examination, the tumor is multicentric within the thyroid gland in at least 20% of cases.[22] Round, laminated calcifications (psammoma bodies) are seen in approximately 25% of cases. The major route of spread of papillary carcinoma is through the lymphatics to nearby cervical lymph nodes. In fact, it is not uncommon for a patient with papillary thyroid cancer to present with enlarged cervical nodes and a palpably normal thyroid gland.[23] Interestingly, the presence of nodal metastasis in the neck does not, in general, appear to adversely alter the prognosis for this malignancy. Distant metastases are very rare (2% to 3% of cases) and occur mostly in the mediastinum and lung. After 20 years, the cumulative mortality from papillary thyroid cancer is typically only 4% to 8%.[23]

Papillary carcinoma has peculiar histologic features (fibrous capsule, microcalcifications) and

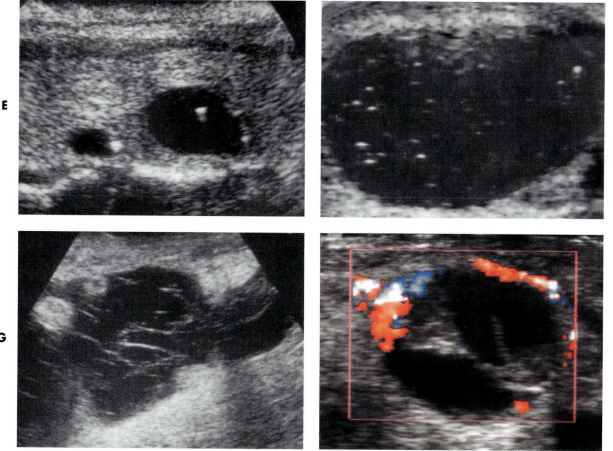

FIG. 21-6, cont'd. Cystic degenerative changes of adenomatous (colloid) nodules. **E** and **F,** Bright echogenic foci (some with comet-tail artifact) in the colloid fluid and wall. **G** and **H,** Intracystic septations of various thickness create multiloculated lesions. Note absence of blood flow in the thick septations.

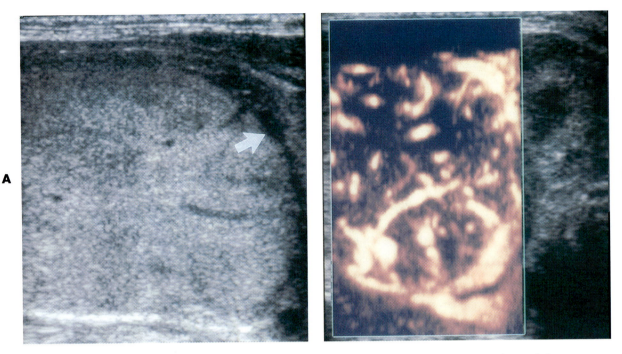

FIG. 21-7. Follicular adenoma. A, Longitudinal scan shows a large, isoechoic solid mass with thick and incomplete peripheral halo *(arrow).* **B,** Power Doppler image shows the intranodular blood supply which creates a spoke-and-wheel-like appearance that is typical of follicular neoplasm.

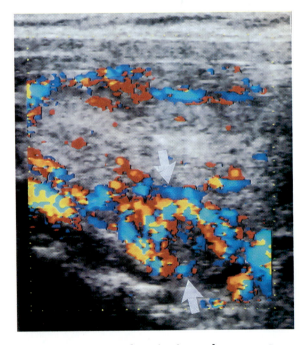

FIG. 21-8. Hyperfunctioning adenoma. Longitudinal color Doppler scan shows intense peripheral and internal vascularity of the nodule *(arrows).*

cytologic features ("ground glass" nuclei, cytoplasmic inclusions in the nucleus, and indentations of the nuclear membrane) which often allow a relatively easy pathologic diagnosis.[24] In particular, microcalcifications, which result from the deposition of calcium salts in the **psammoma bodies,** are present with a high incidence in both the primary tumor and the cervical lymph node metastases.[25] Papillary "microcarcinoma" is a nonencapsulated sclerosing tumor measuring 1 cm or less in diameter. In 80% of cases, the patient presents with enlarged cervical nodes and a palpably normal thyroid gland.[23,24]

Similar to the pathologic features, **sonographic characteristics of papillary carcinoma** are relatively distinctive in most cases:

- hypoechogenicity (in 90% of cases) due to closely packed cell content, with minimal colloid substance (Fig. 21-9, *A*);
- microcalcifications that appear as tiny, punctate hyperechoic foci, either with or without acoustic shadows (Fig. 21-9, *A*, *B*);[14,26,27]
- hypervascularity (in 90% of cases) with disorganized vascularity, mostly in well-encapsulated forms (Fig. 21-10);[28]
- cervical lymph node metastasis which may contain tiny, punctate echogenic foci due to microcalcifications. Occasionally, metastatic nodes may be cystic as a result of extensive degeneration (Fig. 21-11,

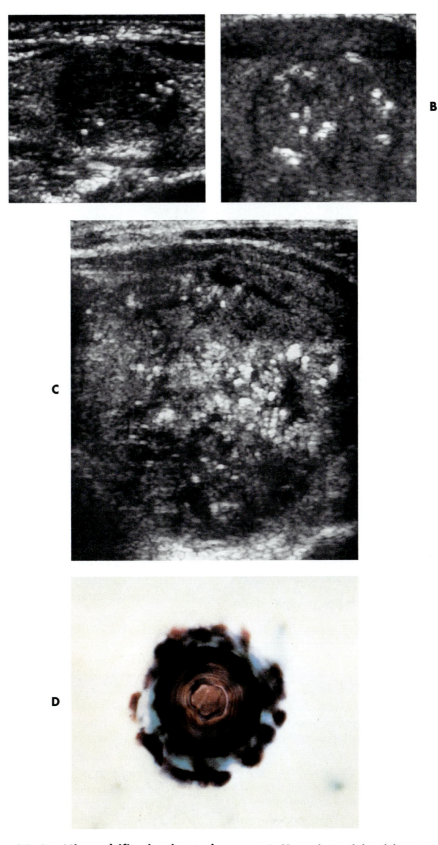

FIG. 21-9. Microcalcification in carcinomas. A, Hypoechoic solid nodule contains multiple tiny, punctate, echogenic foci. This is the classic appearance of papillary carcinoma. B, Isoechoic solid nodule contains multiple punctate echogenic foci. This was papillary carcinoma. C, Heterogeneous solid nodule contains multiple small and echogenic foci. This was medullary carcinoma. D, Calcified psammoma body from pathologic specimen of papillary carcinoma.

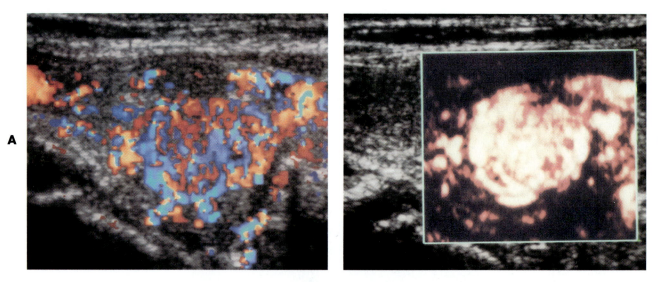

FIG. 21-10. Hypervascular medullary carcinoma. A, Longitudinal color Doppler and **B,** power Doppler images show hypervascularity which is intranodular (internal).

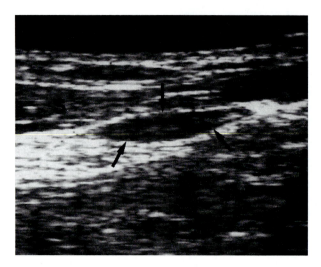

FIG. 21-11. Normal cervical lymph node. Longitudinal view shows typical benign cervical lymph node *(arrows)* with an elongated, slender configuration. Linear echogenic band centrally represents the fatty hilum of the node. S, sternocleidomastoid muscle.

Fig. 21-12). Cystic lymph node metastases in the neck occur almost exclusively in association with papillary thyroid carcinoma but occasionally may occur in nasopharyngeal carcinomas.[29]

Follicular carcinoma is the second subtype of well-differentiated thyroid cancer. It accounts for 5% to 15% of all cases of thyroid cancer, affecting females more often than males.[12] There are two variants of follicular carcinoma and they differ greatly in histology and clinical course.[21,24] The **minimally invasive** follicular carcinomas are encapsulated and only the histologic demonstration of focal invasion of capsular blood vessels of the fibrous capsule itself

> **TYPICAL APPEARANCE OF PAPILLARY THYROID CARCINOMA**
>
> Solid hypoechoic mass
> Tiny echogenic foci due to microcalcifications
> Hypervascularity on color Doppler
> Cervical lymph node metastases

permits differentiation from follicular adenoma. The **widely invasive** follicular carcinomas are not well encapsulated, and invasion of the vessels and the adjacent thyroid is more easily demonstrated. Both variants of follicular carcinoma tend to spread via the bloodstream rather than via lymphatics, and distant metastases to bone, lung, brain, and liver are more likely than metastases to cervical lymph nodes. The widely invasive variant metastasizes in about 20% to 40% of cases and the minimally invasive in only 5% to 10% of cases. Mortality due to follicular carcinoma is approximately 20% to 30% at 20 postoperative years.[12,23]

There are no unique sonographic features that allow differentiation of follicular carcinoma from adenoma, which is not surprising, given the cytologic and histologic similarities of these two tumors. Features that suggest follicular carcinoma include irregular tumor margins, a thick, irregular halo, and a tortuous or chaotic arrangement of internal blood vessels on color Doppler (Fig. 21-13).[16,29]

Medullary carcinoma accounts for only about 5% of all malignant thyroid disease. It is derived from the parafollicular cells, or C cells, and typically secretes the hormone calcitonin, which can be a

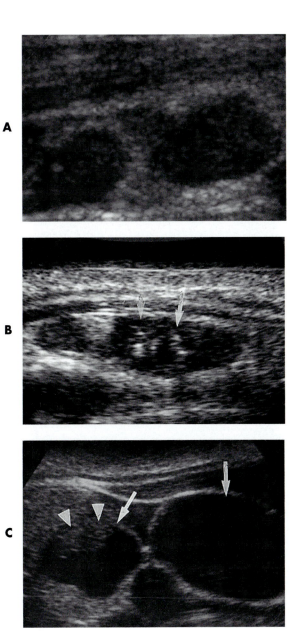

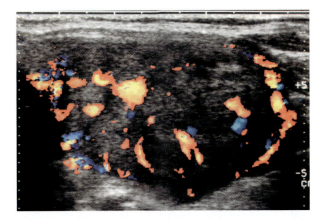

FIG. 21-13. Large follicular carcinoma. Longitudinal scan demonstrates a heterogeneous solid mass with peripheral and internal blood flow.

SONOGRAPHIC FEATURES OF FOLLICULAR THYROID CARCINOMA

Irregular tumor margins
Thick, irregular halo
Tortuous or chaotic arrangement of internal blood vessels

FIG. 21-12. Metastasis to cervical lymph nodes from papillary carcinoma. **A,** Two rounded and hypoechoic nodes. This is the typical appearance of metastasis to cervical nodes. **B,** Heterogeneous oval nodes containing microcalcifications *(arrows)*. **C,** Cystic nodes *(arrows)*. One node contains solid nodules *(arrowheads)* arising from the wall.

---

useful serum marker. This cancer is frequently familial (20%) and is an essential component of the **multiple endocrine neoplasia (MEN) type II syndromes.**[30] The disease is multicentric and/or bilateral in about 90% of the familial cases.[12] There is a high incidence of metastatic involvement of lymph nodes, and the prognosis for patients with medullary cancer is considered to be somewhat worse than that for follicular cancer.

The sonographic appearance of medullary carcinoma is similar to that of papillary carcinoma. Local invasion and metastasis to cervical nodes occur more frequently in patients with medullary carcinoma than in patients with papillary carcinoma (Fig. 21-14). Bright, punctate, echogenic foci caused by nests of amyloid or calcification are detectable in 80% to 90% of medullary carcinomas.[31] These foci can be seen not only in the primary tumor, but also in lymph node metastases and even in hepatic metastases.

Anaplastic thyroid carcinoma is typically a disease of the elderly; it represents one of the most lethal of solid tumors. Although it accounts for less than 5% of all thyroid cancers, it carries the worst prognosis, with a 5-year mortality rate of more than 95%.[32] The tumor typically presents as a rapidly enlarging mass extending beyond the gland and invading adjacent structures. It is often inoperable at the time of presentation.

Anaplastic carcinomas may often be associated with papillary or follicular carcinomas, presumably representing a dedifferentiation of the neoplasm. They tend not to spread via the lymphatics but instead are prone to aggressive local invasion of muscles and vessels.[24] Sonographically these carcinomas are usually hypoechoic and are often seen to encase or invade blood vessels and invade neck muscles (Fig. 21-15). Often these tumors cannot be adequately examined by ultrasound because of their large size. Instead, a CT or MRI scan of the neck usually demonstrates more accurately the extent of the disease.

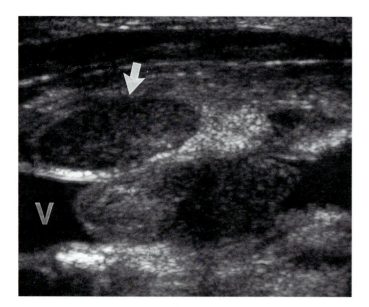

FIG. 21-14. Jugular vein tumor thrombus and adenopathy. Longitudinal scan demonstrates adenopathy *(arrow)* and tumor thrombus from high-grade carcinoma within the jugular vein (V).

SONOGRAPHIC FEATURES OF ANAPLASTIC THYROID CARCINOMA

Hypoechoic masses
Encase or invade blood vessels
Invade neck muscles

Lymphoma. Lymphoma accounts for approximately 4% of all thyroid malignancies. It is mostly of the non-Hodgkin's type and usually affects older females. The typical clinical sign is a rapidly growing mass which may cause symptoms of obstruction such as dyspnea and dysphagia.[33] In 70% to 80% of cases, lymphoma arises from a preexisting chronic lymphocytic thyroiditis (Hashimoto's disease) with subclinical or overt hypothyroidism. The prognosis is highly variable and depends on the stage of the disease. The 5-year survival rate may range from nearly 90% in early-stage cases to less than 5% in advanced, disseminated disease.

Sonographically, lymphoma of the thyroid appears as a hypoechoic, lobulated mass that is nearly avascular. Large areas of cystic necrosis may occur, as well as encasement of adjacent neck vessels.[34] The adjacent thyroid parenchyma may be heterogeneous due to associated chronic thyroiditis.[35]

Clinical Workup

Once a thyroid nodule has been detected, the fundamental problem is to determine if it is benign or malignant. Short of surgical excision, several methods for nodule characterization are in common use, including radionuclide imaging, sonography, and fine-needle aspiration (FNA) biopsy. Each of these techniques has

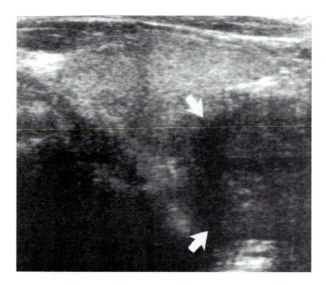

FIG. 21-15. Anaplastic carcinoma. Longitudinal image shows solid hypoechoic mass *(arrows)* arising from the posteroinferior portion of the thyroid and extending into the upper mediastinum.

advantages and limitations and the one(s) chosen in any specific clinical setting depends to a large extent on available instrumentation and expertise.

It is now generally recognized that **FNA biopsy** is the most effective method for diagnosing malignancy in a thyroid nodule.[36-38] In many clinical practices, FNA under direct palpation is the first diagnostic examination performed on any clinically palpable nodule. Neither isotope nor sonographic imaging is used routinely. Instead, they are reserved for special situations or difficult cases. FNA has had a substantial impact on the management of thyroid nodules because it provides more direct information

TABLE 21-1
DIAGNOSTIC YIELD OF THYROID FINE-NEEDLE ASPIRATION (FNA)

Series	No. of Cases	FN Rate %	FP Rate %	Sensitivity %	Specificity %
Hawkins et al.[41]	1399	2.4	4.6	86	95
Khafagi et al.[42]	618	4.1	7.7	87	72
Hall et al.[43]	795	1.3	3.0	84	90
Altavilla et al.[44]	2433	6.0	0.0	71	100
Gharib et al.[40]	10971	2.0	0.7	98	99
Ravetto et al.[45]	2014	11.2	0.7	89	99

FN = false negative; FP = false positive

Modified from Gharib H., Goellner JR. Fine-needle aspiration biopsy of the thyroid: an appraisal. *Ann Intern Med* 1993; 118:282–289.

than any other available diagnostic technique. It is safe, inexpensive, and results in better selection of patients for surgery. The successful use of FNA in clinical practice, however, depends heavily on the presence of an experienced aspirationist and an expert cytopathologist.

Fine-needle thyroid aspirates are classified by the cytopathologist into one of four categories:

- negative (no malignant cells);
- positive for malignancy;
- suspicious for malignancy; or
- nondiagnostic.

If a nodule is classified in either of the first two categories, the results are highly sensitive and specific.[39] The major limitation of the technique is the lack of specificity in the group whose results are suspicious for malignancy, primarily because of the inability to distinguish follicular or Hürthle cell adenomas from their malignant counterparts. In these cases, surgical excision is required for diagnosis. In addition, up to 20% of aspirates may be nondiagnostic, approximately half of which are so because of cystic lesions from which an adequate cell sample was not obtained. In these cases, repeat FNA under sonographic guidance can be performed with the goal of selectively sampling the solid elements of the mass. In the world literature, FNA of thyroid nodules has a sensitivity range of 65% to 98% and specificity of 72% to 100%, with a false-negative rate of 1% to 11% and a false-positive rate of 1% to 8% (Table 21-1).[40] In our practice, the overall accuracy of FNA exceeds 95% and therefore it is currently the most accurate and cost-effective method for initial evaluation of patients with nodular thyroid disease. Since the introduction of FNA into routine clinical practice, the percentage of patients undergoing thyroidectomy has significantly decreased (to approximately 25%) and the cost of thyroid nodule care has decreased by 25%.[40]

The evaluation of thyroid nodules primarily by FNA is common in North America and northern Europe. In other European countries and Japan, the evaluation often relies on radionuclide and sonographic imaging.

BASIC USES OF SONOGRAPHY FOR EVALUATION OF NODULAR THYROID DISEASE

Determine location of palpable neck mass (e.g., thyroid or extra thyroid)
Characterize benign vs. malignant nodule features
Detect occult nodule in patient with history of head and neck irradiation or MEN-II syndrome
Determine extent of known thyroid malignancy
Detect residual, recurrent, or metastatic carcinoma
Guide fine needle aspiration of thyroid nodule or cervical lymph nodes

Sonographic Applications

Although FNA has become the primary diagnostic method for evaluating clinically palpable thyroid nodules, high-resolution sonography has three primary clinical applications:[46-48]

- detection of thyroid and other cervical masses before and after thyroidectomy;
- differentiation of benign from malignant masses on the basis of their sonographic appearance; and
- FNA guidance.

Detection. A basic and practical use of sonography is to establish the precise anatomic location of a palpable cervical mass. The determination of whether such a mass is within or adjacent to the thyroid cannot always be made on the basis of the physical examination alone. Sonography can readily differentiate thyroid nodules from other cervical masses, such as cystic hygromas, thyroglossal duct cysts, or enlarged lymph nodes. Alternatively, sonography may help to confirm the presence of a thyroid nodule when the findings on physical examination are equivocal.

Sonography may be used to detect occult thyroid nodules in patients who have a history of **head and neck irradiation** during childhood as well as for those with a **family history of MEN-II syndrome** because both groups have a known increased risk for

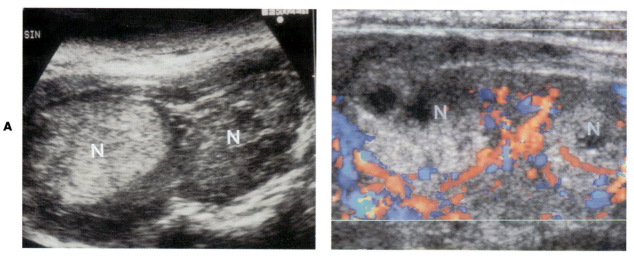

FIG. 21-16. Multinodular goiter. **A,** Longitudinal scan demonstrates hyperechoic and isoechoic nodules (N) which, on color Doppler (**B**), exhibit blood flow peripherally.

development of thyroid malignancy. If a nodule is discovered, a biopsy can be performed under sonographic guidance. It is unknown, however, whether the detection of a thyroid cancer before it becomes clinically palpable will change the ultimate clinical outcome for a given patient.

In the past, when thyroid nodules were evaluated primarily with isotope scintigraphy, it was generally accepted that a "solitary cold" nodule carried a probability of malignancy of between 15% and 25%, whereas a "cold" nodule in a multinodular gland was malignant in less than 1% of cases.[49] However, benign goiter is multinodular in 70% to 80% of cases, and it has recently been demonstrated that 70% of nodules considered solitary on scintigraphy or physical examination are actually multiple when assessed with high-frequency ultrasound (Fig. 21-16).[18,50]

It has been suggested, therefore, that sonography may be used to detect additional occult nodules in patients with clinically solitary lesions, thereby implying that the dominant palpable mass is benign. Such a conclusion is unwarranted, however, in view of the fact that, pathologically, benign nodules often coexist with malignant nodules. In a recent series of 1500 consecutive patients operated on for papillary carcinoma, 33% had coexistent benign nodules at the time of surgery.[51] In addition, papillary thyroid cancer is recognized to be multicentric in at least 20% of cases and occult (i.e., less than 1.5 cm in diameter) in up to 48% of cases.[22,51] In a recent series, almost two thirds (64%) of patients with thyroid cancer had at least one nodule in addition to the probable dominant nodule that was detected sonographically.[52] Pathologically, these extra nodules can be either benign or malignant. Therefore, in patients with a clinically solitary nodule, the sonographic detection of a few additional nodules is not a reliable sign for excluding malignancy.

In patients with known thyroid cancer, sonography can be useful **to determine the extent of disease,** both preoperatively and postoperatively. In most instances a sonographic examination is not performed routinely prior to thyroidectomy, but it can be useful in patients with large cervical masses for evaluation of nearby structures such as the carotid artery and internal jugular vein for evidence of direct invasion or encasement by the tumor. Alternatively, in patients who present with cervical lymphadenopathy caused by papillary thyroid cancer but in whom the thyroid gland is palpably normal, sonography may be used preoperatively to detect an occult, impalpable primary focus within the gland.

After partial or near-total thyroidectomy for carcinoma, sonography is the preferred method for **detecting residual, recurrent, or metastatic disease in the neck.**[53] In patients who have had subtotal thyroidectomy, the sonographic appearance of the remaining thyroid tissue may serve as an important factor in deciding whether complete thyroidectomy is recommended. If a mass is identified, its nature can be determined by ultrasound-guided FNA (Fig. 21-17). If no masses are seen, the clinician may choose to follow the patient with periodic sonographic studies. For patients who have had total or near-total thyroidectomy, sonography has proved to be more sensitive than physical examination in detecting recurrent disease within the thyroid bed or metastatic disease in cervical lymph nodes.[54] Patients with a history of thyroid cancer often undergo periodic sonographic examinations of the neck to detect impalpable recurrent or metastatic disease. When a mass is identified, FNA under sonographic guidance can establish a diagnosis of malignancy and help in surgical planning.

Differentiation. Currently, no single sonographic criterion distinguishes benign thyroid nodules from ma-

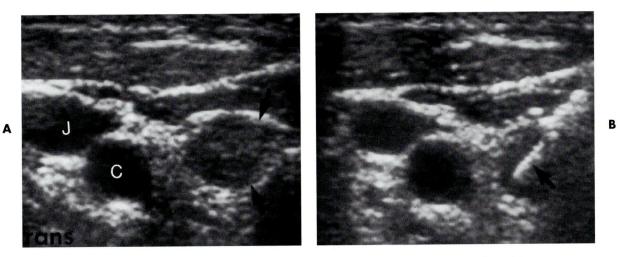

FIG. 21-17. **Recurrent papillary carcinoma in thyroid bed after thyroidectomy.** **A,** Transverse scan of the right side of the neck shows a 1 cm solid mass *(arrows)* medial to carotid artery (C) and jugular vein (J). **B,** Sonographically guided FNA with needle seen within mass *(arrow)*.

lignant nodules with complete reliability.[29,55] Nevertheless, certain sonographic features have been described that are seen more commonly with one type of histology or the other, thus establishing general diagnostic trends (Table 21-2).[29] The fundamental anatomic features of a thyroid nodule on high-resolution sonography are:

- internal consistency (solid, mixed solid and cystic, or purely cystic);
- echogenicity relative to the adjacent thyroid parenchyma;
- margin;
- presence and pattern of calcification;
- peripheral sonolucent halo; and
- presence and distribution of blood flow signals.

Internal Contents. In our experience, approximately 70% of thyroid nodules are solid, whereas the remaining 30% exhibit various amounts of cystic change. A nodule that has a significant cystic component is usually a benign **adenomatous (colloid) nodule** that has undergone degeneration or hemorrhage. When detected by older, lower-resolution ultrasound machines, these lesions were called cysts because the presence of internal debris and a thick wall could not be appreciated. Pathologically, a true epithelium-lined, simple thyroid cyst is extremely rare. Virtually all cystic thyroid lesions seen with high-resolution ultrasound equipment demonstrate some wall irregularity and internal solid elements or debris caused by nodule degeneration (Fig. 21-6). **Comet-tail artifacts** are frequently encountered in cystic thyroid nodules and they are likely to be related to the presence of colloid substance (Fig. 21-6, *E*). In a recent published series of 100 patients presenting with this feature, FNA biopsy was benign in all cases.[19] These comet-tail artifacts can be located in the cyst walls and internal septations or in the cyst fluid. When a more densely echogenic fluid is gravitationally layered in the posterior portion of a cystic cavity, the likelihood of hemorrhagic debris is very high (Fig. 21-6, *C, D*). Frequently, patients with hemorrhagic debris present clinically with a rapidly growing, often tender, neck mass.

Papillary carcinomas may rarely exhibit varying amounts of cystic change and appear almost indistinguishable from benign cystic nodules.[56] However, in cystic papillary carcinomas, the frequent sonographic detection of a solid projection (1 cm or more in size with blood flow signals and/or microcalcifications) into the lumen can lead to suspicion for malignancy (Fig. 21-18). Cervical metastatic lymph nodes from either a solid or a cystic primary papillary cancer may also demonstrate a purely cystic pattern; such an occurrence, although rare, is likely to be pathognomonic of malignant adenopathy (Fig. 21-12).

Echogenicity. Thyroid cancers are usually hypoechoic relative to the adjacent normal thyroid parenchyma (Fig. 21-9). Unfortunately, many benign thyroid nodules are also hypoechoic. In fact most **hypoechoic nodules** are benign because benign nodules are so much more common than malignant nodules. A predominantly **hyperechoic nodule** is more likely to be benign (Fig. 21-5, *B*).[18] The **isoechoic nodule** (visible because of a peripheral sonolucent rim that separates it from the adjacent normal parenchyma) has an intermediate risk of malignancy (Fig. 21-5, *A*).

Halo. A peripheral sonolucent halo that completely or incompletely surrounds a thyroid nodule may be present in 60% to 80% of benign nodules and 15% of thyroid cancers.[18,57] Histologically, it is thought to represent the capsule of the nodule, but hyperplastic nodules that have no capsule often have

TABLE 21-2

RELIABILITY OF SONOGRAPHIC FEATURES IN THE DIFFERENTIATION OF BENIGN FROM MALIGNANT THYROID NODULES*

Feature	Pathologic Diagnosis	
	Benign	**Malignant**
Internal Contents		
Purely cystic content	++++	+
Cystic with thin septa	++++	+
Mixed solid and cystic	+++	++
Comet-tail artifact	+++	+
Echogenicity		
Hyperechoic	++++	+
Isoechoic	+++	++
Hypoechoic	+++	+++
Halo		
Thin halo	++++	++
Thick incomplete halo	+	+++
Margin		
Well defined	+++	++
Poorly defined	++	+++
Calcification		
Eggshell calcification	++++	+
Coarse calcification	+++	+
Microcalcification	++	++++
Doppler		
Peripheral flow pattern	+++	++
Internal flow pattern	++	+++

+ = rare (<1%)

++ = low probability (<15%)

+++ = intermediate probability (16% to 84%)

++++ = high probability (>85%)

*Based on authors' experience and literature data

this sonographic feature. The hypothesis that it represents compressed normal thyroid parenchyma seems to be quite acceptable, especially for rapidly growing thyroid cancers, which often have thick, irregular halos (Fig. 21-19) that are hypovascular or avascular on color Doppler scans. Color and power Doppler imaging have demonstrated that the thin, complete peripheral halo, which is strongly suggestive of benign nodules, represents blood vessels coursing around the periphery of the lesion (the "basket pattern").

Margin. Benign thyroid nodules tend to have sharp, well-defined margins, whereas malignant lesions tend to have irregular or poorly defined margins. For any given nodule, however, the appearance of the outer margin cannot be relied on to predict the histologic features because many exceptions to these general trends have been identified.

Calcification. Calcification can be detected in about 10% to 15% of all thyroid nodules but the location and pattern of the calcification have more predictive value in distinguishing benign from malignant

lesions.[18] **Peripheral, or eggshell-like, calcification** is perhaps the most reliable feature of a benign nodule, but unfortunately, it occurs in only a small percentage of benign nodules (Fig. 21-20). Scattered echogenic foci of calcification with or without associated acoustic shadows are more common. When these calcifications are **large and coarse**, the nodule is more likely to be benign. When the calcifications are **fine and punctate,** however, malignancy is more likely. Pathologically, these fine calcifications may be caused by psammoma bodies, which are commonly seen in papillary cancers (Fig. 21-9).

Medullary thyroid carcinomas often exhibit bright echogenic foci either within the primary tumor or within metastatically involved cervical lymph nodes.[31] The larger echogenic foci are usually associated with acoustic shadowing. Pathologically, these densities are caused by reactive fibrosis and calcification around amyloid deposits, which are characteristic of medullary carcinoma. In the appropriate clinical setting (e.g., MEN-II syndrome or a patient with an increased serum calcitonin level), the finding of echogenic foci within a hypoechoic

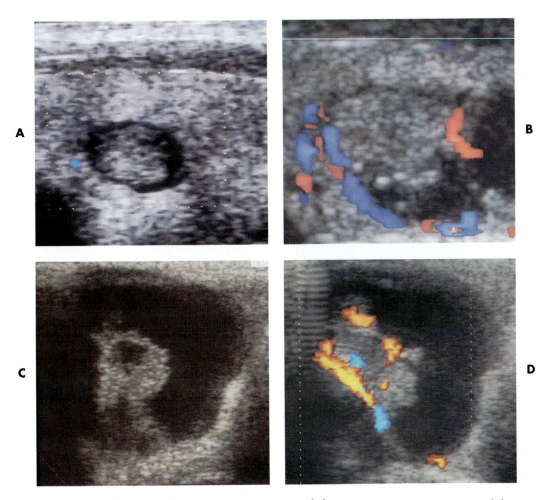

FIG. 21-18. Doppler exam of cystic nodules. **A** and **B** demonstrate a nodule within a cystic lesion. On color Doppler there was no flow within the nodule; this was a degenerated adenomatous colloid nodule. **C** and **D** demonstrate a nodule within a cystic lesion but this nodule has flow within it. This appearance suggests the rare cystic form of papillary carcinoma, which was confirmed.

thyroid nodule or a cervical node can be highly suggestive of medullary carcinoma (Fig. 21-9, *C*).

Based on personal experience and literature data, of the various sonographic features, microcalcifications show the highest accuracy (76%), specificity (93%), and positive predictive value (70%) for malignancy as a single sign; however, sensitivity is low (36%) and insufficient to be reliable for detection of malignancy.[26,27,58]

Doppler Flow Pattern. It is well known from histological studies that most hyperplastic nodules are hypovascular lesions and are less vascular than normal thyroid parenchyma. On the contrary, most **well-differentiated thyroid carcinomas** are generally hypervascular, with irregular tortuous vessels and arteriovenous shunting (Fig. 21-10). **Poorly differentiated and anaplastic carcinomas** are often hypovascular due to extensive necrosis associated with their rapid growth.

Since quantitative analysis of flow velocities is not accurate in differentiating benign from malignant, the only Doppler feature that may be useful is the distribu-

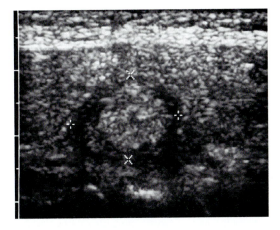

FIG. 21-19. Occult papillary carcinoma. 1.3 cm isoechoic nodule *(calipers)* with thick and irregular halo.

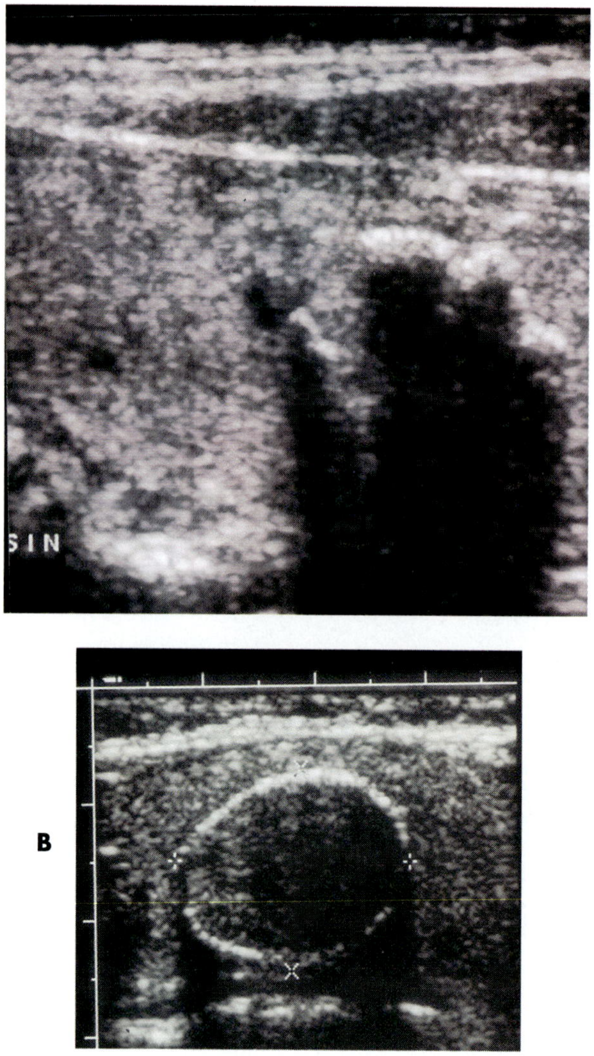

FIG. 21-20. Benign calcification. A, Peripheral coarse calcification casting an acoustic shadow. **B,** Peripheral egg-shell calcification.

tion of vessels. With current technology, no thyroid nodule appears totally avascular on color and power Doppler. The two main categories of vessel distribution are nodules with peripheral vascularity and nodules with internal vascularity (with or without a peripheral component).[16,17,59] It has been demonstrated that 80% to 95% of hyperplastic, goitrous, and adenomatous nodules display **peripheral vascularity** (Fig. 21-16), while 70% to 90% of thyroid malignancies display **internal vascularity, with or without a peripheral component** (Fig. 21-10).[16,28,60,61] There is significant disagreement in the world literature as to the role of color and power Doppler in the diagnosis of thyroid nodules. According to some reports,[62,63] color Doppler is not a reliable aid in the sonographic diagnosis of thyroid nodules, while others think that it does have a diagnostic role.[16,28,60] It is likely that the upcoming generation of Doppler instruments, which have extremely high sensitivity to blood flow, may significantly in-

crease the confusion because internal flow will be found in more benign nodules, thereby decreasing the reliability of this finding. It is not known whether the use of ultrasound contrast agents can improve the diagnostic accuracy of Doppler sonography (Fig. 21-21, 21-22).

Several articles in recent years have reported on the reliability of sonography (gray scale and color/power Doppler) in the differentiation of benign versus malignant thyroid nodules (Table 21-3). Even though no sonographic feature is pathognomonic for malignancy, the high rates of sensitivity, specificity, and accuracy indicate that sonography can be complementary to FNA.

Biopsy Guidance. Sonographically guided percutaneous needle biopsy of cervical masses has become an important technique in many clinical situations. Its main advantage is that it affords continuous real-time visualization of the needle, a crucial requirement for the biopsy of small lesions. Most physicians use a 25-gauge needle using either capillary action or minimal suction with a syringe. There are recent reports of the usefulness of large-gauge, automated, cutting needles for improved pathologic diagnosis.[68,69] The technique of sonographically guided biopsy is described in detail in Chapter 17.

Thyroid nodules that are palpable generally undergo biopsy without imaging guidance. There are three settings, however, in which sonographically guided biopsy of a thyroid nodule is usually indicated. The first is the questionable or inconclusive physical examination when a nodule is suspected but cannot be palpated with certainty. In these patients sonography is used to confirm the presence of a nodule and to provide guidance for accurate biopsy. The second setting is in the patient who is at high risk for developing thyroid cancer and who has a normal gland by physical examination but in whom sonography demonstrates a nodule. Included in this group are patients with a previous history of head and neck irradiation, those who have a positive family history for MEN-II syndrome, and those who have, in the past, undergone subtotal thyroid resection for malignancy. The third group of patients includes those who have had a previous nondiagnostic or inconclusive biopsy performed under direct palpation. Usually about 20% of specimens obtained by palpation guidance are cytologically inconclusive, most often because of the aspiration of nondiagnostic fluid from cystic lesions. Sonography may be used in these cases to selectively guide the needle into a solid portion of the mass (Fig. 21-23).

In patients who have undergone a previous thyroid resection for carcinoma, sonographically guided FNA has become an important method in the early diagnosis of recurrent or metastatic disease in the neck. In our experience with 54 consecutive biopsies of cervical masses, the accuracy of sonographically guided FNA was 94%. Of these 54 sonographically visible masses, 44 were not palpable by clinical examination.[54] In patients who have undergone hemithy-

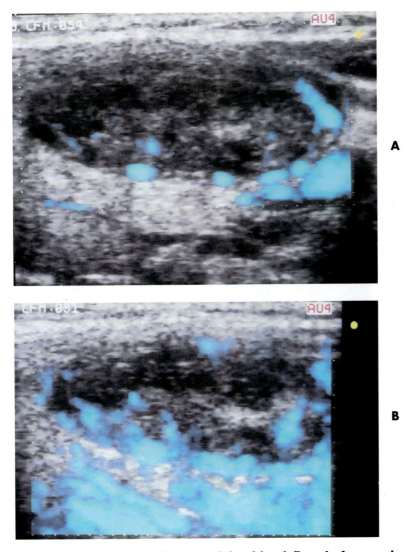

FIG. 21-21. Benign pattern of perinodular blood flow before and after contrast material. **A,** Power Doppler demonstrates predominant flow at the periphery of this benign adenomatous nodule. **B,** After contrast material (microbubbles), the predominant peripheral perinodular flow is enhanced.

TABLE 21-3
ACCURACY OF SONOGRAPHY IN DIFFERENTIATING BENIGN FROM MALIGNANT THYROID NODULES

Author	Sensitivity	Specificity	Accuracy
Jones[64] (1990)	75%	61%	—
Watters et al.[65] (1992)	74%	83%	—
Okamoto et al.[66] (1994)	63%	78%	80%
Leenhardt et al.[67] (1994)	75%	83%	—
Kerr[5] (1994)	87%	95%	94%
Solbiati[28] (1995)	77%	95%	88%

roidectomy for a benign nodule with the detection of one or more foci of occult malignant tumor in the surgical specimen, an ultrasound evaluation of the contralateral lobe is of value to exclude the existence of a worrisome residual nodule.

Cervical lymph nodes, both normal and abnormal, can be readily visualized by high-resolution sonography. They tend to lie along the internal jugular chain, extending from the level of the clavicles to the angle of the mandible, or to be in the region of the thyroid bed.

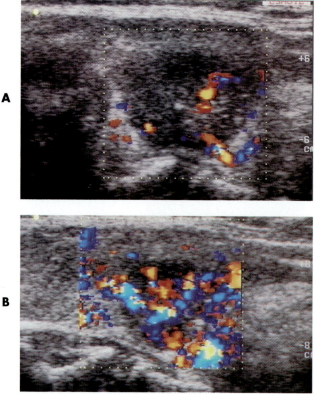

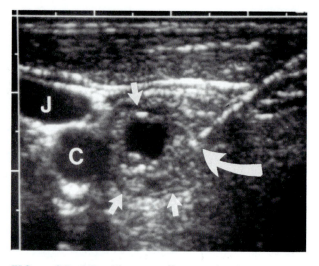

FIG. 21-23. Fine-needle aspiration (FNA). Transverse scan of the right lobe of thyroid demonstrates a nodule *(arrows)* that contains small cystic area. The needle *(curved arrow)* was inserted into the solid portions of the mass where the cytologic yield is higher than in areas of cystic change. This was benign.

FIG. 21-22. Intranodular blood flow in papillary carcinoma before and after contrast material. **A,** Hyperechoic nodule with internal blood flow pattern. **B,** There is an increase in the intranodular vascularity 2 minutes after IV contrast material (Levovist®).

Benign cervical nodes usually have a slender, oval shape and often exhibit a central echogenic band that represents the fatty hilum (Fig. 21-11). **Malignant nodes,** on the other hand, are usually rounder and have no echogenic hilum, presumably because of obliteration by tumor infiltration (Fig. 21-12). Although malignant nodes are often hypoechoic, they may be diffusely echogenic. Because these distinctions are not always clear, FNA under sonographic guidance is often used to confirm malignancy. In our experience, biopsy can be done with a high degree of accuracy in cervical nodes that are as small as 0.5 cm in diameter.

The Incidentally Detected Nodule

Although using high-resolution sonography to detect small, impalpable thyroid nodules may be beneficial in some clinical settings, it may actually introduce problems in other settings. What should one do about the many thyroid nodules detected incidentally during the course of carotid, parathyroid, or other sonographic examinations of the neck? The goal should be to avoid extensive and costly evaluations in the majority of patients with benign disease, without missing the minority of patients who have clinically significant thyroid cancer. By clinical palpation, the prevalence of

thyroid nodules in the United States is 4% to 7% of the general population, but high-resolution sonography has detected thyroid nodules in approximately 40% of hypercalcemic populations.[8,70] Previous studies have shown that patients with hyperparathyroidism have statistically no more nodular thyroid disease than age-matched and sex-matched autopsy controls.[71] Of 1000 consecutive hypercalcemic patients, 410 (41%) had sonographically visible nodules, of which only 80 (8%) were clinically palpable. A similarly high prevalence of sonographically detected thyroid abnormalities was recently reported in Finland.[50] In this study of 101 women with no previous thyroid or parathyroid disease, 36% had one or more sonographically visible nodules. A somewhat higher prevalence of thyroid nodules has been detected at autopsy in patients who had clinically normal thyroid glands; 49.5% had one or more grossly visible nodules.[72] Thus, high-resolution sonography can detect almost as many nodules as are demonstrated by careful pathologic examination, and both studies showed a direct relationship between the prevalence of thyroid nodules and patient age (Fig. 21-24).

Although these studies have shown a high prevalence of thyroid nodules detected by autopsy and sonography, the prevalence of thyroid malignancy reported in them was only 2% and 4%, respectively, with most (90%) being occult (<1.5 cm) papillary cancers (Table 21-4).[70,72] The papillary type of thyroid cancer represents approximately 90% of all thyroid cancers diagnosed in the midwestern United States since 1970.[12,21] The vast majority of patients with occult papillary thyroid cancer have an excellent prognosis, with essentially no reduction in life ex-

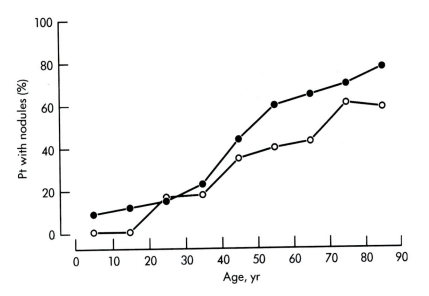

FIG. 21-24. **Comparison of prevalence of thyroid nodules detected by autopsy and sonography.** Autopsy, solid circles; on average 49% in 1955. Sonography, open circles; on average 41% in 1985, as a function of patient age. (Modified from Horlocker TT, Hay JE, James EM et al. Prevalence of incidental nodular thyroid disease detected during high-resolution parathyroid ultrasonography. In: Medeiros-Neto G, Gaitan E, eds. *Frontiers in Thyroidology*, vol. 2. New York: Plenum Medical Book Co; 1986.)

TABLE 21-4
PREVALENCE OF THYROID NODULES

Method of Detection	Patients (%)
Autopsy	49
Sonography	41
Palpation	7
Occult cancer (autopsy)	2
Cancer incidence (annual)	0.005

EVALUATION OF NODULES INCIDENTALLY DETECTED BY SONOGRAPHY

Nodules under 1.5 cm
   Followed by palpation at time of next physical examination
Nodules over 1.5 cm
   Evaluation (usually by FNA)
Nodules that have malignant features
   Evaluation by FNA

pectancy and no morbidity from appropriate surgical therapy. Further evidence that most subclinical thyroid cancers have a benign natural history is the fact that the annual incidence of clinically detected thyroid cancer is only 0.005% (5 per 100,000 persons).[12,21]

If nearly 50% of the United States population has subtle evidence of nodular thyroid disease that can be revealed by sonography, yet the annual incidence rate of clinically apparent thyroid carcinoma is only 0.005%, it is clear that only a small minority of patients with thyroid nodules have a risk of harboring clinically significant thyroid cancer (Table 21-4). Furthermore, if 90% of those cancers are papillary and therefore eminently curable after they become clinically apparent, it seems both impractical and imprudent to pursue for diagnosis all of the small nodules detected incidentally by high-resolution sonography.

Accordingly, for impalpable nodules that are incidentally detected by sonography, two imaging criteria may be used to determine the need for further diagnostic work-up.

Size. Most nodules exceeding 1.5 cm in maximum diameter should be further evaluated (usually by FNA), irrespective of physical and sonographic features. Nodules under 1.5 cm may be followed by palpation at the time of the patient's next physical examination.[73]

Sonographic Appearance. Nodules that have malignant sonographic features (microcalcifications, irregular margin, thick halo, internal flow pattern) should undergo ultrasound-guided FNA (Fig. 21-19).[74]

In most cases of incidentally detected nodules, we recommend the simple follow-up of neck palpation at the time of the patient's next physical examination. Follow-up sonographic examination, radionuclide imaging, FNA, or surgical excision of such incidental nodules is rarely necessary in our practice.

DIFFUSE THYROID DISEASE

Several thyroid diseases are characterized by diffuse rather than focal involvement. This usually results in generalized enlargement of the gland (goiter) and no palpable nodules. Specific conditions that commonly produce such diffuse enlargement include **chronic autoimmune lymphocytic (Hashimoto's) thyroiditis, colloid or adenomatous goiter**, and **Graves' disease.** Diagnosis of these conditions is usually made on the basis of clinical and laboratory findings and, on occasion, by FNA. Sonography is seldom indicated. One clinical setting in which high-resolution sonography can be helpful is when the underlying diffuse disease causes asymmetric thyroid enlargement, which raises the possibility of there being a mass in the larger lobe. The sonographic finding of generalized parenchymal abnormality may alert the clinician to consider diffuse thyroid disease as the underlying cause. FNA, with sonographic guidance if necessary, can be performed if a nodule is detected. Recognition of diffuse thyroid enlargement on sonography can often be facilitated by noting the thickness of the isthmus. Normally, it is a thin bridge of tissue measuring only a few millimeters in anteroposterior dimension. With diffuse thyroid enlargement, the isthmus may be up to 1 cm or more in thickness.

There are several different types of thyroiditis, including acute suppurative thyroiditis, subacute granulomatous thyroiditis (also called de Quervain's disease), and chronic lymphocytic thyroiditis (also called Hashimoto's disease).[75] Each disease has distinctive clinical and laboratory features. **Acute suppurative thyroiditis** is a rare inflammatory disease that is usually caused by bacterial infection. Sonography can be useful in selected cases to detect the development of a frank thyroid abscess. **Subacute granulomatous thyroiditis** is a spontaneously remitting inflammatory disease that is probably caused by viral infection. The clinical findings include fever, enlargement of the gland, and pain on palpation. Sonographically the gland may appear enlarged and hypoechoic with normal or decreased vascularity due to diffuse edema of the gland.[50,76,77] Although usually not necessary, sonography can be used to assess evolution of the disease following medical therapy (Fig. 21-25).

The most common type of thyroiditis is **chronic autoimmune lymphocytic (Hashimoto's) thyroiditis.** It typically occurs as a painless, diffuse enlargement of the thyroid gland in a young or middle-aged woman, often associated with hypothyroidism. The typical sonographic appearance of Hashimoto's thyroiditis is diffuse glandular enlargement with a homogeneous but coarsened parenchymal echo texture, generally more hypoechoic than a normal thyroid

DIFFUSE THYROID DISEASE

Acute suppurative thyroiditis
Subacute granulomatous thyroiditis
Hashimoto's (chronic lymphocytic) thyroiditis
Adenomatous or colloid goiter
Painless (silent) thyroiditis
Graves' disease
Invasive fibrous thyroiditis

(Fig. 21-26, *A*).[78] Fibrotic septations may produce a pseudolobulated appearance of the parenchyma (Fig. 21-26, *B*). Multiple, discrete hypoechoic micronodules from 1 to 6 mm in diameter have been described as strongly suggestive of chronic thyroiditis (Fig. 21-26, *C*). Histologically, they represent lobules of thyroid parenchyma which have been infiltrated by lymphocytes and plasma cells. These lobules are surrounded by echogenic fibrous strands. Micronodulation is a highly sensitive sign of chronic thyroiditis with a positive predictive value of 94.7%.[78] Both benign and malignant thyroid nodules may coexist with chronic lymphocytic thyroiditis, and FNA is often necessary to establish the final diagnosis.[79] Occasionally, hypervascularity similar to the "thyroid inferno" of Graves' disease occurs (Fig. 21-26, *D*). A recent study suggests that hypervascularity occurs when hypothyroidism develops.[80] Not infrequently, cervical lymphadenopathy is present, especially affecting the Delphian node above the thyroid isthmus. The end-stage of chronic thyroiditis is atrophy when the thyroid gland is small, with ill-defined margins and heterogeneous texture due to progressive increase of fibrosis. Blood flow signals are absent. Occasionally, discrete nodules occur, and FNA is needed to establish the diagnosis.[79]

Painless (silent) thyroiditis has the typical histologic and sonographic pattern of chronic autoimmune thyroiditis (hypoechogenicity, micronodulation, and fibrosis), but clinical findings resemble classical subacute thyroiditis, with the exception of node tenderness. Moderate hyperthyroidism with thyroid enlargement usually occurs in the early phase, followed sometimes by hypothyroidism of variable degrees. In postpartum thyroiditis, the progression to hypothyroidism is more frequent. In most circumstances, the disease spontaneously remits within 3 to 6 months, and the gland may return to a normal appearance.

Although the appearance of diffuse parenchymal inhomogeneity and micronodularity is quite typical of Hashimoto's thyroiditis, other diffuse thyroid diseases, most commonly **adenomatous goiter,** may have a similar sonographic appearance. Some patients with adenomatous goiter have multiple discrete nodules separated

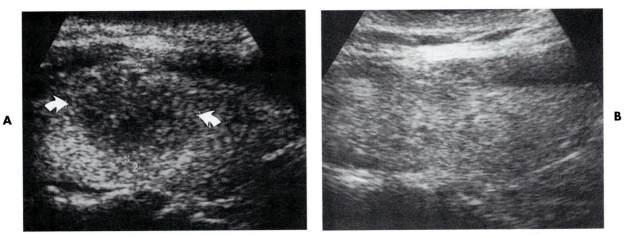

FIG. 21-25. Focal area of subacute thyroiditis. A, Longitudinal image shows an ill-defined hypoechoic area *(arrows)*. **B,** Thyroid gland returns to normal after 4 weeks of medical treatment.

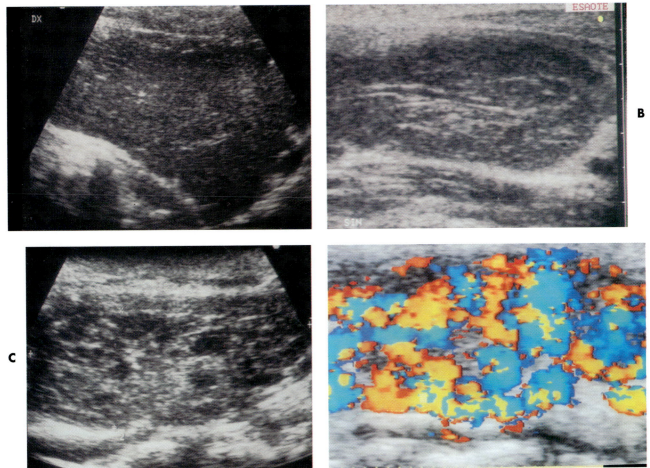

FIG. 21-26. Various appearances of Hashimoto's thyroiditis. A, Enlarged and hypoechoic gland. **B,** Pseudolobulation and coarse fibrous strands. **C,** Multiple hypoechoic micronodules. **D,** Hypervascularity on color Doppler.

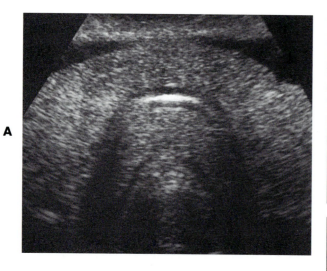

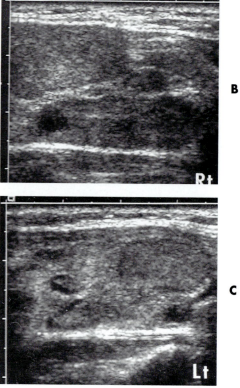

FIG. 21-27. Diffuse goiters. A, Transverse scan shows diffuse enlargement of the isthmus and both lobes without focal nodule. **B** and **C,** Longitudinal scans of the right and left thyroid lobes; a different patient shows a heterogeneous gland containing multiple nodules.

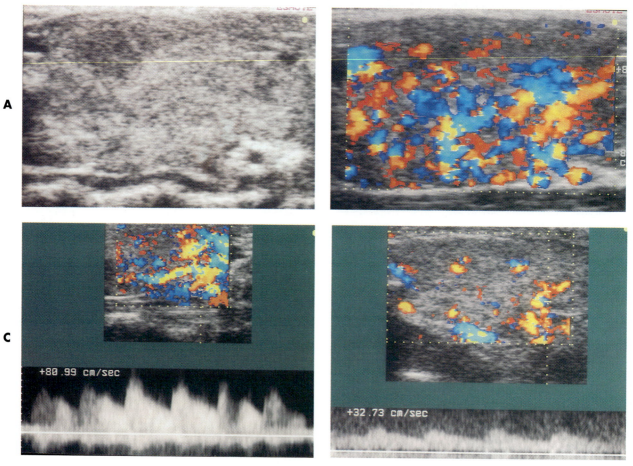

FIG. 21-28. Graves' disease. A, Longitudinal image shows heterogeneous parenchyma. **B,** Color Doppler demonstrates diffuse hypervascularity. **C,** Spectral Doppler demonstrates peak systolic velocity of 80 cm/sec. **D,** Following medical therapy the vascularity and peak systolic velocity return to normal.

by otherwise normal-appearing thyroid parenchyma; others have enlargement with rounding of the poles of the gland, diffuse parenchymal inhomogeneity, and no recognizable normal tissue (Fig. 21-27).

Graves' disease is a common diffuse abnormality of the thyroid gland and is usually biochemically characterized by hyperfunction (thyrotoxicosis). The echo texture may be more inhomogeneous than it is in diffuse goiter, mainly because of the presence of numerous large intraparenchymal vessels. Furthermore, especially in young patients, the parenchyma may be diffusely hypoechoic because of the extensive lymphocytic infiltration or because of the predominantly cellular content of the parenchyma which becomes almost devoid of colloid substance. Color Doppler study often demonstrates a hypervascular pattern referred to as the **"thyroid inferno"** (Fig. 21-28). Spectral Doppler will often demonstrate peak systolic velocities exceeding 70 cm/sec, which is the highest velocity found in thyroid disease. There is no correlation between the degree of thyroid hyperfunction assessed by laboratory studies and the extent of hypervascularity or blood flow velocities. Recent studies have shown that Doppler analysis can be used to monitor therapeutic response in patients with Graves' disease.[81] A significant decrease in flow velocities in the superior and inferior thyroid arteries following medical treatment has been reported.

The rarest type of inflammatory thyroid disease is **invasive fibrous thyroiditis,** also called **Riedel's struma.**[75] This disease affects primarily women and often tends to progress inexorably to complete destruction of the gland. Some cases may be associated with mediastinal or retroperitoneal fibrosis or sclerosing cholangitis. In the few cases of invasive fibrous thyroiditis examined sonographically, the gland was diffusely enlarged and had an inhomogeneous parenchymal echo texture. The primary reason for sonography was to check for extrathyroid extension of the inflammatory process with encasement of the adjacent vessels. Such information can be particularly useful in surgical planning. Open biopsy is generally required to distinguish this condition from anaplastic thyroid carcinoma. The sonographic findings in these two diseases may be identical.

REFERENCES

Anatomy

1. Rogers WM. Anomalous development of the thyroid. In: Werner SC, Ingbar SH, eds. *The Thyroid.* New York: Harper & Row; 1978:416-420.
2. Toma'P, Guastalla PP, Carini C, Lucigrai G. [Collo] In: Fariello G, Perale R, Perri G, Toma'P, eds. Ecografia Pediatrica. Milano: Ambrosiana; 1992:139-162.
3. Solbiati L. La tiroide e leáratiroidi. In: Rizzatto G, Solbiati L, eds. Anatomia Ecografica: Quadri Normali, Varianti e Limiti con il Patologico. Milano: Masson; 1992:35-45.

4. Jarlov AE, Hegedus L, Gjorup T, Hansen JEM. Accuracy of the clinical assessment of thyroid size. *Dan Med Bull* 1991;38:87-89.
5. Kerr L. High-resolution thyroid ultrasound: the value of color Doppler. *Ultrasound Quart* 1994;12:21-43.
6. Yokoyama N, Nagayama Y, Kakezono F et al. Determination of the volume of the thyroid gland by a high-resolutional ultrasonic scanner. *J Nucl Med* 1986;27:1475-1479.
7. Ueda D, Mitamura R, Suzuki N et al. Sonographic imaging of the thyroid gland in congenital hypothyroidism. *Pediatr Radiol* 1992;22:102-105.

Nodular Thyroid Disease

8. Rojeski MT, Gharib H. Nodular thyroid disease: evaluation and management. *N Engl J Med* 1985;313:428-236.
9. Van Herle AJ, Rich P, Ljung B-ME et al. The thyroid nodule. *Ann Intern Med* 1992;96:221-232.
10. Favus MJ, Schneider AB, Stachura ME et al. Thyroid cancer occurring as a late consequence of head-and-neck irradiation: evaluation of 1056 patients. *N Engl J Med* 1976;294:1019-1025.
11. Degroot LJ, Reilly M, Pinnameneni K et al. Retrospective and prospective study of radiation-induced thyroid disease. *Am J Med* 1983;74:852-862.
12. Grebe SKG, Hay ID. Follicular cell-derived thyroid carcinoma. In: Arnold A, ed. *Cancer Treatment and Research. Endocrine Neoplasms.* Norwell, Mass.: Kluwer Academic; 18:91-140.
13. Hennemann G. Non-toxic goitre. *Clin Endocrinol Metab* 1979;8:167-179.
14. Solbiati L, Cioffi V, Ballarati E. Ultrasonography of the neck. *Radiol Clin North Am* 1992;30:941-954.
15. Muller HW, Schroder S, Schneider C, Seifert G. Sonographic tissue characterization in thyroid gland diagnosis. *Klin Wochenschr* 1985;63:706-710.
16. Lagalla R, Caruso G, Midiri M, Cardinale AE. Echo Doppler-couleur et pathologie thyroidienne. *JEMU* 1992; 13:44-47.
17. Solbiati L, Ballarati E, Cioffi V. Contribution of color-flow mapping to the differential diagnosis of the thyroid nodules [abstract] Presented at Radiological Society of North America Meeting 1991.
18. Solbiati L, Volterrani L, Rizzatto G et al. The thyroid gland with low uptake lesions: evaluation by ultrasound. *Radiology* 1985;155:187-191.
19. Ahuja A, Chick W, King W, Metreweli C. Clinical significance of the comet-tail artifact in thyroid ultrasound. *J Clin Ultrasound* 1996;24:129-133.
20. Lagalla R, Caruso G, Cardinale AE. Analisi flussimetrica nelle malattie tiroidee: ipotesi di integrazione con lo studio qualitativo con color-Doppler. *Radiol Med* 1993;85:606-610.
21. Hay ID. Thyroid cancer. *Curr Ther Int Med* 1991;3:931-935.
22. Black BM, Kirk TA Jr, Woolner LB. Multicentricity of papillary adenocarcinoma of the thyroid: influence on treatment. *J Clin Endocrinol Metab* 1960;20:130-135.
23. McConahey WM, Hay ID, Wollner LB et al. Papillary thyroid cancer treated at the Mayo Clinic, 1946 through 1970: initial manifestations, pathologic findings, therapy, and outcome. *Mayo Clin Proc* 1986;61:978-996.
24. Pilotti S, Pierotti MA. Classificazione istologica e caratterizzazione molecolare dei tumori dell'epitelio follicolare della tiroide. *Argomenti di Oncologia* 1992;13:365-380.
25. Holtz S, Powers WE. Calcification in papillary carcinoma of the thyroid. *Radiology* 1958;80:997-1000.
26. Brkljacic B, Cuk V, Tomic-Brzac H, Bence-Zigman Z, Delic-Brkljacic D, Drinkovic I. Ultrasonic evaluation of benign and malignant nodules in echographically multinodular thyroids. *J Clin Ultrasound* 1994;22:71-76.
27. Solbiati L, Ballarati E, Cioffi V. Contribution of color-flow mapping to the differential diagnosis of the thyroid nodules [abstract] Presented at Radiological Society of North America Meeting 1990.

28. Solbiati L, Ierace T, Lagalla R et al. Reliability of high-frequency US and color Doppler US of thyroid nodules: Italian multicenter study of 1,042 pathologically confirmed cases. Which role for scintigraphy and biopsy? [abstract] Presented at Radiological Society of North America Meeting 1995.

29. Solbiati L, Livraghi T, Ballarati E et al. Thyroid gland. In: Solbiati L, Rizzatto G, eds. *Ultrasound of superficial structures.* Edinburgh: Churchill Livingstone;1995:49-85.

30. Chong GC, Beahrs OH, Sizemore GW et al. Medullary carcinoma of the thyroid gland. Cancer 1975;35:695-704.

31. Gorman B, Charboneau JW, James EM et al. Medullary thyroid carcinoma: role of high-resolution ultrasound. *Radiology* 1987;162:147-150.

32. Nel CJC, van Heerden JA, Goellner JR et al. Anaplastic carcinoma of the thyroid: a clinicopathologic study of 82 cases. *Mayo Clin Proc* 1985;60:51-58.

33. Hamburger JI, Miller JM, Kini SR. Lymphoma of the thyroid. *Ann Intern Med* 1983;99:685-693.

34. Kasagi K, Hatabu H, Tokuda Y et al. Lymphoproliferative disorders of the thyroid gland: radiological appearances. *Br J Radiol* 1991;64:569-575.

35. Takashima S, Morimoto S, Ikezoe et al. Primary thyroid lymphoma: comparison of CT and US assessment. *Radiology* 1989;171:439-443.

36. Feld S, Barcia M, Baskic HJ et al. AACE clinical practice guidelines for the diagnosis and management of thyroid nodules. *Endocr Pract* 1996;2:78-84.

37. Miller JM. Evaluation of thyroid nodules: accent on needle biopsy. *Med Clin North Am* 1985;69:1063-1077.

38. Hamberger B, Gharib H, Melton LJ III et al. Fine-needle aspiration biopsy of thyroid nodules: impact on thyroid practice and cost of care. *Am J Med* 1982;73:381-384.

39. Goellner JR, Gharib H, Grant CS et al. Fine-needle aspiration cytology of the thyroid, 1980 to 1986. *Acta Cytol* 1987;31:587-590.

40. Gharib H, Goellner JR. Fine-needle aspiration biopsy of the thyroid: an appraisal. *Ann Intern Med* 1993;118:282-289.

41. Hawkins F, Bellido D, Bernai C et al. Fine-needle aspiration biopsy in the diagnosis of thyroid cancer and thyroid disease. *Cancer* 1987;59:1206-1209.

42. Khafagi F, Wright G, Castles H et al. Screening for thyroid malignancy: the role of fine-needle biopsy. *Med J Aust* 1988;149:302-303, 306-307.

43. Hall TL, Layfield LJ, Philippe A et al. Sources of diagnostic error in fine-needle aspiration of the thyroid. *Cancer* 1989;63:718-725.

44. Altavilla G, Pascale M, Nenci I. Fine-needle aspiration cytology of thyroid gland diseases. *Acta Cytol* 1990;34:251-256.

45. Ravetto C, Spreafico GL, Colombo L. L'esame citologico con agoaspirato nella diagnosi precoce delle neoplasie tiroidee. *Rec Progr Med* 1977;63:258-267.

46. James EM, Charboneau JW. High-frequency (10 MHz) thyroid ultrasonography. *Semin Ultrasound, CT, MR* 1985;6:294-309.

47. Scheible W, Leopold GR, Woo VL et al. High-resolution real-time ultrasonography of thyroid nodules. *Radiology* 1979;133:413-417.

48. Simeone JF, Daniels GH, Mueller PR et al. High-resolution real-time sonography of the thyroid. *Radiology* 1982;145:431-435.

49. Brown CL. Pathology of the cold nodule. *Clin Endocrinol Metab* 1981;10:235-245.

50. Brander A, Viikinkoski P, Nickels J et al. Thyroid gland: US screening in middle-aged women with no previous thyroid disease. *Radiology* 1989;173:507-510.

51. Hay ID. Papillary thyroid carcinoma. *Endocrinol Metab Clin North Am* 1990;19:545-576.

52. Hay ID, Reading CC, Weiland LH et al. Clinicopathologic and high-resolution ultrasonographic evaluation of clinically suspicious or malignant thyroid disease. In: Medeiros-Neto G, Gaitan E, eds. *Frontiers in Thyroidology*, vol. 2. New York: Plenum Medical Book Co; 1986.

53. Simeone JF, Daniels GH, Hall DA et al. Sonography in the follow-up of 100 patients with thyroid carcinoma. *AJR* 1987;148:45-49.

54. Sutton RT, Reading CC, Charboneau JW et al. Ultrasound-guided biopsy of neck masses in postoperative management of patients with thyroid cancer. *Radiology* 1988;168:769-772.

55. Katz JF, Kane RA, Reyes J et al. Thyroid nodules: sonographic-pathologic correlation. *Radiology* 1984;151:741-745.

56. Hammer M, Wortsman J, Folse R. Cancer in cystic lesions of the thyroid. *Arch Surg* 1982;117:1020-1023.

57. Propper RA, Skolnick ML, Weinstein BJ et al. The nonspecificity of the thyroid halo sign. *J Clin Ultrasound* 1980;8:129-132.

58. Takashima S, Fukuda H, Kobayashi T. Thyroid nodules: clinical effect of ultrasound-guided fine-needle aspiration biopsy. *J Clin Ultrasound* 1994;22:535-542.

59. Fobbe F, Finke R, Reichenstein E et al. Appearance of thyroid diseases using colour-coded duplex sonography. *Eur J Radiol* 1989;9:29-31.

60. Argalia G, D'Ambrosio F, Lucarelli F et al. L' eco color Doppler nella caratterizzazione della patologia nodulare tiroidea. *Radiol Med* 1995;89:651-657.

61. Spiezia S, Colao A, Assanti AP et al. Utilita' dell'eco color Doppler con power Doppler nella diagnostica dei noduli tiroidei ipoecogeni: work in progress. *Radiol Med* 1996;91:616-621.

62. Clark KJ, Cronan JJ, Scola FH. Color Doppler sonography: anatomic and physiological assessment of the thyroid. *J Clin Ultrasound* 1995;23:215-223.

63. Shimamoto K, Endo T, Ishigaki T et al. Thyroid nodules: evaluation with color Doppler ultrasonography. *J Ultrasound Med* 1993;11:673-678.

64. Jones AJ, Aitman TJ, Edmonds CJ et al. Comparison of fine-needle aspiration cytology, radioisotopic and ultrasound scanning in the management of thyroid nodules. *Postgrad Med J* 1990;66:914-917.

65. Watters DAK, Ahuja AT, Evans RM et al. Role of ultrasound in the management of thyroid nodules. *Am J Surg* 1992;164:654-657.

66. Okamoto T, Yamashita T, Harasawa A et al. Test performances of three diagnostic procedures in evaluating thyroid nodules: physical examination, ultrasonography and fine-needle aspiration cytology. *Endocr J* 1994;41:243-247.

67. Leenhardt L, Tramalloni J, Aurengo H et al. Echographie des nodules thyroidiens: l'echographiste face aux exigences du clinicien. *Presse-Med* 1994;23:1389-1392.

68. Quinn SF, Nelson HA, Demlow TA. Thyroid biopsies: fine-needle aspiration biopsy versus spring-activated core biopsy needle in 102 patients. *JVIR* 1994;5:619-623.

69. Taki S, Kakuda K, Kakuma K et al. Thyroid nodules: evaluation with US-guided core biopsy with an automated biopsy gun. *Radiology* 1997;202:874-877.

70. Horlocker TT, Hay JE, James EM et al. Prevalence of incidental nodular thyroid disease detected during high-resolution parathyroid ultrasonography. In: Medeiros-Neto G, Gaitan E, eds. *Frontiers in Thyroidology*, vol. 2. New York: Plenum Medical Book Co; 1986:1309-1312.

71. Lever EG, Refetoff S, Straus FH II et al. Coexisting thyroid and parathyroid disease: are they related? *Surgery* 1983;94:893-900.

72. Mortensen JD, Woolner LB, Bennett WA. Gross and microscopic findings in clinically normal thyroid glands. *J Clin Endocrinol Metab* 1955;15:1270-1280.

73. Giuffrida D, Gharib H. Controversies in the management of cold, hot, and occult thyroid nodules. *Am J Med* 1995;99:642-650.

74. Tan GH, Gharib H, Reading CC. Solitary thyroid nodule: comparison between palpation and ultrasonography. *Arch Intern Med* 1995;155:2418-2423.

Diffuse Thyroid Disease

75. Hay ID. Thyroiditis: a clinical update. *Mayo Clin Proc* 1985;60:836-843.
76. Adams H, Jones NC. Ultrasound appearances of de Quervain's thyroiditis. *Clin Radiol* 1990;42:217-218.
77. Birchall IWJ, Chow CC, Metreweli C. Ultrasound appearances of de Quervain's thyroidits. *Clin Radiol* 1990;41:57-59.
78. Yeh HC, Futterweit W, Gilbert P. Micronodulation: ultrasonographic sign of Hashimoto's thyroiditis. *J Ultrasound Med* 1996;15:813-819.
79. Takashima S, Matsuzuka F, Nagareda T et al. Thyroid nodules associated with Hashimoto's thyroiditis: assessment with US. *Radiology* 1992;185:125-130.
80. Lagalla R, Caruso G, Benza I et al. Echo-color Doppler in the study of hypothyroidism in the adult. *(Ital) Radiol Med* 1993;86:281-283.
81. Castagnone D, Rivolta R, Rescalli S et al. Color Doppler sonography in Graves' disease: value in assessing activity of disease and predicting outcome. *AJR* 1996;166:203-207.

CHAPTER 22

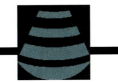

The Parathyroid Glands

•

C. Richard Hopkins, M.D.
Carl C. Reading, M.D.

High-frequency sonography is a well-established, noninvasive imaging method used in the evaluation of patients with parathyroid disease. Sonography is most commonly used for the accurate preoperative localization of enlarged parathyroid glands in patients with hyperparathyroidism. It can also be used to guide the percutaneous biopsy of suspected parathyroid adenomas, particularly in the setting of persistent or recurrent hyperparathyroidism, and for the intraoperative localization of abnormal parathyroid glands. In selected patients, sonography can be used to guide the percutaneous ethanol ablation of parathyroid adenomas as an alternative to surgical treatment.

EMBRYOLOGY AND ANATOMY

The paired superior and inferior parathyroid glands have different embryologic origins, and a knowledge of their development aids in understanding their ultimate anatomic locations.[1-3] **The superior parathyroid glands** arise from the fourth branchial cleft pouch, along with the thyroid gland. Minimal migration occurs during fetal development, and the bilateral superior parathyroids remain close to the posterior aspect of the thyroid's mid to upper portion. The majority of superior parathyroid glands (80%) are found at autopsy within an approximate area of 2 cm, located just superior to the crossing of the recurrent laryngeal nerve and the inferior thyroid artery.[4] The **inferior parathyroid glands** arise from the third branchial cleft pouch, along with the thymus.[2] During fetal development these "parathymus glands" migrate caudally along with the thymus in a more anterior track than their superior counterparts, bypassing the superior glands to become the inferior parathyroid glands.[3] The inferior glands are more variable in location than the superior parathyroids, but usually (over 60%) come to rest at or just inferior to the posterior aspect of the thyroid lower pole (Fig. 22-1).[4] About 25% of the inferior glands will fail to dissociate from the thymus and will continue to migrate lower in the neck tissues or into the mediastinum, usually within the thyrothymic ligament.

A significant percentage of parathyroid glands lie in relatively or frankly ectopic locations in the neck or mediastinum. The inferior parathyroid gland is more frequently ectopic than its superior counterpart. Symmetry to fixed landmarks occurs in 70% to 80%, so side-to-side comparisons can usually be made.[3,4] The ectopic superior parathyroid gland usually lies far posteriorly in the tracheoesophageal groove or has enlarged and has continued its descent from the posterior neck into the posterosuperior mediastinum.[5,6] Superior glands are found less commonly higher in the neck or near the superior extent of the thyroid lobe, or are rarely found surrounded by thyroid tissue within the thyroid capsule.[4] The ectopic inferior parathyroid gland usually has continued to migrate in an anterocaudal direction and is in the low neck or anterosuperior mediastinum, associated with the thymus. Less common ectopic positions of the inferior parathyroid glands include an undescended position high in the neck with a remnant of thymus near the carotid bifurcation, or lower in the neck along the carotid sheath.[7] In other rare cases, ectopic glands have been reported low in the mediastinum within the aortopulmonic window, posterior to the carina, posterior to the esophagus, within the pericardium, or within the posterior triangle of the neck.

Most adults have four parathyroid glands (two superior and two inferior), each measuring about 5 mm by 3 mm by 1 mm and weighing on average 35 to 40 mg (range 10 to 78 mg).[3,8] Supernumerary "fifth" glands are present in up to 13% of the popu-

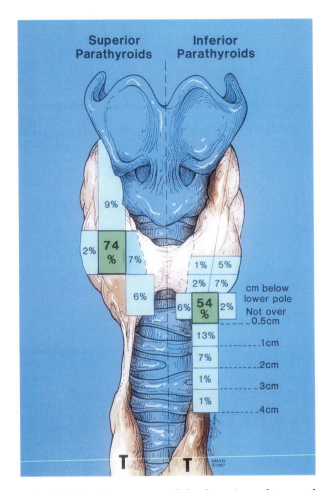

FIG. 22-1. **Frequency of the location of normal superior and inferior parathyroid glands** from 527 autopsies; anatomic drawing. *T*, Thymus. (Adapted from Gilmour JR. The gross anatomy of the parathyroid glands. *J Pathol* 1938;46:133-148.)

lation[3] and may result from the separation of parathyroid remnants when the parathyroid glands pull away from the pouch structures during the embryologic branchial complex phase.[9,10] These supernumerary glands are often associated with the thymus in the anterior mediastinum, suggesting a relationship in their development with the inferior parathyroid glands.[11]

The normal parathyroid gland varies from a yellow to a red-brown color, depending on the amount of parenchymal yellow fat and chief cell content. It is generally oval or bean-shaped, but may be spherical, elongated, or lobulated. Normal glands can be seen occasionally with high-frequency ultrasound, especially in young patients, but sonographic visualization of a normal parathyroid gland in a patient without hyperparathyroidism is not an indication for surgery.[12]

PRIMARY HYPERPARATHYROIDISM

Prevalence

Primary hyperparathyroidism is now recognized as a common endocrine disease, with a prevalence in the United States of 100 to 200 per 100,000 population.[13] Women are affected two to three times more frequently than men, particularly after menopause. More than half of the patients with this disease are over 50 years old, and cases are rare before 20 years of age.

Diagnosis

Hyperparathyroidism is usually suspected because an increased serum calcium level is detected on routine biochemical screening. Hypophosphatasia or increased urine calcium levels may be further biochemical clues to the disease. A serum parathyroid hormone (PTH) level that is "inappropriately high" for the prevailing serum calcium level confirms the diagnosis. Even when the PTH level is within the upper limits of the "normal range" in a hypercalcemic patient, the diagnosis of primary hyperparathyroidism should still be suspected since hypercalcemia from other nonparathyroid causes should suppress the gland's function and decrease the serum PTH level. Because of earlier detection by increasingly routine lab exams, the later "classic" signs of hyperparathyroidism, such as "painful bones, renal stones, abdominal groans, and psychic moans" are often not present. Most patients have no gross manifestations of hyperparathyroidism such as nephrolithiasis, osteopenia, subperiosteal resorption, and osteitis fibrosis cystica. However, subtle nonspecific symptoms, such as muscle weakness, malaise, constipation, dyspepsia, polydipsia, and polyuria, often are elicited from these otherwise asymptomatic patients by more specific questioning.

Pathology

Primary hyperparathyroidism is caused by a single adenoma in 80% to 90% of cases, by multiple gland enlargement in 10% to 20%, and by carcinoma in less than 1% (see box).[14,15] A solitary adenoma may involve any one of the four glands with equal frequency.[16] Multiple gland enlargement is most commonly due to primary parathyroid hyperplasia, but less commonly to multiple adenomas. Hyperplasia usually involves all four glands asymmetrically whereas multiple adenomas involve two or possibly three glands. Because of this inconsistent pattern of gland involvement and the fact that distinguishing hyperplasia from multiple adenomas is difficult pathologically, these two entities are often histologically considered together as "multiple gland disease."[17]

Multiple parathyroid gland enlargement occurs in more than 90% of patients with **multiple endocrine neoplasia, type I (MEN I)**.[18,19] This condition is an uncommon inherited autosomal dominant trait with a high penetrance, which causes adenomatous parathyroid hyperplasia. Most MEN I patients present with hypercalcemia before their third or fourth decade of life. Though not all of the parathyroid glands may be grossly enlarged at the time of the MEN I patient's initial operation, it is likely that all of them will ultimately be involved with hyperplasia.

Carcinoma is a rare cause of primary hyperparathyroidism. The histologic distinction from adenoma is difficult to establish with certainty because both carcinomas and atypical adenomas can exhibit mitotic activity and cellular atypia.[20] The diagnosis usually is made during surgery in a patient with a high calcium level (> 14 mg/dl) when the surgeon discovers an enlarged, firm, fibrous gland adherent to the surrounding tissues by local invasion.[21-24] A thick, fibrotic capsule is often present. Treatment consists of en bloc resection without entering the capsule to prevent seeding, but in many cases cure may not be possible because of the cancer's invasive and metastatic nature. Generally death occurs not from tumor spread but from complications associated with the unrelenting hyperparathyroidism.[16]

Treatment

In symptomatic patients with primary hyperparathyroidism, the treatment of choice is surgical excision of the involved parathyroid gland or glands. Some controversy exists as to whether asymptomatic patients with minimal hypercalcemia should be treated surgically or followed medically with frequent renal function, bone density, and serum calcium levels. In one prospective study of clinical follow-up of 147 asymptomatic patients with a provisional diagnosis of hyperparathyroidism and serum calcium levels less than 11 mg/dl, 20% of the patients needed surgery within 5 years because of progression of their disease.[25,26] Other studies demonstrate that surgical cure rates by an experienced surgeon are greater than 95%, and the morbidity and mortality rates are extremely low.[16,27] Therefore surgical treatment is now usually advised as the most definitive treatment of hyperparathyroidism for both asymptomatic and symptomatic patients.[28,29]

CAUSES OF PRIMARY HYPERPARATHYROIDISM

Single adenoma	80%-90%
Multiple gland enlargement	10%-20%
Carcinoma	< 1%

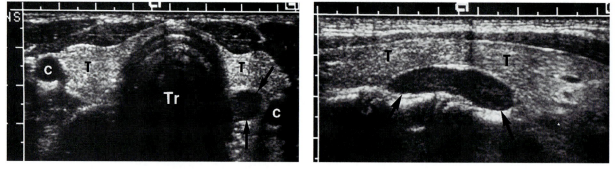

FIG. 22-2. Typical parathyroid adenoma. A, Transverse and, **B,** longitudinal sonograms of a typical oval adenoma *(arrows)* located adjacent to the posterior aspect of the thyroid, *T. Tr,* Trachea; *C,* common carotid artery.

SONOGRAPHIC APPEARANCE

Shape

Parathyroid adenomas are most commonly oval (Fig. 22-2). As parathyroid glands enlarge, they dissect between longitudinally oriented tissue planes in the neck and acquire a characteristic oblong shape. If this process is exaggerated, they can become more elongated and tubelike or even bilobar. There often is asymmetry in the enlargement, and either the cephalic end or caudal end can be more bulbous, producing a triangular, tapering, or teardrop shape.[16,30-32]

Echogenicity

The characteristic hypoechoic echogenicity of parathyroid adenomas is due to the uniform hypercellularity of the gland, which leaves few interfaces for reflecting sound. The echogenicity of the vast majority of parathyroid adenomas is substantially less than that of thyroid tissue (see Fig. 22-2). Four cases of rare functioning parathyroid lipoadenoma have been reported, which are more echogenic than the adjacent thyroid gland because of their high fat content.[33]

Internal Architecture

The vast majority of parathyroid adenomas are homogeneously solid. About 2% have internal cystic components that are due to cystic degeneration (most commonly) or true simple cysts (less commonly) (Fig. 22-3).[32,34-36] Rare adenomas may contain focal internal calcification. Color flow Doppler sonography of an enlarged parathyroid gland may demonstrate a hypervascular pattern with prominent diastolic flow (Fig. 22-4). A vascular arc enveloping between 90 and 270 degrees of the mass, arising from inferior thyroid artery branches, has also been described as a typical finding in parathyroid adenomas.[37] While this arc of flow has not been shown to increase the sensitivity for initially detecting a parathyroid adenoma, it may allow for differentiation from lymph nodes, which have a central hilar flow pattern.[37-39]

Size

Most parathyroid adenomas are 0.8 to 1.5 cm long and weigh 500 to 1000 mg. The smallest adenomas can be minimally enlarged glands that appear virtually normal during surgery but are found to be hypercellular on pathologic examination. The largest adenomas can be 5 cm or more long and weigh more than 10 g. Preoperative serum calcium levels are usually higher in patients with larger adenomas (Fig. 22-5).[25,32]

Multiple Gland Disease

Multiple gland disease can be due to hyperplasia or to multiple adenomas. Individually, these enlarged glands have the same sonographic and gross appearance as other parathyroid adenomas (Fig. 22-6).[16] However, the glands may be inconsistently and asymmetrically enlarged, and the diagnosis of multiple gland disease often is difficult to make sonographically. The appearance may be misinterpreted as solitary adenomatous disease, or the diagnosis may be missed altogether if the glandular enlargement is minimal.

Carcinoma

Sonographically, carcinomas usually are larger than adenomas. The average carcinoma measures more than 2 cm, in contrast to about 1 cm for adenomas. Carcinomas also frequently have a lobulated contour, heterogeneous internal architecture, and internal cystic components; however, large adenomas also can have these features.[40] In most cases, prospective carcinomas are indistinguishable sonographically from large benign adenomas.[41] Gross evidence of invasion of adjacent structures, such as vessels or muscles, is the only reliable preoperative sonographic criterion for diagnosis of malignancy, but this is an uncommon finding.

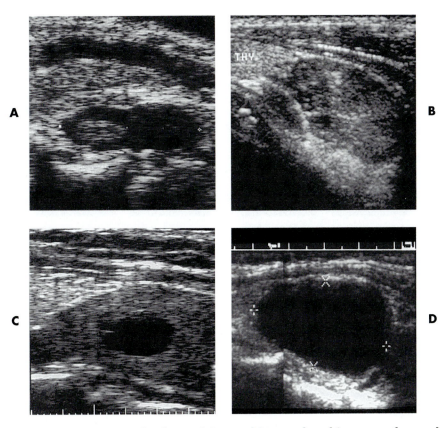

FIG. 22-3. **Spectrum of echogenicity and internal architecture of parathyroid adenomas.** **A,** Mixed hypoechoic and hyperechoic echogenicity. Longitudinal sonogram shows adenoma that is hyperechoic in its cranial portion and hypoechoic in its caudal portion. **B,** Heterogeneous echogenicity. Longitudinal sonogram shows adenoma that is diffusely heterogeneous. **C,** Longitudinal sonogram shows 3 cm adenoma that is partially cystic centrally. **D,** Longitudinal sonogram shows 4 cm adenoma that is predominantly cystic.

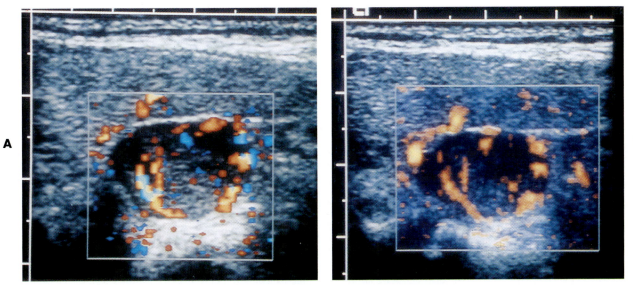

FIG. 22-4. **Typical vascularity of parathyroid adenoma.** **A,** Longitudinal color flow Doppler sonogram shows parathyroid adenoma that has increased blood flow relative to the normal thyroid. **B,** Longitudinal color flow Doppler energy sonogram shows increased vascularity of the adenoma relative to the thyroid.

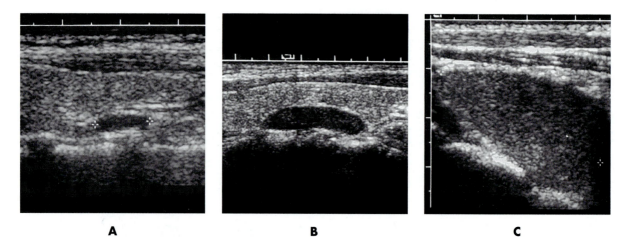

| **A** | **B** | **C** |

FIG. 22-5. Spectrum of size of parathyroid adenomas. **A,** Longitudinal sonogram of a minimally enlarged, 0.6 × 0.2 cm, 150 mg parathyroid adenoma. **B,** Typical midsize, 3 × 0.8 cm, 800 mg adenoma. **C,** Large, 4 × 2 cm, 2500 mg adenoma.

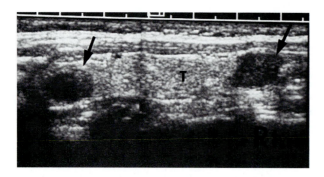

FIG. 22-6. Multiple parathyroid gland enlargement. Longitudinal sonogram of the right neck shows superior and inferior parathyroid enlargement *(arrows). T,* Thyroid.

ADENOMA LOCALIZATION

Sonographic Examination

The sonographic examination of the neck for parathyroid adenoma localization is performed with the patient in a supine position. The patient's neck is hyperextended by a pad centered under the scapulae, and the examiner usually sits at the patient's head. High-frequency (7.5 or 10 MHz) real-time transducers are used to provide optimal spatial resolution and visualization in most patients. In obese patients with thick necks or with large multinodular thyroid goiters, use of a 5-MHz transducer may be necessary to obtain adequate depth of penetration.

Typical Locations

The pattern of the sonographic survey of the neck for adenoma localization can be considered in terms of the pattern of dissection and visualization that the surgeon uses in a thorough neck exploration. The examination is initiated on one side of the neck in the re-

gion of the thyroid gland. The typical **superior parathyroid adenoma** usually is adjacent to the posterior aspect of the midportion of the thyroid (Fig. 22-7). The location of the typical **inferior parathyroid adenoma** is more variable, but usually it lies close to the caudal tip of the lower pole of the thyroid (Fig. 22-8). Most of these inferior adenomas are adjacent to the posterior aspect of the thyroid, and the rest are in the soft tissues 1 to 2 cm inferior to the thyroid. After one side of the neck has been surveyed, a similar survey is conducted of the opposite side (Fig. 22-9). However, 1% to 3% of parathyroid adenomas are ectopic and will not be found in typical locations adjacent to the thyroid. The four most common ectopic locations will be considered separately.

Ectopic Locations

Retrotracheal Adenoma. The most common location of an ectopic superior adenoma is deep in the neck, posterior or posterolateral to the trachea (Fig. 22-10). Superior adenomas tend to enlarge between posterior tissue planes that extend toward the posterior mediastinum. Acoustic shadowing from air in the trachea can make evaluation of this area difficult. Often the adenoma protrudes slightly from behind the trachea, and a portion of the mass will be visible. Turning the patient's head to the opposite side will accentuate the protrusion and provide better accessibility to the retrotracheal area. The transducer should be angled medially to visualize the tissues posterior to the trachea. This process is then repeated from the other side of the neck to visualize the contralateral aspect of the retrotracheal area. This process is analogous to the procedure in which the surgeon runs a fingertip behind the trachea in an attempt to palpate a retrotracheal adenoma.

Maximal turning of the head also often causes the esophagus to move to the opposite side of the trachea

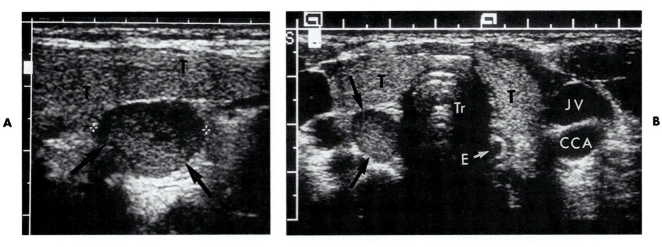

FIG. 22-7. Superior parathyroid adenoma. A, Longitudinal and, **B,** transverse sonograms show 2 cm adenoma *(arrows)* adjacent to the posterior aspect, midportion of the right lobe of the thyroid, *T. Tr,* Trachea; *CCA,* common carotid artery; *JV,* internal jugular vein; *E,* esophagus.

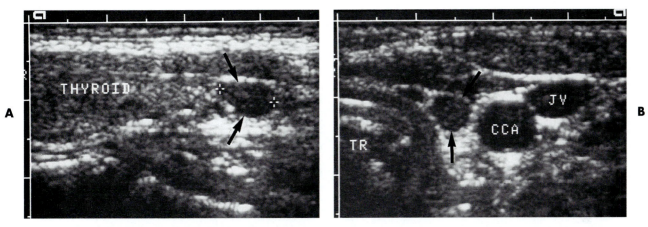

FIG. 22-8. Inferior parathyroid adenoma. A, Longitudinal and, **B,** transverse sonograms show 1 cm adenoma *(arrows)* inferior to the caudal tip, lower pole of the left lobe of the thyroid. *Tr,* Trachea; *CCA,* common carotid artery; *JV,* internal jugular vein.

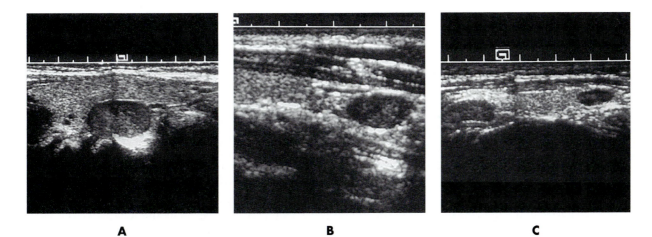

FIG. 22-9. Spectrum of locations of typical parathyroid adenomas. A, Superior adenoma. Longitudinal sonogram shows adenoma posterior to midportion of thyroid. **B,** Inferior adenoma. Longitudinal sonogram shows adenoma 1 cm caudal to lower pole of thyroid. **C,** Hyperplasia. Longitudinal sonogram shows enlarged superior and inferior parathyroid glands.

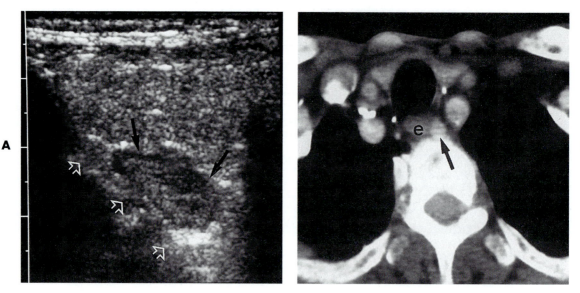

FIG. 22-10. Ectopic adenoma—tracheoesophageal groove. A, Longitudinal angled parasagittal sonogram shows 2 cm ectopic superior parathyroid adenoma *(arrows)* deep in the low neck/upper mediastinum adjacent to the cervical spine *(arrowheads)* with posterior acoustic shadowing. B, CT scan of the low neck/upper mediastinum shows ectopic adenoma *(arrow)* in the left tracheoesophageal groove adjacent to the esophagus, *e*.

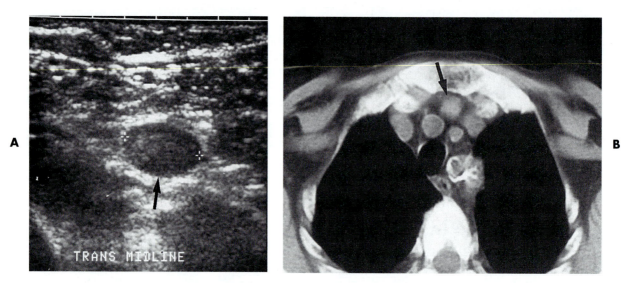

FIG. 22-11. Ectopic adenoma—anterosuperior mediastinum. A, Transverse sonogram angled caudal to the clavicles shows 1 cm ectopic inferior oval parathyroid adenoma *(arrow)* in the soft tissues of the anterosuperior mediastinum. B, CT scan of the upper mediastinum shows the ectopic adenoma *(arrow)* in the anterosuperior mediastinum deep to the manubrium adjacent to the great vessels.

as it becomes compressed between the trachea and the cervical spine. If the radiologist sees the esophagus move completely to protruding from behind one side of the trachea to protruding from the opposite side during maximal head turning, it has effectively "swept" the retrotracheal space and would have pushed any parathyroid adenoma in this location out from behind the trachea.

Mediastinal Adenoma. The most common location for ectopic inferior parathyroid adenomas is low within the neck or in the anterosuperior mediastinum (Fig. 22-11).[42] Parathyroid adenomas are sufficiently hypoechoic that they usually can be visualized as discrete structures separate from the thymus and surrounding tissues. To visualize this area optimally, the patient's neck is hyperextended maximally.

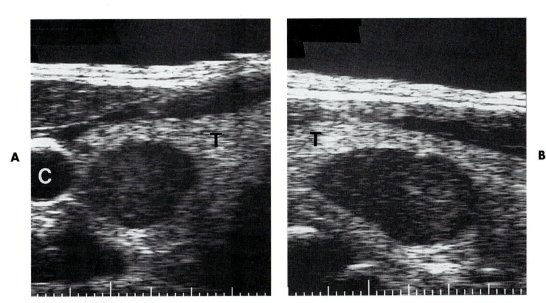

FIG. 22-12. Ectopic adenoma—intrathyroid adenoma. A, Transverse and, **B,** longitudinal sonograms of the right neck show 2 cm oval intrathyroid parathyroid adenoma completely surrounded by thyroid tissue. This occult adenoma was not palpable at the time of two failed neck operations. *T,* Thyroid; *C,* common carotid artery.

With this technique and the transducer angled posteriorly and caudally to the clavicular heads, sonographic visualization is often possible inferiorly to the level of the innominate veins. If the adenoma lies caudally to this level or far anteriorly, just deep to the sternum, it cannot be visualized sonographically.

When an ectopic superior adenoma lies in the mediastinum, it usually is in the posterosuperior region. These adenomas tend to stay in a more posterior plane than the inferior adenomas and lie deep in the low neck or upper mediastinum, requiring use of a 5-MHz transducer for maximal penetration. These adenomas may be intimately associated with the posterior aspect of the trachea, and the head-turning maneuver described for retrotracheal adenomas can be applied here as well. With the patient's neck hyperextended and the transducer angled caudally, the posterior mediastinum sometimes can be visualized to the level of the apex of the arch of the aorta. Adenomas lying caudally to this level cannot be visualized sonographically.

Intrathyroid Adenoma. Intrathyroid adenomas are uncommon and may represent either superior or inferior gland adenomas.[4,43-45] Most intrathyroid adenomas are in the posterior half of the middle to lower pole of the thyroid, are completely surrounded by thyroid tissue, and are oriented with their greatest dimension in the cephalad-caudad direction (Fig. 22-12). Intrathyroid adenomas may be overlooked at the time of operation because they are soft and are similar to surrounding thyroid on palpation. A thyroidotomy or subtotal lobectomy may be needed to find an intrathyroid adenoma. Sonographically, however, parathyroid adenomas usually are well visualized be-

cause they are hypoechoic, in contrast to the echogenic thyroid parenchyma. The internal architecture and appearance of these adenomas are the same as those of adenomas elsewhere in the neck. Sonographically, intrathyroid parathyroid adenomas can be similar to thyroid nodules in appearance, and percutaneous biopsy often is necessary to distinguish between these entities.

Some superior and inferior adenomas may lie under the pseudocapsule or sheath that covers the thyroid gland or within a sulcus of the thyroid, but these are not usually considered to be true intrathyroid adenomas. These adenomas may be difficult for the surgeon to visualize at the time of surgery unless this sheath is opened.[8,43] Sonographically, these adenomas appear the same as other parathyroid adenomas that lie immediately adjacent to the thyroid.

Carotid Sheath/Undescended Adenoma.
Rare ectopic adenomas can lie in a high position superior and lateral in the neck, near the carotid bifurcation at the level of the hyoid bone or attached to the carotid sheath along the course of the common carotid artery (Fig. 22-13).[46-48] These adenomas probably arise from inferior glands that are embryologically undescended or partially descended and come to reside within or adjacent to the carotid sheath that surrounds the carotid artery, jugular vein, and vagus nerve. These adenomas frequently are overlooked during surgery unless the surgeon specifically opens the carotid sheath and dissects within it.[6,7,49] Sonographically, these masses can appear similar to mildly enlarged lymph nodes in the jugular chain, and percutaneous biopsy often is necessary for confirmation.

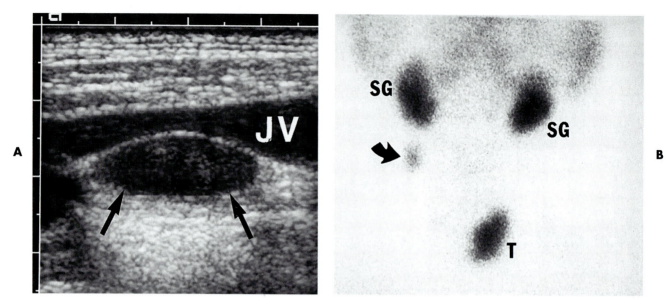

FIG. 22-13. Ectopic adenoma—carotid sheath. A. Longitudinal sonogram of the right side of the neck shows 2 cm ectopic parathyroid adenoma *(arrows)* posterior to the internal jugular vein, *JV.* **B,** Nuclear medicine scan using technetium-99m sestamibi shows focal area of activity in right lateral neck. The right lobe of the thyroid had been surgically removed in previous unsuccessful operation to localize a right ectopic parathyroid adenoma. *T,* Thyroid; *SG,* salivary gland. (From Hopkins CR, Reading CC. Thyroid and parathyroid imaging. *Sem US CT MRI* 1995;6:279-295.)

PERSISTENT OR RECURRENT HYPERPARATHYROIDISM

Persistent hyperparathyroidism is persistence of hypercalcemia after previous failed parathyroid surgery. This is frequently due to an undiscovered ectopic parathyroid adenoma or unrecognized multiple gland enlargement and failure to resect all of the hyperfunctioning tissue during surgery. Persistent postoperative hypercalcemia has been reported in the range of 3% to 10% in many series.[50] Recurrent hyperparathyroidism is defined as hypercalcemia occurring after a 6-month interval of normocalcemia, resulting from the development of a hyperfunctioning parathyroid gland or glands from previously normal glands.[51] Recurrent hyperparathyroidism is often seen in patients with unrecognized MEN I.

In reoperated patients the surgical cure rate is approximately 10% to 30% lower than initial surgery. Because of neck scarring and fibrosis from the previous operation, the morbidity of severe postoperative hypocalcemia and recurrent laryngeal nerve damage is up to 20 times higher.[52-58] During sonographic evaluation of reoperated patients, specific attention is paid to the most likely ectopic parathyroid locations—those associated with a gland that was not discovered at the initial neck dissection.

Imaging prior to reoperation is beneficial, and most care strategies recommend liberal use of studies in this situation.[16,59,60] For most surgeons the preferred approach prior to reoperation is to use the simplest, most sensitive, and least expensive imaging technology, that of ultrasound, as the first imaging method. Sonography has demonstrated some of the highest sensitivities of all modalities for adenoma detection in the reoperative setting.[59] Ultrasound imaging may be followed, as needed, by scintigraphy or magnetic resonance imaging (MRI) when sonographic findings are ambiguous or the risk is high.[60,61] This approach has been shown to turn the nonimaged reoperation procedure with only a 62% success rate into a significantly shorter and less expensive procedure with a success rate of near 90%.[59]

A small subgroup of patients in whom recurrent hyperparathyroidism develops postoperatively has undergone previous autotransplantation of parathyroid tissue in conjunction with previous total parathyroidectomy, usually for complications of chronic renal failure.[62,63] In this procedure a parathyroid gland is sliced into fragments that are inserted into surgically prepared intramuscular pockets in the forearm or sternocleidomastoid muscle. Up to 20% to 33% of patients with parathyroid autotransplantation will develop graft-dependent hypercalcemia.[63,64] Usually these autotransplanted fragments are too small and too similar in echotexture to the surrounding muscle to be visualized adequately on sonographic examination, but occasionally they can be identified. Graft-dependent

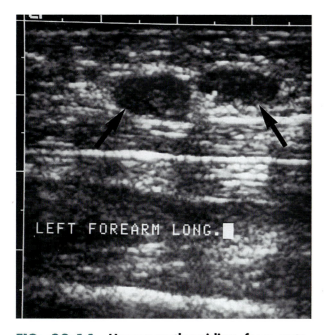

FIG. 22-14. Hyperparathyroidism from auto-transplanted parathyroid tissue. Longitudinal sonogram of left forearm shows two 1 cm hypoechoic nodules *(arrows)* from hyperplasia of autotransplanted parathyroid tissue.

recurrent hyperparathyroidism has a similar appearance to adenomas in the neck of oval, sharply marginated, hypoechoic portions of this autotransplanted tissue, measuring 5 to 11 mm (Fig. 22-14).[64,65] Regardless of the success of preoperative localization studies, the autotransplanted fragments usually are readily found by the surgeon while the patient is under local anesthesia, and a portion of the grafted tissue can be excised to cure the hypercalcemia.

SECONDARY HYPERPARATHYROIDISM

Secondary hyperparathyroidism characteristically is found in patients with chronic renal failure. These patients are unable to synthesize the active form of vitamin D and therefore have chronic hypocalcemia, which results in parathyroid hyperplasia. If untreated, secondary hyperparathyroidism can result in bone demineralization, soft tissue calcification, and acceleration of vascular calcification. Surgical treatment for secondary hyperparathyroidism is uncommon because of the success of dialysis therapy; however, in symptomatic patients who are refractory to dialysis and medical therapy, subtotal parathyroidectomy or total parathyroidectomy with autotransplantation is indicated.[66-69]

In patients with secondary hyperparathyroidism, multiple enlarged glands are present. Individually, these enlarged glands have the same sonographic ap-

pearance as other parathyroid adenomas (see Fig. 22-6). However, the glands may be asymmetrically enlarged. Imaging is not usually necessary, although sonography can be used as a screening tool for the evaluation of the severity of secondary hyperparathyroidism, which can be measured by the amount of gland enlargement.[70] Patients with sonographically enlarged glands have significantly worse symptoms, laboratory values, and radiographic signs of secondary hyperparathyroidism than patients without gland enlargement. Sonography can also be used to aid in localization of the enlarged parathyroid glands prior to surgical resection for secondary hyperparathyroidism.[71]

PITFALLS IN INTERPRETATION

False-Positive Examination

Normal cervical structures, such as small veins adjacent to the thyroid, the esophagus, and the longus colli muscles of the neck, can simulate parathyroid adenomas, producing false-positive results during neck sonography (see box above).

Many **small veins** lie immediately adjacent to the posterior and lateral aspects of both lobes of the thyroid, and when one is tortuous or segmentally dilated, it can simulate a small parathyroid adenoma. Scanning maneuvers that help to establish that the structure in question is a vein, not an adenoma, include: (1) use of real-time imaging in multiple transverse, longitudinal, and oblique planes to show the tubular nature of the vein; (2) Valsalva's maneuver by the patient, which may cause transient engorgement of the vein; and (3) spectral or color flow Doppler imaging to show flow within the vein (Fig. 22-15).

The **esophagus** may partially protrude from behind the posterolateral aspect of the trachea and simulate a large parathyroid adenoma.[72] Turning the patient's head to the opposite side will accentuate the protrusion. Careful inspection of this structure in the transverse plane will show that it has the typical concentric ring appearance of bowel, with a peripheral hypoechoic muscular layer and a central echogenic mu-

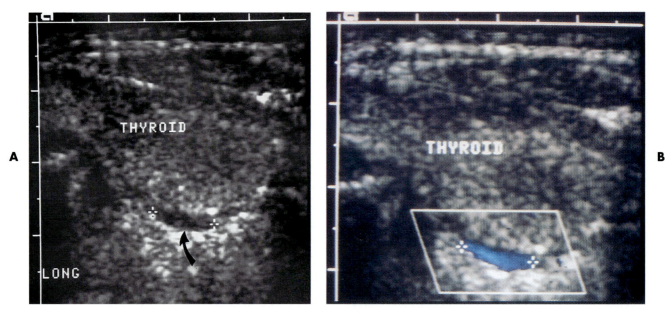

FIG. 22-15. Vein adjacent to thyroid simulates parathyroid adenoma. **A,** Longitudinal sonogram shows 1 cm oval hypoechoic structure *(arrow)* adjacent to the posterior aspect of the thyroid; the structure is suspected to be a parathyroid adenoma. **B,** Color flow Doppler sonogram shows flow throughout the lumen of the structure, demonstrating that it is a vein.

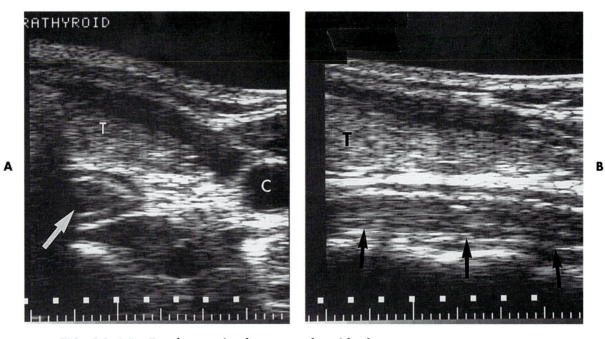

FIG. 22-16. Esophagus simulates parathyroid adenoma. **A,** Transverse sonogram of the left neck shows 1 cm oval hypoechoic structure *(arrow)* located posterior to the thyroid, *T. C,* Common carotid artery. The structure could be a parathyroid adenoma. **B,** Left parasagittal sonogram shows the structure is tubular *(arrows)* and contains fluid in its lumen and therefore is the esophagus.

cosal/intraluminal contents layer. Using a longitudinal scan plane helps to demonstrate the tubular nature of this structure (Fig. 22-16). Real-time imaging while the patient swallows will cause a stream of brightly echogenic mucus and microbubbles to flow through the lumen, which confirms that the structure is esophagus.

The **longus colli muscle** lies adjacent to the anterolateral aspect of the cervical spine. If viewed in the transverse plane, it appears as a hypoechoic triangular mass that can simulate a large parathyroid adenoma located posterior to the thyroid gland. However, scanning in the longitudinal plane will show that this

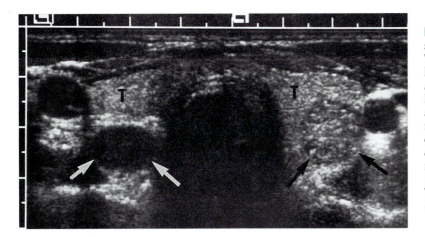

structure is long and flat and contains longitudinal echogenic striations typical of skeletal muscle. Real-time imaging while the patient swallows can be useful because swallowing will cause movement of the thyroid gland and perithyroid structures, such as a parathyroid adenoma, but the longus colli muscle, which is attached to the spine, will remain stationary. Finally, comparison with the opposite side of the neck will demonstrate similar symmetric findings because the longus colli muscles are paired structures located on both sides of the cervical spine.

Pathologic structures that are potential causes of false-positive results include **thyroid nodules** and **cervical lymph nodes**.[32,73] Thyroid nodules can be visualized sonographically in up to 40% of patients undergoing sonographic examination of the neck for parathyroid disease.[74] If a thyroid nodule protrudes from the posterior aspect of the thyroid, it can simulate a mass in the location of a parathyroid adenoma. One sign that can be useful in this situation is a thin echogenic line that separates the parathyroid adenoma (which arises outside of the thyroid gland) from the thyroid gland itself. Thyroid nodules, which arise from within the thyroid gland, do not show this tissue plane of separation.[75] Morphologically, thyroid nodules, unlike parathyroid adenomas, are often partially cystic and some are calcified. Also, thyroid nodules often are of a heterogeneous, mixed echogenicity whereas parathyroid adenomas are of a homogeneous, hypoechoic echogenicity (Fig. 22-17). When a parathyroid adenoma cannot be distinguished from a thyroid nodule by imaging criteria, percutaneous biopsy may be necessary.

Enlarged **cervical lymph nodes** have an oval, hypoechoic appearance like parathyroid adenomas, but they often also have a central echogenic band or hilum composed of fat, vessels, and fibrous tissue, which is a feature that distinguishes them from parathyroid adenomas.[76] Sonographically visible cervical lymph nodes usually lie laterally in the neck in the internal jugular chain adjacent to the jugular vein away from the thyroid. Occasionally, however, parathyroid adenomas can

be found laterally in the neck in the carotid sheath, particularly in the reoperative setting, and percutaneous biopsy may be necessary to distinguish parathyroid adenoma from abnormal lymph node. At least two cases of enlarged lymph nodes containing sarcoid granulomas causing hypercalcemia and false-positive scintigraphic and sonographic examinations have been described.[77]

False-Negative Examination

The three major situations in which examinations give false-negative results are minimally enlarged adenomas, adenomas displaced posteriorly and obscured by a markedly enlarged thyroid goiter, and ectopic adenomas (see box above).

Minimally enlarged adenomas are a common cause of error because these small masses can be difficult to distinguish from thyroid and adjacent soft tissues. **Multinodular thyroid goiters** interfere with parathyroid adenoma detection in two ways. First, the thyroid gland enlargement displaces structures located adjacent to the thyroid posteriorly, away from the transducer. This can necessitate the use of 5-MHz transducers rather than 7.5-MHz transducers to obtain the necessary penetration; this decreases spatial resolution. Second, thyroid goiters have a multinodular contour and irregular echotexture, which hinders the detection of adjacent parathyroid gland enlargement. Some **ectopic adenomas**, such as retrotracheal adenomas or adenomas located deep in the mediastinum, will be inaccessible and nonvisible because of acoustic shadowing from the overlying air and bone.

ACCURACY

Ultrasound

The sensitivity of sonographic parathyroid adenoma localization in primary hyperparathyroidism varies by institution, but most reports range between 70% and 80%.[32,60,75,78-86] Specificity may be improved with ultrasound by using fine-needle aspiration (FNA). As described in detail later (see "Percutaneous Biopsy" section), FNA is a valuable adjunct to ultrasound examination. For a suspected adenoma mass, aspirate specimens can be sent for cytologic analysis as well as PTH assay.[60,87-90]

In persistent or recurrent hyperparathyroidism, the sensitivity of sonography in adenoma localization has been reported to be between 36% and 63%.[60,61,91-95] Ultrasound augmented by FNA and PTH assay can lead to a specificity approaching 100%.[95] It is important to understand that in most large clinical series, 70% to 80% of parathyroid adenomas are found in the neck or are accessible through the neck in patients undergoing reoperation for hyperparathyroidism.[54,56,57] Therefore a thorough ultrasound examination of the neck is important in these reoperative patients. If the adenoma is not visible sonographically, then ectopic mediastinal locations should be considered.[60,95,96]

Other Imaging Modalities

Other methods that have been used commonly for parathyroid adenoma localization are MRI[97-100] and scintigraphy using technetium-99m sestamibi.[101-107] Current less commonly used methods are computed tomography (CT), angiography, and venous sampling.[108-113] Initial studies to evaluate both transesophageal ultrasound[114] and positron emission tomography[115] have shown success in some patients. In the patient being considered for reoperation, sestamibi scintigraphy or MRI may be useful if sonography is negative, particularly for evaluation of the portion of the mediastinum and retrotracheal areas that are not well seen by sonography. Angiography and venous sampling are more invasive, more expensive, and more technically demanding than the imaging modalities mentioned above. These procedures also can be associated with an unacceptably high incidence of complications and are being used in a decreasing number of centers. Studies evaluating the sensitivities of multiple combined preoperative imaging exams describe improved overall accuracy as compared with a single modality examination prior to surgery.[82] When multiple studies are used, at most institutions ultrasound is a good choice as the initial imaging exam when preoperative imaging is used because of its noninvasiveness, low cost, competitive sensitivity, and accuracy.

Discussion: To Image or Not To Image in Primary Hyperparathyroidism

The indications for preoperative imaging of the parathyroid glands in patients with primary hyperparathyroidism vary by institution. In some medical centers where an experienced surgeon is available, routine preoperative parathyroid imaging is not performed.[116] This is because normocalcemia is restored postoperatively in over 95% to 98% of patients and because morbidity is rare when parathyroidectomy is performed by an experienced surgeon.[59,117,118] Except in the settings of diagnostic difficulties or the high-risk patient, it is unlikely that preoperative imaging in primary hyperparathyroidism is cost effective enough to improve the high reported rate of surgical success.[116,117]

There are, however, many proponents of preoperative imaging in primary hyperparathyroidism. These investigators point out that a more rapid and conservative approach of unilateral neck exploration with preoperative imaging guidance has an identical cure rate of a bilateral neck dissection.[96] With localized exploration, benefits may include a significant reduction in operating time as well as reductions in hospital stay, complication risks, and tissue trauma.[50,96] Although a potentially higher rate of persistent hypercalcemia with unilateral parathyroidectomy is present if preoperative imaging misses a contralateral second adenoma, double and triple adenomas have an incidence of well less than 5%, with some studies quoting incidences of less than 1%.[16,96] If the first adenoma was found with imaging, chances are good that any unlikely second contralateral tumors will also be noted. Proponents of preoperative imaging in primary hyperthyroidism also note that some adenomas are found low in the mediastinum and that the operative approach may be changed or optimized if imaging shows tumor near the thymus.[50]

Accurate preoperative localization is particularly helpful to decrease morbidity in the high-risk patient, such as patients with severe cardiac or pulmonary disease.[119-122] Sonography can also shorten the evaluation necessary prior to urgent surgery in a patient with a severe life-threatening hypercalcemic crisis.[122] Finally, when the biochemical diagnosis of hypercalcemia is not clear, the imaging of an adenoma helps to confirm the likely diagnosis of hyperparathyroidism.

In persistent or recurrent hyperparathyroidism, localization studies are clearly indicated because of the lower surgical success rate and the higher morbidity of reoperations.[16] Preoperative localization studies in recurrent hyperparathyroidism contribute to both the success and speed of the repeat operation. In a series of 157 patients who had undergone reexploration for persistent or recurrent hyperparathyroidism, the surgical cure rate was 89%, and it was thought that prospective localization studies contributed to this high rate of success.[94] Also, when the adenoma was localized preoperatively, the time of operation was decreased.

Because most persistent and recurrent parathyroid adenomas are accessible in the neck or upper mediastinum via a cervical incision rather than a sternotomy,[106] sonographic examination of the neck is often the initial localizing procedure of choice in the setting of recurrent or persistent hyperparathyroidism.[93,123]

INTRAOPERATIVE SONOGRAPHY

Intraoperative sonography occasionally can be a useful adjunct in the surgical detection of parathyroid adenomas, particularly in the reoperative setting.[124,125] Intraoperative scanning can be performed with a conventional, high-frequency (7.5 to 10 MHz) transducer draped with a sterile plastic sheath or with a dedicated sterilized intraoperative transducer. Intraoperative sonography appears to be best suited for the localization of inferior and intrathyroid abnormal parathyroid glands. Superior abnormal glands are more difficult to detect.[125] If intraoperative sonography detects an abnormal parathyroid gland, operative time can be shortened. In most studies, however, intraoperative sonography has not affected the outcome of the operation.

PERCUTANEOUS BIOPSY

Sonographically guided percutaneous biopsy is being used with increasing frequency for preoperative confirmation of suspected abnormal parathyroid glands, particularly in the patient who is a candidate for reoperation.[87-90,126-128] This technique has increased the specificity of sonography by permitting the reliable differentiation of parathyroid adenomas from other pathologic structures, such as thyroid nodules and cervical lymph nodes. In addition to its value to the surgeon, a positive biopsy reassures the reluctant reoperative patient.

If the suspected parathyroid adenoma is in a location remote from the thyroid gland, then the main differential diagnostic consideration is a lymph node. Percutaneous biopsy is performed by using a small-caliber, noncutting needle, such as a 25-gauge standard injection needle, to obtain an aspirate that shows either parathyroid cells or lymphocytes (Fig. 22-18).[129] If the suspected parathyroid adenoma lies adjacent to the thyroid gland, a larger specimen (histologic rather than cytologic specimen) may be necessary to differentiate parathyroid tissue from thyroid tissue.[130] A histologic specimen can be obtained with a small-caliber (21- to 25-gauge) cutting needle. Cutting needles are sometimes difficult to insert through the tough, superficial, soft-tissue planes of the neck. However, such a needle can be readily placed through a larger, short, noncutting needle inserted as an "introducer" through the superficial tissues. In addition to cytologic and histologic analyses, the aspirated fluid and blood can be diluted with 1 ml saline and analyzed for PTH by radioimmunoassay.* High concentrations of PTH are unequivocal evidence of parathyroid tissue. There have been no reported complications of percutaneous needle biopsy of suspected parathyroid adenomas.

The accuracy of percutaneous biopsy in the differentiation of parathyroid gland from other structures was 87% in one series of 52 cases.[127] Biopsy failures were due to inadequate recovery of parathyroid tissue.

---

*References 60, 87, 88, 90, 131, 132.

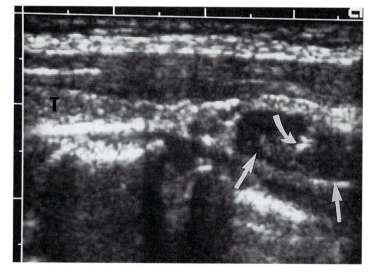

FIG. 22-18. Percutaneous needle biopsy of parathyroid adenoma. Longitudinal sonogram shows 1.5 cm oval parathyroid adenoma *(straight arrows)* in the soft tissues of the low neck in a patient with recurrent hyperparathyroidism. Needle *(curved arrow)* biopsy obtained parathyroid cells, confirming that this mass was a parathyroid adenoma. *T*, Thyroid.

ALCOHOL ABLATION

Sonography has been used to guide percutaneous injection of ethanol into abnormally enlarged parathyroid glands for chemical ablation.[133-140] Currently, alcohol ablation is not used routinely in the treatment of patients with primary hyperparathyroidism, but it is reserved as an alternative therapy for patients who are not surgical candidates, who refuse surgery, or who present with life-threatening malignant hypercalcemia in an emergency situation.[141] Some dialysis patients with recurrence of parathyroid adenomas after previous subtotal surgery or with resistance to calcitriol therapy as well as rare autograft patients with recurrent hyperparathyroidism may also be candidates.[136,142-145] Adenomatous hyperplasia with autonomously functioning glands (tertiary hyperparathyroidism) has also been successfully treated with ultrasound-guided alcohol injection to reduce gland mass.[146]

Alcohol ablation is performed under local anesthesia after a percutaneous biopsy has confirmed the presence of parathyroid tissue or an increased PTH content in the tissue. A small (22- to 25-gauge) needle is inserted into multiple regions of the mass, and 96% ethanol is injected in a volume equal to approximately half the volume of the mass. Under real-time visualization, the tissue becomes highly echogenic at the moment of injection. This echogenicity slowly disappears over a period of approximately 1 minute. There is also a marked decrease in vascularity of the parathyroid adenoma after alcohol injection, presumably secondary to thrombosis and occlusion of the parathyroid vessels (Fig. 22-19). The injections are repeated every day or every other day until the serum calcium level

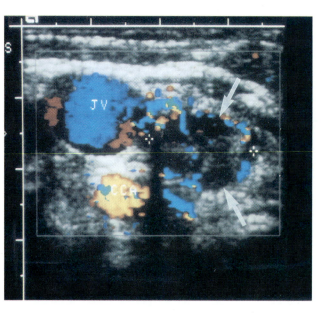
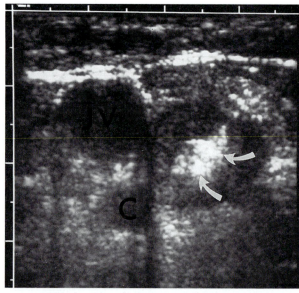
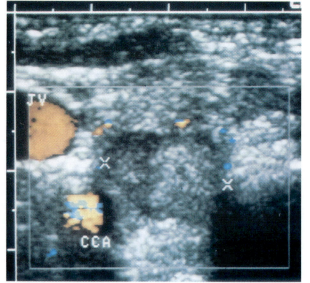

FIG. 22-19. Alcohol ablation of parathyroid adenoma. A, Transverse color sonogram shows 1.5 cm round parathyroid adenoma *(straight arrows)* low in the right neck in a patient with recurrent hyperparathyroidism who was not a surgical candidate because of poor cardiac function. Large amount of blood flow within and surrounding the adenoma. *JV,* Jugular vein; *CCA,* common carotid artery. **B,** Under sonographic guidance, ethanol was injected into multiple areas of the adenoma, which caused the tissues adjacent to the needle tip to become transiently brightly echogenic *(curved arrows).* **C,** One day after alcohol ablation transverse color sonogram of right neck shows that the mass and surrounding tissues show minimal flow. Blood flow is markedly decreased when compared with prealcohol injection image. (From Reading CC. Ultrasound-guided percutaneous ethanol ablation of solid and cystic masses of the liver, kidney, thyroid, and parathyroid. *Ultrasound Q* 1994;12:67-68.)

reaches the normal range. In some cases, three to five injections are necessary.

The results of alcohol injection as a treatment for hyperparathyroidism have been promising. In a series of 18 patients with primary hyperparathyroidism who underwent percutaneous alcohol ablation, two thirds were cured or showed improvement in their biochemical or clinical status at 6 months or more after the procedure.[135] In one series of 12 patients[136] with secondary hyperparathyroidism, 7 had clinical and biochemical improvement. The adverse effects from ethanol ablation in these two series with a total of 30 patients were limited to transient vocal cord paralysis in 4 patients and permanent vocal cord paralysis in 1 patient.

REFERENCES

Embryology and Anatomy

1. Gilmour JR. The gross anatomy of the parathyroid glands. *J Pathol* 1938;46:133-148.
2. Weller GL Jr. Development of the thyroid, parathyroid and thymus glands in man. *Carnegie Institution of Washington: Contributions to Embryology* 1933;24(141):93-139.
3. Mansberger AR, Wei JP. Surgical embryology and anatomy of the thyroid and parathyroid glands. *Surg Clin North Am* 1993;73:727-746.
4. Akerstrom G, Malmaeus J, Bergstrom R. Surgical anatomy of human parathyroid glands. *Surgery* 1984;95:14-21.
5. Edis AJ. Surgical anatomy and technique of neck exploration for primary hyperparathyroidism. *Surg Clin North Am* 1977;57:495-504.
6. Thompson NW, Eckhauser FE, Harness JK. The anatomy of primary hyperparathyroidism. *Surgery* 1982;92:814-821.
7. Edis AJ, Purnell DC, van Heerden JA. The undescended "parathymus." An occasional cause of failed neck exploration for hyperparathyroidism. *Ann Surg* 1979;190:64-68.
8. Wang C-A. The anatomic basis of parathyroid surgery. *Ann Surg* 1976;183:271-275.
9. Norris EH. The parathyroid glands and the lateral thyroid in man: their morphogenesis, histogenesis, topographic anatomy and prenatal growth. *Carnegie Institution of Washington: Contributions to Embryology* 1937;26(159):247-294.
10. Castleman B, Roth SI. Tumors of the parathyroid glands. In: *Atlas of Tumor Pathology*. Fascicle 14, 2nd series. Washington, DC: Armed Forces Institute of Pathology;1978.
11. Russell CF, Grant CS, van Heerden JA. Hyperfunctioning supernumerary parathyroid glands: an occasional cause of hyperparathyroidism. *Mayo Clin Proc* 1982;57:121-124.
12. Hopkins CR, Reading CC. Thyroid and parathyroid imaging. *Sem US CT MRI* 1995;16:279-295.

Primary Hyperparathyroidism

13. Heath H III, Hodgson SF, Kennedy MA. Primary hyperparathyroidism: incidence, morbidity, and potential economic impact in a community. *N Engl J Med* 1980;302:189-193.
14. Van Heerden JA, Beahrs OH, Woolner LB. The pathology and surgical management of primary hyperparathyroidism. *Surg Clin North Am* 1977;57:557-563.
15. Wang CA. Surgery of the parathyroid glands. *Adv Surg* 1966;5:109-127.
16. Kaplan EL, Yashiro T, Salti G. Primary hyperthyroidism in the 1990s. Choice of surgical procedures for this disease. *Ann Surg* 1992;215:300-317.
17. Black WC III, Utley JR. The differential diagnosis of parathyroid adenoma and chief cell hyperplasia. *Am J Clin Pathol* 1968;49:761-775.
18. Prinz RA, Gamvros OI, Sellu D et al. Subtotal parathyroidectomy for primary chief cell hyperplasia of the multiple endocrine neoplasia type I syndrome. *Ann Surg* 1981;193:26-29.
19. Van Heerden JA, Kent RB III, Sizemore GW et al. Primary hyperparathyroidism in patients with multiple endocrine neoplasia syndromes. *Arch Surg* 1983;118:533-535.
20. Weiland LH. Practical endocrine surgical pathology. In: van Heerden JA, ed. *Common Problems in Endocrine Surgery*. Chicago: Year Book Medical Publishers; 1989.
21. Schantz A, Castleman B. Parathyroid carcinoma: a study of 70 cases. *Cancer* 1973;31:600-605.
22. Castleman B, Roth SI. Tumors of the parathyroid glands. In: *Atlas of Tumor Pathology*. Fascicle 14, 2nd series. Washington, DC: Armed Forces Institute of Pathology; 1978.
23. Shane E, Bilezikian JP. Parathyroid carcinoma: a review of 62 patients. *Endocrinol Rev* 1982;3:218-226.
24. Holmes EC, Morton DL, Ketcham AS. Parathyroid carcinoma: a collective review. *Ann Surg* 1969;169:631-640.
25. Purnell DC, Smith LH, Scholz DA et al. Primary hyperparathyroidism: a prospective clinical study. *Am J Med* 1971;50:670-678.
26. Purnell DC, Scholz DA, Smith LH et al. Treatment of primary hyperparathyroidism. *Am J Med* 1974;56:800-809.
27. Clark OH, Duh QY. Primary hyperparathyroidism: a surgical perspective. *Endocrinol Metab Clin North Am* 1989;18:701-714.
28. Kaplan RA, Snyder WH, Stewart A et al. Metabolic effects of parathyroidectomy in asymptomatic primary hyperparathyroidism. *J Clin Endocrinol Metab* 1976;42:415-426.
29. Gaz RD, Wang CA. Management of asymptomatic hyperparathyroidism. *Am J Surg* 1984;147:498-501.

Sonographic Appearance

30. Graif M, Itzchak Y, Strauss S et al. Parathyroid sonography: diagnostic accuracy related to shape, location and texture of the gland. *Br J Radiol* 1987;60:439-443.
31. Randel SB, Gooding GAW, Clark OH et al. Parathyroid variants: ultrasound evaluation. *Radiology* 1987;165:191-194.
32. Reading CC, Charboneau JW, James EM et al. High-resolution parathyroid sonography. *AJR* 1982;139:539-546.
33. Obara T, Fujimoto Y, Ito Y et al. Functioning parathyroid lipoadenoma—report of four cases: clinicopathological and ultrasonographic features. *Endocrinol Jpn* 1989;36:135-145.
34. Lack EF, Clark MA, Buck DR et al. Cysts of the parathyroid gland: report of two cases and review of the literature. *Am Surg* 1978;44:376-381.
35. Krudy AG, Doppman JL, Shawker TH et al. Hyperfunctioning cystic parathyroid glands: computed tomography and sonographic findings. *AJR* 1984;142:175-178.
36. Sistrom CL, Hanks JB, Feldman PS. Supraclavicular mass in a woman with hyperparathyroidism. *Invest Radiol* 1994;2:244-247.
37. Wolf RJ, Cronan JJ, Monchik JM. Color Doppler sonography: an adjunctive technique in assessment of parathyroid adenomas. *J Ultrasound Med* 1994;13:303-308.
38. Calliada F, Bergonzi M, Passamonti C et al. Il contributo del color Doppler nello studio ecografico delle ghiandole paratiroidi iperplasiche. *Radiol Med (Torino)* 1989;78(6):607-611.
39. Gooding GAW, Clark OH. Use of color Doppler imaging in the distinction between thyroid and parathyroid lesions. *Am J Surg* 1992;164:51-56.
40. Daly BD, Coffey SL, Behan M. Ultrasonographic appearances of parathyroid carcinoma. *Br J Radiol* 1989;62:1017-1019.

41. Edmonson GR, Charboneau JW, James EM et al. Parathyroid carcinoma: high-frequency sonographic features. *Radiology* 1986;161:65-67.

Adenoma Localization

42. Clark OH. Mediastinal parathyroid tumors. *Arch Surg* 1988;123:1096-1099.
43. Thompson NW. The techniques of initial parathyroid exploration and re-operative parathyroidectomy. In: Thompson NW, Vinik AI, eds. *Endocrine Surgery Update*. New York: Grune & Stratton; 1983.
44. Al-Suhaili AR, Lynn J, Lavender JP. Intrathyroidal parathyroid adenoma: preoperative identification and localization by parathyroid imaging. *Clin Nucl Med* 1988;13:512-514.
45. Spiegel AM, Marx SJ, Doppman JL et al. Intrathyroidal parathyroid adenoma or hyperplasia; an occasionally overlooked cause of surgical failure in primary hyperparathyroidism. *JAMA* 1975;234:1029-1033.
46. Fraker DL, Doppman JL, Shawker TH et al. Undescended parathyroid adenoma: an important etiology for failed operations for primary hyperparathyroidism. *World J Surg* 1990;14:342-348.
47. Doppman JL, Shawker TH, Krudy AG et al. Parathymic parathyroid: computed tomography, ultrasound and angiographic findings. *Radiology* 1985;157:419-423.
48. Doppman JL, Shawker TH, Fraker DL et al. Parathyroid adenoma within the vagus nerve. *AJR* 1994;163:943-945.
49. Kurtay M, Crile G Jr. Aberrant parathyroid gland in relationship to the thymus. *Am J Surg* 1969;117:705.

Persistent or Recurrent Hyperparathyroidism

50. Irvin GL, Prudhomme DL, Deriso GT et al. A new approach to parathyroidectomy. *Ann Surg* 1994;219:574-581.
51. Clark OH, Way LW, Hunt TK. Recurrent hyperparathyroidism. *Ann Surg* 1976;184:391-399.
52. Levin KE, Clark OH. The reasons for failure in parathyroid operations. *Arch Surg* 1989;124:911-914.
53. Cheung PSY, Borgstrom A, Thompson NW. Strategy in re-operative surgery for hyperparathyroidism. *Arch Surg* 1989;124:676-680.
54. Palmer JA, Rosen IB. Re-operative surgery for hyperparathyroidism. *Am J Surg* 1982;144:406-410.
55. Prinz RA, Gamvros OI, Allison DJ et al. Re-operations for hyperparathyroidism. *Surg Gynecol Obstet* 1981;152:760-764.
56. Grant CS, Charboneau JW, James EM et al. Re-operative parathyroid surgery. *Wien Klin Wochenschr* 1988;100:360-363.
57. Wells SA. Advances in the operative management of persistent hyperparathyroidism. *Mayo Clin Proc* 1991;66:1175-1177.
58. Brennan MF, Marx SJ, Doppman J et al. Results of re-operation for persistent and recurrent hyperparathyroidism. *Ann Surg* 1981;194:671-676.
59. Grant CS, van Heerden JA, Charboneau JW et al. Clinical management of persistent and/or recurrent primary hyperparathyroidism. *World J Surg* 1986;10:555-565.
60. Rodriquez JM, Tezelman S, Siperstein AE et al. Localization procedures in patients with persistent or recurrent hyperparathyroidism. *Arch Surg* 1994;129:870-875.
61. Higgins CB. Role of magnetic resonance imaging in hyperparathyroidism. *Radiol Clin North Am* 1993;31:1017-1028.
62. Brunt LM, Sicard GA. Current status of parathyroid autotransplantation. *Sem Surg Oncol* 1990;6:115-121.
63. Brunt LM, Wells SA Jr. Parathyroid transplantation: indications and results. In: van Herrden JA, ed. *Common Problems in Endocrine Surgery*. Chicago: Year Book Medical Publishers; 1989.

64. Winkelbauer F, Ammann ME, Langle F et al. Diagnosis of hyperparathyroidism with US after autotransplantation: results of a prospective study. *Radiology* 1993;186:255-257.
65. Hergan K, Neyer U, Doringer W et al. MR imaging in graft-dependent recurrent hyperparathyroidism after parathyroidectomy and autotransplantation. *Mag Res Imag* 1995;5:541-544.

Secondary Hyperparathyroidism

66. Wilson RE, Hampers CL, Bernstein DS et al. Subtotal parathyroidectomy in chronic renal failure: a seven-year experience in a dialysis and transplant program. *Ann Surg* 1971;174:640-652.
67. Diethelm AG, Adams PL, Murad TM et al. Treatment of secondary hyperparathyroidism in patients with chronic renal failure by total parathyroidectomy and parathyroid autograft. *Ann Surg* 1981;193:777-791.
68. Reid DJ. Surgical treatment of secondary and tertiary hyperparathyroidism. *Br J Clin Pract* 1989;43:68-70.
69. Leapman SB, Filo RS, Thomalla JV et al. Secondary hyperparathyroidism: the role of surgery. *Am Surg* 1989;55:359-365.
70. Gladziwa U, Ittel TH, Dakshinamurty KV et al. Secondary hyperparathyroidism and sonographic evaluation of parathyroid gland hyperplasia in dialysis patients. *Clin Nephrol* 1992:38;162-166.
71. Takebayashi S, Matsui K, Onohara Y et al. Sonography for early diagnosis of enlarged parathyroid glands in patients with secondary hyperparathyroidism. *AJR* 1987;148:911-914.

Pitfalls in Interpretation

72. Ngo C, Sarti DA. Simulation of the normal esophagus by a parathyroid adenoma. *J Clin Ultrasound* 1987;15:421-424.
73. Karstrup S, Hegedus L. Concomitant thyroid disease in hyperparathyroidism: reasons for unsatisfactory ultrasonographical localization of parathyroid glands. *Eur J Radiol* 1986;6:149-152.
74. Funari M, Campos Z, Gooding GAW et al. MRI and ultrasound detection of asymptomatic thyroid nodules in hyperparathyroidism. *J Comput Assist Tomogr* 1992;16:615-619.
75. Scheible W, Deutsch AL, Leopold GR. Parathyroid adenoma: accuracy of preoperative localization by high-resolution real-time sonography. *J Clin Ultrasound* 1981;9:325-330.
76. Sutton RT, Reading CC, Charboneau JW et al. US-guided biopsy of neck masses in postoperative management of patients with thyroid cancer. *Radiology* 1988;168:769-772.
77. Nabriski D, Bendahan J, Shapiro MS et al. Sarcoidosis masquerading as a parathyroid adenoma. *Head Neck* 1992;14:384-386.

Accuracy

78. Simeone JF, Mueller PR, Ferrucci JT Jr et al. High-resolution real-time sonography of the parathyroid. *Radiology* 1981;141:745-751.
79. Kobayashi S, Miyakawa M, Kasuga Y et al. Parathyroid imaging comparison of 201 TI-99mTc subtraction scintigraphy, computed tomography, and ultrasonography. *Jpn J Surg* 1987;17:9-13.
80. Buchwach KA, Mangum WB, Hahn FW Jr. Preoperative localization of parathyroid adenomas. *Laryngoscope* 1987;97:13-15.
81. Attie JN, Khan A, Rumancik WM et al. Preoperative localization of parathyroid adenomas. *Am J Surg* 1988;156:323-326.
82. Erdman WA, Breslau NA, Weinreb JC et al. Noninvasive localization of parathyroid adenomas: a comparison of x-ray, computed tomography, ultrasound, scintigraphy and magnetic resonance imaging. *Mag Res Imag* 1989;7:187-194.

83. Summers GW, Dodge DL, Kammer H. Accuracy and cost-effectiveness of preoperative isotope and ultrasound imaging in primary hyperparathyroidism. *Otolaryngol Head Neck Surg* 1989;100:210-217.

84. Kohri K, Ishikawa Y, Kodama M et al. Comparison of imaging methods for localization of parathyroid tumors. *Am J Surg* 1992;164:140-145.

85. Gooding GA. Sonography of the thyroid and parathyroid. *Radiol Clin North Am* 1993;31:967-989.

86. Weinberger MS, Robbins KT. Diagnostic localization studies for primary hyperparathyroidism: a suggested algorithm. *Arch Otolaryngol Head Neck Surg* 1994;120:1187-1189.

87. Bergenfelz A, Forsberg L, Hederstrom E et al. Preoperative localization of enlarged parathyroid glands with ultrasonically guided fine needle aspiration for parathyroid hormone assay. *Acta Radiol* 1991;32:403-405.

88. Sacks BA, Pallotta JA, Cole A et al. Diagnosis of parathyroid adenomas: efficacy of measuring parathormone levels in needle aspirates of cervical masses. *AJR* 1994;163:1223-1226.

89. MacFarlane MP, Fraker DL, Shawker TH et al. Use of preoperative fine-needle aspiration in patients undergoing re-operation for primary hyperparathyroidism. *Surgery* 1994;116:959-965.

90. Sardi A, Bolton JS, Mitchell WT et al. Immunoperoxidase confirmation of ultrasonically guided fine needle aspirates in patients with recurrent hyperparathyroidism. *Surg Gynecol Obstet* 1992;175:563-568.

91. Levin KE, Gooding GAW, Okerlund M et al. Localizing studies in patients with persistent or recurrent hyperparathyroidism. *Surgery* 1988;102:917-924.

92. Miller DL, Doppman JL, Shawker TH et al. Localization of parathyroid adenomas in patients who have undergone surgery. PI. Noninvasive imaging methods. *Radiology* 1987;162:133-137.

93. Reading CC, Charboneau JW, James EM et al. Postoperative parathyroid high-frequency sonography: evaluation of persistent or recurrent hyperparathyroidism. *AJR* 1985;144:399-402.

94. Grant CS, van Heerden JA, Charboneau JW et al. Clinical management of persistent and/or recurrent primary hyperparathyroidism. *World J Surg* 1986;10:555-565.

95. Kairaluoma MV, Kellosalo J, Makarainen H et al. Parathyroid re-exploration in patients with primary hyperparathyroidism. *Ann Chirurg Gyn* 1994;83:202-206.

96. Pearl AJ, Chapnik JS, Freeman JL et al. Pre-operative localization of 25 consecutive parathyroid adenomas: a prospective imaging/surgical correlative study. *J Otolaryngol* 1993;22:301-306.

Other Imaging Methods

97. Yao M, Jamieson C, Blend R. Magnetic resonance imaging in preoperative localization of diseased parathyroid glands: a comparison with isotope scanning and ultrasonography. *Can J Surg* 1993;36:241-244.

98. Stevens SK, Chang J, Clark OH et al. Detection of abnormal parathyroid glands in postoperative patients with recurrent hyperparathyroidism: sensitivity of MR imaging. *AJR* 1993;160:607-612.

99. Kang YS, Rosen K, Clark OH et al. Localization of abnormal parathyroid glands of the mediastinum with MR imaging. *Radiology* 1993;189:137-141.

100. Wright AR, Goddard PR, Nicholson S et al. Fat-suppression magnetic resonance imaging in the preoperative localization of parathyroid adenomas. *Clin Radiol* 1992;46:324-328.

101. Lee VS, Wilkinson RH, Leight GS et al. Hyperparathyroidism in high-risk surgical patients: evaluation with double-phase technetium-99m sestamibi imaging. *Radiology* 1995;195:624-633.

102. Billy HT, Rimkus DR, Hartzman S et al. Technetium-99m sestamibi single agent localization versus high-resolution ultrasonography for the preoperative localization of parathyroid glands in patients with hyperparathyroidism. *Am Surg* 1995;61:882-888.

103. Schurrer ME, Seabold JE, Gurll NJ et al. Sestamibi SPECT scintigraphy for detection of postoperative hyperfunctioning parathyroid gland. *AJR* 1996;166:1471-1474.

104. Mazzeo S, Caramella D, Lencioni R et al. Comparison among sonography double-tracer subtraction scintigraphy, and double-phase scintigraphy in the detection of parathyroid lesions. *AJR* 1996;166:1465-1470.

105. Burke GJ, Wei JP, Binet EF. Parathyroid scintigraphy with iodine-123 and ^{99m}Tc-sestamibi: imaging findings. *AJR* 1993;161:1265-1268.

106. Thompson GB, Mullan BP, Grant CS et al. Parathyroid imaging with technetium-99m sestamibi: an initial institutional experience. *Surgery* 1994;116:966-973.

107. Oates E. Improved parathyroid scintigraphy with Tc-99m MIBI, a superior radiotracer. *Appl Radiol* March 1994:37-40.

108. Sommer B, Welter HF, Spelsberg F et al. Computed tomography for localizing enlarged parathyroid glands in primary hyperparathyroidism. *J Comput Assist Tomogr* 1982;6:521-526.

109. Stark DD, Gooding GAW, Moss AA et al. Parathyroid imaging: comparison of high-resolution computed tomography and high-resolution sonography. *AJR* 1983;141:633-638.

110. Okerlund MD, Sheldon K, Corpuz S et al. A new method with high sensitivity and specificity for localization of abnormal parathyroid glands. *Ann Surg* 1984;200:381-387.

111. Ferlin G, Borsato N, Camerani M et al. New perspectives in localizing enlarged parathyroids by technetium-thallium subtraction scan. *J Nucl Med* 1983;24:438-441.

112. Krudy AG, Doppman JL, Miller DL et al. Work in progress: abnormal parathyroid glands: comparison of nonselective arterial digital arteriography, selective parathyroid angiography, and venous digital arteriography as methods of detection. *Radiology* 1983;148:23-29.

113. Krudy AG, Doppman JL, Miller DL et al. Detection of mediastinal parathyroid glands by nonselective digital arteriography. *AJR* 1984;142:693-695.

114. Henry J, Audiffret J, Denizot A et al. Endosonography in the localization of parathyroid tumors: a preliminary study. *Surgery* 1990;108:1021-1025.

115. Hellman P, Ahlstrom H, Bergstrom M et al. Positron emission tomography with ^{11}C-methionine in hyperparathyroidism. *Surgery* 1994;116:974-981.

Discussion: To Image or Not To Image in Primary Hyperparathyroidism

116. Wei JP, Burke GJ, Mansberger AR. Preoperative imaging of abnormal parathyroid glands in patients with hyperparathyroid disease using combination Tc-99m-pertechnetate and Tc-99m-sestamibi radionuclide scans. *Ann Surg* 1994;219:568-573.

117. Roe SM, Burns RP, Graham LD et al. Cost-effectiveness of preoperative localization studies in primary hyperparathyroid disease. *Ann Surg* 1994;219:582-586.

118. Shaha AR, La Rosa CA, Jaffe BM. Parathyroid localization prior to primary exploration. *Am J Surg* 1993;166:289-293.

119. Wu DTD, Shaw JHF. The use of pre-operative scan prior to neck exploration for primary hyperparathyroidism. *Aust NZ J Surg* 1988;58:35-38.

120. Brewer WH, Walsh JW, Newsome HH Jr. Impact of sonography on surgery for primary hyperparathyroidism. *Am J Surg* 1983;145:270-272.

121. Russell CFJ, Laird JD, Ferguson WR. Scan-directed unilateral cervical exploration for parathyroid adenoma: a legitimate approach? *World J Surg* 1990;14:406-409.

122. Windeck R, Olbricht TH, Littmann K et al. Halessonographie in der hypercalamischen Krise. *Dtsch Med Wochenschr* 1985;110:368-370.

123. Wang CA. Parathyroid re-exploration: a clinical and pathological study of 112 cases. *Ann Surg* 1977;186:140-145.

Intraoperative Sonography

124. Kern KA, Shawker TH, Doppman JL et al. The use of high-resolution ultrasound to locate parathyroid tumors during re-operations for primary hyperparathyroidism. *World J Surg* 1987;11:579-585.

125. Norton JA, Shawker TH, Jones BL et al. Intraoperative ultrasound and reoperative parathyroid surgery: an initial evaluation. *World J Surg* 1986;10:631-638.

Percutaneous Biopsy

126. Gooding GAW, Clark OH, Stark DD et al. Parathyroid aspiration biopsy under ultrasound guidance in the postoperative hyperparathyroid patient. *Radiology* 1985;155:193-196.

127. Solbiati L, Montali G, Croce F et al. Parathyroid tumors detected by fine-needle aspiration biopsy under ultrasonic guidance. *Radiology* 1983;148:793-797.

128. Charboneau JW, Grant CS, James EM et al. High-resolution ultrasound-guided percutaneous needle biopsy and intraoperative ultrasonography of a cervical parathyroid adenoma in a patient with persistent hyperparathyroidism. *Mayo Clin Proc* 1983;58:497-500.

129. Glenthoj A, Karstrup S. Parathyroid identification by ultrasonically guided aspiration cytology. Is correct cytological identification possible? *APMIS* 1989;97:497-502.

130. Karstrup S, Glenthoj A, Hainau B et al. Ultrasound-guided, histological, fine-needle biopsy from suspect parathyroid tumors: success-rate and reliability of histological diagnosis. *Br J Radiol* 1989;62:981-985.

131. Doppman JL, Krudy AG, Marx SJ et al. Aspiration of enlarged parathyroid glands for parathyroid hormone assay. *Radiology* 1983;148:31-35.

132. Winkler B, Gooding GAW, Montgomery CK et al. Immunoperoxidase confirmation of parathyroid origin of ultrasound-guided fine needle aspirates of the parathyroid glands. *Acta Cytologica* 1987;31:40-44.

Alcohol Ablation

133. Charboneau JW, Hay ID, van Heerden JA. Persistent primary hyperparathyroidism: successful ultrasound-guided percutaneous ethanol ablation of an occult adenoma. *Mayo Clin Proc* 1988;63:913-917.

134. Karstrup S, Holm HH, Glenthoj A et al. Nonsurgical treatment of primary hyperparathyroidism with sonographically guided percutaneous injection of ethanol: results in a selected series of patients. *AJR* 1990;154:1087-1090.

135. Karstrup S, Transbol I, Holm HH et al. Ultrasound-guided chemical parathyroidectomy in patients with primary hyperparathyroidism: a prospective study. *Br J Radiol* 1989;62:1037-1042.

136. Solbiati L, Giangrande A, DePra L et al. Percutaneous ethanol injection of parathyroid tumors under ultrasound guidance: treatment for secondary hyperparathyroidism. *Radiology* 1985;155:607-610.

137. Verges BL, Cercueil JP, Jacob D et al. Results of ultrasonically guided percutaneous ethanol injection into parathyroid adenomas in primary hyperparathyroidism. *Acta Endocrinol* 1993;129:381-387.

138. Karstrup S, Hegedus L, Holm HH. Acute change in parathyroid function in primary hyperparathyroidism following ultrasonically guided ethanol injection into solitary parathyroid adenomas. *ACTA Endocrinol* 1993;129:377-380.

139. Karstrup S. Ultrasonically guided localization, tissue verification, and percutaneous treatment of parathyroid tumors. *Danish Med Bull* 1995;42:175-191.

140. Reading CC. Ultrasound-guided percutaneous ethanol ablation of solid and cystic masses of the liver, kidney, thyroid, and parathyroid. *Ultrasound Q* 1994;12:67-68.

141. Karstrup S, Lohela P, Apaja-Sarkkinen M et al. Non-operative hypercalcemic crisis. *Acta Med Scand* 1988;224:187-188.

142. Takeda S, Michigishi T, Takazakura E. Ultrasonically guided percutaneous ethanol injection to parathyroid autografts for recurrent hyperparathyroidism. *Nephron* 1993;65:651-652.

143. Takeda S, Michigishi T, Takazakura E. Successful ultrasonically guided percutaneous ethanol injection for secondary hyperparathyroidism. *Nephron* 1992;62:100-103.

144. Kitaoka M, Fukagawa M, Ogata E et al. Reduction of functioning parathyroid cell mass by ethanol injection in chronic dialysis patients. *Kidney Int* 1994;46:1110-1117.

145. Giangrande A, Castiglioni A, Solbiati L et al. Ultrasound-guided percutaneous fine-needle ethanol injection into parathyroid glands in secondary hyperparathyroidism. *Nephrol Dial Transplant* 1992;7:412-421.

146. Cintin C, Karstrup S, Ladefoged S et al. Tertiary hyperparathyroidism treated by ultrasonically guided percutaneous fine-needle ethanol injection. *Nephron* 1994;68:217-220.

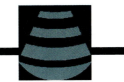

CHAPTER 23

The Breast

•

Ellen B. Mendelson, M.D.

Conventional x-ray mammography is currently the most important breast imaging method. Other diagnostic studies include sonography, spectral and color flow Doppler imaging, magnetic resonance imaging (MRI), computed tomography (CT), radionuclide imaging with agents such as 99 mTc sestamibi for cancers and 99 mTc sulfur colloid for sentinel node labeling, and digital mammography.[1] Computer-aided diagnosis (CAD) is being developed to bolster pattern recognition for interpretation. With the exception of ultrasound (US), most of these techniques have limited applications. In the last two decades, sonography has secured an important place in the diagnosis and management of breast disease.

There are two different levels of approach to breast evaluation:

- Screening for breast carcinoma; and
- Diagnosis and management of benign and malignant breast disease.

The sole purpose of screening is the identification of breast carcinoma: early detection has resulted in a decreased mortality.[2-4] The effectiveness of screening programs relies on the sensitivity and accuracy of the examinations, which should be widely available, affordable, and of documented high benefit and low risk.

Breast sonography is unsuited to breast cancer screening, as many studies using both older as well as current, state-of-the-art automated and hand-held equipment suggest.[5,6] Microcalcifications, an important sign of early breast cancer, accounting for up to 50% of nonpalpable, mammographically-detected breast cancers, are depicted inconsistently.[7] As a screening examination for masses, breast sonography is highly operator- and technique-dependent, time consuming, and, therefore, costly.[5] Most important will be the results of prospective studies of the usefulness of high-resolution US for detecting occult, nonpalpable breast carcinomas.

The breast symptoms of pain and mass are frequently manifestations of normal cyclical changes and benign disease such as cysts, adenosis, and inflammatory processes. These symptoms are often due to physiologic changes and become more worrisome as women enter the age of higher incidence of breast carcinoma. Here, ultrasound makes its greatest contribution in diagnosis and management of breast disorders. Sonography augments the specificity of mammography and is invaluable in characterizing masses as cystic or solid.

When used in conjunction with mammography and clinical examination, breast sonography is indispensable in the diagnosis and management of benign and malignant processes. In addition to the identification of cysts, advances in instrumentation, higher resolution probes, and improvement in scanning techniques have promoted characterization of solid masses and assignment of levels of suspicion to them. In addition, patient comfort and real-time visualization of the needle's path have made US an increasingly preferred imaging technique to guide interventional procedures.

Breast imaging facilities should have state-of-the-art equipment, and the staff should have the time and ability to integrate mammographic and sonographic findings to complete the diagnostic breast evaluation expeditiously. The mammographic study should be monitored and supplemented with ultrasound and interventional procedures as appropriate. In deciding to use ultrasound or perform a sonographically guided interventional procedure, the radiologist must consider its potential to enhance the mammographic interpretation or alter patient management.[8,9]

INDICATIONS FOR BREAST SONOGRAPHY[10]

To characterize mammographic or palpable masses as cystic or solid

To evaluate palpable masses in young (under the age of 30 years), pregnant, and lactating patients

To identify an abscess in a patient with mastitis (Fig. 23-1)

To evaluate nonpalpable abnormalities for which the mammographic diagnosis is uncertain

To help exclude a mass thought to be the cause of an area of mammographic asymmetric density

To confirm or better visualize a lesion seen incompletely or on only one mammographic projection (e.g., near the chest wall)

To guide interventional procedures such as cyst aspiration, large-needle core biopsy, fine-needle aspiration biopsy, abscess drainage, presurgical localization, and galactography

---

INDICATIONS

These uses for breast sonography are also applicable to the postsurgical patient and to the male breast (see box). Sonography is not currently advised for screening a dense breast in its entirety for a possible mass because of its uncertain error rate in these patients.[5]

EQUIPMENT

Breast sonography was used as long ago as 1951 when Wild and Reid imaged a 2- to 3-mm tumor with a 15 MHz A-mode transducer.[8] B-mode studies of the breast were subsequently performed with transducers of lower frequency. Two types of instruments for breast sonography evolved: automated and hand-held.

Fear that the ionizing radiation of mammography would induce cancer led to a demand for alternate methods of breast cancer screening, and automated breast ultrasound units were offered in response.[10] Both prone and supine versions were developed, having transducer frequencies between 4.0 and 7.5 MHz.[11] Advantages of automated breast scanning units include the more reliable display of multiple lesions, which makes comparison with previous examinations easier, and the lower level of operator dependency.

The use of automated breast US instruments has nearly ceased, primarily because of the recognition of their inadequacies as a screening technique. Bassett reported in 1989 that 53% of 319 radiologists surveyed used breast sonography in their practices. Of this group, 93% used hand-held transducers and only

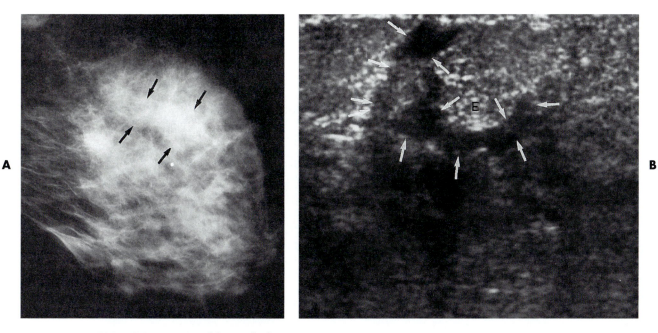

FIG. 23-1. **Mastitis and abscess.** **A,** In a 43-year-old woman with pain and fever, mediolateral oblique mammogram shows dense tissue. Mild edema and irregular areas of parenchyma *(arrows)* in superior breast. **B,** Sonogram shows bright area of echogenicity (E) signifying edema caused by mastitis within which is a C-shaped focal abscess collection *(arrows)* drained with US guidance.

7% used the more costly, cumbersome, and labor-intensive automated scanners.[12] Since that time, the use of breast sonography has increased and all practices offering complete breast imaging would be expected to utilize US.

Hand-held transducers are better suited for the characterization of masses, and the examination is performed more rapidly than with automated units. Guidance of interventional procedures is also more easily accomplished with hand-held transducers. These transducers vary widely in their specifications, design, and quality. Dynamically focused phased array, linear array, and annular array transducers of 7 to 10 MHz are available. Standard-sized transducers and the smaller, intraoperative probes are both appropriate for breast sonography, although the standard-sized probes may be more efficient for general breast scanning purposes. The focal zones of these high-frequency transducers are 3 cm or less, optimizing the resolution of superficial masses. If the transducer is not properly focused in the midportion of the lesion, artifactual echoes may occur with cysts (Fig. 23-2). Even with high-resolution transducers, use of an offset acoustic pad often improves the resolution of subcutaneous and very superficial, near-field lesions.[12,13] Probes of even higher frequency will be soon offered by various manufacturers for breast use. Color flow and spectral Doppler sonography have also been used in breast diagnosis, although their value in differentiating benign from malignant solid masses has not been established.[14-18] Studies are under way to ascertain the value of intravenous contrast agents such as microphilized albumin in increasing the sensitivity and specificity of color flow imaging and power Doppler in tumor detection and categorization of masses as benign or malignant.[19]

EXAMINATION TECHNIQUE

The US study provides an opportunity for physical as well as sonographic examination of the breast, and the mammograms should be available for correlation with the sonographic findings. Sonography of the outer breast is most easily performed with the patient in a supine-oblique position. The patient's shoulder and torso of the side to be examined are elevated by a wedge to minimize the thickness of the upper, outer-quadrant breast tissue. The ipsilateral arm is elevated and flexed at the elbow with the hand resting comfortably under the neck. The contralateral arm remains at the patient's side. In this supine-oblique position, the bulk of breast tissue falls to the contralateral side. Adequate sonographic penetration is assured if the underlying pectoral muscles and ribs are visualized.

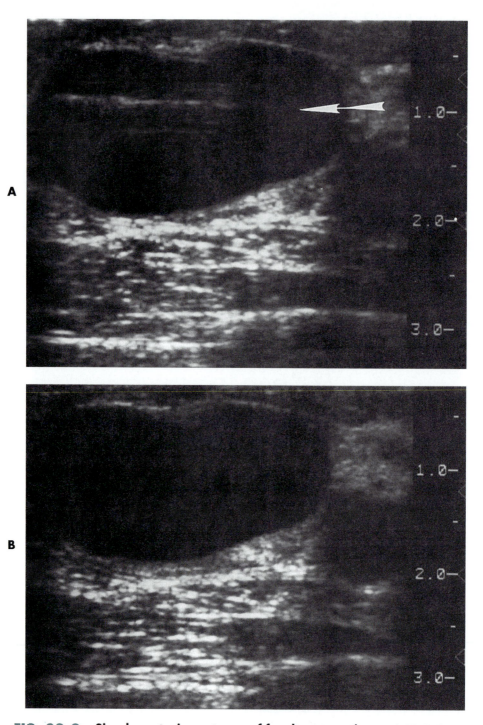

FIG. 23-2. Simple cysts: importance of focal zone settings. **A,** With the most anterior focal zone placed superficially, near-field reverberation artifact *(arrow)* occurs. **B,** Downward shift in the focal zone settings, with the most anterior placed at the midplane of the lesion, is effective in establishing the anechogenicity of the cyst.

For imaging areas other than the upper outer, quadrant, it is preferable to place the patient in the supine position, with her arms at her sides or behind her head. If the purpose of the examination is to evaluate a palpable abnormality and if the lesion is felt only when the patient is seated or standing, the patient should assume that position and locate the site of concern with her fingers. Scanning then should be directed to the region in question.

Radial and orthogonal antiradial approaches to scanning the breast have been proposed as most appropriate anatomically for the branching ducts, segmentally arranged in the conical breast.[13] To depict the breast in its entirety, this scanning technique is almost intuitive. Generally, a quadrant or area is scanned in sagittal and transverse planes. Suspected abnormalities should be viewed orthogonally (with two views at right angles) so that a pseudomass will be recognized and not misinterpreted as a true lesion. For example, a fat lobule may appear similar to an oval fibroadenoma in one view, but when the transducer is rotated 90°, the fat lobule often appears elongated rather than rounded.

Imaging the nipple areolar complex requires special technical maneuvers.[20,21] The nipple creates abrupt changes in surface contour that may result in poor visualization of the deeper tissues. Posterior acoustic shadowing results from air gaps that form between the irregular skin surface and the transducer surface. Fibrous elements within the nipple may also cause shadowing that obscures the retroareolar region. The tissues beneath the nipple may be imaged by placing the transducer adjacent to the nipple and angling into the retroareolar area. If abnormalities are suspected in the skin or superficial subcutaneous tissues, an offset pad or fluid-filled bag can be placed on the skin to improve the resolution of the near field structures.

Sonographic evaluation of multiple lesions may be confusing because a lesion may be counted more than once if viewed from different angles and locations. One approach to counting masses is to try to isolate a lesion manually, pushing it outside of the scanning field. The surrounding parenchyma is then imaged to identify possible additional cysts or masses.

The positioning of the patient during mammography is different from the positioning during sonography, and that affects anatomic relationships. When women are supine, the breast flattens, and the distance between the skin and the chest wall is diminished, as compared with mammographic depiction of the breast with the woman upright. To aid in establishing mammographic-sonographic concordance, if the breast is scanned with the woman upright as she is positioned mammographically, the anatomic relationships are preserved.

If uncertainty exists when correlating the mammographic or palpable findings with sonographic abnormalities, a small radiopaque marker can be placed on the skin over the lesion as it is evaluated initially. The area is then restudied with the woman upright (Fig. 23-3). Finding the marker in the expected location will confirm that the identical lesion is being imaged. If concordance of mammographic and sonographic findings remains in doubt, a needle can be placed in the lesion and then the mammography can be repeated. Another way to establish concordance is by aspiration, with mammographic confirmation of disappearance of the lesion if it is a cyst. Injection of a small amount of air into the region of a solid abnormality and repetition of the mammogram can also confirm that the masses are the same. While these maneuvers are unnecessary in most cases, they can be helpful.

It is most important that US examination of the breast not be reduced to "lumpography." Note should be made of the anatomic landscape of the breast surrounding the lesion so that follow-up examinations can be performed with reidentification of the area of concern by the depth of the lesion and its surrounding pattern of fat lobules, Cooper's ligaments, and fibroglandular interfaces.

DOCUMENTATION

The sonographic findings can be recorded on film, videotape, digitized systems, or any other enduring device.[22] As for mammography, image labeling should be consistent. Although there is no universally accepted method for labeling, the image should show the patient's name, medical record number and/or birth date, the laterality of the breast (right or left), the location of the area depicted, using clock notation, diagram, or other easily understood and reproducible system, and the position of the probe with respect to the breast or lesion (transverse or longitudinal). It may also be useful to describe whether the lesion is

1. retroareolar;
2. in the anterior third of the breast;
3. in the middle portion of the breast;
4. in the posterior third of the breast; or
5. in the axilla or axillary tail of the breast.

To measure the lesion accurately, the longest dimension of a mass should be sought and measured as the *longitudinal axis*. The dimension perpendicular to this is the *short axis* of the mass. In the orthogonal plane, the third dimension of the mass can be measured. If a benign mass such as a probable fibroadenoma is to be followed or if the response of a carcinoma to chemotherapy is to be assessed, the three dimensions of the mass permit volumetric calculations to be made. Consistent, uniform labeling makes find-

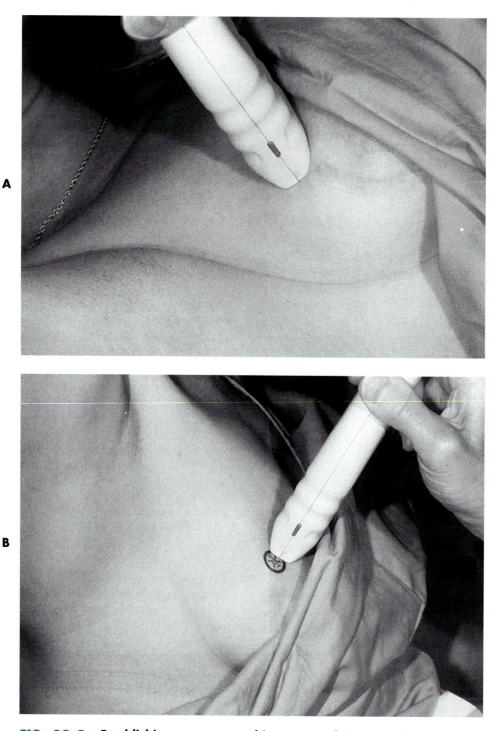

FIG. 23-3. Establishing mammographic-sonographic concordance. A, Once an abnormality is found when scanning in supine or supine-oblique position, the patient can be helped to assume an upright position as the transducer remains on the breast. **B,** A radiopaque marker is then placed at the site, and mammography is performed to confirm concordance of the mammographic and sonographic findings.

ings easier to reproduce on subsequent studies and easier to communicate to clinical colleagues.

SONOGRAPHIC ANATOMY

The anatomic components of the breast and surrounding structures (skin, ducts, adipose tissue, parenchyma, nipple, blood vessels, retromammary muscles, and ribs) have characteristic sonographic features. The **skin complex** is seen as two thin, echogenic lines demarcating a narrow hypoechoic band, the dermis (Fig. 23-4).[23] The normal skin measures up to 0.2 cm in thickness but may be thicker in the lower breast near the inframammary fold.

Fat lobules are oval in one plane of view and elongated in the orthogonal plane. They are hypoechoic relative to the surrounding glandular tissue[24] and may have a central echogenic focus of connective tissue. Subcutaneous fat lobules and those within the breast are usually larger than fat lobules located in the prepectoral area.

The **breast glandular parenchyma** usually appears homogeneously echogenic as compared with fat lobules but may have hypoechoic zones caused by fatty tissue. Not infrequently, the glandular tissue is interlaced with small hypoechoic mammary ducts. The wide range of normal glandular parenchyma seen mammographically can also be appreciated sono-graphically. Areas of asymmetric density seen by mammography may be due to fibroglandular tissue or a mass. In general, fibroglandular tissue appears echogenic, whereas most masses appear as hypoechoic or anechoic structures. Found in patients of all ages but characteristic of the breasts of the very young, extensive homogeneously echogenic tissue often corresponds to mammographically dense breasts, within which radiographic identification of discrete masses may be difficult.

Cooper's ligaments provide the connective tissue support for the breast. With US they appear as thin, echogenic arcs. Particularly in the lower breast, the intersection of curved Cooper's ligaments with fibroglandular tissue can cause alarming posterior acoustic shadowing. Changing the probe angle with respect to the breast or varying the pressure applied to the breast can eliminate the shadowing to allow unimpeded visualization of the breast tissue.

The **terminal duct lobular units** (TDLUs) are important anatomic units from which many benign (cysts, adenosis, fibroadenomas) and malignant processes originate.[25] The TDLUs may enlarge or involute, reflecting age and physiologic differences and proliferating in pregnancy, for example, as the breast readies itself for lactation. Hyperplastic TDLUs are hypoechoic areas that can be recognized on a US image;[26] a small, normal TDLU may not be identified as a discrete anatomic structure even with high-resolution breast ultrasound. Spatial resolution of ultrasound transducers, even with frequencies of up to 12 MHz, may limit recognition of this important unit.

The **mammary ducts,** which are radially arrayed in 7 to 20 segments around the nipple, demonstrate progressive luminal enlargement as they converge on the nipple. The ducts are visible as tubular structures that measure 0.1 to 0.8 cm in diameter (Fig. 23-5).[27] These ducts become smaller and arborize in the peripheral portions of the breast.

The **nipple** is of medium-level echogenicity and attenuates sound, resulting in a posterior acoustic shadow. Scanning obliquely behind the nipple or using an offset pad will allow the area posterior to the nipple to be visualized (Fig. 23-6). The normal nipple may sometimes appear as a well-defined hypoechoic oval structure resembling a superficial adenoma if imaged from an oblique angle.

The mammary tissue is enclosed within a **fascial envelope** composed of a superficial and a deep layer.[27] These fascial layers may be identified as thin lines, although they are not usually visible. The superficial layer is sometimes seen below the dermis, and the deep layer lies over the retromammary fat and pectoralis muscle. The two layers are straddled by Cooper's ligaments. Visualization of the **pectoralis muscle** assures that the breast parenchyma has been

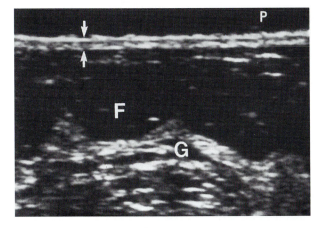

FIG. 23-4. Normal skin. 7.5 MHz image using standoff pad (P) demonstrates two echogenic lines *(arrows)* with thin hypoechoic layer between them. Skin is normally 0.2 cm or less in thickness except in the inframammary fold, where it is slightly thicker. Scalloped hypoechoic subcutaneous fat lobules (F) are seen. Echogenic layer posterior to fat represents fibroglandular parenchyma (G). Linear hypoechoic branching structures within fibroglandular tissue represent ducts, and the G is superimposed over the branch point. Echogenic areas curving slightly in the subcutaneous fat are Cooper's ligaments.

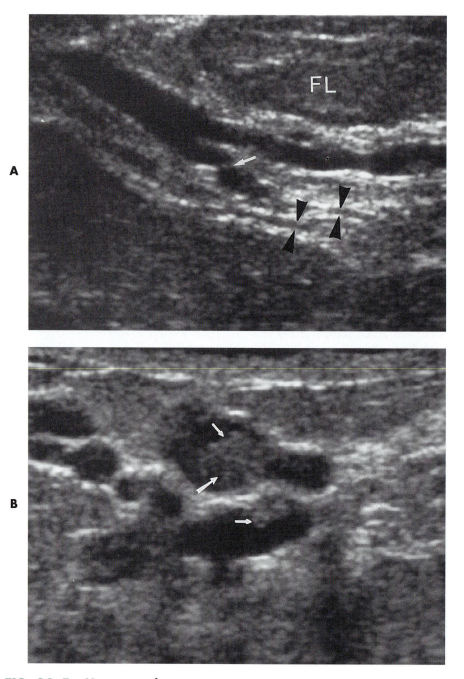

FIG. 23-5. Mammary ducts. A, Two large, normally branching ducts join as they approach the nipple. The deeper of the two ducts makes a bend *(arrow)*. In the glandular tissue are many smaller ducts *(arrowheads)*. Fat lobule, FL. **B,** Beaded, ectatic ducts with cystic dilatation and mural nodules *(arrows)* that represent intraductal papillomas.

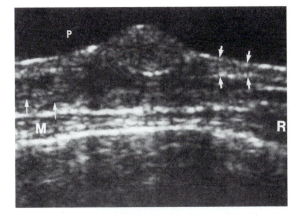

FIG. 23-6. Nipple-areolar complex. Using offset pad (P) and angling transducer into retroareolar area, tissue beneath nipple can be visualized. Unless probe is angled, its contact with nipple often produces acoustic shadow, obscuring retroareolar area. Periareolar skin is thicker near nipple *(thick arrows)* and thinner near periphery. Small black tubular structures represent mammary ducts *(thin arrows)*. R indicates rib; M, pectoralis muscle.

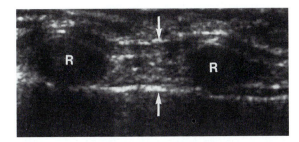

FIG. 23-7. Ribs. Longitudinal scan shows oval ribs (R), hypoechoic sharply marginated structures that attenuate sound. Intercostal muscles *(arrows)* are identified between ribs.

adequately penetrated at that site. The ribs are oval, hypoechoic, periodic structures behind the pectoralis muscles (Fig. 23-7). They attenuate sound, causing a posterior acoustic shadow.

The **axillary vessels** present as tubular structures, which are often seen pulsating during the real-time examination. Duplex Doppler or color flow Doppler imaging can provide confirmation of their vascular nature, particularly of benefit when needle biopsies of lymph nodes or axillary masses are planned.

Lymph nodes may be seen in the axilla as well as within the breast parenchyma.[27,28] Normal lymph nodes are often reniform and may have an echogenic fatty hilus (Fig. 23-8). Sonographically, small normal lymph nodes may resemble fat lobules or cysts and be indistinguishable from small fibroadenomas.[29,30] In depicting the fatty hilus within a lymph node, US is not reliable in excluding malignancy in a woman with breast cancer. Normal-sized

---

SONOGRAPHIC DESCRIPTORS OF BREAST MASSES

Location
Number
Size
Shape
    Round
    Oval
    Irregular
Margins
    Smooth
    Microlobulated
    Macrolobulated
    Irregular or spiculated
    Poorly defined
Orientation
Internal contents
    Solid
    Cystic
    Mixed
Echogenicity
    Anechoic
    Hypoechoic
    Hyperechoic
Heterogeneity
    Homogeneous
    Heterogeneous
Parenchymal interface
    Thin linear
    Echogenic rim
    Irregular
Posterior sound transmission
    Enhancement
    Shadow
    No change
Associated secondary findings
    Skin changes
    Ductal dilatation
    Cooper's ligament straightening or thickening
    Compressibility
Doppler characteristics

---

lymph nodes that are infiltrated with tumor may appear identical to normal nodes, and a previous study may be necessary to show that the hilar fat has been encroached upon, although not yet obliterated. Similarly, enlarged hyperplastic lymph nodes may appear identical to metastatic lymph nodes. On occasion, a hypoechoic cortical focus or an irregular cortical margin may be found in a lymph node, suggesting a metastatic deposit. Ultrasound can be useful to confirm a lymph node by depicting the fatty hilus of a lymph node that may be obscured by fibroglandular tissue on the mammogram.

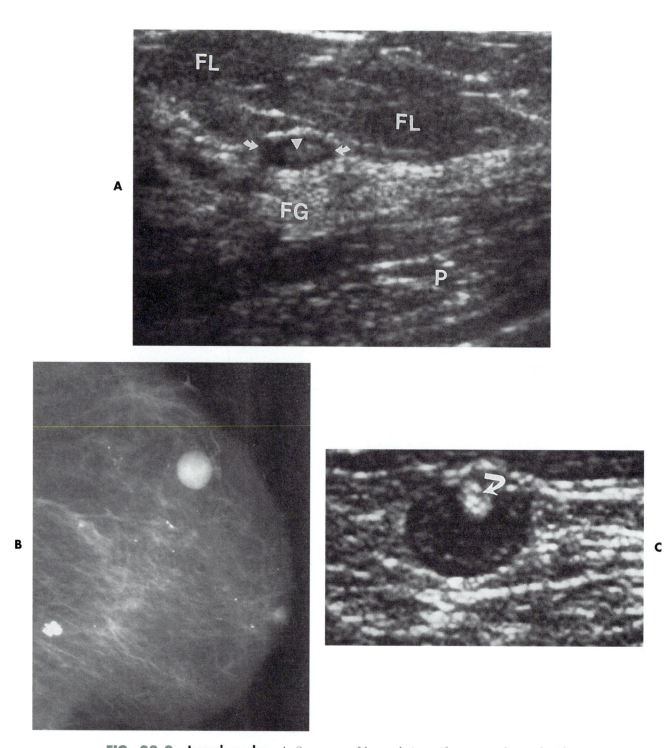

FIG. 23-8. Lymph nodes. A, Sonogram of hypoechoic reniform mass *(arrows)* with central echogenic fat *(arrowhead)* confirms identity of a small breast nodule as an intramammary lymph node. Hypoechoic subcutaneous fat lobules (FL) are anterior to the lymph node, and more echogenic fibroglandular parenchyma (FG) is beneath. Pectoral muscle, P. **B,** Mammogram shows rounded nodule in upper breast in patient with leukemia. **C,** US shows the mass to be an enlarged lymph node with eccentric echogenic focus *(curved arrow)*. Leukemic infiltration was found at biopsy.

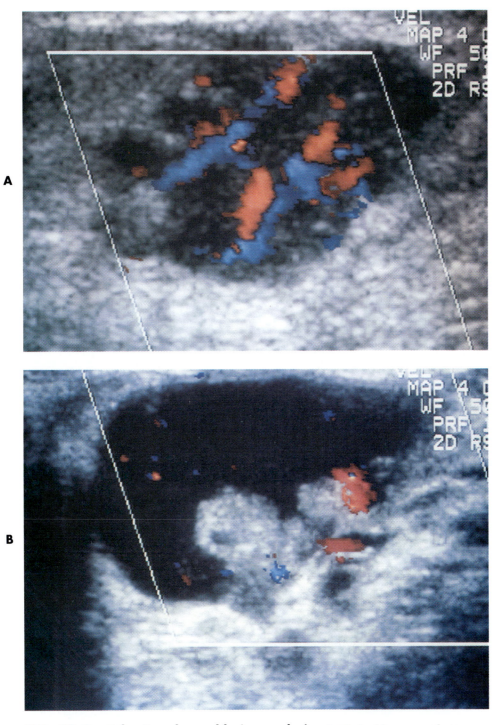

FIG. 23-9. Color Doppler and lesion analysis. A, Marked hypervascularity augments mammographic and US high levels of suspicion for malignancy based on morphology. Histology: undifferentiated infiltrating ductal carcinoma. **B,** Complex cystic mass with mural nodules containing flow. Histology: benign intracystic papillomas. In general, hyper- and neovascularity support a higher level of suspicion, but low or absent flow cannot exclude malignancy if features of the mass are suggestive.

AN APPROACH TO EVALUATING MASSES

For many years, it has been thought that US might not be helpful in analyzing masses smaller than 1.0 cm in diameter. Experience with high-resolution transducers has confirmed that cysts of 0.2 to 0.3 cm in diameter can be detected as can solid lesions of 0.5 cm in diameter or even smaller, depending upon the frequency of the transducer and its resolution, the location of the masses within the breast, the nature of the surrounding parenchyma, and the scanning technique.[5] Although the sonographic appearances of many solid masses are frequently nonspecific, there has been progress in characterization of solid masses, and it is an oversimplification to say that the sole use of ultrasound is merely to differentiate cysts from solid masses. Although spiculation is the most important single feature, combinations of features are better predictors of malignancy than is any single characteristic of a mass.[13,31] Lesion analysis (see the box on page 759), in the context of clinical history, mammographic and physical findings, patient's age, and risk factors for malignancy, can often suggest a level of suspicion (Fig. 23-10). This is similar to the American College of Radiology's BI-RADS categorization of mammographic abnormalities as

1. negative;
2. benign finding;
3. probably benign finding (short-term interval follow-up suggested);
4. suspicious abnormality (consider biopsy); and
5. highly suggestive of malignancy.[32]

Based on this assessment, a number of satisfactory, conservative management approaches can be offered. These management strategies include percutaneous invasive techniques to increase diagnostic specificity, thereby minimizing the need for surgical biopsy.

CYSTS

Breast cysts are common in women in the perimenopausal years of approximately 35 to 50 years of age. Of 593 well-circumscribed mammographic masses over 1 cm evaluated by Moskowitz, 50% were cysts.[33] Following menopause, cysts usually disappear gradually, although they may persist, flourish, or develop in women receiving estrogen or estrogen-progesterone hormonal replacement therapy.

One of the most important contributions of breast sonography is the confident diagnosis of a simple cyst. No further clinical action is needed when a mass meets the sonographic criteria of a simple cyst unless the patient has pain, the mass interferes with clinical or self-examination, or other symptoms are of concern.[21]

Diagnostic criteria, which should be strictly applied, are the same as those for cysts elsewhere in the body. The lesion should

- be anechoic;
- be round or oval;
- be sharply marginated (particularly the posterior walls); and
- demonstrate acoustic enhancement posteriorly.[10,21]

If a cyst is not under tension, pressure applied to it with the transducer may alter its shape. If there is any doubt regarding the diagnosis of a cyst, aspiration is indicated. Lesions of greater compressibility are more likely to be benign than malignant.[34]

For dependable diagnosis of cysts, all aspects of sonographic technique require attention.[12] Gain and power settings must be adjusted for each unit and reset for each patient. Focal-zone placement must be appropriate (Fig. 23-2), with a standoff pad used for superficial lesions. To demonstrate features of a cyst in lesions deeply seated in the breast or in larger breasts, compression and positional alterations may be neces-

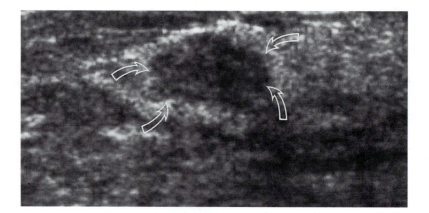

FIG. 23-10. Indeterminate solid mass. At first glance, mass appears fairly well circumscribed and suggestive of fibroadenoma. The mass has heterogeneous echotexture and is hypoechoic with respect to surrounding glandular tissue. Careful scrutiny, however, shows margins to be irregular laterally and posteriorly *(curved arrows)*, elevating level of suspicion. Histology of core biopsy specimens was infiltrating ductal carcinoma.

sary. With increased power or time gain compensation (TGC) settings, the anterior portion of a cyst will fill in, but the posterior wall will remain well-defined. If all of the criteria are fulfilled, the diagnosis of a cyst can be made with nearly 100% accuracy and only routine follow-up will be necessary.[21] In our experience, up to 30% of simple cysts may have low-level internal echoes (Fig. 23-11). The management of these cysts is difficult, and if all of the other criteria are fulfilled except for presence of internal echoes, and there are several such similar-appearing lesions present at sonography, aspiration may be unnecessary and follow-up imaging may suffice.

SOLID AND MIXED MASSES

Sonographic Features and Levels of Suspicion

Carcinoma of the breast is the leading cause of cancer in women in the United States. Until recently, the incidence has been increasing, with 180,300 cases anticipated this year.[35] Early detection offers survival benefits.[1] Ideally, breast imaging should be accurate in the diagnosis of carcinoma. Although certain mammographic and/or sonographic findings allow specific diagnoses of some malignant and benign abnormalities, there is a wide range of sonographic appearances

manifested by neoplastic and nonneoplastic breast lesions. Combinations of sonographic features are better predictors of malignancy than are any one feature.

Although virtually all sonographically visible carcinomas are hypoechoic (relative to adjacent breast parenchyma or fat), many other masses also appear hypoechoic.[5,24] In our experience, we have never seen a carcinoma that is uniformly as echogenic as fibroglandular tissue. With meticulous scanning, although a thick echogenic rim may be seen (Fig. 23-12), a small hypoechoic area is present. The relative echogenicity of lesions is somewhat dependent on dynamic range. In breast sonography, lesions are better depicted within a setting of subtle variations in the gray scale; a high-contrast, black-white image will impede tissue differentiation and lesion characterization.

Although the **shape** of a mass and its **borders** are the most important predictors of benign or malignant nature, overlap remains. Although fibroadenomas are commonly oval, carcinomas may also be elongated as well as rounded. While carcinoma typically has irregular margins, benign lesions, such as abscesses, hematomas, and fat necrosis, may also have jagged margins. Smooth margins, expected with fibroadenomas, may also be a sonographic finding in some primary breast carcinomas as well as in metastases to the breast (Fig. 23-13).[13,31,37]

Posterior acoustic shadowing, which may represent the fibrous response incited by the tumor's presence, may be seen in 40% to 60% of carcinomas (Fig. 23-12).[37-39] Benign neoplasms, such as fibroadenomas, may also exhibit posterior acoustic shadowing, and therefore the finding is not specific for malignancy.[5,11] In our experience, posterior acoustic shadows unrelated to calcification occurred in up to 30% of fibroadenomas, particularly in those fibroadenomas that are hyalinized (Fig. 23-14).[40] Posterior acoustic shadows are also seen in association with fat necrosis, postsurgical and traumatic scarring, radial

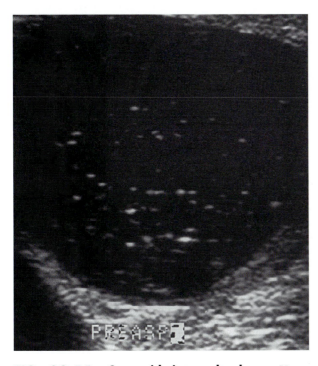

FIG. 23-11. Cyst with internal echoes. Up to 30% of cysts in our experience may have low-level internal echoes, scattered as here, or more homogeneously hypoechoic. Aspiration of these lesions often yields clear, yellowish, or turbid greenish fluid.

ULTRASOUND FEATURES OF A TYPICAL BREAST CARCINOMA

Irregular borders
Round shape or orientation of long axis perpendicular to skin[13,36]
Hypoechogenicity relative to adjacent fibroglandular and/or fatty tissues
Heterogeneous echotexture
Posterior acoustic shadowing
An echogenic rim of variable thickness that may represent tumor extension, desmoplasia, or compressed breast tissue

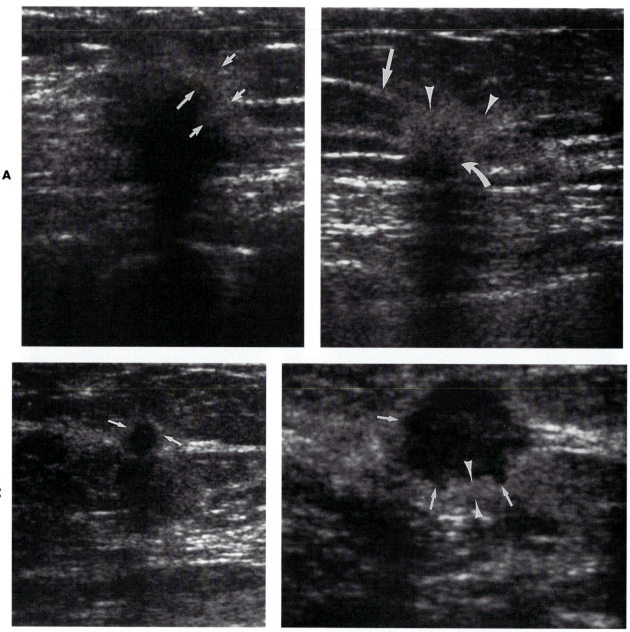

FIG. 23-12. Variable sonographic appearances of infiltrating ductal carcinomas. **A,** Irregularly shaped, poorly marginated mass that is hypoechoic with respect to the surrounding fat lobules. Long axis of mass is perpendicular to skin. A thick echogenic rim *(arrows)* calls attention to the irregular protrusions of the mass into the adjacent disrupted tissue. Posterior acoustic shadowing is intense. **B,** Small hypoechoic mass *(curved arrow)* surrounded by echogenic corolla *(arrowheads)*. The desmoplastic response is drawing a thickened Cooper's ligament *(arrow)* into the mass. Posterior acoustic shadowing is present. **C,** 0.5 cm carcinoma, irregularly shaped, spiculated *(arrows)* and predominantly round in its orientation. Posterior acoustic shadowing is intense. **D,** Microlobulated mass, rounded, heterogeneous internal echogenicity, and echogenic rim *(arrowheads)* are highly suspicious for malignancy. Note absence of posterior acoustic shadowing. Microlobulations *(arrows)*. (**A** and **B** from Goldberg BB, Pettersson H, ed. *The NICER Year Book 1996: Ultrasonography.* Olso: The NICER Institute; 1996.)

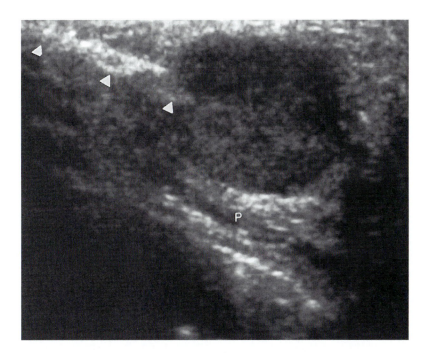

FIG. 23-13. Metastasis to breast from rare placental site tumor. Hypoechoic, solid, superficial mass with mild marginal irregularity prior to firing 14-gauge needle *(arrowheads)* for core biopsy sampling. Metastases to the breast are not uncommonly solitary and well-circumscribed. Pectoral muscle, P.

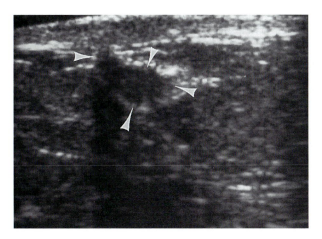

FIG. 23-14. Hyalinized fibroadenoma. Canoeshaped, well-defined mass *(arrowheads)* with macrolobulation anteriorly. Posterior acoustic shadowing is present, seen in up to 30% of noncalcified fibroadenomas, which are often hyalinized, in our experience. Although the mass is isoechoic with respect to adjacent fat lobules, it is oriented differently from the adjacent tissue.

scars, granular cell tumors, focal sclerosing adenosis and fibrosis, diabetic fibrosis, and air-containing abscesses.[41-43] Normal tissues may also cause posterior acoustic shadowing as the transducer passes over the curved tissue planes with multiple interfaces of Cooper's ligaments and other connective tissue septa, fat lobules, and breast parenchyma.

Skin thickening and edema may signify inflammatory breast cancer but it may also occur with mastitis, breast abscess, irradiation therapy, and systemic processes such as congestive heart failure (Fig. 23-15). Although ultrasound does not permit a specific cause to be identified, skin thickening is easy to quantitate with high-resolution sonography. The deeper of the two parallel skin lines usually seen is sometimes interrupted or lost. The thickened dermis—infiltrated, fibrotic, or edematous—often becomes more echogenic compared with the expected hypoechogenicity of this tissue layer. Occasionally, the randomly distributed, engorged lymphatics or interstitial fluid collections can be seen with ultrasound. Progressive decrease in skin thickness can be confirmed sonographically in the patient undergoing radiation therapy whose breast might be difficult to compress fully for mammography.[44,45] If skin thickening and breast edema are unresolved or cannot otherwise be explained, as in patients with radiation-treated breast carcinoma, breast biopsy with inclusion of dermal lymphatics is indicated to exclude inflammatory carcinoma.[25,46] In our experience, US can often demonstrate a mass embedded within the edematous tissue of women with inflammatory breast cancer. The histologic diagnosis can then be made with US-guided core biopsy, and the tumor is most often found to be an infiltrating ductal carcinoma.[25,46]

Asymmetric ductal dilation, a sign of low specificity for malignancy, may represent a carcinoma but more often represents a benign lesion such as intra-

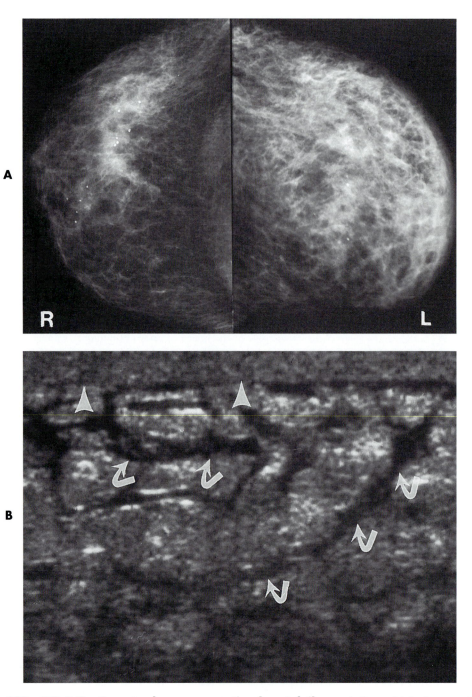

FIG. 23-15. Breast edema: congestive heart failure. A, Interstitial edema and skin thickening, left (L) greater than right (R) on craniocaudal mammographic views of the breasts. **B,** Skin thickening *(arrowheads)* with branched, anechoic linear fluid collections in nonductal pattern *(curved arrows)* representing engorged lymphatics or interstitial fluid collections in 73-year-old woman with congestive heart failure. The bright echogenicity of the tissue containing the interstitial fluid collections is a characteristic of edema. Follow-up imaging after completion of medical therapy showed complete resolution of edema. (**A** and **B** from Goldberg BB, Pettersson H, ed. *The NICER Year Book 1996: Ultrasonography.* Olso: The NICER Institute; 1996.)

ductal papilloma. Unless there has been a change since previous examinations or there is a nipple discharge, interval follow-up rather than biopsy would be recommended.[47]

Macrocalcifications are well depicted sonographically as echogenic foci, often with posterior acoustic shadowing. Popcorn-like clumps of calcification are visualized in fibroadenomas. Coarse calcifications are also seen in fat necrosis, in areas of scarring, in lymph nodes involved with granulomatous disease, and in other lesions.

Microcalcifications, when pleomorphic and irregularly clustered, are the most important mammographic marker for nonpalpable cancers, especially intraductal carcinoma.[4,7,48] The diameter of an individual microcalcification measures 0.1 to 0.4 mm. Occasionally, with high-resolution ultrasound equipment, microcalcifications may be seen, especially when they are located within a mass (Fig. 23-16).[5,37] Microcalcifications, visualized inconsistently, appear as tiny echogenic flecks in the breast parenchyma and are often difficult to distinguish from the many other echogenic surfaces. These microcalcifications usually do not produce acoustic shadows. Determination of the morphologic features of microcalcifications is beyond the resolution capabilities of current instruments, and estimates of the number and extent of microcalcifications are unreliable.

Malignant Masses

Ductal Carcinoma. Infiltrating ductal carcinoma accounts for up to 80% of breast cancers.[49] Arising from the ductal epithelium of smaller and medium-sized ductal elements, infiltrating ductal carcinoma may also occur with other histologic types, such as tubular or invasive lobular carcinoma.[49]

On palpation, these masses feel larger than they appear mammographically and sonographically. This well-known clinical phenomenon can be explained by the desmoplastic reaction incited by the tumor. At mammography, these tumors often have irregular and poorly defined margins that reflect infiltrative behavior of the tumor and fibrous response to its presence. Similarly, most infiltrating ductal carcinomas seen sonographically have irregular, ill-defined borders.[13,50] These tumors are usually heterogeneous, hypoechoic, solid masses that attenuate the acoustic beam. There is, however, a wide range of sonographic appearances of this common type of malignancy. For example, some infiltrating ductal carcinomas have well-defined margins and do not attenuate sound. In our experience, many of these are poorly differentiated histologically (see Fig. 23-16).

Infiltrating Lobular Carcinoma. Second in frequency of occurrence but far less common than infiltrating ductal carcinoma is the infiltrating lobular carcinoma, contributing 8% to 10% of breast cancers.[51] This tumor's propensity for bilaterality and multicentricity ranges from 6% to 36%.[52] Although infiltrating lobular carcinoma may be indistinguishable mammographically from the spiculated masses of infiltrating ductal carcinoma, a common presentation is that of a poorly demarcated, asymmetric, increased density that may be wispy, shaggy, and of low density.[53-56] The tumor cells travel in a linear pattern through the breast parenchyma without a central tumor nidus. The mammographic appearance reflects these histologic characteristics. Particularly in dense breasts or breasts in which the tumor presents as a subtle area of architectural derangement, ultrasound can be valuable in confirming an infiltrative mass, sometimes large, that can be hidden mammographically but suspected clinically as a vague area of induration (Fig. 23-17). At sonography, these hypoechoic tumors are irregularly shaped, have ill-defined margins, sometimes with an echogenic corolla, demonstrate posterior acoustic shadowing, and cause distortion of the surrounding tissues.

Medullary Carcinoma. The medullary carcinoma comprises approximately 5% of breast cancers.[49] It occurs with greater frequency in women under the age of 50 years.[49] Mammographically, these tumors, which may be large, are often fairly well circumscribed. The sharp margins and homogeneous internal architecture of the medullary carcinoma may result in a sonographic appearance similar to that of a cyst, and meticulous attention to focal zone and gain settings may help to avoid misinterpretation. Medullary tumors may be round, lobulated, homogeneous, or hypoechoic and may demonstrate posterior acoustic enhancement.[37,38,53] Low-level internal echoes of the carcinoma that are most evident at higher-gain settings separate these lesions from simple cysts. Some of the margins of the mass may be irregular rather than smooth (Fig. 23-18). These findings may be subtle, and aspiration will be necessary to differentiate a medullary carcinoma from a cyst or abscess.

Mucinous (Colloid) Carcinoma. Another uncommon form of breast carcinoma, mucinous, or colloid, constitutes approximately 1% to 2% of breast cancers.[38] Mucinous carcinoma has a better prognosis than does infiltrating ductal carcinoma.[25] This tumor appears similar to the medullary carcinoma both sonographically and mammographically, but it usually occurs in older women.[49] The sonographic appearance is of a fairly well-defined hypoechoic mass with a homogeneous, low-level internal echogenicity and a lack of significant posterior acoustic attenuation (Fig. 23-19). These features may reflect the large amount of mucin seen microscopically.

Tubular Carcinoma. Occurring approximately as frequently as the mucinous carcinoma, in pure form

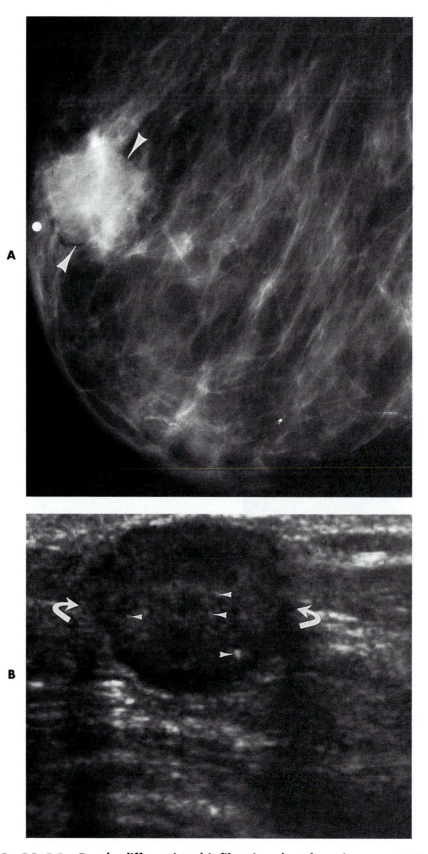

FIG. 23-16. Poorly differentiated infiltrating ductal carcinoma. A, Palpable mass signified by radiopaque marker is lobulated, rounded, but has well-defined angular margins *(arrowheads)* on lateral mammography. **B,** Sonogram shows a heterogeneous, hypoechoic solid mass *(curved arrows)* that is well-marginated and lobulated. Posterior acoustic enhancement is striking in this poorly differentiated infiltrating ductal carcinoma. Microcalcifications, seen embedded in mass, are denoted by arrowheads.

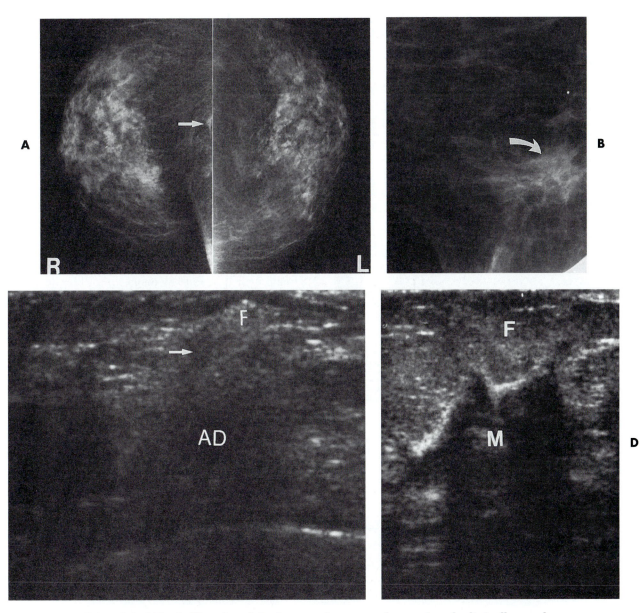

FIG. 23-17. **Infiltrating lobular carcinoma: often missed clinically and mammographically.** **A,** Craniocaudal view of both breasts shows portion of nodular density *(arrow)* in posterior central right breast. **B,** Spot compression magnification view shows wispy area *(arrow)* of parenchymal density in the inframammary fold corresponding to the nodule on the craniocaudal view. **C,** Sonogram of area of mammographic abnormality shows hypoechoic, ill-defined area of architectural distortion (AD) with infiltration *(arrow)* into the adjacent fibroglandular parenchyma (F). US-guided core biopsy confirmed diagnosis of infiltrating lobular carcinoma. **D,** In another patient with vague thickening on self-examination, a mammogram showed dense glandular tissue but no focal mass. Ultrasound demonstrates an extensive hypoechoic angular mass (M) occupying nearly two thirds of the breast. Fibroglandular tissue, F.

these uncommon neoplasms have an excellent prognosis. Mammographically and sonographically, these neoplasms may appear small, with varying degrees of marginal irregularity. Occasionally on the mammogram, long spicules are seen in association with the small mass, but sonographic features are nonspecific (Fig. 23-20).[54,55] An association between the tubular carcinoma and the benign radial scar has been postulated.[56]

Papillary Carcinoma. Occurring most commonly in postmenopausal women, these rare tumors, which may be well-circumscribed mammographically, have a good prognosis, one similar to that of mucinous

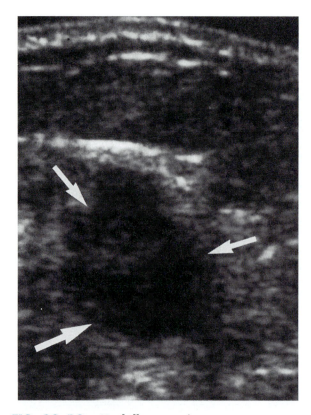

FIG. 23-18. Medullary carcinoma. Sonogram depicts lobulated mass *(arrows)* with ill-defined margins, low-level internal echoes, and a small amount of posterior acoustic enhancement.

or tubular carcinomas.[57-59] Papillary carcinomas may be entirely intraductal or may have areas of invasion.[60] They may be suspected clinically when a bloody nipple discharge is seen, although this sign most often signifies the presence of a benign intraductal papilloma (see Fig. 23-5, *B*). Sonographically, the papillary carcinoma may appear as a solid or complex mass or with solid tissue projecting into a cyst (Fig. 23-21).[61-63]

Benign Masses

Fibroadenoma. Although fibroadenomas are encountered at all ages, the most common mass in a woman under 30 or 35 years old is a fibroadenoma.[59] Fibroadenomas are multiple in 10% to 20% of cases[64,65] and bilateral in approximately 3% or more. Although ductal and lobular carcinomas have been found in or near fibroadenomas, most fibroadenomas do not increase significantly the risk of developing breast cancer.[66] However, complex fibroadenomas containing cysts, sclerosing adenosis, and papillary apocrine changes increase the relative risk by three to four times.[66]

The sonographic features of a fibroadenoma are variable, but in general, fibroadenomas are hypoechoic relative to the fibroglandular parenchyma and isoechoic with fat lobules in the breast (Fig. 23-22).[67] Most of the mass is homogeneous, but, in our experience, heterogeneous regions are commonly present. Usually the mass is oval and sharply marginated, and

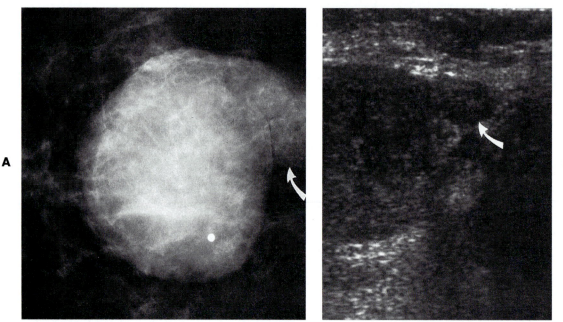

FIG. 23-19. Mucinous (colloid) carcinoma. A, Spot compression mammographic view of palpable (denoted by radiopaque marker) circumscribed mass. A satellite nodule suggestive of a diverticulum is seen laterally *(curved arrow)*. **B,** Sonography of a portion of the mass corresponds well with the mammogram: margins are well defined, and the diverticulum-like satellite *(curved arrow)* is easily seen. This homogeneous mass shows posterior acoustic enhancement.

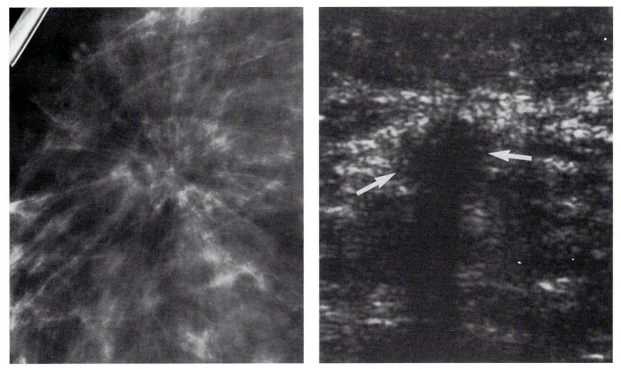

FIG. 23-20. **Tubular carcinoma.** **A,** Magnified mammographic view shows mass with central radiolucent areas and very long radiating spiculations, suggesting radial scar. **B,** Sonogram depicts 0.7-cm, solid, hypoechoic mass with irregular, poorly defined margins *(arrows)* and posterior acoustic attenuation, common features of carcinoma.

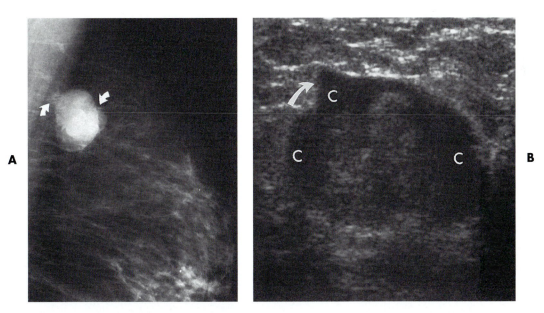

FIG. 23-21. **Papillary carcinoma.** **A,** Mediolateral oblique view of the left breast shows well-circumscribed mass containing area of increased density. Slight marginal irregularity is seen *(arrows)*. **B,** Circumscribed complex mass with anterior protuberance *(curved arrow)*. Central area of echogenicity is surrounded circumferentially by what most likely represents the cystic component (C) of this in situ papillary carcinoma with stromal invasion.

it often has a macrolobulated contour.[13,36] In the 50 fibroadenomas we reviewed retrospectively, all were oval in at least one projection; no fibroadenoma was round in both projections.[41] The long axis of the fibroadenoma has been noted to lie parallel to the skin surface.[13,36] The acoustic attenuation pattern is also variable; most fibroadenomas show some posterior acoustic enhancement, but approximately 30% demonstrate posterior acoustic shadowing that is not caused by calcification.[68]

The clinical management of masses thought to be fibroadenomas depends on the level of clinical concern.[10,69] In a young patient or older woman in whom the mass is not new and who is comfortable with the high probability of benign etiology, observation with short-term, interval follow-up studies (e.g., in 6 months) may be suggested as preferable to excision. The follow-up study may utilize US rather than mammography. Management decisions must involve the patient and consideration of her level of anxiety. If the patient is uneasy, fine-needle aspiration or large-needle core biopsy may increase the level of confidence if the specimen is interpreted as "fibroadenoma" or "consistent with fibroadenoma." A pathologic report of "no malignant cells" may not have the same benign implication because a technical failure, such as missing the mass, can result in the same report.

Phyllodes Tumor. A large, well-circumscribed, lobular mass with rapid growth that occurs in a patient over 30 years of age suggests the possibility of phyllodes tumor. In over 40% of patients, fibroadenomas are also present.[65] Malignant forms of phyllodes tumors, which may metastasize, are identified histologically by mitotic rates exceeding 5 to 10 per high-power field.[65] This solid mass has a nonspecific appearance sonographically. Internal heterogeneity of echogenicity, posterior acoustic enhancement, and hypoechoic clefts may be seen.[70]

Giant Fibroadenoma. These uncommon neoplasms are defined by their large size, typically 5 to 10 cm in diameter.[59,65] If these masses occur in pubescent

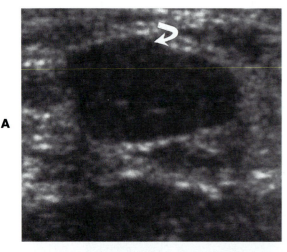

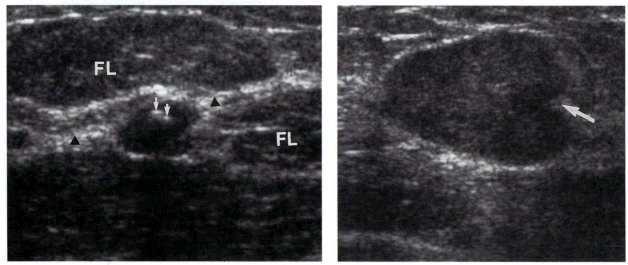

FIG. 23-22. Fibroadenomas: variety of appearances.
A, Oval, hypoechoic mass, long axis parallel to skin. Margins are sharp and thin with mild undulation anteriorly *(curved arrow)*. A few small foci of echogenicity are present internally. No enhancement or shadowing is seen posteriorly. This lesion demonstrates features of a majority of fibroadenomas. **B,** Small fibroadenoma containing calcifications *(arrows)* surrounded by fat lobules (FL) with a small area of fibroglandualr tissue *(arrowheads)* adjacent. Fibroadenoma and fat lobules are isoechoic and similarly shaped; the calcifications aid in distinguishing the mass from the normal fatty tissue. **C,** Typical fibroadenoma with thin, echogenic capsule, orientation parallel to skin, cleft *(arrow)*, slight posterior acoustic enhancement, and mild heterogeneity of internal echoarchitecture. Overall, the fibroadenoma and fat lobules around it are of similar echogenicity.

girls or young women, they may be called juvenile fibroadenomas. These tumors are differentiated from the phyllodes tumor by the younger age of patients (11 to 20 years of age) and the lack of malignant potential, despite very rapid growth that may suggest malignancy. Although they may be multiple and bilateral, one tumor is often dominant. The sonographic appearance is similar to that of a large fibroadenoma with low to medium internal echogenicity and pencil-sharp margins (Fig. 23-23).

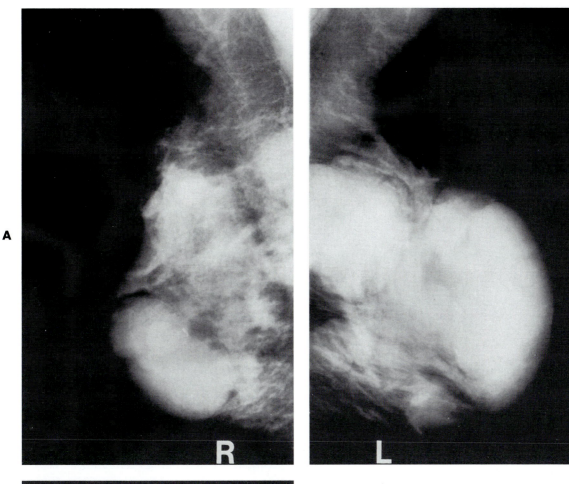

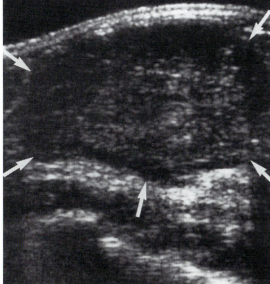

FIG. 23-23. **Giant (juvenile) fibroadenoma in 15-year-old patient.** A and B, Bilateral mammograms show multiple, large, sharply marginated oval masses and small areas of benign-appearing calcification. C, Sonogram of one of the masses demonstrates large, oval, hypoechoic mass *(arrows)* with low-level internal echoes and small amount of posterior acoustic enhancement with normal thickness of the overlying skin.

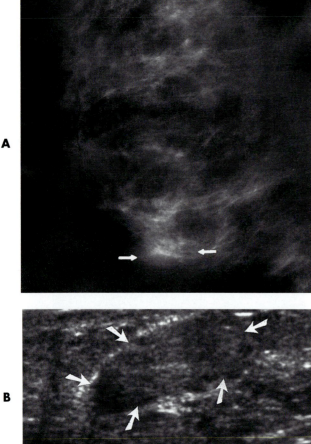

FIG. 23-24. Focal fibrosis. A, Mediolateral oblique mammographic view shows discoid density in the lower breast *(arrows)*. **B,** At sonography, the mass *(arrows)* is also discoid, has benign features, and resembles a fibroadenoma.

Focal Fibrosis. Focal fibrosis is an uncommon, discrete abnormality that is 10% as common as carcinoma.[71] The cause of focal fibrosis is unknown but may relate to postinflammatory or vascular changes. Mammographically, the lesion is a discoid, well-defined soft tissue density. Often one of its margins is angular, and another seems to merge with the adjacent breast parenchyma (Fig. 23-24).[72] Of the eight cases we reviewed, most appeared sonographically as elliptical, hypoechoic, well-defined lesions with no change in posterior acoustic sound transmission.[72] Five or six more recent cases have had similar features. Another author has reported a case of focal fibrosis that is echogenic with posterior acoustic shadowing.[73] Focal fibrosis must be distinguished from **diabetic fibrosis** occurring in long-term-insulin-dependent diabetics. Diabetic fibrosis, at sonography, mimics malignancy and is characterized by hypoechoic masses with jagged, irregular margins and posterior acoustic shadowing.[74]

Hamartoma (Fibroadenolipoma). The hamartoma, or fibroadenolipoma, is a rare benign mass composed of fibrous, epithelial, and lipomatous tissues.[75] Large hamartomas may have a lobulated, cauliflower-like appearance at mammography. Smaller lesions may be oval and well-circumscribed and may contain foci of fatty tissue. A mammogram that shows an encapsulated and partly or fully radiolucent mass is diagnostic of a fat-containing benign tumor such as hamartoma or lipoma. At sonography, hamartomas are heterogeneous with echogenic components representing fat, and they may show posterior acoustic attenuation (Fig. 23-25).[76]

Lipoma. Lipomas occur most frequently in older women, and mammographically, they are radiolucent, thinly encapsulated masses. Unless there is rapid

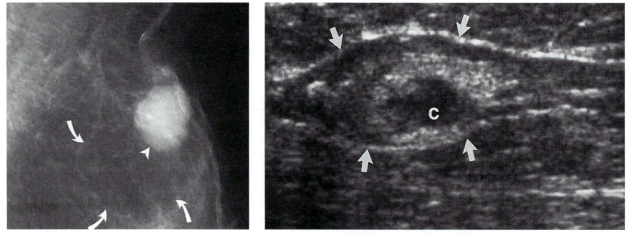

FIG. 23-25. Hamartoma. A, Mammogram of upper breast shows faintly encapsulated *(arrows)* fatty mass containing a benign-appearing component of soft-tissue density *(open arrow)*. **B,** Well-circumscribed, heterogeneous mass *(arrows)* at sonography with echogenic components representing fat. Cysts (C) and other benign entities may also be present. (From Goldberg BB, Pettersson H, ed. *The NICER Year Book 1996: Ultrasonography.* Olso: The NICER Institute; 1996.)

growth, discomfort, or other clinical concerns, fat-containing benign masses such as lipomas and hamartomas require only routine follow-up. Medium-level, homogeneous echoes, and thin capsules characterize these lipomas at US (Fig. 23-26), although sonography is unnecessary in the diagnostic evaluation of lipoma or other fat-containing masses.

Sebaceous (Inclusion) Cysts. Sebaceous cysts, which are sometimes called epidermal inclusion cysts, are usually asymptomatic unless they grow or become infected. They often occur in the inframammary fold, axillary area, or most medial portion of the breasts. On physical examination, an umbilication may be seen in the skin where the tract communicates with the fatty, subcutaneous collection. Mammographically, these lesions are sharply defined and of high radiographic density, and they require removal and capsulectomy. Sonographically, these hypoechoic masses are very well defined, and they have scattered low-level internal echoes and posterior acoustic enhancement (Fig. 23-27). In some cases a central clump of echogenic material is seen. Infected sebaceous cysts may demonstrate marginal irregularity and may be associated with skin thickening. They may resemble superficial carcinomas.

Papilloma. A papilloma is a neoplasm resulting from epithelial proliferation within a lactiferous duct, and papillomas are the most frequent cause of bloody nipple discharge.[77] Solitary intraductal papillomas are not thought to increase the risk of breast cancer significantly.[25] Mammographically, papillomas may be recognized as circumscribed soft-tissue densities often associated with beaded, dilated ducts in the retroareolar area. Sonographically, they may be well-circumscribed solid masses or cystic masses containing solid tissue, similar in appearance to a cystic papillary carcinoma (see Figs. 23-5, *B* and 23-9, *B*).

Galactocele. Galactoceles are cystic masses that contain milk. They are cystic dilatations of ducts that occur during or after lactation, and clinical history offers a clue to the diagnosis.[78] Mammographically, they are well-circumscribed masses of combined soft-tissue density and radiolucency that may represent the fatty nature of the milk. A fat-fluid layer may be seen on a (horizontal beam) 90° lateral mammographic view. The sonographic appearance is nonspecific and reports have described galactoceles variably as echogenic lesions and cystic masses with less through-transmission than expected in simple cysts.[73,79] In our experience, galactoceles have demonstrated fluid-

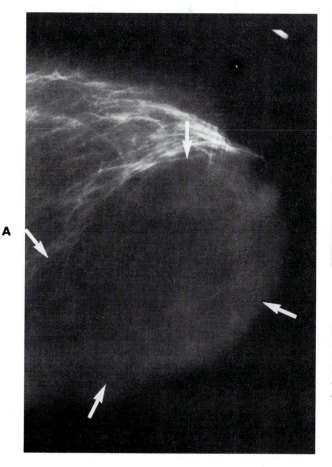

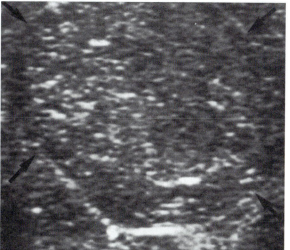

FIG. 23-26. Lipoma. A, Mammogram, which is diagnostic of lipoma, shows large radiolucent mass *(arrows)* over which a few mammary parenchymal elements are draped. **B,** Sonogram shows large, homogeneous, echogenic mass *(arrows)* that is surrounded by thin echogenic capsule.

fluid levels, low-level internal echoes, and debris falling to the lowermost aspect of otherwise simple cysts (Fig. 23-28).

Abscess. Abscesses most frequently occur in the lactating patient, and *Staphylococcus aureus* is the most common offending organism.[80] Abscesses may be found in older women as manifestations of periductal mastitis or as infected cysts. Abscesses are most commonly located in the retroareolar region, but they may also occur away from the nipple or in women with underlying predisposing abnormalities such as diabetes, corticosteroid administration, and other (Fig. 23-29) immunosuppressive conditions. Skin excoriation in severe eczema may provide an entry site for the infectious agent. Sonographic features vary from complex masses with irregular margins to fairly well-circumscribed oval lesions with low-level internal echoes and posterior acoustic enhancement. Needle aspiration can confirm an abscess as well as evacuate it, and follow-up sonography after treatment

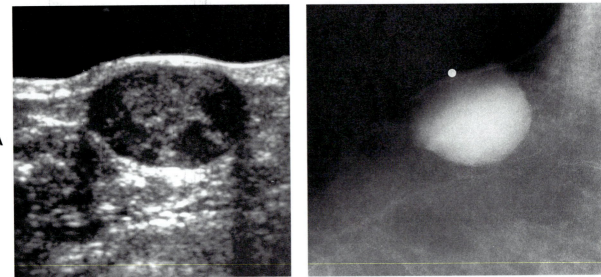

A   B

FIG. 23-27. **Sebaceous or epidermal inclusion cyst.** **A,** Smooth, sharp margins, oval shape, orientation parallel to skin, and very superficial location along with clinical correlation help identify this complex mass with clumped internal echoes and bright posterior acoustic enhancement as a sebaceous cyst. **B,** Mammogram is also characteristic in showing well-defined, circumscribed, high-density mass just beneath the skin. Radiopaque marker indicates that it is palpable.

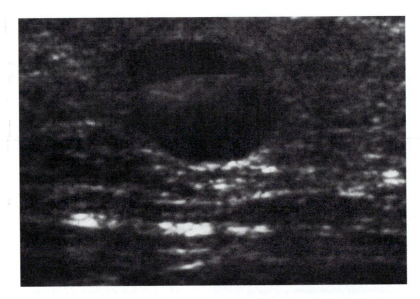

FIG. 23-28. **Galactocele.** Fluid-fluid level is shown in this circumscribed, cystic, milk-filled, painless, mobile mass. Complete evacuation was accomplished with US-guided aspiration. (From Mendelson EB, Tobin CE. US-guided interventions: fine-needle aspiration and large-core needle biopsy. *RSNA Categorical Course in Breast Imaging*; 1995:139-149.)

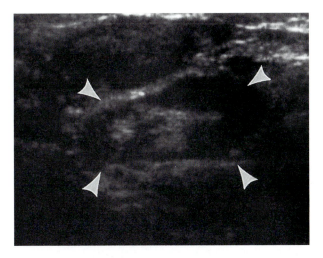

FIG. 23-29. Abscess. Complex mass *(arrowheads)* developed behind nipple in a young woman who attempted to pierce her areola. Percutaneous US-guided aspiration and antibiotic therapy resulted in complete resolution.

should establish resolution. If the lesion has not resolved, biopsy may be indicated to exclude underlying carcinoma.

Radial Scar. A radial scar which, when large, is known as a **complex sclerosing lesion,** is nonpalpable on physical examination, may range in size from microscopic to many centimeters, and at mammography and US mimics spiculated breast carcinoma.[25] Microcalcifications may be present. Mammographically, these elastotic lesions, which entrap ducts centrally, may have central radiolucent areas that suggest the diagnosis. With US, the radial scar may have an irregular margin and posterior acoustic shadowing (Fig. 23-30).[81] These lesions, which may contain a conglomeration of proliferative histologies, have been associated with tubular carcinomas.[56,82] Atypical ductal hyperplasia and ductal carcinoma in situ have also been reported in radial scars, which should be completely excised surgically rather than sampled.[25]

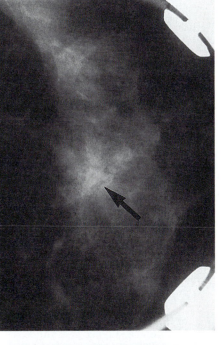

a
A

FIG. 23-30. Radial scar. A, Spot compression magnification craniocaudal view shows suspicious spiculated area *(arrow)* with some radiolucencies. **B,** Irregular margins and shape *(curved arrows)* as well as mild posterior acoustic shadowing suggestive of primary breast carcinoma are seen. **C,** Core biopsy was performed and pathologic results suggested radial scar. Needle *(arrows)* is seen within lesion. Because of the wide variety of proliferative lesions, DCIS or tubular carcinoma must be excluded. These lesions should be excised in their entirety rather than sampled because core biopsies and FNABs may miss significant portions of these complex lesions.

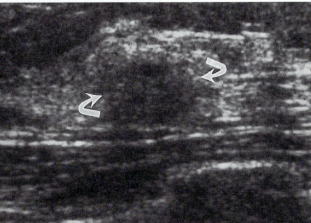

B

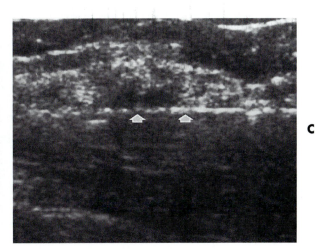

C

INTERVENTIONAL PROCEDURES

Indications and General Principles

Any solitary nonpalpable lesion that may represent a cyst but does not fulfill all of the sonographic cri-

---

INDICATIONS FOR US ASPIRATION OF CYSTS AND CYSTIC MASSES

Masses not fulfilling criteria for simple cysts (Fig. 23-31)

Symptomatic, nonpalpable cysts and some palpable cysts where documentation of evacuation is desirable (Fig. 23-32)

Suspected abscess or infected cyst

Palpable or nonpalpable cysts where imaging guidance is required to avoid complications (e.g., augmented breast or lesion near chest wall)

---

teria should be aspirated using sonographic guidance (see box). Low-level echoes are often present in cysts, and although the lesion will be recognized as a cyst in many instances, aspiration may be required to confirm the diagnosis. If movement of the low-level echogenic contents is observed when pressure is applied or when the patient changes position, a more confident diagnosis of a cyst can be made. Symptomatic relief may be provided by aspiration of cysts causing pain or under tension.[21]

There is debate about the need for ultrasound characterization of palpable masses as well as about the need for guidance when aspirating palpable masses that may be cysts.[83] Proponents of aspiration using palpation suggest that placing a needle into the mass may be more cost-effective, in that both diagnosis and therapy can be provided (see Fig. 23-32). Advocates of imaging guidance cite the importance of documenting complete evacuation of a cyst as well as the importance of continuous visualization of the needle,

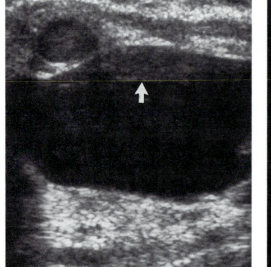

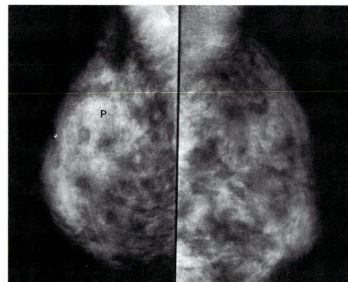

FIG. 23-31. Simple vs. complex cysts: importance of technique. A, Larger cyst fulfills criteria for a simple cyst. The anterior band of echoes *(arrow)* is recognizable as a reverberation artifact. With the focal zone set in the near field, the smaller anterior mass could be interpreted as a complex cyst or solid lesion. At aspiration, it proved to be a simple cyst whose internal echoes were attributable to technical factors. **B,** Bilateral mediolateral oblique mammogram shows dense nodular tissue. Palpable abnormality is in upper right breast (P). **C,** Sonogram of area shows a complex focus of tissue with ducts *(arrowheads)* and small cysts (C) surrounded by echogenic glandular tissue *(arrows)*. Overall impression was that the mass was probably benign. Although aspiration and core biopsies were diagnostic, the patient requested surgical removal and the histology included chronic cystic disease, ductal hyperplasia, and sclerosing adenosis.

which helps to insure safety. Imaging guidance is especially important for lesions located near the chest wall, in the far medial and far lateral aspects of breasts, and near the axilla, and for cysts in patients who have undergone augmentation with silicone prostheses. Symptomatic nonpalpable cysts should be aspirated using US or other imaging guidance. Postaspiration sonography will document complete evacuation or presence of any residual fluid. Should the lesion prove to be solid on attempted evacuation, the aspirate should be sent for cytologic evaluation or large-needle core biopsy should be considered. Core biopsy of solid masses that are probably benign (BI-RADS Category 3)[32] may be performed when short-term, interval follow-up is unacceptable to patient or referring physician.

Percutaneous tissue sampling may be performed for diagnosis of solid masses with indeterminate features and other indications (see box).

Percutaneous procedures may be selected in preference to surgical biopsies when the total number of procedures will be reduced or when the morbidity and cost of a needle biopsy are less than those of open biopsy, and the reliability is as great.[84] If a spiculated mass is found at mammography in a patient who has had no previous surgical procedure or trauma in that area, and the presumptive diagnosis is infiltrating carcinoma, the patient and surgeon may elect definitive breast-conserving therapy without prior histologic diagnosis by using frozen section. Here a needle biopsy would add to, rather than reduce, the overall number of procedures. Where there is greater doubt about the diagnosis or multicentric distribution of malignancy would render the patient ineligible for breast conser-

---

INDICATIONS FOR PERCUTANEOUS SAMPLING OF SOLID MASSES

As a replacement for surgical biopsy for diagnosis only
Lesions highly suggestive of malignancy (BI-RADS™ Category 5)[49] so that definitive treatment options can be determined
Multiple suspicious or indeterminate masses to establish or exclude multicentricity
Suspicious masses (BI-RADS™ Category 4)[49]
   Most important group with broad range in chance of malignancy (e.g., 25% to 90%) (see Fig. 23-10)
Probably benign masses (BI-RADS™ Category 3)[49] when patient anxiety is high and procedure is requested to confirm benign etiology

---

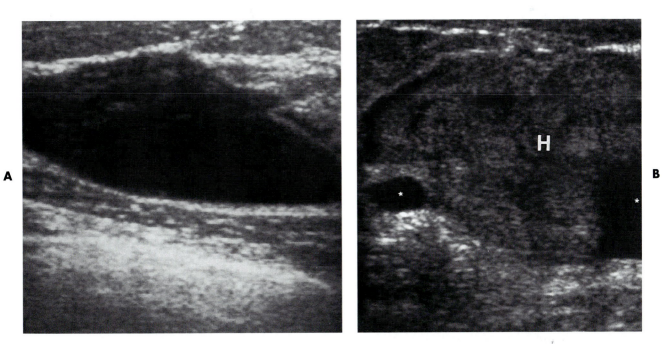

FIG. 23-32. Hematoma after cyst aspiration. **A,** Painful, simple cyst was aspirated with US guidance. **B,** Cyst refilled within a few minutes despite pressure applied to the area. The fresh hemorrhage (H) mimics a solid mass. Two cystic components (*) remain. A hematoma may require 2 weeks to resolve, interfering with the diagnosis of a simple cyst. To avoid such anxiety-producing diagnostic ambiguities (which may also result in additional unnecessary interventions), masses should be imaged prior to rather than after aspiration.

COMPLICATIONS OF US-GUIDED INTERVENTIONAL PROCEDURES

Bleeding

Action: Obtain a history of anticoagulation, chronic aspirin use, or blood dyscrasias; discuss brief interruption of medication (e.g., coumadin) with referring physicians; obtain laboratory assays in individual cases.

Infection

Action: Mention infection to patient as a potential but uncommon complication of breast interventional procedures (antibiotic prophylaxis for patients with rheumatic heart disease or mitral valve prolapse has not been deemed necessary).

Localized Pain

Action: Inform patient that tenderness and ecchymosis are common and are ordinarily self-limited; tell her to expect discoloration of the skin of the breast and some discomfort that may be treated with a nonsteroidal antiinflammatory drug or acetaminophen; provide patient with an ice pack immediately after the procedure.

Pneumothorax

Action: Use technique of needle entry from the short axis of the transducer, in which the needle passes through the acoustic beam along the long axis of the probe (see Fig. 23-33); avoid steep approaches in the medial aspect of the breast, near the chest wall, where the pleura is only a short distance from the aspirating needle.

From Mendelson EB, Tobin CE. US-guided interventions: fine-needle aspiration and large-core needle biopsy. *RSNA Categorical Course in Breast Imaging;* 1995:139-149.

vation, large-needle core biopsy or fine-needle aspiration biopsy would be justified.

Patient Preparation, Equipment, and Technique

Once need for an interventional procedure has been established, the efficiency, safety, comfort, and cost of the particular method should be considered. There is no single correct method for performing procedures, and free-hand, sonographically-directed needle placement utilizes the same principles for fine-needle aspiration of cysts and solid lesions, presurgical localization, and core biopsy. The initial steps for all percutaneous procedures are the same, as are the mechanics of freehand US-guided needle passage.

The patient's informed consent is obtained before any of the procedures is performed.[85] The procedure and its purpose should be described and the complications mentioned (see box above). Although minor bleeding may occur, to date we have had no significant hematomas attributable to large-needle core biopsy.

The patient should indicate her understanding of what will follow.

After the patient assumes the appropriate position for the procedure, the breast should be cleansed with alcohol and Betadine (povidone iodine; Purdue Frederick, Norwalk, Conn.). The probe should be disinfected with alcohol; however, it should not be soaked in alcohol. If the manufacturer suggests that alcohol not be used with a particular probe, a solution such as Cidex (Johnson and Johnson, Arlington, Tex.) can be painted on the transducer face and the probe housing. Although some radiologists prefer to cover the probe with a sterile plastic sheath or wrap, it is not necessary to sheath a transducer if it is carefully prepared, as above.[86] Sheathing the probe may degrade the image and impair manual control of the breast and instrument, making the procedure more difficult to accomplish. The operator and any assistant must wear gloves at all times, primarily for their own protection.

Techniques of Percutaneous Needle Passage. No single correct method exists for performing these procedures, and freehand US-directed needle placement uses the same principles for fine-needle aspiration of cysts and solid lesions, presurgical localization, and core biopsy. Selection of a technique to guide the procedure should reflect the location and nature of the lesion and the particular procedure being performed (Fig. 23-33). It may be easier to perform aspiration, biopsy, or localization of a deeply situated small mass in a large, fatty breast with mammographic (fenestrated compression plate or stereotaxic) guidance than with US guidance. For safe, US-guided aspiration of lesions near the chest wall or adjacent to the implant shell of an augmented breast, the needle shaft must be visualized during the entire procedure.

With this technique, in which the needle enters from the short axis of the transducer (parallel to the sound beam), the mass can be positioned anywhere along the length of the transducer (see Fig. 23-33, *A*). The more horizontal the plane of entry, the better the needle shaft will be seen. It is important that the needle tip not veer from the narrow acoustic beam. If the needle angles to the right or to the left instead of remaining midplane, its tip will no longer be seen. If the lesion is deep, it is best to position the lesion at some distance from the entry point of the needle so a more horizontal approach can be used. Superficial lesions can be positioned near the end of the transducer, and the needle can be directed more vertically into the lesion.

If the lesion is far from the chest wall and the breast is stabilized, presurgical localization and cyst aspiration can sometimes be performed with a more steeply vertical approach from the midportion of the long axis of the transducer (see Fig. 23-33, *B*). This route of entry may offer the shortest distance to the lesion, which the surgeon may prefer. The use of this second technique is limited; the approach diagrammed in Fig.

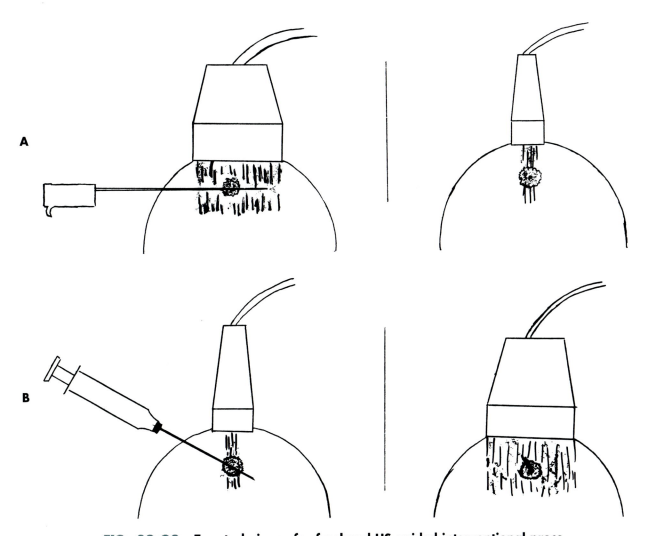

FIG. 23-33. Two techniques for freehand US-guided interventional procedures. **A,** The principal method for these procedures is a horizontal or shallow-angled approach from the end of the linear transducer which minimizes the risk of complications. This technique is suited for core biopsy, fine-needle aspiration biopsy, lesions near the chest wall or an implant shell, or at any other time when it is necessary to visualize the needle shaft and tip during passage and lesion entry. To be visualized, the needle must remain within the scan plane issuing from the central portion of the transducer as shown. **B,** Presurgical localization and some cyst aspirations may also be performed with a more direct vertical approach in which only an echogenic dot is seen as the acoustic beam transects the needle. The needle shaft is not seen, but the distance between the skin entry site and the lesion may be shorter and thus preferred by the surgeon. Here, the lesion is imaged at the midpoint of the long axis of the transducer face, and its depth can be measured. The angle required for the needle's passage can be estimated fairly accurately after only a little experience. (From Mendelson EB, Tobin CE. US-guided interventions: fine-needle aspiration and large-core needle biopsy. *RSNA Categorical Course in Breast Imaging*; 1995:139-149.)

23-1 should, in general, be selected because of its safety and its ability to allow visualization of the needle shaft during the entire procedure.

Linear transducers of 7.0 MHz or greater frequency are best for freehand procedures. Needle guides are offered with some transducers, but we have not found that these guides decrease the difficulty of the procedure or increase its accuracy.

Difficulties with visualization of the needle tip have led to the development of coated, pitted, or scored needle tips to increase echogenicity. We have found no

significant advantage in using these needles. For visualization, the needle must pass within the scan plane; if it remains in the scan plane, an ordinary needle of any caliber will be seen.

A number of options exist for staffing these procedures. One person may hold the probe and perform the procedure. Assistants may help to hold the probe. If an assistant scans, the radiologist performing the procedure has both hands available for use.

One of the most important requirements for success is immobilizing the lesion under the transducer. A second requirement is placement of the probe to allow the direction of needle entry and its passage to be monitored in relation to the anticipated path of the acoustic beam.

Techniques for Specific Procedures

Cyst Aspiration. The area of the cyst should be fixed manually so the needle will penetrate the wall of the lesion instead of pushing it out of the scan plane. Initially, a needle of small caliber may be selected. If the contents of the cyst are of low viscosity, evacuation of the cyst will be rapid and successful. If a tough, fibrous rind encases the cyst, the needle may be deflected. A stiffer, larger-bore needle will be required to enter thick-walled lesions that resist needle penetration. If the first attempt to aspirate with a 21-gauge needle proves unsuccessful, a second attempt should be made with an 18-gauge needle. Alternatively, 19- or 18-gauge needles may be used at the outset to avoid a second needle puncture.

If the cyst is very large, use of a 20-mL syringe and connecting tubing is efficient for cyst evacuation. For smaller cysts, a hypodermic needle and syringe, aspirating gun, and vacuum tube of the type used for venipuncture work well.

We aspirate during continuous scanning, without removing the probe from the site until the procedure is complete. US images are recorded on film before and immediately after the procedure, usually with the needle still in place. After aspiration, a lateral mammogram or other view that best shows the concordance of mammographic and US abnormalities is obtained.

With respect to disposition of cyst fluid, many radiologists and clinicians discard yellow or serous aspirates and greenish fluids suggestive of fibrocystic change. Any blood or other unusual cyst aspirate must be analyzed cytologically. If the aspirate appears purulent, microbiologic study (culture and sensitivity) should be requested in addition to cytologic study. Lesions should be evacuated, and drainage catheters may be placed in abscesses if considerable residuum is present after incomplete aspiration.

Large-Core Needle Biopsy. Large-core needle biopsy has become an important breast diagnostic procedure in the last several years. Cytopathologic expertise in the United States varies; the result is that insufficient samples have been reported in up to 25% of cases in some series. Therefore, for nonsurgical tissue sampling, percutaneous large-core needle biopsy is being used with increasing frequency.[87] Both stereotaxic mammography and US have proved to be accurate in guiding needle placement, and each has advantages. Investigations have shown reliability of large-core needle sampling as a substitute for surgical biopsy.[88] Currently, core biopsies are being performed with spring-activated guns and a 14-gauge needle. For the fatty-fibroglandular consistency of breast tissue, samples obtained with 14-gauge and larger needles have greater cohesiveness for histopathologic analysis than do specimens obtained with 18-gauge and smaller needles, which are less satisfactory.[89] Large-core needle biopsies are also performed with mechanized 11-gauge and 14-gauge cutting needles (Fig. 23-34). Entry of the specimen into the collecting chamber is facilitated by vacuum.

US-guided large-core needle biopsy has the same general advantages as other US-guided procedures. There is choice in positioning the patient. The supine or supine-oblique position used for the procedure may be more comfortable for the patient than the prone or seated position required for stereotaxic mammographic core biopsies. Real-time observation of needle passage and its entry into the lesion cannot be achieved with stereotaxic methods, and US procedures may be accomplished more quickly than stereotaxically guided biopsies, even when the latter are digitally assisted.

Questions have arisen regarding the possibility of needle-tract seeding after large-core needle biopsy. One case of needle-tract seeding of a mucinous carcinoma after core biopsy has been reported.[90] Viability of tumor cells in the needle tract is unknown, and the spread of disease or carcinomatosis has not been an issue with percutaneous biopsy of the lungs and abdominal organs, which has been performed for many years.

The general technique for US-guided core biopsy is diagrammed (see Fig. 23-33, A) and has been described above. Approximately 2 to 5 mL of 1% lidocaine is used. A lidocaine or saline channel from the skin to the lesion can be used to indicate the angle of entry of the 14-gauge needle and to ease the initial passage of the 14-gauge or larger needle, which is sometimes associated with resistance. Bicarbonate mixed with the lidocaine may prevent the burning sensation associated with the local anesthetic.[91]

A small skin nick is made, wide enough to allow a 14-gauge needle to pass without catching at the skin. Ordinarily only one skin nick is necessary. The US-guided needle can be directed to sample areas of the mass. Coaxial systems for use with US-guided core biopsies are also available.[92]

With US visualization of its passage, the needle should be directed toward the lesion. The gun should be fired at a distance from the mass that takes into account the size of the lesion, the location of the sampling area (0.4 cm from the tip of the needle), the 1.7-cm to 1.9-cm length of the sampling area, and the thrust of the needle when the gun is fired (2.2 to 2.3 cm with the "long throw" needles that are currently preferred).[93]

Place each specimen into jars of 5% formalin fixative. Do not immerse the needle tip in formalin if the needle will be used to obtain additional samples. The number of passes required to yield a definitive diagnosis can be determined by working with the pathology department. For masses, four to six passes

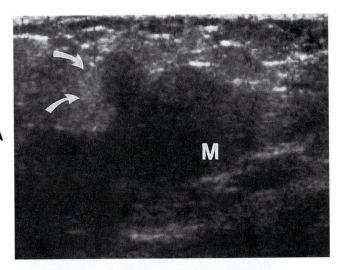

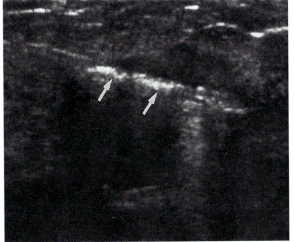

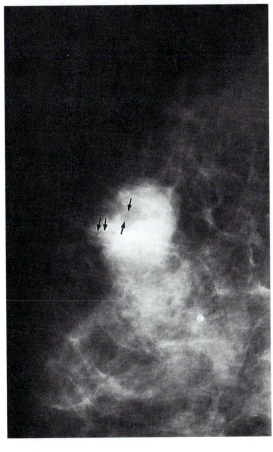

FIG. 23-34. Large-needle core biopsy. A, Suspicious mass (M) with echogenic rim *(curved arrow)* and protuberant knobby satellite. **B,** To obtain a histologic diagnosis prior to selection of definitive therapy, large-needle core biopsy with a 14-gauge needle (vacuum technique) was performed. Cutting edge of needle *(arrows)* within mass is brightly echogenic. **C,** Post–core-biopsy lateral view mammogram shows mass with minimal postprocedural stranding and a small foci of air *(arrows)* at sampling site. No hematoma is present.

are ordinarily made. A greater number of passes are made for microcalcifications.[94] Core biopsies for microcalcifications are often performed stereotaxically, although some microcalcifications, particularly when embedded in a mass, can be seen and targeted with US.

Fine-Needle Aspiration Biopsy. If no fluid is obtained from a mass that might have represented a complex cyst, a slide should be made of the needle contents for cytopathologic evaluation. If the cytologic preparation is inadequate or the interpretation not definitive, a new solid mass should undergo core biopsy or be excised surgically.

The success of fine-needle aspiration biopsy (FNAB) depends on the following six factors:
1. Familiarity with the US appearance of many breast lesions;
2. Experience with the use of US to guide procedures;
3. Accurate placement of the needle into the periphery, the center, or any other area of the lesion desired;
4. Effective aspiration technique to obtain sufficient cellular material unadulterated with blood;
5. Immediate preparation of slides according to the preferences of the cytopathologist (if a cytopathologist or cytotechnologist is present, the sufficiency

of the samples can be confirmed prior to the conclusion of the procedure); and

6. Experience of the cytopathologist in evaluating breast lesions, which should at least match that of the radiologist doing the procedure.

By means of one of the two freehand approaches described above, short excursions into the lesion should be made with a 21- to 23-gauge needle and syringe guided by US, by applying negative pressure. These brief but numerous up-and-down excursions should allow material from the mass to enter the needle. If blood is seen, the pass should be concluded and the slide made.

A modification of this technique involves the use of an aspirating gun. Many of these guns take 10-mL syringes, are easy to use, and allow even the smallest hand to exert sufficient negative pressure to collect the aspirate.

Another method involves use of a 23- or 25-gauge needle without a syringe. The same short excursions are made into the lesion, and they cause cells to enter the needle through capillary action.[95] A syringe containing a few milliliters of air should then be attached to the needle and the contents of the needle expelled onto a slide to be prepared as described above.

Still another technique makes use of a coaxial needle apparatus with a 19-gauge outer cannula placed at the edge of the lesion. A smaller (21-gauge) aspirating needle is then introduced through the longer cannula to sample the lesion.

FNAB performed by experienced mammographers or sonologists and interpreted by seasoned cytopathologists should provide reliable diagnoses of malignancy, with no false-positive findings. To avoid sampling error and false-negative results, certain fibrotic lesions, infiltrating lobular carcinomas, and abnormalities in areas of prior radiation are better sampled with large-needle core biopsy.

Presurgical Localization. An important procedure that can also be performed with US guidance is presurgical localization of needle hook wires (Fig. 23-35).[96] US has several advantages over the use of a fenestrated mammographic plate for this procedure. The patient is often in a supine-oblique or supine position, as for surgery, and frequently the US approach uses the shortest distance from the skin to the lesion, an approach ordinarily preferred by surgeons. Either of the two methods described (see Fig. 23-33) can be used.

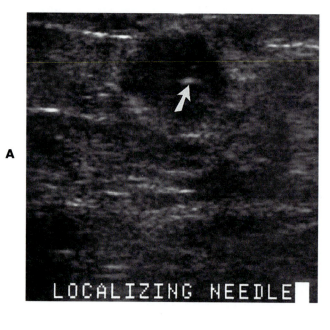

A

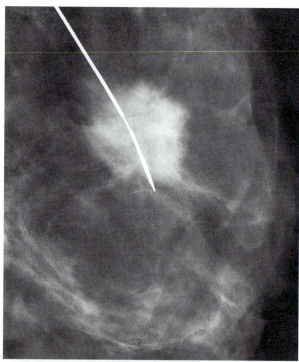

B

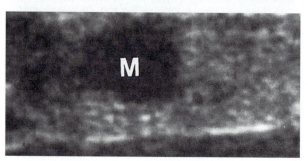

C

FIG. 23-35. US-guided presurgical localization.
A, Using the more vertical method of needle passage (see Fig. 23-33, *B*), only a portion of the hook wire *(arrow)* is visible in the malignant-appearing mass. **B,** Specimen radiography shows spiculated mass with tip of hook wire projecting over cancer. **C,** Specimen sonography can also be performed to document presence of the mass, M, within the excised tissue. Linear echoes are from bottom of specimen container.

US guidance is indicated for lesions that are inaccessible to mammographic fenestrated-plate localization, such as those that are high in the axillary tail of the breast or situated far posteriorly and for any masses or other lesions that can be imaged with US. The patient need not be supine or in an oblique position. The patient may be seated or standing if the lesion is best seen and approached in those positions. If the lesion is well circumscribed and hypoechoic and might represent an atypical cyst, it is better to remove the hook wire from the needle before the needle is placed. If fluid emerges from the needle, a syringe can be attached and the lesion evacuated.

If one is certain that the needle has been correctly placed, the hook wire can be deployed in the tissue. Alternatively, mammographic confirmation of the location of the needle can be obtained before the wire is hooked.

Fully labeled, craniocaudal and lateral mammograms that show the location of the hook wire are to be obtained and sent to the surgeon.

As is true of all nonpalpable lesions localized prior to surgery, an image of the specimen is essential. Mammographic localization requires a radiograph of the specimen. With US, images of the specimen can be obtained with mammography or US or both. Even if the lesion is not seen at mammography, a radiograph of the specimen may be helpful. With the tighter compression and better magnification that is possible for a tissue specimen, an abnormality can sometimes be seen that was not perceptible on preoperative mammograms. Specimen findings should be reported to the surgeon in the operating room prior to closure of the incision.

Dexterity with US guidance of breast interventional procedures will allow the radiologist to be flexible and versatile when selecting nonsurgical alternatives for diagnosis and management of breast conditions. The expected result should be an improvement in the efficiency and cost-effectiveness of patient care.[84]

TRAUMA AND POSTOPERATIVE ALTERATIONS

In breast trauma for which mammography cannot be performed because of breast contusion and pain, sonography can depict the complex collections of varying echogenicity, depending on the acuteness of injury. The outlines of the hemorrhagic areas may be rounded or oval but are often jagged where bleeding has dissected the tissue planes. If there is need to image the patient, the changes can be tracked sonographically until a mammogram can be performed without severe discomfort. As hematomas resolve, areas of scarring and fat necrosis may develop.

Sonography is of particular benefit in the patient who has had **surgical augmentation**. Mammography may be limited, and ultrasound can be a useful supplement.[44,45] In addition to parenchymal abnormalities, defects, loculations, leakages, and contractures involving the prosthesis may be diagnosed with ultrasound. Extracapsular rupture or rupture into the breast substance or axilla is seen as amorphous echogenicity, "echogenic noise," or a "snowstorm" pattern of echoes (Fig. 23-36).[97,98] For diagnosis of intracapsular rupture, MRI has greater sensitivity and

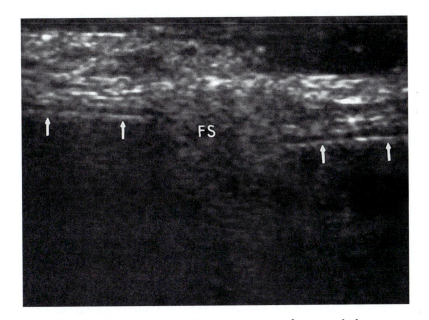

FIG. 23-36. Extracapsular implant rupture: characteristic appearance. Amorphous focus of free silicone (FS) lying in the tissues outside of the shell *(arrows)* of the single lumen silicone prosthesis. Although the echogenicity of the silicone diminishes distally, the silicone obscures visualization of deeper structures.

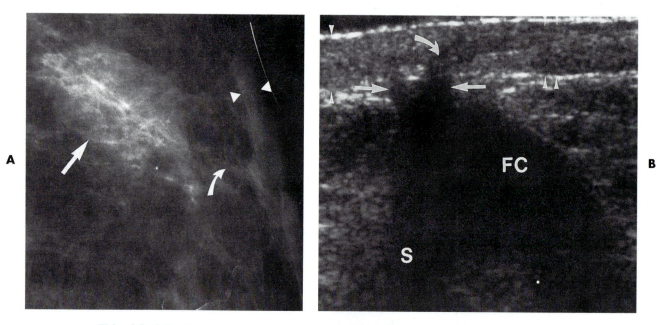

FIG. 23-37. **Breast conservation therapy: postoperative fluid collection.** A, 18 months after lumpectomy and radiation therapy for infiltrating ductal carcinoma, a tangential magnified mammographic view shows thickened skin *(arrowheads)* at the incision site (wire taped to skin) and an elliptical soft-tissue density at the site of tumor removal *(arrow)*. Tract from incision site to tumor bed *(curved arrow)* is seen. B, Correlative sonogram shows fluid collection (FC) with some marginal irregularity *(arrows)* where fibrotic change is occurring *(arrows)*. Thickened skin related to the radiation therapy can be appreciated with US *(arrowheads)*. These collections resolve slowly within a year or two and are replaced by scarring, which is associated with posterior acoustic shadowing (S). Tract from incision site to tumor bed *(curved arrow)* is seen.

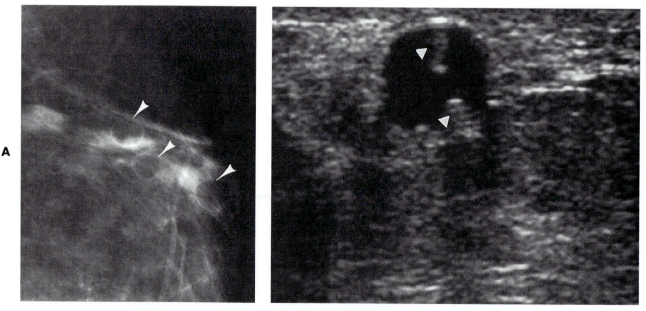

FIG. 23-38. **Oil cysts and fat necrosis after breast surgery.** A, Mammographic view of circumscribed, round radiolucent areas *(arrowheads)* developing following procedure. These oil cysts will resorb, calcify, or become areas of fibrosis and fat necrosis. B, Typical sonographic appearance of an oil cyst, here containing some debris *(arrowheads)*. The cystic lesion will develop irregular margins and posterior acoustic shadowing as fat necrosis and scarring develop.

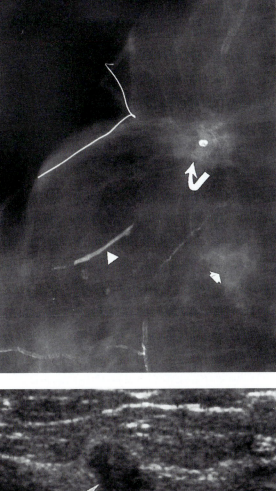

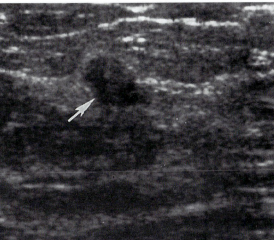

FIG. 23-39. Tumor recurrence of infiltrating ductal carcinoma 5 years after lumpectomy and radiation therapy. A, Mammographic tangential view shows incision site marked with wire, lumpectomy site with scarring and benign calcification *(curved arrow)*, a sutural calcification *(arrowhead)*, and a small density near the lumpectomy site *(short arrow)*. **B,** Sonogram of small density depicts irregularly shaped hypoechoic mass *(arrow)* situated among fat lobules. US-guided core biopsy established tumor recurrence.

specificity than US[99] although US has a high negative predictive value for rupture.[100]

Along with mammography, sonography is also sometimes used to evaluate the site of a lumpectomy for breast carcinoma.[44] The clinical and mammo-

graphic signs of recurrent carcinoma can be similar to postoperative and postirradiation changes, including mass, edema, skin thickening, and calcification.[45] The cavity left by the tumor's removal often fills with fluid. These fluid collections resolve over a period of 6 to 18 months, and sonography can be used to confirm that a palpable or mammographic mass is fluid-filled as well as to document its reduction over time (Fig. 23-37).[44,45,101] Later, with the maturation of fat necrosis (Fig. 23-38) and other postsurgical changes, as scarring occurs, the margins of a postoperative collection will become irregular and an acoustic shadow will originate from the region.[44,45] Once the scar has developed, the detection of a new, enlarging, or more nodular mass at that site suggests the possibility of local tumor recurrence (Fig. 23-39).

REFERENCES

1. Adler DD, Wahl RL. New methods for imaging the breast: techniques, findings and potential. *AJR* 1995;164:19-30.
2. Tabar L, Fagerberg CJG, Gad A et al. Reduction in mortality from breast cancer after mass screening with mammography. *Lancet* 1985;1:829-832.
3. Feig SA. Methods to identify benefit from mammographic screening of women aged 40-49 years. *Radiology* 1996;201:309-316.
4. Kopans DB. Mammography screening and the controversy concerning women aged 40 to 49. *Radiol Clin North Am* 1995;33:1273-1290.
5. Jackson VP. The current role of ultrasonography in breast imaging. *Radiol Clin North Am* 1995;33:1161-1168.
6. Jackson VP. Role of US in breast imaging. *Radiology* 1990;177:305-311.
7. Monsees BS. Evaluation of breast microcalcifications. *Radiol Clin North Am* 1995;33:1109-1121.
8. Dempsey PJ. Breast sonography: historical perspective, clinical applications and image interpretation. *Ultrasound Q* 1988;6:69-90.
9. Rubin E, Dempsey PJ, Pile NS et al. Needle-localization biopsy of the breast: impact of a selective core needle biopsy program on yield. *Radiology* 1995;195:627.

Indications

10. Feig SA. The role of ultrasound in a breast imaging center. *Semin US CT MR* 1989;10:90-105.

Equipment

11. Jackson VP, Kelly-Fry E, Rothschild PA et al. Automated breast sonography using a 7.5 MHz PVDF transducer: preliminary clinical evaluation. *Radiology* 1986;159:679-684.
12. Bassett LW, Kimme-Smith C. Breast sonography: technique, equipment and normal anatomy. *Semin US CT MR* 1989;10:82-89.
13. Stavros AT, Thickman D, Rapp CL et al. Solid breast nodules: use of sonography to distinguish between benign and malignant lesions. *Radiology* 1995;196:123-134.
14. Cosgrove DO, Bamber JC, Davey JB et al. Color Doppler signals from breast tumors. Work in progress. *Radiology* 1990;176:175.
15. Cosgrove DO, Kedar BP, Bamber JC et al. Breast diseases: color Doppler US in differential diagnosis. *Radiology* 1993;189:99.

16. McNicholas MMJ, Mercer PM, Miller JC et al. Color Doppler sonography in the evaluation of palpable breast masses. *AJR* 1993;161:765.

17. Minasian H, Bamber JC. A preliminary assessment of an ultrasonic Doppler method for the study of blood flow in human breast cancer. *Ultrasound Med Biol* 1982;8:357.

18. Schoenberger SG, Sutherland CM, Robinson AE. Breast neoplasms: duplex sonographic imaging as an adjunct in diagnosis. *Radiology* 1988;168:665-668.

19. Kedar RP, Cosgrove D, McCready VR et al. Microbubble contrast agent for color Doppler US: effect on breast masses. Work in progress. *Radiology* 1996;198:679-686.

Examination Technique

20. Rubin E, Miller VE, Berland LL et al. Hand-held real-time breast sonography. *AJR* 1985;144:623-627.

21. Hilton SVW, Leopold GR, Olson LK et al. Real-time breast sonography: application in 300 consecutive patients. *AJR* 1986;147:479-486.

Documentation

22. *ACR Standard for Performance of the Breast Ultrasound Examination.* Reston, Va: American College of Radiology; 1995:209-211.

Sonographic Anatomy

23. Kopans DB, Mever JE, Proppe KH. Double line of skin thickening on sonograms of the breast. *Radiology* 1981;141:485-487.

24. Spencer GM, Rubens DJ, Roach DJ. Hypoechoic fat: sonographic pitfall. *AJR* 1995;164:1277.

25. Sewell CW. Pathology of benign and malignant breast disorders. *Radiol Clin North Am* 1995;33:1067-1080.

26. Tobin CE, Hendrix TM, Geyer SJ et al. Breast imaging case of the day. *Radiographics* 1996;16:1225-1226.

27. Rosen PP. *Breast Pathology* Philadelphia: Lippincott-Raven; 1997:1-15.

28. Yang WT, Ahuja A, Tang A et al. Ultrasonographic demonstration of normal axillary lymph nodes: a learning curve. *J Ultrasound Med* 1995;14:823-827.

29. Gordon PB, Gilks B. Sonographic appearance of normal intramammary lymph nodes. *J Ultrasound Med* 1988;7:545-548.

30. Chan INV, Troupin RH, Yeh I-T. Solid axillary masses: attempts at sonographic differentiation of an axillary lymph node from fibroadenoma. *Breast Dis* 1989;2:187-194.

An Approach to Evaluating Masses

31. Mendelson EB, Tobin CE, Merritt CRB et al. Marginal analysis of breast masses with high resolution US. *Radiology* 1994;193(P)(suppl):177.

32. *Breast Imaging Reporting and Data System (BI-RADS™).* Reston, Va: American College of Radiology; 1993:15.

Cysts

33. Moskowitz M. Predictive value of certain mammographic signs in screening for breast cancer. *Cancer* 1983;51:1007-1011;(ab) 149:888.

34. Garra BS, Cespedes EI, Ophir J et al. Elastography of breast lesions: initial clinical results. *Radiology* 1997;202:79-86.

Solid and Mixed Masses

35. *The American Cancer Society: Breast Cancer Facts and Figures 1996.* Atlanta: American Cancer Society; 1996:1.

36. Fornage BD, Lorigan JG, Andry E. Fibroadenoma of the breast: sonographic appearance. *Radiology* 1989;172:671.

37. Jackson VP. Sonography of malignant breast disease. *Semin US CT MR* 1989;10:119-131.

38. Cole-Beuglet C, Soriano RZ, Kurtz AB et al. Ultrasound analysis of 104 primary breast carcinomas classified according to histopathologic type. *Radiology* 1983;147:191-196.

39. Cole-Beuglet C. Sonographic manifestation of malignant breast disease. *Semin Ultrasound* 1982;3:51-57.

40. Mendelson EB, Bohm-Velez M, Bhagwanani DG et al. Sonographic spectrum of fibroadenomas: a guide to clinical management. Paper presented at the Radiological Society of North America Annual Meeting. Chicago; 1988.

41. Harper AP, Kelly-Fry E, Noe JS et al. Ultrasound in the evaluation of solid breast masses. *Radiology* 1983;146:731-736.

42. Logan WW, Hoffman HY. Diabetic fibrous disease. *Radiology* 1989;172:667-670.

43. Tobin CE, Hendrix TM, Geyer SJ et al. Breast imaging case of the day. *Radiographics* 1996;16:983-985.

44. Mendelson EB. Imaging the post-surgical breast. *Semin US CT MR* 1989;10:154-170.

45. Mendelson EB. Evaluation of the postoperative breast. *Radiol Clin North Am* 1992;30:107-138.

46. Tavassoli FA. *Pathology of the Breast.* Norwalk, Conn.: Appleton and Lange; 1992:399-403.

47. Sickles EA. Management of lesions appearing probably benign at mammography. In: *Radiological Diagnosis of Breast Diseases.* Berlin: Springer-Verlag; 1997:168.

48. Lanyi M. Differential Diagnosis of Microcalcifications. In: Friedrich M, Sickles EA, eds. *Radiological Diagnosis of Breast Diseases.* Berlin: Springer-Verlag; 1997:89-136.

49. Tavassoli FA. *Pathology of the Breast.* Norwalk, Conn.: Appleton and Lange; 1992:294-347.

50. Mendelson EB, Tobin CE, Merritt CRB et al. Marginal analysis of breast masses with high resolution US (abstract). *Radiology* 1994;193(P):177.

51. Howell A, Harris M. Infiltrating lobular carcinoma of the breast. *Br Med J* 1985;291:1371.

52. Dixon JM, Anderson TJ, Page DL et al. Infiltrating lobular carcinoma of the breast: incidence and consequence of bilateral disease. *Br J Surg* 1983;70:513-516.

53. Meyer JE, Amin E, Lindfors KK et al. Medullary carcinoma of the breast: mammographic and sonographic appearance. *Radiology* 1989;170:79-82.

54. Feig SA, Shaber GS, Patchefsky AS et al. Tubular carcinoma of the breast. *Radiology* 1978;129:311-314.

55. Elson BC, Helvie MA, Frank FS et al. Tubular carcinoma of the breast: mode of presentation, mammographic appearance, and frequency of nodal metastases. *AJR* 1993;161:1173-1178.

56. Fisher ER, Palekar AS, Kotwal N et al. A non-encapsulating sclerosing lesion of the breast. *Am J Clin Pathol* 1979;71:239-246.

57. Baker, RR. Unusual lesions and their management. *Surg Clin North Am* 1990;70:963-975.

58. Page DL, Anderson TJ. *Diagnostic Histopathology of the Breast.* Edinburgh: Churchill Livingstone; 1987:186-187.

59. Hughes LE, Mansel RE, Webster DJT et al. *Benign Disorders and Diseases of the Breast.* London: Bailliere Tindal; 1988:59-73.

60. Rosen PP. *Breast Pathology.* Philadelphia: Lippincott-Raven; 1997:335-353.

61. Tobin CE, Hendrix TM, Resnikoff LB et al. Breast imaging case of the day. *Radiographics* 1996;16:720-722.

62. Mitnick JS, Vazquez MF, Harris MN et al. Invasive papillary carcinoma of the breast: mammographic appearance. *Radiology* 1990;177:803-806.

63. Reuter K, D'Orsi CJ, Reale F. Intracystic carcinoma of the breast: the role of ultrasonography. *Radiology* 1984;153:233-234.

64. Fechner RE, Mills SE. *Breast Pathology* Chicago: ASCP Press; 1990:30.

65. Rosen PP. *Breast Pathology.* Philadelphia: Lippincott-Raven; 1997:143-155.

66. Dupont WD, Page DL, Parl FF et al. Long-term risk of breast cancer in women with fibroadenoma. *N Eng J Med* 1994;331:10-15.
67. Jackson VP, Rothschild PA, Kreipke DL et al. The spectrum of sonographic findings of fibroadenoma of the breast. *Invest Radiol* 1986;21:31-40.
68. Mendelson EB, Bohm-Velez M, Bhagwanani DG et al. Sonographic spectrum of fibroadenomas: a guide to clinical management. Paper presented at the Radiological Society of North America Annual Meeting, Chicago; 1988.
69. Sickles EA. Management of probably benign breast lesions. *Radiol Clin North Am* 1995;33:1123-1130.
70. Jackson VP. Benign breast lesions. In: Bassett LW, Jackson VP, Jahan R, Fu YS, Gold RH, ed. *Diagnosis of Diseases of the Breast*. Philadelphia: WB Saunders Co; 1997:429-435.
71. Haagensen CD. *Diseases of the Breast, 3rd ed*. Philadelphia: WB Saunders Co; 1986:267-312.
72. Mendelson EB, Bohm-Velez M, Lamas C et al. Focal breast fibrosis: mimic of breast carcinoma. Paper presented at the American Roentgen Ray Society Annual Meeting, New Orleans; 1989.
73. Adler DD. Ultrasound of benign breast conditions. *Semin US CT MR* 1989;10:106-118.
74. Logan WW, Hoffman NY. Diabetic fibrous disease. *Radiology* 1989;172:667-670.
75. Rosen PP. *Breast Pathology*. Philadelphia: Lippincott-Raven; 1997:676-679.
76. Adler DD, Jeffries DO, Helvie MA. Sonographic features of breast hamartomas. *J Ultrasound Med* 1990;9:85-90.
77. Rosen PP. *Breast Pathology* Philadelphia: Lippincott-Raven; 1997:67-75.
78. Jackson VP. Benign breast lesions. In: Bassett LW, Jackson VP, Jahan R, Fu YS, Gold RH, eds. *Diagnosis of Diseases of the Breast*. Philadelphia: WB Saunders Co; 1997:402.
79. Gomez A, Mata JM, Donoso L et al. Galactocele: three distinctive radiographic appearances. *Radiology* 1986;158:43-44.
80. Bland KI. Inflammatory, infectious, and metabolic disorders of the mamma. In: Bland KI, Copeland EM, eds. *The Breast: Comprehensive Management of Benign and Malignant Diseases*. Philadelphia: WB Saunders Co; 1991:87-112.
81. Vega A, Garijo F. Radial scar and tubular carcinoma: mammographic and sonographic findings. *ACTA Radiol* 1993; 34:43-47.
82. Rosen PP. *Breast Pathology*. Philadelphia: Lippincott-Raven; 1997:420-424.

Interventional Procedures
83. Evans WP. Breast Masses. *Radiol Clin North Am* 1995;33: 1085-1108.
84. Lindfors KK, Rosenquist CJ. Needle core biopsy guided with mammography: a study of cost-effectiveness. *Radiology* 1994;190:217-222.

85. ACR Standard for the Performance of Ultrasound-Guided Percutaneous Breast Interventional Procedures. Reston, Va: American College of Radiology; 1996.
86. Reading CC, Charboneau JW. Ultrasound-guided biopsy of the abdomen and pelvis. In: Rumack CM, Wilson Sr, Charboneau JW, eds. *Diagnostic Ultrasound*. St. Louis: Mosby-Year Book; 1991:429.
87. Fajardo LL, Jackson VP, Hunter TB. Interventional procedures in diseases of the breast: needle biopsy, pneumocystography, and galactography. *AJR* 1992;158:1231.
88. Parker SH, Burbank F, Jackman RJ et al. Percutaneous large-core breast biopsy: a multi-institutional study. *Radiology* 1994;193:359-364.
89. Dowlatshahi K, Yaremko ML, Kluskens LF et al. Nonpalpable breast lesions: findings of stereotaxic needle-core biopsy and fine-needle aspiration cytology. *Radiology* 1991;181:745-750.
90. Harter LP, Curtis JS, Ponto G et al. Malignant seeding of the needle track during stereotaxic core needle breast biopsy. *Radiology* 1992;185:713-714.
91. Parker SH, Lovin JD, Jobe WE et al. Stereotactic breast biopsy with a biopsy gun. *Radiology* 1990;176:741-747.
92. Kaplan SS, Racenstein MJ, Wong WS et al. US-guided core biopsy of the breast with a coaxial system. *Radiology* 1995;194:573.
93. Hendrick RE, Parker SH. Stereotactic imaging. In: *Syllabus: a categorical course in physics: technical aspects of breast imaging*. Oak Brook, Ill: Radiological Society of North America; 1992:233-243.
94. Liberman L, Dershaw DD, Rosen PP et al. Stereotaxic 14-gauge breast biopsy: how many core biopsy specimens are needed? *Radiology* 1994;192:793-795.
95. Fornage BD. Interventional ultrasound of the breast. In: McGahan JP, ed. *Interventional Ultrasound*. Baltimore: Williams & Wilkins; 1990:71.
96. D'Orsi CJ, Mendelson EB. Interventional breast ultrasonography. *Semin US CT MR* 1989;10:132.

Trauma and Postoperative Alterations
97. Levine RA, Collins TL. Definitive diagnosis of breast implant rupture by ultrasonography. *Plast Reconst Surgery* 1991; 87:1126-1128.
98. Harris KM, Ganott MA, Shestak KC et al. Silicone implant rupture: detection with US. *Radiology* 1993;187:761-768.
99. Gorczyca DP, DeBruhl ND, Ahn CY. Silicone breast implant ruptures in an animal model: comparison of mammography, MR imaging, US, and CT. *Radiology* 1994;190:227-232.
100. Venta LA, Salomon SG, Filsak ME et al. Sonographic signs of breast implant rupture. *AJR* 1996;166:1413-1419.
101. Balu-Maestro C, Bruneton J-N, Geoffray A. Ultrasonographic post-treatment follow-up of breast cancer patients. *J US Med* 1991;10:1-8.

CHAPTER 24

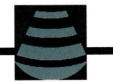

The Scrotum

•

Timothy J. Dambro, M.D.

Rhonda R. Stewart, M.D.

Barbara A. Carroll, M.D.

Many imaging modalities have supplemented physical examination in the evaluation of scrotal disease, including scrotal ultrasound, which has proven to be an accurate means of evaluating many scrotal diseases. Technical advancements in high-resolution real-time and color flow Doppler sonography have led to an increase in the clinical applications of scrotal sonography.

IMAGING TECHNIQUE

Thorough palpation of the scrotal contents and history taking should precede the sonographic examination. A direct contact scan is most commonly performed, but a water bath approach may also be used. Any acoustic coupling gel may be used. The patient is examined in the supine position. The scrotum is elevated with a towel draped over the thighs, and the penis is placed on the patient's abdomen and covered with a towel. Alternatively, the scrotal sac may be supported by the examiner's hand. Patients are asked to localize painful sites and palpable nodules within the scrotum. Palpation of these areas by the sonographer during the examination is often useful. A 7.5- or 10-MHz transducer is commonly used because it provides increased resolution of the scrotal contents. If greater penetration is needed, a 5-MHz transducer may be used, or with marked scrotal swelling, a 3.5-MHz transducer may be used. Images of both testes are obtained in transverse and sagittal planes. If possible, a transverse scan demonstrating both testes for comparison is obtained. Additional views may also be obtained in the coronal or oblique planes, with the patient upright, or performing Valsalva's maneuver when necessary. Color flow and power mode Doppler examination may also be performed to evaluate testicular blood flow in normal and pathologic states.

ANATOMY

The adult testes are ovoid glands measuring 3 to 5 cm in length, 2 to 4 cm in width, and 3 cm in anteroposterior dimension. Their weight ranges from 12.5 to 19 g. Their size and weight decrease with age.[2,8,9] The testes are surrounded by a dense white fibrous capsule, the tunica albuginea. Multiple thin septations (septula) arise from the innermost aspect of the tunica albuginea and converge posteriorly to form the **mediastinum testis** (Fig. 24-1). The mediastinum testis forms the support for the entering and exiting testicular vessels and ducts. As the septula proceed posteriorly from the tunica albuginea, they form 250 to 400

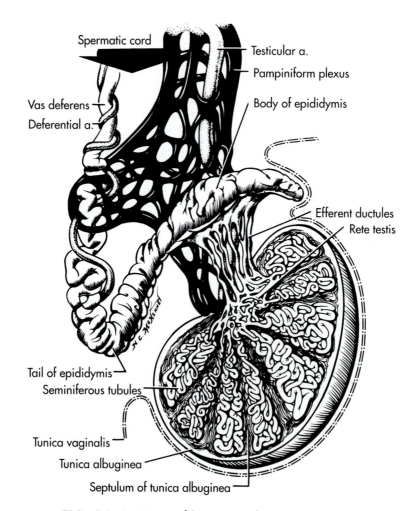

Spermatic cord

Testicular a.

Pampiniform plexus

Body of epididymis

Vas deferens

Deferential a.

Efferent ductules

Rete testis

Tail of epididymis

Seminiferous tubules

Tunica vaginalis

Tunica albuginea

Septulum of tunica albuginea

FIG. 24-1. **Normal intrascrotal anatomy.**

wedge-shaped lobuli that contain the seminiferous tubules. There are approximately 840 tubules per testis. As the tubules course centrally, they join other seminiferous tubules to form 20 to 30 larger ducts, known as the tubuli recti. The tubuli recti enter the mediastinum testis, forming a network of channels within the testicular stroma, called the rete testis. The rete terminate in 10 to 15 efferent ductules at the superior portion of the mediastinum, which carry the seminal fluid from the testis to the epididymis.

Sonographically the **normal testis** has a homogeneous granular echo texture composed of uniformly distributed medium-level echoes, similar to that of the thyroid. The mediastinum testis is sometimes seen as a linear echogenic band extending craniocaudally within the testis (Fig. 24-2). Its appearance varies according to the amount of fibrous and fatty tissue present. It is best visualized after age 15 and before age 60.[9] The tunica albuginea is not normally visualized as a separate structure. The **septula testis** may be seen as linear echogenic or hypoechoic structures (Fig. 24-3). The rete testis may be visualized as a hypoechoic or septated cystic area adjacent to the head of the epididymis.

The **epididymis** is a curved structure measuring 6 to 7 cm in length lying posterolateral to the testis. It is composed of a head, a body, and a tail. The head of the epididymis, also known as the globus major, is located adjacent to the superior pole of the testis and is the largest portion of the epididymis. It is formed by 10 to 15 efferent ductules from the rete testis joining together to form a single convoluted duct, the ductus epididymis. This duct forms the body and the majority of the tail of the epididymis. It measures approximately 600 cm in length and follows a very convoluted course from the head to the tail of the epididymis. The body or corpus of the epididymis lies adjacent to the posterolateral margin of the testis. The tail or globus minor is loosely attached to the lower pole of the testis by areolar tissue. The ductus epididymis forms an acute angle at the inferior aspect of the globus minor and courses cephalad on the medial aspect of the epididymis to the spermatic cord. The appendix testis, a remnant of the Müllerian duct, is a small ovoid structure located beneath the head of the epididymis. The appendix epididymis, representing a detached efferent duct, is a small stalk projecting off the epididymis, which may be duplicated. Rarely, other appendages, the paradidymis and the superior and inferior vas aberrans of Haller, may be seen.[10]

Sonographically the **epididymis** is normally isoechogenic or slightly more echogenic than the testis, and its echo texture may be coarser. The **globus**

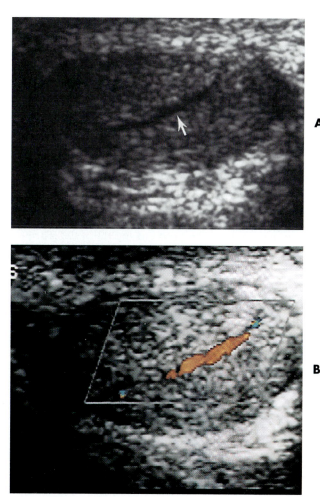

FIG. 24-3. Normal testicular band. A, Transverse scan of the testis demonstrates a hypoechoic linear intratesticular band. **B,** Color flow Doppler depicts the vascular nature of this band.

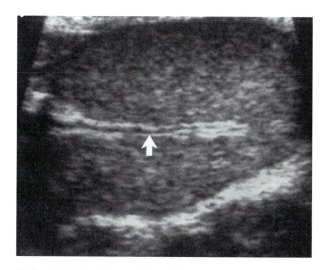

FIG. 24-2. Normal mediastinum testis. Longitudinal scan demonstrates the mediastinum testis *(arrow)*, which is seen as an echogenic fibrofatty tissue surrounding an anechoic vascular structure.

major normally measures 10 to 12 mm in diameter and lies lateral to the superior pole of the testis (Fig. 24-4). The **body** tends to be isoechoic or slightly less echogenic than the globus major and testis. The normal body measures less than 4 mm in diameter, averaging 1 to 2 mm. The **tail, appendix epididymis,** and **appendix testis** are most often identified sonographically as separate structures when a hydrocele is present.

Knowledge of the arterial supply of the testis is important for interpretation of color flow Doppler sonography of the testis. **Testicular blood flow** is supplied primarily by the **deferential, cremasteric (external spermatic),** and **testicular arteries.** The deferential artery originates from the inferior vesical artery and courses to the tail of the epididymis, where it divides and forms a capillary network. The cremasteric artery arises from the inferior epigastric artery. It courses with the remainder of the structures of the spermatic cord through the inguinal ring, continuing to the surface of the tunica vaginalis, where it anastomoses with capillaries of the testicular and deferential arteries. The testicular arteries arise from the anterior aspect of the aorta just below the origin of the renal arteries. They course through the inguinal canal with the spermatic cord to the posterosuperior aspect of the testis. Upon reaching the testis, the testicular artery divides into branches, which pierce the tunica albuginea and arborize over the surface of the testis in a layer known as the tunica vasculosa. Centripetal branches arise from these capsular arteries; these branches course along the septula to converge on the mediastinum. From the mediastinum, these branches form recurrent rami that course centrifugally within the testicular parenchyma, where they branch into arterioles and capillaries.[7] In roughly half of normal testes a trans-

mediastinal artery supplies the testis, entering through the mediastinum and coursing toward the periphery of the gland. These arteries may be unilateral or bilateral, single or multiple, and are frequently seen as a hypoechoic band in the midtestis.

The **velocity waveforms of the normal capsular and intratesticular arteries** show high levels of antegrade diastolic flow throughout the cardiac cycle, reflecting the low vascular resistance of the testis (Fig. 24-5).[3] Supratesticular arterial waveforms vary in appearance. Two main types of waveforms exist: a low-resistance waveform like the capsular and intratesticular arteries, and a high-resistance waveform with sharp, narrow systolic peaks and little or no diastolic flow (Fig. 24-6).[3] This high-resistance waveform is believed to reflect the **high vascular resistance of the extratesticular tissues.** The deferential and cremasteric arteries within the spermatic cord primarily supply the epididymis and extratesticular tissues, but also supply the testis via anastomoses with the testicular artery.

A hypoechoic **intratesticular band** has been described in 10% of normal testes (see Fig. 24-3).[11] This well-circumscribed band is most commonly visualized in the middle third of the testicle, nearly perpendicular to the mediastinum on sagittal scans. It measures up to 3 mm in diameter and 3 cm in length. Pulsed

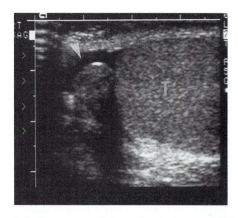

FIG. 24-4. Normal head of the epididymis. Longitudinal scrotal scan demonstrates the head of the epididymis *(cursors)* lying superior to the testis, *T*. A small, normal amount of fluid is seen between the layers of the tunica vaginalis *(arrowhead)*.

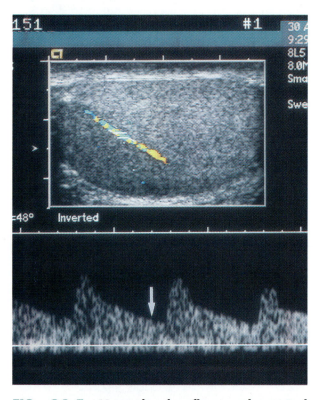

FIG. 24-5. Normal color flow and spectral Doppler of the testicular artery. There are characteristic low-impedance arterial waveforms with a large amount of end-diastolic flow *(arrow)*.

wave Doppler sonography of the band demonstrates a low-resistance waveform characteristic of the normal intratesticular arterial waveform in half the cases. Venous waveforms are usually not obtained from this region, but it is believed that the vein also contributes to the thickness of the hypoechoic band.

The **spermatic cord** consists of the vas deferens; the cremasteric, deferential, and testicular arteries; a pampiniform plexus of veins; the lymphatics; and the nerves of the testis. Sonographically the normal spermatic cord lies just beneath the skin and is difficult to distinguish from the adjacent soft tissues of the inguinal canal.[12] It may be visualized within the scrotum when a hydrocele is present or with the use of color flow Doppler sonography.

The **dartos,** a layer of muscle fibers lying beneath the scrotal skin, is continuous with the scrotal septum, which divides the scrotum into two separate chambers. The walls of the chambers are formed by the fusion of the three fascial layers.

The **tunica vaginalis** is the space between these scrotal fascial layers and the tunica albuginea of the testis. During embryologic development, the tunica vaginalis arises from the **processus vaginalis,** an outpouching of fetal peritoneum that accompanies the testis in its descent into the scrotum. The upper portion of the processus vaginalis, extending from the internal inguinal ring to the upper pole of the testis, is normally obliterated. The lower portion, the tunica vaginalis, remains as a closed pouch folded around the testis. Only the posterior aspect of the testis, the site of attachment of the testis and epididymis, is not in continuity with the tunica vaginalis. The inner or visceral layer of the tunica vaginalis covers the testis, epididymis, and lower portion of the spermatic cord. The outer or parietal layer of the tunica vaginalis lines the walls of the scrotal pouch and is attached to the fascial coverings of the testis. A small amount of fluid is normally present between these two layers, especially in the polar regions and between the testicle and epididymis.

The scrotal covering layers are normally inseparable by sonography and are visualized as a single echogenic stripe. If any type of fluid is present in the scrotal wall, the tunica vaginalis may be identified as a separate structure.[2]

SCROTAL MASS

Ultrasound of the scrotum can detect intrascrotal masses with a sensitivity of nearly 100%.[13] It plays a major role in the evaluation of scrotal masses because its accuracy is 98% to 100% in differentiating intratesticular and extratesticular pathology.[5,14] This distinction is important in patient management because most extratesticular masses are benign, but the majority of intratesticular lesions are malignant.[1,9] Virtually all intratesticular masses should be considered malignant until proven otherwise.[2]

Most malignant testicular neoplasms are more hypoechoic than normal testicular parenchyma; however, hemorrhage, necrosis, calcification, or fatty changes can produce areas of increased echogenicity within these tumors. Uniformly echogenic masses are more often benign processes resulting from infectious or vascular abnormalities. Nevertheless, even echogenic lesions must still be considered potentially malignant, as most benign testicular processes, hypoechoic or hyperechoic, are nonspecific in appearance.

Testicular neoplasms account for 1% to 2% of all malignant neoplasms in men and are the fifth most frequent cause of death in men aged 15 to 34 years.[15] Approximately 65% to 94% of patients with testicular neoplasms present with painless unilateral testicular masses or diffuse testicular enlargement and from 4% to 14% present with symptoms of metastatic disease.[2,16,17] Primary testicular tumors are 90% to 95% of germ cell origin and are generally highly malig-

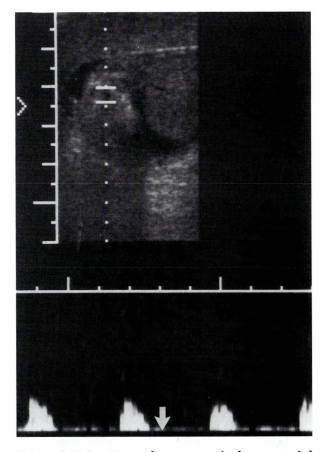

FIG. 24-6. Normal extratesticular arterial Doppler tracings. The cremasteric and deferential arteries of the spermatic cord demonstrate a high-resistance waveform without evidence of significant diastolic flow *(arrow).*

nant.[18] Only 60% of testicular germ cell tumors are of a single histologic type, and the remainder contain two or more histologic types. Gonadal stromal tumors, arising from Sertoli's cells or Leydig's cells, account for 3% to 6% of testicular masses,[2,9,17] and the majority of these mesenchymal neoplasms are benign (see box).

Malignant Tumors

Germ Cell Tumors. **Pure seminoma** is the most common single-cell type of testicular tumor in adults, accounting for 40% to 50% of all germ cell neoplasms. It is also a common component of mixed germ cell tumors, occurring in 30% of these tumors. Seminomas occur in a slightly older age group when compared with other testicular neoplasms, demonstrating a peak incidence in the fourth and fifth decades of life.[2,13,19-21] They rarely occur before puberty. They are less aggressive than other testicular tumors and are commonly confined within the tunica albuginea at presentation with only 25% of patients with metastases at diagnosis. As a result of the radiosensitivity and chemosensitivity of the primary tumor and its metastases, seminomas have the most favorable prognosis of the malignant testicular tumors. A second primary synchronous or metachronous germ cell tumor occurs in 1% to 2.5% of patients with seminomas.

Seminoma is the most common tumor type in **cryptorchid testes.** Between 8% and 30% of patients with seminoma have a history of undescended testes.[17,20,21] The risk of developing a seminoma is substantially increased in an undescended testis, even after orchiopexy. There is also an increased risk for developing malignancy in the contralateral normally located testis; therefore sonography is sometimes used to screen for an occult tumor in the remaining testis.

Macroscopically, seminoma is a homogeneously solid, firm, round or oval tumor that varies in size from a small nodule in a normal-size testis to a large mass causing diffuse testicular enlargement.[15] The sonographic features of **pure seminoma** parallel this homogeneous macroscopic appearance (Fig. 24-7). They are composed predominantly of uniform, low-level echoes without calcification or cystic areas.[22] These tumors may be smoothly marginated or ill defined, but are generally very hypoechoic compared with normally echogenic testicular parenchyma.

Embryonal cell carcinoma is the second most common testicular germ cell neoplasm. It often occurs in combination with other neoplastic germ cell elements, particularly yolk sac tumor and teratoma. It constitutes 20% to 25% of all primary germ cell malignancies. These tumors occur in a younger age group than do seminomas, with a peak incidence during the latter part of the second and third decades of life. It is uncommon before puberty and after the age of 50

PATHOLOGIC CLASSIFICATION OF TESTICULAR TUMORS

Germ cell tumors
Tumors of one histologic type
    Seminoma
        Classical
        Spermatocystic
    Embryonal cell carcinoma
        Adult type
        Infantile type
        Endodermal sinus tumor
    Teratoma
        Mature
        Immature
        With malignant transformation
        Choriocarcinoma
Tumors of more than one histologic type
    Teratoma and embryonal cell carcinoma (teratocarcinoma)
    Choriocarcinoma and any other type
    Other combinations

Tumors of gonadal stroma
Leydig's cell tumors
Sertoli's cell, granulosa cell, theca cell tumors
Tumors of primitive gonadal stroma
Mixtures of the above

Modified from Mostofi FK, Price EB Jr. Tumors of the male genital system. In: *Atlas of Tumors Pathology*. Fascicle 8, 2nd series. Washington, DC: Armed Forces Institute of Pathology; 1973.

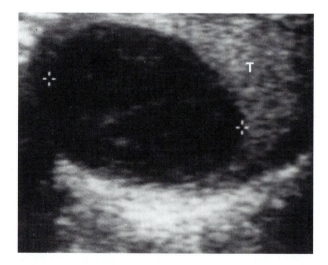

FIG. 24-7. Seminoma. A well-circumscribed, predominantly hypoechoic, intratesticular mass *(cursors)* with echogenicity markedly less than that of the normal adjacent testis, *T*, is characteristic of seminoma.

years. These malignancies are usually small, but may replace part or all of the testis without producing pronounced enlargement. Despite their small size, they tend to be more aggressive than seminomas, frequently invading the tunica albuginea, resulting in distortion of the testicular contour (Fig. 24-8). They frequently cause visceral metastases.[2,21] The infantile form, **endodermal sinus** or **yolk sac tumor,** is the most common germ cell tumor in infants, accounting for 60% of testicular neoplasms in this age group, commonly occurring before the age of 2 years. It is associated with elevated alphafetoprotein levels in 95% of infants. Both embryonal cell carcinoma and endodermal sinus tumor are less radiosensitive and chemosensitive than seminomas and have a reported 5-year survival rate of 25% to 35%.[21]

The sonographic features of embryonal cell carcinoma parallel its histology. It is generally more inhomogeneous and poorly marginated than the seminoma. Invasion of the tunica may occur, resulting in distortion of the testicular contour. Cystic areas are present in one third of tumors,[13] and echogenic foci, with or without acoustic shadowing, are not uncommon.

Teratomas constitute approximately 5% to 10% of primary testicular neoplasms.[21] They are defined according to the World Health Organization classification on the basis of the presence of derivatives of the different germinal layers (endoderm, mesoderm, ectoderm). There are three categories of teratomas according to this classification: mature, immature, and teratoma with malignant transformation.[17] One third of teratomas will metastasize, usually via a lymphatic route, within 5 years.[2,21] The reported 5-year survival rate is 70%. The peak age incidence is infancy and early childhood, with another peak in the third decade of life. In infants and young children, teratomas are the second most common testicular tumor and are most commonly mature, well differentiated, and benign. Occasional cases may contain immature elements, but metastases are rare.[20] After puberty teratomas commonly contain immature and mature elements admixed with other germ cell types. Teratomas in adults are usually malignant.

Sonographically the teratoma is commonly a well-defined, markedly inhomogeneous mass containing cystic and solid areas of various sizes. Dense echogenic foci causing acoustic shadowing are common, resulting from focal calcification, cartilage, immature bone, fibrosis, and noncalcific scarring (Fig. 24-9).[22]

Choriocarcinoma is the rarest type of germ cell tumor, constituting only 1% to 3% of malignant primary testicular tumors.[21] It rarely occurs in its pure form; only 18 cases were encountered among more than 6000 testicular tumors registered at the Armed Forces Institute of Pathology.[23] Approximately 23% of mixed germ cell tumors contain a component of choriocarcinoma.[20] The peak incidence is in the second and third decades of life. These tumors are highly malignant and metastasize early via hematogenous and

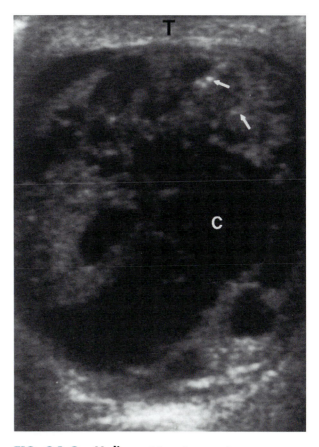

FIG. 24-9. Malignant teratoma. A transverse testicular scan demonstrates a large malignant teratoma replacing most of the testis. Cystic, *C*, and solid elements with small echogenic foci *(arrows)* from small calcifications are present. *T*, Residual normal testis.

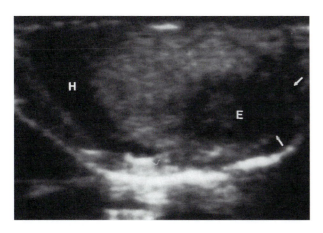

FIG. 24-8. Embryonal cell carcinoma. An aggressive, poorly marginated, embryonal cell carcinoma, *E*, is seen to invade through the layers of the tunica *(arrows)*. A small hydrocele is also present, *H*.

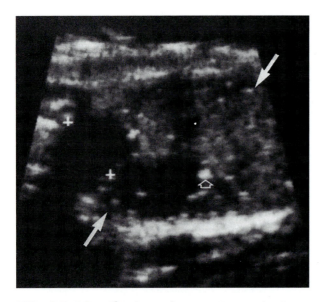

FIG. 24-10. Choriocarcinoma. Longitudinal scan demonstrates a testis diffusely involved by choriocarcinoma *(arrows)*. There are large cystic areas of necrosis *(cursors)* and areas of increased echogenicity corresponding to hemorrhage and calcification *(open arrow)*.

lymphatic routes. Patients often have symptoms resulting from hemorrhagic metastases: hemoptysis, hematemesis, and CNS symptoms. Gynecomastia is common because of the high levels of circulating chorionic gonadotropins.[17] Metastases may be present without any evidence of choriocarcinoma in the testicle. Sonography demonstrates a mass of mixed echogenicity containing areas of hemorrhage, necrosis, and calcification (Fig. 24-10).

Mixed germ cell tumors contain different neoplastic germ cell elements in various combinations. They are the second most common primary testicular malignancy after seminoma, constituting 40% of all germ cell tumors. They occur in the same age group as nonseminomatous germ cell tumors. The combined teratoma and embryonal cell carcinoma is the most frequent mixed germ cell tumor, previously called **teratocarcinoma.** It commonly contains both solid and cystic elements with a sonographic appearance similar to a pure teratoma.

Stromal Tumors. Gonadal stromal tumors account for 3% to 6% of all testicular neoplasms. Approximately 20% of these tumors occur in children.[15] The term **gonadal stromal tumor** refers to a neoplasm containing Leydig's, thecal, granulosa, or lutein cells and fibroblasts in various degrees of differentiation. These tumors may contain single or multiple cell types because of the totipotentiality of the gonadal stroma.[17] Gonadal stromal tumors in conjunction with germ cell tumors are called gonadoblastomas. The majority of gonadoblastomas occur in

males with cryptorchidism, hypospadia, and female internal secondary sex organs.[20]

The majority of stromal tumors are **Leydig's cell tumors.** They account for 1% to 3% of all testicular neoplasms and occur predominantly between the ages of 20 and 50 years.[19,20,24] Patients most commonly present with painless testicular enlargement or a palpable mass. Approximately 15% of patients present with gynecomastia resulting from the secretion of androgens, estrogens, or a combination. Impotence, loss of libido, or precocious virilization may also occur in young men. The tumor is bilateral in 3% of cases. From 10% to 15% of tumors demonstrate malignant behavior, invading the tunica at diagnosis. Foci of hemorrhage and necrosis are present in 25% of tumors.[19,24] These gonadal tumors are usually small, solid, and hypoechoic on ultrasound (Fig. 24-11). Cystic spaces resulting from hemorrhage and necrosis are occasionally seen in larger lesions.[25]

The Occult Primary Tumor. Ultrasound plays an important role in patients with a normal physical examination who present with mediastinal, retroperitoneal, or supraclavicular metastases resulting from metastatic testicular carcinoma.[26-28] The detection of the occult primary tumor is important in patient management because if it is not removed, metastases will continue. Ultrasound has been shown to be able to detect impalpable testicular neoplasms. The primary testicular tumor may regress despite widespread advancing metastatic disease resulting in an echogenic fibrous and possibly calcific scar. It has been theorized that this regression is due to the high metabolic rate of the tumor and vascular compromise from the tumor outgrowing its blood supply. Usually no viable tumor cells are identifiable on histologic section in these cases.[15,16] The affected testis is often normal size or small. The sonographic finding of an echogenic focus with or without posterior acoustic shadowing is not specific for a **"burned-out" tumor**, but is strongly suggestive of this diagnosis in the context of histologically proven testicular metastases (Fig. 24-12).[29]

Approximately 95% of primary testicular neoplasms larger than 1.6 cm in diameter show increased vascularity on color flow Doppler ultrasound examinations. However, the color flow Doppler findings do not appear to play a major role in the evaluation of adult testicular tumors.[30] Conversely, preliminary work suggests that pediatric testicular tumors may be isoechoic with the normal testicular parenchyma and may be more readily appreciated using color flow Doppler ultrasound.[31] Focal diffuse inflammatory lesions cannot be distinguished from neoplasms based on color flow Doppler appearance or pulsed Doppler findings.

Nonpalpable testicular tumors have also been detected in patients presenting with infertility.[18] In these

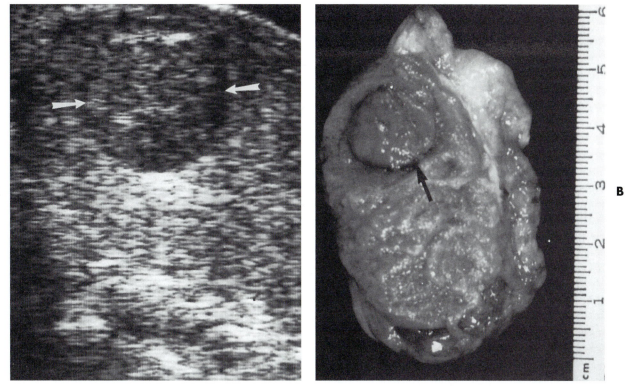

FIG. 24-11. Leydig's cell tumor. A, Longitudinal scan of the superior half of the testis demonstrates a small, solid, homogeneous, and well-circumscribed mass *(arrows)*. B, Gross pathologic specimen confirms the well-circumscribed nature of this Leydig's cell tumor *(arrow)*. (Courtesy of J. William Charboneau, M.D., Mayo Clinic, Rochester, Minn.)

cases, sonography is also important in surgical localization for intraoperative diagnosis since testicle-sparing resection may be performed if the lesion is benign. Incidentally discovered nonpalpable lesions are usually benign.[32] Many believe that if tumor markers and the chest radiograph are normal, patients can undergo an excisional testicular biopsy using an inguinal, organ-sparing approach. If the frozen section demonstrates a benign lesion, the organ can be spared. Ultrasound follow-up of an incidentally detected lesion is only recommended if there is strong clinical suggestion that the lesion is nonneoplastic (i.e., a recent history of trauma or infection).

Testicular Metastases

Metastases, Leukemia, and Lymphoma.
Leukemia and **lymphoma** are the most common metastatic testicular tumors. **Malignant lymphoma** is the most common secondary testicular neoplasm. It accounts for 1% to 8% of all testicular tumors and is the most common testicular tumor in men over age 60; still, testicular involvement occurs in only 0.3% of patients with lymphoma.[17,33] The peak age at diagnosis is between 60 and 70 years; 80% of patients are over the age of 50 years at diagnosis. Malignant lym-

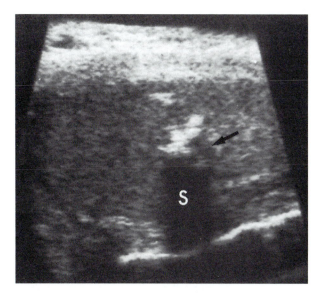

FIG. 24-12. Regressed "burned-out" tumor. Longitudinal scrotal scan demonstrates 0.7 cm, solid, echogenic, calcified mass with acoustic shadowing, *S*, in the midportion of the testis. A small, hypoechoic component *(arrow)* represents either viable residual embryonal cell carcinoma or "burned-out" tumor.

phoma is the most common bilateral testicular tumor, occurring bilaterally either in a synchronous or, more commonly, metachronous manner in 6% to 38% of cases. One half of bilateral testicular neoplasms are malignant lymphoma.[17,19]

Testicular lymphoma may occur as a site of primary extranodal disease, in association with disseminated disease, or as the initial manifestation of occult nodal disease. Approximately 10% of patients have lymphoma localized to the testis.[17,33] This form of testicular lymphoma has a better prognosis, but systemic lymphoma develops in 25% of patients soon after presentation or after orchiectomy. The remainder of patients with testicular involvement have a uniformly poor prognosis. The 5-year survival rate is 5% to 20%. The median survival is 9.5 to 12 months.[34,35]

Most patients with malignant lymphoma present with a painless testicular mass or diffuse testicular enlargement. Approximately 25% of patients have constitutional symptoms of lymphoma, such as fever, weakness, anorexia, or weight loss.[33]

Most malignant lymphomas of the testicle are of the non-Hodgkin's type. Using the Rappaport classification, diffuse histiocytic lymphoma is the most common type of testicular lymphoma, followed by poorly differentiated lymphocytic lymphoma.[17] Hodgkin's lymphoma is extremely rare; only four cases have been reported.[36]

Lymphoma of the testis is often large at diagnosis. The tunica vaginalis is usually intact, but extension into the epididymis and spermatic cord is common, occurring in up to 50% of cases.[19] The scrotal skin is rarely involved. Grossly, the tumor is not encapsulated but compresses the parenchyma to the periphery. The majority of malignant lymphomas are homogeneous, hypoechoic, and diffusely replace the testis.[17,33] However, focal hypoechoic lesions can occur (Fig. 24-13). Hemorrhage and necrosis are rare.

Leukemia is the second most common metastatic testicular neoplasm. Primary testicular leukemia is rare, but leukemic infiltration of the testicle during bone marrow remission is common in children.[17,37] It is believed that the testis acts as a sanctuary site for leukemic cells during chemotherapy because of a "blood-gonad barrier" that inhibits concentration of chemotherapeutic agents.[37] The highest frequency of testicular involvement is found in patients with acute leukemia (64%). Approximately 25% of patients with chronic leukemia have testicular involvement.[38] Most cases of testicular involvement occur within 1 year of discontinuation of long-term remission maintenance chemotherapy. The rate of relapse in this setting is nearly 13%.[37]

The sonographic appearance of lymphoma and leukemia is nonspecific. Diffuse infiltration, producing diffusely enlarged, hypoechoic testes, is the

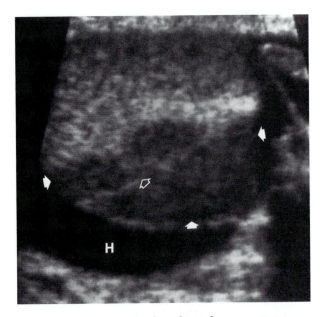

FIG. 24-13. Testicular lymphoma. Transverse scrotal scan demonstrates a focal hypoechoic lymphomatous mass *(arrows)* in a patient with diffuse histiocytic lymphoma metastatic to the testis. A small branch of the septula testis is seen *(open arrow)* encased by this lymphomatous mass. *H*, Hydrocele.

most frequent presentation for both processes (Fig. 24-14). Focal, sharply marginated, anechoic masses with through-sound transmission and occasional low-level internal echoes have been described in chronic lymphocytic leukemia.[38] Although color flow Doppler imaging shows increased vascularity in testicular lymphoma and leukemia, differentiation cannot be made from diffuse inflammatory processes.[39]

Other Metastases. Nonlymphomatous metastases to the testes are uncommon, representing only 0.02% to 5% of all testicular neoplasms.[40,41] The most frequent primary sites are the **lung** and **prostate.**[19] Other frequent primary sites for metastatic neoplasms include **kidney, stomach, colon, pancreas,** and **melanoma.**[40,42] Most metastases are clinically silent, being discovered incidentally at autopsy or after orchiectomy for prostatic carcinoma (Fig. 24-15). Testicular metastases are most common during the sixth and seventh decades of life and are more frequent than primary germ cell tumors after age 50.[2,35] They are commonly multiple and are bilateral in 15% of cases.[19] Since primary germ cell tumors may also be multicentric and bilateral, these features are not helpful in distinguishing primary from metastatic testicular neoplasms. Widespread systemic metastases are usually present at diagnosis.[39] Possible routes of metastases to the testis include retrograde venous, hematogenous, retrograde lymphatic, and direct tumor invasion.[33,34] Sites remote from the testis, such as the lung and skin, most likely spread via the

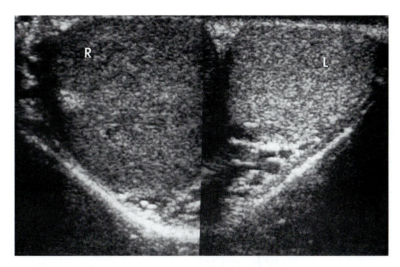

FIG. 24-14. Testicular leukemia. Transverse scan shows both the right, *R*, and left, *L*, testes and demonstrates diffuse hypoechoic enlargement of the right testis resulting from leukemic infiltrate.

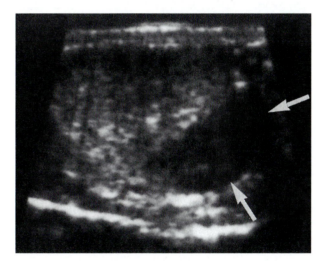

FIG. 24-15. Testicular metastasis. Transverse testicular scan demonstrates a hypoechoic lung carcinoma metastasis *(arrows)* to the testis.

TESTICULAR METASTASES

Lymphoma
Mostly non-Hodgkin's
10% localized to testis

Leukemia
Second most common
64% acute leukemia
Sanctuary site

Nonlymphoma metastases
Lung and prostate most common
Kidney, stomach, colon, pancreas, melanoma

hematogenous route. Retrograde venous extension through the spermatic vein has been shown to occur in renal cell carcinoma and may also occur in **bladder** and **prostate** tumors.[43] Neoplasms with metastases to the periaortic lymph nodes may involve the testis through retrograde lymphatic extension. Colorectal carcinoma may also directly invade the testes. Sonographic features of nonlymphomatous testicular metastases vary. They are often hypoechoic, but may be echogenic or complex in appearance.[2]

Benign Intratesticular Lesions

Cysts. Testicular cysts are discovered incidentally on ultrasound in 8% to 10% of the population.[44,45] Cystic testicular lesions are not uniformly benign because testicular tumors may undergo cystic degeneration because of hemorrhage or necrosis. The differentiation between a benign cyst and a cystic neo-

plasm is of utmost clinical importance. Benign cysts of the testicle have received much attention in the literature, but cystic neoplasms are not widely reported. Of the 34 cystic testicular masses discovered by ultrasound by Hamm et al.,[44] 16 were neoplastic. Teratomas are the most common tumors to contain both cystic and solid components.

Cysts of the tunica albuginea are located within the tunica, usually on the anterior and lateral aspects of the testis. They vary in size from 2 to 5 mm and are well defined. They may be solitary or multiple, unilocular or multilocular. They are discovered in patients in their fifth and sixth decades of life and are commonly asymptomatic. Histologically, they are simple cysts lined with cuboid or low columnar cells and filled with serous fluid (Fig. 24-16).[46-48] Complex tunica albuginea cysts may simulate a testicular neoplasm.[49] Careful scanning in multiple planes and possibly MRI may help identify the benign nature of a tunica albuginea cyst.

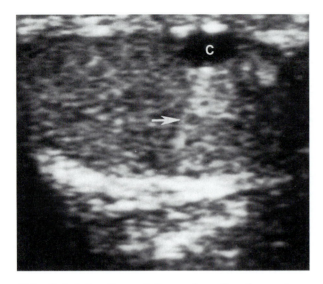

FIG. 24-16. Cyst of the tunica albuginea. Longitudinal scrotal scan demonstrates a well-circumscribed peripheral tunica albuginea cyst, *C*, with posterior acoustic enhancement *(arrow)*.

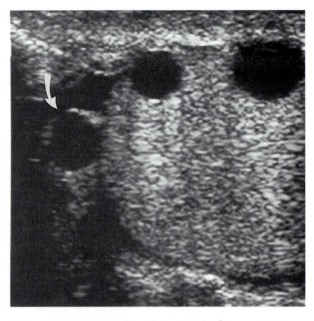

FIG. 24-17. Benign intratesticular cysts. Longitudinal scan demonstrates two intratesticular cysts and an epididymal cyst *(arrow)*.

Intratesticular cysts are simple cysts filled with clear serous fluid that vary in size between 2 and 18 mm.[50,51] Sonographically they are well-defined, anechoic lesions with thin, smooth walls and posterior acoustic enhancement. Hamm et al.[44] reported that in all 13 of their cases, the cysts were located near the mediastinum testis, supporting the theory that they originate from the rete testis, possibly secondary to posttraumatic or postinflammatory stricture formation (Fig. 24-17).[44,46]

Tubular Ectasia of the Rete Testis. Tubular ectasia of the rete testis can be mistaken for a testicular neoplasm.[52-57] This tubular ectasia is usually associated with epididymal obstruction secondary to inflammatory or traumatic lesions. Variable-sized cystic lesions in the region of the mediastinum testis with no associated soft-tissue abnormality and no flow on color flow Doppler imaging are seen (Fig. 24-18). A large number of these abnormalities are bilateral and are usually associated with an ipsilateral spermatocele. The characteristic ultrasound appearance and location should make it possible to distinguish this benign condition from a malignancy, thus avoiding an orchiectomy. Characteristic MRI findings include intratesticular abnormal signal intensity similar to that of water in the region of the mediastinum testis.[54]

Cystic Dysplasia. Cystic dysplasia is a rare congenital malformation, usually occurring in infants and young children, although one case has been reported in a 30-year-old man.[58] Only eight cases have been described.[59] This lesion is believed to result from an embryologic defect preventing connection of the tubules of the rete testis and the efferent ductules. Pathologically the lesion consists of multiple, interconnecting cysts of various sizes and shapes, separated by fibrous septae.[59] This lesion originates in the rete testis and extends into the adjacent parenchyma, resulting in pressure atrophy of the adjacent testicular parenchyma. The cysts are lined by a single layer of flat or cuboidal epithelium. Renal agenesis or dysplasia frequently coexists with testicular cystic dysplasia.[59]

Epidermoid Cysts. The epidermoid cyst is a benign tumor of germ cell origin, representing approximately 1% of all testicular tumors. These tumors may occur at any age, but are most common during the second to fourth decades of life.[19,60,61] Patients usually present with a painless testicular nodule; one third are discovered incidentally on physical examination. Diffuse painless testicular enlargement occurs in 10% of cases.[60,62] These lesions are generally well-circumscribed, solid tumors lying beneath the tunica albuginea. Pathologically the tumor wall is composed of fibrous tissue with an inner lining of squamous epithelium. The cyst is filled with flaky, cheesy-white keratin.

Epidermoid cysts are believed to represent monomorphic or monodermal development of a teratoma along the line of ectodermal cell differentiation.[60,62,63] These benign lesions can only be differentiated from premalignant teratomas through histologic examination. By definition, epidermoid cysts contain no teratomatous elements, and thus have no malignant potential.

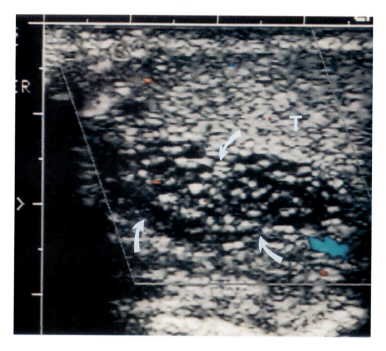

FIG. 24-18. Ectasia of rete. Longitudinal image shows tubular cystic change *(arrows)* in the posterior portion of the testis, *T*.

Sonographically, epidermoid cysts are generally well-defined, solid, hypoechoic masses, which occasionally are internally hyperechoic. The mass typically has an echogenic capsule (Fig. 24-19).[61,62] Although this appearance is relatively characteristic, malignancy cannot be completely excluded on sonographic findings alone. The proper treatment of these lesions is still debated. A conservative testicle-sparing approach with local excision (enucleation) or simple or radical orchiectomy can be performed.[60,64] Differentiation from a teratoma can only be made by careful pathologic examination of the cyst wall and adjacent testis.[60] Orchiectomy results in 100% survival, and no further treatment is necessary.

Abscess. Testicular abscesses are usually a complication of epididymo-orchitis; they may also result from missed testicular torsion, gangrenous or infected tumor, or primary pyogenic orchitis. Common infectious causes of abscess formation are **mumps, smallpox, scarlet fever, influenza, typhoid, sinusitis, osteomyelitis, appendicitis,** and many others.[65] The testicular abscess may rupture through the tunica vaginalis, resulting in pyocele formation or fistulous formation to the skin.

Sonography demonstrates, most commonly, an enlarged testicle containing a predominantly fluid-filled mass with hypoechoic or mixed echogenic areas visualized (Fig. 24-20). An atypical appearance has been described in which there was disruption of the testicular architecture with hyperechoic striations sepa-

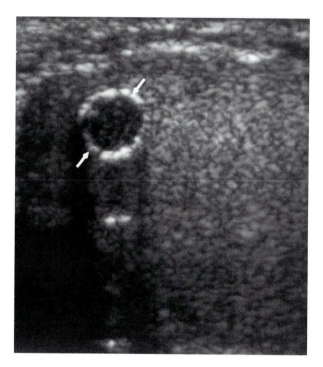

FIG. 24-19. Benign epidermoid cyst. Longitudinal testicular scan demonstrates well-circumscribed epidermoid "keratin" cyst with smooth echogenic walls *(arrows)* and echogenic material within it. At surgery a well-encapsulated, benign epidermoid cyst that contained cheesy material was found with calcifications in the capsule. The benign sonographic appearance resulted in testicular sparing. (Courtesy of Ben Hollenberg, M.D., Presbyterian Hospital, Charlotte, NC.)

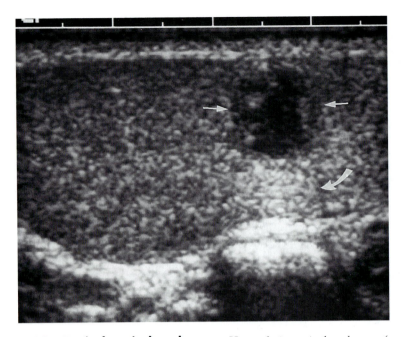

FIG. 24-20. Typical testicular abscess. Hypoechoic testicular abscess *(arrows)* is indistinguishable from a tumor. However, enhanced posterior sound transmission *(curved arrow)* suggests that the mass is primarily fluid.

TESTICULAR CYSTIC LESIONS

Benign
Tunica albuginea cysts
Intratesticular cysts
Tubular ectasia of rete testis
Cystic dysplasia
Epidermoid cysts
Abscess

Malignant
Teratocarcinoma
Yolk sac tumors
Necrosis/hemorrhage in tumor
Tubular obstruction by tumor
Lymphoma

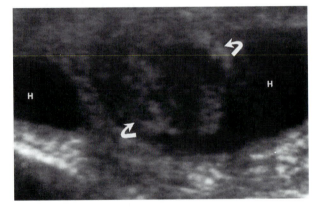

FIG. 24-21. Atypical testicular abscess. Atypical appearance of a testicular abscess *(curved arrows)* is noted with echogenic and hypoechoic components. *H,* Bilateral hydroceles.

rating hypoechoic spaces (Fig. 24-21).[66] The striations were believed to represent fibrous septa that separate the hypoechoic, necrotic testicular parenchyma. There are no diagnostic sonographic features of testicular abscesses, but they can often be differentiated from tumors by clinical symptoms.

In patients with acquired immunodeficiency syndrome (AIDS), differentiation of abscess from a neoplastic process is difficult on ultrasound examination. Clinical findings may be helpful; however, orchiectomy is frequently necessary to obtain a histologic diagnosis.[67,68]

Infarction. Testicular infarction may follow torsion, trauma, bacterial endocarditis, polyarteritis nodosa, leukemia, hypercoagulable states, and Henoch-Schönlein purpura.[69,70,71] Spontaneous infarction of the testis is rare. The sonographic appearance depends on the age of the infarction. Initially, an infarct is seen as a focal, hypoechoic mass or as a diffusely hypoechoic testicle of normal size. The focal hypoechoic mass cannot be distinguished from a neoplasm based on its appearance.[72,73] These lesions should be largely avascular, depending on the age of the infarction. If a well-circumscribed, nonpalpable, relatively

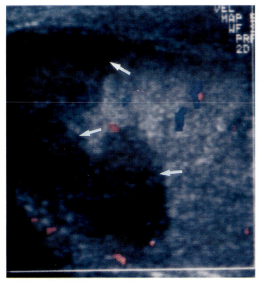

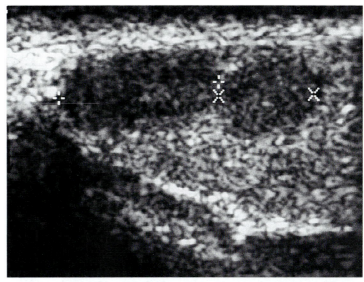

FIG. 24-22. Testicular infarcts. A, Longitudinal scrotal ultrasound shows a peripheral, well-demarcated, hypoechoic mass with no apparent blood flow *(arrows)*. **B,** Repeat exam shows that the masses *(++, XX)* and the entire testes have decreased in size. **C,** Power mode Doppler shows no definite flow in these testicular infarcts *(arrows)*.

peripheral, hypoechoic mass demonstrates complete lack of vascularity on power mode Doppler imaging or following the administration of ultrasound contrast agent, it may be possible to distinguish such benign infarctions from neoplasm in patients with appropriate clinical presentations (Fig. 24-22). However, a larger experience is required to substantiate this hypothesis. With time, the hypoechoic mass or entire testicle often decreases in size and develops areas of increased echogenicity because of **fibrosis or dystrophic calcification** (Fig. 24-23).[9,66,70] The early sonographic appearance may be difficult to differentiate from a testicular neoplasm, but infarcts substantially decrease in size whereas tumors characteristically enlarge with time.[2,73]

Sarcoidosis. Sarcoidosis may involve the epididymis and, less commonly, the testis. Genital in-

volvement occurs in less than 1% of patients with systemic sarcoidosis.[2,9] The clinical presentation is one of acute or recurrent epididymitis or painless enlargement of the testis or epididymis. Sonographically, sarcoid lesions are irregular, hypoechoic solid masses in the testis or epididymis (Fig. 24-24).[5,74] Occasionally, hyperechoic calcific foci with acoustic shadowing may be seen.[3] Differentiation from an inflammatory process or neoplasm is difficult on sonography alone. Resection or orchiectomy may be necessary for definitive diagnosis.

Adrenal Rests. **Congenital adrenal hyperplasia** is an autosomal recessive disease involving an adrenal cortical enzyme defect. This disease may become clinically obvious early in life or in early adulthood. The clinical presentation is often that of a testicular mass or testicular enlargement, presenting with precocious puberty with or without salt wasting.

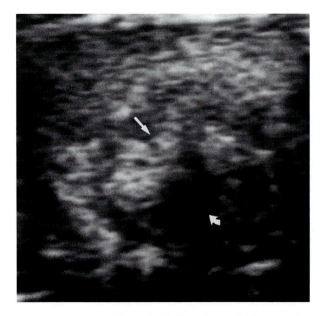

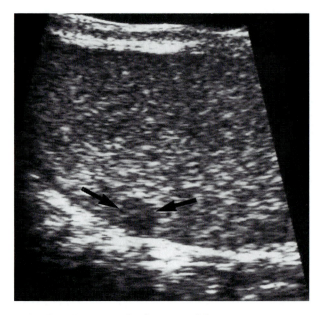

FIG. 24-23. Chronic infarction of the testis. Transverse scan through a testis with chronic infarction demonstrates areas of both increased *(arrow)* and decreased *(curved arrow)* echogenicity, which is indistinguishable from the appearance of malignancy.

FIG. 24-24. Testicular sarcoid. Longitudinal scan of the testis demonstrates a small, hypoechoic, solid mass *(arrows)* representing sarcoidosis. (Courtesy of J. William Charboneau, M.D., Mayo Clinic, Rochester, Minn.)

Adrenal rests arise from aberrant adrenal cortical cells that migrate with gonadal tissues in fetal life. They can form tumorlike masses in response to elevated levels of circulating adenocorticotropic hormone (ACTH) in congenital adrenal hyperplasia and Cushing's syndrome and may rarely undergo malignant transformation. On sonography, these lesions are multifocal hypoechoic lesions. Occasionally, posterior acoustic shadowing has been described (Fig. 24-25). Many adrenal rests demonstrate spokelike vascularity with multiple peripheral vessels radiating toward a central point within the mass. If the patient is known to have the appropriate hormonal abnormalities associated with congenital adrenal hyperplasia, and if ultrasound demonstrates the appropriate findings, no further work-up is necessary in most instances.[75,76]

Scrotal Calcifications. Scrotal calcifications may be seen within the parenchyma of the testicle, on the surface of the testicle, or freely located in the fluid between the layers of the tunica vaginalis. Large, smooth, curvilinear calcifications without an associated soft-tissue mass suggest a large cell, calcifying, Sertoli's cell tumor, although occasionally "burned-out" germ cell tumors may have a similar appearance.[77] Scattered calcifications may be found in tuberculosis, filariasis, and scarring from regressed germ cell tumor or trauma.

Testicular microlithiasis is an uncommon condition in which calcifications are present within the seminiferous tubules.[9] These calcifications occur in normal

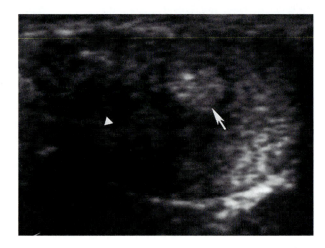

FIG. 24-25. Adrenocortical rest cell tumors. Longitudinal scrotal scan demonstrates multiple echogenic *(arrow)* and hypoechoic *(arrowhead)* focal masses in the testis. This appearance is indistinguishable from other malignancies and similar to rest cell tumors in the epididymis or spermatic cord.

and cryptorchid testes and have been reported in **Klinefelter's syndrome, male pseudohermaphroditism,** and **testicular neoplasms.**[78-80] It is postulated that microlithiasis results from calcification of corpora-amylacea-like bodies that may be found in the seminiferous tubules of both cryptorchid and normally descended testes.[81] Sonography demonstrates innumerable small, hyperechoic foci diffusely scattered

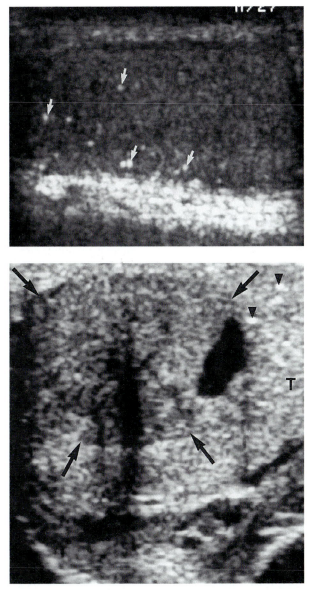

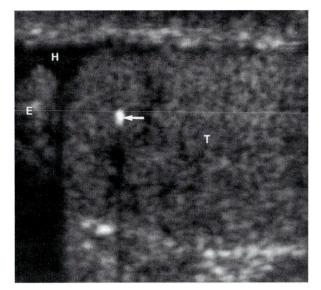

FIG. 24-27. **Testicular calcification.** Longitudinal scrotal scan of an asymptomatic patient reveals a normal-appearing testis, *T*, and epididymis, *E*, as well as a small hydrocele, *H*. A well-circumscribed focal calcification *(arrow)* was incidentally detected and was probably related to prior inflammatory change or sperm cell granuloma formation because there was no change in 6 months.

FIG. 24-26. **Testicular microlithiasis preceding testicular carcinomas.** **A,** Scan of 27-year-old man with a history of mild scrotal pain demonstrates testicular microlithiasis *(arrows)*. **B,** Follow-up scan 1 year later reveals development of a mixed seminoma-embryonal cell carcinoma *(arrows)*. *T,* Normal testis. Microlithiasis *(arrowheads)*.

SCROTAL CALCIFICATIONS

Testicular
Solitary; postinflammatory granulomatous, vascular
Microlithiasis
"Burned-out" germ cell tumor
Large cell calcifying Sertoli's cell tumor
Teratoma/teratocarcinomas
Sarcoid
Tuberculosis
Infarct—chronic

Extratesticular
Tunica vaginalis "scrotal pearls"
Chronic epididymitis
Schistosomiasis

throughout the testicular parenchyma, which rarely shadow and occasionally show a comet-tail appearance. Bilateral involvement may occur (Fig. 24-26).

Initially it was felt that testicular microlithiasis was a benign process with a characteristic sonographic appearance that did not require further evaluation.[82] However, recent reports have shown a significant occurrence of coexisting primary testicular neoplasm and testicular microlithiasis.[83,84] Forty percent of 42 patients with testicular microlithiasis demonstrated associated neoplasm in one series.[83] It appears that testicular microlithiasis can no longer be regarded as

a benign incidental observation. A recent case at our institution demonstrated development of a primary germ cell tumor a year and a half after the initial observation of "tumor-free" microlithiasis. At present, routine ultrasound follow-up of patients with testicular microlithiasis is indicated probably at 6-month intervals, with appropriate tumor marker evaluation.

Isolated microlithiasis involving fewer than five simple calcifications per testes is a more common, probably benign condition usually related to inflammatory, granulomatous, or vascular calcifications (Fig. 24-27). At present, if there are fewer than five microliths per cross-sectional image, the diagnosis of testicular microlithiasis is unwarranted, and follow-up of these patients is probably not necessary.

Extratesticular scrotal calculi arise from the surface of the tunica vaginalis and may break loose to migrate about between the two layers of the tunica (Fig. 24-28). They have been called fibrinoid loose bodies or scrotal pearls because of their macroscopic appearance, which is usually round, pearly white, and rubbery. Histologically they consist of fibrinoid material deposited around a central nucleus of hydroxyapatite.[85] They may result from inflammation of the tunica vaginalis or torsion of the appendix testis or epididymis. Secondary hydroceles are common because of inhibition of the normal secretion and absorption by the tunica vaginalis, usually as a result of inflammation. Hydrocele formation facilitates the sonographic diagnosis of scrotal calculi (Fig. 24-29).

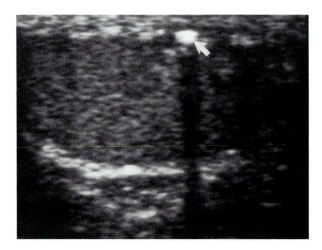

FIG. 24-28. Calcified plaque from the tunica vaginalis. Longitudinal scan demonstrates calcification of the tunica vaginalis *(arrow)*.

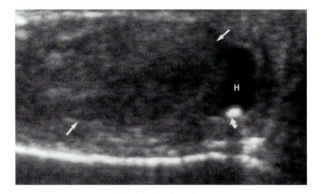

FIG. 24-29. Scrotal calculus. Longitudinal scrotal scan demonstrates an inhomogeneous-appearing testis *(arrows)* in a patient with multiple bouts of acute and chronic epididymitis. A small reactive hydrocele, *H*, contains an echogenic, free-floating, scrotal calculus *(curved arrow)*. This palpable calculus was the reason for the sonogram.

Extratesticular Pathology
Hydrocele, Hematocele, and Pyocele.
Serous fluid, blood, pus, or urine may accumulate in the space between the parietal and visceral layers of the tunica vaginalis lining the scrotum. These fluid collections are confined to the anterolateral portions of the scrotum because of the attachment of the testis to the epididymis and scrotal wall posteriorly (the bare area) (Fig. 24-30).

The normal scrotum contains a few milliliters of serous fluid between the layers of the tunica vaginalis. Approximately 85% of asymptomatic subjects who underwent scrotal ultrasound had minimal amounts of fluid in one hemiscrotum.[86]

Hydrocele is an abnormal accumulation of serous fluid, which is the most common cause of painless scrotal swelling[3] and may be congenital or acquired. The congenital type results from incomplete closure of the processus vaginalis, with persistent open communication between the scrotal sac and the peritoneum, usually resolving by 18 months of age.

Acquired hydroceles are the result of trauma in 25% to 50% of cases. Large hydroceles result uncommonly from neoplasms whereas small hydroceles occur in 60% of patients with testicular tumors.[2,4,87] Other causes of secondary hydroceles include epididymitis, epididymo-orchitis, and torsion.[9,21]

Sonography plays an important role as it can detect a potential cause of the hydrocele and permit evaluation of the testicle when a large hydrocele hampers

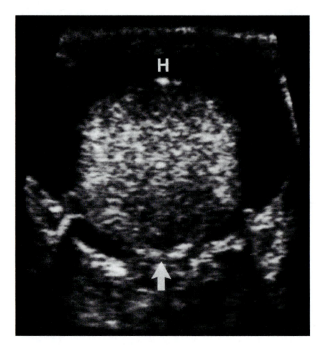

FIG. 24-30. Hydrocele. Transverse scrotal scan demonstrates a hydrocele, *H*, surrounding all parts of the testis except the posterior portion *(arrow)* where the testis is attached directly to the scrotal wall.

palpation. Hydroceles are characteristically anechoic collections with good sound transmission surrounding the anterolateral aspects of the testis, providing an excellent acoustic window for imaging the testis. Low-level to medium-level echoes from fibrin bodies or cholesterol crystals may occasionally be visualized moving freely within a hydrocele.[4,13]

Hematoceles and **pyoceles** are less common than simple hydroceles. Hematoceles result from trauma, surgery, diabetes, neoplasms, torsion, or atherosclerotic disease.[88] Pyoceles result from rupture of an abscess into an existing hydrocele or directly into the space between the layers of the tunica vaginalis. Both hematoceles and pyoceles contain internal septations and loculations (Fig. 24-31).

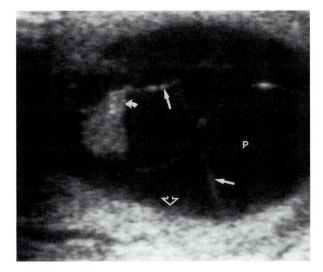

FIG. 24-31. Pyocele. Transverse scan through the superior aspect of the right hemiscrotum in a patient with epididymitis and testicular abscess formation demonstrates a pyocele, *P*, with multiple internal septations *(arrows)* and dependent debris *(open arrow)*. An enlarged appendix epididymis is also seen *(curved arrow)*.

Thickening of the scrotal skin and calcifications may be seen in chronic cases.

Varicocele. A varicocele is a collection of abnormally dilated, tortuous, and elongated veins of the pampiniform plexus located posterior to the testis, accompanying the epididymis and vas deferens within the spermatic cord (Fig. 24-32).[3,4,9,89] The veins of the pampiniform plexus normally range from 0.5 to 1.5 mm in diameter, with a main draining vein up to 2 mm in diameter.

There are two types of varicoceles: primary (idiopathic) and secondary. The **idiopathic varicocele** is caused by incompetent valves in the internal spermatic vein, which permit retrograde passage of blood through the spermatic cord into the pampiniform plexus. It is the most common correctable cause of male infertility, occurring in 21% to 39% of men attending infertility clinics.[90-92] Idiopathic varicoceles occur on the left side in 98% of cases and are usually detected in men between 15 and 25 years of age.[9] The left-sided predominance is believed to be due to the fact that the venous drainage on the left side is into the renal vein, as opposed to the right spermatic vein, which drains directly into the vena cava. Idiopathic varices normally distend when the patient is upright or performs Valsalva's maneuver and may decompress when the patient is supine. Primary varicoceles are bilateral in up to 70% of cases.[93]

Secondary varicoceles result from increased pressure on the spermatic vein or its tributaries by marked hydronephrosis, an enlarged liver, abdominal neoplasms, or venous compression by a retroperitoneal mass.[4,21] A search for neoplastic obstruction of gonadal venous return must be undertaken in cases of a right-sided, nondecompressible, or newly discovered varicocele in a patient over age 40, as these cases are rarely idiopathic.[3] The appearance of secondary varicoceles is not affected by patient position.

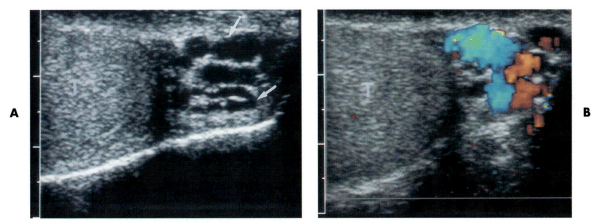

FIG. 24-32. Varicocele. **A,** Longitudinal scan demonstrates a large serpiginous varix *(arrows)*. **B,** Color flow Doppler image shows flow within varicocele. *T,* Testis.

In infertile men, sonography aids in the diagnosis of clinically palpable and subclinical varicoceles. There is no correlation between the size of the varicocele and the degree of testicular tissue damage leading to infertility. Therefore early detection and treatment of subclinical varicoceles are important.[92]

Sonographically the varicocele consists of multiple, serpiginous, anechoic structures more than 2 mm in diameter, creating a tortuous multicystic collection located adjacent or proximal to the upper pole of the testis and head of the epididymis. Occasionally the varicocele may appear similar to a small, septated spermatocele. Differentiation between varicocele and spermatocele may be accomplished using duplex or color flow Doppler sonography. Similarly, dilated veins in the mediastinum testes can be distinguished from tubular ectasia of the rete testes by use of color flow or pulsed wave Doppler ultrasound. A high-frequency transducer in conjunction with low-flow Doppler settings should be used to optimize slow-flow detection within varices. Slowly moving red blood cells may be visualized with high-frequency transducers, even when flow is too slow to be detected by Doppler imaging (see Fig. 24-32). Venous flow can be augmented with the patient in the upright position or during Valsalva's maneuver. In addition, varicoceles, unlike spermatoceles, follow the course of the spermatic cord into the inguinal canal and are easily compressed by the transducer.[2,4,21]

Scrotal Hernia. A scrotal hernia is another common paratesticular mass. Although scrotal hernias are usually diagnosed on the basis of clinical history and physical examination, sonography is useful in the evaluation of atypical cases. The hernia may contain small bowel, colon, and/or omentum.[94] The presence of bowel loops within the hernia may be confirmed by the visualization of valvulae conniventes or haustrations and detection of peristalsis on real-time examination. If these features are absent, differentiation from other extratesticular multicystic masses, such as hematocele and pyocele, may be difficult. The presence of highly echogenic material within the scrotum may be due to a hernia-containing omentum or other fatty masses (Fig. 24-33). Sonographic examination of the inguinal canal must also be performed to identify the extension of omentum or bowel loops from the inguinal canal into the scrotum.[21,94]

Tumors. Extratesticular neoplasms are rare and usually involve the epididymis. The most common extratesticular neoplasm is the **adenomatoid tumor,** representing 32% of these tumors.[16,95] It is most frequently located in the epididymis, especially in the globus minor, but may also arise in the spermatic cord or testicular tunica (Fig. 24-34).[18] This neoplasm may occasionally invade adjacent testicular parenchyma. It may occur at any age, but is most commonly found in

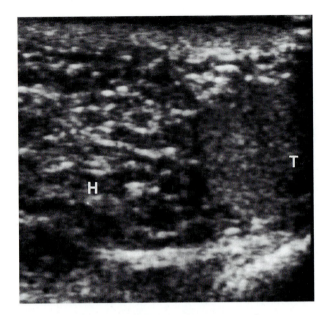

FIG. 24-33. Herniated mesenteric fat, *H,* lies superior to the right testes, *T.*

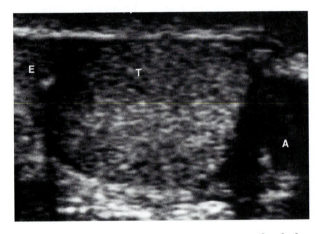

FIG. 24-34. Adenomatoid tumor, tail of the epididymis. Longitudinal scrotal scan demonstrates a normal testis, *T,* and head of the epididymis, *E,* with a large, well-circumscribed, hypoechoic mass, *A,* in the tail of the epididymis.

patients age 20 to 50 years.[2,18,96] It is generally unilateral, solitary, well defined, and round- or oval-shaped, rarely measuring greater than 5 cm in diameter. Occasionally it may appear plaquelike and ill defined. Sonography usually demonstrates a solid, well-circumscribed mass with echogenicity equal to or greater than that of the testis.[2] It may also be hypoechoic.

Other benign extratesticular tumors are rare and include **fibromas, hemangiomas, lipomas, leiomyomas, neurofibromas,** and **cholesterol granulomas.**[18] **Adrenal rests** may also be encountered in the spermatic cord, testis, epididymis, rete testis, and tunica albuginea in approximately 10% of infants.[18]

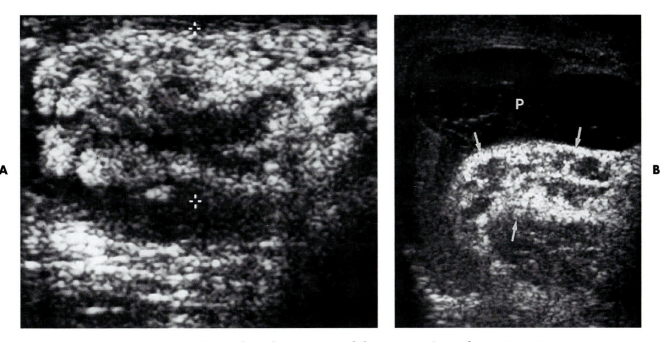

FIG. 24-35. Primary lymphosarcoma of the spermatic cord. A, A large, firm, palpable mass proved to be a heterogeneous, tubular extratesticular mass *(++)* in the distribution of the spermatic cord. **Severe epididymo-orchitis and a pyocele,** *P.* **B,** A strikingly similar appearance of the spermatic cord *(arrows)*, which is frequently enlarged and heterogeneous in epididymo-orchitis, but there should not be a firm palpable mass and the findings should improve with treatment.

Papillary cystadenomas of the epididymis may be seen in patients with Hippel-Lindau disease.[74] Primary extratesticular scrotal malignant neoplasms include **fibrosarcoma, liposarcoma,** and, less commonly, **malignant histiocytoma** and **lymphoma** in adults, and **rhabdomyosarcoma** in children (Fig. 24-35).

Metastatic tumors to the epididymis are also rare. The most common primary sites include the testicle, stomach, kidney, prostate, colon, and, less commonly, pancreas.[74,95,97,98] Sonography demonstrates focal, echogenic areas of thickening within the epididymis commonly in association with a hydrocele.

Epididymal Lesions

Cystic lesions. Spermatoceles are more common than epididymal cysts. They were both seen in 20% to 40% of all asymptomatic patients studied by Leung et al.,[86] and 30% were multiple cysts. Both epididymal cysts and spermatoceles are believed to result from dilation of the epididymal tubules, but the contents of these masses differ.[3,74] Cysts contain clear serous fluid whereas spermatoceles are filled with spermatozoa and sediment-containing lymphocytes, fat globules, and cellular debris, giving the fluid a thick, milky appearance.[2,74] Both lesions may result from prior episodes of epididymitis or trauma. Spermatoceles and epididymal cysts appear identical on ultrasound: anechoic, well-circumscribed masses with no or few internal echoes (Fig. 24-36). Loculations and septa-

tions are commonly seen (Fig. 24-37), and differentiation between spermatocele and epididymal cyst is rarely clinically important. Spermatoceles almost always occur in the head of the epididymis whereas epididymal cysts arise throughout the length of the epididymis.

EXTRATESTICULAR TUMORS

Benign
Adenomatoid tumor
Fibroma
Lipoma
Hemangioma
Leiomyoma
Neurofibroma
Cholesterol granuloma
Adrenal rest
Papillary cystadenoma

Malignant
Fibrosarcoma
Liposarcoma
Rhabdosarcoma
Histiocytoma
Lymphoma
Metastases

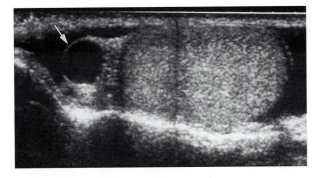

FIG. 24-36. Epididymal cyst. Longitudinal scrotal scan demonstrates an epididymal cyst *(arrow)* involving the head of the epididymis, indistinguishable in appearance from a spermatocele.

Sperm granuloma. Sperm granulomas are believed to arise from extravasation of spermatozoa into the soft tissues surrounding the epididymis, producing a necrotizing granulomatous response.[2,9,99,100] These lesions are usually asymptomatic but are frequently associated with prior epididymal infection or trauma. They are most often found in patients after vasectomy. The typical sonographic appearance is that of a solid, hypoechoic mass that is usually located within the epididymis, although they may simulate an intratesticular lesion.[99]

Postvasectomy changes in the epididymis. Sonographic changes in the epididymis have been reported in 45% of patients after vasectomy. These findings include epididymal enlargement and inhomogeneity and the development of sperm granulomas and cysts. It is theorized that vasectomy produces increased pressure in the epididymal tubules, causing tubular rupture with subsequent formation of sperm granulomas. This tubular rupture may protect the testis from the effects of increased back pressure. These sonographic findings are nonspecific and may be seen in patients who have epididymitis.[101] Postorchiectomy sonographic findings include hematomas, local tumor recurrence, secondary primary tumor, and the sonographic appearance of testicular prosthesis.[102]

Chronic epididymitis. Patients with incompletely treated acute bacterial epididymitis usually present with a chronically painful scrotal mass. Patients with chronic granulomatous epididymitis due to spread of tuberculosis from the genitourinary tract complain of a hard, nontender scrotal mass.[3] Sonography most commonly demonstrates a thickened tunica albuginea and a thickened, irregular epididymis. Calcification may be identified within the tunica albuginea or epididymis.[2,103] Untreated granulomatous epididymitis will spread to the testes in 60% to 80% of cases.[9] Focal testicular involvement may simulate the appearance of

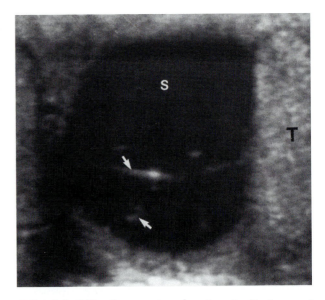

FIG. 24-37. Spermatocele. Longitudinal scan of the head of the epididymis demonstrates a spermatocele, *S,* which contains septations *(open arrows). T,* Testicle.

a testicular neoplasm on sonography whereas diffuse testicular involvement results in an enlarged, irregular testis with diffuse homogeneous hypoechogenicity.

ACUTE SCROTUM

Torsion

There is a wide differential diagnosis of an acutely painful and swollen scrotum, including torsion of the spermatic cord and testis, torsion of a testicular appendage, epididymitis and/or orchitis, acute hydrocele, strangulated hernia, idiopathic scrotal edema, Henoch-Schönlein purpura, abscess, traumatic hemorrhage, hemorrhage into a testicular neoplasm, and scrotal fat necrosis. Torsion of the spermatic cord and acute epididymitis or epididymo-orchitis are the most common causes of an acute scrotum. These entities cannot be distinguished by physical examination or laboratory tests in up to 50% of cases.[104] Torsion is more common in children, but represents only 20% of acute scrotal pathology in postpubertal men.[2] Prompt diagnosis is necessary since torsion requires immediate surgery to preserve the testis. The testicular salvage rate is 80% to 100% if surgery is performed within 5 to 6 hours of the onset of pain, 70% if surgery is performed within 6 to 12 hours, and only 20% if surgery is delayed for more than 12 hours.[105] Immediate surgical exploration has been advised in boys and young men with acute scrotal pain unless a definitive diagnosis of epididymitis/orchitis can be made. This aggressive approach has resulted in an increased testicular salvage rate but also an increase in unnecessary surgical procedures.[106] Radionuclide testicular imaging, real-time sonography, and Doppler sonography have been used to increase the accuracy of differentiation between infection and torsion.[107] Currently ultrasound, using color flow and/or power mode Doppler, is the imaging study of choice to diagnose the cause of acute scrotal pain in adults.

There are two types of testicular torsion: intravaginal and extravaginal. **Intravaginal torsion** is the most common type, occurring most commonly at puberty. It results from anomalous suspension of the testis by a long stalk of spermatic cord, resulting in complete investment of the testis and epididymis by the tunica vaginalis. It has been likened to a "bell and clapper." There is a tenfold greater incidence of torsion in undescended testes after orchiopexy.[108] Anomalous testicular suspension is also present in 50% to 80% of the contralateral testes.[21]

Extravaginal torsion occurs most commonly in newborns without the "bell and clapper" deformity. It is believed to be due to the motility of the entire vaginalis, resulting in torsion of the testis and its tunica at the level of the external ring. The more compliant veins are obstructed before the arteries in both forms of torsion, resulting in early vascular engorgement and edema of the testicle.

A spectrum of gray-scale sonographic changes has been reported **in the acute phase of torsion** within 1 to 6 hours.[104,109] The testicle becomes enlarged, inhomogeneous, and hypoechoic as compared with the contralateral normal testis (Fig. 24-38). Common extratesticular findings include an enlarged epididymis containing foci of increased and decreased echogenicity, skin thickening, and reactive hydrocele formation. Occasionally, the testicle may have normal echogenicity.[110-112] Generalized testicular hyperechogenicity has been reported in two cases of acute torsion in the absence of histologic changes of testicular hemorrhage or infarction.[104-113]

During the **subacute phase of torsion** (1 to 10 days), the degree of testicular hypoechogenicity and enlargement increases within the first 5 days, then diminishes over the next 4 to 5 days. The epididymis remains enlarged but is often echogenic. Hydroceles are common in cases of **chronic torsion.**[109] In a recent report by Vick et al.,[113] large echogenic or complex extratesticular masses caused by hemorrhage within the tunica vaginalis, epididymis, or other extratesticular locations were visualized in cases of **missed torsion.** The gray-scale findings of acute and subacute torsion are not specific and may be seen in testicular infarction secondary to epididymitis, epididymo-orchitis, and traumatic testicular rupture or infarction.[114,115]

Pulsed wave and color flow Doppler examination of the spermatic cord and testicular vessels have been

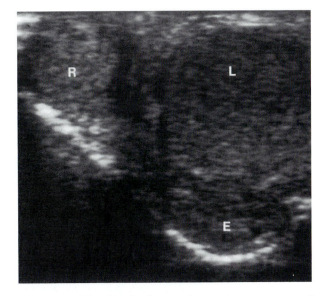

FIG. 24-38. **Testicular torsion.** Transverse scan of the scrotum demonstrates that the left testis, *L*, and epididymis are markedly enlarged and hypoechoic relative to the normal right testis. Similar findings could be seen in a severe case of epididymitis-epididymo-orchitis.

used to help differentiate torsion from epididymo-orchitis (Fig. 24-39).[104,111,115,116] The presence of normal or increased blood flow within the testicle would theoretically exclude the diagnosis of acute torsion. Meticulous scanning of the testicular parenchyma and the use of low-flow detection Doppler techniques are required because testicular vessels are small and have low flow velocities.

The diagnosis of **testicular ischemia** depends on the ability to unequivocally demonstrate the presence of normal blood flow in the normal, contralateral, asymptomatic testicle. Several recent series have reported color flow Doppler findings in testicular ischemia.[116,117] One of these reported 86% sensitivity, 100% specificity, and 97% accuracy in the diagnosis of testicular torsion using color flow Doppler sonography.[117] In addition, torsion of the testicular appendage was correctly diagnosed in five patients so that conservative treatment was undertaken, sparing unnecessary surgery.[116] This series reported a single false-negative study with intra-testicular blood flow detected in a testis that was subsequently shown at surgery to be torsed. Interestingly, only a 360-degree torsion of the spermatic cord was present, suggesting at least 540 degrees of torsion is necessary to completely occlude testicular blood flow.[118,119] Thus with lesser degrees of spermatic cord torsion, minimal residual flow may exist within the testis. With progressive torsion, the normal arterial waveforms can become progressively tardus-parvus, resembling pulsatile venous traces.[119]

Color flow Doppler sonography shows a higher sensitivity in demonstrating decreased testicular flow in

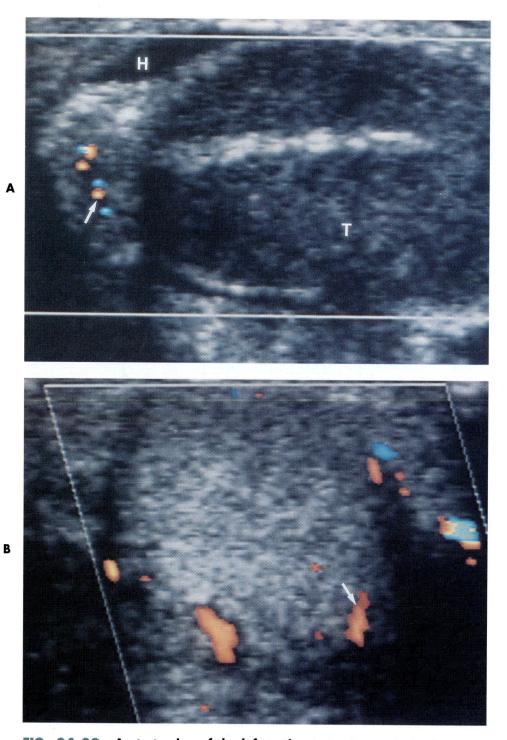

FIG. 24-39. **Acute torsion of the left testis.** **A,** An absence of color flow in the testis, *T*, and a small amount of flow in the region of the head of the epididymis *(arrow)*. Parenchymal echogenicity is decreased. *H,* Hydrocele. **B,** Asymptomatic right testis demonstrates color flow within the testis *(arrow)* and normal parenchymal echogenicity.

incomplete torsion[120] than does nuclear scintigraphy. While color flow Doppler sonography is useful in the initial evaluation of suspected torsion in pediatric patients, testicular scintigraphy has been advocated to corroborate ultrasound findings when intratesticular flow cannot be demonstrated using color flow Doppler.[121] Recent advances have been made in the detection of testicular ischemia with the use of power mode Doppler sonography, which has increased the ability to detect slower blood flow within smaller caliber vessels. Research with intravascular contrast agents for use in ultrasound shows promise for increasing the sensitivity of detecting blood flow in the scrotum.

In cases of **subacute or chronic torsion,** color flow Doppler demonstrates absent intratesticular flow and increased flow in the peritesticular tissues, including the epididymis-cord complex and dartos fascia (Fig. 24-40). In cases of **detorsion,** color flow Doppler may demonstrate increased testicular and peritesticular flow or normal flow.[116,118] It is important to remember that reactive hyperemia of the testicle, resulting from the resolution of intermittent torsion, may mimic hyperreactive blood flow in epididymo-orchitis on color flow Doppler sonography. However, clinical findings should help differentiate intermittent torsion and epididymo-orchitis in the acute setting.

Torsion of the testicular appendage has been described as an avascular hypoechoic mass adjacent to a normally perfused testis and surrounded by an area of increased color flow Doppler perfusion.[116] However, other investigators have described a different appearance, specifically that of an echogenic extratesticular mass situated between the head of the epididymis and the upper pole of the testis.[122]

Epididymitis and Epididymo-orchitis

Epididymitis is the most common cause of the acute scrotum in postpubertal men, representing 75% of all acute intrascrotal inflammatory processes. It usually results from a lower urinary tract infection and is less commonly hematogenous or traumatic in origin. The common causative organisms are *Escherichia coli*, *Pseudomonas*, and *Aerobacter*.[123] Sexually transmitted organisms causing urethritis, such as *Gonococcus* and *Chlamydia*, are common causes of epididymitis in young men. Less commonly, epididymitis may accompany mumps or syphilitic orchitis. The peak age incidence is between 40 and 50 years. Classically, patients present with the insidious onset of pain, which increases over a period of 1 to 2 days. Fever, dysuria, and urethral discharge may also be present.

Sonography characteristically demonstrates thickening and enlargement of the epididymis, most com-

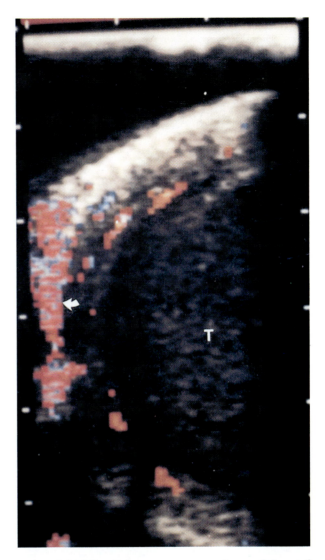

FIG. 24-40. Subacute traumatic avulsion of the spermatic cord shows absent testicular flow, *T*, with soft-tissue reactive hyperemia *(curved arrow).*

monly involving the head (Fig. 24-41).[13] The entire epididymis is involved in 50% of cases. The echogenicity of the epididymis is usually decreased, and its echo texture is often coarse and heterogeneous, probably because of edema and/or hemorrhage. Reactive hydrocele formation is common, and associated skin thickening may be seen.

Color flow Doppler ultrasound usually demonstrates increased blood flow in the epididymis and/or testis as compared with the asymptomatic side (see Fig. 24-41).[124] Direct extension of epididymal inflammation to the testicle, called epididymo-orchitis, occurs in up to 20% of patients with acute epididymitis. Isolated orchitis may also occur. In such cases, increased blood flow would be localized to the testis (Fig. 24-42). Testicular involvement may be focal or diffuse. Characteristically, **focal orchitis** produces a hypoechoic area adjacent to an enlarged portion of the

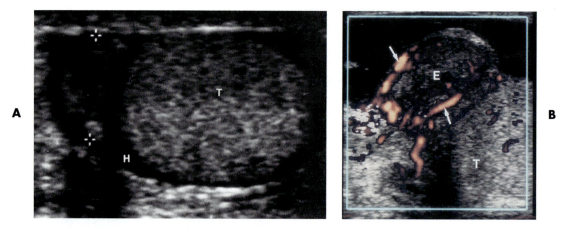

FIG. 24-41. Acute epididymitis. A, Longitudinal scan in a patient with acute epididymitis shows a hypoechoic, enlarged, epididymal head *(cursors)* and a small, reactive hydrocele, *H. T,* Testis. **B,** Power mode Doppler shows increased flow *(arrows)* in the enlarged hypoechoic head of the epididymis, *E.* Testicular flow is not as increased, *T.*

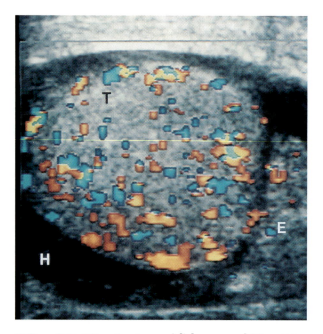

FIG. 24-42. Acute epididymo-orchitis. Color flow Doppler demonstrates an "inferno" of testicular color signal, *T. H,* Hydrocele; *E,* epididymis.

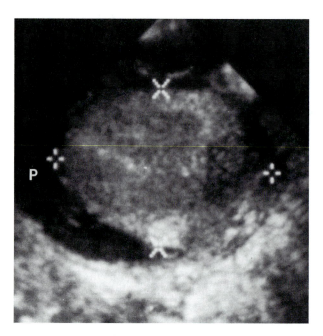

FIG. 24-43. Chronic epididymo-orchitis (unresponsive to antibiotic therapy). A diffusely inhomogeneous testis *(cursors)* surrounded by a pyocele, *P,* containing septations and purulent debris. At surgery multiple areas of orchitis and abscess formation were noted within the testis.

epididymis. If left untreated, the entire testicle may become involved, appearing hypoechoic and enlarged (Fig. 24-43). Testicular involvement may also result from secondary effects of epididymal inflammation. Occasionally, marked edema associated with acute epididymitis may result in occlusion of the testicular blood supply, resulting in ischemia and subsequent infarction. If vascular disruption is extremely severe, resulting in **complete testicular infarction,** changes would be indistinguishable from those seen in testicular torsion. In such instances, increased blood flow would be seen proximal to the area of vascular disruption because of swelling and edema. The hyperemic blood flow in the dartos and proximal spermatic cord would be in striking contrast to the avascular scrotal contents distal to the point of vascular occlusion. Resultant ischemia associated with severe epididymitis also predisposes the testicle to infection, which may be in the form of focal orchitis, abscess formation, or diffuse gangrenous **epididymo-orchitis.** In most cases of epididymo-orchitis, the testicle retains its ovoid and smooth contour. Color flow Doppler sonography may demonstrate focal areas of reactive hyperemia and increased blood flow associated with relatively avascular areas of infarction in both the testis and epididymis in cases of severe epididymo-orchitis. Diastolic flow reversal in the arterial waveforms of the testis is an ominous finding associated with testicular infarction in cases of severe epididymo-orchitis.[125]

TRAUMA

Prompt diagnosis of a **ruptured testis** is of utmost importance because of the direct relationship between early surgical intervention and testicular salvageability. Approximately 90% of testicles can be saved if surgery is performed within the first 72 hours whereas only 45% may be salvaged after 72 hours.[126,127] Clinical diagnosis is often impossible because of marked scrotal pain and swelling. Jeffrey et al.[126] correctly identified 12 out of 12 cases of testicular rupture using sonography. Sonographic features include focal areas of altered testicular echogenicity corresponding to areas of hemorrhage or infarction, and hematocele formation in 33% of patients. A discrete fracture plane was identified in only 17% of cases (Fig. 24-44). The testicular contour is often irregular. Although these features are not specific for a ruptured testicle, they may suggest the diagnosis in the appropriate clinical setting, prompting immediate surgical exploration. Vascular disruption may also be demonstrated by color flow Doppler sonography (Fig. 24-45). Care should be taken to avoid mistaking a complex intrascrotal hematoma from apparent testicular rupture. Use of Doppler and color flow Doppler imaging may aid in separating the normal vascularized testis from a complex hematoma.[128] Ultrasound can also be used to discern the severity of scrotal trauma due to bullet wounds. Hematomas and hematoceles can be distinguished from testicular rupture, and foreign bodies can be localized.[129] A careful grayscale and color flow Doppler evaluation of the epididymis should be performed in all exams done for blunt trauma. Traumatic epididymitis may be an isolated finding that should not necessarily be confused with an infectious process.[130]

CRYPTORCHIDISM

The testes normally begin their descent through the inguinal canal into the scrotal sac at approximately 36 weeks of gestation. The gubernaculum testis is a fibromuscular structure that extends from the inferior pole of the testis to the scrotum and guides the testis

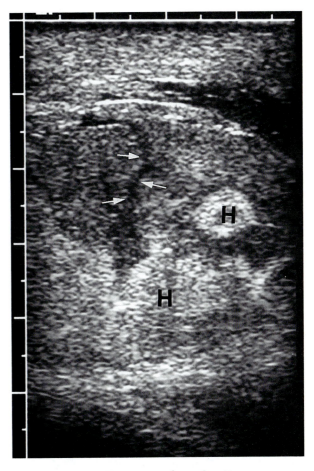

FIG. 24-44. **Fracture of testis.** Transverse scan demonstrates a heterogeneous testicle with a linear band *(arrows)* representing fracture. *H,* Testicular hematoma.

ACUTE SCROTUM

Torsion of the testes
Epididymo-orchitis
Testicular appendage torsion
Strangulated hernia
Idiopathic scrotal edema
Trauma
Henoch-Schönlein purpura

in its descent, which is normally completed at birth.[9] Undescended testis is one of the most common genitourinary anomalies in male infants. At birth, 3.5% of male infants weighing more than 2500 g have an undescended testis; 10% to 25% of these cases are bilateral. This figure decreases to 0.8% by age 1 year since the testes descend spontaneously in most infants. The incidence of undescended testes increases to 30% in premature infants, approaching 100% in neonates who weigh less than 1 kg at birth.[131,132] Complete descent is necessary for full testicular maturation.[131,132]

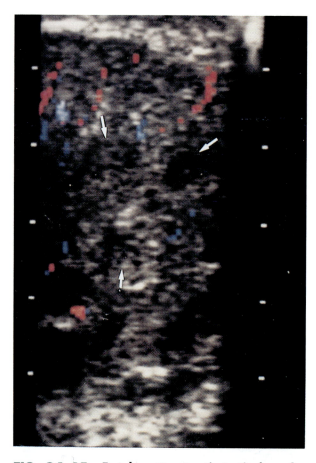

FIG. 24-45. Focal posttraumatic testicular edema and hypovascularity. Color flow Doppler scan through the lower pole of a testis posttrauma demonstrates an area of hypoechogenicity *(arrows)* that is relatively avascular.

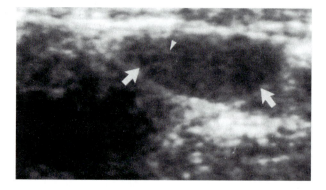

FIG. 24-46. Atrophic testis in inguinal canal. Longitudinal scan through the inguinal canal demonstrates an elliptical, small, cryptorchid testis *(arrows)* with an echogenic band, representing the mediastinum testis *(arrowhead).*

Malpositioned testes may be located anywhere along the pathway of descent from the retroperitoneum to the scrotum. The majority (80%) of undescended testes are palpable, lying at or below the level of the inguinal canal. Anorchia occurs in 4% of the remaining patients with impalpable testes.[132]

Localization of the undescended testis is important for the prevention of two potential **complications of cryptorchidism: infertility** and **cancer.** Infertility results from progressive pathologic changes that develop in both the undescended and contralateral normal testis after the age of 1 year.[132-134] The undescended testis is 48 times more likely to undergo malignant change than the normally descended testis.[2] It is believed that the hormonal deficiency resulting in failure of testicular descent predisposes the patient to malignancy. Approximately 0.04% of patients with an undescended testis will develop carcinoma annually. The lifetime risk of death from a testicular malignancy in men of any age with an undescended testis is approximately 9.7 times the risk in normal men.[133]

The most common malignancy is seminoma. The risk of malignancy is increased in both the undescended testis after orchiopexy and the normally descended testis. Therefore careful serial examinations of both testes are essential.

Because of the superficial location of the inguinal canal in children, sonography of the undescended testis should be performed with a high-frequency transducer and a standoff pad to avoid reverberation artifacts. Sonographically the **undescended testis** is often smaller and slightly less echogenic than the contralateral normally descended testis (Fig. 24-46). A specific diagnosis of an undescended testis may be made if the mediastinum testis is identified. A large lymph node or the pars infravaginalis gubernaculi (PIG), which is the distal bulbous segment of the gubernaculum testis, has been mistaken for the testis, but theoretically, neither of these should contain an internal echogenic band. In reality, visualization of the mediastinum testis in undescended testes is often difficult. In addition, echogenic foci may be visualized within the PIG and lymph nodes, which may lead to a misdiagnosis of undescended testis. After completion of testicular descent, the PIG and gubernaculum normally atrophy. If the testis remains undescended, both structures persist. The PIG is located distal to the undescended testis, usually in the scrotum, but may be found in the inguinal cord. Sonographically the PIG is hypoechoic, a cordlike structure of echogenicity similar to the testis, with the gubernaculum leading to it.[135]

The success of sonography in the localization of undescended testes varies among series. Wolverson et al.[136] reported a sensitivity of 88%, specificity of 100%, and accuracy of 91% in the sonographic localization of undescended testes. In a later study, Weiss et al.[137] reported a sensitivity of 70% for palpable testes and 13% for nonpalpable testes. MRI has sensitivity and specificity similar to ultrasound in the evaluation of cryptorchidism.[138,139] MRI shares two main advantages with ultrasound: noninvasiveness and lack of ionizing radiation. An additional advantage of MRI is the ability to obtain multiplanar images of the retroperitoneum and inguinal region. Undescended testes are characteristically hypointense with respect to fat on short TR/TE sequences and hyperintense or isointense with respect to fat on long TR/TE sequences. These signal characteristics of undescended testes are identical to those of scrotal testes. Disadvantages of MRI include cost, long scanning time, frequent need for sedation, and lack of a bowel contrast agent in evaluation of abdominal testes. Because of sonography's lack of ionizing radiation, lower cost, and shorter scanning time, and the fact that it does not require sedation or oral contrast, it should be the initial method of evaluation of cryptorchidism. Nonvisualization of an undescended testis on ultrasound or MRI does not exclude its presence, and therefore laparoscopy or surgical exploration should be performed if clinically indicated.

REFERENCES

1. Carroll BA, Gross DM. High-frequency scrotal sonography. *AJR* 1983;140:511-515.
2. Krone KD, Carroll BA. Scrotal ultrasound. *Radiol Clin North Am* 1985;23:121-139.
3. Middleton WD, Thorne DA, Melson GL. Color Doppler ultrasound of the normal testis. *AJR* 1989;152:293-297
4. Hricak H, Filly RA. Sonography of the scrotum. *Invest Radiol* 1983;18:112-121.
5. Rifkin MD, Kurtz AB, Pasto ME et al. The sonographic diagnosis of focal and infiltrating intrascrotal lesions. *Urol Radiol* 1984;6:20-26.
6. Rifkin MD. Scrotal ultrasound. *Urol Radiol* 1987;9:119-126.
7. Middleton WD, Bell MW. Analysis of intratesticular arterial anatomy with emphasis on transmediastinal arteries. *Radiology* 1993;189:157-160

Anatomy
8. Trainer TD. Histology of the normal testis. *Am J Surg Pathol* 1987;11:797-809.
9. Rifkin MD, Foy PM, Goldberg BB. Scrotal ultrasound: acoustic characteristics of the normal testis and epididymis defined with high resolution superficial scanners. *Med Ultrasound* 1984;8:91-97.
10. Allen TD. Disorders of the male external genitalia. In: Kelalis PP, King LR, eds. *Clinical Pediatric Urology*, Philadelphia: WB Saunders Co; 1976:636-668.
11. Fakhry J, Khoury A, Barakat K. The hypoechoic band: a normal finding on testicular sonography. *AJR* 1989;153:321-323.
12. Gooding GAW. Sonography of the spermatic cord. *AJR* 1988;151:721-724.

The Scrotal Mass
13. Benson CB, Doubilet PM, Richie JP. Sonography of the male genital tract. *AJR* 1989;153:705-713.
14. Rifkin MD, Kurtz AB, Pasto ME et al. Diagnostic capabilities of high-resolution scrotal ultrasonography: prospective evaluation. *J Ultrasound Med* 1985;4:13-19.

15. Grantham JG, Charboneau JW, James EM et al. Testicular neoplasms: 29 tumors studied by high-resolution ultrasound. *Radiology* 1985;775-780.
16. Kirschling RJ, Kvols LK, Charboneau JW et al. High-resolution ultrasonographic and pathologic abnormalities of germ cell tumors in patients with clinically normal testes. *Mayo Clin Proc* 1983;58:648-653.
17. Javadpour N. *Principles and Management of Testicular Cancer*. New York: Thieme Inc; 1986.
18. Goldfinger SS, Rothberg R, Buckspan MB et al. Incidental detection of impalpable testicular neoplasm by sonography. *AJR* 1986;146:349-350.
19. Talerman A, Roth LM. *Pathology of the Testis and Its Adnexa*. New York: Churchill Livingstone; 1986.
20. Jacobsen GK, Talerman A. *Atlas of Germ Cell Tumors*. Copenhagen: Munksgaard; 1989.
21. Ruzal-Shapiro C, Newhouse JH. Genitourinary ultrasound. In: Taveras JM, Ferrucci JT, eds. *Radiology: Diagnosis-Imaging Intervention*. Philadelphia: JB Lippincott Co; 1986:4.
22. Schwerk WB, Schwerk WNM, Rodeck G. Testicular tumors: prospective analysis of real-time ultrasound patterns and abdominal staging. *Radiology* 1987;164:369-374.
23. Mostofi FK, Price EB Jr. Tumors of the male genital system. In: *Atlas of Tumor Pathology*, Fascicle 8, 2nd series. Washington, DC: Armed Forces Institute of Pathology; 1973.
24. Emory TH, Charboneau JW, Randall RV et al. Occult testicular interstitial-cell tumor in a patient with gynecomastia: ultrasonic detection. *Radiology* 1984;151:474.
25. Cunningham JJ. Echographic findings in Sertoli cell tumor of the testis. *J Clin Ultrasound* 1981;9:341-342.
26. Glazer HS, Lee JKT, Melson GL et al. Sonographic detection of occult testicular neoplasms. *AJR* 1981;138:673-675.
27. Bockrath JJ, Schaeffer AJ, Kies JS et al. Ultrasound identification of impalpable testicular tumor. *J Urol* 1981;130:355-356.
28. Moudy PC, Makhija JS. Ultrasonic demonstration of a nonpalpable testicular tumor. *J Clin Ultrasound* 1983;11:54-55.
29. Shawker TH, Javadpour N, O'Leary T, et al: Ultrasonographic detection of "burned-out" primary testicular germ cell tumors in clinically normal testes. *J Ultrasound Med* 1983;2:477-479.
30. Horstman WG, Melson GL, Middleton WD et al. Testicular tumors: findings with color Doppler US. *Radiology* 1992;185:733-737.
31. Luker GD, Siegel MJ. Pediatric testicular tumors: evaluation with gray-scale and color Doppler US. *Radiology* 1994;191:561-564.
32. Horstman WG, Haluszka MM, Burkhard TK. Management of testicular masses incidentally discovered by ultrasound. *J Urol* 1994;151:1263-1265.
33. Doll DC, Weiss RB. Malignant lymphoma of the testis. *Am J Med* 1986;81:515-523.
34. Tepperman BS, Gospodarowicz M, Bush RS et al. Non-Hodgkin lymphoma of the testis. *Radiology* 1982;142:203-208.
35. Paladugu RP, Bearman RM, Rappaport H. Malignant lymphoma with primary manifestation in the gonad: a clinicopathologic study of 38 patients. *Cancer* 1980;45:561-571.
36. Hamlin JA, Kagan AR, Friedman NB. Lymphomas of the testicle. *Cancer* 1972;29:1532-1536.
37. Rayor RA, Scheible W, Brock WA et al. High resolution ultrasonography in the diagnosis of testicular relapse in patients with lymphoblastic leukemia. *J Urol* 1982;128:602-603.
38. Phillips G, Kumari-Subaiya S, Sawitsky A. Ultrasonic evaluation of the scrotum in lymphoproliferative disease. *J Ultrasound Med* 1987;6:169-175.

39. Mazzu D, Jeffrey RB Jr, Ralls PW. Lymphoma and leukemia involving the testicles: findings on gray-scale and color Doppler sonography. *AJR* 1995;164:645-647.

40. Dahnert WF, Rifkin MD, Kurtz AB. Ultrasound case of the day. *RadioGraphics* 1989;9:554-558.

41. Grignon DJ, Shum DT, Hayman WP. Metastatic tumors of the testes. *Can J Surg* 1986;29:359-361.

42. Werth V, Yu G, Marshall FF. Nonlymphomatous metastatic tumor to the testis. *J Urol* 1981;127:142-144.

43. Hanash KA, Carney JA, Kelalis PP. Metastatic tumors to testicles: routes of metastasis. *J Urol* 1969;102:465-468.

44. Hamm B, Fobbe F, Loy V. Testicular cysts: differentiation with ultrasound and clinical findings. *Radiology* 1988;168:19-23.

45. Gooding GAW, Leonhardt W, Stein R. Testicular cysts: US findings. *Radiology* 1987;163:537-538.

46. Becker J, Arger PH, Wein AJ et al. Inclusion cyst of the tunica albuginea: demonstration by ultrasound. *Urol Radiol* 1983;5:127-129.

47. Turner WR, Derrick FC, Sanders P et al. Benign lesions of the tunica albuginea. *J Urol* 1977;117:602-604.

48. Warner KE, Noyes DT, Ross JS. Cysts of the tunica albuginea testis: a report of 3 cases with a review of the literature. *J Urol* 1984;132:131-132.

49. Poster RB, Spirt BA, Tamsen A et al. Complex tunica albuginea cyst simulating an intratesticular lesion. *Urol Radiol* 1991;13:129-132.

50. Takihari H, Valvo JR, Tokuhara M et al. Intratesticular cysts. *Urology* 1982;20:80-82.

51. Rifkin MD, Jacobs JA. Simple testicular cyst diagnosed preoperatively by ultrasound. *J Urol* 1983;129:982-983.

52. Fisher JE, Jewett TC, Nelson SJ et al. Ectasia of the rate testis with ipsilateral renal agenesis. *J Urol* 1982;128:1040-1043.

53. Nistal M, Regadera J, Paniagua R. Cystic dysplasia of the testis. *Arch Pathol Lab Med* 1984;104:579-583.

54. Tartar VM, Trambert MA, Balsara ZN et al. Tubular ectasia of the testicle: sonographic and MR imaging appearance. *AJR* 1993;160:539-542.

55. Brown DL, Benson CB, Doherty FJ et al. Cystic testicular mass caused by dilated rete testis: sonographic findings in 31 cases. *AJR* 1992;158:1257-1259.

56. Weingarten BJ, Kellman GM, Middleton WD et al. Tubular ectasia within the mediastinum testis. *J Ultrasound Med* 1992;11:349-353.

57. Older RA, Watson LR. Tubular ectasia of the rete testis: a benign condition with a sonographic appearance that may be misinterpreted as malignant. *J Urol* 1994;152:477-478.

58. Cho CS, Kosek J. Cystic dysplasia of the testis: sonographic and pathologic findings. *Radiology* 1985;156:777-778.

59. Keetch DW, McAlister WH, Manley CB et al. Cystic dysplasia of the testis—sonographic features with pathologic correlation. *Pediatr Radiol* 1991;21:501-503.

60. Shah KH, Maxted WC, Dhun B. Epidermoid cysts of the testis: a report of three cases and an analysis of 141 cases from the world literature. *Cancer* 1981;47:577-582.

61. Caravelli JF, Peters BE. Sonography of bilateral testicular epidermoid cysts. *J Ultrasound Med* 1984;3:273-274.

62. Buckspan MB, Skeldon SC, Klotz PG et al. Epidermoid cysts of the testicle. *J Urol* 1985;134:960-961.

63. Malek RS, Rosen JS, Farrow GM. Epidermoid cyst of the testis: a critical analysis. *Br J Urol* 1986;58:55-59.

64. Eisenmenger M, Lang S, Donner CH et al. Epidermoid cysts of the testis: organ-preserving surgery following diagnosis by ultrasonography. *Br J Urol* 1993;71:955-957.

65. Hermansen JC, Dhusid MJ, Sty MR. Bacterial epididymo-orchitis in children and adolescents. *Clin Pediatr* 1980;19:812-815.

66. Mevorach RA, Lerner RM, Dvoretsky PM et al. Testicular abscess: diagnosis by ultrasonography. *J Urol* 1986;136:1213-1216.

67. Korn RL, Langer JE, Nisenbaum HL et al. Non-Hodgkin's lymphoma mimicking a scrotal abscess in a patient with AIDS. *J Ultrasound Med* 1994;13:715-718.

68. Smith FJ, Bilbey JH, Filipenko JD et al. Testicular pseudotumor in the acquired immunodeficiency syndrome. *Urology* 1995;45:535-537.

69. Vick CW, Bird LI, Rosenfield AT et al. Scrotal masses with a uniformly hyperechoic pattern. *Radiology* 1983;148:209-211.

70. Blei L, Sihelnik S, Bloom D et al. Ultrasonographic analysis of chronic intratesticular pathology. *J Ultrasound Med* 1983;2:17-23.

71. Wu VH, Dangman BC, Kaufman RP Jr. Sonographic appearance of acute testicular venous infarction in a patient with a hypercoagulable state. *J Ultrasound Med* 1995;14:57-59.

72. Flanagan JJ, Fowler RC. Testicular infarction mimicking tumour on scrotal ultrasound—a potential pitfall. *Clin Radiol* 1995;50:49-50.

73. Einstein DM, Paushter DM, Singer AA et al. Fibrotic lesions of the testicle: sonographic patterns mimicking malignancy. *Urol Radiol* 1992;14:205-210.

74. Rifkin MD, Kurtz AB, Goldberg BB. Epididymis examined by ultrasound: correlation with pathology. *Radiology* 1984;151:187-190.

75. Avila NA, Premkumar A, Shawker TH et al. Testicular adrenal rest tissue in congenital adrenal hyperplasia: findings at gray-scale and color Doppler US. *Radiology* 1996;198:99-104.

76. Vanzulli A, DelMaschio A, Paesano P et al. Testicular masses in association with adrenogenital syndrome: US findings. *Radiology* 1992;183:425-429.

77. Gierke CL, King BF, Bostwick DG et al. Large-cell calcifying Sertoli cell tumor of the testis: appearance at sonography. *AJR* 1994;163:373-375.

78. Doherty FJ, Mullins TL, Sant GR et al. Testicular microlithiasis: a unique sonographic appearance. *J Ultrasound Med* 1987;6:389-392.

79. Nistal M, Paniagua R, Diez-Pardo JA. Testicular microlithiasis in 2 children with bilateral cryptorchidism. *J Urol* 1979;121:535-537.

80. Vegni-Talluri M, Bigliardi E, Vanni MG et al. Testicular microliths: their origin and structure. *J Urol* 1980;124:105-107.

81. Breger RC, Passarge E, McAdams AJ. Testicular intratubular bodies. *J Clin Endocrinol Metab* 1965;25:1340-1346.

82. Janzen DL, Mathieson JR, March JI et al. Testicular microlithiasis: sonographic and clinical features. *AJR* 1992;158:1057-1060.

83. Backus ML, Mack AL, Middleton WD et al. Testicular microlithiasis: imaging appearances and pathologic correlation. *Radiology* 1994;192:781-785.

84. Patel MD, Olcott EW, Kerschmann RL et al. Sonographically detected testicular microlithiasis and testicular carcinoma. *J Clin Ultrasound* 1993;21:447-452.

85. Linkowski GD, Avellone A, Gooding GAW. Scrotal calculi: sonographic detection. *Radiology* 1985;156:484.

86. Leung ML, Gooding GAW, Williams RD. High-resolution sonography of scrotal contents in asymptomatic subjects. *AJR* 1984;143:161-164.

87. Worthy L, Miller EI, Chin DH. Evaluation of extratesticular findings in scrotal neoplasms. *J Ultrasound Med* 1986;5:261-263.

88. Cunningham JJ. Sonographic findings in clinically unsuspected acute and chronic scrotal hematoceles. *AJR* 1983;140:749-752.

89. Wolverson MK, Houttuin E, Heiberg E et al. High-resolution real-time sonography of scrotal varicocele. *AJR* 1983;141:775-779.

90. Belker AM. The varicocele and male infertility. *Urol Clin North Am* 1981;8:41-44.

91. Gonda RL, Karo JJ, Forte RA et al. Diagnosis of subclinical varicocele in infertility. *AJR* 1987;148:71-75.

92. Hamm G, Fobbe F, Sorensen R et al. Varicoceles: combined sonography and thermography in diagnosis and post-therapeutic intervention. *Radiology* 1986;160:419-424.

93. McClure RD, Hricak H. Scrotal ultrasound in the infertile man: detection of subclinical unilateral and bilateral varicoceles. *J Urol* 1986;135:711-714.

94. Subramanyam BR, Balthazar EJ, Raghavendra BN et al. Sonographic diagnosis of scrotal hernia. *AJR* 1982;139:535-538.

95. Faysal MH, Strefling A, Kosek JC. Epididymal neoplasms: a case report and review. *J Urol* 1983;129:843-844.

96. Pavone-Macaluso M, Smith PH, Bagshaw MA. *Testicular Cancer and Other Tumors of the Genitourinary Tract.* New York: Plenum Press; 1985.

97. Smallman LA, Odedra JK. Primary carcinoma of sigmoid colon metastasizing to epididymis. *Urology* 1984;23:598-599.

98. Wachtel TL, Mehan DJ. Metastatic tumors of the epididymis. *J Urol* 1970;103:624-626.

99. Dunner PS, Lipsit ER, Nochomovitz LE. Epididymal sperm granuloma simulating a testicular neoplasm. *J Clin Ultrasound* 1982;10:353-355.

100. Ramanathan K, Yaghoobian J, Pinck RL. Sperm granuloma. *J Clin Ultrasound* 1986;14:155-156.

101. Jarvis LJ, Dubbins PA. Changes in the epididymis after vasectomy: sonographic findings. *AJR* 1989;152:531-534.

102. Eftekhari F, Smith JK. Sonography of the scrotum after orchiectomy: normal and abnormal findings. *AJR* 1993;160:543-547.

103. Fowler RC, Chennells PM, Ewing R. Scrotal ultrasonography: a clinical evaluation. *Br J Radiol* 1987;60:649-654.

Acute Scrotum

104. Mueller DL, Amundson GM, Rubin SZ et al. Acute scrotal abnormalities in children: diagnosis by combined sonography and scintigraphy. *AJR* 1988;150:643-646.

105. Hricak H, Lue T, Filly RA et al. Experimental study of the sonographic diagnosis of testicular torsion. *J Ultrasound Med* 1983;2:349-356.

106. Donahue RE, Cass BP, Veeraraghavan K. Immediate exploration of the unilateral acute scrotum in young male subjects. *J Urol* 1978;124:829-832.

107. Chen DCP, Holder LE, Kaplan GN. Correlation of radionuclide imaging and diagnostic ultrasound in scrotal diseases. *J Nucl Med* 1986;27:1774-1781.

108. Williamson RCN. Torsion of the testis and allied conditions. *Br J Surg* 1976;63:465-476.

109. Finkelstein MS, Rosenberg HK, Snyder HM et al. Ultrasound evaluation of scrotum in pediatrics. *Urology* 1986;27:1-9.

110. Bird K, Rosenfield AI, Taylor KJW. Ultrasonography in testicular torsion. *Radiology* 1983;147:527-534.

111. Middleton WD, Melson GL. Testicular ischemia: color Doppler sonographic findings in five patients. *AJR* 1989;152:1237-1239.

112. Chinn DH, Miller EI. Generalized testicular hyperechogenicity in acute testicular torsion. *J Ultrasound Med* 1985;4:495-496.

113. Vick CW, Bird K, Rosenfield AT et al. Extratesticular hemorrhage associated with torsion of the spermatic cord: sonographic demonstration. *Radiology* 1986;158:401-404.

114. Bird K, Rosenfield AT. Testicular infarction secondary to acute inflammatory disease: demonstration by B-scan ultrasound. *Radiology* 1984;152:785-788.

115. Margin B, Conte J. Ultrasonography of the acute scrotum. *J Clin Ultrasound* 1987;15:37-44.

116. Lerner RM, Mevorach RA, Hulbert WC et al. Color Doppler ultrasound in the evaluation of acute scrotal disease. *Radiology* 1990;176:355-358.

117. Burks DD, Markey BJ, Burkhard TK et al. Suspected testicular torsion and ischemia: evaluation with color Doppler sonography. *Radiology* 1990;175:815-821.

118. Middleton WD, Siegel BA, Melson GL et al. Acute scrotal disorders: prospective comparison of color Doppler US and testicular scintigraphy. *Radiology* 1990;177:177-181.

119. Bude RO, Kennelly MJ, Adler RS et al. Nonpulsatile arterial waveforms: observations during graded testicular torsion in rats. *Acad Radiol* 1995;2:879-882.

120. Fitzgerald SW, Erickson S, DeWire DM et al. Color Doppler sonography in the evaluation of the adult acute scrotum. *J Ultrasound Med* 1992;11:543-548.

121. Atkinson Jr GO, Patrick LE, Ball TI Jr et al. The normal and abnormal scrotum in children: evaluation with color Doppler sonography. *AJR* 1992;158:613-617.

122. Hesser U, Rosenberg M, Gierup J et al. Gray-scale sonography in torsion of the testicular appendages. *Pediatr Radiol* 1993;23:529-532.

123. Berger RE, Alexander ER, Harnisch JP et al. Etiology, manifestations and therapy of acute epididymitis: prospective study of 50 cases. *J Urol* 1979;121:750-754.

124. Horstman WG, Middleton WD, Melson GL. Scrotal inflammatory disease: color Doppler US findings. *Radiology* 1991;179:55-59.

125. Sanders LM, Haber S, Dembner A et al. Significance of reversal of diastolic flow in the acute scrotum. *J Ultrasound Med* 1994;13:137-139.

Trauma

126. Jeffrey RB, Laing FC, Hricak H et al. Sonography of testicular trauma. *AJR* 1983;141:993-995.

127. Lupetin AR, King W, Rich PJ et al. The traumatized scrotum: ultrasound evaluation. *Radiology* 1983;148:203-207.

128. Cohen HL, Shapiro ML, Haller JO et al. Sonography of intrascrotal hematomas simulating testicular rupture in adolescents. *Pediatr Radiol* 1992;22:296-297.

129. Learch TJ, Hansch LP, Ralls PW. Sonography in patients with gunshot wounds of the scrotum: imaging findings and their value. *AJR* 1995;165:879-883.

130. Gordon LM, Stein SM, Ralls PW. Traumatic epididymitis: evaluation with color Doppler sonography. *AJR* 1996;166:1323-1325.

Cryptorchidism

131. Elder JS. Cryptorchidism: isolated and associated with other genitourinary defects. *Pediatr Clin North Am* 1987;34:1033-1053.

132. Harrison JH et al. *Campbell's Urology.* 4th ed. Philadelphia: WB Saunders Co; 1979.

133. Friedland GW, Chang P. The role of imaging in the management of the impalpable undescended testis. *AJR* 1988;151:1107-1111.

134. Kogan SJ. Cryptorchidism and infertility: an overview. *Dialog Pediatr Urol* 1982;4:2-3.

135. Rosenfield AT, Blair DN, McCarthy S et al. The pars infravaginalis gubernaculi: importance in the identification of the undescended testis. *AJR* 1989;153:775-778.

136. Wolverson MK, Houttuin E, Heiberg E et al. Comparison of computed tomography with high-resolution real-time ultrasound in the localization of the impalpable undescended testis. *Radiology* 1983;146:133-136.

137. Weiss R, Carter AR, Rosenfield AT. High-resolution real-time ultrasound in the localization of the undescended testis. *J Urol* 1986;135:936-938.

138. Fritzsche PJ, Hricak H, Kogan BA et al. Undescended testis: value of magnetic resonance imaging. *Radiology* 1987;169-173.

139. Kier R, McCarthy S, Rosenfield AT et al. Nonpalpable testes in young boys: evaluation with magnetic resonance imaging. *Radiology* 1988;169:429-433.

CHAPTER 25

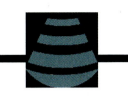

The Penis

•

Bernard F. King, Jr., M.D.

The penis is the male genital organ; it has the dual functions of erection and of providing a route for the excretion of urine and semen. Imaging of the penis has been limited in the past to plain films, urethrography, and cavernosography. Computed tomography and magnetic resonance imaging have also been advocated as a means of evaluating penile pathology.[1–3] Recently, however, high-resolution ultrasound of the penis with Doppler analysis of the penile blood vessels has offered detailed analysis of the anatomic and vascular structures of the penis. Ready availability and

lack of ionizing radiation make ultrasound one of the most promising modalities in evaluating penile pathology.

Sonography can be used reliably for evaluation of penile masses, trauma, and urethral strictures. Peyronie's disease and congenital anomalies of the penis can also be adequately evaluated with high-resolution penile sonography.

The most exciting developments in penile sonography have been in the area of impotence. Not only can one obtain gray-scale images of the penis, but in addition, Doppler analysis of blood flow within the penile arteries can be assessed. This anatomic information and estimation of blood flow within the vessels can aid in the diagnostic evaluation of patients who may have vasculogenic impotence.

ANATOMY

The anatomy of the penis is unique and complex (Fig. 25-1). The penis is composed of three cylindric structures of cavernous tissue. **Two corpora cavernosa** lie in the dorsal two-thirds of the penis and a **single corpus spongiosum** lies in the ventral one-third of the penis. The two corpora cavernosa are the main erectile structures of the penis. Both of the corpora cavernosa and the corpus spongiosum are enveloped in a thick fascial sheath, the **tunica albuginea.** The urethra travels through the center of the corpus spongiosum. Distally, the penis exhibits a conical extremity, the glans penis. The **glans penis** is

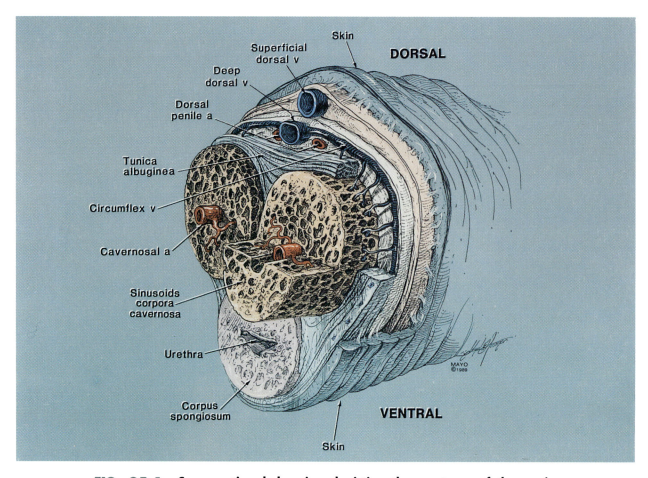

FIG. 25-1. Cross-sectional drawing depicting the anatomy of the penis.
(From Quam JP, King BF, James EM et al. Duplex and color Doppler sonographic evaluation
of vasculogenic impotence. *AJR* 1989;153:1141-1147.)

formed by an expansion of the corpus spongiosum, which fits over the blunt terminations of the corpora cavernosa. The corpora cavernosa and corpus spongiosum are composed of sinusoidal spaces lined by smooth muscle and endothelium. There is a septum dividing both corpora cavernosa that contains many fenestrations, allowing for multiple anastomotic channels that connect the sinusoidal spaces of both corpora cavernosa. These small sinusoidal spaces in the corpora cavernosa distend with blood during an erection. The corpus spongiosum also becomes engorged during erection but adds little to the erectile state of the penis.

The blood supply to the penis comes primarily from the right and left internal pudendal arteries, which originate from the right and left internal iliac arteries. Each internal pudendal artery gives off a perineal branch, a bulbar branch, and a very small urethral artery before continuing as the artery of the penis. The **right and left penile arteries** enter the base of the penis and branch into cavernosal arteries and dorsal arteries. The cavernosal arteries are the

primary source of blood flow to the erectile tissue of the penis (Fig. 25-2). Each **cavernosal artery** travels near the center of each corpus cavernosum as it sends off small helicine arteries that communicate directly with the sinusoidal spaces, which are not visible sonographically. The paired **dorsal arteries** supply blood primarily to the skin and glans of the penis. However, anastomotic branches occur between the dorsal penile arteries and the deep cavernosal arteries.

Venous drainage of the erectile tissue of the penis occurs primarily via emissary veins, which are not visible sonographically. These emissary veins perforate the thick tunica albuginea and empty into circumflex veins that ultimately travel to the dorsal aspect of the penis and empty into the **deep dorsal penile vein,** which is sonographically visible (Fig. 25-3). The deep dorsal vein then empties into the retropubic venous plexus. Venous drainage of the corpus cavernosum also occurs through crural veins at the base of the penis. The skin and glans are drained through the superficial dorsal veins.

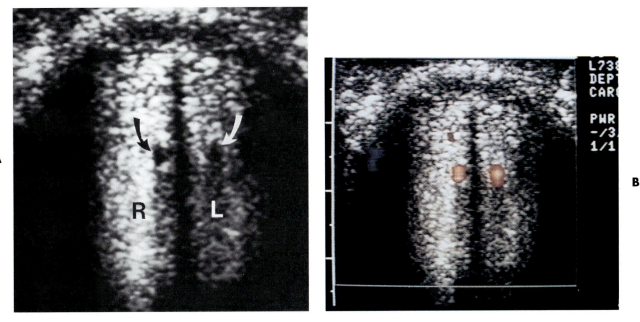

FIG. 25-2. **Corpora cavernosa.** **A.** Transverse sonogram of the penis depicting the right (R) and left (L) corpora cavernosa. The cavernosal arteries *(arrows)* are seen near the midline of each corpus cavernosum. **B.** Color Doppler sonogram more clearly demonstrates the cavernosal arteries.

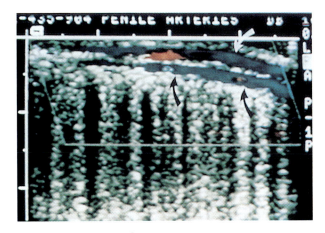

FIG. 25-3. **Dorsal veins.** Longitudinal color Doppler sonogram of the dorsal surface of the penis depicting the damp dorsal penile vein *(black arrows)* that drains the erectile tissue of the penis. Also note the superficial dorsal penile vein *(white arrow)* that drains the skin and glans of the penis.

PHYSIOLOGY

Penile erection results from smooth muscle relaxation in the walls of the sinusoids and the helicine and cavernosal arteries of each corpora cavernosa. As sinusoidal muscle tone diminishes and the sinusoids distend with blood, the small emissary veins become compressed between the peripheral sinusoids and the unyielding peripheral tunica albuginea. This activates a veno-occlusive mechanism that maintains sinusoidal distention and limits venous outflow from the sinusoidal spaces (Fig. 25-4). With continued arterial inflow and limited venous outflow, the sinusoidal spaces distend to such a degree that the cavernosal tissue becomes rigid.[4–15]

The chemical mediators of **sinusoidal relaxation** are poorly understood. Adrenergic mediators appear to inhibit sinusoidal smooth muscle relaxation in the baseline flaccid state. When a psychoerotic stimulus occurs, parasympathetic nerve terminals, mediated by acetylcholine, are stimulated. These cholinergic effects suppress the adrenergic fibers, thus allowing for smooth-muscle relaxation. In addition, acetylcholine appears to indirectly stimulate endothelial cells lining the sinusoidal spaces. This cholinergic effect on the endothelial cells is thought to result in the production of **endothelium-derived relaxing factor (EDRF)** which, in turn, is believed to cause relaxation of the smooth muscle lining the sinusoidal spaces via nitrous oxide.[16,17] When the psychoerotic stimulus subsides, the smooth-muscle relaxation and dilatation of the blood vessels supplying the penis diminish. The sinusoids then shrink, resulting in less compression of the emissary veins and thus allowing venous outflow to again occur unimpeded. The penis then becomes flaccid.[18,19]

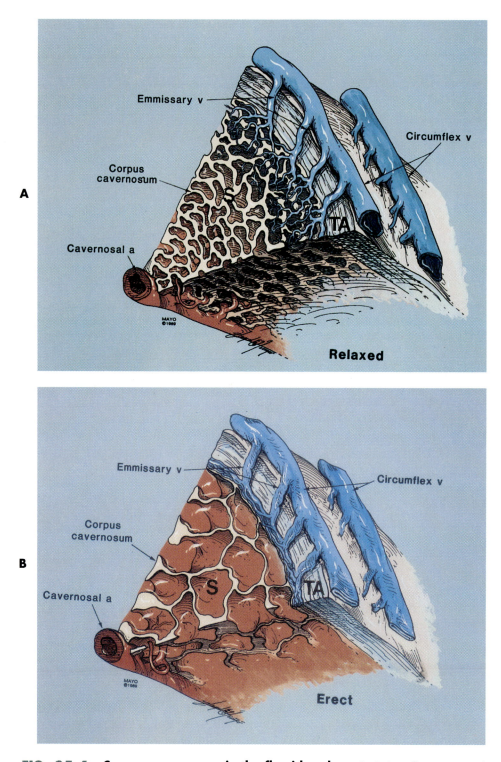

FIG. 25-4. **Corpus cavernosum in the flaccid and erect state.** Cross-sectional wedge drawings of the corpus cavernosum in the flaccid (**A**) and erect (**B**) states. During the erectile process, the cavernosal arteries and sinusoids *(S)* distend with blood and compress the draining venules against the thick and rigid tunica albuginea *(TA)*. The compression and near occlusion of these draining venules prevent venous efflux from the cavernosal tissues and allow for prolonged maximal distention of the cavernosal sinusoids, resulting in an erection.

EXAMINATION TECHNIQUE

Penile sonographic examination is performed with the patient supine with the penis lying on the anterior abdominal wall (Fig. 25-5). High frequency (7.5 to 10.0 MHz) linear array ultrasound transducers provide high-resolution images of the penis. The transducer is placed transversely on the ventral surface starting at the level of the glans and moving down to the base of the penis. The two corpora cavernosa are easily identified on transverse images as circular structures adjacent to each other, separated by the septum penis. The cavernosal arteries are visualized near the medial portion of the corpora cavernosa (Fig. 25-2). Rarely, one may see collateral vessels crossing the septum penis from one cavernosal artery to another or from the dorsal penile artery to the cavernosal artery. The two dorsal penile arteries are smaller than the cavernosal arteries and can sometimes be visualized if the dorsal surface of the penis is scanned transversely using color Doppler. The corpus spongiosum is often compressed and difficult to visualize when scanning the ventral aspect of the penis. However, by applying a generous amount of acoustic gel and with gentle compression by the transducer, one can adequately visualize the corpus spongiosum.

The echotexture of the corporal structures should be uniform throughout. **The fascial planes,** including the tunica albuginea, will be seen as hyperechoic regions surrounding the periphery of the corporal structures. The penis should be scanned to exclude the possibility of excessive amounts of fibrosis within the corporal bodies and/or in the fascial layers around the corporal bodies. Palpable abnormalities (i.e., Peyronie's plaques) should be scanned to assess the sonographic features of the masses and their exact location with respect to the corporal bodies.

Longitudinal evaluation of each corporal body of the penis should also be obtained from the ventral surface. The cavernosal arteries are seen as small tubular structures with echogenic walls in the center of the corpora cavernosa (Fig. 25-6). Evaluation of the corpus spongiosum and urethra is also performed from the ventral aspect of the penis. Copious amounts of acoustic gel or an acoustic pad on the surface of the penis can be used to optimize visualization and to avoid excessive compression by the transducer. Visualization of the **penile urethra** is optimally performed by distending it. This can be accomplished while the patient is voiding or by injecting the urethra with a viscous lidocaine gel in a retrograde fashion (Fig. 25-7). The latter method is preferred because of optimal distention that can be maintained over a longer period of time. This is accomplished by inserting a tapered-tip syringe containing viscous lidocaine jelly into the urethral meatus and then applying a distal penile clamp to maintain distention of the penile urethra.

IMPOTENCE

Until recently it was thought that psychological factors accounted for most causes of impotence.[20] However, studies using nocturnal penile tumescence have revealed that a majority of cases of impotence

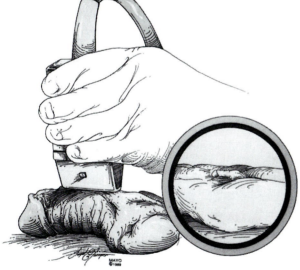

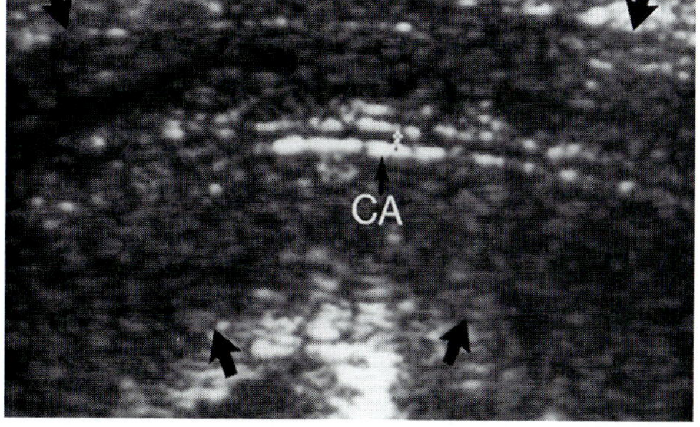

FIG. 25-5. Technique of penile sonography. Drawing depicting the technique of penile sonography. The penis is in the anatomic position, lying on the anterior abdominal wall. The transducer is placed on the ventral surface of the penis. (From Hattery RR, King BF, Lewis RW et al. Vasculogenic impotence: duplex and color Doppler. *Radiol Clin North Am* 1991;29:629-645.)

FIG. 25-6. Left corpus cavernosum. Longitudinal sonogram of the left corpus cavernosum *(arrows)*. Echogenic walls of the cavernosal artery *(CA)* are seen near the middle of the corpora.

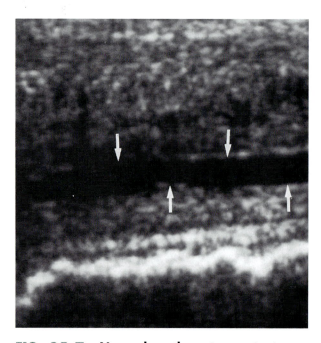

FIG. 25-7. Normal urethra. Longitudinal sonourethrogram from the dorsal surface of the penis depicts the normal urethra *(arrows)* distended with lidocaine gel. (Courtesy of Carol B. Benson, M.D., Boston.)

have organic causes.[21-25] Subsequent studies have shown that vasculogenic impotence is one of the most frequent causes of erectile failure (Fig. 25-8).[24-28] Vasculogenic impotence may be due to poor arterial inflow into the penis (arteriogenic impotence) or excessive venous leakage of blood from the penis (venogenic impotence), or both.

Noninvasive and Invasive Tests

Many examinations, invasive and noninvasive, have been used to evaluate arterial inflow into the penis and to look for possible excessive venous leakage from erectile tissue.[29-73] Arteriography with selective internal iliac angiography is considered the gold standard in the evaluation of arteriogenic impotence.[27,29,30,38,43,44,50,54,63,66] However, this technique is invasive and is therefore not suitable as a screening examination. Many patients are currently screened for vasculogenic impotence by measuring their clinical response to an intracavernosal injection of a vasodilating pharmacologic agent.[5,22,33,34,57,58,74] Many vasodilating medications have been used, including papaverine, phentolamine, and prostaglandin E-1. By injecting these vasodilators intracavernosally, one can bypass the psychoerotic and neurologic pathways that normally initiate an erection. Most investigators believe that the arterial inflow and veno-occlusive mechanisms are intact if the patient develops an erection after the intracavernosal injection of these vasodilators. Thus, a full erection after the intracavernosal injection of a vasodilating agent should indicate an ad-

equate vascular system. Since this method is easy to perform and is reproducible, it offers many advantages as a screening test for vasculogenic impotence. However, the technique fails to differentiate arteriogenic from venogenic impotence. This differentiation is important because the treatment for arteriogenic impotence is markedly different from the treatment for venogenic impotence.

The **penile-brachial index (PBI)** was once a very popular screening test to identify patients who might have arteriogenic impotence.[27,63] The penile-brachial index is calculated by dividing the mean systolic pressure in the penile arteries by the mean systolic pressure in the brachial artery. In general, a value of less than 0.7 suggests arteriogenic impotence. However, studies have shown that there is considerable overlap between normal and abnormal patients, based on PBI results.

Duplex Doppler Examination

The desire for a more accurate noninvasive test of arterial inflow into the penis led to the development of duplex Doppler sonography of the cavernosal arteries of the penis. **Duplex sonography was more accurate** than continuous wave sonography because of its ability to allow visualization of the deep cavernosal artery and obtain a reliable pulsed Doppler signal from it. Using real-time gray-scale sonographic visualization, Lue et al. showed that precise Doppler sampling and blood velocity measurements of the deep cavernosal arteries could be performed before and after intracavernosal injections of vasodilating agents.[36] In addition, changes in diameter of the cavernosal artery could be obtained before and after administration of the vasodilating agent. With knowledge of the blood velocity and change in diameters of the cavernosal arteries after the intracavernosal injection of a vasodilating agent, one can estimate the amount of arterial blood flow available for the corporal erectile tissue of the penis during an artificially induced erection.

The **technique of duplex sonography of the penis** in the evaluation of vasculogenic impotence continues to evolve. The examination should take place in a quiet room with minimal distractions and interruptions. Too many external distractions could affect the patient's response to the vasodilating agent and thus alter the velocity parameters. Longitudinal examination of the corpora cavernosa is best accomplished in a parasagittal plane from a ventral approach (Fig. 25-9). In the flaccid state the cavernosal artery can follow a tortuous course and can be seen intermittently on longitudinal scans. In the erect state, the cavernosal artery assumes a straighter course. Near the base of the penis, the cavernosal artery can be difficult to appreciate on gray-scale imaging. Color

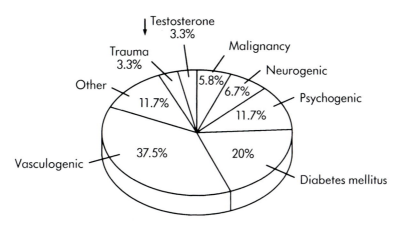

FIG. 25-8. Causes of impotence. Pie graph displaying the relative frequencies of the various causes of impotence. (Modified from Quam JP, King BF, James EM et al. Duplex and color Doppler ultrasound evaluation of vasculogenic impotence science exhibit. *Radiol Soc North Am*. Chicago; 1989.)

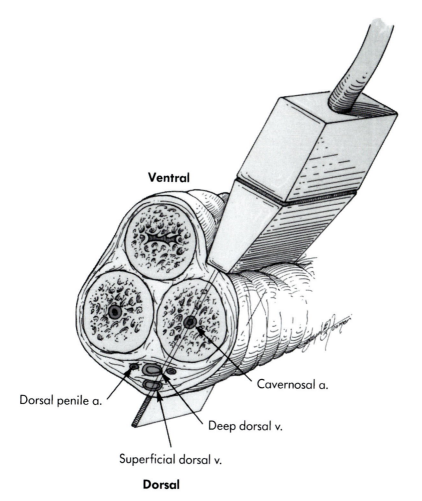

FIG. 25-9. Transducer position for Doppler examination of the cavernosal artery. Position on the ventral aspect of the penis. Drawing depicts the medially directed position of the transducer. (From King BF Jr, Hattery RR, James EM, Lewis RW. Duplex sonography in the evaluation of impotence: current techniques. *Semin Intervent Radiol* 1990;7:215-221.)

Doppler can aid in the identification of the cavernosal artery in this region (Fig. 25-10).

The diameters of the cavernosal arteries can be obtained by measuring the internal lumen (Fig. 25-6). In some patients the cavernosal arteries are too small to measure accurately before the injection of a vasodilating agent. Because of the wide variability, multiple measurements on each side should be obtained and averaged.

Following the measurement of the diameters of the cavernosal arteries, a vasodilating agent is injected. The types and doses of commonly used vasodilating agents vary widely. Initially, many investigators use 60 mg of papaverine in 2 ml of solution injected into either the left or right corpus cavernosum.[36] The vasodilating agent easily diffuses from one corpus cavernosum to the other because of the many fenestrations of the septum separating the corpora cavernosa. Other investigators have used a lower dose of papaverine (40 mg) along with a second agent such as phentolamine (2.5 mg). Phentolamine is an alpha adrenergic blocking agent that potentiates the smooth-muscle relaxation effects of papaverine. Prostaglandin E-1 has also been used alone as a smooth-muscle relaxer. Others have used a triple agent consisting of papaverine 4.4 mg, phentolamine 0.15 mg, and prostaglandin E-1 1.5 µg in 0.25 ml to minimize the

possibility of priapism, which may occur in 2% to 8% of the patients.[72,75] It is thought that small doses of these vasodilating agents used together result in an additive effect that allows one to use minimal doses of the vasodilating agent with optimal response and minimal discomfort.

It is important to inject the vasodilating agent into the dorsal two-thirds of the penile shaft accurately so that the agent does not enter into the corpus spongiosum or urethra (Fig. 25-11). Care must also be taken to avoid injecting the vasodilating agent into the subcutaneous tissue, which could result in massive swelling of the skin and possible necrosis. All patients should be informed that if a painful erection occurs or if the erection does not subside after 1 hour, the patient should contact his referring physician or go directly to an emergency room for evaluation and treatment of priapism. Pharmacologic-induced priapism is persistent painful erection of the penis 1 to 3 hours after the intracavernosal injection of a vasodilating agent. Persistent priapism (greater than 1 to 3 hours) could result in ischemic necrosis of cavernosal tissue and resulting fibrosis of this erectile tissue. Patients who are prone to priapism include those who have a history of neurogenic impotence, those with sickle cell disease or trait, and patients on heparin therapy. Small doses or avoidance of vasodilating agents may be warranted in these patients.[74-81]

Treatment of priapism usually consists of aspirating approximately 20 ml of blood from a corpus cavernosum. If this fails to relieve the priapism, then 200 µg of phenylephrine HCl (Neosynephrine) diluted in 1 ml of normal saline can be injected intracavernosally to facilitate mild vasoconstriction and cessation of the erection. Treatment of priapism should be carried out by trained and experienced physicians.[72]

Following the intracavernosal injection of a vasodilating agent, the diameters of the cavernosal arteries

---

CAVERNOSAL ARTERIES

Normal Doppler Measurements

Peak systolic velocity > 30 cm/s
End diastolic velocity < 3 cm/s
Artery diameter increase 70%

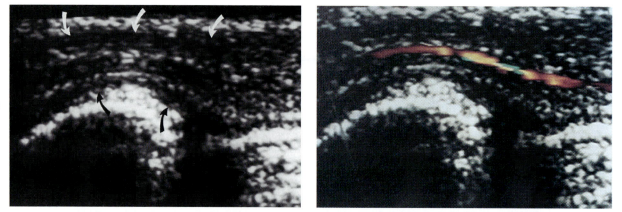

FIG. 25-10. Cavernosal artery. A, Longitudinal gray-scale sonogram of the corpus cavernosum *(outlined by arrows)*. The cavernosal artery is not identified. **B,** With the addition of color Doppler, the cavernosal artery *(red)* is easily identified.

are again measured, and velocity measurements are obtained in these cavernosal arteries. Doppler analysis of blood flow in the cavernosal artery is optimally obtained near the base of the penis where the Doppler angle is the smallest. The smaller the Doppler angle, the more accurate the velocity measurements will be. Spectral Doppler analysis of cavernosal arteries enables one to take **peak systolic** and **end-diastolic velocity** measurements.

Maximal effect of the vasodilating agents is reached about 5 to 20 minutes after the injection in most patients, but the time is highly variable. Therefore, most investigators feel that velocity measurements in the cavernosal arteries should begin approximately 5 minutes after injection. Velocity measurements should then be obtained continuously or at 5-minute intervals for at least 20 to 30 minutes after injection (Fig. 25-12).[2,21,22] Peak systolic velocities (PSVs) and end-diastolic velocity measurements should be obtained in both cavernosal arteries at each 5-minute interval. The **postinjection cavernosal artery diameter** measurements should be obtained 5 minutes after injection. The effects of the vasodilating agents may begin to wear off as early as 20 to 30 minutes after the injection, and some patients may require a second or third injection in order to achieve normal velocities.

There appear to be five phases of spectral waveforms in the cavernosal arteries after the intracavernosal injection of vasodilating agents in normal males (Fig. 25-13).[42] These five phases in normal men occur within approximately 5 to 20 minutes after the intra-

cavernosal injection of a vasodilating agent. However, abnormal patients with vasculogenic impotence may never complete all normal phases because of abnormal arterial inflow or because of an impaired veno-occlusive mechanism.

Arteriogenic Impotence. Peak systolic velocities following the intracavernosal injection of a vasodilating agent appear to be the most valuable parameter when evaluating patients for potential arteriogenic impotence. In a study of normal male volunteers, it was found that the **normal average peak systolic velocity** following the intracavernosal injection of a vasodilating agent is approximately 30 to 40 cm/sec.[42] Lue et al. found that the majority of patients who have a moderate-to-good response to papaverine clinically have peak systolic velocities of 25 cm/sec or greater.[36] In addition, no patients in their study who had a poor response to papaverine injection had peak systolic velocities of 25 cm/sec or greater. Collins et al. also have found that patients who responded sonographically to papaverine had average peak systolic velocities of 26.8 cm/sec.[38] We reported a series of 12 patients with suspected arteriogenic impotence who underwent pelvic arteriography.[40] All five patients with abnormal findings on arteriography also had abnormal peak systolic velocities of less than 25 cm/sec. Six out of seven patients with normal arteriograms had peak systolic velocities in their cavernosal arteries of 25 cm/sec or greater. These studies indicate that when comparing sonographic response to a vasodilating agent with arteriography, a peak systolic

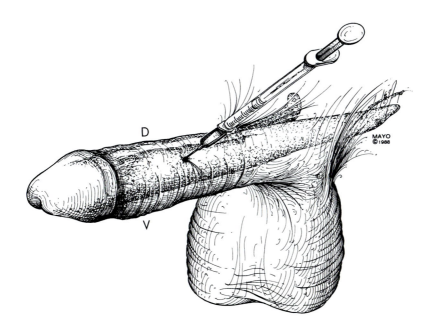

FIG. 25-11. Vasodilating agent. Drawing of the penis depicting the injection of a vasodilating agent. Care must be taken to inject the vasodilating agent into the dorsal two-thirds of the shaft of the penis. *D*, dorsal; *V*, ventral.

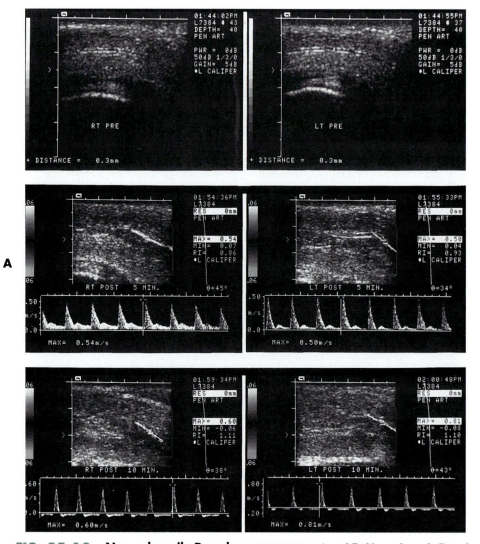

FIG. 25-12. Normal penile Doppler sonogram. A and B. Normal penile Doppler sonogram of both cavernosal arteries at 5, 10, 15, and 20 minutes after the injection of a vasodilating agent. Pre- and postcavernosal artery diameter measurements are also made.

Continued.

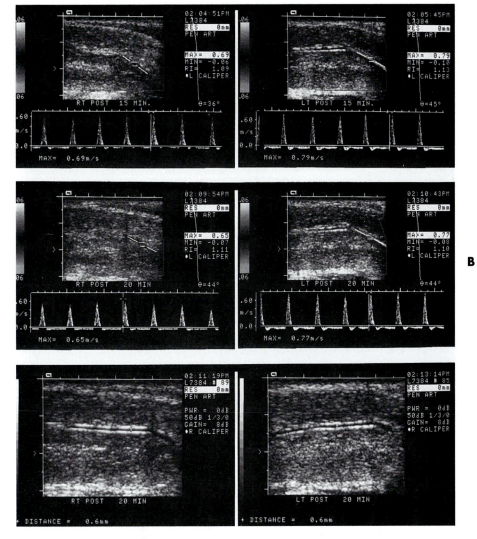

B

FIG. 25-12, cont'd.   For legend see opposite page.

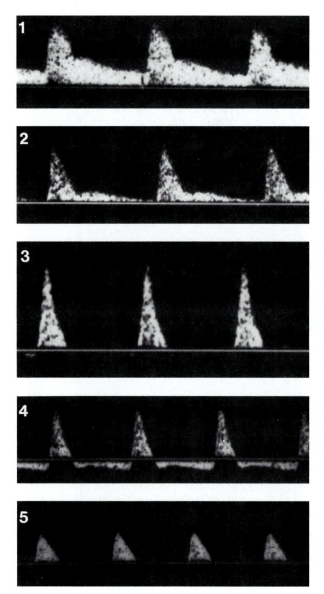

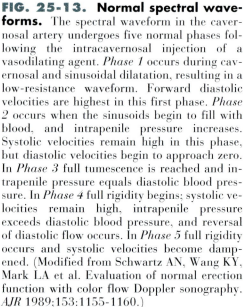

FIG. 25-13. Normal spectral waveforms. The spectral waveform in the cavernosal artery undergoes five normal phases following the intracavernosal injection of a vasodilating agent. *Phase 1* occurs during cavernosal and sinusoidal dilatation, resulting in a low-resistance waveform. Forward diastolic velocities are highest in this first phase. *Phase 2* occurs when the sinusoids begin to fill with blood, and intrapenile pressure increases. Systolic velocities remain high in this phase, but diastolic velocities begin to approach zero. In *Phase 3* full tumescence is reached and intrapenile pressure equals diastolic blood pressure. In *Phase 4* full rigidity begins; systolic velocities remain high, intrapenile pressure exceeds diastolic blood pressure, and reversal of diastolic flow occurs. In *Phase 5* full rigidity occurs and systolic velocities become dampened. (Modified from Schwartz AN, Wang KY, Mark LA et al. Evaluation of normal erection function with color flow Doppler sonography. *AJR* 1989;153:1155-1160.)

velocity of 25 cm/sec or less suggests inadequate arterial inflow to allow for moderate or good erections.

Benson et al. have grouped impotent patients into three subgroups based on Doppler ultrasound data.[41] The first subgroup of patients were considered normal and were found to have average peak systolic velocities of 47 cm/sec The second group of patients, who were felt to have mild-to-moderate arterial insufficiency, had an average peak systolic velocity of 35 cm/sec, and the third group, who had severe arterial insufficiency, were found to have an average peak systolic velocity of 7 cm/sec. The investigators concluded that a cut-off value for normal individuals of 40 cm/sec peak systolic velocity should be used. Other studies of normal men have found an average peak systolic velocity of 37 cm/sec.[79] These investigators went on to state that a peak systolic velocity of 30 cm/sec could correctly distinguish all patients with normal cavernosal arteries from those with severe arterial disease.

Arterial blood flow is not only a function of the velocity in a particular vessel but also a function of the cross-sectional area of the lumen of the vessel. Because of this, investigators have advocated measuring the change in diameter of the cavernosal arteries after the injection of a vasodilating agent. These investigators feel that the initial size of the artery is probably not a good indicator of arterial disease and that arterial compliance and ability to dilate are more important.[36] They feel that a 75% increase in vessel diameter is a good indication of normal arterial inflow into the cavernosal artery. However, because of the small size of the cavernosal arteries and the potential error in diameter measurement, one cannot rely totally on diameter changes.

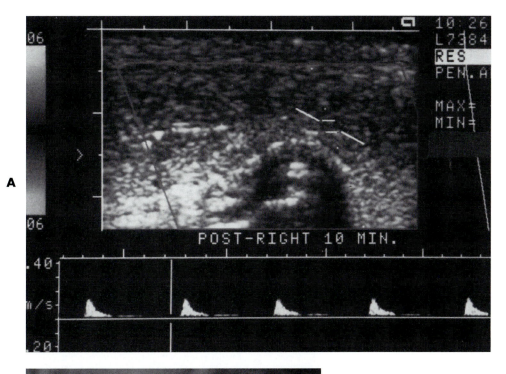

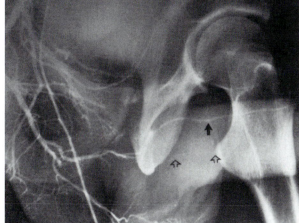

FIG. 25-14. Arteriogenic impotence. A, Duplex sonogram of the right cavernosal artery following the intracavernosal injection of 60 mg papaverine revealed a decreased arterial velocity of approximately 15 cm/sec. **B,** Pelvic arteriogram demonstrates no opacification of the cavernosal artery *(open arrows)*. The normal dorsal artery is identified *(black arrow)*.

From these data it seems logical to assume that **peak systolic velocities in cavernosal arteries of less than 25 cm/sec after administration of a vasodilating agent should suggest arterial disease** and should lead to a more definite evaluation with selective internal pudendal arteriography, if clinically warranted (Fig. 25-14). Values between 25 and 30 cm/sec should be considered borderline. **Peak systolic velocity measurements greater them 30 cm/sec should be considered normal.** However, several exceptions exist. If there is a marked discrepancy between the velocities of the two cavernosal arteries (greater than 10 cm/sec difference), **unilateral arterial disease of the penis** may be present. Adequate blood flow through one cavernosal artery may be all that is needed for adequate erections; however, unilateral arterial disease of the penis may be

significant in certain individuals, and appropriate arteriography may need to be pursued. Another exception occurs when the peak systolic velocity is greater than 100 cm/sec. This high velocity has been seen in patients with **diffuse vascular spasm and/or small vessel disease.** Such patients demonstrate little or no change in cavernosal arterial diameter measurements before and after the injection of a vasodilating agent. Therefore, if extremely high velocities in the cavernosal arteries (greater than 100 cm/sec) are detected, one should closely evaluate the caliber of the cavernosal arteries. If the caliber does not significantly increase following the vasodilating agent, the patient may have diffuse small vessel disease (i.e., **diabetes**) or diffuse vasospasm (**nicotine abuse, medications**).

The direction of blood flow in the cavernosal artery may be reversed. It has been shown that reversal of diastolic flow is a normal phenomenon in the latter stages of erection. However, one should **never** encounter reversal of blood flow during systole. Reversal of systolic blood flow is often caused by **proximal penile artery occlusion** with collateral flow in a retrograde fashion into the affected cavernosal artery.[70] Proximal penile artery occlusion can result from **trauma, corporal fibrosis,** or **atherosclerotic vessel disease.**

Collateral vessels to the cavernosal artery may be a normal variant. However, collateral vessels from the contralateral cavernosal artery or the dorsal penile artery may indicate proximal vessel disease in the affected artery. These collateral vessels can often be seen with color Doppler sonography.

Particular attention should be given to the presence of arterial sinusoidal fistulas or arterial venous fistulas within the corporal tissue of the penis in patients who have developed erectile dysfunction following trauma. Color Doppler evaluation can often locate the fistula. Partial priapism is often an accompanying sign in arterial sinusoidal fistulas.

Venogenic Impotence. Vasculogenic impotence may also be due to excessive venous leakage from the corporal bodies of the penis. Although the exact cause of excessive venous leakage is unknown, it is believed by many investigators to be secondary to a stretching of the thick tunica albuginea. This stretching prevents the compression of the emissary veins draining the sinusoids during the erection process. Because of the lack of compression of the emissary veins, venous outflow continues to occur rapidly from the corporal tissues and an erection is never fully obtained.

Traditionally, venogenic impotence has been evaluated with cavernosometry and cavernosography.[47-51,55,60] However, these examinations are invasive and are not suitable for screening purposes. Therefore, duplex sonography has been used recently as a screening examination for venogenic impotence.

Duplex Doppler Examination of the Cavernosal Arteries in the Normal Patient. During the examination there is an increase in diastolic and systolic velocities immediately following the intracavernosal injection of a vasodilating agent. This corresponds to the physiologic dilatation of the cavernosal artery, helicine arteries, and sinusoidal spaces. As the sinusoidal spaces are dilating and filling, resistance in the cavernosal artery is low, and forward diastolic flow increases. However, when the veno-occlusive mechanism engages, the sinusoids become maximally distended, and intracavernosal pressure increases. At this point, vascular resistance increases, and diastolic flow ceases or even reverses. If a patient's veno-occlusive mechanism is not intact, excessive venous leakage will persist, and intracavernosal pressures will remain low. The Doppler spectral waveform will

continue to exhibit the prominent forward diastolic flow of a low-resistance vascular bed throughout the examination. Therefore, patients who continue to have high end-diastolic velocities (over 3 cm/sec) late in the examination (15 to 20 minutes postinjection), despite normal arterial inflow (peak systolic velocities of 30 cm/sec), may have venogenic impotence[40] (Fig. 25-15). Cavernosometry and cavernosography should be considered for these patients. Patients who demonstrate reversal of diastolic flow in both cavernosal arteries should have an intact veno-occlusive mechanism.

The deep dorsal penile vein drains the majority of venous efflux from the corpora cavernosa. Some investigators have recommended velocity measurements in the deep dorsal penile vein as a means of detecting excessive venous leakage. However, early results reveal that normal patients and patients with excessive venous leakage may both have high, deep dorsal vein velocities.[71] In addition, it has also been found that some patients who have excessive venous leakage on cavernosometry and cavernosography may leak primarily via the crural veins near the base of the penis and not via the deep dorsal penile vein. Therefore, it appears that measuring deep dorsal vein velocities may not be a very helpful parameter for detecting venogenic impotence.

Pitfalls in Duplex Doppler Sonography for Impotence

Time of Velocity Measurements. Early investigators recommended that velocity measurements be obtained 5 to 10 minutes after injection. However, recent studies have indicated that the response to the intracavernosal vasodilating agent varies among individuals.[72,82-84] Peak systolic velocity in normal males can occur at any time from 5 to 30 minutes after injection. Therefore, in order to detect maximum velocities, the peak systolic velocity measurements should be measured at 5, 10, 15, and 20 minutes after injection.

Because normal individuals will have high end-diastolic velocities early in the examination (5 to 10 minutes after injection), many investigators feel that end-diastolic velocity measurements at the 15-, 20-, and 30-minute points should be used in screening patients who may have venogenic impotence. Persistent low-resistance spectral waveforms at these later times (high diastolic velocities greater than 5 cm/sec) indicate persistent and excessive venous leakage as a cause of venogenic impotence.

Although intracavernosal injection of vasodilating agents is supposed to bypass the psychological stimulus needed for erection, **excessive psychological overlay** may result in impaired response to these vasodilating agents. Suboptimal peak systolic velocities (< 25 cm/sec) can occur in normal patients with excessive anxiety and alpha-adrenergic tone.[85,86]

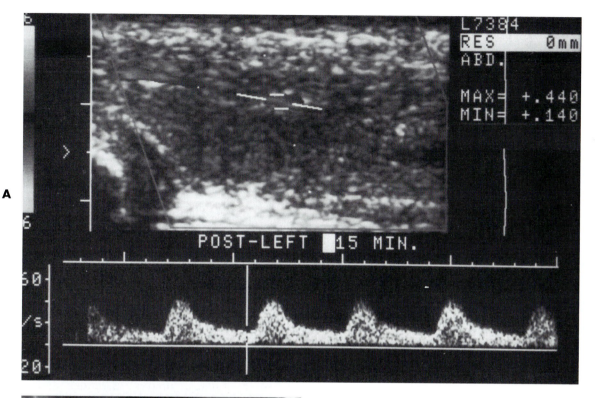

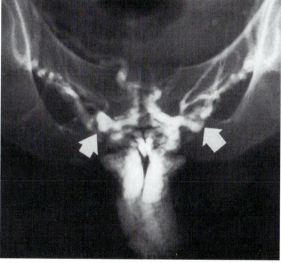

FIG. 25-15. Venogenic impotence. A. Duplex sonogram of a left cavernosal artery 15 minutes following injection demonstrates a normal peak systolic velocity of 44 cm/sec. However, there is persistent high end-diastolic velocity of 14 cm/sec suggestive of excessive venous leakage. B. Cavernosogram reveals massive venous leak into the retropubic venous plexus *(arrows)*.

Occasionally, patients become very anxious about an injection into the penis and/or an ultrasound evaluation of the penis. Because of this anxiety, the response to the vasodilating agent may be inhibited. We have found that 26% of patients who do not respond (PSV < 30 cm/s) to the first injection will respond to a second or third injection. Because of this, we routinely reinject at 20 minutes if patients have not responded to the first injection. If, after 10 minutes, the patient has not responded to the second injection, we will administer a third injection. If, after the third injection, the patient has not responded, we stop and conclude the patient has poor arterial inflow. Each patient should be counseled about the safety of the technique, and professional standards should be maintained during the examination. A quiet darkened room may help to allay fears in certain patients.

Improper Injection of Vasodilating Agents. If the vasodilating agent is injected into the corpus spongiosum, the agent will not be available to the sinusoidal tissue in the corpora cavernosa and erection will not occur. In addition, the injection of the vasodilating agent could enter the urethra and be expelled through the urethral meatus.

PEYRONIE'S DISEASE

Peyronie's disease is fibrosis of the fibrous sheaths covering the corpora cavernosa. It occurs without known cause, usually in men over 45 years of age. This fibrotic area sometimes does not permit lengthening of the related surface during erection, so the erect penis bends toward that area. The fibrotic area usually involves the dorsum of the penis but can involve the septum penis and/or the lateral aspects of the penis. The bend of the penis toward the area of fibrotic plaque results in a deformity known as a **chordee**. In the early stages of erection it is accompanied by pain, and eventually the degree of curvature may preclude coitus. It is believed that the process begins as a vasculitis of the connective tissue beneath the tunica albuginea and then extends to adjacent structures. This leads to fibrosis and, at times, calcification or even ossification.

Palpation of the shaft reveals a well-demarcated raised plaque of fibrosis that is usually in the midline of the dorsum near the base of the penis, although it may be placed more laterally or distally. Plain film evaluation of the penis may reveal areas of calcification within the indurated area.

Sonographically, the plaques of Peyronie's disease appear as dense, hyperechoic areas near the peripheral margin of the corpus cavernosum, usually along the dorsal aspect of the penis.[1,3,53,87-95] In one study, 22% of the plaques identified sonographically were not clinically palpable. In approximately 33% of the patients, these plaques cast an acoustic shadow that is most likely related to the presence of calcification (Fig. 25-16). In rare instances the plaques of Peyronie's disease will be evident as hypoechoic lesions that appear as an enlargement of the pericavernous tissue. This latter presentation is found in the earliest stages of the disease, when fibrosis is scarce and interstitial edema is present. The fibrosis and plaque may extend into the corpus cavernosum and occlude the cavernosal artery. Occlusion of the cavernosal artery may result in arteriogenic impotence.

Sonography can assess the size and location of the plaque for preoperative evaluation. Sonography may be used to follow some patients undergoing medical treatment for evaluating regression of the plaques.

PENILE URETHRA

The male urethra consists of the posterior urethra, which includes the prostatic and membranous urethra, and the anterior urethra, which includes the bulbous and penile urethra. The sonographic evaluation of the posterior urethra can be performed using a transrectal ultrasound approach. The anterior urethra can be studied by placing the transducer on the

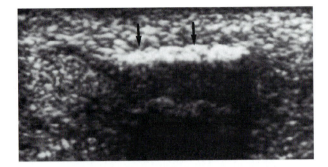

FIG. 25-16. Penile plaque. Longitudinal sonogram of the medial aspect of the right corpus cavernosum depicting an echogenic plaque *(arrows)* with posterior acoustic shadow.

surface of the penis and distending the urethra with fluid or gel.

The indications for sonography of the penile urethra include the evaluation of urethral strictures and the detection and localization of foreign bodies or stone material. Sonography has also been used for the evaluation of traumatic urethral disruption and urethral diverticula.[96-100]

Urethral strictures occur most commonly secondary to gonococcal urethritis or trauma. Sonographic evaluation of urethral strictures has several advantages over radiographic studies. Ultrasound does not use ionizing radiation, which is important for younger patients with strictures, who may require multiple examinations. During transverse and longitudinal real-time ultrasound the three-dimensional nature of the urethra can be appreciated. The soft tissues surrounding the urethra can also be examined for scarring and other abnormalities. The disadvantage of sonography of the penile urethra is its inability to visualize the posterior prostatic urethra without the use of a transrectal approach. Fortunately, most strictures occur in the anterior urethra.

The normal urethral lumen measures 4 mm or less in diameter and has smooth, thin walls. A stricture of the anterior urethra appears as a segment of narrowed lumen with irregularity and thickening of the urethral wall due to fibrosis and scarring (Fig. 25-17). The length of the stricture can be accurately measured, and dilatation of the urethra proximal to the stricture can also be appreciated. Sonographic guidance of stricture dilatation can be performed when indicated.

Nonradiopaque foreign bodies or **radiopaque stones** may be found in the urethra during ultrasonic evaluation. When looking for a urethral foreign body, the bulbous and penile urethra should be scanned before distention of the urethra to locate the foreign object, as it may be dislodged during retrograde filling.

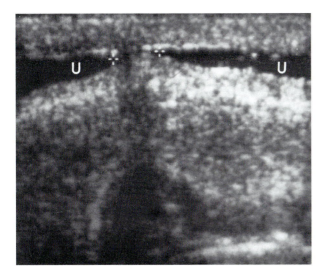

FIG. 25-17. Urethral stricture. Longitudinal sonourethrogram depicting a focal urethral stricture *(cursors)*. *U*, urethra. (Courtesy of Carol B. Benson, M.D., Boston.)

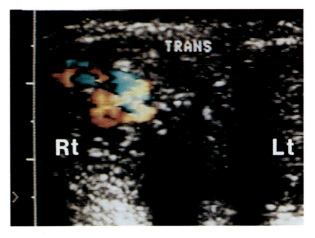

FIG. 25-18. Arteriosinusoidal fistula. Transverse color Doppler sonogram shows an area of increased color flow involving a large portion of the right cavernosal tissue consistent with an arteriosinusoidal fistula. (From Hattery RR, King BF et al. Vasculogenic impotence: duplex and color Doppler. *Radiol Clin North Am* 1991;29:629-645.)

Urethral diverticula in the penile urethra are rare but can occur as a result of previous urethritis. These diverticula appear as fluid-filled outpouchings adjacent to the urethra. Those diverticula that do not fill on retrograde urethrography can be seen sonographically.

PENILE CARCINOMA

Almost all tumors of the penis are of epithelial origin and they almost always involve the distal portion of the penis.[93,101,102] The incidence of penile carcinoma is lower in those populations in which circumcision is common. Stage I carcinoma of the penis involves a lesion limited to the glans or foreskin. Stage II tumors invade the shaft or corpora cavernosa. Stage III tumors are those that invade the shaft and have lymph node involvement. Stage IV tumors have distant metastases.

Approximately 50% of patients are likely to have metastases in the regional inguinal lymph node chain at the time of recognition because the disease is painless and often hidden within the nonretractable foreskin. Early diagnosis of metastatic nodal involvement remains the best available means for establishing appropriate management and prognosis. Ultrasound-guided fine-needle aspiration biopsy of enlarged inguinal lymph nodes can aid in the preoperative assessment in these patients.[102]

High-resolution sonography visualizes the extent of the primary tumor and its involvement in the corporal tissues. Penile cancer can appear hypoechoic or hyperechoic. The margins of the tumor are easily appreciated, and the involvement of the corporal tissues can be nicely demonstrated.[85] In penile cancers, a 2-cm margin of tumor-free tissue proximal to the tumor is a prerequisite for penile amputation.

PENILE TRAUMA

Penile trauma can be classified as either penetrating (e.g., knife or bullet) or blunt.[103] Injury to the penis following blunt trauma usually occurs when the penis is erect. Fracture of the penis occurs when there is disruption of the tunica albuginea and corpora cavernosa.[104,105] Penile fractures are often associated with a urethral tear. Although the findings may be clinically obvious, sonography can be helpful for vascular evaluation.[106] In some individuals, arterial sinusoidal fistulas occur following straddle injuries. These rare arterial sinusoidal fistulas result in partial tumescence of a portion of the penis.[65,106] Gray-scale sonography of this area may reveal a hypoechoic area due to hematoma in the corpus cavernosum. Color flow Doppler will often more clearly demonstrate an arteriovenous fistula of the cavernosal tissues (Fig. 25-18).

REFERENCES
Anatomy

1. Rollandi GA, Tentarelli T, Vespier M. Computed tomographic findings in Peyronie's disease. *Urol Radiol* 1985;7: 153-156.

2. Fisher M, Kricum M. Imaging of the Pelvis. Rockville, Md: Aspen Publishers, Inc.; 1989.

3. Hricak H, Marotti M, Gilbert TJ et al. Normal penile anatomy and abnormal penile conditions: evaluation with MR imaging. *Radiology* 1988;169:683-690.

Physiology

4. Aboseif SR, Lue TF. Hemodynamics of penile erection. *Urol Clin North Am* 1988;15:1-7.

5. Stackl W, Hasun R, Marberger M. Intracavernous injection of prostaglandin El in impotent men. *J Urol* 1988;140:66.

6. Fujita T, Shirai M. Mechanism of erection. *J Clin Exp Med* 1989;148:249.

7. Shirai M, Ishii N. Hemodynamics of erection in man. *Arch Androl* 1981;6:27.

8. Tudoriu T, Bourmer H. The hemodynamics of erection at the level of the penis and its local deterioration. *J Urol* 1983; 129:741-745.

9. Saenz de Tejada IS, Goldstein I, Krane RJ. Local control of penile erection: nerves, smooth muscle and endothelium. *Urol Clin North Am* 1988;15:9-15.

10. Newman HF, Northup JD, Delvin J. Mechanism of human penile erection. *Invest Urol* 1963;1:350-353.

11. Lue T, Tanagho E. Physiology of erection and pharmacologic management of impotence. *J Urol* 1987;137:829.

12. Saenz de Tejada IS, Goldstein I, Krane RJ. Local control of penile erection: nerve, smooth muscle and endothelium. *Urol Clin North Am* 1988;15:9-15.

13. Shirai M, Ishii N, Mitsukawa S et al. Hemodynamic mechanism of erection in the human penis. *Arch Androl* 1978; 1:345-349.

14. Beutler LE, Gleason DM. Integrating the advances in the diagnosis and treatment of male potency disturbance. *J Urol* 1981;126:338-342.

15. Collins WE, McKendry JBR, Silverman M et al. Multidisciplinary survey of erectile dysfunction. *Can Med Assoc J* 1982;128:1393-1399.

16. Hirsch IH, Smith RL, Chancellor MB et al. Use of intracavernous injection of prostaglandin E1 for neuropathic erectile dysfunction. *Paraplegia* 1994;32:661-664.

17. Pickard RS, King P, Zar MA et al. Corpus cavernosal relaxation in impotent men. *Br J Urol* 1994;74:485-491.

18. Lug TF, Tanagho EA. Physiology of erection and pharmacological management of impotence. *J Urol* 1987;137:829-836.

19. Lue TF, Zeineh RA, Schmidt RA et al. Physiology of erection. *World J Urol* 1983;1:194-196.

Impotence

20. Masters WH, Johnson VE. *Human Sexual Inadequacy.* New York: Little, Brown, & Co Inc; 1970.

21. Karacan I, Salis PJ, Williams RL. The role of the sleep laboratory in the diagnosis and treatment of impotence. In: William RL, Karacan I, Frazier SH, eds. *Sleep Disorders: Diagnosis and Treatment.* New York: John Wiley & Sons Inc; 1978.

22. Abber IC, Lue TF, Orvis BR et al. Diagnostic tests for impotence: a comparison of papaverine injection with the penile-brachial index and nocturnal penile tumescence monitoring. *J Urol* 1986;3-28.

23. Karacan I, Moore CA. Nocturnal penile tumescence: an objective diagnostic aid for erectile dysfunction. In: Bennett AH, ed. *Management of Male Impotence.* Baltimore: Williams & Wilkins; 1982.

24. Krane RJ, Goldstein I, Saenz de Tejada I. Medical progress: impotence. *N Engl J Med* 1989;321:1648-1659.

25. Shabsigh R, Fishman IJ, Scott FB. Evaluation of erectile impotence. *Urology* 1988;32:83-90.

26. Mueller SC, Lue TF. Evaluation of vasculogenic impotence. *Urol Clin North Am* 1988;15:65-76.

27. Chiu RC, Lidstone D, Blundell PE. Predictive power of penile brachial index in diagnosing male sexual impotence. *J Vasc Surg* 1986;4:251-256.

28. Wagner G, Uhrenholdt A. Blood flow by clearance in the human corpus cavernosum in the flaccid and erect states. In: Zorgniotti AW, Rossi G, eds. *Vasculogenic Impotence: Proceedings of the First International Conference on Corpus Cavernosum Revascularization.* Springfield, Ill: Charles C. Thomas, Publisher; 1980.

29. Forsberg L, Olsson AM, Neglen P. Erectile function before and after aorto-iliac reconstruction: a comparison between measurements of Doppler acceleration ratio, blood pressure and angiography. *J Urol* 1982;127:379-382.

30. Velcek D, Sniderman KW, Vaughan ED et al. Penile flow index utilizing a Doppler pulse wave analysis to identify penile vascular insufficiency. *J Urol* 1980;123:669-672.

31. Bookstein JJ. Penile vascular catheterization in the diagnosis and treatment of impotence. *Cardiovasc Intervent Radiol* 1988;11(special issue):183-261.

32. Bookstein JJ, Valji K, Parsons L, Kessler W. Pharmaco-arteriography in the evaluation of impotence. *J Urol* 1987; 137:333-337.

33. Virag R, Frydman D, Legman M et al. Intracavernous injection of papaverine as a diagnostic and therapeutic method in erectile failure angiology. *J Vasc Dis* 1984;35:79-87.

34. Buvat J, Bervat-Hertaut M, Dehaene JL et al. Is intravenous injection of papaverine a reliable screening test for vasculogenic impotence? *J Urol* 1986;135:476-478.

35. Robinson LQ, Woodcock JP, Stephenson TP. Duplex scanning in suspected vasculogenic impotence: a worthwhile exercise? *Br J Urol* 1989;63:432-436.

36. Lue TF, Hricak H, Marich KW et al. Vasculogenic impotence evaluated by high-resolution ultrasonography and pulsed Doppler spectrum analysis. *Radiology* 1985;155:777-781.

37. Desai KM, Gingell JC, Skidmore R et al. Application of computerized penile arterial waveform analysis in the diagnosis of arteriogenic impotence: an initial study in potent and impotent men. *Br J Urol* 1987;60:450-456.

38. Collins JP, Lewandowski BJ. Experience with intracorporeal injection of papaverine and duplex ultrasound scanning for assessment of arteriogenic impotence. *Br J Urol* 1987;59:84-88.

39. Krysiewicz S, Mellinger BC. The role of imaging in the diagnostic evaluation of impotence. *AJR* 1989;153:1133-1139.

40. Quam JP, King BF, James EM et al. Duplex and color Doppler sonographic evaluation of vasculogenic impotence. *AJR* 1989;153:1141-1147.

41. Benson CB, Vickers MA. Sexual impotence caused by vascular disease: diagnosis with duplex sonography. *AJR* 1989;153: 1149-1153.

42. Schwartz AN, Wang KY, Mack LA et al. Evaluation of normal erectile function with color flow Doppler sonography. *AJR* 1989;153:1155-1160.

43. Paushter DM. Role of duplex sonography in the evaluation of sexual impotence. *AJR* 1989;153:1161-1163.

44. Lue TF, Hricak H, Marich KW et al. Evaluation of arteriogenic impotence with intracorporeal injection of papaverine and the duplex ultrasound scanner. *Semin Urol* 1985;3:43-48.

45. Gall H, Barhren W, Scherb W et al. Diagnostic accuracy of Doppler ultrasound technique of the penile arteries in corre-

lation to selective arteriography. *Cardiovasc Intervent Radiol* 1988;11:225-231.

46. Bookstein JJ. Penile angiography: the last angiographic frontier. *AJR* 1988;150:47-54.

47. Lue TF, Hricak H, Schmidt RA et al. Functional evaluation of penile veins by cavernosography in papaverine-induced erection. *J Urol* 1986;135:479-482.

48. Lewis RW. This month in investigative urology: venous impotence. *J Urol* 1988;140:1560.

49. Bookstein JJ. Cavernosal veno-occlusive insufficiency in male impotence: evaluation of degree and location. *Radiology* 1987;164:175-178.

50. Malhotra CM, Balko A, Wincze JP et al. Cavernosonography in conjunction with artificial erection for evaluation of venous leakage in impotent men. *Radiology* 1986;161:799-802.

51. Lewis RW. Venous surgery for impotence. *Urol Clin North Am* 1988;15:115-121.

52. Rajfer J, Canan VP, Dorey FJ et al. Correlation between penile angiography and duplex scanning of cavernous arteries in impotent men. *J Urol* 1990;143:1128-1130.

53. Montague D. *Noninvasive Vascular Evaluation in Disorders of Male Sexual Function.* Chicago: Year Book Medical Publishers Inc; 1988.

54. Vickers M, Benson C, Richie J. High-resolution ultrasonography and pulsed wave Doppler for detection of corporovenous incompetence in erectile dysfunction. *J Urol* 1990;143:1125-1127.

55. Datta NS. Corpus cavernosography in conditions other than Peyronie's disease. *J Urol* 1977;118:588-590.

56. Gray R, Keresteci A, St Louis E et al. Investigation of impotence by internal pudendal angiography: experience with 73 cases. *Radiology* 1982;144:773-780.

57. Lakin M, Montague D, Medendorp S et al. Intracavernous injection therapy: analysis of results and complications. *J Urol* 1990;143:1138-1141.

58. Virag R, Frydman D, Legman M et al. Intracavernous injection of papaverine as a diagnostic and therapeutic method in erectile failure. *Angiology* 1984;35:79.

59. Goldstein I, Siroky M, Nath R et al. Vasculogenic impotence: role of the pelvic steal test. *J Urol* 1982;128:300.

60. Fournier G, Juenemann K, Lue T et al. Mechanisms of venous occlusion during canine penile erection: an anatomic demonstration. *J Urol* 1987;137:163.

61. Mellinger BC, Vaughan ED Jr, Thompson SL et al. Correlation between intracavernous papaverine injection and Doppler analysis in impotent men. *Urology* 1987;416-419.

62. Virag R, Bouilly P, Frydman D. Is impotence an arterial disorder? A study of arterial risk factors in 440 impotent men. *Lancet* 1985;1:181-184.

63. Abelson D. Diagnostic value of the penile pulse and blood pressure: a Doppler study of impotence in diabetics. *J Urol* 1975;113:636-639.

64. Nessi R, de Flaviis L, Bellizoni G et al. Digital angiography of erectile failure. *Br J Urol* 1987;59:584-589.

65. Ginestie JP, Romieu A. *Radiologic Exploration of Impotence.* Boston: Nijhoff; 1978.

66. Puyau FA, Lewis FW. Corpus cavernosography: pressure, flow and radiography. *Invest Radiol* 1983;18:517-522.

67. Delcour C, Wespes E, Vandenbosch G et al. Impotence: evaluation with cavernosography. *Radiology* 1986;161:803-806.

68. Maatman TJ, Montague DK, Martin LM. Cost-effective evaluation of impotence. *Urology* 1986;27:132-135.

69. Hattery RR, King BF, Lewis RW et al. Vasculogenic impotence: duplex and color Doppler. *Radiol Clin North Am* 1991;29:629-645.

70. Hattery RR, King BF Jr, James EM et al. Vasculogenic impotence: duplex and color Doppler imaging. *AJR* 1991;156:189-195.

71. Quam JP, King BF, James EM et al. Duplex and color Doppler ultrasound evaluation of vasculogenic impotence (scientific exhibit). *Radiol Soc North Am*, 1989.

72. King BF Jr, Hattery RR, James EM, Lewis RW. Duplex sonography in the evaluation of impotence: current techniques. *Semin Intervent Radiol* 1990;7:215-221.

73. King BF Jr. Color Doppler flow imaging evaluation of the deep dorsal penile vein in vascular impotence (abstract). *Radiol Soc North Am* 1989;371.

74. Tanaka T. Papaverine hydrochloride in peripheral blood and the degree of penile erection. *J Urol* 1990;143:1135-1137.

75. Broderick GA, Harkaway R. Pharmacologic erection: time-dependent changes in the corporal environment. *Int J Impot Res* 1994;6:9-16.

76. Burkhalter J, Morano J. Partial priapism: the role of computed tomography in its diagnosis. *Radiology* 1985;156:159.

77. Abozeid M, Juenemann K, Luo J et al. Chronic papaverine treatment: the effect of repeated injections on the simian erectile response and penile tissue. *J Urol* 1987;138:1263.

78. Summers J. Pyogenic granuloma: an unusual complication of papaverine injection therapy for impotence. *J Urol* 1990;143:1227-1228.

79. Virag R. About pharmacologically induced prolonged erection (letter to the editor). *Lancet* 1985;1:519.

80. Hu K, Burks C, Christy W. Fibrosis of the tunica albuginea: complication of long-term intracavernous pharmacological self-injection. *J Urol* 1987;138:404.

81. Kiely E, Williams C, Goldie L. Assessment of the immediate and long-term effects of pharmacologically induced penile erections in the treatment of psychogenic and organic impotence. *Br J Urol* 1987;59:164.

82. Govier FE, Asase D, Hefty TR et al. Timing of penile color flow duplex ultrasonography using a triple drug mixture. *J Urol* 1995;153:1472-1475.

83. Kim SH, Paick JS, Lee SE et al. Doppler sonography of deep cavernosal artery of the penis: variation of peak systolic velocity according to sampling location. *J of Ultrasound Med* 1994;13:591-594.

84. Fitzgerald SW, Erickson SJ, Foley WD et al. Color Doppler sonography in the evaluation of erectile dysfunction: patterns of temporal response to papaverine. *AJR* 1991;157:331-336.

85. Lee B, Sikka SC, Randrup ER et al. Standardization of penile blood flow parameters in normal men using intracavernous prostaglandin E1 and visual sexual stimulation. *J Urol* 1993;149:49-52.

86. Knispel HH, Andresen R. Color-coded duplex sonography in impotence: significance of different flow parameters in patients and controls. *Eur Urol* 1992;21:22-26.

Peyronie's Disease

87. Balconi G, Angeli E, Nessi R et al. Ultrasonographic evaluation of Peyronie's disease. *Urol Radiol* 1988;10:85-88.

88. Metz P, Ebbehoj J, Uhrenholdt A et al. Peyronie's disease and erectile failure. *J Urol* 1983;30:1103-1104.

89. Altraffer LF, Jordan JH. Sonographic demonstration of Peyronie's plaques. *Urology* 1981;17:292-295.

90. Fleischer AC, Rhamy RK. Sonographic evaluation of Peyronie's disease. *Urology* 1981;17:290-291.

91. Gelbard M, Sarti D, Kanfman J. Ultrasound imaging of Peyronie's plaques. *J Urol* 1981;125:44-45.

92. Merkle W. Cause of deviation of the erectile penis after urethral manipulations (Kelami syndrome): demonstration of ultrasound findings and case reports. *Urol Int* 1990;45:183-185.

93. Rifkin M. Urethra and penis. In: *Diagnostic Imaging of the Lower Genitourinary Tract.* New York: Raven Press; 1985.

94. Vermooten V. Metaplasia in the penis: the presence of bone, bone marrow and cartilage in the glans. *N Engl J Med* 1933;209:368-369.

95. Frank R, Gerard P, Wise G. Human penile ossification: a case report and review of the literature. *Urol Radiol* 1989;11:179-181.

Penile Urethra

96. Benson CB. Sonography of the male urethra. Current status of prostate and lower urinary tract imaging course. AIUM Annual Meeting; March 3-4, 1990; New Orleans.

97. McAninch JW, Laing FC, Jeffrey RB. Sonourethrography in the evaluation of urethral strictures: a preliminary report. *J Urol* 1988;139:294-297.

98. Gluck CD, Bundy AL, Fine C et al. Sonographic urethrogram: a comparison to roentgenographic techniques in 22 patients. *J Urol* 1988;140:1404-1408.

99. Kauzlaric D, Barmeir E, Peyer P et al. Sonographic appearances of urethral diverticulum in the male. *J Ultrasound Med* 1988;7:107-109.

100. Merkle W, Wagner W. Sonography of the distal male urethra-a new diagnostic procedure for urethral stricture: results of a retrospective study. *J Urol* 1988;140:1409-1411.

Penile Carcinoma

101. Sufrin G, Huben R. Benign and malignant lesions of the penis. In: Gillenwater J, Grayhack I, Howards S et al, eds. *Adult and Pediatric Urology*. Chicago: Year Book Medical Publishers Inc; 1987.

102. Scappini P, Piscioli F, Pusiol T, Hofstetter A et al. Penile cancer: aspiration biopsy cytology for staging. *Cancer* 1986;58:1526-1533.

Penile Trauma

103. Smith D. *General Urology: Injuries to the Genitourinary Tract*. Los Altos, Calif: Lange Medical Books, 1978:233-252.

104. Grosman H, Gray R, St Louis E et al. The role of corpus cavernosography in acute "fracture" of the penis. *Radiology* 1982;144:787-788.

105. Ames ES, Newhouse JH, Cronan JJ. Radiology of male periurethral structures. *AJR* 1988;151:321-324.

106. Dierks PR, Hawkins H. Sonography and penile trauma. *J Ultrasound Med* 1983;2:417-419.

CHAPTER 26

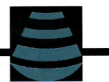

The Rotator Cuff

•

Marnix T. van Holsbeeck, M.D.

Laurence A. Mack, M.D.

Frederick A. Matsen III, M.D.

Keith Y. Wang, Ph.D., M.D.

Shoulder pain has many causes. Tendinitis, cuff strain, and partial- or full-thickness tear may cause pain and weakness on elevation of the arm.[1] The pain in rotator cuff disease is often worse at night and might keep the patient awake for prolonged periods of time. Underlying these symptoms in many patients over 40 years of age is rotator cuff fiber failure.[2] The supraspinatus tendon fibers typically fail first. The subscapularis and infraspinatus tendons, two other tendons of the **rotator cuff**, fail when the tear extends. The teres minor, the fourth component of the rotator cuff, is rarely affected. Calcific tendinitis, cervical radiculopathy, and acromioclavicular arthritis may mimic rotator cuff pathology. Contrast arthrography has long been the premier radiologic examination used to diagnose full-thickness tears of the rotator cuff.[3] Two competing noninvasive imaging techniques, ultrasound and magnetic resonance imaging (MRI), are taking over the role of arthrography. High-resolution real-time ultrasound has been shown to be a cost-effective means of examining the rotator cuff.[4-8] Ultrasound is the modality of choice in our institution. In the last 5 years we performed over 6000 shoulder ultrasound studies.

CLINICAL CONSIDERATIONS

Rotator cuff fiber failure is[1] the most common cause of shoulder pain and dysfunction in the patient over age 40. Epidemiologic studies by Codman, DePalma, and others have demonstrated the frequency of rotator cuff fiber failure increases with age.[9-11] This aging of tendons has been shown in imaging studies as well.[12-15] The earliest changes are often located in the substance of the tendon, resulting in so-called "delamination" of the cuff. Fiber failure is a step-by-step process from partial-thickness tear, almost always first in the supraspinatus, to massive tears involving multiple cuff tendons.

Rotator cuff tear may occur insidiously and, in fact, unnoticed by the patient, a process termed by some as **"creeping tendon ruptures."**[16] Asymptomatic tears affect a fraction of the population as large as 30% in the group over age 60.[12] When a larger group of fibers fails at one time, the shoulder demonstrates pain at rest and accentuation of pain on use of the rotator cuff (e.g., extension, abduction or external rotation). When even greater numbers of fibers fail at one time, a process known as "acute extension" of the shoulder may demonstrate sudden onset of substantial weakness in flexion, abduction, and external rotation.

As we age, our rotator cuff becomes increasingly susceptible to tearing with less severe amounts of applied force. Thus, although a major force is required to tear the usual rotator cuff of a 40-year-old person, a relatively trivial force may result in tear of the rotator cuff of the average 60-year-old individual. This is analogous to the predisposition of older women to femoral neck fractures. Although differences of the acromial shape, abnormalities of the acromial clavicular joint, and other factors may also affect the susceptibility of the rotator cuff to fiber failure, age-related deterioration and loading of the rotator cuff seem to be the dominant factors in determining the failure patterns of the cuff tendons.

Symptoms of rotator cuff fiber failure in the acute phase usually include pain at rest and on motion. Later, subacromial crepitance occurs when the arm is rotated in the partially flexed position, and, finally, arm weakness occurs. When the rotator cuff fails, shoulder instability can result and so-called internal impingement may then manifest itself. The humeral head is no longer stabilized and may impinge on the tissues in between the head and the acromion. This process leads to sclerosis and remodeling of the acromion, and it may result in a traction spur along the coracoacromial ligament.[17]

TECHNICAL CONSIDERATIONS

Mechanical sector scanners with frequencies between 5 and 10 MHz have been used in the shoulder successfully in the early literature of rotator cuff sonography. The use of these mechanical sector scanners is now outdated. The utility of these transducers is limited by several factors: near-field artifact, narrow superficial image field, and **tendon anisotropy.** This last named artifact is caused by the anisotropic structure of tendons. Parallelism of collagenous structures results in peculiar imaging characteristics: the echogenicity of the tendon depends on the angle of the transducer relative to the tendon during tendon interrogation. The curved footprint of the mechanical sector scanners will result in heterogeneous appearance of the tendons. Even with optimal perpendicular technique, the center of the image will appear hyperechoic while the side lobes will be hypoechoic. This hypoechogenicity can be mistaken for pathology by the unexperienced reader.

State-of-the-art imaging of the cuff should be done with a high-resolution linear array transducer. Transducers of high frequency, 7 or 7.5 MHz, are preferable to those of lower frequency. In patients with a thin subcutaneous layer we now routinely use a 10-MHz linear array transducer. These transducers demonstrate marked improvement in near resolution when compared with other devices. In addition, the broad superficial field of view is helpful to improve the near-field image.

TECHNIQUE

Understanding the complex three-dimensional rotator cuff anatomy during sonography is crucial to successful rotator cuff sonography. The bone might limit the examination of the inexperienced examiner. For those who start in shoulder ultrasound but who have experience in arthrography, we would recommend performing a quick ultrasound examination before and after each arthrogram. This allows the examiner to test his or her diagnostic abilities instantaneously. When we started, we did the arthrograms in single contrast; this enabled us to repeat the exam and correct our mistakes in those cases in which we failed to make the diagnosis of a tear. Those who have no experience with arthrography can scan in the operating room or in the anatomy laboratory. Surgical exploration or dissection may teach the most valuable lessons. Those initial steps are necessary to improve knowledge of the anatomy, which is essential in mastering the technique and accelerating the learning curve.

The bony landmarks guide the examination (Fig. 26-1). The fingers of the examiner can palpate the acromion, the scapular spine, and the coracoid and acromioclavicular joints. Transducer orientation relative to those landmarks will be essential in making corrections to the technique in viewing complex shoulder pathology. External bony landmarks are important in shoulder imaging when scanning a patient with significant pathology and loss of normal soft tissue landmarks.

The patient is scanned while seated on a rotating stool without armrests. The examiner sits comfortably

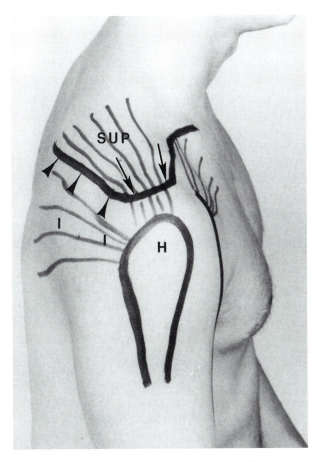

FIG. 26-1. General anatomic landmarks. Lateral photograph shows the bony structure, which limits the acoustic window for the examination of the cuff. *Sup,* Supraspinatus muscle and tendon; *I,* infraspinatus muscle and tendon; *arrowheads,* scapular spine; *arrows,* acromion; *H,* humerus.

5 cm above the patient on a stool, preferably with wheels, to enhance mobility. Both shoulders, starting with the less symptomatic one, should be examined if the examiner is a beginner. The following technique is used at our institution.[8]

Transverse images through the long biceps are obtained with the arm and forearm on the patient's thigh, the hand palm pronated (Fig. 26-2). The **bicipital groove** serves as the anatomic landmark to differentiate the subscapularis tendon from the supraspinatus tendon. The groove is concave; bright echoes reflect off the bony surface of the humerus. The tendon of the long head of the biceps is visualized as a hyperechoic oval structure within the bicipital groove on the transverse images. The tendon courses through the rotator cuff interval and divides the subscapularis from the supraspinatus tendon. Scanning should begin with the proximal long biceps tendon above the biceps tendon groove. The intracapsular biceps shows more obliquely in the shoulder capsule. The biceps is then followed throughout its course in the bicipital groove; the scan should extend as far down as the musculotendinous junction. This allows detection of the smallest fluid collections in the medial triangular recess at the distal end of the tendon sheath.[18] Such small biceps sheath collections are a very sensitive indicator of joint fluid. A 90-degree rotation of the transducer into a longitudinal view will ascertain the intactness of the biceps tendon.[19] The transducer must be carefully aligned along the biceps groove (Fig. 26-3). Gentle pressure on the distal aspect of the transducer is necessary to parallel align the transducer and tendon to avoid artifact due to anisotropy.

The transducer position is then returned to the transverse plane and moved proximally along the humerus to visualize the **subscapularis** tendon, which appears as a band of medium-level echoes deep to the subdeltoid fat and bursa. The subscapularis tendon is viewed parallel to its axis (Fig. 26-4); scanning during passive and external rotation may be helpful in assessing the integrity of the subscapularis tendon, which may be disrupted in patients with chronic anterior shoulder dislocation. External rotation is also necessary to diagnose subluxation of the long biceps tendon, especially if only present intermittently.[20]

The normal **subdeltoid bursa** is recognized as a thin, hypoechoic layer in between deltoid muscle on one side and the rotator cuff tendons and biceps tendon on the deep side. Hyperechoic peribursal fat surrounds the outer aspect of the synovial layer.[21]

The **supraspinatus** tendon is scanned perpendicular to its axis (transversely) by moving the transducer laterally posteriorly. The sonographic window is very narrow, and careful transducer positioning is essential (Fig. 26-5). The supraspinatus tendon is visualized as a band of medium-level echoes deep to the subdeltoid bursa and superficial to the bright echoes originating from the bone surface of the greater tuberosity.

The rest of the examination is done with the arm adducted and hyperextended and the shoulder in moderate internal rotation[5,7,22] (Fig. 26-6). This position can best be explained to the patient by asking him or her to reach to the opposite back pocket. Both longitudinal sections along the course of the supraspinatus tendon and images transverse to the tendon insertion and perpendicular to the humeral head are obtained. Correct orientation is achieved when an imaging plane shows crisp bone surface definition and sharp outline of the cartilage of the humeral head. During longitudinal scanning, the transducer overlays the acromion medially and the lateral aspect of the greater tuberosity laterally. The transducer sweeps around the humeral head circumferentially; the transducer should be held perpendic-

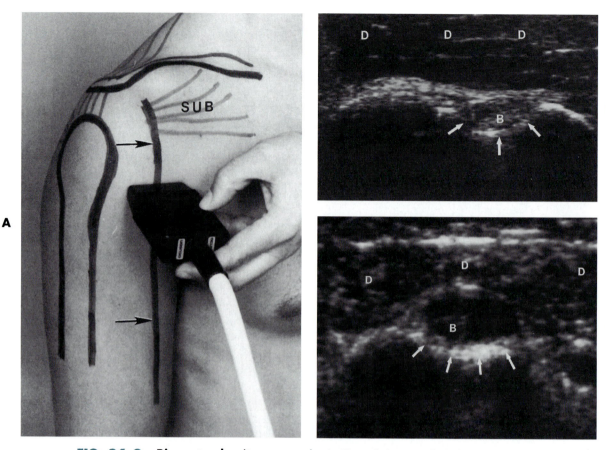

FIG. 26-2. **Biceps tendon (transverse).** **A,** Clinical photograph. **B,** Sonogram shows the biceps tendon, *B,* as a hyperechoic oval structure within the bicipital groove *(arrows)*. **C,** Scan in the same location demonstrates a hypoechoic biceps tendon, *B,* surrounded anteriorly by fluid in a different patient with joint effusion and rotator cuff tear. *D,* Deltoid muscle; *SUB,* subscapularis tendon; *arrows,* bicipital groove. (From Mack LA, Nyberg DA, Matsen FA. Sonographic evaluation of rotator cuff. *Radiol Clin North Am* 1988:26:161-177.)

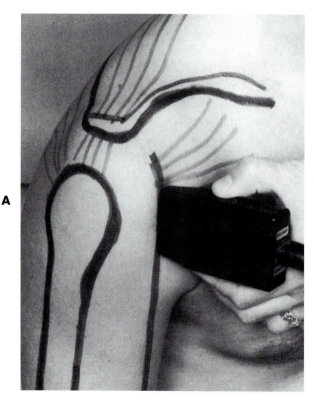

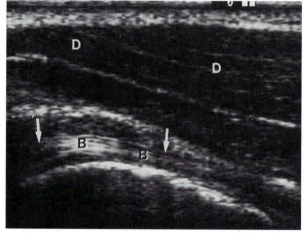

FIG. 26-3. **Biceps tendon (longitudinal).** **A,** Clinical photograph. **B,** Scan shows the biceps tendon, *B.* Note that the tendon *(arrows)* becomes artifactually hypoechoic as the angle it makes with the transducer diverges from 180 degrees. *D,* Deltoid tendon.

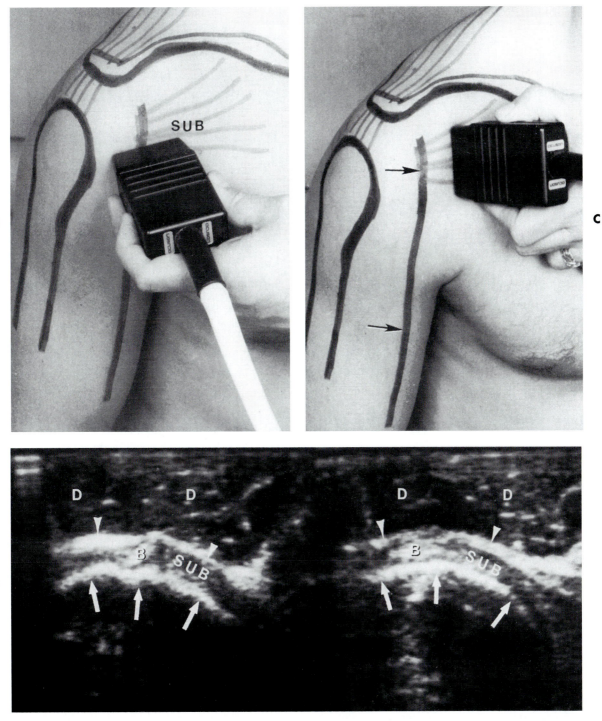

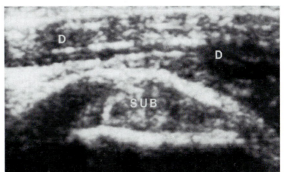

FIG. 26-4. Subscapularis tendon. A, Clinical photograph and, B, dual image show the subscapularis tendon, *SUB*, parallel to its axis (longitudinal in internal and external rotation) viewed as a band of medium-level echoes deep to the subdeltoid bursa *(arrowheads)*. D, Deltoid muscle; *B*, biceps tendon; *arrows*, humeral surface. C and D, Clinical photograph and scan perpendicular to the axis of the subscapularis tendon. *Arrows*, Biceps tendon; *SUB*, subscapularis tendon; *D*, deltoid muscle. (A and B From Mack LA, Nyberg DA, Matsen FA. Sonographic evaluation of rotator cuff. *Radiol Clin North Am* 1988;26:161-177.)

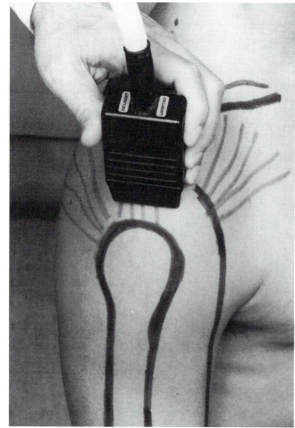

A

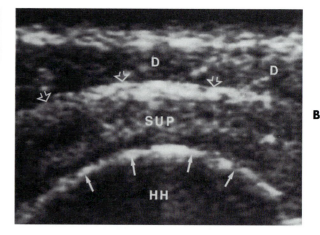

B

FIG. 26-5. Supraspinatus tendon (transverse).
A and **B,** Clinical photograph and scan show the
supraspinatus tendon, *SUP,* as a band of medium-level
echoes deep to the subdeltoid bursa *(open arrows). Arrows,*
Humeral surface; *D,* deltoid muscle; *HH,* humeral head. (**B**
From Mack LA, Nyberg DA, Matsen FA. Sonographic evaluation of rotator cuff. *Radiol Clin North Am* 1988;26:161-
177.)

ular to the humeral head surface at all times. This
sweeping motion through the supraspinatus tendon
starts anteriorly next to the long biceps tendon; we
cover an area of approximately 2.5 cm lateral to the
long biceps tendon. Infraspinatus tendon is scanned
beyond this point. The musculotendinous junction
shows as hypoechoic muscle surrounding hyperechoic
infraspinatus tendon. The transverse scan starts just
lateral to the acromion and translates downward over
the supraspinatus tendon and the greater tuberosity.
The critical zone is that portion of the tendon that begins approximately 1 cm posterolateral to the biceps
tendon. Failure to adequately visualize this area may
cause a false-negative result.[5]

Scanning of the supraspinatus tendon is followed
by the visualization of the infraspinatus and teres
minor tendons by moving the transducer posteriorly
and in the plane parallel to the scapular spine. The
infraspinatus tendon appears as a beak-shaped
soft-tissue structure as it attaches to the posterior aspect of the greater tuberosity (Fig. 26-7).[6] Internal
and external shoulder rotation may be helpful in the
examination of the infraspinatus tendon. This maneuver relaxes and contracts the infraspinatus tendon
in alternating fashion. At this level, a portion of the
posterior glenoid labrum is seen as a hyperechoic, triangular structure. The fluid of the infraspinatus re-

cess surrounds the labrum. The hypoechoic articular
cartilage of the humeral head, which shows lateral to
the labrum, contrasts significantly with the hyperechogenicity of the fibrocartilage. Scanning is extended medially to encompass the spinoglenoid notch
and the suprascapular vessels and nerve. The transversely oriented transducer is moved distally, and the
teres minor is then visualized. The **teres minor** has a
trapezoidal structure (Fig. 26-8). It is differentiated
from the infraspinatus tendon by its broader and
more muscular attachment. Tears of this tendon are
rare, and we have not encountered isolated teres
minor tears in the 6000 symptomatic shoulders we
have scanned. Despite this, we scan this region to ensure ourselves that the infraspinatus tendon has been
scanned in its entirety. Small joint effusions will also
easily show in this location.[23] Demonstration of this
helps distinguish articular processes such as rheumatoid arthritis and septic arthritis, which will cause effusion. In rotator cuff disease it is rare to find fluid in
this location.

Coronal images through the acromioclavicular
joints are obtained at the end of the examination.
Right-left comparison can show degenerative or traumatic pathology that can mimic or cause impinge-
ment-like symptoms. The superior glenoid labrum
can be shown with the transducer aligned posterior to

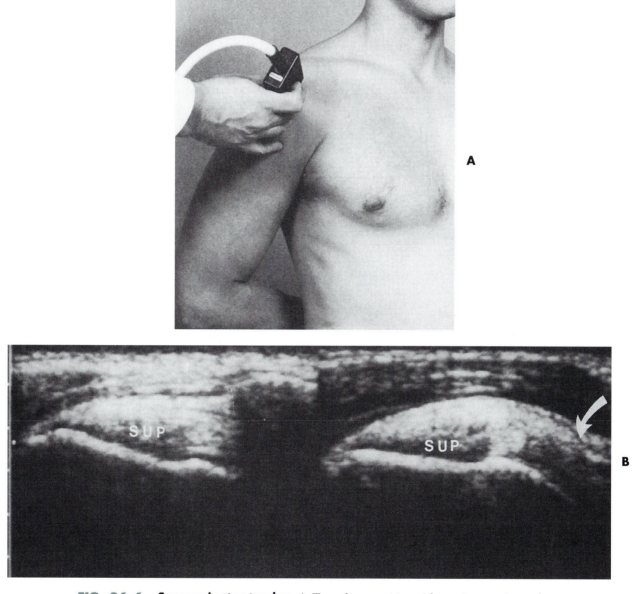

FIG. 26-6. **Supraspinatus tendon.** **A,** Transducer position with arm in extension and internal rotation. **B,** Paired longitudinal views of supraspinatus tendon with arm in neutral and extension with internal rotation demonstrate improved visualization of the supraspinatus tendon *(arrow).*

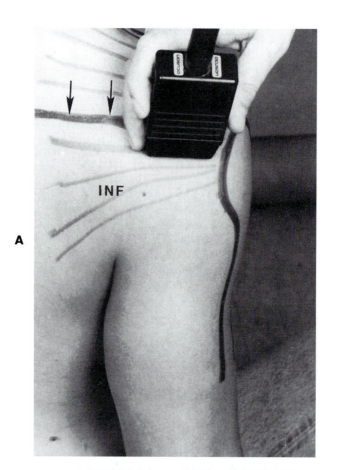

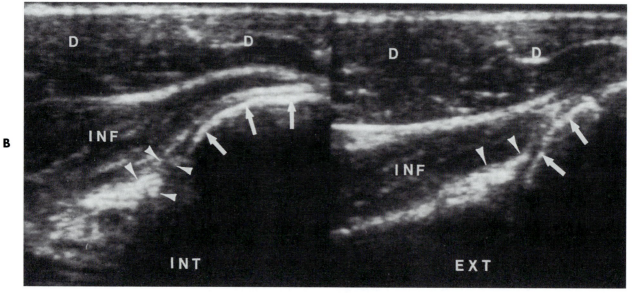

FIG. 26-7. Infraspinatus tendon. A, Clinical photograph. B, Dual image of the infraspinatus tendon, *INF*, in internal, *INT*, and external, *EXT*, rotation. *Black arrows*, Scapular spine; *white arrows*, humeral surface; *D*, deltoid muscle; *arrowheads*, posterior glenoid labrum. (B From Mack LA, Nyberg DA, Matsen FA. Sonographic evaluation of rotator cuff. *Radiol Clin North Am* 1988;26:161-177.)

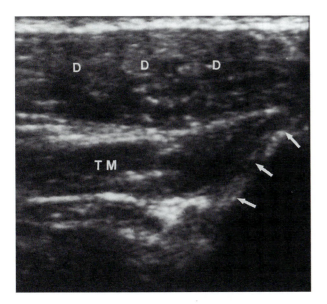

FIG. 26-8. **Teres minor.** The teres minor, *TM*, is visualized as a trapezoidal structure. *Arrows*, Humerus; *D*, deltoid muscle. (From Mack LA, Nyberg DA, Matsen FA. Sonographic evaluation of rotator cuff. *Radiol Clin North Am* 1988;26:161-177.)

the acromioclavicular joint and oriented perpendicular to the superior glenoid. A curved linear array transducer will be necessary if diagnosis of superior labral detachment (SLAP lesions) is desired.

THE NORMAL CUFF

The Cuff in the Adolescent

The rotator cuff **tendons** are hyperechoic relative to the deltoid muscle bellies (see Fig. 26-6). The cuff tendons are enveloped in a thin synovial layer that is normally thinner than 1.5 mm and appears hypoechoic relative to the tendons. The thickness of this bursal layer does not change; the subacromial-subdeltoid **bursa** is as thick over the long biceps tendon as it is over the subscapularis, supraspinatus, and infraspinatus tendons. A correctly performed examination will show a neatly defined bursa that shows as a hypoechoic stripe thinner than the thickness of the hypoechoic hyaline cartilage over the humeral head. This extraarticular bursa is a virtual space, it contains lubricant synovial fluid; this fluid cannot be distinguished on a routine shoulder ultrasound study. The bursa is hoof-shaped in cross section, and it often extends from the coracoid anteriorly around the lateral shoulder and posteriorly past the glenoid. The pleural space and the bursal synovial space share a number of similarities, including the virtual space (which can become distended in effusions), the thin lubricating layer of fluid in their

lumen, and the extensive network of capillary vessels and lymph vessels in their wall. Those vessels are not visible with color flow Doppler studies in patients with normal rotator cuff anatomy, but they have been shown in the power color flow Doppler studies of patients with inflamed cuffs.[24] The boundary between the bursa and the deltoid muscle consists of the so-called peribursal fat. This layer appears hyperechoic, and its thickness is remarkably uniform; body habitus seems to have little influence on the thickness of this fat layer.

Rotator cuff pathology is rare in young patients. Bursal and labral pathology can occur. Some of these conditions can mimic tendon tears. It is important to know that the adolescent cuff consists of more muscle than the aging cuff. The relative length of tendon to muscle increases with age.[25] Hypoechoic areas in the cuff in patients under age 20 may simply represent muscle, and the finding should not easily be attributed to a tear.

Age-Related Changes

The cuff in individuals under age 30 is watertight. Arthrography studies show that there should not be a communication with the subacromial-subdeltoid bursa.[18] Postmortem and cadaver studies have shown a high prevalence of rotator cuff tears in aging shoulders. Keyes[26] examined 73 unselected cadavers and found full-thickness tears of the supraspinatus in 13.4% of shoulders. Full-thickness tears were not recorded for those younger than 50 years in age; the prevalence over 50 years of age was 31%. Wilson and Duff[27] examined an unselected series of 74 bodies at postmortem and 34 dissecting-room cadavers over age 30 years. They found full-thickness tears of the supraspinatus tendon in 11% and partial-thickness tears in 10% of the shoulders. Fukuda et al.[28] reported a 7% prevalence of complete tears and a 13% prevalence of incomplete tears in a study of cadavers that included no details on age. With such high percentages of rotator cuff tears in cadaver studies, how many of these tears would have been asymptomatic? A study we conducted recently showed that ultrasound can detect **asymptomatic tears.**

Ninety volunteer subjects (47 women and 43 men) in a population who had never sought medical attention for shoulder disease underwent shoulder sonography; 77% (69 of 90) were Caucasian, 13% (12 of 90) were African-American, 9% (8 of 90) were Asian, and 1% (1 of 90) was Hispanic. Eighteen subjects were between the ages of 30 and 39 years; 18 were between ages 40 and 49 years; 18 were between ages 50 and 59 years; 13 were between ages 60 and 69 years; 13 were between ages 70 and 79 years; and 10 were between ages 80 and 99 years.

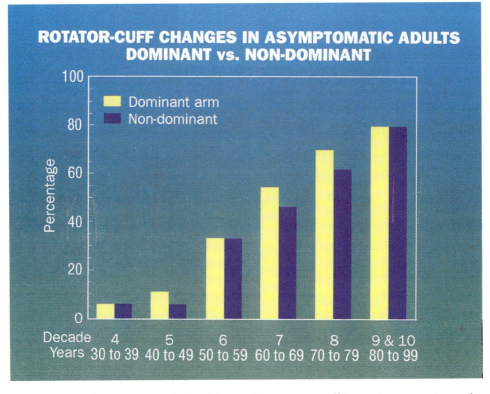

FIG. 26-9. Percentage of shoulders with rotator cuff tears in asymptomatic adults in different age groups. Chart shows comparison between dominant and non-dominant arms.

The proportion of women to men was nearly equal for each decade.

No statistically significant differences were found in the prevalence of rotator cuff lesions in each gender for either the dominant or nondominant arm (Fig. 26-9). We found no statistically significant differences in the incidence of rotator lesions related to gender or reported level of exertional activities. But the prevalence of rotator cuff tears in both the dominant and nondominant arms showed a linear increase after the fifth decade of life. This difference was statistically very significant between the third, fourth, and fifth decades and above.[12] The cumulative percentage of partial- and full-thickness tears was approximately 33% between the ages of 50 and 59 years, 55% between 60 and 69 years, 70% between 70 and 79 years, and as high as 78% above age 80 (see Fig. 26-9; Fig. 26-10).

A total of 26 full-thickness and 15 partial-thickness tears were found. Sixteen individuals or 64% of the patients with tears had **bilateral rotator cuff tears**. The youngest subject with a partial-thickness tear was 35 years old. The youngest subject with a full-thickness tear was 54 years old. The age range for partial-thickness tears was from 35 to 80 years of age. The age range of full-thickness tears was from 54 to

92 years of age. The average age in the partial-thickness group was 56 years. The average age in the full-thickness group was 63 years.

In 19 cases (46%) the rotator cuff tears had associated intrasynovial fluid. In 15 cases the fluid was located in the biceps tendon sheath, and in the remaining 4 cases it was located in the subacromial-subdeltoid bursa. There were two individuals with tears and fluid in the biceps tendon sheath and in the bursa simultaneously. The infraspinatus recess appeared normal in all of our patients. Eleven effusions were noted in the long biceps tendon sheath in subjects who did not have tears of the cuff. There was never excess fluid in the subacromial-subdeltoid bursa in the absence of rotator cuff tear. Shallow erosion or irregularity of the bone surface under the tear was noted in 90% of tears; bone changes were present in all but 4 partial-thickness tears. Greater tuberosity irregularity was noted in 37 shoulders or in 21% of shoulders in this study. Twelve shoulders showed irregular greater tuberosities and no rotator cuff tear. A statistically significant correlation between asymptomatic rotator cuff tears and irregularity of the greater tuberosity was found (Fig. 26-11).

Twenty of the full-thickness tears were considered large and involved more than one tendon. Three

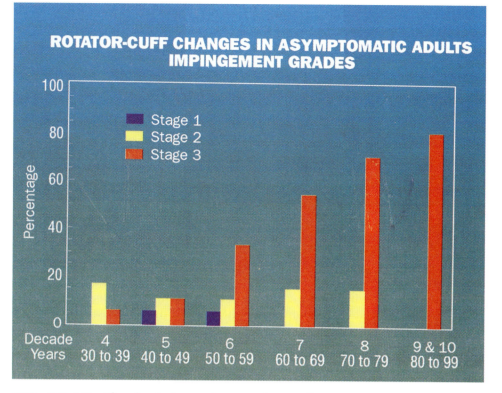

FIG. 26-10. **The chart shows the prevalence of stage 1 to stage 3 impinge-ment for the dominant arm in different age groups.** Abnormalities in the subacromial space were staged sonographically as follows: stage 1 if bursal thickness from 1.5 to 2 mm; stage 2 if bursal thickness over 2 mm; stage 3 if partial- or full-thickness rotator cuff tear.

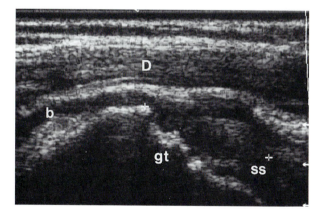

FIG. 26-11. Asymptomatic full-thickness rotator cuff tear. The longitudinal scan through the supraspinatus tendon, *ss*, shows retraction of tissue *(calipers)*. The bone surface of the uncovered greater tuberosity, *gt*, is irregular. The subdeltoid bursa, *b*, is filled with fluid. *D*, Deltoid muscle.

tears were massive and over 4 cm in diameter, and three tears were small and under 2 cm in width when measured over the base of the greater tuberosity.

Ten partial-thickness tears were mixed echogenicity, and five were hypoechoic. Nine mixed echogeni-city lesions and two hypoechoic tears exhibited bone change in the greater tuberosity.

Our results indicate that the finding of a rotator cuff abnormality or an effusion in the biceps tendon sheath can be compatible with normal and pain-free mobility of the shoulder. Rotator cuff findings should be interpreted with care over the age of 50. A rotator cuff tear is not necessarily the cause of the pain in an aging shoulder and can be an incidental finding. Degenerative rotator cuff changes may be regarded as a natural correlate of aging, with a statistically significant linear increase after the fifth decade of life. Clinical judgment must be used to distinguish asymptomatic from symptomatic rotator cuff tears. On the other hand, finding a rotator cuff tear should not stop the clinician from searching for other causes of shoulder pain. Our shoulder ultrasound reading is done in conjunction with the reading of the initial shoulder radiographic evaluation. It is not uncommon that we find missed primary or secondary neoplasms of bone, myeloma, or Pancoast's tumors using this careful approach. Limited and painful shoulder elevation can be due to a number of diseases, of which rotator cuff disease is the most common. Simultaneous occurrence of a full-thickness tear with a tumor in or around the shoulder is not rare in our experience.

PREOPERATIVE APPEARANCES

Criteria of Rotator Cuff Tears

Previously published sonographic criteria for rotator cuff pathology can be categorized into four groups[29]: nonvisualization of the cuff, localized absence or focal nonvisualization, discontinuity, and focal abnormal echogenicity.

Nonvisualization of the Cuff. Direct contact of the humeral head with the acromion is an indication of massive cuff tear. In this situation, the ultrasound image shows deltoid muscle directly on top of the humeral head (Fig. 26-12). In some cases, thickened bursa and fat will be noted between the deltoid muscle and the surface of the humeral head. This tissue layer is more hypoechoic and patchy in texture. The thickness of this layer will depend on the location of the tear, but generally it will be thinner and more irregular than the normal cuff layer. Some bursae have been noted to be up to 5 mm thick. This synovial layer has been mistaken for normal cuff by the inexperienced sonographer. With massive tears, exceeding 4 cm, the humeral head may ascend through the defect because of pulling of the deltoid muscle. The supraspinatus tendon is retracted under the acromion, and, as a rule, surgical reattachment will be impossible at this stage (Fig. 26-13). The extent of tear should be reported because multiple tendons are often involved. The diagnosis of these tears can be predicted on shoulder radiographs. Some centers use radiographs with comparison views during active shoulder abduction or anteroposterior supine views of the subacromial space to counteract the gravitational pull on the humerus.[30] As a rule, the subacromial space should not be smaller than 5 mm.

Focal Nonvisualization of the Cuff. Smaller tears will appear as localized absence of supraspinatus tendon or, in rare cases, local absence of subscapularis tendon. The most common tear pattern is caused by disease at the tendon-bone junction.

The tendon will retract from the bone surface, leaving a bare area of bone (Fig. 26-14). This finding has been reported in the past as the **"naked tuberosity"** sign.[31] The bone surface of the greater tuberosity and anatomic neck of the humerus are irregular in approximately 79% of these tears. The vast majority of such tears will occur anteriorly in the supraspinatus tendon and in the critical zone. Characteristically, a small amount of tissues will be preserved surrounding the biceps tendon. Ideally, such tears can be confirmed in two perpendicular scan planes. Sometimes this will not be possible because the tear may show full thickness in one plane but not be identified as such in the orthogonal plane. This phenomenon has been attributed to partial volume averaging in tears that are smaller than the footprint of the transducers. Small **horizontal tears** typically appear on longitudinal images but can be missed on transverse images.[31] A helpful finding is the **"infolding" of bursal and peribursal fat** tissue into the focal defect. With few exceptions, this folding is a sign of a full-thickness tear. If the tear is larger, bursal and peribursal tissue will approximate the bone surface (see Fig. 26-14).

Focal nonvisualization should not be confused with segmental thinning of cuff after rotator cuff surgery. This thinning is normal after most tendon-bone reimplantations. In those cases, a bony trough is detected as a rounded or V-shaped defect in the humeral contour. The tendon is brought down into this narrow slit. The tendon is not repaired onto the tuberosity anatomically with a broad insertion but with a tapered end. It is well known that a number of those reconstructions fail to be watertight even after successful surgery. The rents in the capsule cause additional focal thinning. In a patient with a negative baseline study, retears can be identified by visualizing anechoic fluid leaking through a tear.

Discontinuity in the Cuff. This term has been used for tears that are located more proximally in the tendon. These tears tend to be of the **vertical type** and are more often traumatic.[31] The patient may have a history of prior shoulder dislocation. Discontinuity is observed when the small defects fill with joint fluid or hypoechoic reactive tissue (Fig. 26-15). Such defects are often accentuated by placing the arm in extension and internal rotation (Fig. 26-16). Often, a small amount of bursal fluid is also present. The sonographer can use this fluid as a natural contrast medium to show the tear in more detail. Manual compression of the subdeltoid bursa can move the fluid through the tear into the joint. This maneuver will show the tear more clearly. A focally bright interface around a segment of hyaline cartilage and deep to hypoechoic tendon is considered a sign of a full-thickness tear (see Fig. 26-15).

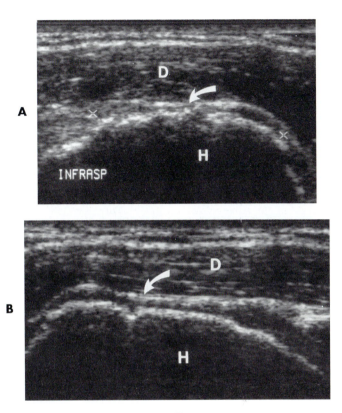

FIG. 26-12. Nonvisualization of cuff. A, Transverse view. The deltoid muscle, *D*, is in direct contact with the humeral head, *H*. A hyperechoic layer *(curved arrow)* of fat shows deep to the deltoid; this layer is interposed between the deltoid and the humerus. B, Longitudinal view through the expected location of the supraspinatus tendon. The supraspinatus tendon is absent. A hyperechoic layer of fat *(curved arrow)* is noted deep to the deltoid, *D. H*, Humeral head.

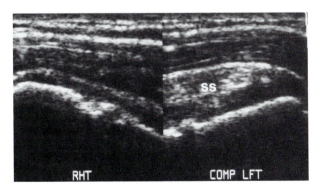

FIG. 26-13. Irreparable rotator cuff tear. Longitudinal right-left comparison shows a significant discrepancy in the thickness of the soft tissues. The supraspinatus tendon, *ss*, appears normal in the asymptomatic left shoulder, *LFT*. The supraspinatus tendon in the right, *RHT*, shoulder retracted out of sight. Arthroscopy showed the torn edge of the supraspinatus tendon withdrawn beyond the glenoid cavity. The rotator cuff defect was deemed irreparable.

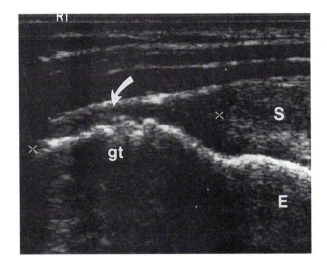

FIG. 26-14. Horizontal full-thickness tear. The longitudinal image through the supraspinatus tendons, *S*, shows 2 cm retraction of the torn tendon (distance between calipers). Bursa and peribursal fat *(curved arrow)* rest directly on the irregular bone surface of the greater tuberosity, *gt. E*, Humeral epiphysis.

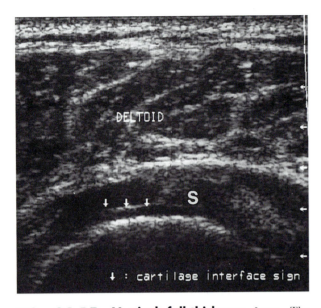

FIG. 26-15. Vertical full-thickness tear. The transverse image through the supraspinatus tendon, *S*, shows an anechoic area of discontinuity within the rotator cuff layer. The cartilage of the humeral head is surrounded by a bright interface and is marked as the "cartilage interface" sign.

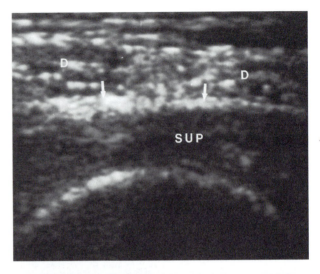

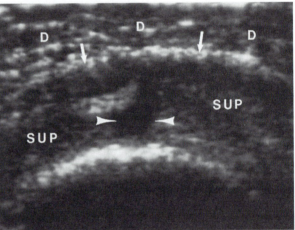

FIG. 26-16. Discontinuity of the cuff. Transverse scans of the supraspinatus tendons, *SUP*, in, **A,** neutral position and, **B,** with the arm in extension and internal rotation show a small tear filled with fluid *(arrowheads)*. Note the tear is only seen with the arm in extension. *D*, Deltoid muscle; *arrows*, subdeltoid bursa.

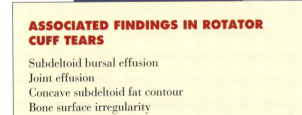

ASSOCIATED FINDINGS IN ROTATOR CUFF TEARS

Subdeltoid bursal effusion
Joint effusion
Concave subdeltoid fat contour
Bone surface irregularity

This sign has been named the **cartilage-interface sign** in an earlier report.[31]

Focal Abnormal Echogenicity. Cuff echogenicity may be diffusely or focally abnormal. Diffuse abnormalities of cuff echogenicity have proven to be unreliable sonographic signs for cuff tear.

Focal abnormal echogenicity has been associated with small full- and partial-thickness tears. An area of increased echogenicity might represent a new interface within the tendon at the site of fiber failure, as has been observed in some partial-thickness tears.[8] The small linear or comma-shaped hyperechoic lesion is often surrounded by edema or fluid and appears as a hypoechoic halo (Fig. 26-17). The partial-thickness tears are similar to the **"rim rents"** that were first ob-

served pathologically by Codman.[9] A slightly different type of partial-thickness tear can appear as an anechoic spot on the articular or bursal side of the tendon.[8] Careful inspection of the synovial surfaces of the tendon is necessary. Only those focal hypoechoic defects that violate the surface may be considered tears (Fig. 26-18). **Intrasubstance lesions** are the most common type of partial lesions and account for almost 50% of the defects. We do not call them tears because they are not considered "tears" by the surgeons who cannot observe them by direct tendon inspection. This poses a diagnostic problem similar to that of intrasubstance lesions of the menisci seen on MRI studies. Associated bone or synovial findings may be helpful if the ultrasound findings are equivocal.

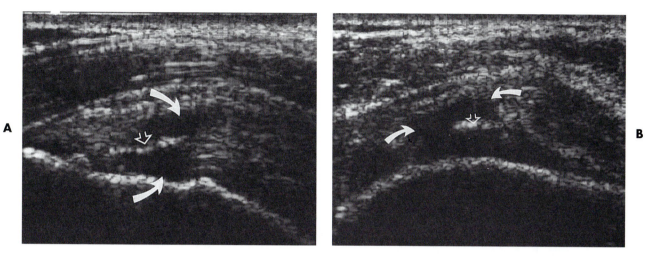

FIG. 26-17. Focal abnormal echogenicity. A, Longitudinal supraspinatus tendon view of an articular side partial-thickness tear, the so-called "rim rent." A linear hyperechoic lesion in the supraspinatus tendon *(open arrow)* is surrounded by hypoechoic edema *(curved arrows)*. B, Transverse supraspinatus tendon view of same partial-thickness defect. The same hyperechoic lesion is noted.

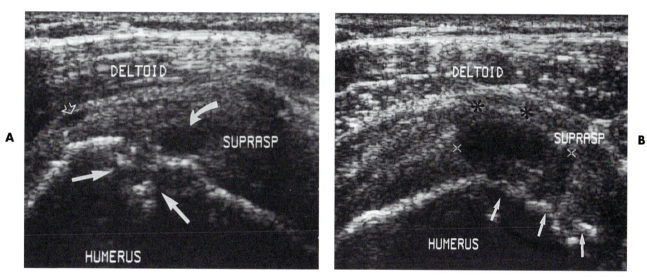

FIG. 26-18. Focal abnormal echogenicity—a hypoechoic rim rent. A, Longitudinal supraspinatus tendon view of an articular side partial-thickness tear. A hypoechoic lesion *(curved arrows)* appears deep in the supraspinatus tendon. The bone surface is irregular *(arrows)*, and a small amount of fluid *(open arrow)* is noted in the subdeltoid bursa. B, Transverse supraspinatus tendon view of the same partial-thickness tear (between calipers). An intact tissue layer *(asterisks)* covers the bursal surface of the tear. The bone surface is irregular *(arrows)*.

Associated Findings

Subdeltoid Bursal Effusion. Visualization of subdeltoid bursal effusion is the most reliable associated finding of rotator cuff tear (Fig. 26-19). It is found in both full- and partial-thickness tears. Anechoic fluid differs from hypoechoic edema of the bursal synovium. Edema is a common finding in shoulder impingement but is only rarely associated with a tear. Edema and fluid can be distinguished from each other using the "transducer compression test." A synovial recess filled with fluid will be emptied by compression; a recess with synovial edema changes little in shape. Other causes for fluid in the bursa include calcium milk with synovitis and septic bursitis. Hollister et al.[32] found the sonographic appearance of bursal fluid to have a specificity of 96% for the diagnosis of rotator cuff tears. Similar results were found by Farin et al.[33] In our prospective study

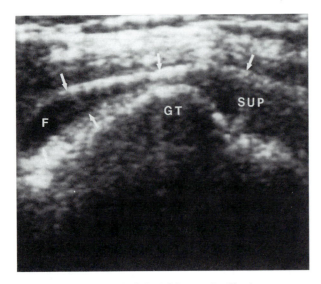

FIG. 26-19. Subdeltoid bursal effusion. Long-itudinal scan of the supraspinatus tendon, *SUP*, with the transducer placed laterally demonstrates a small subdeltoid bursal effusion. *F. Arrows,* Subdeltoid bursa; *GT,* greater tuberosity.

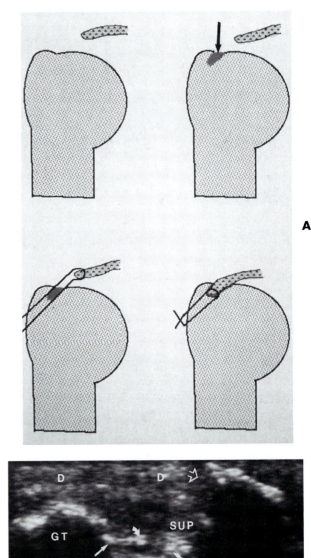

FIG. 26-20. Rotator cuff repair-sonographic appearances. A, Drawing demonstrating the surgical technique for cuff reimplantation with creation of trough *(arrow)* in the humeral head, reimplantation of the residual tendon within that trough, and characteristic method of suture placement. **B,** Longitudinal supraspinatus tendon, *SUP,* image shows characteristic appearances of reimplantation trough *(arrows)*. Acromioplasty defect *(open arrows)* is also visualized. *GT,* Greater tuberosity; *curved arrow,* reimplantation suture; *D,* deltoid muscle. (From Mack LA, Nyberg DA, Matsen FA et al. Sonography of the post-operative shoulder. *AJR* 1988;150:1089-1093.)

of rotator cuff disease,[8] all patients with fluid in the bursa had a rotator cuff tear.

Joint Effusion. Joint fluid can be found in the joint recesses, including the infraspinatus, subcoracoid, and axillary recesses. In a patient who sits in the upright position, most fluid will accumulate in the biceps tendon sheath. Approximately half of these effusions are associated with rotator cuff tears.[6] The other half roughly will be due to a variety of articular causes of shoulder disease. When a large fluid collection is found in the infraspinatus recess without fluid in the subdeltoid bursa, inflammatory or infectious causes of joint disease should always be excluded.[23]

Concave Subdeltoid Fat Contour. In the normal patient, the bright linear echoes from the subdeltoid bursal fat are convex upward. Concavity of the subdeltoid contour may be noted in medium and large tears, reflecting the absence of cuff tendon. It may be possible to approximate the deltoid and the humeral surface even in smaller tears using transducer compression at the site of the tear.

Bone Surface Irregularity. Only recently[8] has bone irregularity been cited as an important and common associated finding in rotator cuff tears. The majority of partial- and full-thickness tears of the distal 1 cm of the rotator cuff are associated with small bone spurs and pits in the bone surface of the greater tuberosity. It is possible that the use of higher-frequency transducers for rotator cuff imaging has made these findings more evident. The

tuberosity abnormality matches the tendon abnormality in location, size, and shape. The cause of the abnormality is unknown. Trauma due to an impaction of the tuberosity on the acromion during shoulder elevation has been considered.

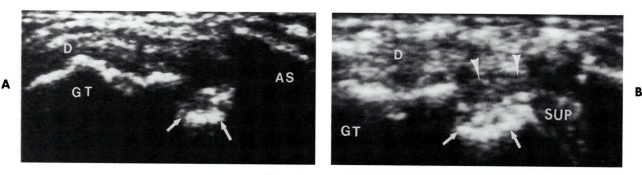

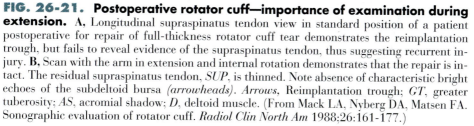

FIG. 26-21. **Postoperative rotator cuff—importance of examination during extension.** **A,** Longitudinal supraspinatus tendon view in standard position of a patient postoperative for repair of full-thickness rotator cuff tear demonstrates the reimplantation trough, but fails to reveal evidence of the supraspinatus tendon, thus suggesting recurrent injury. **B,** Scan with the arm in extension and internal rotation demonstrates that the repair is intact. The residual supraspinatus tendon, *SUP,* is thinned. Note absence of characteristic bright echoes of the subdeltoid bursa *(arrowheads).* *Arrows,* Reimplantation trough; *GT,* greater tuberosity; *AS,* acromial shadow; *D,* deltoid muscle. (From Mack LA, Nyberg DA, Matsen FA. Sonographic evaluation of rotator cuff. *Radiol Clin North Am* 1988;26:161-177.)

POSTOPERATIVE APPEARANCES

Recent reports in the literature suggest that sonography can play an important role in the postoperative follow-up after rotator cuff repair.[34,35] Because surgery may distort sonographic landmarks, sonography in the postoperative patient is rendered more difficult than in the preoperative patient. It is important therefore to understand the surgical procedures used in acromioplasty and cuff repair.

In acromioplasty, the anterior inferior aspect of the acromion is surgically removed. Sonographically, this appears as disruption of the normal, rounded, smooth acromial contour. After surgery, the acromion appears pointed (Fig. 26-20). Because the inferior aspect of the acromion is removed, a greater extent of the supraspinatus tendon may be visualized.

Repair of a cuff tear creates unique sonographic landmarks. The cuff tendons are reimplanted into a trough made perpendicular to the axis of the supraspinatus tendon. The reimplantation trough is placed in the humeral head at a site that provides optimal tendon tension. The trough appears sonographically as a defect in the humeral contour best viewed with the transducer longitudinal to the supraspinatus tendon (see Fig. 26-20). Suture material may be seen deep in the trough as specular echoes. Scanning the arm in extension and internal rotation may be necessary to visualize this site of tendon reimplantation, especially when it is medially placed (Fig. 26-21). Failure to scan in this position may lead to a false-positive diagnosis. Such a maneuver, however, should be used with care, especially in the immediate postoper-

ative period, to avoid reinjury of the friable, newly reimplanted tendons.

Sonographic appearances of the cuff tendons never return to normal in the postoperative patient. Tendons, especially the supraspinatus tendon, are often echogenic and thinned when compared with the contralateral shoulder. Joint effusions are common and best visualized along the biceps tendon. Because resection of the subdeltoid bursa removes an important landmark, dynamic scanning is especially important in distinguishing a thin, hyperechoic cuff from adjacent deltoid muscle.

Recurrent Tear

Sonographically, recurrent tears most often appear as absence of the cuff. Fluid filling a defect in a rotator cuff repair or loose sutures are other indications of recurrent tear (Fig. 26-22). Unless baseline scans are available in the postoperative period, it may be difficult to differentiate small recurrent tears from the appearances created when only a small amount of cuff tendon remains to be reattached. Thinning of the tendon is useless as a criterion, and bone irregularity is the rule in the postoperative patient. Recurrent tears are common. They occur in up to 40% of patients in whom a small defect was repaired and in 80% of those patients who had large tears preoperatively.

PITFALLS

Inadequate transducer positioning is the most common error in scanning the rotator cuff. False-posi-

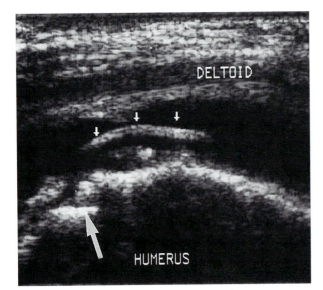

FIG. 26-22. Recurrent tear—postoperative ultrasound exam. Longitudinal scan along the deltoid muscle in the region of the reimplantation trough *(arrow)*. A loose suture *(small arrows)* is noted within a subdeltoid bursal effusion. The proximal humerus has an abnormal round appearance. The anatomic neck has disappeared.

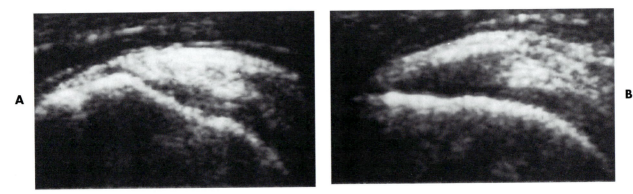

FIG. 26-23. Artifactual changes in tendon echogenicity. **A** and **B,** Two views of the same supraspinatus tendon demonstrate considerable changes in echogenicity that may be artifactually created by transducer position and orientation.

tive and false-negative results may be produced in this manner. For example, scanning the supraspinatus tendon transversely with the transducer placed laterally may artifactually mimic a rotator cuff tear. An oblique transverse scan of the supraspinatus tendon can be falsely reported as thinning of the cuff. The examiner must therefore view the cuff in two orthogonal planes. Visualization of neatly depicted bony contour will help in avoiding those pitfalls.

A cause of tendon heterogeneity is the geometric relationship of the tendon to the transducer. As demonstrated by Crass et al.[36] and Fornage,[37] failure to orient the transducer parallel to the fibers of the tendon may result in artifactual areas of decreased echogenicity (Fig. 26-23). When only a small area of the tendon is parallel to the transducer, a focal area of increased echogenicity may be produced, mimicking a small partial- or full-thickness tear. This artifact is especially pronounced with sector transducers.

REFERENCES

1. Matsen FA, Arntz CT. Subacromial impingement. In: Rockwood CA, Matsen FA III. eds. *The Shoulder. Vol II.* Philadelphia: W.B. Saunders Co; 1990.
2. Neviaser RJ, Neviaser TJ. Observations on impingement. *Clin Orthop* 1990;254:60-63.
3. Resnick D. Shoulder arthrography. *Radiol Clin North Am* 1981; 19:243-252.
4. Mack LA, Matsen FA, Kilcoyne JF et al. Ultrasound evaluation of the rotator cuff. *Radiology* 1985;157:205-209.
5. Mack LA, Gannon MK, Kilcoyne RF et al. Sonographic evaluation of the rotator cuff. Accuracy in patients without prior surgery. *Clin Orthop* 1988;234:21-27.
6. Middleton WD, Reinus WR, Totty WF et al. Ultrasonographic evaluation of the rotator and biceps tendon. *J Bone Joint Surg* 1986;68:440-450.
7. Crass JR, Craig EV, Feinberg SB. Ultrasonography of rotator cuff tears: a review of 500 diagnostic cuffs. *J Clin Ultrasound* 1988;16:313-327.
8. van Holsbeeck MT, Kolowich PA, Eyler WR et al. Ultrasound depiction of partial-thickness tear of the rotator cuff. *Radiology* 1995;197:443-446.

Clinical Considerations
9. Codman EA. *The Shoulder*, 2nd ed. Boston: Thomas Todd; 1934.
10. DePalma AF. *Surgery of the Shoulder*, 2nd ed. Philadelphia: JB Lippincott; 1973.
11. Refior HJ, Kroedel A, Melzer C. Examinations of the pathology of the rotator cuff. *Arch Orthop Trauma Surg* 1987;106:301-308.
12. Milgrom C, Schaffler M, Gilbert S et al. Rotator-cuff changes in asymptomatic adults. The effect of age, hand dominance and gender. *J Bone Joint Surg* 1995;77(B):296-298.
13. Sher JS, Uribe JW, Posada A et al. Abnormal findings on magnetic resonance images of asymptomatic shoulders. *J Bone Joint Surg* 1995; 77(A):10-15.
14. Raven PB. Asymptomatic tears of rotator cuff are commonplace. *Sports Med Dig* 1995;17:11-12.
15. Miniaci A, Dowdy PA, Willits KR et al. Magnetic resonance imaging evaluation of the rotator cuff tendons in the asymptomatic shoulder. *Am J Sports Med* 1995;23:142-145.
16. Petterson G. Rupture of the tendon aponeurosis of the shoulder joint in anterior inferior dislocation. *Acta Chir Scand Suppl* 1942;77:1-184.
17. Neer CS. Anterior acromioplasty for the chronic impingement syndrome in the shoulder, a preliminary report. *J Bone Joint Surg* 1972:54A:41-51.

Technique
18. Rakofsky M. *Fractional Arthrography of the Shoulder.* Stuttgart: Gustav Fisher; 1987.
19. Ptasznik R. Hennessy OF. Abnormalities of the biceps tendon of the shoulder: sonographic findings. *AJR* 1995;164:409.

20. Farin PU, Jaroma H, Harju A et al. Medial displacement of the biceps brachii tendon: evaluation with dynamic sonography during maximal external rotation. *Radiology* 1995;195:845.
21. van Holsbeeck M, Strouse PJ. Sonography of the shoulder: evaluation of the subacromial-subdeltoid bursa. *AJR* 1993;160: 561-564.
22. Crass JR, Craig EV, Feinberg SB. The hyperextended internal rotation view in rotator cuff ultrasound. *J Clin Ultrasound* 1987;15:416-420.
23. van Holsbeeck M, Introcaso J, Hoogmartens M. Sonographic detection and evaluation of shoulder joint effusion. *Radiology* 1990;177(P):214.

The Normal Cuff
24. Newman JS, Adler RS, Bude RO et al. Detection of soft tissue hyperemia: value of power Doppler sonography. *AJR* 1994; 163:385-389.
25. Petersson CJ. Ruptures of the supraspinatus tendon. Cadaver dissection. *Acta Orthop Scand* 1984;55:52-56.
26. Keyes EL. Observations on rupture of the supraspinatus tendon. *Ann Surg* 1933;97:849-856.
27. Wilson CL, Duff GL. Pathological study of degeneration and rupture of the supraspinatus tendon. *Ann Surg* 1943;47:121-135.
28. Fukuda H, Mikasa M, Yamanaka K. Incomplete thickness rotator cuff tears diagnosed by subacromial bursography. *Clin Orthop* 1987;223:51-58.

Postoperative Appearances
29. Middleton WD. Status of rotator cuff sonography. *Radiology* 1989;173:307-309.
30. Bloom RA. Active abduction view: a new maneuver in the diagnosis of rotator cuff tears. *Skeletal Radiol* 1991;20:255.
31. van Holsbeeck M, Introcasco J. Ultrasound of tendons. Patterns of disease. *Instruction Course Lectures* 1993;47:475-481.
32. Hollister MS, Mack LA, Pattern RM et al. Association of sonographically detected subacromial/subdeltoid bursal effusion and intraarticular fluid with rotator cuff tear. *AJR* 1995; 165:605-608.
33. Farin PU, Jaroma H, Jarju A et al. Shoulder impingement syndrome: sonographic evaluation. *Radiology* 1990;176:845-849.

Postoperative Appearances
34. Mack LA, Nyberg DA, Matsen FA III et al. Sonography of the postoperative shoulder. *AJR* 1988;150:1089-1093.
35. Crass JR, Craig EV, Feinberg SB. Sonography of the postoperative rotator cuff. *AJR* 1988;148:561-564.

Pitfalls
36. Crass JB, Van de Vegte GL, Harkavy LA. Tendon echogenicity: ex vivo study. *Radiology* 1988;169:791-794.
37. Fornage BD. The hypoechoic normal tendon: a pitfall. *J Ultrasound Med* 1987;6:19-22.

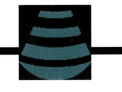

CHAPTER 27

The Tendons

•

Bruno D. Fornage, M.D.

The tendons of the extremities are particularly well suited for examination by high-frequency (7.5 to 13 MHz) or even very high-frequency (15 to 20 MHz) ultrasound transducers because of their superficial location. The vast majority of tendon disorders are related to trauma and inflammation and are associated with athletic or occupational activities that result in overuse of the tendon, mostly through excessive tension or repetitive microtrauma.

ANATOMY

Tendons are made of dense connective tissue and are extremely resistant to traction forces.[1] The densely packed collagen fibers are separated by a small amount of ground substance with a few elongated fibroblasts and are arranged in parallel bundles. The peritenon is a layer of loose connective tissue that wraps around the tendon and sends intratendinous septa between the bundles of collagen fibers.

At the musculotendinous junction, there is an interdigitation between the muscle fibers and the collagen fibrils. The bony insertion of tendons is usually markedly calcified and characterized by the presence of cartilaginous tissue. Tendons usually attach to tuberosities, spinae, trochanters, processes, or ridges.

Blood supply to tendons is poor, and nutritional exchanges occur mostly via the ground substance. With aging, the amount of ground substance and the number of fibroblasts decrease while the number of fibers and amount of fat within the tendon increase.

In certain areas of mechanical constraint, tendons are associated with additional structures that provide mechanical support or protection. Fibrous sheaths keep certain tendons close to bony pieces and prevent bowstringing; examples include the flexor and extensor retinacula at the wrist, the fibrous sheaths of the flexor tendons in the fingers, and the peroneal and flexor retinacula at the foot. Sesamoid bones are intended to reinforce a tendon's strength. **Synovial sheaths** are double-walled tubular structures that surround some tendons; the inner wall of the sheath is in intimate contact with the tendon. The two layers are in continuity with each other at both ends. A minimal amount of synovial fluid allows the tendon to glide smoothly within its sheath. **Synovial bursae** are small, fluid-filled pouches that are found in particular locations and act as bolsters to facilitate the play of tendons.

TECHNIQUE OF EXAMINATION

Because of their wider field of view and their better resolution in the near field, **linear array electronic transducers** are the best choice for tendon sonography; significant artifacts related to the obliquity of the ultrasound beam in relation to the tendon fibers are generated by mechanical or phased array sector scanners and convex array transducers, except in the central portion of the scan. Images of exquisite resolution are obtained with the 7.5- or 10-MHz linear array transducers available on current state-of-the-art scanners, although new machines with mechanical transducers ranging from 13 to 20 MHz are now commercially available. The field of view of the 7.5- or 10-MHz probes is usually restricted to a width of 3 to 4 cm and even less as the frequency increases. Most scanners allow splitting of the screen on the monitor to obtain a montage of two contiguous scans. However, there is always a risk of some overlapping between the two views, so measurements of lesions that straddle the

two half-screens may be inaccurate. An alternative is to use a lower-frequency (e.g., 5-MHz) transducer with a wider field of view. Recently, image-processing software has been developed that allows the field of view of the real-time, linear array probe to be stretched up to about 50 cm by simply dragging the probe in a fashion similar to the compound scanning used in the 1970s. By offering a panoramic view of the structures examined, this new technique removes a long-standing limitation of real-time ultrasound (Fig. 27-1).

A **standoff pad** is useful for placing very superficial tendons (e.g., extensor tendons of the fingers at the dorsum of the hand) in the optimal focal zone and for evaluating tendons in regions with uneven surface.[2] When a standoff pad is used, care should be taken to maintain the ultrasound beam strictly perpendicular to the region being examined to avoid artifacts.[3]

A combination of longitudinal and transverse scans provides a three-dimensional approach to tendon examination. A valuable reference for normal anatomy of the region being examined is obtained by scanning the same area in the contralateral extremity or region, although the rare possibility of bilateral tendon disorders should be kept in mind.

When examining tendons, the clinician should take full advantage of sonography's real-time capability by examining the tendon at rest and during active and passive mobilization through **flexion and extension maneuvers** or by performing palpation under real-time monitoring.[3]

NORMAL SONOGRAPHIC APPEARANCE

All normal tendons are echogenic and display a characteristic **fibrillar echotexture** on longitudinal scans (see Fig. 27-1).[3] When tendons are scanned at 13 to 20 MHz, the fibrillar pattern becomes even finer (Fig. 27-2). The fine echogenic lines have been shown to correspond to the interfaces between the collagen bundles and the endotenon.[4] Although they are easily seen when they are surrounded by hypoechoic muscles, tendons are less well demarcated when they are surrounded by echogenic fat. A key step in the identification of tendons is their mobilization under real-time sonographic monitoring on longitudinal scans. On transverse sections, the reflective bundles of fibers give rise to a finely punctate echogenic pattern (see Fig. 27-2; Fig. 27-3). Transverse scans provide the most accurate measurements of tendon thickness.[3]

Sesamoid bones appear as hyperreflective structures associated with acoustic shadowing. **Synovial sheaths** are barely seen at 7.5 MHz. However, at frequencies of 15 MHz and above, they appear as a thin, hypoechoic underlining of the tendon (Fig. 27-4). The

---

TECHNIQUE OF EXAMINATION

Use linear array transducer
Use highest frequency available
Use a standoff pad for very superficial structures
Avoid false hypoechogenicity artifacts due to
     improper angling of the probe
Always combine longitudinal and transverse scans
Check contralateral tendon for reference
Perform dynamic examination during flexion and
     extension maneuvers
Also use color flow (power mode) Doppler imaging

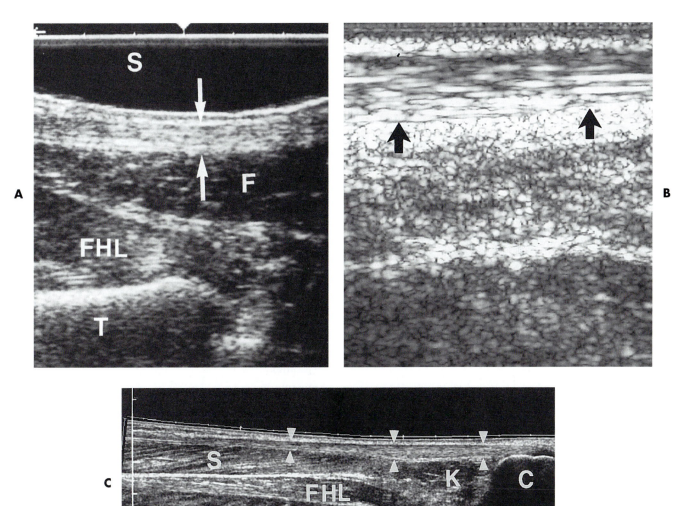

FIG. 27-1. Normal Achilles tendon. A, Longitudinal scan obtained with a 5-MHz transducer shows the echogenic, fibrillar texture of the tendon *(arrows)*. *F,* Kager's fatty triangle; *FHL,* flexor hallucis longus; *S,* standoff pad; *T,* tibia. **B,** Longitudinal scan obtained with a 10-MHz transducer shows the fibrillar echotexture of the tendon better *(arrows)*. Note the reduced field of view compared with **A. C,** Longitudinal scan obtained with extended field of view (Siescape®, Siemens) shows the entire length of the Achilles tendon *(arrowheads)* from its origin to its insertion into the calcaneus. *C,* Calcaneus; *F,* Kager's fatty triangle; *FHL,* flexor hallucis longus; *S,* termination of the soleus muscle; *T,* tibia.

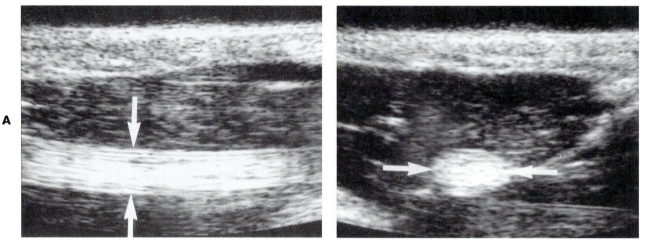

FIG. 27-2. Normal hand, thenar region. A, Longitudinal sonogram at 20 MHz shows the echogenic tendon of the flexor pollicis longus muscle *(arrows).* **B,** Transverse scan shows the echogenic oval cross section of the tendon *(arrows).*

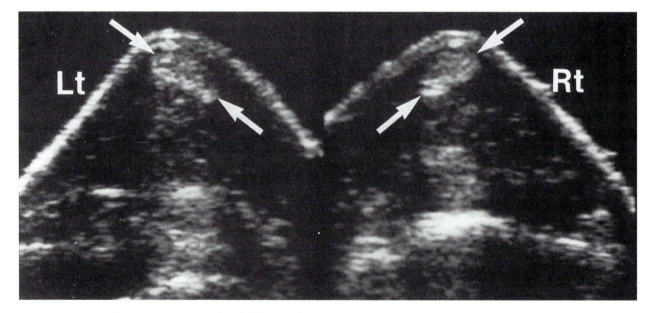

FIG. 27-3. Normal Achilles tendons. Transverse scans of the normal echogenic left and right Achilles tendons *(arrows)* with the patient in the prone position demonstrate the oblique orientation of the tendon plane.

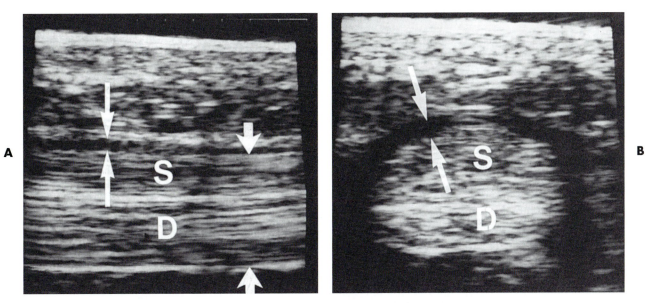

FIG. 27-4. **Normal flexor tendons of the third finger in the palm examined with a 15-MHz transducer.** **A,** Longitudinal sonogram shows the echogenic superficial, *S*, and deep, *D*, flexor tendons *(short arrows)* with a prominent fibrillar texture. Long arrows indicate the synovial sheath. **B,** Transverse scan shows the echogenic cross section of the tendons, *S* and *D*. The arrows point to the synovial sheath.

largest **synovial bursae** (deep infrapatellar, retrocalcanear) can be seen on sonograms as flattened, fluid-filled structures that are only a few millimeters thick (Fig. 27-5).[5]

The most significant artifact associated with tendon sonography is a **false hypoechogenicity** resulting from an oblique ultrasound beam. The optimal display of the echogenic fibrillar texture of a tendon requires that the ultrasound beam be strictly perpendicular to the tendon axis. The slightest obliquity causes scattering of the beam, which results in an artifactual hypoechogenicity.[6] Early erroneous descriptions of hypoechoic normal tendons, in particular of the rotator cuff, were due to this artifact. This artifact constantly affects scans obtained with sector transducers—phased array, mechanical, or curved array transducers—with which only the midline portion of the scan is free of artifacts and displays the normal tendon echogenicity (Fig. 27-6). When a linear array transducer is used, the artifact occurs whenever the tendon is not parallel to the surface of the transducer. When the artifact is caused by a tendon's curved course, changing the position of the probe or suppressing the curvature of the tendon through muscle contraction clears the artifact (Fig. 27-7). When a standoff pad is used, it is crucial to verify constantly that the footprint of the transducer is parallel to the tendon's axis. Transverse scans are equally affected by false hypoechogenicity artifacts (Fig. 27-8).

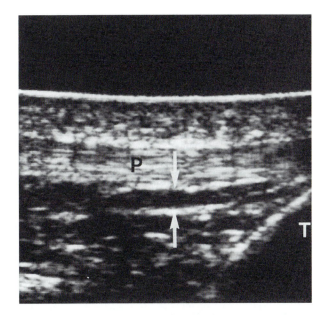

FIG. 27-5. **Normal infrapatellar bursa.** Longitudinal scan of the knee shows the deep infrapatellar bursa *(arrows)* posterior to the distal patellar tendon. *T*, Tibia; *P*, patellar tendon.

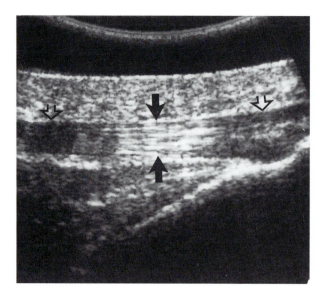

FIG. 27-6. False hypoechogenicity of normal patellar tendon caused by curved array transducer. On this longitudinal scan of the distal patellar tendon obtained with a 10-MHz curved array sector transducer, the tendon exhibits normal echogenicity *(arrows)* only in the narrow midportion of the scan, where the beam is perpendicular to the tendon. On either side, the obliquity of the beam is responsible for the artifactual tendon hypoechogenicity *(open arrows)*.

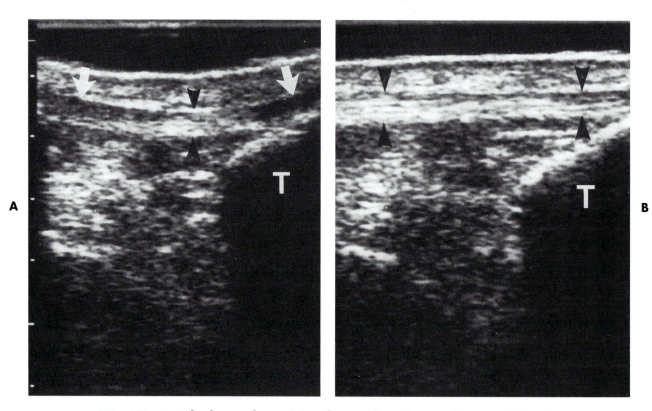

FIG. 27-7. False hypoechogenicity of normal patellar tendon caused by the tendon's curved course at rest. **A.** Longitudinal scan at rest shows the curved tendon *(arrowheads)* with the artifact affecting the segments of the tendon that are oblique to the beam *(arrows)*. **B.** Contraction of the quadriceps straightens the tendon *(arrowheads)*, which now exhibits normal echogenicity. *T*, Tibia.

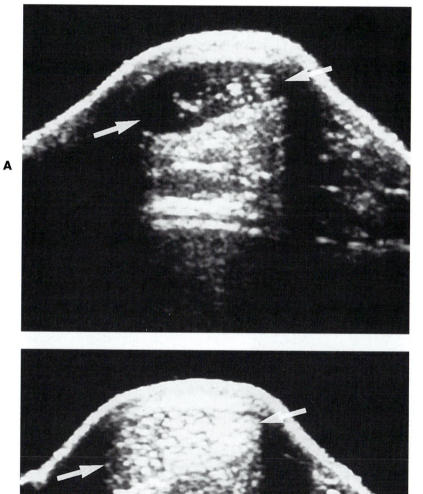

A

B

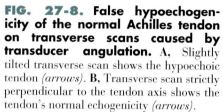

FIG. 27-8. **False hypoechogenicity of the normal Achilles tendon on transverse scans caused by transducer angulation.** **A,** Slightly tilted transverse scan shows the hypoechoic tendon *(arrows)*. **B,** Transverse scan strictly perpendicular to the tendon axis shows the tendon's normal echogenicity *(arrows)*.

Shoulder

Sonography of the rotator cuff and the rest of the shoulder is discussed in Chapter 26.

Elbow

With the elbow flexed at an angle of 90 degrees, the tendon of the triceps brachii muscle is readily identified on both longitudinal and transverse scans. The common tendons of the flexor and extensor muscles of the forearm, inserting into the medial and lateral epicondyles, respectively, can also be demonstrated (Fig. 27-9). The tendon of the biceps brachii muscle can be appreciated at its insertion into the radial tuberosity.

Hand and Wrist

In the carpal tunnel, the echogenic **flexor tendons of the fingers** are surrounded by the hypoechoic ulnar bursa and are best seen when the wrist is moderately flexed (Fig. 27-10). The **median nerve** courses anterior to the flexor tendons of the second finger outside the ulnar bursa. On transverse scans, the flexor tendons are seen to move dramatically during contraction of the fist. The median nerve is also subject to marked changes in shape during these transverse displacements of the tendons. The median nerve is slightly less echogenic than the tendons. Actually, with the use of very-high-frequency transducers, the median nerve, like other major peripheral nerves, appears to comprise multiple, thin, hypoechoic tubules, with the interfaces between them being the origin of the overall hyperechogenicity of the nerve (see Fig. 27-10, *B*).[7]

In the palm, the pairs of superficial and deep flexor tendons of the fingers are clearly identified. On longitudinal scans, the play of the tendons of a given finger

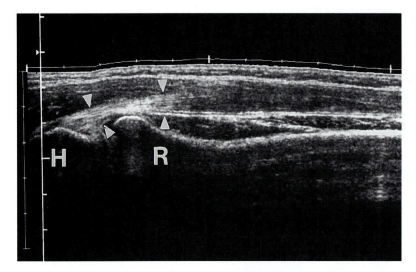

FIG. 27-9. Normal elbow. Coronal scan of the lateral aspect of the elbow obtained with extended field of view (Siescape®, Siemens) shows the entire length of the normal echogenic common tendon of the extensor muscles of the forearm *(arrowheads)* inserting into the lateral epicondyle. *H*, Humerus; *R*, radius.

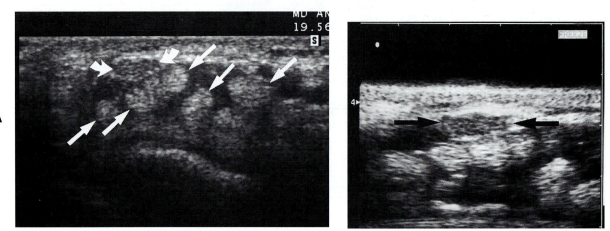

FIG. 27-10. Normal wrist. A, Transverse scan at 7.5 MHz with the wrist in moderate flexion shows the normal echogenic cross sections of the superficial and deep flexor tendons of the fingers *(arrows)*, which lie in the hypoechoic ulnar bursa. *Curved arrows*, Median nerve. **B,** Transverse scan at 20 MHz shows the median nerve *(arrows)*, which is less echogenic than the underlying flexor tendons.

is appreciated in real-time during flexion and extension of that finger. On transverse scans, the pairs of deep and superficial flexor tendons appear as echogenic rounded structures adjacent to the corresponding hypoechoic lumbrical muscles (Fig. 27-11).

In the fingers, the flexor tendons follow the concavity of the phalanges and therefore are affected by a hypoechoic artifact along most of their course, with the exception of the segments that are strictly perpendicular to the ultrasound beam (Fig. 27-12).[8,9]

Knee

Sonography is an excellent technique with which to visualize the extensor tendons of the knee.[10,11]

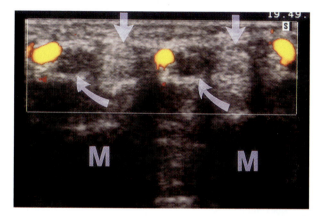

FIG. 27-11. Normal palm of hand. Transverse scan shows the normal echogenic, rounded, superficial and deep flexor tendons of the third and fourth fingers *(arrows)* adjacent to the hypoechoic lumbrical muscles *(curved arrows)*. Power mode Doppler imaging demonstrates flow in the common palmar digital arteries. *M,* Metacarpal bones.

Because both the quadriceps and the patellar tendons may be slightly concave anteriorly when the knee is extended and at rest, scans should be obtained during contraction of the quadriceps muscle or with the knee flexed, which straightens the tendons and eliminates the hypoechoic artifact (see Fig. 27-7).

The **quadriceps tendon** comprises four tendons (the tendons of the rectus femoris, vastus lateralis, vastus medialis, and vastus intermedius muscles), which are not usually distinguished sonographically as separate structures. The quadriceps tendon lies underneath the subcutaneous fat and anterior to a fat pad and to the collapsed suprapatellar bursa (Fig. 27-13). On transverse scans, the quadriceps tendon is oval.

The **patellar tendon** extends from the patella to the tibial tuberosity (Fig. 27-14), over a length of 5 to 6 cm. On transverse sections, the patellar tendon has a convex anterior and flat posterior surface. At its midportion, the tendon is about 4 to 5 mm thick and 20 to 25 mm wide.[11] The subcutaneous prepatellar and infrapatellar bursae are not visible. The deep infrapatellar bursa may appear as a flattened, anechoic structure 2 to 3 mm thick (see Fig. 27-5).

Sonography has been used in the evaluation of **collateral ligaments,** but normal ligaments are not always easily delineated from the articular capsule and from the surrounding subcutaneous tissues.[12] A few reports claim good results in the evaluation of the **cruciate ligaments.**[13,14] However, the sonographic examination of these tendons is limited by the fact that it is virtually impossible to scan them otherwise than obliquely—which results in an artifactual hypoechoic appearance. It is therefore difficult to evaluate them for other than gross rupture. As a rule, the cruciate

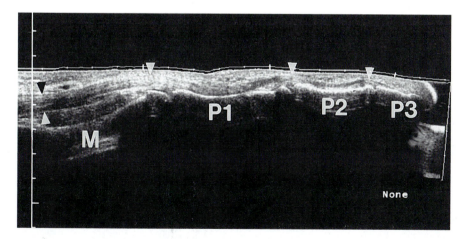

FIG. 27-12. Normal finger. Longitudinal scan obtained with extended field of view (Siescape®, Siemens) shows the normal superficial and deep flexor tendons *(arrowheads)* coursing along the phalanges. Note that the tendons exhibit normal echogenicity only in the segments that are parallel to the linear array transducer; the tendons are falsely hypoechoic in the segments that lie oblique to the beam. *M,* Metacarpal; *P1,* first phalanx; *P2,* second phalanx; *P3,* third phalanx.

ligaments are far better assessed with magnetic resonance imaging (MRI).

Foot and Ankle

The **Achilles tendon** is formed by the fusion between the aponeuroses of the soleus and gastrocnemius muscles. It inserts into the posterior surface of the calcaneus. In the absence of artifacts, the Achilles tendon is echogenic and exhibits a characteristic fibrillar texture on longitudinal scans (see Fig. 27-1).[15] The termination of the hypoechoic soleus muscle is easily identified anterior to the origin of the tendon. The fatty Kager's triangle, which lies anterior to the distal half of the tendon, is usually echogenic, but may show some variation in echogenicity among individuals. More anteriorly lie the hypoechoic flexor hallucis longus muscle and the echogenic posterior surface of the tibia. The flattened, hypoechoic **subtendinous**

calcaneal bursa is sometimes seen in the angle formed by the tendon and the calcaneus. The tendon fibers at the bony insertion have a short oblique course that causes an artifactual hypoechogenicity (Fig. 27-15). This pattern should not be misdiagnosed as the subcutaneous calcaneal bursa, which is not normally seen. Recently, a sonographic study performed at 10 and 15 MHz revealed the presence of two tendinous portions of different echogenicity representing the portions arising from the soleus and the gastrocnemius muscles.[16]

On transverse sonograms, the cross section of the tendon is grossly elliptical and tapers medially. The tendon plane is remarkable in that it is oblique forward and medially (see Fig. 27-3). Because of this configuration, there is a risk of overestimating the thickness of the tendon on strictly sagittal scans, and measurements should therefore be taken from transverse scans. At 2 to 3 cm above its insertion, the Achilles tendon is 5 to 7 mm thick and 12 to 15 mm wide.[15] A correlation has been found between the tendon's thickness and the subject's height.[17] Another study showed that the Achilles tendon is wider in athletes than in control subjects and suggested that long-term training results in tendon enlargement.

In the ankle, sonography readily demonstrates the tendons of the peroneus longus and brevis muscles laterally and of the tibialis posterior muscle medially. The tendons of the flexor digitorum longus and flexor hallucis longus muscles can also be identified behind the medial malleolus whereas the tendons of the tibialis anterior, extensor hallucis longus, and extensor digitorum longus muscles are seen at the anterior aspect of the ankle joint. Dynamic examination during specific flexion and extension maneuvers of the ankle and foot helps identify individual tendons. The ankle tendons are enveloped in synovial sheaths. In a recent study, a small amount of fluid was found in the posterior tibial tendon sheath and in the common peroneal

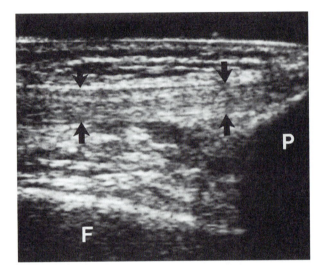

FIG. 27-13. Normal quadriceps tendon. Longitudinal scan shows the echogenic tendon *(arrows)* surrounded by fat. *F*, Femur; *P*, patella.

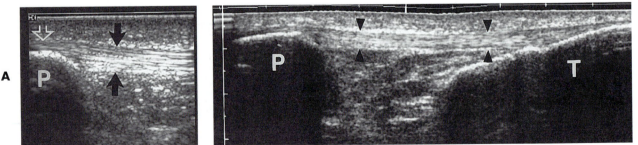

FIG. 27-14. Normal patellar tendon. A, Longitudinal scan obtained with a 10-MHz transducer shows the fibrillar echotexture of the tendon *(arrows)*. Note the prepatellar fibers *(open arrow)*. *P*, Patella. **B,** Longitudinal scan obtained with extended field of view (Siescape®, Siemens) shows the entire tendon *(arrowheads)* extending from the patella to the tibial tuberosity. The tendon is about 4 mm thick. *P*, Patella; *T*, tibia.

tendon sheath in 71% and 12% of ankles in asymptomatic volunteers, respectively.[18]

In the foot, the examination technique and normal sonographic appearance of the flexor and extensor tendons of the toes do not differ significantly from those of the tendons of the fingers.[9]

PATHOLOGY

Tendon disorders result most often from trauma (tears) or inflammation (tendinitis).

Tears

Tears usually occur on tendons that have been rendered fragile by such factors as aging, presence of calcifications, general or local corticosteroid therapy, and underlying systemic diseases (rheumatoid arthritis, lupus erythematosus, diabetes mellitus, and gout).[19-22]

SONOGRAPHIC SIGNS OF TENDON TEARS

Discontinuity of fibers (partial or complete)
Hematoma of variable size, usually small
Bone fragment in case of bone avulsion
Nonvisualization of the retracted tendon in case of complete tear

---

In the absence of those predisposing factors, biopsy specimens taken in the vicinity of the rupture site often demonstrate degenerative changes, sometimes described as "tendinosis."

Complete Tears. Recent **complete tendon tears** are often correctly diagnosed clinically. However, if physical examination is delayed, it may be indeterminate because of inflammatory changes. Sonography can show the full-thickness discontinuity of the tendon. The gap between the torn tendon fragments is filled with hypoechoic hemorrhagic fluid (or clot) or granulomatous tissue, depending on the lesion's age (Fig. 27-16). The gap varies in length, and when the torn fragments are separated by a long distance, the tendon may not be visualized at all. This nonvisualization may occur in complete ruptures of the rotator cuff and of the flexor tendons of the fingers.[23] With the exception of ruptures of the Achilles tendon, in which a hematoma can develop around the whole tendon, ruptures are usually associated with minimal focal hemorrhage. In the case of avulsion of the tendon from the bone, a **bone fragment** may appear as a bright echogenic focus with an acoustic shadow (Fig. 27-17).

Incomplete Tears. **Incomplete tears** are difficult to diagnose clinically and to differentiate from focal tendinitis. Accurate sonographic diagnosis is important because early diagnosis and treatment of a partial tear will prevent a subsequent complete rupture. A sensitivity of 94% has been reported for sonography in the diagnosis of partial tears of the Achilles

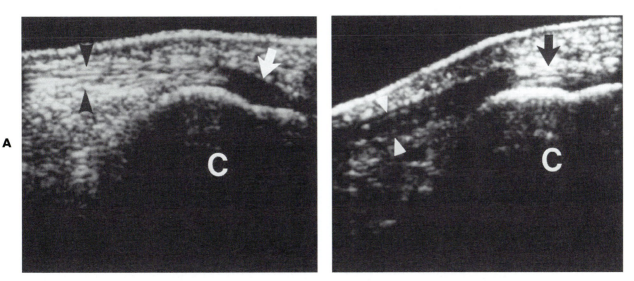

A   **B**

FIG. 27-15. False hypoechogenicity of the normal Achilles tendon at its insertion into the calcaneus. A, Longitudinal scan with the linear array transducer parallel to the tendon *(arrowheads)* shows the markedly hypoechoic distal extremity of the tendon *(arrow),* whose course is oblique to the beam. **B,** Placing the transducer parallel to the distal tendon clears the artifact *(arrow),* while the rest of the tendon *(arrowheads)* is now falsely hypoechoic. *C,* Calcaneus.

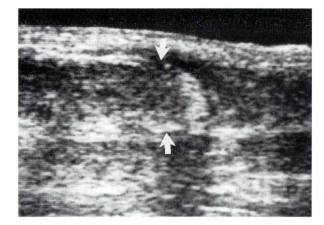

FIG. 27-16. **Complete tear of the Achilles tendon.** Longitudinal scan shows the retracted, swollen upper fragment *(arrows)*.

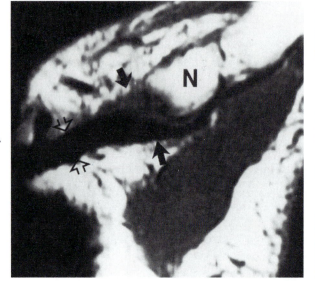

A

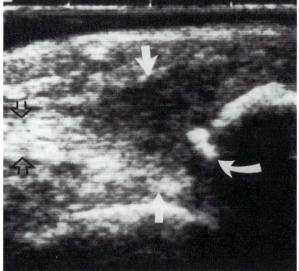

B

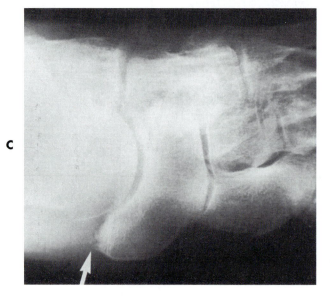

C

FIG. 27-17. **Complete tear of the posterior tibial tendon at its insertion into the navicular bone.** A, MRI scan of the foot (oriented to compare with the sonogram) shows the torn ligament *(arrows)*. The open arrows indicate the normal tendon. *N,* navicular bone. B, Coronal sonogram shows the hypoechoic focal hemorrhage and the tendon discontinuity *(arrows)*. The open arrows indicate the normal tendon. The curved arrow points to the avulsed bone fragment. C, Radiograph confirms the bone avulsion at the tendon's insertion *(arrow)* into the navicular bone.

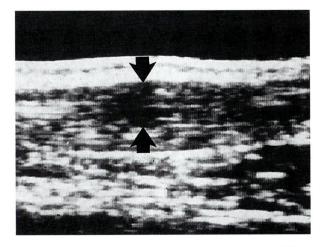

FIG. 27-18. Partial rupture of the Achilles tendon. Longitudinal scan of the tendon shows a focal discontinuity of fibers *(arrows)* at the posterior aspect of the tendon.

SONOGRAPHIC SIGNS OF TENDINITIS

Thickening of the tendon
Decreased echogenicity
Blurred margins
Increased vascularity on color flow Doppler imaging
Calcifications in chronic tendinitis

---

tendon.[24] Other studies have reported the superiority of MRI over sonography in the diagnosis of incomplete Achilles tendon tears.[25,26]

Sonographically, recent partial ruptures appear as focal hypoechoic defects in the tendon or at its attachment (Fig. 27-18).[5,24,27] The three-dimensional evaluation of partial ruptures requires a combination of longitudinal and transverse scans.

When the patellar tendon is partially detached from the patellar apex, longitudinal scans show the tendon fibers' discontinuity whereas transverse scans below the patellar apex demonstrate the round defect in the midline of the tendon (Fig. 27-19).

Inflammation

Edema associated with inflammation of tendons and/or surrounding structures is responsible for the thickening and decreased echogenicity of the tendons involved. The increased vascularity associated with inflammation can now be depicted using **color flow (power mode) Doppler imaging.** When the objective quantification of hypervascularity on color flow Doppler imaging becomes routinely available, it will permit follow-up of patients with inflammatory lesions and documentation of the response to therapy.[28]

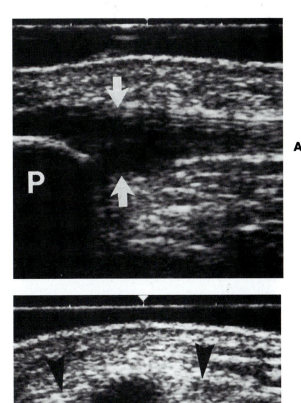

FIG. 27-19. Partial detachment of the superior portion of the patellar tendon. A, Midsagittal scan shows the hematoma and the tendon discontinuity *(arrows)* at the upper insertion of the tendon. *P,* patella. **B,** Transverse scan shows the well-defined, round, hypoechoic midline hematoma *(arrow). Arrowheads,* Tendon's margins.

Tendinitis. Tendinitis is mostly associated with athletic or occupational activities. At pathologic examination, there are degenerative changes often associated with the presence of microcysts. The increased vascularity and edema are responsible for the increased volume of the tendon. Calcifications may be present in chronic tendinitis. Tendinitis may affect the whole or only part of the tendon. In the patellar tendon, focal tendinitis usually involves the upper insertion, but focal involvement of the distal insertion may occur after transposition of the tibial tuberosity.

In **acute tendinitis,** the tendon is thickened and the margins are often ill defined. There is also a diffuse decrease in echogenicity (Fig. 27-20).[11,15]

Because improper scanning may result in a falsely hypoechoic tendon, the examination technique must be flawless. Comparison with sonograms of the unaffected contralateral tendons is often valuable.

In **chronic tendinitis,** the contours of the tendon may be deformed with a bumpy appearance. High-frequency sonography has proved accurate in the detection of minute intratendinous calcifications, which appear as bright foci with or without acoustic shad-

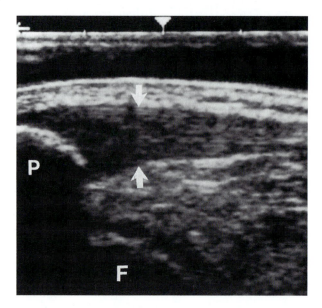

FIG. 27-20. Acute patellar tendinitis. Longitudinal scan shows thickening and decreased echogenicity of the upper two thirds of the tendon *(arrows). F,* Femoral condyle; *P,* patella.

owing, occasionally with a comet-tail artifact (Fig. 27-21, *A*). However, the size and shape of these calcifications are better appreciated on low-kilovoltage radiographs, preferably obtained with the use of a mammographic unit (Fig. 27-21, *B*).[29]

Sonography with color flow (power mode) Doppler imaging can demonstrate the focal or diffuse increase in vascularity (Fig. 27-22). The presence of flow in a focal area of markedly decreased echogenicity helps confirm the diagnosis of focal tendinitis and rules out an acute partial tear because blood flow is not expected to be present in the blood-filled defect resulting from the tear (Fig. 27-23). Color flow Doppler imaging can also be used to monitor a patient's **response to anti-inflammatory therapy.** A decrease in size of the tendon and a return to a normal level of echogenicity and very low vascularity indicate healing.

Peritendinitis. In **peritendinitis,** inflammation is limited to the peritenon, the layer of connective tissue that wraps around the tendon. This condition is frequently found in the Achilles tendon. Sonographically, peritendinitis is characterized by a hypoechoic thickening of the peritenon, with the tendon remaining grossly unaffected. Color flow (power mode) Doppler imaging often demonstrates increased vascularity (Fig. 27-24).

Tenosynovitis. Tenosynovitis is defined as the inflammation of a tendon sheath. Any tendon surrounded by a synovial sheath, especially tendons in the hand, wrist, and ankle, can be affected. Trauma, including repeated microtrauma, and pyogenic infection are most commonly responsible for acute tenosynovitis.

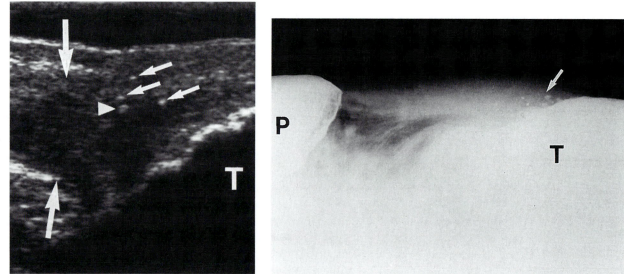

FIG. 27-21. Chronic calcified patellar tendinitis. A, Longitudinal scan of the lower attachment of the tendon shows a markedly thickened, hypoechoic tendon *(long arrows)* with blurred contours and tiny hyperechoic calcifications *(short arrows),* one with a comet-tail artifact *(arrowhead).* **B,** Lateral low-kilovoltage radiograph obtained with a mammographic unit shows the swollen patellar tendon and the small calcifications *(arrow). T,* Tibia; *P,* patella.

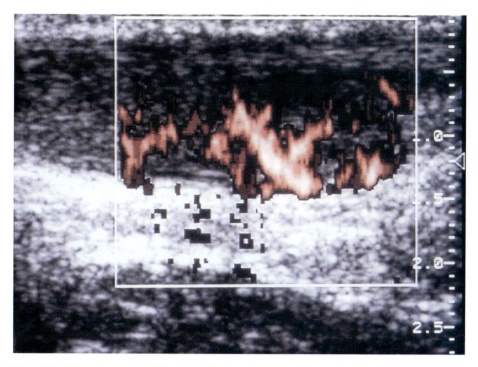

FIG. 27-22. Acute Achilles tendinitis. Longitudinal power mode color Doppler scan shows marked hypervascularity in the deep aspect of the tendon. Note the markedly decreased echogenicity of the tendon. (Courtesy of Dr. D. H. Touche.)

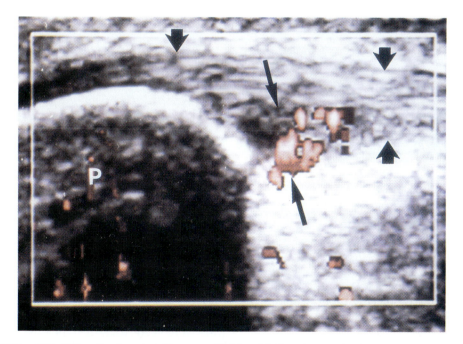

FIG. 27-23. Acute patellar tendinitis. Midline longitudinal power mode color Doppler scan shows a focal increase in tendon vascularity in an area of decreased echogenicity *(arrows)* close to the apex of the patella. Short arrows delineate the patellar tendon. *P,* Patella. (Courtesy of Dr. D. H. Touche.)

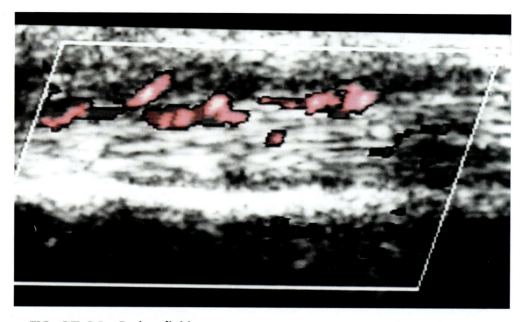

FIG. 27-24. Peritendinitis. Longitudinal power mode Doppler scan of Achilles tendon shows hypervascularity of the swollen hypoechoic peritenon posteriorly. (Courtesy of Dr. D. H. Touche.)

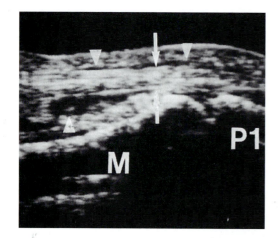

FIG. 27-25. Tenosynovitis of the flexor tendons of a finger. Longitudinal scan of the volar aspect of the metacarpophalangeal joint shows the tendon sheath distended by a small amount of fluid *(arrowheads)*. The flexor tendons are normal *(arrows)*. *M,* Metacarpal; *P1,* first phalanx.

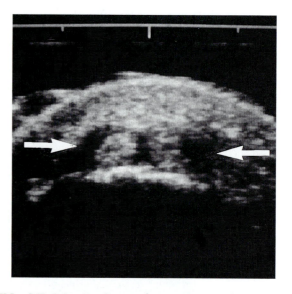

FIG. 27-26. De Quervain's tenosynovitis. Transverse scan of the wrist shows the thickened, hypoechoic synovial sheath *(arrows)* surrounding the tendons of the abductor pollicis longus and extensor pollicis brevis muscles.

Cases of tenosynovitis caused by a foreign body retained within a tendon sheath in the hand have been reported.[30] Sonographically, the diagnosis of acute tenosynovitis is made when fluid in the sheath, even a minimal quantity, is identified (Fig. 27-25).[31,32] Internal echoes representing debris can be seen in suppurative tenosynovitis, a serious condition that can rapidly involve the tendon.[33]

Chronic tenosynovitis is characterized by a hypoechoic thickening of the synovial sheath, most often with little or no fluid. The thickening of the sheath may impair the movement of tendons in narrow passages. In **De Quervain's tenosynovitis,** the tendons of the abductor pollicis longus and extensor pollicis brevis muscles are constricted by the thickened sheath in the pulley over the radial styloid process. Sonography can demonstrate the hypoechoic thickening of the tendon sheath (Fig. 27-26).[9,34] Color flow Doppler imaging may demonstrate increased vascularity in the tissues involved. Sonography can

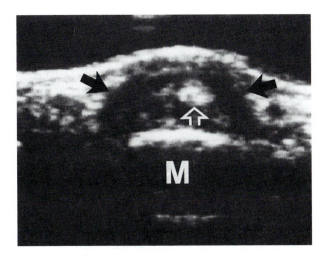

FIG. 27-27. Rheumatoid tenosynovitis of the extensor tendon of a finger at the dorsum of the hand. Transverse scan shows the hypoechoic pannus *(arrows)* surrounding the tendon *(open arrow)*. *M,* Metacarpal.

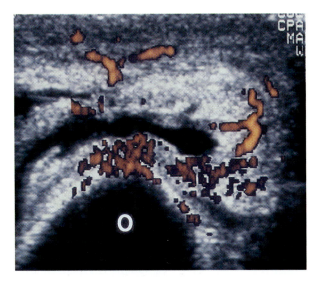

FIG. 27-28. Bursitis. Transverse scan of the posterior aspect of the elbow shows the thick-walled, fluid-containing olecranal bursa. Power mode color Doppler imaging shows the bursa's hypervascularity. *O,* Olecranon.

be used to guide the injection of contrast medium into the sheath for **tenography,** a study that silhouettes the sheath wall but cannot demonstrate its thickness.[35] Sonography has also been used to guide injection of steroids into the synovial sheath of the posterior tibial tendon in patients with chronic inflammatory arthropathy.[36]

Rheumatoid arthritis has a predilection for synovial tissues, including tendon sheaths in the distal extremities. Sonography has proved effective in the diagnosis of **rheumatoid tenosynovitis** in the hand.[37] The tendon sheath involved by the pannus is markedly hypoechoic (Fig. 27-27), and, occasionally, fluid is also present in the sheath. Color flow Doppler imaging shows significant hypervascularity of the pannus. Sonographic findings of tendon involvement include thickening and inhomogeneity of the tendon, whose margins appear jagged.[38] At a later stage, sonography can demonstrate a marked thinning of the tendon or a partial or complete rupture.[39]

Bursitis. **Bursitis** occurs most often in the subdeltoid, olecranal, radiohumeral, patellar, and calcaneal bursae. Trauma and, more important, repeated microtrauma are believed to play an important role in bursitis, although no initiating factor can be found in many cases. Interestingly, transient accumulation of fluid in the subacromial bursa has been demonstrated on sonograms of the shoulder for up to 16 to 20 hours after handball training.[40] In the early acute stage of bursitis, when the bursa is filled with fluid, sonograms demonstrate a sonolucent, fluid-filled collection with ill-defined margins. Prepatellar bursitis is a common

finding in carpet layers.[41] At the chronic stage, a complex sonographic appearance with internal echogenic debris results from the presence of granulomatous tissue, precipitated fibrin, and, occasionally, calcification. Color flow Doppler imaging often shows increased vascularity in the thickened wall of the bursa (Fig. 27-28).

Nonarticular Osteochondroses. Osgood-Schlatter and Sinding-Larsen-Johansson diseases are both nonarticular osteochondroses of the knee that occur in ossification centers subjected to traction stress. Both conditions occur in adolescents, typically in boys involved in athletic activities. Although the diagnosis is strongly suggested by the clinical history, radiographic studies are often performed to confirm the diagnosis. Recently, high-resolution sonography has been used in the evaluation of these two conditions.[42]

Osgood-Schlatter disease is osteochondrosis of the tibial tuberosity. In a study of 70 cases, sonography revealed swelling of the anechoic cartilage in 100% of cases, fragmentation of the echogenic ossification center of the anterior tibial tuberosity in 75% of cases, diffuse thickening of the patellar tendon in 22% of cases, and deep infrapatellar bursitis in 17% of cases.[43]

Sinding-Larsen-Johansson disease is osteochondrosis of the accessory ossification center at the lower pole of the patella. In this rare disease, sonography can demonstrate the fragmented, echogenic ossification center and the swollen, hypoechoic cartilage and surrounding soft tissues, including the origin of the patellar tendon.[44]

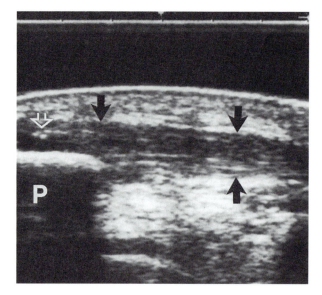

FIG. 27-29. Postoperative pattern. Longitudinal scan of the patellar tendon performed 15 months after surgery for tendinitis shows a diffusely thickened, heterogeneous, hypoechoic tendon *(arrows)* with ill-defined margins and minute calcifications *(open arrow)*. P, Patella.

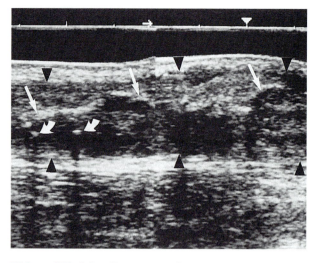

FIG. 27-30. Postoperative pattern. Longitudinal scan of the Achilles tendon shows a markedly thickened tendon *(arrowheads)* that contains an echogenic band associated with shadowing, representing synthetic surgical reinforcement material (polydioxanone sulfate) *(arrows)*. Note the bright echoes representing sutures *(curved arrows)*.

Postoperative Patterns

After surgical repair, tendons appear enlarged and heterogeneous with blurred, irregular margins on sonograms (Fig. 27-29).[5,45] This postoperative pattern may last for several months or years; therefore sonography cannot reliably differentiate recurrent tears and tendinitis from postoperative changes. Occasionally, sonography can detect bright echogenic foci caused by residual synthetic suture material or calcification (Fig. 27-30). Doppler studies may demonstrate residual hypervascularization in tendons postoperatively.

Tumors and Pseudotumors

Benign tumors of tendons or their sheaths include **giant cell tumors** and **osteochondromas.** The giant cell tumor of tendon sheaths is believed to represent a circumscribed form of pigmented villonodular synovitis. It involves preferentially the flexor surface of the fingers and is usually found in young and middle-aged women. Local recurrences may occur after incomplete excision. Sonographically, giant cell tumors appear as hypoechoic masses, sometimes with lobulated contours.[9]

Malignant tumors are rare. **Synovial sarcomas** may arise from a tendon sheath. They appear as a hypoechoic lobulated mass that sometimes contains calcifications.

In patients with **familial hypercholesterolemia,** sonography demonstrates multiple hypoechoic **xanthomas** in the Achilles tendon in 95% of patients and can detect early focal xanthomas in not yet enlarged tendons.[46] In a group of 30 adults with familial hypercholesterolemia, the mean thickness of the Achilles tendon was 11.1 mm versus 4.5 mm in normal subjects and 4.9 mm in a group with nonfamilial hypercholesterolemia.[47] It has also been shown that sonography can detect hypoechoic infiltration of the Achilles tendon in 38% of children affected with familial hypercholesterolemia.[48] In contrast, another study did not show significant abnormalities in secondary (nonfamilial) hypercholesterolemia.[49] Sonography can be used to monitor the effect of therapy on the Achilles tendon's thickness and echotexture.

Intratendinous rheumatoid nodules appear on sonograms as hypoechoic nodules.[37] In contrast, **intratendinous tophi** appear as highly echogenic foci with acoustic shadowing, which allows their differentiation from intratendinous rheumatoid nodules.[50]

In **dialysis-related amyloidosis,** joint synovia and capsules and tendons (e.g., the supraspinatus tendon) may be thickened, with the thickening increasing with the duration of dialysis.[51]

Ganglion cysts most commonly occur in the hand but can develop from any joint or tendon sheath. Sonography demonstrates the oval fluid collection adjacent to the joint space or tendon (Fig. 27-31). Occasionally, chronic cysts or cysts containing a viscous fluid have internal echoes, causing the cyst to appear similar to a hypoechoic solid tumor.

Another cyst that commonly occurs adjacent to a joint is the **popliteal cyst.** Popliteal cysts are caused by an abnormal distention of the gastrocnemio-semimembranosus bursa, which frequently commu-

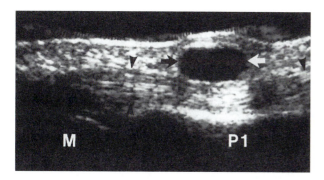

FIG. 27-31. Ganglion cyst on the volar aspect of the first phalanx of the second finger. Longitudinal scan shows a well-defined, 0.8 cm cystic structure *(arrows)* anterior to the flexor tendons of the finger *(arrowheads)*. Note the distal acoustic enhancement. *M*, Metacarpal; *P1*, first phalanx.

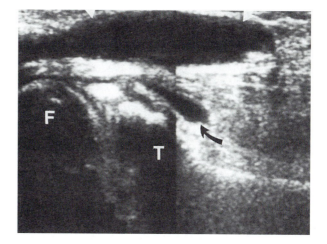

FIG. 27-32. Popliteal cyst. Longitudinal scan demonstrates a teardrop-shaped cystic mass *(arrow)* in the soft tissues posterior to the knee joint with a smaller portion *(curved arrow)* anterior to the gastrocnemius medialis muscle. Note the internal echoes due to hypertrophied synovium. *F*, Femoral condyle; *T*, tibia.

nicates with the knee joint through a slit-shaped opening at the posteromedial aspect of the joint capsule. They are frequently found in association with pathologic conditions that cause an increase in the intraarticular pressure through overproduction of synovial fluid, capsular sclerosis, or synovial hypertrophy; among these conditions, rheumatoid arthritis is the most common. Popliteal cysts present clinically as asymptomatic or symptomatic popliteal masses. Large cysts dissecting into the calf or ruptured cysts produce a swollen, painful limb that mimics thrombophlebitis.

A popliteal cyst typically appears sonographically as a fluid-filled collection.[52-54] Occasionally, longitudinal scans demonstrate a second anechoic area anterior to the tendon of the gastrocnemius muscle. Transverse scans readily confirm that both areas represent sections of the same cyst, which surrounds the tendon of the muscle (Fig. 27-32). Internal echoes representing fibrinous strands or debris and synovial thickening can be seen in inflamed or infected cysts. In patients with rheumatoid arthritis, a popliteal cyst may be completely filled with pannus, thus mimicking a solid mass. **Osteochondromatosis** can also develop in a popliteal cyst, giving rise to hyperechoic loose bodies that cast acoustic shadows when calcified.[55] In a recently ruptured cyst, sonography can demonstrate the leak as a subcutaneous fluid collection extending distally to the lower calf. However, when the examination is deferred, sonographic diagnosis may be more problematic because the leaking fluid has been resorbed and only an ill-defined hypoechoic residual area remains.[53]

SONOGRAPHY VERSUS OTHER IMAGING MODALITIES

For many decades, low-kilovoltage radiography and xeroradiography were the only imaging techniques applicable to tendons. Although they can silhouette tendons, particularly when the tendons are surrounded by fat, these techniques fail to demonstrate the structure of the tendons. However, they are still the best modalities with which to document unequivocally calcifications in tendons or bursae.

Tenography is performed by injecting contrast medium into the sheath. This somewhat neglected imaging technique provides detailed global views of the inner wall of the sheath but cannot appreciate the thickness of the wall as sonography does.[56,57]

Because computed tomography (CT) is limited to transverse scans of the extremities in routine practice and does not provide sufficient contrast resolution, it has rarely been used in the evaluation of tendons.[58,59]

MRI has emerged as an accurate modality for soft-tissue imaging and appears to be a direct competitor of high-frequency sonography in the field of tendon imaging.[60] However, high-frequency sonography is currently the only real-time cross-sectional imaging technique. Sonograms can be quickly obtained along virtually any orientation, and very-high-frequency transducers now provide exquisite spatial and contrast resolution. In addition, the cost of sonography is low, and equipment is widely available. However, because of the small size of the structures being examined and the possibility of technique-related artifacts, tendon sonography is operator-dependent and requires experience to yield accurate results.

REFERENCES

Anatomy

1. McMaster PE. Tendon and muscle ruptures. Clinical and experimental studies on the causes and location of subcutaneous ruptures. *J Bone Joint Surg* 1933;15:705-722.

Technique of Examination

2. Fornage BD, Touche DH, Rifkin MD. Small parts real-time sonography: a new "water-path." *J Ultrasound Med* 1984; 3:355-357.

3. Fornage BD. *Ultrasonography of Muscles and Tendons. Examination Technique and Atlas of Normal Anatomy of the Extremities.* New York: Springer-Verlag; 1988.

Normal Sonographic Appearance

4. Martinoli C, Derchi LE, Pastorino C et al. Analysis of echotexture of tendons with US. *Radiology* 1993;186:839-843.

5. Fornage BD, Rifkin MD. Ultrasound examination of tendons. *Radiol Clin North Am* 1988;26:87-107.

6. Fornage BD. The hypoechoic normal tendon: a pitfall. *J Ultrasound Med* 1987;6:19-22.

7. Silvestri E, Martinoli C, Derchi LE et al. Echotexture of peripheral nerves: correlation between US and histologic findings and criteria to differentiate tendons. *Radiology* 1995;197:291-296.

8. Fornage BD, Rifkin MD. Ultrasound examination of the hand. *Radiology* 1986;160:853-854.

9. Fornage BD, Rifkin MD. Ultrasonic examination of the hand and foot. *Radiol Clin North Am* 1988;26:109-129.

10. Dillehay GL, Deschler T, Rogers LF et al. The ultrasonographic characterization of tendons. *Invest Radiol* 1984; 19:338-341.

11. Fornage BD, Rifkin MD, Touche DH et al. Sonography of the patellar tendon: preliminary observations. *AJR* 1984;143:179-182.

12. De Flaviis L, Nessi R, Leonardi M et al. Dynamic ultrasonography of capsulo-ligamentous knee joint traumas. *J Clin Ultrasound* 1988;16:487-492.

13. Röhr E. Die sonographische Darstellung des hinteren Kreuzbandes. *Röntgenblatter* 1985;38:377-379.

14. Scherer MA, Kraus M, Gerngross H et al. Importance of ultrasound in postoperative follow-up after reconstruction of the anterior cruciate ligament (in German). *Unfallchirurg* 1993; 96:47-54.

15. Fornage BD. Achilles tendon: ultrasound examination. *Radiology* 1986;159:759-764.

16. Bertolotto M, Perrone R, Martinoli C et al. High resolution ultrasound anatomy of normal Achilles tendon. *Br J Radiol* 1995;68:986-991.

17. Koivunen-Niemela T, Parkkola K. Anatomy of the Achilles tendon (tendo calcaneus) with respect to tendon thickness measurements. *Surg Radiol Anat* 1995;17:263-268.

18. Nazarian LN, Rawool NM, Martin CE et al. Synovial fluid in the hindfoot and ankle: detection of amount and distribution with US. *Radiology* 1995;197:275-278.

Pathology

19. Downey DJ, Simkin PA, Mack LA et al. Tibialis posterior tendon rupture: a cause of rheumatoid flat foot. *Arthritis Rheum* 1988;31:441-446.

20. Ismail AM, Balakrishnan R, Rajakumar MK. Rupture of patellar ligament after steroid infiltration. Report of a case. *J Bone Joint Surg* 1969;51B:503-505.

21. Kricun R, Kricun ME, Arangio GA et al. Patellar tendon rupture with underlying systemic disease. *AJR* 1980;135:803-807.

22. Morgan J. McCarty DJ. Tendon ruptures in patients with systemic lupus erythematosus treated with corticosteroids. *Arthritis Rheum* 1974;17:1033-1036.

23. Souissi M, Giwerc M, Ebelin M et al: Exploration échographique des tendons fléchisseurs des doigts de la main. *Presse Med* 1989;18:463-466.

24. Kalebo P, Allenmark C, Peterson L et al. Diagnostic value of ultrasonography in partial ruptures of the Achilles tendon. *Am J Sports Med* 1992;20:378-381.

25. Weinstabl R. MR and ultrasound study of Achilles tendon injury (in German). *Unfallchirurgie* 1992;18:213-217.

26. Neuhold A, Stiskal M, Kainberger F et al. Degenerative Achilles tendon disease: assessment by magnetic resonance and ultrasonography. *Eur J Radiol* 1992;14:213-220.

27. Leekam RN, Salsberg BB, Bogoch E et al. Sonographic diagnosis of partial Achilles tendon rupture and healing. *J Ultrasound Med* 1986;5:115-116.

28. Newman JS, Laing TJ, McCarthy CJ et al. Power Doppler sonography of synovitis: assessment of therapeutic response—preliminary observations. *Radiology* 1996;198:582-584.

29. Fornage B, Touche D, Deshayes JL et al. Diagnostic des calcifications du tendon rotulien. Comparaison échoradiographique. *J Radiol* 1984;65:355-359.

30. Howden MD. Foreign bodies within finger tendon sheaths demonstrated by ultrasound: two cases. *Clin Radiol* 1994;49:419-420.

31. Middleton WD, Reinus WR, Totty WG et al. Ultrasound of the biceps tendon apparatus. *Radiology* 1985;157:211-215.

32. Gooding GAW. Tenosynovitis of the wrist. A sonographic demonstration. *J Ultrasound Med* 1988;7:225-226.

33. Jeffrey RB Jr, Laing FC, Schechter WP et al. Acute suppurative tenosynovitis of the hand: diagnosis with ultrasound. *Radiology* 1987;162:741-742.

34. Marini M, Boni S, Pingi A et al. De Quervain's disease: diagnostic imaging. *Chir Organi Mov* 1994;79:219-223.

35. Fornage BD. *Ultrasound of the Extremities* (in French). Paris: Vigot; 1991.

36. Brophy DP, Cunnane G, Fitzgerald O et al. Technical report: ultrasound guidance for injection of soft tissue lesions around the heel in chronic inflammatory arthritis. *Clin Radiol* 1995;50:120-122.

37. Fornage BD. Soft-tissue changes in the hand in rheumatoid arthritis: evaluation with ultrasound. *Radiology* 1989;173: 735-737.

38. Grassi W, Tittarelli E, Blasetti P et al. Finger tendon involvement in rheumatoid arthritis. Evaluation with high-frequency sonography. *Arthritis Rheum* 1995;38:786-794.

39. Coakley FV, Samanta AK, Finlay DB. Ultrasonography of the tibialis posterior tendon in rheumatoid arthritis. *Br J Rheumatol* 1994;33:273-277.

40. Kruger-Franke M, Fischer S, Kugler A et al. Stress-related clinical and ultrasound changes in shoulder joints of handball players (in German). *Sportverletz Sportschaden* 1994;8:166-169.

41. Myllymaki T, Tikkakoski T, Typpo T et al. Carpet-layer's knee. An ultrasonographic study. *Acta Radiol* 1993;34:496-499.

42. De Flaviis L, Nessi R, Scaglione P et al. Ultrasonic diagnosis of Osgood-Schlatter and Sinding-Larsen-Johansson diseases of the knee. *Skeletal Radiol* 1989;18:193-197.

43. Bergami G, Barbuti D, Pezzoli F. Ultrasonographic findings in Osgood-Schlatter disease (in Italian). *Radiol Med (Torino)* 1994;88:368-372.

44. Barbuti D, Bergami G, Testa F. Ultrasonographic aspects of Sinding-Larsen-Johansson disease (in Italian). *Pediatr Med Chir* 1995;17:61-63.

45. Blei CL, Nirschl RP, Grant EG. Achilles tendon: ultrasonic diagnosis of pathologic conditions. *Radiology* 1986;159:765-767.

46. Bude RO, Adler RS, Bassett DR et al. Heterozygous familial hypercholesterolemia: detection of xanthomas in the Achilles tendon with US. *Radiology* 1993;188:567-571.

47. Ebeling T, Farin P, Pyorala K. Ultrasonography in the detection of Achilles tendon xanthomata in heterozygous familial hypercholesterolemia. *Atherosclerosis* 1992;97:217-228.

48. Koivunen-Niemela T, Viikari J, Niinikoski H et al. Sonography in the detection of Achilles tendon xanthomata in children with familial hypercholesterolaemia. *Acta Paediatr* 1994;83:1178-1181.

49. Kainberger F, Seidl G, Traindl O et al. Ultrasonography of the Achilles tendon in hypercholesterolemia. *Acta Radiol* 1993; 34:408-412.

50. Tiliakos N, Morales AR, Wilson CH Jr. Use of ultrasound in identifying tophaceous versus rheumatoid nodules (letter). *Arthritis Rheum* 1982;25:478-479.

51. Jadoul M, Malghem J, Van de Berg B et al. Ultrasonographic detection of thickened joint capsules and tendons as marker of dialysis-related amyloidosis: a cross-sectional and longitudinal study. *Nephrol Dial Transplant* 1993;8:1104-1109.

52. McDonald DG, Leopold GR. Ultrasound B-scanning in the differentiation of Baker's cyst and thrombophlebitis. *Br J Radiol* 1972;45:729-732.

53. Gompels BM, Darlington LG. Evaluation of popliteal cysts and painful calves with ultrasonography: comparison with arthrography. *Ann Rheum Dis* 1982;41:355-359.

54. Bouffard A, van Holsbeck M. The knee. In: Fornage BD, ed. *Musculoskeletal Ultrasound*. New York: Churchill Livingstone; 1995.

55. Moss GD, Dishuk W. Ultrasound diagnosis of osteochondromatosis of the popliteal fossa. *J Clin Ultrasound* 1984;12:232-233.

Sonography Versus Other Imaging Modalities

56. Engel J, Luboshitz SW, Israeli A et al. Tenography in DeQuervain's disease. *Hand* 1981;13:142-146.

57. Gilula LA, Oloff L, Caputi R et al. Ankle tenography: a key to unexplained symptomatology. Part II: Diagnosis of chronic tendon disabilities. *Radiology* 1984;151:581-587.

58. Mourad K, King J, Guggiana P. Computed tomography and ultrasound imaging of jumper's knee: patellar tendinitis. *Clin Radiol* 1988;39:162-165.

59. Rosenberg ZS, Feldman F, Singson RD et al. Ankle tendons: evaluation with computed tomography. *Radiology* 1988;166: 221-226.

60. Beltran J, Mosure JC. Magnetic resonance imaging of tendons. *Crit Rev Diagn Imaging* 1990;30:111-182.

CHAPTER 28

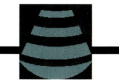

The Extracranial Cerebral Vessels

•

Kelly S. Freed, M.D.
Linda K. Brown, M.D.
Barbara A. Carroll, M.D.

Stroke secondary to atherosclerotic disease is the third leading cause of death in the United States. Many stroke victims survive the catastrophic event with some degree of neurologic impairment.[1] More than 500,000 new cases of cerebrovascular accidents are reported annually.[2] Ischemia from severe, flow-limiting stenosis due to atherosclerotic disease involving the extracranial carotid arteries is implicated in approximately 20% to 30% of strokes.[2] An estimated 80% of strokes are thromboembolic in origin, often with carotid plaque as the embolic source.[3]

Carotid atherosclerotic plaque with resultant stenosis usually involves the internal carotid artery within 2 cm of the carotid bifurcation. This location is readily amenable to examination by sonography as well as surgical intervention. Carotid endarterectomy (CEA) has been proven to be more beneficial than medical therapy in symptomatic patients with greater than 70% carotid stenosis.[4-7] Recent data have also demonstrated that CEA produces a reduction in ipsilateral stroke in asymptomatic patients with greater than 60% stenosis.[2,8] Accurate diagnosis of hemodynamically significant stenosis is critical to identify those patients who would benefit from surgical intervention. Sonography can also assess plaque morphology such as hemorrhagic plaque, which is a source of increased risk for thromboembolic events.[9]

The diagnostic work-up of carotid disease has changed dramatically over the past two decades. Carotid sonography has largely replaced angiography as the most noninvasive and cost-effective screening method to assess suspected extracranial carotid atherosclerotic disease. Gray-scale, color flow Doppler, power mode Doppler, and pulsed wave Doppler imaging techniques are routinely used in the evaluation of patients with neurologic symptoms and suspected extracranial cerebral disease. Magnetic resonance angiography (MRA) is also becoming more widely available as a screening tool for the identification of carotid bifurcation disease, as well as for clarification of ultrasound findings. Angiography is often now reserved for those patients in whom the ultrasound or MRA examination is equivocal or inadequate.

Other carotid ultrasound applications include evaluation of carotid bruits, monitoring progression of known atherosclerotic disease,[10] assessment during or after endarterectomy,[11] preoperative screening prior to major vascular surgery, and evaluation after detection of retinal cholesterol emboli.[12] Nonatherosclerotic carotid diseases can also be evaluated, including follow-up of carotid dissection,[13-15] examination of fibromuscular dysplasia or Takayasu's arteritis, assessment of malignant carotid artery invasion,[16,17] and work-up of pulsatile neck masses and carotid body tumors.[18,19]

CAROTID ARTERY ANATOMY

The first major branch of the aortic arch is the innominate or brachiocephalic artery, which divides into the right subclavian and right common carotid arteries. The second major branch is the left common carotid artery, which is generally separate from the third major branch, the left subclavian artery (Fig. 28-1).

The common carotid arteries (CCA) ascend into the neck posterolateral to the thyroid gland and lie deep to the jugular vein and sternocleidomastoid muscle. At the carotid bifurcation, they divide into the external carotid artery (ECA) and the internal carotid artery (ICA). The ICA usually has no branching vessels in the neck. The ECA, which supplies the facial musculature, has multiple branches in the neck. The

ICA may demonstrate an ampullary region of mild dilatation just beyond its origin.

CAROTID SONOGRAPHIC TECHNIQUE

Carotid artery examinations are performed with the patient supine, the neck slightly extended, and the head turned away from the side being examined. Some operators prefer to perform the examination at the patient's side, and others prefer to sit at the patient's head. A 5- to 10-MHz transducer is used for imaging, and a 3- to 7-MHz for Doppler, the choice depending on the patient's body habitus and technical characteristics of the ultrasound machine. Color flow Doppler imaging and power mode Doppler imaging may be performed with 5- to 10-MHz transducers. In cases of critical stenosis, the Doppler parameters should be optimized to detect very slow flow.

Gray-scale examination begins in the transverse projection. Scans are obtained along the entire course of the cervical carotid artery from the supraclavicular

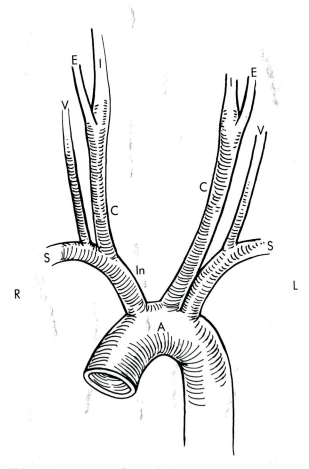

FIG. 28-1. Branches of the aortic arch and extracranial cerebral arteries. A, Aortic arch; *In*, innominate artery; *C*, common carotid artery; *V*, vertebral artery; *S*, subclavian artery; *I*, internal carotid artery; *E*, external carotid artery; *R*, right side; *L*, left side.

INDICATIONS FOR CAROTID ULTRASOUND

Evaluation of patients with TIAs, CVA
Evaluation of carotid bruits
Follow-up of known disease
Monitoring of endarterectomy results
Preoperative screening prior to major vascular surgery
Evaluation of potential source of retinal emboli
Evaluation of pulsatile neck mass
Follow-up of carotid dissection

notch cephalad to the angle of the mandible (Fig. 28-2). Inferior angulation of the transducer in the supraclavicular area images the CCA origin. The left CCA origin is deeper and more difficult to image consistently than the right. The carotid bulb is identified as a mild widening of the CCA near the bifurcation. Transverse views of the carotid bifurcation establish the orientation of the external and internal carotid arteries and help define the optimal longitudinal plane in which to perform Doppler spectral analysis. When the transverse ultrasound images demonstrate occlusive atherosclerotic disease, the percentage of diameter stenosis or area stenosis can be calculated directly using electronic calipers and software analytic algorithms available on most duplex instruments.

The examination plane necessary for optimal longitudinal scans of the carotid artery is determined by the course of the vessels demonstrated on the transverse study. In some patients the optimal longitudinal orientation will be nearly coronal, and in others it will be almost sagittal. In the majority of cases the optimal longitudinal scan plane will be oblique, somewhere between sagittal and coronal. In approximately 60% of patients, both vessels above the carotid bifurcation and the CCA can be imaged in the same plane (Fig. 28-3); in the remainder, only a single vessel will be imaged in the same plane as the CCA. Images are obtained to display the relationship of both branches of the carotid bifurcation to the visualized plaque disease, and the cephalocaudal extent of the plaque is measured. Several anatomic features differentiate the ICA from the ECA. In about 95% of patients, the ICA is posterior and lateral to the ECA. This may vary considerably, however.[11] The ICA frequently has an ampullary region of dilatation just beyond its origin and is usually larger than the ECA. One reliable distinguishing feature of the ECA is identification of branching vessels. The superior thyroidal artery is often seen as the first branch of the ECA after the bifurcation of the CCA. Occasionally an aberrant superior thyroidal artery branch will arise from the distal CCA. The ICA usually has no branches in the neck. In some patients a considerable amount of the ICA will be visible, but in others only the immediate origin of the vessel will be accessible. Rarely, the bifurcation may not be visible at all.[20] A useful method to identify the ECA is the tapping of the superficial temporal artery in the preauricular area. The pulsations are transmitted back to the ECA where they cause a "sawtooth" appearance of the spectral waveform.

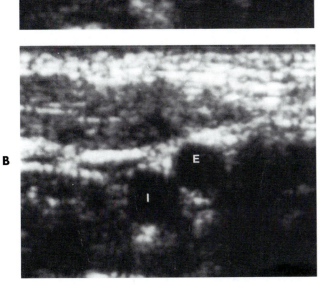

FIG. 28-2. Carotid sonographic anatomy.
A, Right transverse images demonstrate the relationship of the common carotid artery, *A*, to the internal jugular vein, *V*, thyroid gland, *T*, and sternocleidomastoid muscle, *M. Tr,* Trachea. **B,** Carotid bifurcation just cephalic to the bulb. External carotid artery, *E,* lies anteromedial to the internal carotid artery, *I.*

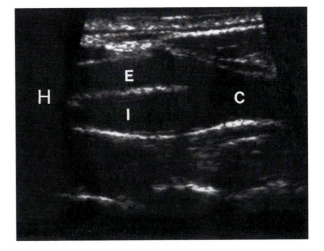

FIG. 28-3. Carotid bifurcation. Longitudinal scan through a normal carotid bifurcation demonstrates the common carotid artery, *C,* internal carotid artery, *I,* and external carotid artery, *E.* External carotid artery is the smaller and more anteromedial of the two vessels above the bifurcation in most individuals. *H,* Head of patient.

CAROTID SONOGRAPHIC INTERPRETATION

Each facet of the carotid sonographic examination is valuable in the final determination of the presence and extent of disease. In most instances the image and Doppler assessments will agree. However, when there are discrepancies between Doppler and image information, every attempt should be made to discover the source of the disagreement. The more closely the image and Doppler findings correlate, the higher the degree of confidence in the diagnosis. Generally speaking, gray-scale and color flow or power mode Doppler images better demonstrate and quantify low-grade stenoses, but high-grade occlusive disease is more accurately defined by Doppler spectral analysis.

Visual Inspection of Gray-Scale Images

Vessel Wall Thickness. Longitudinal views of the layers of the normal carotid wall demonstrate **two nearly parallel echogenic lines,** separated by a hypoechoic to anechoic region (Fig. 28-4). The first echo, bordering the vessel lumen, represents the lumen-intima interface; the second echo is caused by the media-adventitia interface. The media is the anechoic/hypoechoic zone between the echogenic lines. The distance between these lines represents the combined thickness of **the intima and media (I-M complex).** Thickening of the I-M complex greater than 0.8 mm is considered abnormal and may represent the

earliest changes of atherosclerotic disease.[21] The thickness of the far wall of the CCA has been shown to correlate with histologic thicknesses of the intima plus the media.[22] This measurement is highly reproducible and may represent a method of monitoring progression or regression of early atherosclerotic changes.[22,23] The mean thickness of the I-M complex is related to cardiovascular risk factors, including age, smoking, and systolic blood pressure. Thickening of the I-M complex or focal plaque correlates with an increased risk for the development of cardiovascular symptoms in asymptomatic patients.[22]

Plaque Characterization. Atheromatous carotid plaques should be carefully evaluated to determine plaque extent, location, surface contour and texture, as well as assessment of luminal stenosis.[24] Embolism is the most common cause of transient ischemic attacks (TIAs) rather than flow-limiting stenosis.[9] Fewer than half of patients with documented TIAs have hemodynamically significant stenosis. It is important to identify low-grade atherosclerotic lesions that may contain hemorrhage or ulceration that can serve as a nidus for emboli that cause both TIAs and stroke.[1] Between 50% and 70% of patients with hemispheric symptoms demonstrate hemorrhagic or ulcerated plaque. Plaque analysis of carotid endarterectomy specimens has implicated intraplaque hemorrhage as an important factor in the development of neurologic symptoms.[24,26-32] However, the relationship between sonographic plaque morphology and onset of symptoms is controversial.

Plaque texture is generally classified as being homogeneous or heterogeneous.* **Homogeneous plaque** has a uniform echo pattern and a smooth surface (Fig. 28-5). The uniform acoustic texture corresponds pathologically to **dense, fibrous, connective tissue.** Calcified plaque produces posterior acoustic shad-

---

*References 9, 25, 28, 33, 34.

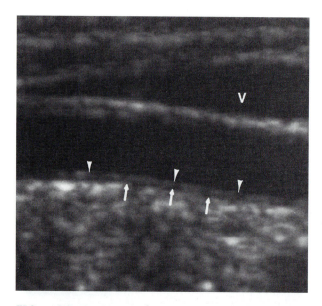

FIG. 28-4. Normal common carotid artery wall thickness. Longitudinal scan shows good definition of the far wall layers. The initial bright echo along the far wall *(arrowheads)* defines the lumen-intima interface. The second echogenic line *(arrows)* represents the media-adventitia interface. *V,* Internal jugular vein. A similar set of echoes parallels the near wall.

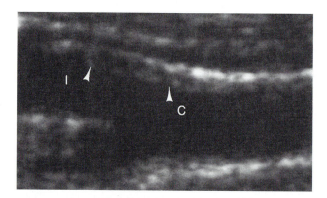

FIG. 28-5. Smooth homogeneous plaque. Longitudinal scan at the bifurcation shows wall thickening extending from the common carotid artery, *C,* up into the internal carotid artery, *I (arrowheads).* The uniform acoustic texture corresponds pathologically to dense fibrous connective tissue.

owing and is common in asymptomatic individuals (Fig. 28-6). **Heterogeneous plaque** has a more complex echo pattern and contains at least one or more focal sonolucent areas (Fig. 28-7). Heterogeneous plaque is characterized pathologically by containing **intraplaque hemorrhage** and/or deposits of lipid, cholesterol, and proteinaceous material.[9] Sonography accurately determines the presence or absence of intraplaque hemorrhage (sensitivity 90% to 94%, specificity 75% to 88%).[26,32,35-37] A "Swiss cheese" plaque appearance with multiple sonolucent areas is characteristic of intraplaque hemorrhage. Virtually all ulcerated plaques are associated with intraplaque hemorrhage. Sonographic findings that suggest **plaque ulceration** include a focal depression or break in the plaque surface or an anechoic area within the plaque, which extends to the plaque surface without an intervening echo between the vessel lumen and the anechoic

plaque region (Fig. 28-8) (see first box below). Some sources suggest classifying plaque according to four types (see second box below). Plaque types 1 and 2 are much more likely to be associated with intraplaque hemorrhage and/or ulceration and are considered unstable and subject to abrupt increase in plaque size following hemorrhage or embolization.[9,33] Types 1 and 2 plaque are typically found in symp-

---

ULTRASOUND FEATURES SUGGESTIVE OF PLAQUE ULCERATION

Focal depression or break in plaque surface
Anechoic region within plaque extending to vessel lumen
Eddies of color within plaque

PLAQUE MORPHOLOGY

Type 1—predominantly echolucent plaque, with a thin echogenic cap
Type 2—substantially echolucent with small areas of echogenicity
Type 3—predominantly echogenic with small areas of echolucency
Type 4—uniformly echogenic

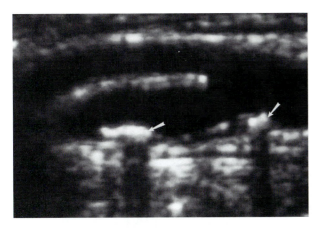

FIG. 28-6. Calcific plaques *(arrows)* with acoustic shadowing are common in the carotid arteries of asymptomatic patients and are generally stable.

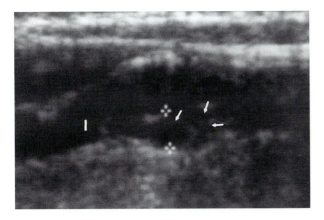

FIG. 28-7. Heterogeneous plaque (between + marks) near the origin of the internal carotid artery, *I*. The plaque contains several sonolucent areas *(arrows)* characteristic of intraplaque hemorrhage.

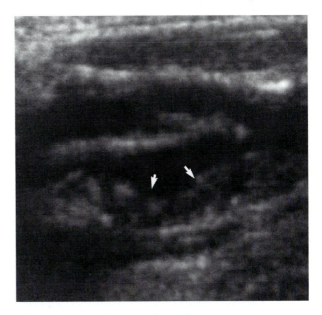

FIG. 28-8. Plaque ulceration. Longitudinal view of the internal carotid artery, *I*, shows a focal contour depression (between white arrows).

tomatic patients with greater than 70% diameter stenosis. Types 3 and 4 plaque are generally composed of fibrous tissue and/or calcification. These are generally more benign, stable plaques that are common in asymptomatic older individuals (see Fig. 28-5).

Although ultrasound reportedly detects intraplaque hemorrhage reliably, in general, neither angiography nor ultrasound has proven highly accurate in identifying ulcerated plaque. However, recent studies suggest that color flow Doppler ultrasound (CDU) and power mode Doppler ultrasound (PDU) can improve sonographic identification of plaque ulceration. CDU or PDU may demonstrate slow-moving eddies of color within an anechoic region in plaque, which suggests ulceration (Fig. 28-9).[38] The demonstration of these flow vortices was 94% accurate in predicting ulcerative plaque at surgery in one study.[39] Preliminary studies suggest that ultrasound contrast agents may further improve the ability to identify plaque surface characteristics.

A potential pitfall in the diagnosis of plaque ulceration may result from a mirror-image duplication artifact producing pseudoulceration of the carotid artery (Fig. 28-10). Highly reflective plaque can produce a CDU ghost artifact simulating ulceration. However, the region of color within the plaque can be recognized

as artifactual as the spectral waveform and color shading within the pseudoulceration are of lower amplitude but otherwise identical to those within the true carotid lumen. Conversely, pulsed wave Doppler traces from within ulcer craters show low-velocity damped waveforms (Fig. 28-11).[38] Although the diagnosis of ulceration is controversial, the ability to reliably predict intraplaque hemorrhage with its associated clinical implications underscores the importance of ultrasound plaque characterization. The presence of heterogeneous, irregular plaque should be noted because hemorrhagic plaque in a stenosis of less than 50% may be considered a "surgical lesion" in the appropriate clinical setting.

Evaluation of Stenosis. Measurements of carotid diameter and area stenosis should be made in the transverse plane perpendicular to the long axis of the vessel.[24] Measurements made on longitudinal scans may overestimate the severity of stenosis by partial voluming through an eccentric plaque. Percentage of diameter stenosis and percentage of area stenosis are not always linearly related. Clinical records should state the type of stenosis measured. Asymmetric stenoses are most appropriately assessed with percentage of area stenosis measurements,[24] although these measurements are often time-consuming and

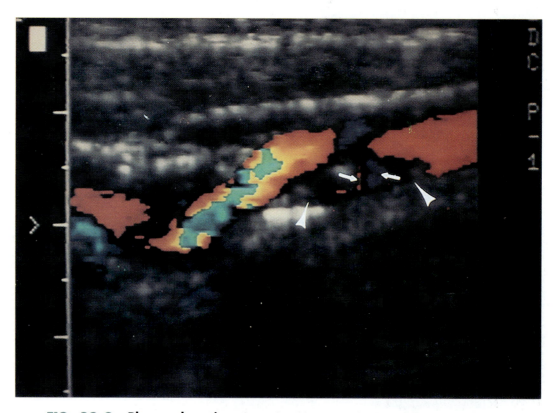

FIG. 28-9. **Plaque ulceration** *(arrowheads)*. Longitudinal color flow Doppler image near the internal carotid artery origin has an irregular contour and contains low-velocity vortices outlined by color *(arrows)*, suggesting abnormal flow in ulcerated areas.

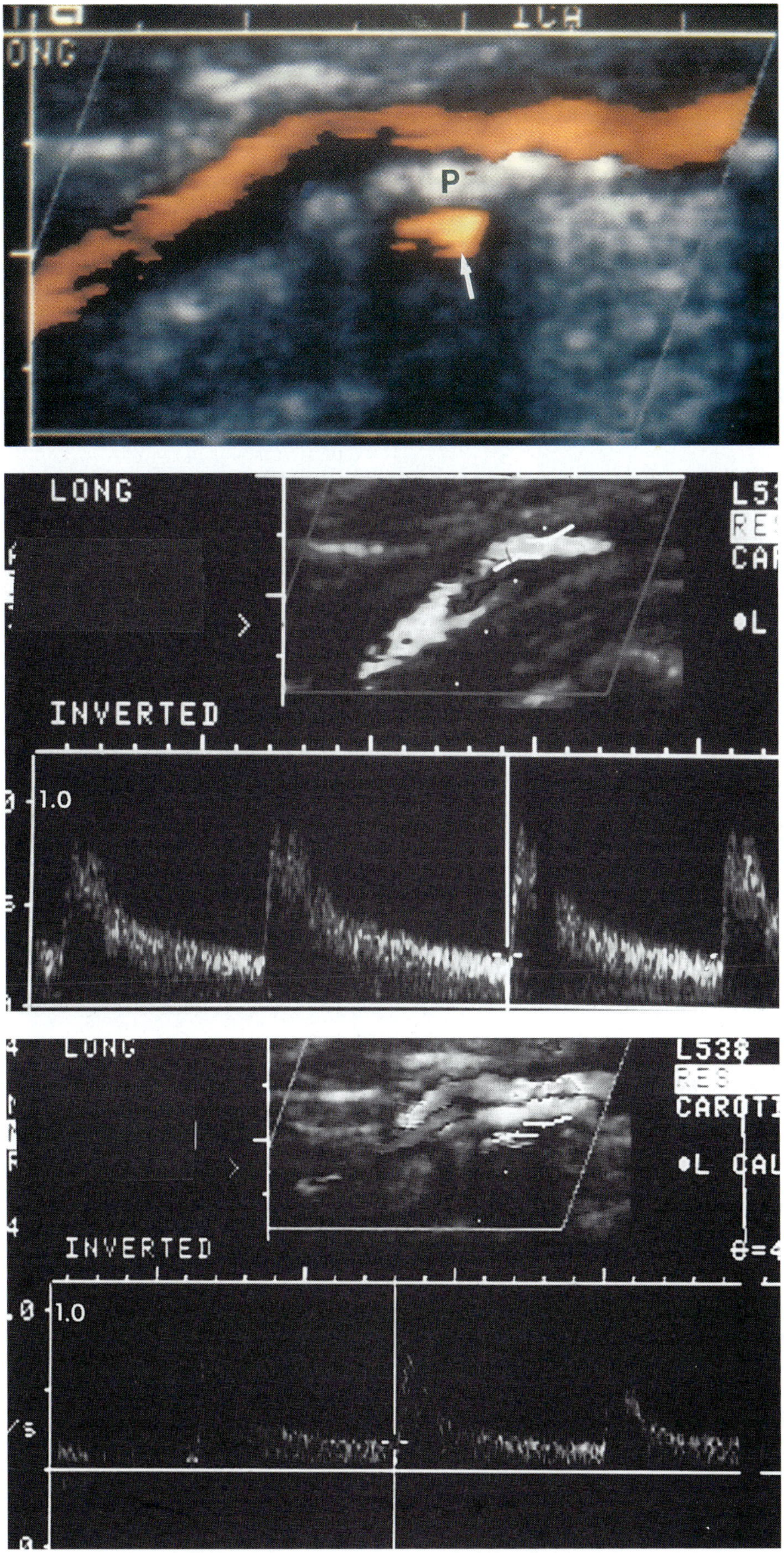

FIG. 28-10. Pseudoulceration A, Longitudinal color flow Doppler image of the proximal left internal carotid artery demonstrates an area of "pseudoulceration" *(arrow)* lying deep to a calcified plaque, *P.* **B,** Pulsed wave Doppler waveforms obtained from the lumen of the internal carotid artery consistent with a less than 50% diameter stenosis. **C,** Pulsed wave Doppler waveforms obtained from the region of the pseudoulcer demonstrate a similar peak systolic velocity. However, the amplitude of the waveform is less than the artery lumen because mirror-image artifacts have weaker signals.

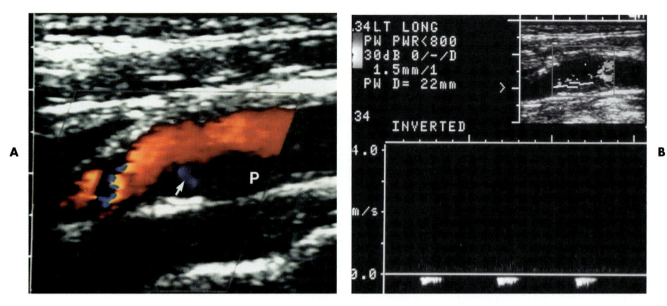

FIG. 28-11. Plaque ulceration with low-velocity reversed flow. A, Longitudinal image of the proximal right internal carotid artery demonstrates hypoechoic plaque, *P*, with an associated area of reversed low-velocity eddy flow within an ulcer *(arrow)*. **B,** Pulsed wave Doppler waveforms obtained in the area of this ulcer crater demonstrate the very damped, low-velocity reversed flow not characteristic of that seen within the main vessel lumen of the ICA.

technically difficult. The cephalocaudal extent and length of plaques should be noted as should the presence of tandem plaques.

As the severity of a stenosis increases, the quality of the real-time image deteriorates.[10,40,41] Several factors work against successful image assessment of high-grade stenosis. Plaque calcification and irregularity produce shadowing, which obscures the vessel lumen. **"Soft plaque"** often has acoustic properties similar to flowing blood, producing anechoic plaques or thrombi that are almost invisible on gray-scale images. In the most extreme cases, vessels can show little visible plaque, yet be totally occluded (Fig. 28-12). Color flow Doppler imaging readily identifies such phenomena. For these reasons, real-time gray-scale ultrasound is best suited for the evaluation of non-rate-limiting lesions, and not for quantifying high-grade stenoses, which are more accurately determined by spectral analysis.[42,43]

Spectral Analysis

Normal Doppler Spectrum. The Doppler spectrum is a quantitative graphic display of the velocities and directions of moving red blood cells present in the Doppler sample volume. Although Doppler assessment of carotid occlusive disease can be performed using frequency data, velocity calculations are preferable.[44] Velocity values are potentially more accurate than frequency shift measurements because the angle of in-

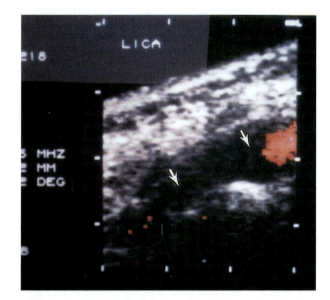

FIG. 28-12. Anechoic thrombus. Longitudinal color flow Doppler image of the internal carotid artery demonstrates proximal flow but no flow distally because of anechoic thrombosis *(arrows)*.

sonation (theta) between the transducer line of sight and the blood flow vector (Fig. 28-13) is used to convert a frequency shift to velocity. Frequency shifts vary according to the angle of insonation (theta) and the incident Doppler frequency; velocity measurements take both these factors into account.

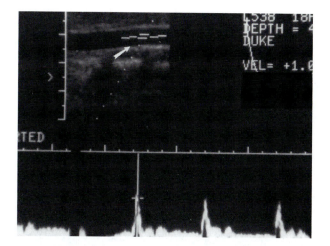

FIG. 28-13. Normal Doppler waveform, common carotid artery. Angle theta *(arrow)* between the transducer line of sight *(dotted line)* and the flow vector indicator bar (aligned parallel to the vascular lumen) should be between 30 and 60 degrees.

The Doppler spectral display represents velocities on the *y*-axis and time on the *x*-axis. By convention, flow toward the transducer is displayed above the zero velocity baseline, and flow away from the transducer is below. For ease of spectral analysis, spectra that project below the baseline are often inverted and placed above the baseline, always keeping in mind the true direction of flow within the vessel. The amplitude of each velocity component (the number of red blood cells with each velocity component) is used to modulate the brightness of the traces. This is also known as a gray-scale velocity plot. In the normal carotid artery, the frequency spectrum is narrow in systole and somewhat wider in early and late diastole. There is usually a black zone between the spectral line and the zero velocity baseline called the "spectral window."[45,46]

The internal carotid and external carotid branches of the common carotid artery have distinctive spectral waveforms (Fig. 28-14). The **ECA** supplies the high-resistance vascular bed of the facial musculature; thus its flow resembles that of other peripheral arterial vessels. Flow velocity rises sharply during systole and falls rapidly in diastole, approaching zero or transiently reversing direction. The **ICA** supplies the low-resistance circulation of the brain and demonstrates flow similar to that in vessels supplying other blood-hungry organs, such as the liver, kidneys, and placenta. The common feature in all low-resistance arterial waveforms is that a large quantity of forward flow continues throughout diastole. The **CCA** waveform is a composite of the internal and external waveforms, but most often the common carotid more closely resembles the internal carotid flow pattern, and diastolic flow is generally above the baseline. Approximately

80% of the blood flowing from the CCA goes through the ICA into the brain whereas 20% goes through the ECA into the facial musculature. The relative decrease in blood flow through the ECA will cause it to have a generally lower-amplitude gray-scale waveform than that found in either the ICA or the CCA.[11]

Doppler Spectral Examination. The extent of the Doppler spectral interrogation required depends on whether CDU is available. If CDU is available, the pulsed wave Doppler sample volume can be placed in the areas of abnormal color. In cases where both gray-scale and color flow Doppler images of an entire carotid artery are normal, only representative spectral tracings from the CCA, ICA, and ECA are necessary to complete the examination.

If CDU is not available, a rapid initial Doppler spectral survey of the entire vessel is made with a wide gate covering the entire width of the vascular lumen. The Doppler gate is then narrowed to a minimum (1.5 mm³), and frequency or velocity spectral analysis is performed. Again, with the advantage of CDU, the time-consuming process of pulsed wave Doppler spectral analysis along the entire course of the vessel can be abbreviated. Blood flow velocities are obtained and spectral analysis performed below, at, and just beyond the region of maximum visible stenosis, and at 1 cm intervals distal to the visualized plaque until the vessel becomes intracranial or the signal can no longer be obtained. Positioning the Doppler angle cursor parallel to the vessel walls determines angle theta, which is used to convert frequency information into velocity values (see Fig. 28-13). Angle theta is defined as the angle between the Doppler transducer line of sight and the direction of blood flow. The ideal angle theta is 0 degrees, as the cosine of this angle is one, thus resulting in the greatest possible detectable frequency shift. However, this angle is rarely achievable in the clinical setting. Therefore a range of angles from 30 to 60 degrees is considered acceptable for carotid spectral analysis. When angle theta exceeds 60 to 70 degrees, the accuracy of velocity/frequency data declines precipitously to the point where virtually no velocity change is detected at angle theta of 90 degrees. The entire course of the CCA and ICA should be interrogated with a consistent angle theta maintained throughout the examination when possible. Generally, only the origin of the ECA is evaluated, as occlusive plaque here is less common than in the ICA and is rarely clinically significant. A stenosis of the ECA should be noted, however, for it may account for a worrisome cervical bruit when the ICA is normal.[20]

Spectral Broadening. Atheromatous plaque projecting into the arterial lumen disturbs the normal smooth laminar flow of erythrocytes. The red blood cells (RBCs) move with a wider range of velocities, so the spectral line becomes wider, filling in the normally

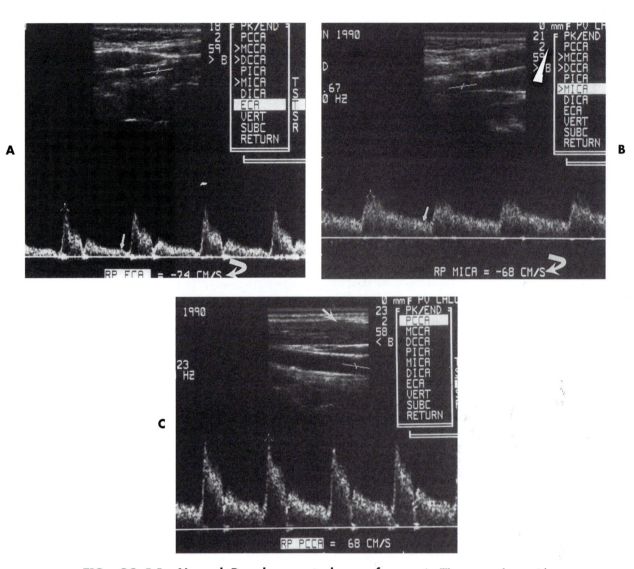

FIG. 28-14. Normal Doppler spectral waveforms. A, The external carotid artery, *ECA,* shows low-velocity flow in diastole *(arrow),* indicating a high-impedance circulation. **B,** The internal carotid artery, *ICA,* has high diastolic flow *(arrow)* associated with the low impedance of the cerebral vasculature. **C,** Common carotid artery, *CCA,* waveform is a composite of the external and internal carotid arteries. Note that in **C,** flow is toward the transducer *(arrow)* and the Doppler spectrum is plotted above the baseline. In **A** and **B,** flow is directed away from the transducer. Although these spectra have been inverted (placed above the baseline), the negative velocity *(curved arrow)* values remind the operator of the true direction of flow away from the transducer.

black spectral window. This phenomenon is termed "spectral broadening" (Figs. 28-15 and 28-16). Spectral broadening increases in proportion to the severity of carotid artery stenosis, and a number of schemes have been derived to measure this parameter.[44,47-49] Some duplex machines allow the operator to measure the spectral spread between the maximum and minimum velocities (bandwidth), and thus quantitate spectral broadening. The validity of these measurements remains to be proven, however, and further correlative studies are needed to document the rela-

tionship of quantitative spectral broadening parameters to specific degrees of stenosis.[49] Nevertheless, a visible "gestalt" of the amount of spectral window obliteration, as well as color flow Doppler heterogeneity, provides a useful, if not quantitative, predictor of the severity of flow disturbance.

Pitfalls. "Pseudospectral broadening" can be caused by technical factors such as a **too high gain setting.** In such instances the background around the spectral waveform often contains noise. Whenever spectral broadening is suspected, the gain should be

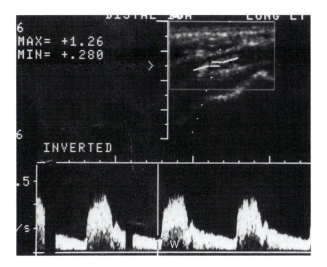

FIG. 28-15. Stenosis of 40% to 59% of the internal carotid artery, *ICA;* High-velocity blood flow patterns in stenotic vessels. High peak systolic velocity (126 cm/s). Diastolic velocity is normal. *W*, Spectral window.

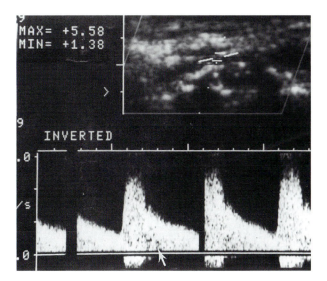

FIG. 28-16. Stenosis of 80% to 99% of the internal carotid artery, *ICA.* Peak systolic velocity is 558 cm/s. Note obliteration of the spectral window *(arrow)* indicating "turbulence" associated with the more severe stenosis. The diastolic velocity (138 cm/s) is also abnormally elevated with this severe stenosis. "Inverted" means flow is directed away from the transducer; the spectrum has been inverted and placed above the baseline for ease of spectral analysis.

lowered to see if the spectral window clears. Similarly, spectral broadening caused by **vessel wall motion** can occur when the Doppler sample volume is too large or positioned too near the vessel wall. Decreasing the size of the sample volume and placing it midstream should eliminate this potential pitfall.

Altered flow patterns can be found **normally at certain sites** in the carotid system. For instance, it is

normal to find flow separation at the **site of branching vessels**, such as where the CCA branches into the ECA and ICA.[50] Flow disturbances also occur at sites where there is an **abrupt change in the vessel diameter.** For instance, spectral broadening may be encountered in a normal carotid bulb where the CCA terminates in a localized area of dilatation as it divides into the ECA and ICA.[11]

The tendency for spectral broadening to occur increases in direct proportion to the velocity of blood flow. For example, it can be observed in normal ECAs, vertebral arteries, and in a CCA that is supplying collateral circulation contralateral to an occluded ICA. **Increased velocity** may also account for the disturbed flow that is sometimes observed in the normal extracranial carotid arteries of young athletes with normal cardiac outputs or in patients in pathologic high cardiac output states. It is also seen in arteries supplying **arteriovenous fistulas** and **arteriovenous malformations**.[11,51] Postoperative spectral broadening may persist for months **after carotid endarterectomy** in the absence of significant residual or recurrent disease. This may be due to changes in wall compliance.

Tortuous carotid vessels can demonstrate spectral broadening and asymmetric high-velocity flow jets in the absence of plaque disease. Other nonatheromatous causes of disturbed blood flow in the extracranial carotid arteries include **aneurysms, arterial wall dissections,** and **fibromuscular dysplasia.**

Spectral broadening suggests vascular disease; however, correlation with gray-scale and color flow Doppler images can define the cause of spectral broadening. An awareness of normal flow spectra combined with appropriate Doppler techniques can obviate many potential diagnostic pitfalls.

High-Velocity Blood Flow Patterns. Carotid stenoses usually begin to cause velocity changes when they exceed 50% diameter (70% cross-sectional area).[1] Velocity elevations generally increase as the severity of the stenosis increases. At critical stenoses (>95%) the velocity measurements may actually decrease and the waveform becomes dampened.[43,52] In these cases, correlation with color flow Doppler or power mode Doppler imaging is essential to correctly diagnose the severity of the stenosis. Velocity increases are focal and most pronounced in and immediately distal to a stenosis, emphasizing the importance of sampling directly in these regions. As one moves further distal from a stenosis, flow begins to reconstitute and assume a more normal pattern, provided a tandem lesion does not exist distal to the initial site of stenosis.

Initial sonographic estimations of ICA diameter stenosis used ranges of 0 to 50%, 50% to 60%, 60% to 80%, and 80% to 99%. Degree of stenosis was based on the gray-scale and pulsed wave Doppler parameters, including ICA peak systolic velocity (**PSV**), ICA end diastolic velocity (**EDV**), CCA PSV, CCA EDV, **peak systolic ICA/CCA ratios**, and **peak end diastolic ICA/CCA ratios**. Peak systolic velocity has proven accurate for quantifying high-grade stenoses.[41,44] The relationship of this parameter to the degree of luminal narrowing is well defined, and it is easily measured.[52,53] At our institution, a rule of thumb is peak systolic ICA velocities less than 125 cm/s are consistent with less than 50% diameter stenosis; 125 to 250 cm/s corresponds with 50% to 75% diameter stenosis; greater than 250 cm/s corresponds with greater than 75% to 80% diameter stenosis. End diastolic velocity ratios have proven useful in distinguishing between degrees of high-grade stenosis.[54] There are no established criteria for grading ECA stenoses. Occlusive plaque involving the ECA is less common than in the ICA and is rarely clinically significant. Similarly, velocity criteria used to grade CCA stenoses have not been well established. However, a rule of thumb we utilize is if we are able to visualize 2 cm proximal and 2 cm distal to a mid CCA stenosis, then a peak systolic velocity ratio obtained 2 cm proximal to the stenosis versus that in the region of the greatest visible stenosis can be used to grade the percent diameter stenosis in a fashion analogous to that used in peripheral artery studies. Therefore a doubling of the peak systolic velocity across a lesion would correspond to at least 50% diameter stenosis, and a velocity ratio in excess of 3.5 corresponds to a greater than 75% stenosis. While duplex sonography remains an accurate method of quantifying ICA stenoses, the addition of color flow Doppler and, more recently, power mode Doppler to the diagnostic regimen has significantly improved diagnostic confidence and reproducibility. Color flow or power mode Doppler may also be used to estimate the percent diameter stenosis in the ECA and CCA.

The degree of carotid stenosis considered clinically significant in the symptomatic or asymptomatic patient is in evolution. Initially it was felt that lesions causing 50% diameter stenosis were significant; this percentage has changed as more information is gathered from clinical trials. Two large multicenter trials, the **North American Symptomatic Carotid Endarterectomy Trial (NASCET) and the European Carotid Surgery Trial (ECST)**, have demonstrated that **carotid endarterectomy is more beneficial than medical therapy in symptomatic patients with 70% to 99% ICA stenosis**.[4,5] The degree of carotid stenosis was determined angiographically in both these studies, using two different sets of criteria. In NASCET, the percent stenosis was determined by comparing the stenotic luminal diameter to the "normal" diameter of the distal cervical ICA.[4,5] In ECST, the "normal" ICA diameter was estimated at the level of the stenosis.

The results of NASCET and ECST have generated reappraisals of the Doppler parameters in an attempt to elicit those velocity parameters that most accurately correspond to 70% or greater stenosis. Attempts have also been made to standardize Doppler criteria or to determine the Doppler parameter or combination of parameters that reliably identify greater than 70% ICA stenosis. Most sources agree the single best parameter is the PSV of the ICA,[55] although other parameters such as the peak systolic ICA/CCA ratio has been postulated as the most sensitive and specific parameter (Table 28-1).[56] However, studies have reported ICA PSVs ranging from 130 cm/s[57] to 325 cm/s,[56] which correlate with greater than 70% ICA stenosis at different institutions. This wide range of PSVs reinforces the fact that individual ultrasound laboratories must determine which Doppler parameters are accurate for their instruments. Correlation of

TABLE 28-1
DOPPLER SPECTRUM ANALYSIS

Diameter Stenosis	ICA/CCA Peak Systolic Velocity Ratio	ICA/CCA Peak End Diastolic Velocity Ratio	Peak Systolic Velocity	Peak End Diastolic Velocity
0—40%	< 1.5	< 2.6	< 110 cm/sec > 25 cm/sec	< 40 cm/sec
41%—59%	< 1.8	< 2.6	> 120 cm/sec	< 40 cm/sec
60%—69%	> 1.8	> 2.6	> 150 cm/sec	> 40 cm/sec
70%—79%	> 3.0	> 3.3	> 210 cm/sec	> 70 cm/sec
80%—99%	> 3.7	> 5.5	> 280 cm/sec < 25 cm/sec	> 100 cm/sec
Occlusion			Unilateral damped flow in CCA. No flow or reversed flow proximal to ICA occlusion.	

the velocity ranges obtained by ultrasound with degrees of stenosis determined by angiography is necessary to achieve accurate, reproducible results for a particular ultrasound laboratory.

Color Flow Doppler Ultrasound

Color flow Doppler ultrasound displays flow information in real time over the entire image or a selected area (Fig. 28-17). Stationary soft-tissue structures, which lack a detectable phase or frequency shift, are assigned an amplitude value and displayed in a gray-scale format with flowing blood in vessels superimposed in color. The mean Doppler frequency shift produced by RBC ensembles pulsing through a selected sample volume is obtained using an autocorrelative method or a time domain processing (speckle motion analysis) method. Color assignments depend on the direction of blood flow relative to the Doppler transducer. Blood flow toward the transducer appears in one color, and flow away from the transducer in another. These color assignments are arbitrary and are generally set up so that arterial flow is depicted as red, and venous flow as blue. Color saturation displays indicate the variable velocity of blood flow. Deeper shades usually indicate low velocities centered around the zero velocity color flow baseline. As velocity increases, the shades become lighter or are assigned a different color hue. Some systems allow selected frequency shifts to be displayed in a contrasting color, such as green. This "green-tag" feature provides a real-time estimation of the presence of high-velocity flow. Setting the color flow Doppler scale can also be used to create an aliasing artifact corresponding to high-velocity flow within areas of the vessel (Fig. 28-18). Color assignments are a function of both the mean frequency shift produced by moving

RBC ensembles and the Doppler angle theta. If the vessel is tortuous or diving, this angle will change along the course of the vessel, resulting in changing color assignments that are unrelated to the change in RBC velocity. Furthermore, the color assignments will reverse in tortuous vessels as their course changes relative to the Doppler transducer even though the absolute direction of flow is unchanged. Portions of a vessel that parallel the Doppler beam when the angle of insonation is 90 degrees will have little or no frequency shift detected and no color will be seen.

Color flow Doppler studies should be performed with optimal flow sensitivity and gain settings. Color flow should fill the entire vessel lumen but not spill over into adjacent soft tissues. The pulse repetition frequency (PRF) and frame rates should be set to allow visualization of flow phenomenon anticipated in a vessel. Frame rates will vary as a function of the width of the area chosen for color flow Doppler display, as well as the depth of the region of interest. The greater the color image area, the slower the frame rate will be. The deeper the posterior boundary of the color image, the slower the PRF. Color flow Doppler sensitivity should be adjusted to detect anticipated velocities such that if slow flow in a preocclusive carotid lesion is sought, low flow settings with decreased sampling rates are employed (see box on p. 898). However, the system will then alias at lower velocities because of the decrease in PRF. In addition to changes in the PRF, **optimization of the Doppler angle, gain and power settings**, a **decrease in the wall filter**, an **increase in persistence**, and an **increase in ensemble or dwell time** can be used to optimize low flow detection.

Flowing blood becomes in effect its own contrast medium with CDU or PDU outlining the patent vessel

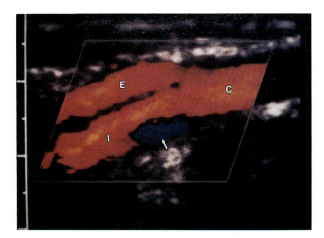

FIG. 28-17. Normal longitudinal color flow Doppler image of the carotid bifurcation. Flow reversal zone blue area *(arrow)* appears at early systole or peak systole and persists variable amounts of time into diastole. *I*, ICA; *C*, CCA; *E*, ECA.

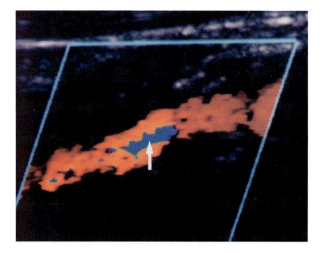

FIG. 28-18. Aliasing within the central lumen of the vessel in the area of fastest laminar flow *(arrow)*. Color flow Doppler image of the internal carotid artery.

OPTIMIZATION OF LOW FLOW VELOCITIES

Decreased sampling rate (i.e., decreased PRF)
Doppler angle as low as possible (60 degrees or less)
Decreased wall filter
Increased persistence
Increase in dwell time
Increase gain
Increased power

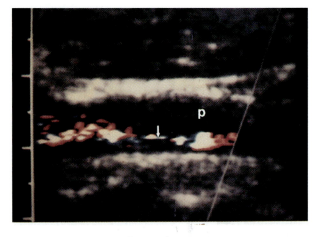

FIG. 28-19. High-grade stenosis. Longitudinal color flow Doppler image of the ICA demonstrates a large amount of plaque, *P*, and a small residual lumen *(arrow)* with white areas indicating high-velocity flow.

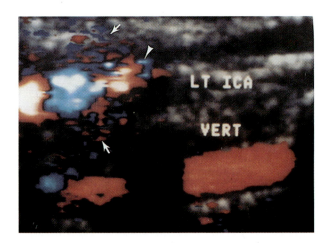

FIG. 28-20. Perivascular color artifact distal to ICA stenosis *(arrowhead).* A random localized mixture of red and blue colors in the perivascular soft tissues *(arrows)* resulting from tissue vibration from "turbulent" intravascular blood flow.

lumen (Fig. 28-19). This allows determination of the true course of the vessel, facilitating positioning of the Doppler cursor, and thus allowing more reliable velocity determinations. Furthermore, CDU facilitates Doppler spectral analysis by rapidly identifying areas of flow abnormalities. The highest velocity shifts can frequently be identified by color flow Doppler aliasing. CDU facilitates placing the pulsed wave Doppler range gate in the region of these most striking color abnormalities. The presence of a stenosis can be determined by color Doppler changes in the vessel lumen as well as by visible luminal narrowing. If a stenosis produces a bruit or thrill, the resultant perivascular tissue vibrations may actually be seen as transient speckles of color in the adjacent soft tissues more prominent during systole (Fig. 28-20).[58,59] Comparisons of CDU with conventional duplex sampling techniques and angiography have shown relatively similar accuracy, sensitivity, and specificity.[60,61] However, CDU offers many valuable benefits (see box on top of page 899). CDU reduces the examination time by pinpointing areas of color flow Doppler abnormality for pulsed wave Doppler spectral analysis. Branches of the ECA are readily detected, facilitating differentiation from the ICA. The real-time flow information over a large cross-sectional area provides a global overview of flow abnormalities and allows the course of a vessel to be readily determined. Furthermore, color flow Doppler improves diagnostic confidence and reproducibility of ultrasound studies and thereby avoids many potential diagnostic pitfalls. The laminar blood flow is disrupted in the region of the carotid bifurcation where there is a **normal transient flow reversal** opposite the origin of the ECA (see Fig. 28-17). Color flow Doppler displays this normal flow separation as an area of flow reversal located along the outer wall of the carotid bulb, which appears either at early systole or in peak systole and persists for a variable amount of time into the diastolic portion of the cardiac cycle.[62,63] This flow reversal can produce some strikingly bizarre pulsed wave Doppler waveforms; however, the color flow Doppler appearance readily discerns the nature of these waveform changes. Furthermore, it has been suggested that the

absence of this flow reversal is abnormal and may represent one of the earliest changes of atherosclerotic disease.[62] The flow reversal seen in the region of the carotid bifurcation is clearly different than that seen with color flow Doppler aliasing. Contiguous saturated areas of red and blue are seen in this low-velocity flow separation as compared with the very different contiguous color hues representing the highest color assignments for forward and reversed flow. Helical flow in the CCA can be an indirect indication of proximal arterial stenosis, but can occur as a normal variant. Color flow Doppler imaging graphically displays the eccentric spiraling of flow up the CCA.

Color flow Doppler imaging may help avoid potential diagnostic pitfalls. Alterations in cardiovascular physiology, tandem lesions, contralateral carotid dis-

ADVANTAGES OF COLOR FLOW DOPPLER IMAGING

Reduction in examination time
Quick identification of areas of stenosis/high velocity, which facilitates spectral analysis
Improved diagnostic reproducibility and confidence
Distinguish occlusion from "string sign" better than pulsed Doppler
Simultaneous hemodynamic and anatomic information
Velocity and directional blood flow information
Improved accuracy in quantitating stenoses
Clarifies pulsed wave Doppler image mismatch

DISADVANTAGES OF COLOR FLOW DOPPLER IMAGING

Angle dependent—prone to artifacts
Resolution less than gray-scale imaging
Less Doppler spectral information
Slower frame rates

ease, arrhythmias, postoperative changes, and tortuous vessels can lead to underestimation or overestimation of the degree of stenosis. In such cases, CDU can provide direct visualization of the patent lumen in a fashion analogous to angiography.[64] In fact, since angiography images only the vessel lumen, not the vessel wall, both color flow and power mode Doppler imaging have the potential to evaluate stenoses even more completely than angiography. Furthermore, since flow patterns are displayed with color flow Doppler imaging, the local hemodynamic consequences of the lesion are readily discerned. CDU appears to have particular value in detecting small residual channels of flow in areas of high-grade carotid stenoses.[60,61,64-66] PDU offers a comparable advantage and has the theoretical potential to be more sensitive for detecting extremely low-amplitude, low-velocity flow. Finally, color flow and power mode Doppler imaging have the potential to clarify mismatches between image and spectral Doppler, further improving diagnostic accuracy and confidence.

Although CDU offers many advantages, it is angle dependent and prone to artifacts such as aliasing.[67] The spatial resolution of CDU is less than that of gray-scale imaging, while the Doppler resolution is inferior to pulsed wave Doppler spectral analysis. The color saturation cannot be equated with velocity.[58] The color image is corrected for only one angle, and thus changes

in color saturation may simply reflect changes in the vessel course and the relative Doppler angle. Color systems generally compute the mean velocity to produce the color pixel in the image. However, the examiner is usually interested in determining the maximal velocity, and therefore pulsed wave Doppler spectral analysis remains necessary for precise quantification of a hemodynamically significant stenosis.

Power Mode Doppler Ultrasound

The color signal in PDU is generated from the integrated power mode Doppler spectrum. The amplitude of the reflected echoes determines the brightness and color tone of the color signal. This amplitude is dependent on the density of RBCs flowing within the sample volume. PDU uses a larger dynamic range with a better signal-to-noise ratio than CDU. Because PDU does not evaluate frequencies but rather amplitude or power, artifacts such as aliasing do not occur. PDU, unlike CDU, is largely angle independent. These features combine to make PDU exquisitely sensitive to detecting a residual string of flow in the region of a suspected carotid occlusion. It is also hypothesized that PDU has better edge definition than CDU. The combination of improved edge definition and relative angle-independent flow imaging offers the potential for better visual assessment of the degree of stenosis using PDU. Better edge definition may also allow PDU to better define plaque surface characteristics (Fig. 28-21). Despite the many potential benefits of PDU, it does not provide velocity or directional flow information.[68] Furthermore, PDU is very motion sensitive.

Pitfalls

Although absolute velocity determinations are valuable in assessing the degree of vascular stenosis, there are times when these measurements are less reliable.[44,69] Variations in cardiovascular physiology may affect carotid velocity measurements.[70] For example, velocities produced by a stenosis in a **hypertensive patient** will be higher than those in a normotensive individual with a comparable narrowing. On the other hand, a **reduction in cardiac output** will diminish both systolic and diastolic velocities. **Cardiac arrhythmias, aortic valvular lesions,** and **severe cardiomyopathies** can cause significant aberrations in the shape of carotid flow waveforms and alter systolic and diastolic velocity readings (Fig. 28-22). Use of an **aortic balloon pump** can also distort the Doppler velocity spectrums. These alterations can invalidate the use of standard Doppler parameters to quantify stenoses. **Bradycardia,** for example, produces increased stroke volume, causing systolic velocities to increase, but prolonged diastolic runoff causes spuriously decreased end diastolic values. Patients with isolated severe or critical aortic stenosis may demonstrate duplex waveform abnormal-

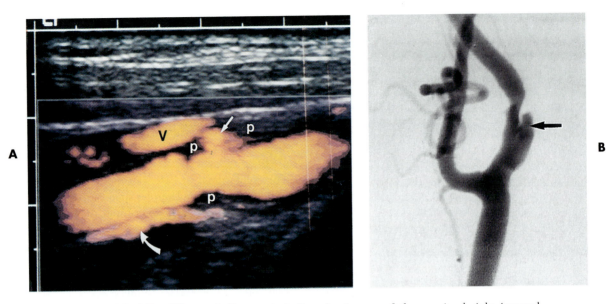

FIG. 28-21. Ulcer. A, Power mode Doppler images of the proximal right internal carotid artery demonstrate an area of ulceration *(arrow)* in the region of a proximal ICA plaque, *P.* Jugular vein, *V,* power mode Doppler mirror-image artifact *(curved arrow).* **B,** Angiogram demonstrating the similar area of proximal right ICA ulceration *(arrow).*

ADVANTAGES OF POWER MODE DOPPLER ULTRASOUND

No aliasing
Potentially increases accuracy of grading stenoses
Aids in distinguishing preocclusive from occlusive
  lesions
Potential superior depiction of plaque surface
  morphology
Increased sensitivity to detecting low-velocity, low-
  amplitude blood flow
Angle independent

DISADVANTAGES OF POWER MODE DOPPLER ULTRASOUND

Does not provide direction or velocity flow
  information
Very motion sensitive (poor temporal resolution)

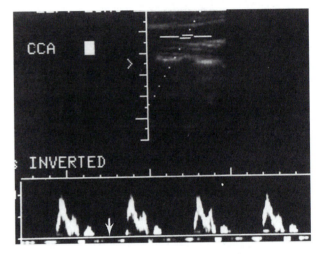

FIG. 28-22. Severe aortic insufficiency, AI. Left CCA spectral analysis demonstrates a grossly disturbed pattern with diastolic flow reversal and absent end diastolic flow *(arrow).*

ities, including prolonged acceleration time, decreased peak velocity, delayed upstroke, and rounded waveforms. However, mild or moderate aortic stenosis usually results in little or no sonographic abnormality.[71] Frequently an **image/Doppler mismatch** alerts the examiner to potential pitfalls.

CDU can be used to overcome diagnostic dilemmas in these situations, particularly when "cine loop" playback capabilities are present. Cine loop allows the computer to store up to 10 seconds of the previous color flow Doppler recording for playback at the real-time rate or frame by frame. This allows assessment of filling of all parts of the vessel lumen. **Obstructive lesions** in one carotid artery can **affect** velocities in the **contralateral vessel.** For example, severe unilateral ICA stenosis or occlusion may cause shunting of increased flow through the contralateral carotid system. This increased flow artificially increases velocity measurements in the contralateral vessel, particularly in areas of stenosis (Fig. 28-23).[72] Conversely, a prox-

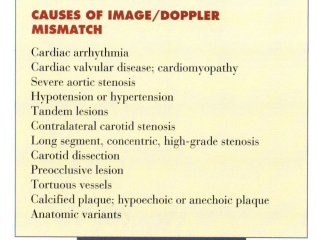

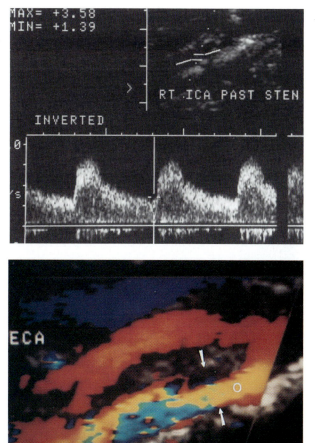

FIG. 28-23. High-grade stenosis in left ICA (contralateral) causes spurious velocity elevation in the right ICA. A, Markedly elevated peak systolic velocity just beyond the right internal carotid artery, *ICA,* stenosis (358 cm/s) corresponds with 80% to 99% stenosis. This velocity value is invalid because the extreme stenosis of the left contralateral ICA increases flow to the right side. **B,** Longitudinal color flow Doppler image of moderate stenosis of the origin of the right ICA, *O,* demonstrates a moderate atheromatous plaque anteriorly and a residual color-filled lumen *(arrows).* Color inhomogeneity beyond the stenotic zone shows "turbulence" associated with stenosis and color aliasing because of high velocities. Angiography confirmed right ICA stenosis (40% to 59% range).

imal CCA or innominate artery stenosis may reduce flow, with consequent reduction of velocity measurements in a stenosis that is distal to the point of obstruction (**tandem lesion**).

Velocity ratios that compare velocity values in the ICA to those in the ipsilateral CCA can help avoid some pitfalls.[44] Of particular value are the peak systolic ratio (PSV in the ICA/PSV in the CCA)[49,73] and the end diastolic ratio (EDV in the ICA/EDV in the CCA).[54] Velocity ratios corresponding to specific degrees of vascular stenosis are listed in Table 28-1.

Values obtained in the ICA should be obtained at or just distal to the point of maximum visible stenosis and/or at the point of greatest color flow Doppler spectral abnormality. Values obtained from the CCA should be obtained proximal to the widening in the region of the carotid bulb. Velocity ratios should always be employed when unusually high or low common carotid velocities or significant asymmetry of common carotid velocities is detected. As discussed in the previous section on spectral broadening, color flow Doppler imaging is invaluable in the avoidance of pitfalls related to spurious Doppler spectral traces.

Although high-grade stenoses usually produce increased velocity in the region of a plaque and distal to it, high-grade intracranial or extracranial occlusive **lesions in tandem may reduce anticipated velocity shifts** and produce an atypical high-resistance ICA waveform. Vessels should be examined as far cephalad as possible to avoid missing a distal "tandem" lesion. Flow immediately distal to stenosis of over 95% is often damped or tardus-parvus and decreased in velocity (Fig. 28-24). High-grade vascular narrowings, particularly those of a circumferential nature, that occur over a long segment of a vessel, may also produce damped waveforms without a high-velocity frequency shift. Although no definite velocity elevations are present in such a long circumferential narrowing, spectral broadening and disturbed flow distal to such a narrowing is usually apparent. In addition, the fusiform narrowing is usually detected with the real-time image, particularly if color flow Doppler is employed.

Another source of error in pulsed wave Doppler ultrasound analysis is **aliasing,** which is caused by the inability to detect the true peak velocity because the Doppler sampling rate (pulse repetition frequency, PRF) is too low. A classic visual example of aliasing can

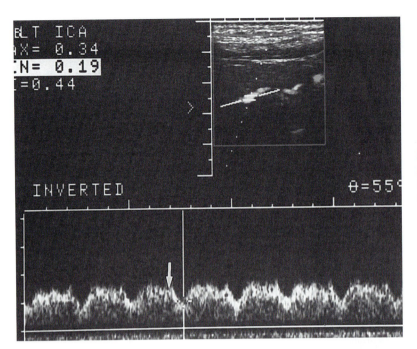

FIG. 28-24. Low-velocity tardus/ parvus waveforms *(arrow)* are seen in a left ICA distal to a greater than 95% diameter stenosis.

be seen in western films, with the apparent reversal of stagecoach wheel spokes when the wagon wheel rotations exceed the film frame rate. The maximum detectable frequency shift can be no greater than half the PRF. With aliasing, the tips of the time velocity spectrum (representing high velocities) are cut off and wrap around to appear below the baseline (Fig. 28-25). If aliasing occurs, **continuous wave probes** used in conjunction with duplex pulsed wave Doppler can readily demonstrate the true peak velocity shift. Aliasing can also be overcome or decreased by **increasing angle theta** (the angle of Doppler insonation), thereby reducing the detected Doppler shift, or by decreasing the insonating sound beam frequency. **Increasing the PRF** increases the detectable frequency shift, but the PRF increase is limited by the depth of the vessel as well as the center frequency of the transducer.[24,46] One can also **shift the zero baseline** and reassign a larger range of velocities to forward flow to overcome aliasing. It is also valid to **add velocity values above and below the baseline** to obtain an accurate velocity value, provided multiple wraparounds do not occur, as seen in extremely high velocities. Aliasing may sometimes be useful in color flow Doppler image interpretation, where color flow Doppler aliasing can accent the severity of flow disturbances as well as define the patent lumen.

Internal Carotid Artery (ICA) Occlusion

Carotid occlusion is diagnosed when no flow is detected in a vessel. Occasionally, transmitted pulsations into an occluded ICA may mimic abnormal flow in a patent vessel. The pulsed wave Doppler cursor should be clearly located in the ICA lumen, and arterial pul-

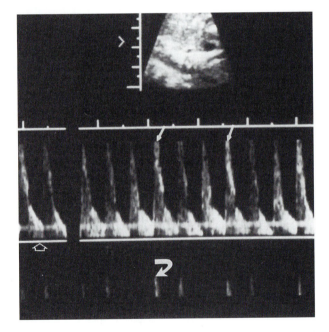

FIG. 28-25. Aliasing. High velocities that exceed one half the pulse repetition frequency (PRF) are cut off *(arrows)* and wrapped around to appear below the baseline *(curved arrow)* in reversed direction. The tips of the aliased signals point toward the baseline *(open arrow)*, which is the opposite of the waveform for a true flow reversal.

satile flow should be identified. Close attention should be paid to the direction of flow and the nature of pulsations. **True center stream sampling** should be documented by transverse scanning, and the sample volume reduced in size as much as possible. Extraneous pulsations should seldom be transmitted to the center of the thrombus.[40]

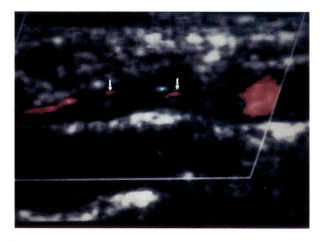

FIG. 28-26. **Residual "string" of flow** *(arrows)* within a long, high-grade ICA stenosis. Longitudinal color flow Doppler scan of the ICA.

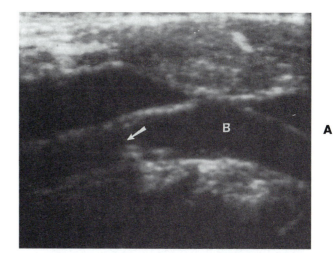

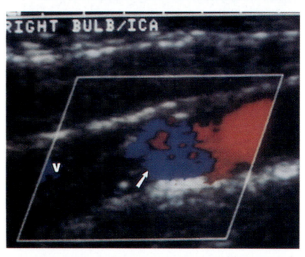

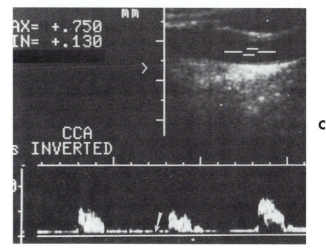

As a high-grade stenosis approaches occlusion, the high-velocity jet is reduced to a mere trickle. It may be difficult to locate the small residual string of flow within a largely occluded lumen using gray-scale imaging alone, particularly if the adjacent plaque or thrombus is anechoic, making the residual lumen invisible during real-time examination, or if there is calcified plaque obscuring visualization.

In critical high-grade stenoses (>95%), standard sensitivity color flow Doppler settings may fail to demonstrate a string of residual flow. Thus it is always prudent to employ the "slow flow" sensitivity settings on color flow Doppler to discriminate between **critical stenoses and occlusions** (Fig. 28-26).[61,64] Alternatively, PDU with its increased sensitivity to detecting low-amplitude, low-velocity signals may be used to visualize a residual string of blood flow. Color flow Doppler imaging is 95% to 98% accurate in distinguishing high-grade stenosis from complete occlusion on angiography when appropriate technical parameters are employed.[74,75]

The presence of a high-grade ICA stenosis or occlusion can often be inferred from inspection of the ipsilateral CCA pulsed wave Doppler waveform or color flow or pulsed wave Doppler image (Fig. 28-27). The pulsed wave Doppler waveforms in the ipsilateral CCA and ICA proximal to a lesion frequently demonstrate an asymmetric, high-resistance signal with decreased, absent, or reversed diastolic flow except when there has been ECA collateralization to the intracranial circulation. Similarly, color flow or power mode Doppler images may show a flash of color flow in systole but a conspicuous decrease or absence of color flow in diastole, which is asymmetric compared with the contralateral side.[74,75] The diagnosis of carotid occlusion versus a "string sign" is made more accurately

FIG. 28-27. **Internal carotid artery (ICA) occlusion.** **A,** Longitudinal gray-scale image of the ICA demonstrates thrombus filling the ICA lumen *(arrow)*, suggesting occlusion. *B,* Bulb. **B,** Color flow Doppler shows flow reversal (blue) immediately proximal *(arrow)* to the lesion with no residual channel of flow in the lesion, indicating occlusion. **C,** Damped spectral waveform in the CCA proximal to the occlusion. Note markedly diminished diastolic flow *(arrow)* indicating high resistance.   *Continued.*

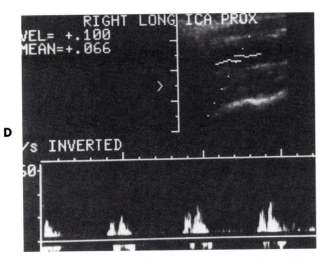

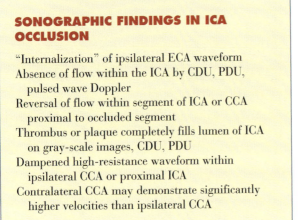

FIG. 28-27, cont'd. D, Damped spectral waveform in ICA proximal to the occlusion, tracing above and below the baseline, indicates bidirectional flow.

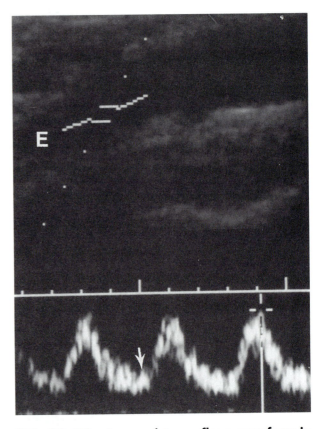

FIG. 28-28. Low-resistance flow waveform in an ECA, *E.* that is providing collateral circulation to the brain around an occluded ICA. Note increased end-diastolic flow *(arrow).*

SONOGRAPHIC FINDINGS IN ICA OCCLUSION

"Internalization" of ipsilateral ECA waveform

Absence of flow within the ICA by CDU, PDU, pulsed wave Doppler

Reversal of flow within segment of ICA or CCA proximal to occluded segment

Thrombus or plaque completely fills lumen of ICA on gray-scale images, CDU, PDU

Dampened high-resistance waveform within ipsilateral CCA or proximal ICA

Contralateral CCA may demonstrate significantly higher velocities than ipsilateral CCA

---

with color flow Doppler and power mode Doppler than with gray-scale duplex scanning, and may obviate the need for angiography to confirm a sonographically diagnosed ICA occlusion.[74,75]

Another pitfall in the diagnosis of a totally occluded ICA is **mistaking a patent ECA or one of its branches for the ICA.** The situation is especially confusing when the ECA/ICA collaterals open in response to longstanding ICA disease and the ECA acquires a low-resistance waveform ("internalization") (Fig. 28-28). One technique that can aid in identifying the ECA is scanning at the origin of the vessel while simultaneously tapping the temporal artery. Percussion of the superficial temporal artery often results in a serrate distortion of the Doppler waveform in the ECA (80% of ECAs percussed in one study) (Fig. 28-29).[76] However, this maneuver should be used with caution, as the temporal tap can also be seen in the CCA and ICA, though less com-

monly (54% and 33%, respectively) than in the ECA.[76] Branching vessels are a unique feature of the ECA that can also be used to differentiate this vessel from the ICA. CDU can facilitate the identification of such branching vessels (Fig. 28-30). Usually the combination of vessel **size, position, waveform shape, the presence of branches,** and the **temporal tap response** can correctly **identify the ECA.**

Although distal propagation of thrombus almost invariably occurs following an ICA occlusion, CCA occlusions are often localized. Flow may be maintained in the ECA and ICA, but must be reversed in one of the two vessels. Ultrasound is the preferred method for evaluating maintenance of flow around the carotid bifurcation following proximal CCA occlusion. Most commonly, retrograde flow in the ECA will supply antegrade flow in the ipsilateral ICA. Occasionally, the opposite flow pattern will be encountered (Fig. 28-31).[40,77,78]

Preoperative Strategies for Patients with Carotid Artery Disease

The preoperative work-up of carotid disease is evolving in response to the results of the NASCET,

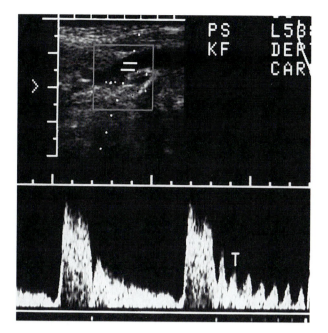

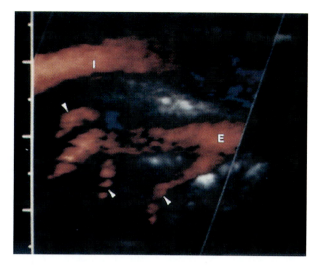

FIG. 28-30. **The ICA, *I*, and ECA, *E*, superior to the bifurcation.** Longitudinal view color flow Doppler facilitates visualization of ECA branches *(arrowheads)*.

FIG. 28-29. **Temporal artery tap.** Spectral Doppler traces of the ECA demonstrate the characteristic serrate Doppler waveform disturbance, *T*, produced by the temporal tap maneuver.

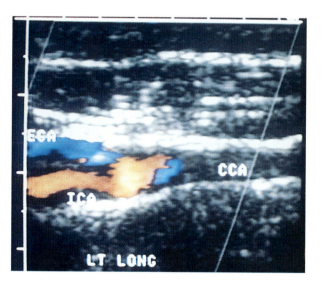

FIG. 28-31. **CCA occlusion.** A longitudinal color flow Doppler image of the left carotid bifurcation demonstrates retrograde flow in the ECA and antegrade flow in the ICA in a patient with a completely occluded CCA.

ECST, and Asymptomatic Carotid Atherosclerosis Study (ACAS),[79] and the development of more accurate and noninvasive imaging techniques. While many still consider angiography the "gold standard," criticisms of this technique include significant intraobserver variability and the fact that angiography may frequently underestimate the degree of stenosis.[80] In

fact, comparisons of angiographic and sonographic estimations of carotid stenosis reveal a closer surgical correlation with the ultrasound measurements.[80] Carotid sonography has proven a highly accurate method of detecting high-grade stenoses as well as differentiating critical stenoses from occlusion, particularly since the advent of CDU and PDU. MRA is cur-

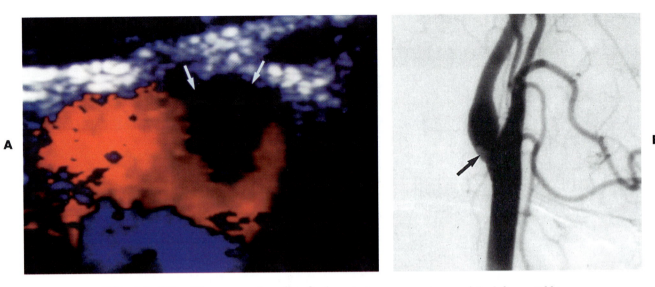

FIG. 28-32. Fibromuscular dysplasia. A, A transverse image of the left carotid bifurcation demonstrates a hypoechoic filling defect *(arrows)* in the region of the carotid bulb without evidence of color flow Doppler aliasing to suggest velocity increases. This hypoechoic mass deformed mildly with blood flow. **B,** An angiogram confirms a small filling defect in the same area *(arrow)* consistent with thrombus associated with possible atypical FMD in a young female. Follow-up ultrasound after 1 month of anticoagulation treatment demonstrated a completely normal-appearing carotid bulb.

rently demonstrating comparable accuracy to ultrasound and angiography for the detection and quantification of carotid stenosis. MRA, like ultrasonography, can depict plaque morphology and can additionally evaluate the intracranial circulation. MRA may be helpful in situations where calcified plaque obscures the underlying carotid lumen from insonification.

Many investigators now suggest replacing preoperative angiography with a combination of carotid sonography and MRA. They advocate using angiography only in cases where MRA and carotid sonography have discordant results or are inadequate.[81,82] Other studies support the use of carotid sonography alone prior to endarterectomy.[83-85] Numerous studies show that greater than 90% of surgical candidates can be adequately screened using clinical assessment and ultrasound alone. However, if aortic arch proximal vessel disease is suspected, or in cases of suspected complete occlusion, some still advocate preoperative angiography.

NONATHEROSCLEROTIC CAROTID DISEASE

Nonatherosclerotic carotid disease is far less common than plaque disease. **Fibromuscular dysplasia (FMD)**, a noninflammatory process with hypertrophy of muscular and fibrous arterial walls separated by abnormal zones of fragmentation, involves the ICA more commonly than other carotid segments. A char-

acteristic "string of beads" appearance has been described on angiography. Only a few reports of the ultrasound features of FMD exist.[86,87] Many patients with FMD have nonspecific or no obvious ultrasound abnormalities demonstrated. FMD may be asymptomatic or can result in carotid dissection or subsequent thrombotic embolic events (Fig. 28-32). **Arteritis** resulting from autoimmune processes such as Takayasu's arteritis or temporal arteritis or radiation changes can produce diffuse concentric thickening of carotid walls, which most frequently involves the CCA.[88]

Cervical trauma can produce carotid **dissections** or aneurysms. Carotid dissections can also occur spontaneously as a sequelae of a vasculopathy or atherosclerotic disease without a discrete history of trauma.[89] The ultrasound examination of a carotid dissection may reveal a mobile or fixed **echogenic intimal flap** with or without thrombus formation. There frequently is a striking image/Doppler mismatch with a paucity of gray-scale abnormalities seen in association with marked flow abnormalities (Fig. 28-33). CDU or PDU may readily clarify the source of this mismatch by demonstrating abrupt tapering of the patent color flow Doppler filled lumen to the point of an ICA occlusion, analogous to the findings commonly seen on angiography. Although the ICA is frequently occluded, demonstrating absent flow with a high-resistance waveform in the proximal ipsilateral CCA, flow in the ICA may demonstrate high velocities associated with luminal narrowing secondary to

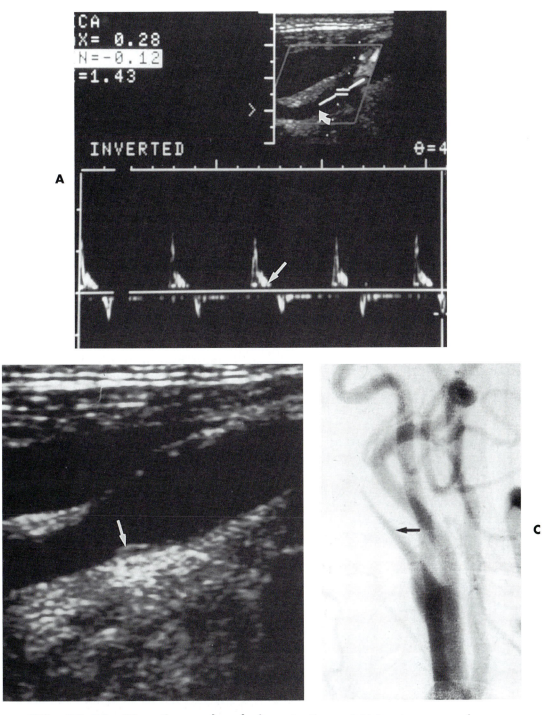

FIG. 28-33. Dissection and occlusion. A, Abnormal high-resistance waveforms *(arrow)* at the origin of the right ICA with no evidence of flow distal to this point *(curved arrow)*. B, Gray-scale evaluation of the vessel in the area of the occlusion demonstrates only a small linear echogenic structure *(arrow)* without evidence of significant atherosclerotic narrowing. C, Subsequent angiogram demonstrates the characteristic tapering to the point of occlusion *(arrow)* associated with carotid artery dissection and thrombotic occlusion.

hemorrhage and thrombus in the area of the false lumen. Accordingly, flow velocity waveforms in the CCA may be normal or demonstrate very damped, high-resistance waveforms. MRA, another noninvasive imaging test, readily demonstrates mural hematoma, confirming the diagnosis of ICA dissection. Although angiography is frequently used to initially diagnose a dissection, ultrasound can be used to follow patients to assess the therapeutic response to anticoagulation therapy. Repeat sonographic evaluation of patients with ICA dissection following anticoagulation therapy reveals recanalization of the artery in as many as 70% of cases.[90-92] It is important to consider the diagnosis of dissection as a cause of neurologic symptoms, particularly when the clinical presentation, age, and patient history are atypical for that of atherosclerotic disease or hemorrhagic stroke.

Carotid body tumors, one of several paragangliomas that involve the head and neck, are usually benign, well-encapsulated masses located at the carotid bifurcation. These tumors may be bilateral and are very vascular, often producing an audible bruit. Some of these tumors produce catecholamines, producing sudden changes in blood pressure intraoperatively or postoperatively. CDU demonstrates an extremely vascular soft-tissue mass at the carotid bifurcation (Fig. 28-34). CDU can also be used to monitor embolization or surgical resection of carotid body tumors. **Extravascular masses** such as lymph nodes, hematomas, or abscesses that compress or displace the carotids can be readily distinguished from primary vascular masses such as aneurysms or pseudoaneurysms. **Posttraumatic pseudoaneurysms** can usually be distinguished from a true carotid aneurysm by demonstrating the characteristic to-and-fro waveforms in the neck of the pseudoaneurysm as well as the internal variability ("ying-yang") characteristic of a pseudoaneurysm (Fig. 28-35).

TRANSCRANIAL DOPPLER SONOGRAPHY

In transcranial Doppler (TCD) sonography, a low-frequency, 2-MHz transducer is used to **evaluate blood flow within the intracranial carotid and vertebrobasilar system and the circle of Willis.** Access

---

SONOGRAPHIC FINDINGS IN ICA DISSECTION

ICA
Absent flow/occlusion
Echogenic intimal flap ± thrombus
Hypoechoic thrombus ± luminal narrowing
Normal appearance

CCA
High resistance waveform
Damped flow
Normal

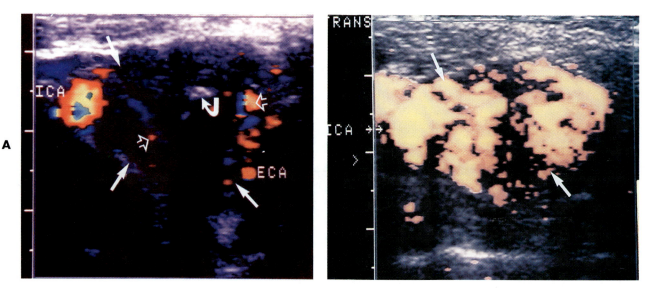

FIG. 28-34. Carotid body tumor. A, Transverse image of the carotid bifurcation that contains a hypoechoic mass *(arrows)* with some calcification *(curved arrow).* The color flow Doppler images at a carotid setting demonstrate only scattered areas of vascularity within this mass *(open arrows).* **B,** Power mode Doppler ultrasound of the same carotid body tumor demonstrates striking increased vascularity *(arrows)* when compared with the standard color flow Doppler carotid settings.

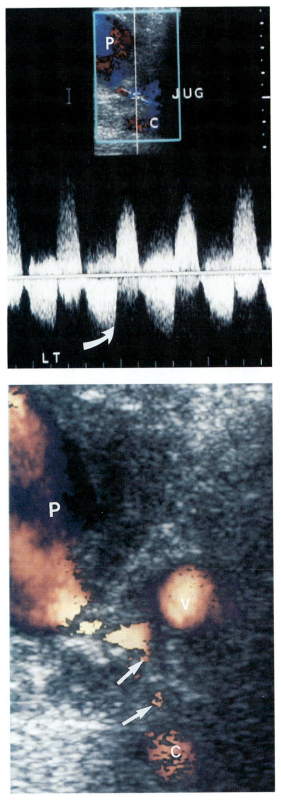

FIG. 28-35. Pseudoaneurysm. A, A transverse image of the left distal CCA, *C*, demonstrates a characteristic to-and-fro waveform *(curved arrow)* in the neck of the large pseudoaneurysm, *P*, which resulted from an attempted central venous line placement. **B,** Power mode Doppler better demonstrates the long neck *(arrows)* that extends from the CCA, *C*, to the pseudoaneurysm, *P. V,* Jugular vein.

is achieved through the orbits, foramen magnum, or, most commonly, the region of temporal calvarial thinning (**transtemporal window**).[93] However, many patients, up to 55% in one series,[94] may not have access for an interpretable TCD examination. Women, particularly African-American women, have a thick temporal bone through which it is difficult to insonate the basal cerebral arteries.[94,95] This difficulty limits the feasibility of TCD imaging as a routine part of the noninvasive cerebrovascular work-up.[94]

By using spectral analysis, various parameters, including mean velocity and peak systolic and end diastolic velocity, and pulsatility and resistive indices of the blood vessels are determined. Color flow (power mode) Doppler can improve velocity determination by providing better angle theta determination and localizing the course of vessels.[93] TCD has many applications, including evaluation of **intracranial stenoses** and **collateral circulation**, detection and follow-up of **vasoconstriction** from subarachnoid hemorrhage, determination of **brain death,** and identification of **arteriovenous malformation**.[95-98] TCD is most reliable in diagnosing stenoses of the middle cerebral artery with sensitivities as high as 91% reported.[95,96] TCD is less reliable for detecting stenoses of the intracranial vertebrobasilar system, anterior and posterior cerebral arteries, and terminal ICA.[95,96] However, TCD is helpful in assessing vertebral artery patency and flow direction when no flow is detected in the extracranial vertebral artery (Fig. 28-36). Diagnosis of an intracranial stenosis is based on an increase in mean velocity of blood flow in the affected vessel compared with the contralateral vessel at the same location.[95,96]

Advantages of TCD sonography also include its availability to be used to monitor patients in the operating room or angiographic suite for potential cerebrovascular complications.[96] Intraoperative TCD monitoring can be performed with the transducer strapped over the transtemporal window, allowing evaluation of blood flow in the MCA during carotid endarterectomy. Adequacy of cerebral perfusion can be assessed while the carotid artery is clamped.[96] TCD is also capable of detecting intraoperative microembolization ("HITS"), which produces high-amplitude "spikes" on the Doppler spectrum.[96,99] The technique can be used for the serial evaluation of vasospasm. This diagnosis is usually based on serial examinations of the relative increase in blood flow velocity and resistive index changes resulting from a decrease in the lumen of the vessel caused by vasospasm.[96]

VERTEBRAL ARTERY

The vertebral arteries supply the majority of the posterior brain circulation. Via the circle of Willis, they also

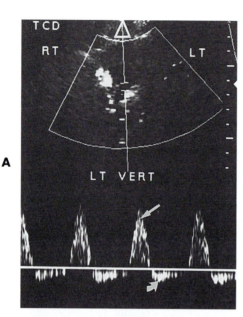

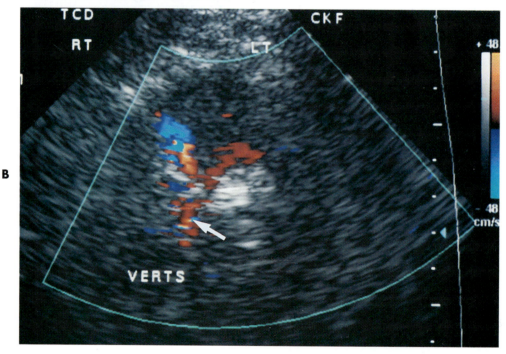

FIG. 28-36. Transcranial Doppler imaging. A, A transcranial duplex scan of the posterior fossa in a patient with an incomplete left subclavian steal syndrome demonstrates retrograde systolic flow *(arrow)* and antegrade diastolic flow *(curved arrow)*. The scan is obtained in a transverse projection from the region of the foramen magnum *(open arrowhead)*. **B,** A color flow Doppler image obtained in the same patient demonstrates that there is not only retrograde flow within the left vertebral artery, but within the basilar artery *(arrow)* as well.

provide collateral circulation to other portions of the brain in cases of carotid occlusive disease. Evaluation of the extracranial vertebral artery seems a natural extension of carotid duplex and color flow Doppler imaging.[100,101] Historically, however, these arteries have not been studied as intensively as the carotid arteries. Symptoms of vertebrobasilar insufficiency also tend to be rather vague and poorly defined, compared with symptoms referable to the carotid circulation. It is often difficult to make an association confidently between a lesion and symptoms. Furthermore, there has been relatively limited interest in surgical correction of vertebral lesions.[20] Finally, the anatomic variability,

small size, deep course, and limited visualization resulting from overlying transverse processes make the vertebral artery more difficult to examine accurately with ultrasound.[101-103] The clinical utility of vertebral duplex scanning remains under investigation. Its role in diagnosing subclavian steal and presteal phenomena is well established.[20,64,104,105] Less clear-cut is the use of vertebral duplex scanning in evaluating vertebral artery stenosis, dissection, or aneurysm.

Anatomy

The vertebral artery is usually the first branch off of the subclavian artery (Fig. 28-37). Variation in the

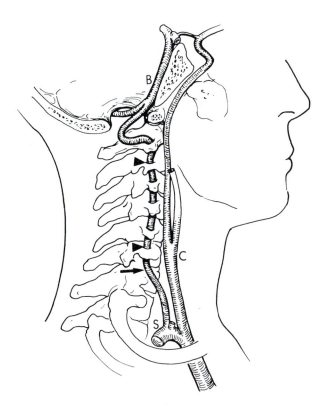

FIG. 28-37. Vertebral artery course *(arrow).* It goes through cervical spine transverse foramina *(arrowheads)* and joins the contralateral vertebral artery to form the basilar artery, *B. C*, Carotid artery; *S*, subclavian artery.

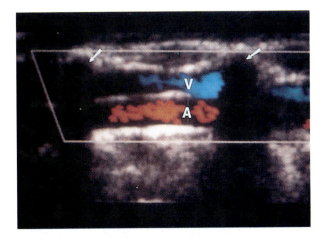

FIG. 28-38. Normal vertebral artery, A, and vein, V. Longitudinal color flow Doppler shows the vertebral artery and vein running between the transverse processes of C2-C3, which are identified by their periodic acoustical shadowing *(arrows).*

origin of the vertebral arteries is common, however. In 6% to 8% of cases, the left vertebral artery arises directly from the aortic arch proximal to the left subclavian artery. In 90% of people, the proximal vertebral artery ascends superomedially, passing anterior to the transverse process of C7, and enters the transverse foramen at the C6 level. The remainder of vertebral arteries enter into the transverse foramina at the C5 or C7 levels and, rarely, at the C4 level. Size of vertebral arteries is variable, with the left larger than the right in 42% of cases, the two vertebral arteries equal in size in 26% of cases, and the right larger than the left in 32% of cases.[106] One vertebral artery may even be congenitally absent.

Technique and Normal Examination

Vertebral artery visualization with Doppler flow analysis can be obtained in 92% to 98% of vessels (Fig. 28-38).[102,107] Color flow Doppler facilitates rapid detection of vertebral arteries, but does not significantly improve this detection rate.[103] Vertebral artery duplex examinations are performed by first locating the CCA in the longitudinal plane. The direction of flow in the CCA and jugular vein is determined. A gradual sweep of the transducer laterally demonstrates the vertebral artery and vein running between the transverse pro-

cesses of C2-C6, which are identified by their periodic acoustic shadowing. Transverse scanning with color flow Doppler allows the examiner to visualize the carotid artery and jugular vein at the same time and use them as references to determine the direction of flow in the vertebral artery.[104]

Angling the transducer caudad allows visualization of the vertebral artery origin in 60% to 70% of the arteries, 80% on the right hand side and 50% on the left. This discrepancy may relate to the fact that the left vertebral artery origin is deeper and that it arises directly from the aortic arch 6% to 8% of the time.[102,108]

The **presence and direction of flow** should be established. Visible plaque disease should be assessed. The vertebral artery supplies blood to the brain and usually has a low-resistance flow pattern similar to that of the CCA, with continuous flow in systole and diastole; however, wide variability in waveform shape has been noted in angiographically normal vessels.[109] Because the vessel is small, flow tends to demonstrate a broader spectrum. The clear spectral window seen in the normal carotid system is usually filled in the vertebral artery (Fig. 28-39).[40]

The vertebral vein (often a plexus of veins) runs parallel and adjacent to the vertebral artery. Care must be taken not to mistake its flow for that of the adjacent artery, particularly if the venous flow is pulsatile. Comparison with jugular venous flow during respiration should readily distinguish between vertebral artery and vein. At times the ascending cervical branch of the thyrocervical trunk can be mistaken for the vertebral artery. This can be avoided by looking for landmark transverse processes that accompany the vertebral artery and also by paying careful attention to the waveform of the visualized vessel. The as-

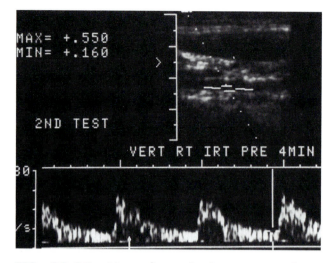

FIG. 28-39. Normal vertebral artery Doppler spectral waveform. A low-resistance flow pattern similar to common and internal carotid arteries. Spectral broadening may fill the clear spectral window *(arrow)*.

cending cervical branch has a high-impedance waveform pattern similar to that of the external carotid artery.[104]

Transcranial Doppler sonographic examination of the vertebrobasilar artery system can be performed as an adjunct to the extracranial evaluation. The examination is conducted with a 2-MHz transducer with the patient sitting, using a suboccipital midline nuchal approach, or with the patient supine, using a retromastoidal approach. Color flow or power mode Doppler facilitates transcranial imaging of the vertebrobasilar system (see Fig. 28-36).[110]

Subclavian Steal

The **subclavian steal phenomenon** occurs when there is **high-grade stenosis** or **occlusion** of the **proximal subclavian or innominate** arteries with patent vertebral arteries bilaterally. The artery of the ischemic limb "steals" blood from the vertebrobasilar circulation via retrograde vertebral artery flow, which may result in symptoms of vertebrobasilar insufficiency (Fig. 28-40). Symptoms are usually most pronounced during exercise of the upper extremity but can be produced by changes in head position. However, there is often poor correlation between vertebrobasilar symptoms and the subclavian steal phenomenon. Usually, flow within the basilar artery is unaffected unless there is severe stenosis of the vertebral artery supplying the steal.[96,110] Additionally, surgical or angioplastic restoration of blood flow may not result in relief of symptoms.[111] The subclavian steal syndrome is most commonly **caused** by **atherosclerotic** disease, although traumatic, embolic, surgical, congenital, and neoplastic factors have also been implicated. While the proximal subclavian stenosis or oc-

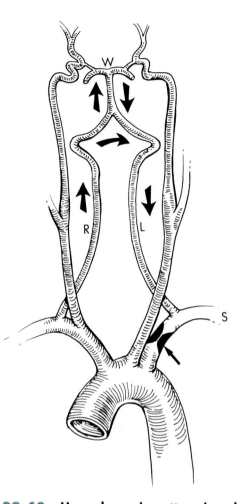

FIG. 28-40. Hemodynamic pattern in subclavian steal syndrome diagram. Proximal left subclavian artery occlusive lesion *(small arrow)* decreases flow to the distal subclavian artery, *S*. This produces retrograde flow *(large arrows)* down the left vertebral artery, *L*, and stealing from the right vertebral artery, *R*, and other intracranial vessels via the circle of Willis, *W*.

clusion may be difficult to image, particularly on the left, the vertebral artery waveform abnormalities correlate with the severity of the subclavian disease.

Doppler evaluation of the vertebral artery reveals four distinct abnormal waveforms that correlate with subclavian or vertebral artery pathology on angiography. These include the complete subclavian steal, partial or incomplete steal, presteal phenomenon, and tardus-parvus vertebral artery waveforms.[112] In a **complete subclavian steal,** there is complete reversal of flow within the vertebral artery (Fig. 28-41). **Incomplete or partial steals** demonstrate transient reversal of vertebral flow during systole (Fig. 28-42).[96,110,113] Incomplete steal suggests high-grade stenosis of the subclavian or innominate artery rather than occlusion. Provocative maneuvers such as exercising the arm for 5 min or 5-min inflation of a sphyg-

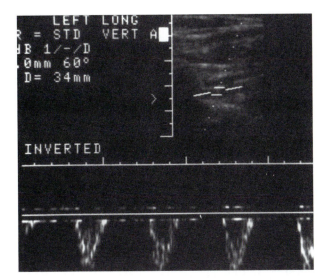

FIG. 28-41. Reversed flow in the vertebral artery, diagnostic of subclavian steal. The Doppler spectrum has been inverted, so cephalic flow should project above the baseline if flow was in the normal direction.

ABNORMAL VERTEBRAL ARTERY WAVEFORMS

Complete subclavian steal

Reversal of flow within the vertebral artery ipsilateral to the stenotic or occluded subclavian or innominate artery

Incomplete or partial subclavian steal

Transient reversal of vertebral artery flow during systole

May be converted into a complete steal by provocative maneuvers

Suggests stenotic, not occlusive, lesion

Presteal phenomenon

"Bunny" waveform: systolic deceleration less than diastolic flow

May be converted into partial steal by provocative maneuvers

Seen with proximal subclavian stenosis

Tardus-parvus or damped waveform

Seen with vertebral artery stenosis

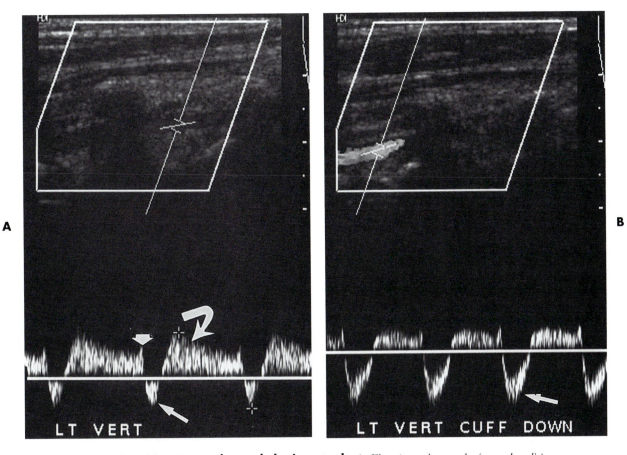

FIG. 28-42. Incomplete subclavian steal. A, Flow in early systole *(arrowhead)* is antegrade; flow in peak systole *(arrow)* is retrograde; and flow in late systole and diastole *(curved arrow)* is again antegrade. **B,** Following provocative maneuvers, the amount of retrograde flow in peak and late systole has increased *(arrow)*.

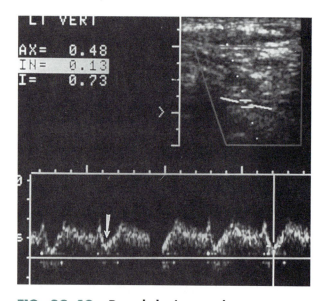

FIG. 28-43. Presubclavian steal. A pulsed wave Doppler trace in the left vertebral artery demonstrates peak systolic deceleration *(arrow)* in a patient with a "presteal" waveform. There was a 50% diameter proximal left subclavian artery stenosis.

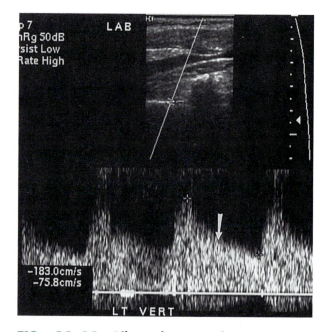

FIG. 28-44. Bilateral ICA occlusion and increased collateral flow into the vertebral artery. A pulsed wave Doppler spectral trace from a left vertebral artery demonstrates strikingly high velocities and disturbed flow *(arrow)*. While this degree of velocity elevation and flow disturbance could be associated with a focal stenosis, in this case there was increased velocity throughout the vertebral artery.

momanometer on the arm to induce rebound hyperemia on the side of the subclavian or innominate lesion can enhance the sonographic findings and may convert an incomplete steal to a complete steal.[86,105]

The presteal or "bunny" waveform shows antegrade flow, but with a striking deceleration of velocity in mid to late systole to a level less than end diastolic velocity and is seen in patients with proximal subclavian stenosis, as with the partial steal waveform (Fig. 28-43).[112] The "bunny" waveform can be converted into a partial steal or complete steal waveform by provocative maneuvers. A damped, tardus-parvus waveform can be seen in patients with high-grade proximal vertebral stenosis.[110]

With subclavian steal, color flow Doppler imaging may show two similarly color-encoded vessels between the transverse processes, representing the vertebral artery and vein.[64] Transverse images of the vertebral artery with color flow Doppler imaging show reversed flow when compared with the CCA.[101] A Doppler spectral waveform must be produced in all such cases to avoid mistaking flow reversal within an artery for flow in a pulsatile vertebral vein.[64,104]

Stenosis and Occlusion

Diagnosis of **vertebral artery stenosis** is more difficult than diagnosis of flow reversal. Most hemodynamically significant stenoses occur at the origin, which is situated deep in the upper thorax and can be seen in only approximately 60% to 70% of patients.[102,107,108] Even if the subclavian vertebral artery

origin is visualized, optimal adjustments of the Doppler angle for accurate velocity measurements may be difficult because of the deep location and vessel tortuosity. No accurate reproducible criteria for evaluating vertebral artery stenosis exist. As flow is normally "turbulent" within the vertebral artery, spectral broadening cannot be used as an indicator of stenosis. Velocity measurements are not reliable as criteria for stenosis because of the wide normal variation in vertebral artery diameter. Although velocities greater than 100 cm/s often indicate stenosis, they can occur in angiographically normal vessels. For instance, high flow velocity may be present in a vertebral artery that is serving as a major collateral pathway for cerebral circulation in cases of carotid occlusion (Fig. 28-44).[108] Thus only a **focal increase in velocity of at least 50%, visible stenosis on gray-scale or color flow Doppler, or a striking tardus-parvus vertebral artery waveform** is likely to indicate significant vertebral stenosis. Variability of resistivity indices in normal and abnormal vertebral arteries precludes the use of this parameter as an indicator of vertebral disease.[109]

Diagnosis of **vertebral artery occlusion** is also difficult. Often, inability to detect arterial flow is due to a small or congenitally absent vertebral artery or a technically difficult examination. Differentiation of severe stenosis from occlusion is difficult for the same reasons. Furthermore, markedly dampened blood flow velocity in high-grade stenoses and a decreased number of RBCs traversing the area evaluated may result in a Doppler signal with amplitude too low to be detected.[103] Power mode Doppler imaging may prove useful in this situation. Visualization of only a vertebral vein is very suggestive of vertebral artery occlusion or congenital absence.

INTERNAL JUGULAR VEIN

The internal jugular veins are the major vessels responsible for return of venous blood from the brain. The most common clinical indication for duplex and color flow sonography of the internal jugular vein is the evaluation of suspected **jugular venous thrombosis.**[114-121] Thrombus formation may be related to central venous catheter placement. Other indications include diagnosis of jugular venous ectasia[122-125] and guidance for internal jugular or subclavian vein cannulation,[126-128] particularly in difficult situations where vascular anatomy is distorted.

Technique

The normal internal jugular vein is easily visualized. The vein is scanned with the neck extended and the head turned to the contralateral side. Longitudinal and transverse scans are obtained with light transducer pressure on the neck to avoid collapsing the vein. A coronal view from the supraclavicular fossa is used to image the lower segment of the internal jugular vein and medial segment of the subclavian vein as they join to form the brachiocephalic vein.

The jugular vein lies lateral and anterior to the CCA, lateral to the thyroid gland, and deep to the sternocleidomastoid muscle (see Fig. 28-2). The vessel has sharply echogenic walls and a hypoechoic or anechoic lumen. Normally a valve can be visualized in its distal portion.[117,119,129] The right internal jugular vein is usually larger than the left.[124]

Real-time sonography demonstrates venous pulsations related to right heart contractions as well as changes in venous diameter that vary with changes in intrathoracic pressure. Doppler examination graphically depicts these flow patterns (Fig. 28-45). On inspiration, negative intrathoracic pressure causes flow toward the heart and the jugular veins to decrease in diameter. During expiration and during Valsalva's maneuver, increased intrathoracic pressure causes a decrease in the blood return and the veins enlarge; little or no flow is noted. Walls of the normal jugular vein collapse completely when moderate transducer pressure is applied. Sudden sniffing reduces intrathoracic pressure, causing momentary collapse of the vein

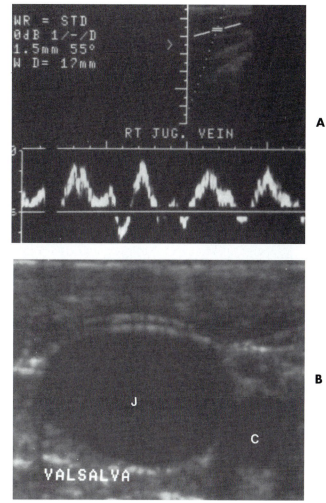

FIG. 28-45. Normal jugular vein. A, Complex venous pulsations in the jugular vein reflect the cycle of events in the right atrium. **B,** During Valsalva's maneuver, increased intrathoracic pressure causes a decrease in the blood return to the heart and the internal jugular vein, *J,* enlarges. *C,* CCA.

on real-time sonography, accompanied by a brief increase in venous flow toward the heart as shown by Doppler examination.[116,118-120]

Thrombosis

Clinical features of jugular venous thrombosis (JVT) include a tender, ill-defined, nonspecific neck mass or swelling. The correct diagnosis may not be immediately obvious.[117] Thrombosis of the internal jugular vein can be completely asymptomatic because of the deep position of the vein and the presence of abundant collateral circulation.[120] This condition was previously diagnosed by venography, an invasive procedure prompted only by a high index of suspicion. With the introduction of noninvasive techniques such as ultrasound, computed tomography (CT),[130] and MRA,[131] JVT is being identi-

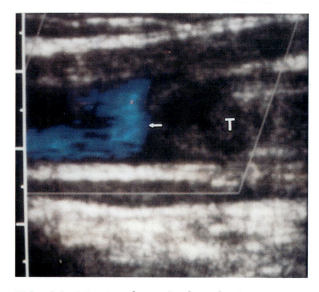

FIG. 28-46. Jugular vein thrombosis. Longitudinal color flow Doppler image demonstrates flow *(arrow)* superior to echogenic thrombus, T.

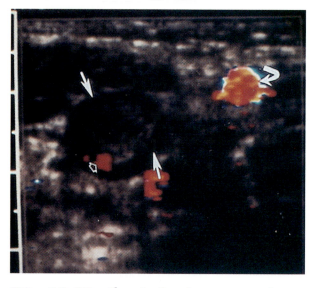

FIG. 28-47. Chronic jugular venous thrombosis with increased venous flow in a collateral vein *(curved arrow).* Transverse color flow Doppler image. Echogenic thrombus *(arrows)* nearly fills the right jugular lumen. A small recanalized channel shows flow *(open arrow).*

fied more frequently. Internal jugular thrombosis most commonly results from complications of **central venous catheterization**.[115,119,120] Other causes include **intravenous drug abuse, mediastinal tumor, hypercoagulable states, neck surgery**, and **local inflammation/adenopathy**.[117] Some cases are idiopathic or spontaneous.[118] Possible complications of JVT include suppurative thrombophlebitis, clot propagation, and pulmonary embolism.[117,121]

Real-time examination[114-121] reveals an enlarged noncompressible vein, which may contain visible echogenic intraluminal thrombus. **Acute thrombus** may be anechoic and indistinguishable from flowing blood; however, characteristic lack of compressibility and absent Doppler or color flow Doppler in the region of a thrombus quickly leads to the correct diagnosis. In addition, there is visible loss of vein response to respiratory maneuvers and venous pulsation. Spectral and color flow Doppler interrogations reveal absent flow (Fig. 28-46). Collateral veins may be identified (Fig. 28-47), particularly in cases of chronic internal JVT. Central liquefaction or other heterogeneity of the thrombus also suggests chronicity. **Chronic thrombi** may be difficult to visualize because they tend to organize and are difficult to separate from echogenic perivascular fatty tissue.[119] Absence of cardiorespiratory phasicity in a patent jugular or subclavian vein can indicate a more central nonocclusive thrombus. Confirmation of bilateral loss of venous pulsations strongly supports a more central thrombus, which can be documented by venography or MRA.

Thrombus related to catheter insertion is often demonstrated at the tip of the catheter, although it may be seen anywhere along the course of the vein. The catheter can be visualized as two parallel echogenic lines separated by an anechoic region. Flow is not commonly demonstrated in the catheter, even if the catheter itself is patent.

Ultrasound has proved to be a reliable means of diagnosing jugular and subclavian vein thrombosis and has the advantage over CT and MRI of being inexpensive, portable, and nonionizing, and requiring no intravenous contrast. Ultrasound has limited access and cannot image all portions of the jugular and subclavian veins, especially those located behind the mandible or below the clavicle. However, knowledge of the full extent of thrombus is not frequently a critical factor in treatment planning.[117,121] Serial sonographic examination to evaluate response to therapy after the initial assessment can be performed safely and inexpensively. Furthermore, ultrasound can document venous patency prior to vascular line placement, facilitating safer and more successful catheter insertion.

REFERENCES

1. Carroll BA. Carotid sonography. *Radiology* 1991;178:303-313.
2. Executive Committee for the Asymptomatic Carotid Atherosclerotic Study. Endarterectomy for asymptomatic carotid artery stenosis. *JAMA* 1995;273(18):1421-1428.
3. Fontenelle LJ, Simper SC, Hanson TL. Carotid duplex scan

versus angiography in evaluation of carotid artery disease. *Am Surg* 1994;60:864-868.

4. North American Symptomatic Carotid Endarterectomy Trial Collaborators. Beneficial effect of carotid endarterectomy in symptomatic patients with high-grade carotid stenosis. *N Engl J Med* 1991;325:445-453.

5. European Carotid Surgery Trialists' Collaborative Group. MRC European Carotid Surgery Trial: interim results for symptomatic patients with severe (70% to 99%) and mild (0 to 29%) carotid stenosis. *Lancet* 1991;337:1235-1243.

6. Neale ML, Chambers JL, Kelly AT et al. Reappraisal of duplex criteria to assess significant carotid stenosis with special reference to reports from the North American Symptomatic Carotid Endarterectomy Trial and the European Carotid Surgery Trial. *J Vasc Surg* 1994;20:642-649.

7. Chang YJ, Golby AJ, Albers GW. Detection of carotid stenosis. *Stroke* 1995;26:1325-1328.

8. Derdeyn CP, Powers WJ, Moran CJ et al. Role of Doppler US in screening for carotid atherosclerotic disease. *Radiology* 1995;197:635-643.

9. Merritt CRB, Bluth EI. The future of carotid sonography. *AJR* 1992;158:37-39.

10. Ricotta JJ. Plaque characterization by B-mode scan. *Surg Clin North Am* 1990;70(1):191-199.

11. Gerlock AJ, Giyanani VL, Krebs C. *Applications of Noninvasive Vascular Techniques.* Philadelphia: WB Saunders Co; 1988:147-159.

12. Taylor KJW. Clinical applications of carotid Doppler ultrasound. In: Taylor KJW, Burns PN, Wells PNT, eds. *Clinical Applications of Doppler Ultrasound.* New York: Raven Press; 1988:120-161.

13. Bluth EI, Shyn PB, Sullivan MA et al. Doppler color flow imaging of carotid artery dissection. *J Ultrasound Med* 1989;8:149-153.

14. Hennerici M, Steinke W, Rautenberg W. High-resistance Doppler flow pattern in extracranial carotid dissection. *Arch Neurol* 1989;46:670-672.

15. Rothrock JF, Lim V, Press G et al. Serial magnetic resonance and carotid duplex examinations in the management of carotid dissection. *Neurology* 1989;39:686-692.

16. Gritzmann N, Grasl MCH, Helmer M et al. Invasion of the carotid artery and jugular vein by lymph node metastases: detection with sonography. *AJR* 1990;154:411-414.

17. Gooding GAW, Langman AW, Dillon WP et al. Malignant carotid artery invasion: sonographic detection. *Radiology* 1989;171:435-438.

18. Steinke W, Hennerici M, Aulich A. Doppler color flow imaging of carotid body tumors. *Stroke* 1989;20:1574-1577.

19. Tihansky DP, Porter PS. Pulsed Doppler-ultrasonic diagnosis of carotid body tumor. *NY State J Med* 1989;89:580-582.

Carotid Sonographic Technique

20. Grant EG, Wong W, Tessler F et al. Cerebrovascular ultrasound imaging. *Radiol Clin North Am* 1988;26:1111-1130.

Carotid Sonographic Interpretation

21. Polak JF, O'Leary DH, Kronmal RA et al. Sonographic evaluation of carotid artery atherosclerosis in the elderly: relationship of disease severity to stroke and transient ischemic attack. *Radiology* 1993;188:363-370.

22. Veller MG, Fisher CM, Nicolaides AN et al. Measurement of the ultrasonic intima-media complex thickness in normal subjects. *J Vasc Surg* 1993;17:719-725.

23. Bort ML, Mulder PGH, Hofman A et al. Reproducibility of carotid vessel wall thickness measurements. The Rotterdam Study. *J Clin Epidemiol* 1994;47(8):921-930.

24. O'Leary DH, Polak JF. High-resolution carotid sonography: past, present, and future. *AJR* 1989;153:699-704.

25. Bluth EI, Stavros AT, Marich KW et al. Carotid duplex sonography: a multicenter recommendation for standardized imaging and Doppler criteria. *RadioGraphics* 1988;8:487-506.

26. Langsfield M, Gray-Weale AC, Lusby RJ. The role of plaque morphology and diameter reduction in the development of new symptoms in asymptomatic carotid arteries. *J Vasc Surg* 1989;9:548-557.

27. Leahy AL, McCollum PT, Feeley TM et al. Duplex ultrasonography and selection of patients for carotid endarterectomy: plaque morphology or luminal narrowing? *J Vasc Surg* 1988;8:558-562.

28. Reilly LM, Lusby RJ, Hughes L et al. Carotid plaque histology using real-time ultrasonography: clinical and therapeutic implications. *Am J Surg* 1983;146:188-193.

29. Persson AV, Robichaux WT, Silverman M. The natural history of carotid plaque development. *Arch Surg* 1983;118:1048-1052.

30. Lusby RJ, Ferrell LD, Ehrenfield WK et al. Carotid plaque hemorrhage: its role in production of cerebral ischemia. *Arch Surg* 1982;117:1479-1488.

31. Edwards JH, Kricheff II, Gorstein F et al. Atherosclerotic subintimal hematoma of the carotid artery. *Radiology* 1979;133:123-129.

32. Imparato AM, Riles TS, Gorstein F. The carotid bifurcation plaque: pathologic findings associated with cerebral ischemia. *Stroke* 1979;10:238-245.

33. Gerovlakas G, Ramaswami G, Nicolaides A et al. Characterization of symptomatic and asymptomatic carotid plaques using high-resolution real-time ultrasonography. *Br J Surg* 1993;80(10):1274-1276.

34. Holdsworth RJ, McCollum PT, Bryce JS et al. Symptoms, stenosis and carotid plaque morphology. Is plaque morphology relevant? *Eur J Vasc Endovasc Surg* 1995;9:80-85.

35. Sterpetti AV, Schultz RD, Feldhaus RJ et al. Ultrasonographic features of carotid plaque and the risk of subsequent neurologic deficits. *Surgery* 1988;104:652-660.

36. Weinberger J, Marks SJ, Gaul JJ et al. Atherosclerotic plaque at the carotid artery bifurcation: correlation of ultrasonographic imaging with morphology. *J Ultrasound Med* 1987;6:363-366.

37. Bluth EI, Kay D, Merritt CRB et al. Sonographic characterization of carotid plaque: detection of hemorrhage. *AJR* 1986;146:1061-1065.

38. Stahl JA, Middleton WD. Pseudoulceration of the carotid artery. *J Ultrasound Med* 1992;11:355-358.

39. Furst H, Hartl WH, Jansen I et al. Color-flow Doppler sonography in the identification of ulcerative plaques in patients with high grade carotid artery stenosis. *AJNR* 1992;13:1581-1587.

40. Grant EG. Duplex sonography of the cerebrovascular system. In: Grant EG, White EM, eds. *Duplex Sonography.* New York: Springer-Verlag; 1988:7-68.

41. Comerota AJ, Cranley JJ, Cook SE. Real-time B-mode carotid imaging in diagnosis of cerebrovascular disease. *Surgery* 1981;89:718-729.

42. Zwiebel WJ, Austin CW, Sackett JF et al. Correlation of high-resolution, B-mode and continuous-wave Doppler sonography with arteriography in the diagnosis of carotid stenosis. *Radiology* 1983;149:523-532.

43. Jacobs NM, Grant EG, Schellinger D et al. Duplex carotid sonography: criteria for stenosis, accuracy, and pitfalls. *Radiology* 1985;154:385-391.

44. Zwiebel WJ. Spectrum analysis in carotid sonography. *Ultrasound Med Biol* 1987;13:623-636.

45. Taylor KJW, Holland S. Doppler ultrasound: Pt I. Basic principles, instrumentation, and pitfalls. *Radiology* 1990;174:297-307.

46. Carroll BA, von Ramm OT. Fundamentals of current Doppler technology. *Ultrasound Q* 1988;6:275-298.

47. Kassam M, Johnston KW, Cobbold RSC. Quantitative estimation of spectral broadening for the diagnosis of carotid arterial disease: method and in vitro results. *Ultrasound Med Biol* 1985;11:425-433.

48. Douville Y, Johnston KW, Kassam M. Determination of the hemodynamic factors which influence the carotid Doppler spectral broadening. *Ultrasound Med Biol* 1985;11:417-423.

49. Garth KE, Carroll BA, Sommer FG et al. Duplex ultrasound scanning of the carotid arteries with velocity spectrum analysis. *Radiology* 1983;147:823-827.

50. Phillips DJ, Greene FM, Langlois Y et al. Flow velocity patterns in the carotid bifurcations of young, presumed normal subjects. *Ultrasound Med Biol* 1983;9:39-49.

51. Lichtman JB, Kibble MB. Detection of intracranial arteriovenous malformation by Doppler ultrasound of the extracranial carotid circulation. *J Ultrasound Med* 1987;6:609-612.

52. Robinson ML, Sacks D, Perlmutter GS et al. Diagnostic criteria for carotid duplex sonography. *AJR* 1988;151:1045-1049.

53. Kohler TR, Langlois Y, Roederer GO et al. Variability in measurement of specific parameters for carotid duplex examination. *Ultrasound Med Biol* 1987;13:637-642.

54. Friedman SG, Hainline B, Feinberg AW et al. Use of diastolic velocity ratios to predict significant carotid artery stenosis. *Stroke* 1988;19:910-912.

55. Hunink MGM, Polak JF, Barlan MM et al. Detection and quantification of carotid artery stenosis: efficacy of various Doppler velocity parameters. *AJR* 1993;160:619-625.

56. Moneta GL, Edwards JM, Chitwood RW. Correlation of North American Symptomatic Carotid Endarterectomy Trial (NASCET) angiographic definition of 70% to 99% internal carotid artery stenosis with duplex scanning. *J Vasc Surg* 1993;17:152-159.

57. Faught WE, Mattos MA, van Bemmelen et al. Color-flow duplex scanning of carotid arteries: new velocity criteria based on receiver operator characteristic analysis for threshold stenoses used in the symptomatic and asymptomatic carotid trials. *J Vasc Surg* 1994;19:818-828.

58. Sumner DS. Use of color-flow imaging technique in carotid artery disease. *Surg Clin North Am* 1990;70:201-211.

59. Middleton WD, Erickson S, Melson GL. Perivascular color artifact: pathologic significance and appearance on color Doppler ultrasound images. *Radiology* 1989;171:647-652.

60. Polak JF, Dobkin GR, O'Leary DH et al. Internal carotid artery stenosis: accuracy and reproducibility of color-Doppler-assisted duplex imaging. *Radiology* 1989;173:793-798.

61. Erickson SJ, Mewissen MW, Foley WD et al. Stenosis of the internal carotid artery: assessment using color Doppler imaging compared with angiography. *AJR* 1989;152:1299-1305.

62. Middleton WD, Foley WD, Lawson TL. Flow reversal in the normal carotid bifurcation: color Doppler flow imaging analysis. *Radiology* 1988;167:207-210.

63. Zierler RE, Phillips DJ, Beach KW et al. Noninvasive assessment of normal carotid bifurcation hemodynamics with color-flow ultrasound imaging. *Ultrasound Med Biol* 1987;13:471-476.

64. Erickson SJ, Middleton WD, Mewissen MW et al. Color Doppler evaluation of arterial stenoses and occlusions involving the neck and thoracic inlet. *RadioGraphics* 1989;9:389-406.

65. Middleton WD, Foley WD, Lawson TL. Color-flow Doppler imaging of carotid artery abnormalities. *AJR* 1988;150:419-425.

66. Merritt CRB. Doppler color flow imaging. *J Clin Ultrasound* 1987;15:591-597.

67. Branas CC, Weingarten MS, Czeredarczuk M et al. Examination of carotid arteries with quantitative color Doppler flow imaging. *J Ultrasound Med* 1994;13:121-127.

68. Griewing B, Driesner F, Kallwellis G et al. Cerebrovascular disease assessed by color-flow and power Doppler ultrasonography. *Stroke* 1996;27:95-100.

69. Taylor DC, Strandness DE. Carotid artery duplex scanning. *J Clin Ultrasound* 1987;15:635-644.

70. Zbornikova V, Lassvik C. Duplex scanning in presumably normal persons of different ages. *Ultrasound Med Biol* 1986;12:371-378.

71. O'Boyle MK, Vibhaker NI, Chung J et al. Duplex sonography of the carotid arteries in patients with isolated aortic stenosis: imaging findings and relation to severity of stenosis. *AJR* 1996;166:197-202.

72. Hayes AC, Johnston W, Baker WH et al. The effect of contralateral disease on carotid Doppler frequency. *Surgery* 1988;103:19-23.

73. Blackshear WM, Phillips DJ, Chikos PM et al. Carotid artery velocity patterns in normal and stenotic vessels. *Stroke* 1980;11:67-71.

74. Berman SS, Devine JJ, Erdoes LS et al. Distinguishing carotid artery pseudo-occlusion with color-flow Doppler. *Stroke* 1995;26:434-438.

75. Görtter M, Niethammer R, Widder B. Differentiating subtotal carotid artery stenoses from occlusions by colour-coded duplex sonography. *J Neurol* 1994;241:301-305.

76. Kliewer MA, Freed KS, Hertzberg BS et al. Temporal artery tap: usefulness and limitations in carotid sonography. In press. *Radiology*.

77. Bebry AJ, Hines GL. Total occlusion of the common carotid artery with a patent internal carotid artery; report of a case. *J Vasc Surg* 1989;10:469-470.

78. Blackshear WM, Phillips DJ, Bodily KC et al. Ultrasonic demonstration of external and internal carotid patency with common carotid occlusion: a preliminary report. *Stroke* 1980;11:249-252.

79. Executive Committee for the Asymptomatic Carotid Atherosclerosis Study. Endarterectomy for asymptomatic carotid artery stenosis. *JAMA* 1995;273:1421-1428.

80. Alexandrov AV, Bladin CF, Maggisano R et al. Measuring carotid stenosis—time for a reappraisal. *Stroke* 1993;24(9):1292-1296.

81. Polak JF, Kalina P, Donaldson MC et al. Carotid endarterectomy: preoperative evaluation of candidates with combined Doppler sonography and MR angiography. *Radiology* 1993;186:333-338.

82. Nicholas GG, Osborne MA, Jaffee JW et al. Carotid artery stenosis: preoperative noninvasive evaluation in a community hospital. *J Vasc Surg* 1995;22:9-16.

83. Mattos MA, Hodgson KJ, Faught WE et al. Carotid endarterectomy without angiography: is color-flow duplex scanning sufficient? *Surgery* 1994;116:776-783.

84. Cartier R, Cartier P, Fontaine A. Carotid endarterectomy without angiography. The reliability of Doppler ultrasonography and duplex scanning in preoperative assessment. *CJS* 1993;36(5):411-415.

85. Fontenelle LJ, Simper SC, Hanson TL. Carotid duplex scan versus angiography in evaluation of carotid artery disease. *Am Surg* 1994;60(11):864-868.

Carotid Sonographic Interpretation

86. Furie DM, Tien RD. Fibromuscular dysplasia of arteries of the head and neck: imaging findings. *AJR* 1994;162:1205-1209.

87. Kliewer MA, Carroll BA. Ultrasound case of the day. *RadioGraphics* 1991;11:504-505.

88. Maeda H, Handa N, Matsumoto M et al. Carotid lesions detected by B-mode ultrasonography in Takayasu's arteritis: "macaroni sign" as an indicator of the disease. *Ultrasound Med Biol* 1991;17(7):695-701.

89. Gardner OJ, Gosink BB, Kallman CE. Internal carotid artery dissections: duplex ultrasound imaging. *J Ultrasound Med* 1991;10:607-614.

90. Sturzenegger M. Spontaneous internal carotid artery dissection: early diagnosis and management in 44 patients. *J Neurol* 1995;242:231-238.

91. Sturzenegger M, Mattle HP, Rivoir A et al. Ultrasound findings in carotid artery dissection: analysis of 43 patients. *Neurology* 1995;45:691-698.

92. Steinke W, Rautemberg W, Scjwartz A et al. Noninvasive monitoring of internal carotid artery dissection. *Stroke* 1994;25(5):998-1005.

Transcranial Doppler

93. Lupetin AR, Davis DA, Beckman J et al. Transcranial Doppler sonography. Pt 1. Principles, technique and normal appearance. *RadioGraphics* 1995;15(1):179-191.

94. Comerota AJ, Katz ML, Hosking JD et al. Is transcranial Doppler a worthwhile addition to screening tests for cerebrovascular disease? *J Vasc Surg* 1995;21:90-97.

95. Rorick MB, Nichols FT, Adams RJ. Transcranial Doppler correlation with angiography in detection of intracranial stenosis. *Stroke* 1994;25:1931-1934.

96. Lupetin AR, Davis DA, Beckman et al. Transcranial Doppler sonography. Pt 2. Evaluation of intracranial and extracranial abnormalities and procedural monitoring. *RadioGraphics* 1995;15:193-209.

97. Lin SU, Ryu SJ, Chu NS. Carotid Doppler and transcranial color coded sonography in evaluation of carotid-cavernous sinus fistulas. *J Ultrasound Med* 1994;13:557-564.

98. Mast H, Mohr JP, Thompson JLP et al. Transcranial Doppler ultrasonography in cerebral arteriovenous malformation. *Stroke* 1995;26:1024-1027.

99. Gaunt ME, Martin PJ, Smith JL et al. Clinical relevance of intraoperative embolization detected by transcranial Doppler sonography during carotid endarterectomy: a prospective study of 100 patients. *Br J Surg* 1994;81:1435-1439.

Vertebral Artery

100. Bendick PJ, Glover JL. Hemodynamic evaluation of vertebral arteries by duplex ultrasound. *Surg Clin North Am* 1990;70:235-244.

101. Lewis BD, James EM, Welch TJ. Current applications of duplex and color Doppler ultrasound imaging: carotid and peripheral vascular system. *Mayo Clin Proc* 1989;64:1147-1157.

102. Visona A, Lusiani L, Castellani V et al. The echo-Doppler (duplex) system for the detection of vertebral artery occlusive disease: comparison with angiography. *J Ultrasound Med* 1986;5:247-250.

103. Davis PC, Nilsen B, Braun IF et al. A prospective comparison of duplex sonography vs angiography of the vertebral arteries. *AJNR* 1986;7:1059-1064.

104. Bluth EI, Merritt CRB, Sullivan MA et al. Usefulness of duplex ultrasound in evaluating vertebral arteries. *J Ultrasound Med* 1989;8:229-235.

105. Walker DW, Acker JD, Cole CA. Subclavian steal syndrome detected with duplex pulsed Doppler sonography. *AJNR* 1982;3:615-618.

106. Elias DA, Weinberg PE. Angiography of the posterior fossa. In: Taveras JM, Ferrucci JT, eds. *Radiology: Diagnosis-Imaging-Intervention.* Philadelphia: JB Lippincott Co; 1989;3:6-7.

107. Bendick PJ, Jackson VP. Evaluation of the vertebral arteries with duplex sonography. *J Vasc Surg* 1986;3:523-530.

108. Ackerstaff RGA, Grosveld WJHM, Eikelboom BC et al. Ultrasonic duplex scanning of the prevertebral segment of the vertebral artery in patients with cerebral atherosclerosis. *Eur J Vasc Surg* 1988;2:387-393.

109. Carroll BA, Holder CA. Vertebral artery duplex sonography (abstract). *J Ultrasound Med* 1990;9:S27-28.

110. deBray JM et al. Effect of subclavian syndrome on the basilar artery. *Acta Neurol Scand* 1994;90:174-178.

111. Thomassen L, Aarli JA. Subclavian steal phenomenon. *Acta Neurol Scand* 1994;90:241-244.

112. Courneya DL, Carroll BA. Vertebral artery pre-steal waveform: the "bunny" waveform. Presented at the 1995 Radiological Society of North America.

113. Branchereau A, Magnon PE, Espinoza H et al. Subclavian artery stenosis: hemodynamic aspects and surgical outcome. *J Cardiovasc Surg* 1991;32:604-611.

Internal Jugular Vein

114. Williams CE, Lamb GHR, Roberts D et al. Venous thrombosis in the neck: the role of real time ultrasound. *Eur J Radiol* 1989;9:32-36.

115. Hubsch PJS, Stiglbauer RL, Schwaighofer BWAM et al. Internal jugular and subclavian vein thrombosis caused by central venous catheters: evaluation using Doppler blood flow imaging. *J Ultrasound Med* 1988;7:629-636.

116. Gaitini D, Kaftori JK, Pery M et al. High-resolution real-time ultrasonography: diagnosis and follow-up of jugular and subclavian vein thrombosis. *J Ultrasound Med* 1988;7:621-627.

117. Albertyn LE, Alcock MK. Diagnosis of internal jugular vein thrombosis. *Radiology* 1987;162:505-508.

118. Falk RL, Smith DF. Thrombosis of upper extremity thoracic inlet veins: diagnosis with duplex Doppler sonography. *AJR* 1987;149:677-682.

119. Weissleder R, Elizondo G, Stark DD. Sonographic diagnosis of subclavian and internal jugular vein thrombosis. *J Ultrasound Med* 1987;6:577-587.

120. De Witte BR, Lameris JS. Real-time ultrasound diagnosis of internal jugular vein thrombosis. *J Clin Ultrasound* 1986;14:712-717.

121. Wing V, Scheible W. Sonography of jugular vein thrombosis. *AJR* 1983;140:333-336.

122. Gribbin C, Raghavendra BN, Ginsburg HB. Ultrasound diagnosis of jugular venous ectasia. *NY State J Med* 1989;9:532-533.

123. Hughes PL, Qureshi SA, Galloway RW. Jugular venous aneurysm in children. *Br J Radiol* 1988;61:1082-1084.

124. Jasinski RW, Rubin JM. Computed tomography and ultrasonographic findings in jugular vein ectasia. *J Ultrasound Med* 1984;3:417-420.

125. Stevens RK, Fried AM, Hood TR. Ultrasonic diagnosis of jugular venous aneurysm. *J Clin Ultrasound* 1982;10:85-87.

126. Lee W, Leduc L, Cotton DB. Ultrasonographic guidance for central venous access during pregnancy. *Am J Obstet Gynecol* 1989;161:1012-1013.

127. Bond DM, Nolan R. Real-time ultrasound imaging aids jugular venipuncture. *Anesth Analg* 1989;68:700-701.

128. Machi J, Takeda J, Kakegawa T. Safe jugular and subclavian venipuncture under ultrasonographic guidance. *Am J Surg* 1987;153:321-323.

129. Dresser LP, McKinney WM. Anatomic and pathophysiologic studies of the human internal jugular valve. *Am J Surg* 1987;154:220-224.

130. Patel S, Brennan J. Diagnosis of internal jugular vein thrombosis by computed tomography. *J Comput Assist Tomogr* 1981;5:197-200.

131. Braun IF, Hoffman JC, Malko JA et al. Jugular venous thrombosis: magnetic resonance imaging. *Radiology* 1985;157:357-360.

CHAPTER 29

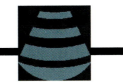

The Peripheral Arteries

•

Joseph F. Polak, M.D., M.P.H.

The arteries of the upper and lower extremities are easily accessible to sonographic imaging. They are free from many of the technical limitations and acoustic interference that normally plague imaging of the abdominal and thoracic vessels. There are enough imaging windows to permit the positioning of the transducer directly over the artery of interest without any loss of signal due to overlying bone. High-resolution imaging transducers with frequencies above 5 MHz can routinely be used since the arteries lie in close proximity to the skin, typically at depths of 6 cm or less.

Real-time gray-scale imaging is useful for evaluating the presence of atherosclerotic plaque or confirming the presence of extravascular masses. Gray-scale imaging is, however, limited in the evaluation of stenosis (Fig. 29-1). The addition of Doppler waveform analysis makes duplex ultrasonography a powerful diagnostic tool for detecting significant atherosclerotic lesions, differentiating significant arterial stenoses from occlusion, and assessing the nature of perivascular masses (e.g., differentiating hematoma from pseudoaneurysm). Color flow Doppler imaging has made it possible to directly image blood flow patterns. When compared with duplex sonography, color flow imaging can survey larger volumes of tissue and longer vascular segments in a more reasonable period of time. Not only does color flow imaging decrease the length of the peripheral arterial examination as compared with duplex sonography alone, it also improves diagnostic accuracy.[1,2] Power mode Doppler imaging, with or without the use of ultrasound contrast agents, may further improve

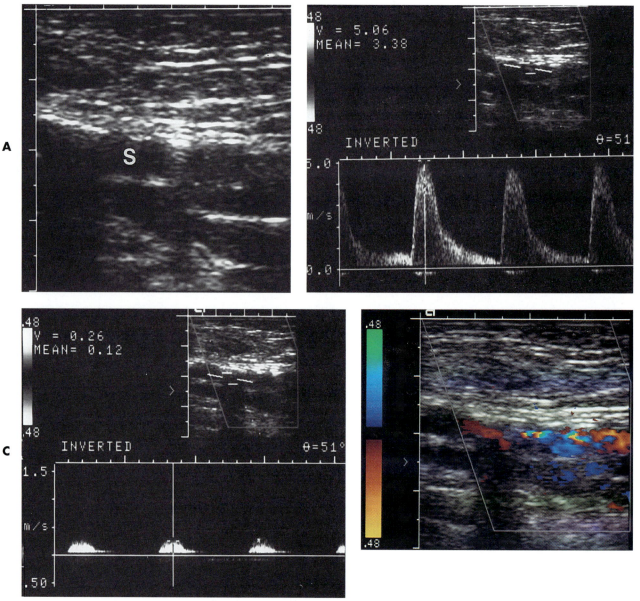

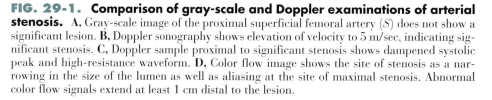

FIG. 29-1. **Comparison of gray-scale and Doppler examinations of arterial stenosis.** **A,** Gray-scale image of the proximal superficial femoral artery (S) does not show a significant lesion. **B,** Doppler sonography shows elevation of velocity to 5 m/sec, indicating significant stenosis. **C,** Doppler sample proximal to significant stenosis shows dampened systolic peak and high-resistance waveform. **D,** Color flow image shows the site of stenosis as a narrowing in the size of the lumen as well as aliasing at the site of maximal stenosis. Abnormal color flow signals extend at least 1 cm distal to the lesion.

the diagnostic accuracy of sonography. It is therefore not surprising that ultrasound imaging is increasingly used to evaluate the patient with suspected or confirmed arterial disease.

When compared to angiography, the sonographic approaches discussed in this chapter have the advantage of being noninvasive, relatively inexpensive, and well suited for serial examinations. Computed tomographic angiography (CTA) can be competitive with sonography, but it is more expensive, involves ionizing radiation, and requires intravenous contrast material.

CTA also has lower resolution than sonography and cannot image small changes in the lumen of arteries less than 5 mm in size. Magnetic resonance angiography (MRA) can be used to detect significant stenoses and arterial occlusions. Magnetic resonance imaging (MRI) can be used to evaluate suspected extravascular processes. In general, CTA and MRA are much less interactive but are often more reproducible than sonography. Whether MRA and CTA will prove to be more cost-effective than sonography for evaluating the peripheral arterial system remains to be seen.

INSTRUMENTATION

Real-Time Gray-Scale Imaging

The peripheral arteries of interest vary in size from 1 to 6 mm. Accurate visualization of the arterial lumen to determine the presence of atherosclerotic lesions requires high-resolution transducers, typically more than 3.5 MHz. Carrier frequencies in the range of 5 to 10 MHz are preferred. A good compromise is a center frequency near 5 MHz since it offers good resolution and depth penetration in larger regions such as the thigh. For detailed visualization of smaller arteries, a central frequency near 7 MHz is preferred. The 10-MHz transducers have limited penetration but are useful for examining very superficial structures such as bypass grafts and small vessels such as the ulnar and radial arteries.

The linear phased array transducer is ideal for imaging the extremity arteries. The transducer has sufficient length to permit rapid coverage of long arterial segments by holding it longitudinal to the artery and by sliding it in a series of nonoverlapping increments. Smaller footprint curved array or sector transducers are useful for imaging deeper vessels such as the iliac arteries and the central portions of the subclavian arteries.

Doppler Sonography

Electronically steered ultrasound transducers have replaced mechanical transducers for simultaneous gray-scale imaging and Doppler analysis. Duplex sonography, which is the simultaneous display of Doppler spectral information and of the gray-scale image, is a necessity for examining the peripheral arteries and arterial bypass grafts.[3] Careful real-time control is needed to position the Doppler sample gate and to accurately detect sites of maximal blood flow velocity in small arteries. The Doppler frequencies used vary between 3 to 10 MHz, tending to be lower than the frequencies used for the simultaneously acquired gray-scale image. A 5 MHz frequency is often used because it allows detection of slowly moving blood and yet avoids aliasing that can occur at sites of rapidly moving blood, such as stenoses or arteriovenous fistulas.

Color flow Doppler imaging is now considered a necessity for peripheral arterial sonography. The simultaneous display of moving blood superimposed on a gray-scale image has made it possible to rapidly survey the flow patterns within long sections of the peripheral arteries and bypass grafts.[4] In general, an efficient approach to peripheral vascular sonography relies on color flow Doppler sonography to rapidly identify zones of flow disturbances and then on duplex sonography with Doppler spectral analysis to characterize the type of flow abnormality present.[1,5] The color Doppler image displays only the mean frequency shift caused by moving structures. Most manufacturers will use lower frequencies for the color flow image than for the gray-scale image. This approach, in part, overcomes early aliasing of the color flow image that occurs at the lower frame rates used for the color display.

Power mode Doppler imaging is a variant of color flow imaging that displays information on the motion of blood. Advantages over color flow imaging are that the blood flow information does not alias, the signal strength is much less angle dependent, and that slowly moving blood is more conspicuous. A disadvantage is the loss of information pertaining to the direction of blood flow.

ARTERIAL DOPPLER FLOW PATTERNS

Normal Arteries

The normal Doppler pattern of arterial flow in the extremity is a high-resistance waveform reflecting constriction of the small vessels of the muscles distally (Fig. 29-2). This is in sharp contrast to the persistent low-resistance profile seen in the internal and common carotid arteries. The typical extremity flow profile is a **triphasic pattern** (Table 29-1). This consists of a strong forward component of blood flow during systole, followed by a short reversal of flow during early diastole. A return to forward flow of lower amplitude normally follows and lasts for a variable length of diastole. The diastolic portion of blood flow is extremely variable, disappearing with vasoconstriction due to cold or increasing with warmth or following exercise.

Stenotic Arteries

The normal high-resistance pattern typically becomes a low-resistance pattern when significant arterial disease is present proximal to the region being sampled. This low-resistance pattern resembles that of the internal carotid artery and reflects the opening of collateral vessels and the loss of the normal arteriolar tone in response to muscle ischemia. It is typically seen distal to an arterial occlusion but can also be seen distal to high-grade stenotic lesions.

A localized increase in velocity occurs at the site of a stenosis. This increase is detected as a shift in Doppler frequency proportional to the lumen diameter narrowing across which the blood is flowing.[6-8] This can be shown as an increase in peak systolic velocity on the Doppler spectral display or by a decrease in color saturation or even aliasing on the color map (see Fig. 29-1). The motion of blood distal to the stenosis becomes less organized and shows a large variation in both direction and velocity, and this effect is maintained over a distance of one or more centimeters. This

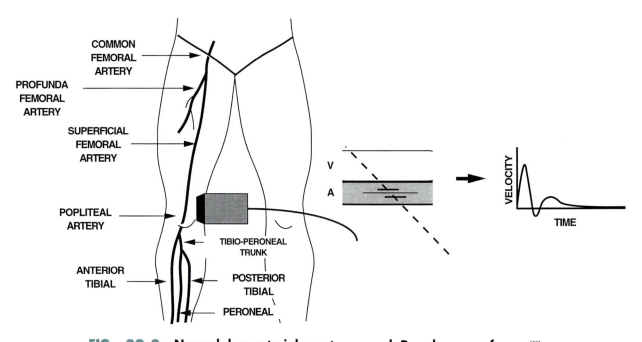

FIG. 29-2. Normal leg arterial anatomy and Doppler waveform. The normal Doppler spectrum of flowing blood in the lower extremity arteries has a triphasic pattern: (1) forward flow during systole, (2) short period of flow reversal in early diastole, and (3) a variable amount of low-velocity flow during the remainder of diastole. Arterial Doppler signals used to measure blood flow velocities should be sampled with the transducer held parallel to the vessel and with the angle between the direction of the ultrasound beam and the direction of blood flow kept at 60 degrees or less.

zone of turbulence is detected on Duplex sonography as a broadening of the spectral window and as increased variance on color flow Doppler imaging.

Arteriovenous Fistulas

Arteriovenous (A-V) fistulas can be classified as **congenital** or **iatrogenic.** Congenital A-V fistulas are the abnormal communications between artery and larger distended venous channels. These are usually obvious clinically and are located close to the skin surface of the involved extremity. These are normally visualized as distended venous channels into which feed single or multiple arterial branches. When small A-V fistulas are distended, veins may not have had a chance to develop, and the abnormality is only seen as increase in venous velocity due to the fistula.

Iatrogenic communications may arise following selective arterial or venous catheterization or other forms of penetrating trauma. The communication can often be visualized as a jet of blood, with the draining vein being abnormally distended when compared with the other side (Fig. 29-3). Blood flow in the recipient vein is often arterialized. The jet of blood has high-velocity signals within it, which can cause a perivascular Doppler artifact which is due to tissue movement (bruit).[9] A common cause of a false-positive sonographic diagnosis of A-V fistula is a hematoma that

causes compression of the vein, resulting in a high-velocity, although not pulsatile, signal in the vein.

Vascular Masses—Pseudoaneurysm

The differential diagnosis of perivascular masses is dramatically aided by the use of both duplex and color flow Doppler ultrasound. The presence of blood flow within a cystic mass contiguous to an artery suggests the diagnosis of **pseudoaneurysm,** which is a complication that sometimes develops following arterial catheterization or penetrating trauma. A typical swirling motion or color "ying-yang" sign is typically seen within the cystic mass.[10,11] With iatrogenic or traumatic pseudoaneurysms, a small diameter neck is seen as a communicating channel between the artery and the cystic mass.[12] The duplex sonographic finding of a **"to-and-fro" sign** is typically detected in the communicating channel of the pseudoaneurysm (Fig. 29-4). The "to" component is due to blood entering during systole as expansion occurs in the pseudoaneurysm (Fig. 29-5). Often, a high-velocity scale (pulse repetition frequency or PRF) is needed for detection since the flow in the channel is of a very high velocity. The "fro" component is seen during diastole as the blood stored in the cavity is ejected back into the artery. The "fro" component is more prominent if the pseudoaneurysm expands efficiently and if there is

TABLE 29-1

ARTERIAL DOPPLER FLOW PATTERNS AND CORRELATES

Flow Pattern	Diagram	Correlate
Triphasic signal		Normal resting signals with early diastolic reversal indicating normal distal arterial bed and sufficient run-off
Biphasic signal with absent diastolic flow		Arterial vasoconstriction or acute arterial obstruction distal to sampling site
Monophasic low-velocity flow with prolonged systolic peak (tardus parvus); absent systolic reversal, continuous antegrade flow throughout cycle		Arterial vasodilatation distal to occlusion or high-grade stenoses
Monophasic high-velocity turbulent continuous flow		Arteriovenous fistula
Forward systolic and reverse diastolic flow classically referred to as "to-and-fro"		Reverse diastolic flow in neck of pseudo-aneurysm due to compliant nature of the pseudoaneurysm

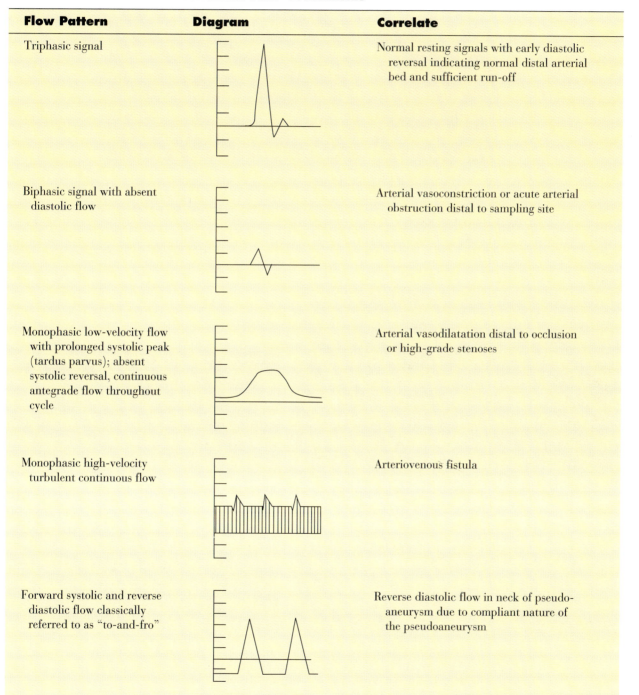

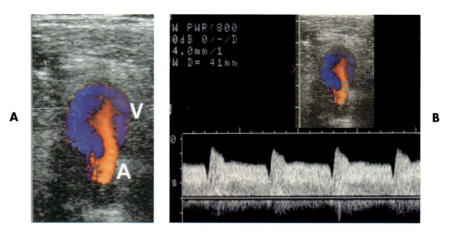

FIG. 29-3. A-V fistula flow pattern. A, This color flow image shows a high velocity jet from the profunda femoral artery, *A,* into the distended common femoral vein, *V.* **B,** The low-resistance arterial-type signals in the communication between artery and vein are typical of an arteriovenous fistula.

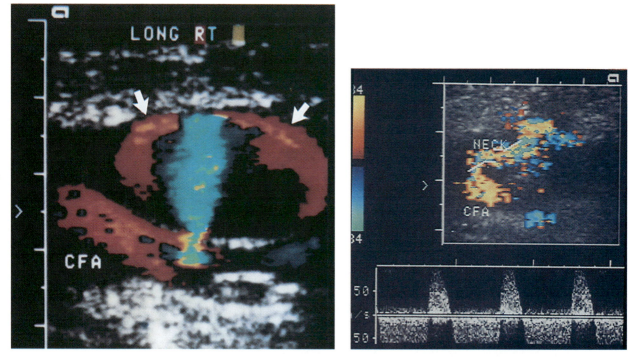

FIG. 29-4. Femoral artery pseudoaneurysms. A, Longitudinal color flow Doppler image of the right common femoral artery 1 day after arteriogram demonstrates an oval mass *(arrows)* anterior to the artery. At real-time the swirling blood is identified and the site of leak is seen as a blue jet of color arising from the anterior surface of the artery. **B,** Transverse Doppler image of the neck of a pseudoaneurysm of a different patient demonstrates the typical "to-and-fro" spectral pattern.

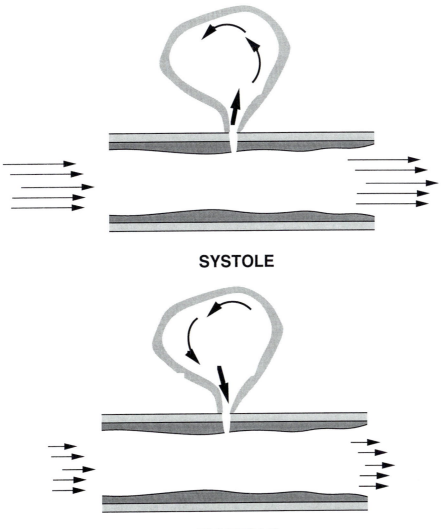

SYSTOLE

DIASTOLE

FIG. 29-5. Pseudoaneurysm flow pattern. The "swirling" motion of blood is identified, as well as a small communicating channel between the artery and the perivascular collection. Blood enters the pseudoaneurysm during systole ("to") when blood pressure is higher in the artery than in the collection. Blood exits during diastole ("fro") when the (pressure) energy that has been stored in the soft tissues surrounding the collection is greater than diastolic pressure.

a wide pulse pressure between systole and diastole. Although usually solitary, pseudoaneurysms can have multiple connecting compartments. Pseudoaneurysms also can occur at the anastomosis of a synthetic graft. The communicating channel is usually wide rather than the narrow communicating channel occurring following arterial catheterization.

A **hyperplastic lymph node** is a perivascular mass that can be mistaken for a pseudoaneurysm because of the arterial and venous signals radiating from the hilum of the node.[13,14] However, a hyperplastic lymph node does not have either a channel communicating to an adjacent artery or a to-and-fro pattern. **Arterial aneurysms** are easily recognized by their typical appearance and location within the confines of

the arterial wall. Although fusiform aneurysms obey this rule, it may be difficult to differentiate a saccular aneurysm from a pseudoaneurysm.[15]

PERIPHERAL ARTERIAL DISEASE

Incidence and Clinical Importance

Peripheral vascular disease is at least as prevalent as coronary artery disease or cerebrovascular disease.[16] The coexistence of these three processes is to be expected since atherosclerosis is a generalized process. The clinical presentation and the development of symptomatic disease are, however, different. Coronary artery disease and carotid artery disease can present in a catastrophic and very noticeable fashion as myocardial infarction or stroke, respectively. Many patients suffer from peripheral arterial disease for years before seeking medical assistance.[17] This is a reflection of the normal development of collateral channels that are often sufficient to maintain perfusion to the extremity of the older patient. This balance between supply and demand is maintained as long as the patient does not exercise or ambulate too vigorously. In general, these patients can go on for years, decreasing their levels of activity as their disease progresses. Disabling claudication is therefore more likely to be a presenting symptom in the younger patient with high levels of daily activity.

Other events that force the patient to seek medical assistance are the development of chronic changes of arterial insufficiency or poor wound healing. Acute embolic events originating from a more proximal arterial lesion, such as from either ulcerated plaques or thrombosing popliteal aneurysms, can cause extensive tissue loss, including loss of the affected limb unless an intervention is performed.

The widespread use of arterial bypass operations has modified the natural history of peripheral arterial disease. The high patency rates for both arterial bypass surgery and angioplasty have made it possible for patients who would previously have had amputations to remain asymptomatic until other causes of mortality intercede. Cardiovascular events are likely causes of death in these preselected patients with progressive generalized atherosclerosis.

Duplex sonography is now well accepted as the primary noninvasive modality for detecting evidence of lower extremity bypass graft dysfunction. It is also increasingly being used to evaluate the success of peripheral angioplasty. Doppler imaging of the leg arteries to determine the extent and nature of arterial lesions has become practical with the aid of color flow Doppler imaging. Although duplex Doppler sonography can be used to determine the presence of significant arterial lesions, the task of evaluating the whole leg is labor and time intensive. It takes 30 to 60 minutes to map out the arterial tree of each leg using Duplex ultrasound.[18] With color flow Doppler mapping, this task can be accomplished in 15 to 20 minutes.[1]

Lower Extremity
Normal Anatomy and Doppler Flow Patterns.
The deep arteries of the leg travel with an accompanying vein. The **common femoral artery** starts at the level of the inguinal ligament and continues for 4 to 6 cm until it branches into the **superficial and deep femoral arteries** (see Fig. 29-2). The deep femoral artery quickly branches to supply the region of the femoral head and the deep muscles of the thigh. With peripheral arterial disease, collateral

pathways often form between this deep femoral artery and the lower portions of the superficial femoral or the popliteal arteries. The superficial femoral artery continues along the medial aspect of the thigh at a depth of 4 to 8 cm until it reaches the adductor canal. It then exits the lower boundary of the adductor canal through the adductor hiatus and continues as the **popliteal artery**. The popliteal artery crosses posterior to the knee and gives off small geniculate branches and terminates as two major branches: the **anterior tibial artery** and the **tibioperoneal trunk**. The anterior tibial artery courses in the anterior compartment of the lower leg after crossing through the interosseous membrane. It finally crosses the ankle joint as the **dorsalis pedis artery**. The tibioperoneal trunk gives off the **posterior tibial** and the **peroneal arteries**, which supply the calf muscles. The posterior tibial artery is more superficial than the peroneal artery and can be followed down to its typical location behind the medial malleolus.

The flow pattern in all of these branches is a triphasic one (see Fig. 29-2). There is an early systolic acceleration in velocity followed by a brief period of low-amplitude flow reversal before returning to antegrade diastolic flow of low velocity. This pattern can be more pulsatile in the profunda femoris artery. Peak systolic velocities vary with the level of the artery, typically at 100 cm/s at the common femoral artery down to 70 cm/s at the popliteal artery. The tibioperoneal arteries have peak systolic velocities of 40 to 50 cm/s. The response to either **exercise or transient ischemia** is a loss of the triphasic pattern and the development of a monophasic pattern (persistent antegrade flow) with loss of the period of flow reversal and prominent antegrade flow during diastole (Fig. 29-6). The peak systolic velocity is decreased in the limb of a patient with ischemic arterial disease; it is increased in a healthy individual following exercise.

Aneurysms—Diagnostic Criteria.
Aneurysms develop as the structural integrity of the arterial wall weakens. A bulge or **focal enlargement of 20%** of the expected vessel diameter constitutes a simple functional definition of an aneurysm. Focal enlargement of the artery is more likely to occur at the level of the popliteal or distal superficial femoral artery. They are often bilateral and can remain asymptomatic for long periods of time. Ultrasound imaging has become a gold standard in itself for confirming this suspected diagnosis.[19,20] While ultrasound can visualize the progressive thrombosis that fills in the aneurysm lumen to the level of the dilated wall, the lumen will typically appear normal at angiography (Fig. 29-7). Ultrasound can be used to follow these aneurysms, as is done for abdominal aortic aneurysm. There are, unfortunately, no strict size criteria that can be used to determine the patient's suitability for operation.

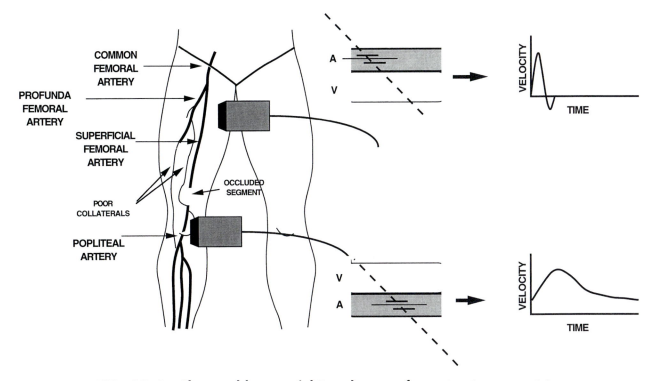

FIG. 29-6. Abnormal leg arterial Doppler waveform. Significant arterial disease alters the Doppler waveform sampled distal to the lesion as follows: arterial signals will resemble the low-resistance pattern normally seen in the internal carotid or renal arteries with antegrade flow during most of diastole. The Doppler waveform sampled proximal to a high-grade stenosis or occlusion shows loss of diastolic flow.

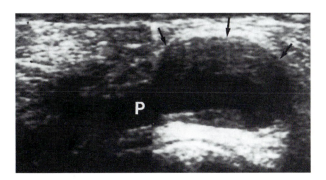

FIG. 29-7. Popliteal artery aneurysm. Longitudinal image of the popliteal space demonstrates a 3 × 4 cm aneurysm *(arrows)*, which contains a large amount of thrombus. *P*, Popliteal artery.

Empirically, a peripheral artery aneurysm of 2 cm or greater usually requires surgical repair.[21] The development of symptoms due to distal embolization by the thrombus accumulating in the lumen is an absolute indication for surgical intervention, irrespective of the size of the aneurysm.[21] Doppler techniques are useful in confirming the continued patency of a channel within the thrombosing aneurysm either at presentation or following surgery.

Aneurysms—Diagnostic Accuracy. Direct pathologic verification of ultrasound-diagnosed aneurysms has shown the technique to be sensitive, specific, and superior to angiography. The accuracy of Doppler techniques for confirming patency or occlusion has yet to be reported.

Stenosis and Occlusions—Diagnostic Criteria. The diagnosis of peripheral disease is often made by noting a change in the flow pattern seen on the Doppler spectrum (Fig. 29-8; Tables 29-2 and 29-3).

Distal to less severe arterial lesions, the period of early diastolic flow reversal (dicrotic notch) decreases and ultimately disappears as the lesion becomes more severe. The diastolic velocity also increases with the severity of the lesion, although on occasion a high-resistance biphasic pattern can be seen (Fig. 29-9). With severe lesions, the flow pattern is mainly that of forward flow with the peak end diastolic velocity approaching the peak systolic velocity. One explanation for the development of this pattern is the progressive dilatation of the arterioles within the distant muscle vascular bed due to the release of metabolites caused by local ischemia. Another is the development of many small collateral vessels that diminish the effective resistance of the more distally located obstructing lesion. This pattern,

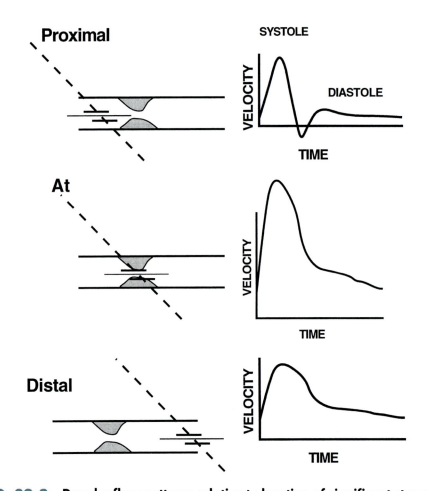

FIG. 29-8. Doppler flow patterns relative to location of significant stenosis.
Proximal to the lesion, the flow pattern is normal. At the stenosis, the peak systolic velocity increases in proportion to the degree of stenosis. Alterations in the diastolic portion of the Doppler waveform sampled at the lesion are dependent on the state of the distal arteries and on lesion severity and geometry; diastolic flow may increase dramatically or be almost absent. Distal to the stenosis, the peak systolic velocity returns to values equal to or lower than those proximal to the stenosis. If the stenosis is severe, peripheral vasodilatation causes an increase in the relative amount of diastolic flow.

TABLE 29-2
STENOSIS: FINDINGS AND CORRELATES

Finding	Correlate
Peak systolic velocity above 200 cm/s	Stenosis of at least 50% diameter
Peak systolic velocity ratio of 2 or greater compared with adjacent normal arterial segment	Stenosis of 50% or more
Decreased peak systolic velocity with high-resistance waveform	Doppler sample just proximal to high-grade stenosis or occlusion
Increased flow velocity—false-positive for stenosis	1. Steep Doppler angle
	2. Vessel kink
	3. Sampling in collateral artery

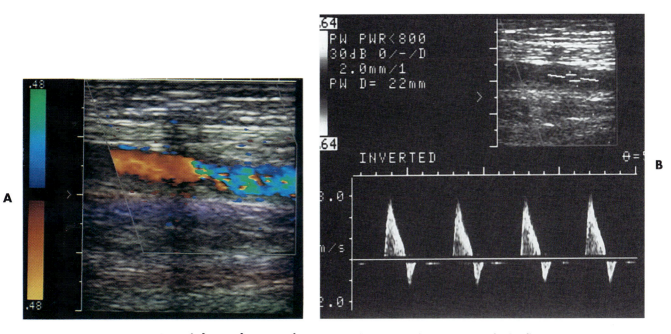

FIG. 29-9. **High-grade stenosis.** **A,** Color flow image shows aliasing of color flow signals in the mid superficial femoral artery. Arteriography confirmed the presence of a high-grade stenosis. **B,** The Doppler waveform sampled at the site where aliasing was seen shows an elevation of the peak systolic velocities to 300 cm/s, yet the early diastolic flow reversal is preserved.

TABLE 29-3
ARTERIAL OCCLUSIONS: FINDINGS AND CORRELATES

Finding	Correlate	
Absent flow signals	1. Occlusion 2. Calcification 3. Near total occlusion 4. Poor sensitivity of Doppler either due to depth or poor instrument settings	} False-positive for occlusion
Echogenic material in artery	Thrombosis associated with occlusion	
Large collateral branches seen during color flow imaging	Indicate high likelihood of more distal occlusion or high-grade stenosis	
Low-amplitude and persistent antegrade flow during systole and diastole	Sampling site is likely distal to occlusion or high-grade stenosis	
Low-amplitude systolic signals in occluded segment (false-negative)	1. Signals due to transmitted pulsations in occluded segment or 2. Inadvertent sampling of collateral branch parallel to occluded segment	

although a general finding, may not be seen on sampling within vessels proximal to high-grade focal lesions or occlusions. Signals in the artery proximal to high-grade lesions often show a **high-resistance pattern** (see Fig. 29-6). Without collateral vessels, forward flow can sometimes only be maintained during systole. Since the **peak systolic velocity** is less affected by vasodilatation, it is the preferred Doppler velocity parameter to be measured from the

Doppler spectrum at the site of a suspected stenosis. A slow-rise, low-amplitude, low-resistance pattern (**tardus parvus**) is often seen distal to segmental occlusions (see Fig. 29-6; Fig. 29-10).

Focal areas of doubling of the peak systolic velocity have been shown to correspond to **lesions of greater than 50% narrowing** in the lumen diameter of the artery.[22] The velocity at the stenosis is divided by the velocity proximal to the stenosis (see Fig. 29-8).

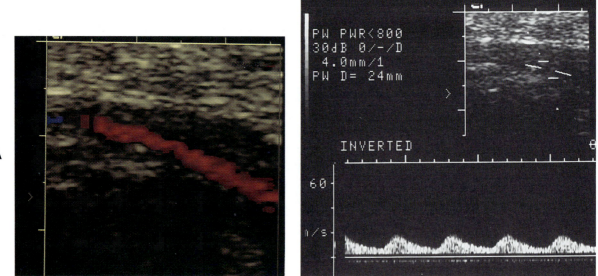

FIG. 29-10. Flow distal to occlusion. A, Color flow image was used to locate and evaluate the popliteal artery distal to a superficial femoral artery occlusion. No diastolic reversal of flow was seen and average velocities were low. **B,** The corresponding pulsed wave Doppler waveform in the popliteal artery shows a low-amplitude (parvus) waveform with a slow systolic rise (tardus). This waveform is typical of what is seen distal to an arterial occlusion.

Stenoses and Occlusions—Diagnostic Accuracy.

The original paper by Kohler et al. reported that Doppler sonography had a diagnostic sensitivity of 82% and a specificity of 92% for detecting segmental arterial lesions of the femoropopliteal arteries.[18] These authors noted, however, that selective sampling had to be performed along the full course of the femoral and popliteal arteries. Since these segments normally measure 30 to 40 cm, it is not surprising that such a survey takes from 1 to 2 hours to perform, especially if the iliac arteries are to be evaluated.

Color flow Doppler sonography has been shown to reduce the time needed to examine the carotid artery for suspected stenosis by 40% when compared with spectral Doppler alone.[5] A similar effect has been shown when using color flow mapping to detect focal lesions in the femoropopliteal artery. The diagnostic accuracy of the examination is slightly better than that of noncolor-assisted duplex sonography.[2,23] When color flow Doppler sonography is used, the examination time is reduced to 30 minutes.[1] Many authors have now reported on the accuracy of color flow imaging of the peripheral arteries. The accuracy is close to 98% for distinguishing occlusions from nonoccluded segments. The accuracy for the detection of stenoses is better than 85% (Table 29-4).[1,24,25] Most of the data pertains to selected imaging of the femoropopliteal arteries, with a few groups including an evaluation of the iliac arteries and "run-off" arteries, which are the anterior and posterior tibial and peroneal arteries.[18,23,26,27] The evaluation of the run-off arteries is not as accurate as for the femoropopliteal system and is especially lower for the peroneal artery.[28,29]

Color flow imaging has been used to triage patients to selected therapy without the use for arteriography in more than half of patients presenting with symptoms of peripheral arterial disease.[30] Doppler sonography can also be used to triage patients likely to need peripheral angioplasty and therefore better manage more expensive imaging resources such as arteriography.[31-33]

The use of color flow Doppler imaging and duplex sonography for the evaluation of sites having undergone percutaneous interventions, such as angioplasty or atherectomy, is of interest. An original report indicated that a measurement made a few days after angioplasty was predictive of lesion recurrence.[34] Subsequent studies have failed to confirm this observation.[35,36] Of greater interest is the likelihood that duplex sonography can be used as an objective end point for the long-term technical success of an intervention. For example, the results following atherectomy show higher incidence of reocclusion than indicated by patients' symptoms.[37] There are concerns that this strategy may be limited since patients' symptoms drive the need for repeat interventions.[38] It appears that serial monitoring of angioplasty sites can predict lesion recurrence.[39]

Upper Extremity

Normal Anatomy and Doppler Flow Patterns.

The arteries of the upper extremity are accompanied by veins: solitary veins at the subclavian

TABLE 29-4

SENSITIVITY OF COLOR DOPPLER SONOGRAPHY AS COMPARED WITH ARTERIOGRAPHY FOR THE DETECTION OF STENOTIC (>50%) ARTERIAL SEGMENTS*

Author	Number of Segments Detected/ Number with Stenoses	Number of Segments in each Limb Studied
Cossman et al.[23]	156/(180)	8
Polak et al.[33]	22/(29)	7
Mulligan et al.[26]	8/(11)	7
Whelan et al.[25]	130/(141)	7
Total	316/(361)=87.5%	

*Refers to the number of segments studied in each femoropopliteal system. The common femoral and the profunda femoral are considered to be one segment each. The superficial femoral artery is typically separated into two or three segments of equal length while the popliteal artery is considered as either one or two segments.

and axillary level, duplicated veins at the brachial levels and distally. The proximal portion of the **subclavian arteries** can be identified by angling caudally using an acoustic window superior to the sternoclavicular joint. The subclavian artery is imaged superficial to the vein when the transducer is placed in the supraclavicular fossa. Near the junction of the mid and proximal third of the clavicle, it is necessary to use a window with the transducer caudal to the clavicle. From this view, the subclavian artery is seen deep to the subclavian vein. The origin of the **axillary artery** is lateral to the first rib, normally near the junction of the cephalic and the axillary vein. The axillary artery can be followed as it courses medially over the proximal humerus to become the **brachial artery**. In most subjects the artery can be followed to the antecubital fossa where it trifurcates into the radial, ulnar, and interosseous branches. The **radial and ulnar arteries** can normally be imaged to the level of the wrist. It is also possible to visualize the smaller digital branches. The normal Doppler flow pattern of the arteries of the arm is triphasic and similar to the pattern seen in the leg.

Pathophysiology and Diagnostic Accuracy.

Most clinical interest in the noninvasive evaluation of the upper extremity arterial branches is directed to the detection of focal stenosis caused by thoracic outlet syndrome, the confirmation of native arterial occlusion secondary to emboli or trauma, the confirmation of pseudoaneurysms, the detection of complications following cardiac catheterization, and the evaluation of dialysis shunts.

There are few reports in the literature of Doppler evaluation of patients with **thoracic outlet syn-**

drome. It is possible to induce stenosis in the subclavian artery by positioning the arm in a position that elicits the patient's symptoms. Symptoms most often occur when their arm is markedly abducted. There is a frequent association between thoracic outlet syndrome and distal arterial embolization. The extent of these acute or chronic occlusions must be mapped out to assess the feasibility of possible bypass surgery before subjecting the patient to angiography. Cases of proximal occlusions associated with vasculitis have also been demonstrated.

Upper extremity arterial occlusion, which may occur as a complication of cardiac catheterization, can be detected by color flow and duplex Doppler sonography. Soft-tissue swelling at the arteriotomy site can be evaluated to differentiate hematoma from pseudoaneurysm.

GRAFTS

Complications of Synthetic Vascular Bypass Grafts

The complications likely to affect the function of synthetic lower extremity bypass grafts are varied and are a function of the **type of bypass graft used** and of the **time since operative placement.**[40,41] In the first and second years following operation, graft stenosis and occlusion can occur either secondary to technical errors or to the development of fibrointimal lesions at the anastomoses. Later graft failure can be due to the progression of atherosclerotic lesions in the native vessels proximal and distal to the graft. The late complication of an anastomotic pseudoaneurysm occurs on average 5 to 10 years following graft placement and preferentially affects the femoral anastomosis of aortofemoral grafts.[5,42] Infection can occur at any time following graft placement and can be associated with the development of an anastomotic pseudoaneurysm.

Pseudoaneurysm Versus Hematoma. Although the diagnostic accuracy of duplex Doppler sonography is above 95% for making the diagnosis of perigraft or vascular **pseudoaneurysms,** no specific spectral waveform patterns from within the cystic mass have been described.[43,44] The addition of color flow Doppler imaging can reveal an almost classic appearance of swirling motion of blood in the perivascular mass.[41] This sign is not specific to a pseudoaneurysm because saccular aneurysms share similar flow patterns (see Fig. 29-5; Figs. 29-11 to 29-13). The diagnosis of pseudoaneurysm is made when the vascular mass is situated beyond the normal lumen of the vessel and the **"to-and-fro" sign** is detected by Doppler spectral analysis of the communication between the perivascular collection and the graft. Although specific, this communication is sometimes

Systole

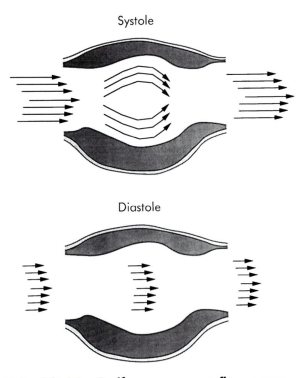

Diastole

FIG. 29-11. Fusiform aneurysm flow pattern.
The flow patterns within the lumen of an aneurysm will vary
during the different stages of its evolution. Here, with minimal
bulging of the wall and a small amount of mural thrombus,
flow eddies are established during late systole (top). During
diastole, a more normal pattern is reestablished (bottom).

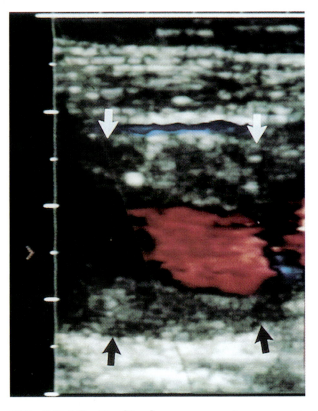

FIG. 29-12. Popliteal aneurysm. Aneurysm with
a large amount of thrombus along its wall (arrows). The
lumen is straight enough so that there are no significant flow
eddies during systole.

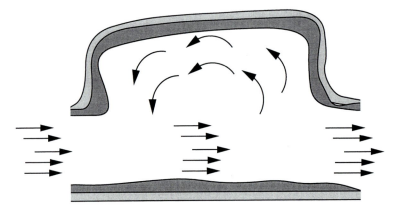

FIG. 29-13. Saccular aneurysm flow pattern. A saccular aneurysm has flow eddies during late systole and the major portion of diastole. This corresponds to a "swirling" pattern. Differentiation between a saccular aneurysm and a pseudoaneurysm, arising at the anastomosis of a synthetic graft, can be difficult.

difficult to find with spectral Doppler and is often absent in anastomotic pseudoaneurysms (see Fig. 29-4;
Fig. 29-14). Color flow Doppler improves the detection of the communicating channel.

Care must be taken to differentiate perivascular
pulsations transmitted within a **hematoma** from
flowing blood within a pseudoaneurysm. Adjustment
of the flow sensitivity of the imaging device to mini-

mize this artifact can help eliminate this error. Setting
the color velocity scale (PRF) to a high value can eliminate this artifact while not hampering the detection of
the communicating channel of a pseudoaneurysm.

Stenosis and Occlusion. An anastomotic
stenosis will typically cause a marked increase in the
Doppler velocity signals sampled at the anastomosis
or beyond. There is, however, a normal tendency for

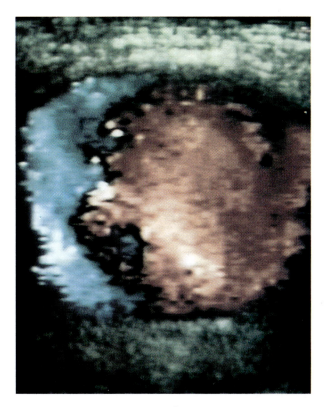

FIG. 29-14. Bypass graft aneurysm. Transverse image of a large anastomotic aneurysm at the distal anastomosis of an aortobifemoral bypass graft has within it a typical swirling pattern of blood flow.

turbulent flow to develop as the graft tapers to the anastomosis. Increases in velocity due to the geometry of the anastomotic connection are common and can cause up to a 100% increase in velocity without being indicative of a pathologic lesion. There are no studies addressing the actual incidence and significance of this finding. Serial monitoring of these sites of disturbed flow may be used with the premise that an increase in velocity over a few months is indicative of a developing stenosis.[45] The absence of Doppler signals within a graft is diagnostic of an occlusion.

Autologous Vein Grafts

Two types of venous bypass grafts are currently used for arterial revascularization: the reversed vein and the in situ vein grafts. The **reversed vein** is a segment of native superficial vein that has been harvested from its normal anatomic location, reversed, and then anastomosed to the native artery segments proximal and distal to the diseased segments. The **in situ** technique typically uses the greater saphenous vein, although the lesser saphenous vein can be used for popliteal to distal tibioperoneal bypass surgery. The vein is left in its native bed. The valves are lysed, and the side branches, which normally communicate with the deep venous system, are ligated. The proximal and distal

portions of the vein are mobilized and anastomosed to the selected arterial segments.

Three different mechanisms are responsible for **bypass graft failure**. Early failures are seen within 1 month following surgery and are normally ascribed to technical errors. These include poor suture line placement, the opening of unsuspected venous channels in the in situ grafts, poor selection of anastomotic sites, and poorly lysed venous valves. During the first 2 years following surgery, fibrointimal or fibrotic lesions can develop either at the anastomosis or within the graft conduit, most often at the site of a venous valve. Late failures, beyond this 2-year period, are thought to be secondary to continued progression of the atherosclerotic process in the native vessels proximal and distal to the anastomoses.

Stenosis. The measurement of graft velocity, either in the early or late postoperative period, can be used to detect grafts with a high likelihood of incipient failure. Bandyk et al. have shown that a peak systolic velocity below 40 or 45 cm/s can be used to identify such grafts.[46,47] This criterion identifies only the more severely diseased grafts.[48] It does not identify the sites of stenoses likely to continue to progress until they become flow restrictive and finally result in graft thrombosis.[49] These lesions are commonly the result of **fibrointimal hyperplasia**, and their existence must be known before they can be monitored for possible progression of severity. Color flow Doppler sonography can be used to survey the length of these bypass grafts, which varies from 30 to 80 cm. The site of a suspected stenosis can be quickly identified and Doppler spectral analysis used to grade the severity of the stenosis with the use of the peak systolic velocity ratio (Fig. 29-15). This ratio is calculated by dividing the peak systolic velocity measured at the suspected stenosis by that measured in the portion of the graft 2 to 4 cm proximal (see Fig. 29-8; Fig. 29-16). Velocity ratios of **2 or greater correspond to 50% diameter stenosis** while ratios of **3 or greater to 75% stenosis**.[18,50] More recent data suggest that a slightly higher velocity ratio would correspond to a 75% diameter stenosis.[51] This method is very accurate for the detection and grading of stenoses.[52-54] Potential limitations are tandem lesions where the flow field of one stenosis overlaps the flow field of another located more distally.[55] It is now recognized that the early lesions develop within 3 months after surgery and are detectable by sonography even before the patient develops symptoms.[56] Intervention, most often surgical revision of the developing stenosis, is indicated since it has been shown that these lesions, if left alone, ultimately progress to cause bypass graft occlusions.[56,57] The issue of an appropriate upper limit for the peak systolic velocity ratio has yet to be decided, although values above 3, and likely 4 or more, warrant intervention.

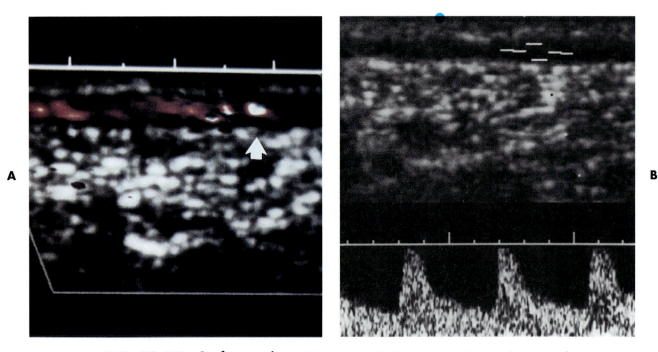

FIG. 29-15. Graft stenosis. A, This portion of a femoroperoneal in situ bypass graft has a small zone of high-flow velocities indicating stenosis *(arrow)*. **B,** The corresponding Doppler spectrum shows a marked increase in flow velocity at the site of color flow disturbance.

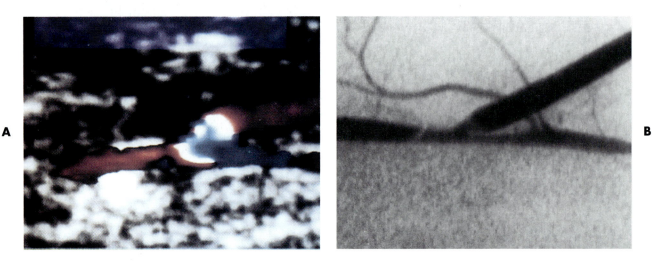

FIG. 29-16. Anastomotic stenosis. A, This longitudinal image of the anastomosis of a bypass graft to a posterior tibial artery shows a zone of color flow Doppler aliasing consistent with a significant narrowing. The relatively normal size of the flow lumen is caused by a misregistration of the color signals because of the relative acceleration of the red blood cells. **B,** The corresponding arteriogram confirms the presence of a distal anastomotic stenosis.

A-V Fistula. This complication is apt to occur with the in situ technique. Small A-V fistulas can easily be missed at operation and open in the few weeks following surgery. Color flow Doppler sonography is a simple and elegant way of documenting their presence. Intraoperative sonography can be used to locate fistulas in need of surgical correction.[46] Color flow Doppler sonography, without the need for angiography, is typically used as the only guide for surgical repair of A-V communication between in situ vein graft and the deep native veins.

Dialysis Fistula

The use of sonography in the evaluation of dialysis A-V fistulae or hemodialysis access grafts is varied.[58,59] The native artery to vein anastomosis, typically done between radial artery and vein (Brescia-Cimino procedure), has almost totally been replaced by bypass grafts (Fig. 29-17). These are typically inserted in the forearm and are either **synthetic** (polytetrafluoroethylene or PTFE) or made of **autologous vein**. Problems common to both types of dialysis access include the development of **microaneurysms, larger aneurysms,**

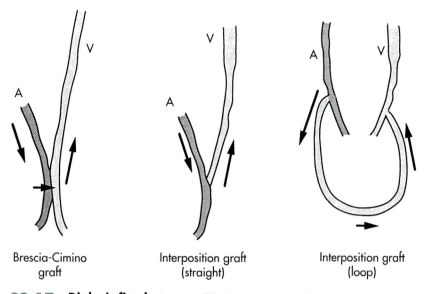

FIG. 29-17. **Dialysis fistula types.** The interposition grafts are more commonly used than the Brescia-Cimino native fistulas. Most stenoses are located at or just beyond the venous anastomosis. The material used for the grafts is typically synthetic, although native vein segments can be used.

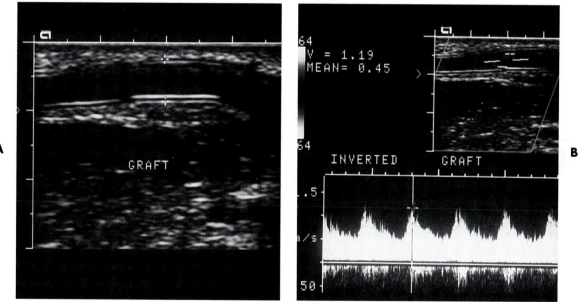

FIG. 29-18. **Normal synthetic graft.** A, Gray-scale image shows a graft made of PTFE, the material used in most dialysis access grafts. The wall typically appears as an echogenic double line. B, This Doppler velocity waveform is typical of a normal dialysis access graft. Peak systolic velocities tend to be above 100 cm/s. Turbulence, seen as a harsh contour of the waveform and filling in of the spectral window, is commonly seen.

pseudoaneurysms, or **stenoses.** Color flow Doppler imaging can readily detect these abnormalities. Duplex sonography can be used to detect and grade stenoses: the accuracy of the technique is estimated at 86% with a sensitivity of 92% and specificity of 84%.[58] The loss in specificity is explained by turbulent flow patterns set up by a very tortuous graft course. The diagnostic accuracy is improved in straight segment grafts to the efferent veins, where the sensitivity increases to 95% for a

specificity of 97%.[58] The addition of color flow Doppler does not seem to improve diagnostic accuracy.[60]

The diagnostic criteria for stenosis of hemodialysis access grafts have been reported by several authors.[61-63] Peak systolic velocities in well-functioning dialysis access grafts are typically between 100 cm/s and 200 cm/s (Fig. 29-18), tending to be higher in the first 6 months after graft placement or shunt creation.[63] Superimposed stenosis can therefore be difficult to de-

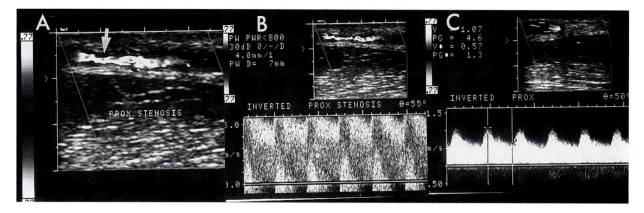

FIG. 29-19. Stenosis at venous side of synthetic graft. **A,** Gray-scale image of a color flow Doppler study shows a narrowed segment *(arrow)* of dialysis graft. **B,** This Doppler waveform shows aliasing and velocities of greater than 500 cm/s at the venous anastomosis of a dialysis access graft. **C,** The normal Doppler velocity waveform is sampled in the graft just proximal to the stenosis.

tect given the high baseline velocities (Fig. 29-19). Elevations of 100% (velocity ratios of 2 or greater) are consistent with **high-grade stenoses.** Low-flow states of 50 cm/s or less are also indicative of high-grade stenoses. Color flow and gray-scale images are also useful for confirming the presence of an anatomic lesion (see Fig. 29-19).[62] Stenotic lesions tend to develop on the venous side of the access fistula in more than 80% of cases.[64] Occasionally, the stenosis can be at the level of the subclavian vein, specifically in individuals who have had temporary hemodialysis access with the aid of indwelling large-diameter catheters.[65]

Complications of Invasive Procedures

The use of duplex or color flow Doppler sonography is common for the screening of patients who have had invasive procedures and in cases where the diagnosis of A-V fistula or pseudoaneurysm is suspected. The findings on the sonographic examination are commonly accepted as conclusive, without the need for preoperative angiography.

A-V Fistula. Fistulous communications following cardiac catheterization or other angiographic procedures can be quickly detected using color flow Doppler imaging.[66,67] In the femoral region, **turbulence** is seen within either the common femoral or profunda femoral vein with **arterialized signals** shown on the Doppler spectrum (see Fig. 29-3). The **fistulous communication** can be seen on color flow Doppler, although it may be difficult to localize with duplex sonography alone (Fig. 29-20). The turbulence associated with the fistula can be confused with turbulent signals due to extrinsic compression of the vein by a hematoma, which is also a common complication following catheterization. Visualization of the communicating channel allows a confident diagnosis of A-V fistula rather than extrinsic venous compression by a hematoma. An indirect sign of the fistula is dilatation

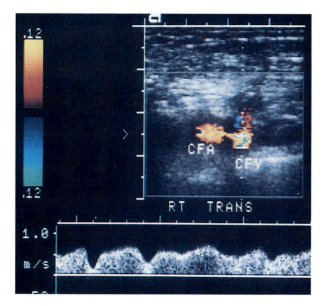

FIG. 29-20. A-V fistula. Transverse color flow image of the right leg shows a communicating channel between the common femoral artery, *CFA*, and common femoral vein, *CFV*. Spectral Doppler from the CFV shows an arterialized turbulent waveform. The patient underwent surgical repair without the need for arteriography because of the clear communication on the color flow Doppler image.

of the vein and a poor Valsalva's response. With small A-V communications, the venous velocity can decrease during Valsalva's maneuver. Complete abolition of the flow signals during Valsalva's maneuver suggests that the fistula is likely to spontaneously occlude over the next few weeks. With larger A-V communications, velocity in the affected vein is not decreased by Valsalva's maneuver when compared with the vein in the normal extremity. Transcutaneus therapy aimed at achieving closure of the fistula has been described using ultrasound monitoring and by applying pressure over the fistula for periods of 20 to

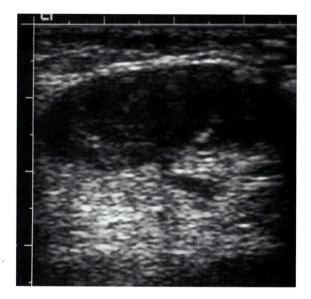

FIG. 29-21. Thrombosed pseudoaneurysm/ hematoma. This heterogeneous, mainly hypoechoic mass is typical of a thrombosed pseudoaneurysm after successful compression therapy. A hematoma may have a similar appearance or present as a diffuse infiltration that only mildly distorts the soft tissues despite the presence of a palpable mass.

60 minutes.[68] Success rates for transcutaneous repair are 30% or lower.[68]

Pseudoaneurysm. This complication may develop following **penetrating trauma** or **arterial catheterization**. As described earlier in this chapter, the swirling blood flow and the direct communication between pseudoaneurysm and arterial lumen should be detectable by color flow imaging. Once considered a relative medical emergency, the management of pseudoaneurysms has significantly been affected by the wide use of sonography. The natural history of pseudoaneurysms is often benign, with spontaneous thrombosis and closure when patients are kept at bed rest (Fig. 29-21).[69] Fellmeth et al. first described the use of **transcutaneous compression therapy** of pseudoaneurysms that resulted from catheterization.[68] They described a simple protocol of applying direct pressure with the ultrasound probe over the neck of the pseudoaneurysm. The probe was positioned in the long axis of the artery as flow into the cavity was obliterated by firm compression. Successful occlusion required 20 minutes of compression. If initial compression was not successful, the procedure was repeated up to three times. Transcutaneous compression therapy was successful in more than 80% of reported cases. Subsequent reports have confirmed the high success rates of the procedure.[70,71] Although initial reports indicated a lower success rate if patients were anticoagulated, a recent report has also shown a high success rate in patients who are anticoagulated.[72] Other reports have described a very high likelihood of success for smaller pseudoaneurysms and those with longer

communicating channels.[73,74] Pseudoaneurysms arising from the axillary or the brachial arteries can also be successfully treated by transcutaneous compression therapy.[75,76] Many authors have remarked on the need for significant analgesia to alleviate discomfort during prolonged firm compression. A potential complication of transcutaneous compression therapy is arterial or venous thrombosis.

It is interesting that there is an apparent increase in the prevalence of pseudoaneurysm as reported by several authors. Kresowik et al. reported incidence rates almost 10 times the 0.5% rate that was reported several decades ago.[77] Plausible explanations for this increase in pseudoaneurysm incidence were the use of more aggressive anticoagulation and the larger-sized catheters used during angioplasty procedures. A recent report emphasized the most important predictor of subsequent pseudoaneurysm formation was limited compression time after femoral artery catheterization.[78]

REFERENCES

1. Polak JF, Karmel MI, Mannick JA et al. Determination of the extent of lower-extremity peripheral arterial disease with color-assisted duplex sonography: comparison with angiography. *AJR* 1990;155:1085-1089.
2. deVries S, Hunink M, Polak JF. Summary receiver operating characteristic curves as a technique for meta-analysis for the diagnostic performance of duplex ultrasonography in peripheral arterial disease. *Acad Radiol* 1996;3:361-369.

Instrumentation
3. Barber FE, Baker DW, Nation AWC et al. Ultrasonic duplex echo Doppler scanner. *IEEE Trans Biomed Engin* 1974; 21:109-113.
4. Kasai C, Namekawa K, Koyano A et al. Real-time two-dimensional blood flow imaging using an autocorrelation technique. *IEEE Trans Sonics Ultrasound* 1985;S32:458-463.
5. Polak JF, Dobkin GR, O'Leary DH et al. Internal carotid artery stenosis: accuracy and reproducibility of color-Doppler-assisted duplex imaging. *Radiology* 1989;173:793-798.

Arterial Doppler Flow Patterns
6. Spencer MP, Reid JM. Quantitation of carotid stenosis with continuous-wave (C-W) Doppler ultrasound. *Stroke* 1979; 10:326-330.
7. Reneman R, Spencer M. Local Doppler audio spectra in normal and stenosed carotid arteries in man. *Ultrasound Med Biol* 1979;5:1-11.
8. Ojha M, Johnston K, Cobbold R et al. Potential limitations of center-line pulsed Doppler recordings: an in-vitro flow visualization study. *J Vasc Surg* 1989;9:515-520.
9. Middleton WD, Erickson S, Melson GL. Perivascular color artifact: pathologic significance and appearance on color Doppler US images. *Radiology* 1989;171:647-652.
10. Wilkinson DL, Polak JF, Grassi CJ et al. Pseudoaneurysm of the vertebral artery: appearance on color-flow Doppler sonography. *AJR* 1988;151:1051-1052.
11. Mitchell DG. Color Doppler imaging: principles, limitations, and artifacts. *Radiology* 1990;177:1-10.
12. Abu-Yousef MM, Wiese JA, Shamma AR. The "to-and-fro" sign: duplex Doppler evidence of femoral artery pseudoaneurysm. *AJR* 1988;150:632-634.

13. Morton MJ, Charboneau JW, Banks PM. Inguinal lymphadenopathy simulating a false aneurysm on color-flow Doppler sonography. *AJR* 1988;151:115-116.

14. Bjork L, Leven H. Intra-arterial DSA and duplex-Doppler ultrasonography in detection of vascularized inguinal lymph node. *Acta Radiol* 1990;31:106-107.

15. Musto R, Roach M. Flow studies in glass models of aortic aneurysms. *Can J Surg* 1980;23:452-455.

Peripheral Arterial Disease

16. Newman AB, Siscovick DS, Manolio TA et al. Ankle-arm index as a marker of atherosclerosis in the Cardiovascular Health Study. *Circulation* 1993;88:837-845.

17. Cronenwett JL, Warner KG, Zelenock GB et al. Intermittent claudication. Current results of nonoperative management. *Arch Surg* 1984;119:430-436.

18. Kohler TR, Nance DR, Cramer MM et al. Duplex scanning for diagnosis of aortoiliac and femoropopliteal disease: a prospective study. *Circulation* 1987;76:1074-1080.

19. Gooding GA, Effeney DJ. Ultrasound of femoral artery aneurysms. *AJR* 1980;134:477-480.

20. MacGowan SW, Saif MF, O'Neil G et al. Ultrasound examination in the diagnosis of popliteal artery aneurysms. *Br J Surg* 1985;72:528-529.

21. Shortell CK, DeWeese JA, Ouriel K et al. Popliteal artery aneurysms: a 25-year surgical experience. *J Vasc Surg* 1991;14:771-779.

22. Jager KA, Phillips DJ, Martin RL et al. Noninvasive mapping of lower limb arterial lesions. *Ultrasound Med Biol* 1985; 11:515-521.

23. Cossman DV, Ellison JE, Wagner WH et al. Comparison of contrast arteriography to arterial mapping with color-flow duplex imaging in the lower extremities. *J Vasc Surg* 1989; 10:522-529.

24. Fletcher FP, Kershaw LZ, Chan A et al. Noninvasive imaging of the superficial femoral artery using ultrasound duplex scanning. *J Cardiovasc Surg* 1990;31:364-367.

25. Whelan FF, Barry MH, Moir JD. Color flow Doppler ultrasonography: comparison with peripheral arteriography for the investigation of peripheral arterial disease. *J Clin Ultrasound* 1992;20:369-374.

26. Mulligan SA, Matsuda T, Lanzer P et al. Peripheral arterial occlusive disease: prospective comparison of MR angiography and color duplex US with conventional angiography. *Radiology* 1991;178:695-700.

27. Moneta GL, Yeager RA, Antonovic R et al. Accuracy of lower extremity arterial duplex mapping. *J Vasc Surg* 1992;15:275-284.

28. Moneta GL, Yeager RA, Lee RW et al. Noninvasive localization of arterial occlusive disease: a comparison of segmental pressures and arterial duplex mapping. *J Vasc Surg* 1993;17:578-582.

29. Karacagil S, Lofberg A, Granbo A et al. Value of duplex scanning in evaluation of crural and foot arteries in limbs with severe lower limb ischemia. A prospective comparison with angiography. *Eur J Vasc Endovasc Surg* 1996;12:300-303.

30. Elsman BH, Legemate DA, van der Heijden FH et al. Impact of ultrasonographic duplex scanning on therapeutic decision making in lower limb arterial disease. *Br J Surg* 1995;82:630-633.

31. Collier P, Wilcox G, Brooks D et al. Improved patient selection for angioplasty utilizing color Doppler imaging. *Am J Surg* 1990;160:171-174.

32. Edwards JM, Goldwell DM, Goldman ML et al. The role of duplex scanning in the selection of patients for transluminal angioplasty. *J Vasc Surg* 1991;13:69-74.

33. Polak JF, Karmel MI, Meyerovitz MF. Accuracy of color Doppler flow mapping for evaluation of the severity of femoropopliteal arterial disease: a prospective study. *JVIR* 1991;2:471-479.

34. Mewissen MW, Kinney EV, Bandyk DF et al. The role of duplex scanning versus angiography in predicting outcome after balloon angioplasty in the femoropopliteal artery. *J Vasc Surg* 1992;15:860-866.

35. Sacks D, Robinson ML, Summers TA et al. The value of duplex sonography after peripheral artery angioplasty in predicting subacute stenosis. *AJR* 1994;162:179-183.

36. Katzenschlager R, Ahmadi A, Minar E et al. Color duplex ultrasound guided transluminal angioplasty of the femoropopliteal artery: initial and 6-months results. *Radiology* 1996;199:331-334.

37. Vroegindeweij D, Tielbeek A, Buth J et al. Directional atherectomy versus balloon angioplasty in segmental femoropopliteal artery disease: two-year follow-up with color-flow duplex scanning. *J Vasc Surg* 1995;21:255-268.

38. Tielbeek A, Rietjens E, Buth J et al. The value of duplex surveillance after endovascular intervention for femoropopliteal obstructive disease. *Eur J Vasc Endovasc Surg* 1996;12:145-150.

39. Spijkerboer A, Nass P, de Valois J et al. Iliac artery stenoses after percutaneous transluminal angioplasty: follow-up with duplex ultrasonography. *J Vasc Surg* 1996;23:691-697.

Grafts

40. Hedgcock MW, Eisenberg RL, Gooding GA. Complications relating to vascular prosthetic grafts. *J Can Assoc Radiol* 1980; 31:137-142.

41. Polak JF, Donaldson MC, Whittemore AD et al. Pulsatile masses surrounding vascular prostheses: real-time US color flow imaging. *Radiology* 1989;170:363-366.

42. Nichols WK, Stanton M, Silver D et al. Anastomotic aneurysms following lower extremity revascularization. *Surgery* 1980;88:366-374.

43. Helvie MA, Rubin JM, Silver TM et al. The distinction between femoral artery pseudoaneurysms and other causes of groin masses: value of duplex Doppler sonography. *AJR* 1988;150:1177-1180.

44. Coughlin BF, Paushter DM. Peripheral pseudoaneurysms: evaluation with duplex US. *Radiology* 1988;168:339-342.

45. Sanchez LA, Suggs WD, Veith FJ et al. Is surveillance to detect failing polytetrafluoroethylene bypasses worthwhile: twelve-year experience with 91 grafts. *J Vasc Surg* 1993;18:981-990.

46. Bandyk DF, Jorgensen RA, Towne JB. Intraoperative assessment of in situ saphenous vein arterial bypass grafts using pulsed Doppler spectral analysis. *Arch Surg* 1986;121:292-299.

47. Bandyk DF, Cato RF, Towne JB. A low flow velocity predicts failure of femoropopliteal and femorotibial bypass grafts. *Surgery* 1985;98:799-809.

48. Mills JL, Harris EJ, Taylor LM Jr. et al. The importance of routine surveillance of distal bypass grafts with duplex scanning: a study of 379 reversed vein grafts. *J Vasc Surg* 1990;12:379-389.

49. Grigg MJ, Nicolaides AN, Wolfe JH. Detection and grading of femorodistal vein grafts stenoses: duplex velocity measurements compared with angiography. *J Vasc Surg* 1988;8:661-666.

50. Hunink MGM, Polak JF. Response to commentary on accuracy of color Doppler flow mapping for evaluation of the severity of femoropopliteal arterial disease: a prospective study. *JVIR* 1991;2:477-478.

51. Ranke C, Creutzig A, Alexander K. Duplex scanning of the peripheral arteries: correlation of the peak velocity ratio with angiographic diameter reduction. *Ultrasound Med Biol* 1992; 18:433-440.

52. Londrey GL, Hodgson KJ, Spadone DP et al. Initial experience with color-flow duplex scanning of infrainguinal bypass grafts. *J Vasc Surg* 1990;12:284-290.

53. Polak JF, Donaldson MC, Dobkin GR et al. Early detection of saphenous vein arterial bypass graft stenosis by color-assisted duplex sonography: a prospective study. *AJR* 1990;154:857-861.

54. Buth J, Disselhoff B, Sommeling C et al. Color-flow duplex criteria for grading stenosis in infrainguinal vein grafts. *J Vasc Surg* 1991;14:716-728.

55. Leng GC, Whyman MR, Donnan PT et al. Accuracy and reproducibility of duplex ultrasonography in grading femoropopliteal stenoses. *J Vasc Surg* 1993;17:510-517.

56. Mills JL, Bandyk DF, Gathan V et al. The origin of infrainguinal vein graft stenosis: a prospective study based on duplex surveillance. *J Vasc Surg* 1995;21:16-25.

57. Idu MM, Blankestein JD, de Gier P et al. Impact of a color-flow duplex surveillance program on infrainguinal vein graft patency: a five-year experience. *J Vasc Surg* 1993;17:42-53.

58. Tordoir JH, de Bruin HG, Hoeneveld H et al. Duplex ultrasound scanning in the assessment of arteriovenous fistulas created for hemodialysis access: comparison with digital subtraction angiography. *J Vasc Surg* 1989;10:122-128.

59. Scheible W, Skram C, Leopold GR. High resolution real-time sonography of hemodialysis vascular access complications. *AJR* 1980;134:1173-1176.

60. Middleton WD, Picus DD, Marx MV et al. Color Doppler sonography of hemodialysis vascular access: comparison with angiography. *AJR* 1989;152:633-639.

61. Koksoy C, Kuzu A, Erden I et al. Predictive value of colour Doppler sonography in detecting failure of vascular access grafts. *Br J Surg* 1995;82:50-52.

62. Dousset V, Grenier N, Douws C et al. Hemodialysis grafts: color Doppler flow imaging correlated with digital subtraction angiography and functional status. *Radiology* 1991;181:89-94.

63. Villemarette P, Hower J. Evaluation of functional longevity of dialysis access grafts using color flow Doppler imaging. *J Vasc Tech* 1992;16:183-188.

64. Kanterman RY, Vesely TM, Pilgram TK et al. Dialysis access grafts: anatomic location of venous stenosis and results of angioplasty. *Radiology* 1995;195:135-139.

65. Schwab SJ, Quarles LD, Middleton JP et al. Haemodialysis-associated subclavian vein stenosis. *Kidney Int* 1988;33:1156-1159.

66. Altin RS, Flicker S, Naidech HJ. Pseudoaneurysm and arteriovenous fistula after femoral artery catheterization: association with low femoral punctures. *AJR* 1989;152:629-631.

67. Roubidoux MA, Hertzberg BS, Carroll BA et al. Color flow and image-directed Doppler ultrasound evaluation of iatrogenic arteriovenous fistulas in the groin. *J Clin Ultrasound* 1990; 18:463-469.

68. Fellmeth BD, Roberts AC, Bookstein JJ et al. Postangiographic femoral artery injuries: nonsurgical repair with US-guided compression. *Radiology* 1991;178:671-675.

69. Kotval PS, Khoury A, Shah PM et al. Doppler sonographic demonstration of the progressive spontaneous thrombosis of pseudoaneurysms. *J Ultrasound Med* 1990;9:185-190.

70. Fellmeth BD, Baron SB, Brown PR et al. Repair of postcatheterization femoral pseudoaneurysms by color flow ultrasound guided compression. *Am Heart J* 1992;123:547-551.

71. Cox GS, Young JR, Gray BR et al. Ultrasound-guided compression repair of postcatheterization pseudoaneurysms: results of treatment in one hundred cases. *J Vasc Surg* 1994; 19:683-686.

72. Dean S, Olin J, Piedmonte M et al. Ultrasound-guided compression closure of postcatheterization pseudoaneurysms during concurrent anticoagulation: a review of seventy-seven patients. *J Vasc Surg* 1996;23:28-35.

73. DiPrete DA, Cronan JJ. Compression ultrasonography: treatment for acute femoral artery pseudoaneurysms in selected cases. *J Ultrasound Med* 1992;11:489-492.

74. Paulson EK, Hertzberg BS, Paine SS et al. Femoral artery pseudoaneurysms: value of color Doppler sonography in predicting which ones will thrombose without treatment. *AJR* 1992;159:1077-1081.

75. Rooker KT, Morgan CA, Haseman MK et al. Color flow guided repair of axillary artery pseudoaneurysm. *J Ultrasound Med* 1992;11:625-626.

76. Skibo L, Polak JF. Compression repair of a postcatheterization pseudoaneurysm of the brachial artery under sonographic guidance. *AJR* 1993;160:383-384.

77. Kresowik TF, Khoury MD, Miller BV et al. A prospective study of the incidence and natural history of femoral vascular complications after percutaneous transluminal coronary angioplasty. *J Vasc Surg* 1991;13:328-335.

78. Katzenschlager R, Ugurluoglu A, Ahmadi A et al. The incidence of pseudoaneurysm after diagnostic and therapeutic angiography. *Radiology* 1995;195:463-466.

CHAPTER 30

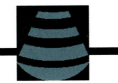

The Peripheral Veins

•

Bradley D. Lewis, M.D.

METHODS

The clinical evaluation of the peripheral venous system is notoriously difficult and inaccurate. Accordingly, numerous imaging and nonimaging methods have been developed to aid clinicians with this diagnostic problem. These methods can be divided arbitrarily into three main categories:

Noninvasive, Nonimaging, Physiologic Methods

Noninvasive, nonimaging, physiologic methods rely on altered venous flow hemodynamics to indirectly infer the presence of venous disease. Examples include plethysmographic techniques and continuous wave Doppler ultrasonography. In general, these techniques are highly operator dependent, subjective, lacking in specificity, and they fail to define the anatomy. However, they are inexpensive and may serve a useful screening function in the hands of competent, experienced clinicians.

Invasive Imaging Methods—Venography

Venography displays the anatomy of the venous system and is the "gold standard" of venous imaging against which all other techniques are measured. However, its high relative cost, invasive nature, and low but finite risk of contrast reaction and postvenographic phlebitis have led to reluctance to use it. It also lacks the ability to give physiologic information.

Noninvasive Imaging Methods—Ultrasound

Real-time imaging with B-mode ultrasound and the addition of duplex Doppler and color flow Doppler ultrasound provides objective anatomic information similar to that of venography as well as physiologic information of venous hemodynamics.

The relatively low cost, noninvasive nature, widespread availability, portability, and proven high accuracy of ultrasound have led to its primary role in the diagnosis of venous thrombosis. Ultrasound has also assumed a role in the evaluation of venous incompetence, preoperative vein mapping, and evaluation of the venous system for patency before the placement of venous catheters.

The peripheral venous system is amenable to evaluation by other imaging techniques, too. Computed tomography (CT) continues to evolve with the availability of helical and, to a lesser extent, electron-beam CT. The reduced imaging times of these techniques allow vascular imaging, which is directed primarily at the arterial system but also allows exquisite depiction of the venous system. Magnetic resonance imaging (MRI) and magnetic resonance angiography (MRA) also continue to evolve and have shown promise in imaging the peripheral venous system. However, with the high accuracy, portability, availability, and cost of ultrasound, it is unlikely that CT or MRI will be used other than in rare problem-solving situations in the peripheral venous system.

INSTRUMENTATION

Gray-Scale Imaging

The relatively superficial location and lack of overlying bowel and skeletal structures allow high-resolution imaging of most of the peripheral veins, with few exceptions. This superficial location favors the use of higher-frequency transducers. In most patients, a 5-MHz, linear, phased array transducer optimizes gray-scale imaging of the femoropopliteal and subclavian veins. In large patients or in instances in which the iliac veins or the inferior vena cava must be evaluated to determine the proximal extent of a thrombus, a 3.5-MHz transducer may be necessary to obtain adequate depth of penetration. Higher-frequency, 7.5-MHz transducers optimize visualization of superficial veins such as the greater and lesser saphenous, brachial, and distal calf veins. As in all areas of sonography, the highest-frequency transducer that gives adequate depth of penetration should be used to optimize spatial resolution.

Doppler Sonography

Doppler sonographic techniques include both quantitative duplex spectral analysis and qualitative color flow Doppler sonography. Both techniques have a pivotal role in identifying and objectively quantifying disease states in the peripheral veins and give sonography the ability to detect altered venous hemodynamics. It is this coupling of anatomic and physiologic information that makes sonography such a powerful tool in the evaluation of vascular disease. The same linear, phased array transducers are coupled with Doppler ultrasound, which typically has a lower frequency. Many phased array transducers have the ability to steer the Doppler beam at angles independent of the imaging beam. Thus, shallower Doppler angles can be used, decreasing error caused by poor Doppler angles. These considerations are even more critical in arterial evaluation. Color flow Doppler sonography is the simultaneous display of flow information in color superimposed on the gray-scale image. This qualitative information demonstrates relative blood velocity, areas of flow disturbance, and direction of blood flow. Color flow Doppler ultrasound has simplified and decreased examination times in many vascular sonographic studies. This technique permits rapid screening of long segments of the venous system and can provide critical information, especially in segments that are not amenable to compression, such as the subclavian veins or the leg veins in very large or obese persons.

LOWER EXTREMITY VEINS

Anatomy

The venous system of the lower extremities is divided into superficial and deep systems. The **superficial system** consists of the greater and lesser saphenous veins and their branches. The **greater saphenous vein** arises from the medial aspect of the common femoral vein in the proximal thigh, inferior to the inguinal ligament but superior to the bifurcation of the common femoral vein (Fig. 30-1). The greater saphenous vein then extends inferiorly to the level of the foot in the subcutaneous tissues of the medial thigh and leg. The normal greater saphenous vein typically is a single vein that is 1 to 3 mm in diameter at the level of the ankle and 3 to 5 mm in diameter at the saphenofemoral junction. These measurements assume importance when this vessel is evaluated before it is harvested for use as an autologous vein graft.

The **lesser saphenous vein** has a variable insertion into the posterior aspect of the proximal or mid popliteal vein. The lesser saphenous vein then travels in the subcutaneous tissues of the dorsal calf to the ankle. The lesser saphenous vein is normally 1 to 2 mm in diameter distally and 2 to 4 mm in diameter at its junction with the popliteal vein and is also suitable for autologous graft material in many patients. Both

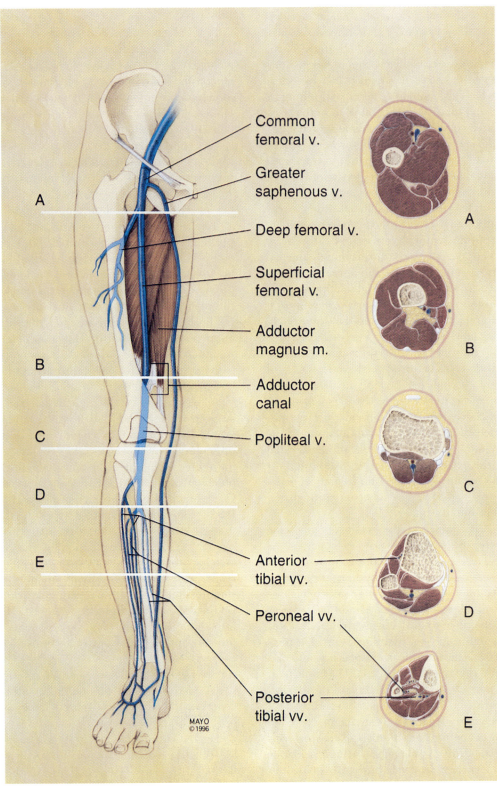

FIG. 30-1. Anatomy of lower extremity veins.

the lesser and greater saphenous veins can become abnormally enlarged or varicose when superficial venous incompetence is present.

Evaluation of the lower extremity veins typically is directed at the **deep system**. The **common femoral vein** begins at the level of the inguinal ligament as the continuation of the external iliac vein and lies just medial and deep to the adjacent common femoral artery (see Fig. 30-1). The common femoral vein bifurcates into the deep and superficial femoral veins in the proximal thigh 6 to 8 cm distal to the inguinal ligament and several centimeters distal to the bifurcation of the common femoral artery. The **deep (profunda) femoral vein** continues to lie medial to its respective artery as it travels deep and laterally to drain the musculature of the thigh. The deep femoral vein typically bifurcates extensively, and only the proximal portion can be evaluated.

The **superficial femoral vein** extends distally in the fascial space deep to the sartorius muscle, medial to the quadriceps muscle group, and lateral to the adductor muscle group. The superficial femoral vein remains medial to the superficial femoral artery until it passes through the adductor canal in the distal thigh. The adductor canal is formed by a separation in the tendinous insertion of the adductor magnus muscle. This canal is deep in the distal thigh and consists of dense aponeurotic and tendinous tissue. This makes visualization and compression of this segment of the distal superficial femoral vein difficult in large patients. The **popliteal vein** is the continuation of the superficial femoral vein as it exits the adductor canal in the popliteal space of the posterior distal thigh. At this level, the popliteal vein lies immediately superficial to the popliteal artery as it passes through the popliteal space into the upper calf.

The first deep branch of the popliteal vein is the paired **anterior tibial vein**, which accompanies the corresponding artery into the anterior compartment of the calf. These veins continue distally along the anterior surface of the interosseous membrane to the dorsal aspect of the foot. Shortly after the origin of the anterior tibial veins, the tibioperoneal venous trunk bifurcates into paired peroneal and posterior tibial veins. The **peroneal veins** lie adjacent to the peroneal artery and medial to the posterior aspect of the fibula. The fibula is an important landmark for the localization of these veins. The **posterior tibial veins** accompany the artery deep in the musculature of the calf, posterior to the tibia. Visualization of the proximal portion of the posterior tibial veins can be difficult in patients with muscular or obese calves. However, these veins are easier to identify as they pass posterior to the medial malleolus and can often be evaluated in a retrograde fashion.

Finally, numerous deep veins drain the musculature of the calf. These gastrocnemial and soleal veins do not have accompanying arteries and vary in size and extent. They are a common site of acute deep venous thrombosis (DVT) in high-risk or postoperative patients. However, their variability often makes complete evaluation and detection of DVT suboptimal.

Deep Venous Thrombosis

Clinical Significance. The true incidence of acute DVT and its major complication, pulmonary embolism, is not known. Approximately 50,000 cases of pulmonary embolism are diagnosed each year in the United States, and autopsy studies have shown that only 19% of pulmonary emboli are suspected clinically.[1] Approximately 200,000 patients are hospitalized each year for the treatment of acute DVT, but the majority of patients with DVT are asymptomatic.[1,2] The difficulty in making the diagnosis is due mainly to the inaccuracy of the clinical evaluation.

The signs and symptoms of acute DVT include **pain, erythema**, and **swelling**. These findings are nonspecific and can be caused by several local or systemic conditions. The presence of a palpable "cord," or thrombosed vein, most commonly is due to superficial thrombophlebitis, which is not usually associated with DVT. These factors contribute to a clinical accuracy of approximately 50% for the diagnosis of acute DVT in symptomatic patients.[2-4] In fact, most hospitalized patients at high risk for developing acute venous thrombosis are asymptomatic.[2] In our vascular laboratory, only 374 (15%) of 2489 patients referred in 1995 for suspected acute DVT had positive findings on sonographic examination. Since untreated acute DVT is a difficult clinical diagnosis and may have severe complications, including pulmonary embolism and postphlebitic syndrome, DVT requires an accurate noninvasive method to establish the diagnosis. Numerous studies and extensive clinical experience have proven that sonography is an ideal technique for this purpose.

Examination. Evaluation of the deep venous system of the leg in patients with suspected acute DVT relies primarily on gray-scale imaging and venous compression in the transverse plane with color flow Doppler frequently added. A 5-MHz linear array transducer is suitable for most patients. With mild pressure applied to the leg by the transducer, a normal vein will collapse completely and the vein walls will coapt (Fig. 30-2). The degree of pressure required varies, depending on the depth and location of the vein, but it is always less than that required to compress the adjacent artery.

The patient is examined in the supine position. The leg is abducted and rotated externally, with slight flexion of the knee. The standard examination begins with the common femoral vein immediately distal to the inguinal ligament. The veins are visualized and compressed in a stepwise fashion every 2 to 3 cm through the level of the distal superficial femoral vein in the adductor canal. The proximal deep femoral vein and greater saphenous vein are also visible in this plane and

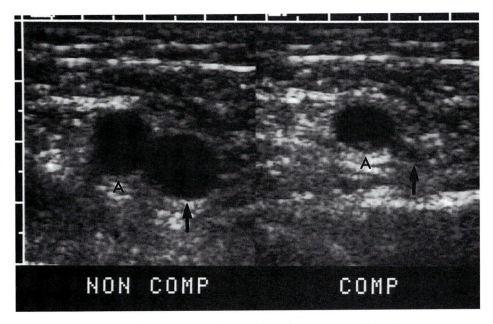

FIG. 30-2. **Normal venous compression ultrasonography.** Transverse image of the right common femoral artery, *A*, and vein *(arrows)* before, *NON COMP*, and after compression, *COMP*, with the ultrasonographic transducer. The normal vein collapses completely with compression.

can be evaluated in most patients. The popliteal vein is evaluated best with the patient prone and the foot resting on a pad to maintain slight knee flexion. The left lateral decubitus position also provides adequate visualization. In these positions, transverse compression sonography can be carried out through the popliteal trifurcation. Many modifications or additions to this standard compression ultrasound examination can be used.

Examination Modifications. Typically, the pelvic venous system is not examined because there is poor visualization because of its depth and frequently overlying bowel gas. However, duplex spectral analysis of the common femoral vein while the patient performs **Valsalva's maneuver** can provide indirect evidence of proximal venous patency in the pelvic veins. In normal subjects, there is constant antegrade venous flow with slight superimposed variation with each respiratory phase. During Valsalva's maneuver, there is a short period of flow reversal, followed by no flow because of increased intraabdominal pressure. With release of Valsalva's maneuver, there is an abrupt increase in forward venous flow, which quickly returns to baseline (Fig. 30-3, *A*). Patients with complete obstruction of the common or external iliac vein will have decreased or absent flow and loss of variation with respiration. There is no change in this spectral pattern with Valsalva's maneuver (Fig. 30-3, *B*). Sluggish venous flow may also be appreciated at standard real-time imaging because echogenic red blood cell rouleaux become visible. Valsalva's maneuver provides indirect "physiologic" evidence of venous patency from the level of the common femoral vein through the inferior vena cava. False-negative exami-

nations may occur with this indirect portion of the examination because of partial, nonoccluding thrombus in the iliac veins and patients with well-developed pelvic venous collaterals. Both of these conditions may result in a normal response to Valsalva's maneuver. In thinner patients, the iliac veins may be visualized directly. A 3.5-MHz transducer with color flow Doppler capability may provide adequate visualization.

The addition of **color flow Doppler sonography** is a useful modification of the standard compression examination. In normal veins, color should fill the vessel lumen from wall to wall, with little or no color aliasing outside the vessel lumen. Venous flow augmentation by squeezing the calf is often necessary to produce complete color filling. Color flow Doppler ultrasound can be helpful in evaluating venous segments that are poorly seen because of the patient's size or the deep location of the segment.[5] Color flow Doppler ultrasound may have some advantages over standard compression techniques in patients with chronic DVT as well.[5,6]

Evaluation of the calf veins is an additional modification of the standard examination that is aided by color flow Doppler techniques.[6-8] However, the clinical value and cost-effectiveness of this evaluation are controversial. In many medical centers, the lower leg is not evaluated because it is rare for the isolated calf DVT to cause significant pulmonary emboli. However, in other medical centers, the calf is evaluated routinely for local symptoms due to the 20% incidence of proximal clot propagation, the increased incidence of postphlebitic syndrome, and significant venous insufficiency after untreated calf thrombus. Given these variables, it is possible to evaluate portions of the deep venous system

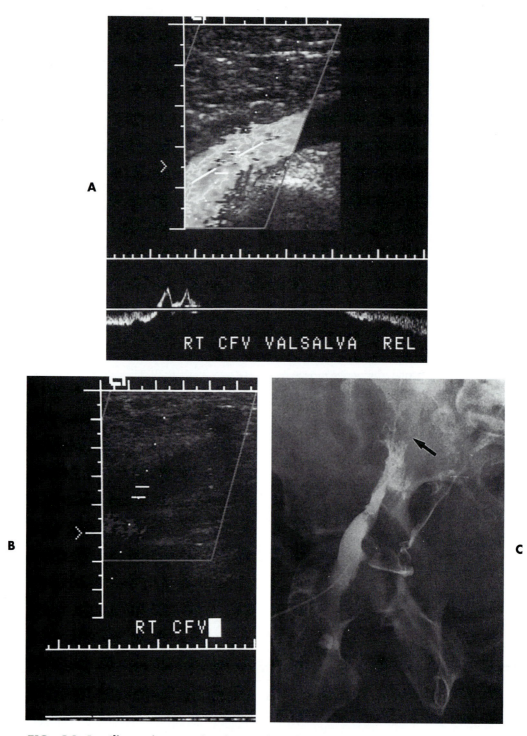

FIG. 30-3. Iliac vein examination with Valsalva's maneuver. A, Normal response—longitudinal image of the common femoral vein, *CFV*, in a normal patient. Duplex spectral analysis shows a normal response to Valsalva's maneuver, with a short period of flow reversal, followed by a period of no flow. With release, *REL*, of Valsalva's maneuver, flow returns. **B,** Abnormal response—spectral analysis of the common femoral vein in another patient shows markedly decreased flow, with no response to Valsalva's maneuver. This vein was compressible (not shown). **C,** Iliocavagram shows obstruction of the right common iliac vein *(arrow)* caused by metastatic adenopathy.

of the calf in many patients with an accuracy approaching that for the femoropopliteal system.[6-8]

Patients can be positioned so they are prone, in the left lateral decubitus position, or in the sitting position. Tilting the examination table into a reverse Trendelenburg position or having the patient sit improves visualization by distending the calf veins. The paired posterior tibial and peroneal veins are imaged with the transducer placed over the posterior calf. Color flow Doppler sonography with augmentation of venous flow is used to confirm venous patency. The anterior tibial veins can be evaluated from an anterior approach. However, thrombus isolated to these veins is rare, and thus anterior examination is not necessary if the peroneal and posterior tibial veins are well seen and normal.[6] The deep veins of the gastrocnemius and soleus muscles are variable in size and visibility and are not amenable to routine complete examination but should be noted when seen.

Finally, a modification of the standard examination has been proposed that would greatly abbreviate the examination.[9] A limited venous compression sonographic examination of only the common femoral and popliteal veins in **symptomatic patients** would result in significant time savings, with a minimal decrease in sensitivity. This can be justified because of the relative rarity of isolated superficial femoral vein or iliac vein thrombosis, because calf vein thrombosis is clinically less important, and because there will be potential cost savings from a shortened examination. Frederick et al.[10] recently reported a 4.6% incidence of isolated thrombosis of the superficial femoral vein. It is doubtful that the cost savings of limited compression ultrasound will justify this reduced accuracy. Complete compression ultrasound from the proximal common femoral vein through the distal popliteal vein remains the standard of care.

Findings. The gray-scale compression sonographic findings of acute DVT are based on direct visualization of the thrombus and lack of venous compressibility (Fig. 30-4). Visualization of thrombus is variable, depending on the extent, age, and echogenicity of the clot. Unfortunately, some acute thrombi may be anechoic, and gray-scale imaging alone can be misleading. Therefore **the lack of complete venous compression** is the hallmark finding of DVT. **Venous distention** by thrombus can be seen acutely in patients but is less common as the clot ages and becomes organized. **Changes in vein caliber with respiration and Valsalva's maneuver are lost** in patients with DVT. However, this finding is presented only in the proximal thigh and is not usually helpful below the bifurcation of the common femoral vein.

Color flow Doppler ultrasound depiction of DVT relies on identifying either a persistent filling defect or thrombus in the color column of the vessel lumen (see Fig. 30-4, *B*) or the absence of flow. Color flow sonography thus depicts the degree of venous obstruction and any residual patent lumen. It is most helpful in deep segments of the thigh, pelvic, and calf veins (Fig. 30-5).

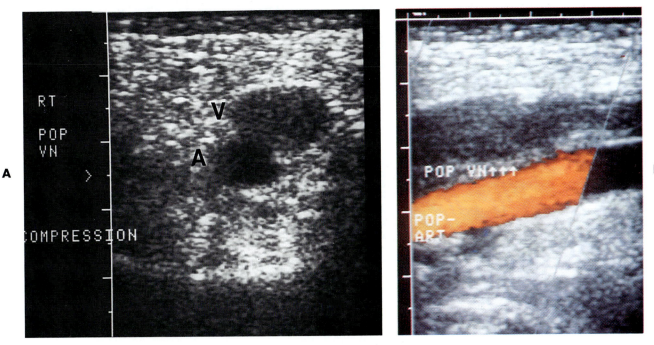

FIG. 30-4. Acute deep venous thrombosis. A, Transverse image of the popliteal vein, *POP VN*, shows lack of venous compressibility and internal echoes caused by deep venous thrombosis. **B,** Longitudinal color flow Doppler ultrasonography shows no flow and internal echoes in the popliteal vein *(arrows)* because of complete thrombosis. *POP ART,* Popliteal artery.

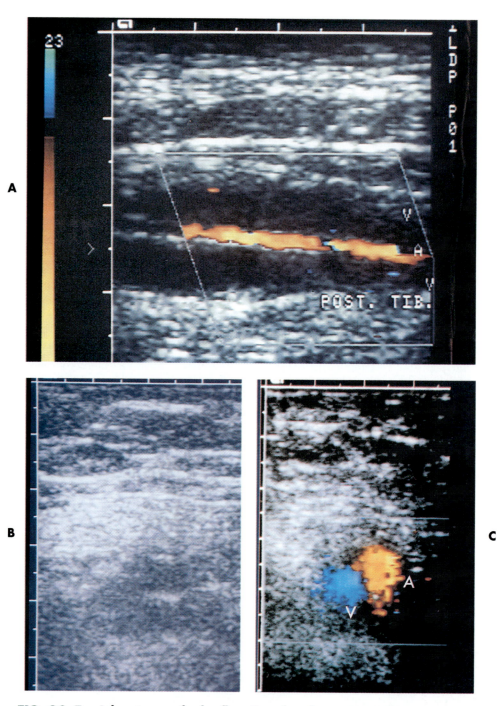

FIG. 30-5. Advantages of color flow Doppler ultrasonography. A, Complete **thrombosis of the paired posterior tibial** *(POST TIB)* **veins** *(V)* on each side of the posterior tibial artery; *(A)* longitudinal color flow Doppler ultrasound of the calf. Color flow Doppler ultrasound is essential for evaluation of the calf veins. **B, Indeterminate** compression ultrasound of the distal superficial femoral vein in the adductor canal. **C, Normal distal superficial femoral artery and vein.** Transverse color flow Doppler ultrasound in the same patient. Color flow Doppler ultrasound aids visualization of deep venous segments in large patients.

Accuracy. The accuracy and clinical utility of sonographic assessment of DVT have been studied extensively. The patient population is of critical importance and should be considered in two broad groups, symptomatic and asymptomatic patients. In **symptomatic** patients, studies comparing venography with compression ultrasonography have shown an average sensitivity of 95% and specificity of 98%.[11] Studies of **asymptomatic,** high-risk, or postoperative patients have shown poorer results. Pooled results of six studies showed an average sensitivity of 59% and specificity of 98% in this patient population.[12] The small size, nonocclusive nature, and higher prevalence of isolated calf thrombi in this group of patients undoubtedly account for the lower sensitivity, since these are more difficult to diagnose with ultrasound as compared with venography. Given these results, the ideal patient for sonographic evaluation has symptoms that extend above the knee.

Chronic DVT. The ability to characterize DVT as acute or chronic is a difficult clinical and imaging problem. Serial studies of patients with acute DVT show that up to 53% of these patients have persistent abnormal findings with compression ultrasound done from 6 to 24 months later.[13,14] These patients may present with postphlebitic syndrome and have symptoms that mimic those of acute DVT. Anticoagulation therapy is not indicated for these patients. Venography

has been the standard imaging method for distinguishing between acute and chronic DVT. However, cost considerations and invasiveness have relegated venography to a problem-solving role in most medical centers. Although ultrasound may be able to help in some cases, currently the role of ultrasound in the diagnosis of chronic DVT is unproven.

As an acute thrombus ages, it undergoes fibroelastic organization, with clot retraction, chronic occlusion, or wall thickening of the involved segment. These changes lead to poor visualization of the clot and incomplete venous compression. Although compression sonography has little role in the diagnosis of chronic DVT, several authors have suggested that color flow Doppler ultrasound may have a role in some patients in differentiating acute DVT from chronic changes.[5,6] Findings suggestive of chronic DVT at color flow Doppler imaging include irregular echogenic vein walls, thickening of the vein walls due to retracted thrombus, decreased diameter of the vein lumina (venous lumina), atretic venous segments, well-developed venous collateral vessels, associated deep venous insufficiency, and absence of distended veins containing hypoechoic or isoechoic thrombus (Fig. 30-6).

Although these findings may be suggestive of chronic DVT and should be familiar to practicing radiologists, the accuracy and role of color flow Doppler ultrasound in patients with chronic DVT are not proven.

Venous Insufficiency
Pathophysiology. In many patients, venous insufficiency is caused by venous valvular damage following DVT. The fibroelastic organization and retraction present in the organizing thrombus secondarily involve any adjacent venous valve. This leads to deep venous insufficiency, which develops in approximately half of the patients with acute DVT. With venous insufficiency there is direct transmission of the hydrostatic pressure of the standing column of fluid in the venous system down to the distal leg. Clinically, this leads to leg swelling, chronic skin and pigmentation changes, woody induration, and, finally, nonhealing venous stasis ulcers.

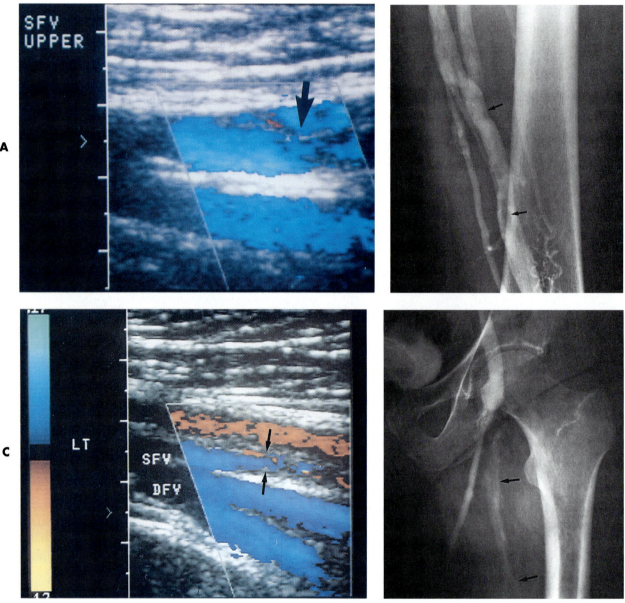

FIG. 30-6. Chronic deep venous thrombosis. A, Longitudinal color flow Doppler ultrasonography of the superficial and deep femoral veins shows an echogenic, weblike, filling defect *(arrow)* in the superficial femoral vein, *SFV*. **B,** Venography confirms changes of chronic DVT *(arrows)*. **C,** Longitudinal color flow Doppler ultrasound in another patient shows irregular thickening of the wall of the proximal superficial femoral vein, with a decrease in luminal diameter *(arrows)*. **D,** Venography confirms findings of chronic DVT *(arrows)*. *DFV,* Deep femoral vein. (From Lewis BD, James EM, Welch TJ et al. Diagnosis of acute deep venous thrombosis of the lower extremities: prospective evaluation of color Doppler flow imaging versus venography. *Radiology* 1994;192:651-655.)

Superficial venous insufficiency leads to distended **subcutaneous varicosities** but has a much better prognosis. Perforating veins communicate from the superficial to the deep system and may also become incompetent, typically because of long-standing deep venous insufficiency.

Examination. The examination is performed with the patient in an upright or semi-upright posi-

tion, with the body's weight supported by the contralateral leg. This positioning is necessary to create the hydrostatic pressure needed to reproduce venous insufficiency. Duplex spectral analysis is obtained at several levels of the deep and superficial venous system during provocative maneuvers. Duplex Doppler tracings in the common femoral vein and proximal greater saphenous vein are obtained during

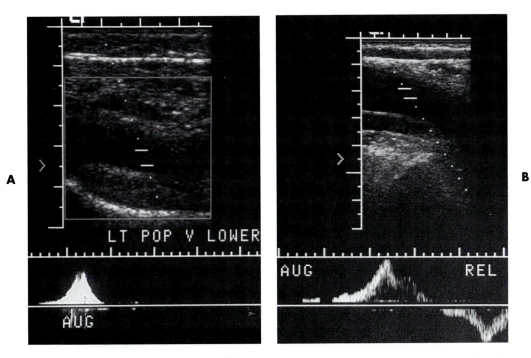

FIG. 30-7. Deep venous insufficiency. A, Duplex spectral analysis of the popliteal vein, *POP V*, shows a normal response to distal venous augmentation, *AUG*. **B,** Duplex spectral analysis in another patient shows marked deep venous insufficiency, with reversed flow equaling forward flow. *REL,* Augmentation released.

Valsalva's maneuver. Several spectral tracings are obtained in the deep and superficial venous system to the level of the popliteal and saphenous veins at the knee. Reverse augmentation by squeezing the thigh above or standard distal venous augmentation by squeezing the calf can be used to assess for insufficiency. However, distal augmentation is more reproducible and easier for a single examiner to perform.

Findings. After brisk distal augmentation, the flow in normal veins is antegrade, with a very short period of flow reversal as returning blood closes the first competent venous valve (Fig. 30-7, *A*). Insufficient veins have a greater degree of reversed flow for a longer period of time (Fig. 30-7, *B*). Quantification schemes have been proposed by evaluating peak flow during venous reflux and measuring the length of time reflux occurs. However, these are not readily reproducible and need to be validated for each laboratory.

Venous Mapping

Vein Harvest for Autologous Grafts. Ultrasound mapping and marking are helpful in many patients before a vein is harvested for autologous graft material. Any superficial vein can be used, but the greater saphenous vein is the most suitable for graft purposes. The examination is performed with the patient in the supine or reverse Trendelenburg position. A tourniquet or blood pressure cuff that is inflated to 40 mm Hg and placed around the proximal thigh can be used to increase venous distention and to aid mapping. The greater saphenous vein is identified and marked from the level of the saphenofemoral junction to as far distally as possible. All major branch points should also be marked to aid the surgeon. A superficial vein typically needs to be larger than 2 mm in diameter, but not varicose, to be suitable graft material. The lesser saphenous vein, basilic vein, and cephalic vein are secondary choices and can be used if the greater saphenous vein has already been harvested or is inadequate.

Insufficient Perforating Vein Marking. Newer surgical techniques of subfascial endoscopic ligation of insufficient perforating veins are being used in some medical centers to treat chronic venous stasis changes and nonhealing venous ulcers. These techniques are aided by accurate localization and marking of insufficient venous perforators. The majority of perforating veins are located below the knee in the medial calf. In an upright patient, distended perforating veins are visible as they pass from the subcutaneous tissues through the fascia into the deep muscles of the calf. These are easily visible on standard gray-scale imaging, and insufficiency can be documented with duplex spectral analysis and flow augmentation (Fig. 30-8). Competent perforating veins are much smaller in caliber and often are difficult or impossible to visualize.

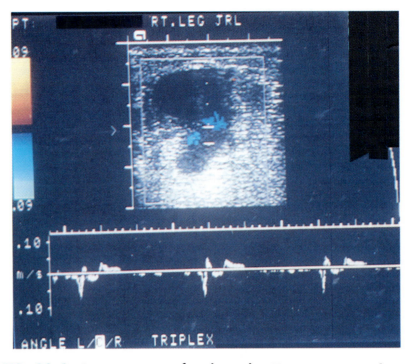

FIG. 30-8. Incompetent perforating vein. Transverse image and spectral analysis of a dilated perforating vein in the medial calf shows to-and-fro flow with distal augmentation. The perforating vein is markedly enlarged and communicates with a large superficial varix.

UPPER EXTREMITY VEINS

Anatomy

Venous return from the arm is primarily through the superficial cephalic and basilic veins. The **cephalic vein** travels in the subcutaneous fat of the lateral aspect of the arm. The cephalic vein joins with the deep venous system at the superior aspect of the axillary or distal subclavian vein (Fig. 30-9). The **basilic vein** is located superficially in the medial aspect of the arm. At the level of the teres major muscle, it joins with the paired deep brachial veins. The **brachial veins** are smaller, deeper, and adjacent to the brachial artery. The level where the brachial and basilic veins join, that is, at the teres major muscle, defines the lateral aspect of the axillary vein. The **axillary vein** is adjacent and superficial to the axillary artery as it passes from the teres major muscle to the first rib through the axilla.

As the axillary vein crosses the first rib, it becomes the lateral portion of the subclavian vein. The subclavian vein is inferior and superficial to the adjacent artery as they pass medially deep to the clavicle. The medial portion of the subclavian vein receives the smaller external jugular vein and the larger internal jugular vein in the base of the neck to form the brachiocephalic vein. The internal jugular vein extends from the jugular foramen in the base of the skull to the confluence with the subclavian vein. The internal jugular vein travels in the carotid sheath and is superficial and lateral to the common carotid artery in the anterior neck. The left and right internal jugular veins are often unequal in size. The brachiocephalic vein is formed by the confluence of the subclavian and internal jugular veins. The right brachiocephalic vein travels along the superficial aspect of the superior right mediastinum. The left brachiocephalic vein is longer and passes from the left superior mediastinum to the right, just deep to the sternum. The right and left brachiocephalic veins join to form the superior vena cava.

Clinical Background

The most common indication for ultrasound evaluation of upper extremity veins is to identify venous thrombosis. The cause and clinical significance of acute DVT of the upper extremity veins differ from those of acute DVT in the legs. Most cases of arm DVT are thought to be due to the presence of a **central venous catheter** or **pacemaker lead**. Of patients with central catheters, 26% to 67% develop thrombosis, although the majority are asymptomatic.[15,16] **Radiation therapy, effort-induced thrombosis,** and **malignant obstruction** are causes of venous obstruction that are more common in the thorax and arm than in the leg. Although the cause of upper extremity DVT differs from that of the lower extremity, the pathophysiology of its evolution is similar.

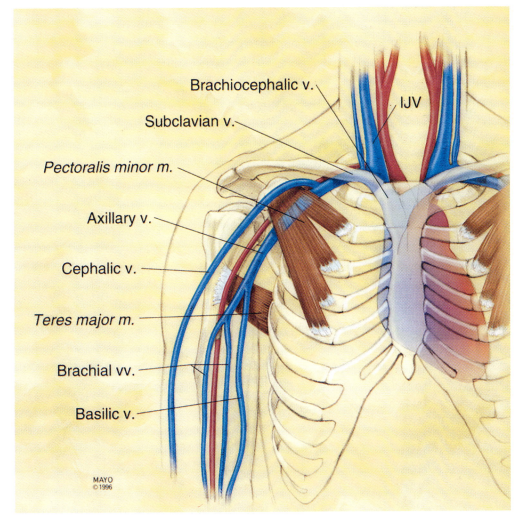

FIG. 30-9. **Anatomy of upper extremity veins.** *IJV*, Internal jugular vein.

The sequelae of upper extremity thrombosis are less severe than those of lower extremity thrombosis. Only 10% to 12% of patients with arm DVT develop pulmonary emboli, and the majority of these are insignificant.[17-19] The development and manifestations of venous stasis and venous insufficiency due to deep venous thrombosis are less common and less severe than in the leg. Chronic swelling, skin changes, and nonhealing venous ulcers are rare in the arm. This is due to two major factors: first, multiple extensive collateral venous pathways usually develop in the arm and upper thorax after an episode of thrombosis or venous obstruction; second, the arm veins are not exposed to the high hydrostatic pressure that leg veins have. Chronic occlusion related to intravenous catheter use and venous thrombosis has made obtaining suitable central venous access difficult in many hospitalized and chronically ill patients. Sonography is ideal for identifying suitable sites for venous access. In difficult cases, direct real-time ultrasonic guidance can be used for placement of venous catheters.

Venous Thrombosis

Examination. Evaluation of the venous system of the upper thorax and arm typically extends from the superior aspect of the brachiocephalic veins through the axillary or brachial veins. The internal jugular veins are also studied. The patient is positioned supine, with the arm to be examined slightly abducted and rotated externally. The patient's head is turned slightly to the opposite side. The highest-frequency transducer that still provides adequate depth of penetration is used. Typically, a 7.5-MHz linear array transducer is used for the internal jugular vein and the arm veins through the axillary vein. A 5-MHz linear array transducer with color flow Doppler ultrasound capability is often necessary to visualize the subclavian vein.

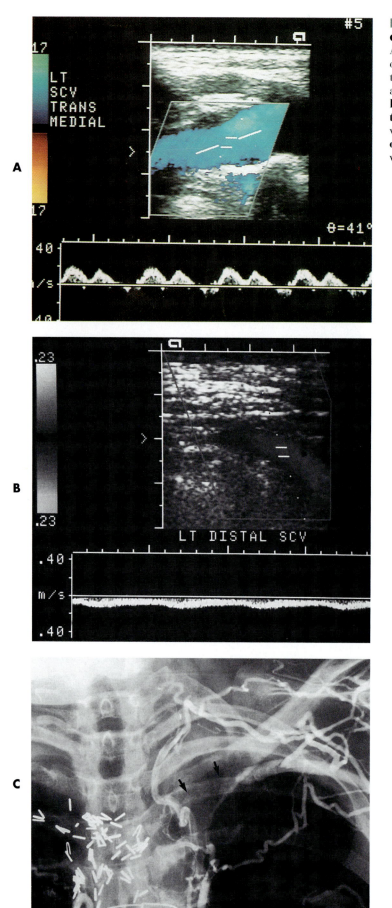

FIG. 30-10. **Comparison of normal and obstructed subclavian veins.** **A, Normal subclavian vein,** *SCV,* transverse color flow Doppler ultrasonography and spectral analysis. There is complete color filling and normal transmitted cardiac pulsations. **B, Loss of the transmitted cardiac pulsations.** Transverse image of the left subclavian vein in another patient. **C, Subclavian vein occlusion** *(arrows)* with numerous collateral vessels on venogram.

Evaluation of the venous system of the upper thorax and arm presents several technical challenges different than the lower extremity. First, the overlying skeletal structures and the lung make direct visualization and examination of the inferior brachiocephalic veins and superior vena cava impossible. Second, the clavicle precludes compression ultrasound of the subclavian vein. Third, the typical development of large venous collateral pathways in patients with venous obstruction can be confusing or lead to false-negative sonographic examination results if they are not recognized as collateral pathways. For these reasons, color flow Doppler sonography, attention to detail, and knowledge of the normal anatomic relationships are crucial.

The internal jugular vein is examined initially with compression sonography in the transverse plane and is followed inferiorly to its junction with the subclavian and upper brachiocephalic veins. An inferiorly angled, coronal, supraclavicular approach with color flow Doppler sonography is necessary to evaluate the superior brachiocephalic vein and the medial portion of the subclavian vein. Duplex Doppler sonographic analysis of the inferior internal jugular vein, superior brachiocephalic vein, and medial subclavian vein is helpful to assess transmitted cardiac pulsatility and respiratory phasicity. Because of the proximity to the heart, duplex Doppler spectral tracings in these sites will show greater transmitted pulsatility than in the leg veins. Loss of this pulsatility may be due to a more central venous obstruction (Fig. 30-10). Comparison of these Doppler ultrasound waveforms with those from the contralateral arm is often helpful to confirm the presence or absence of venous obstruction. Response to Valsalva's maneuver or a brisk inspiratory sniff can also be observed and may also help evaluate venous patency. If the patient sniffs, the internal jugular vein or subclavian vein will decrease in diameter, and spectral analysis will show an increase in blood velocity. Patients with central brachiocephalic vein or superior vena cava obstruction lose this response.

The **subclavian vein** is difficult to visualize completely. A coronal, supraclavicular, inferiorly angled approach is used medially, and a coronal, infraclavicular, superiorly angled approach is used laterally. The venous segment deep to the clavicle often is imaged incompletely. Because of the overlying clavicle, color flow Doppler sonography is necessary to confirm complete venous patency. The examiner should also

---

FINDINGS IN VENOUS THROMBOSIS OF THE UPPER EXTREMITY

Incomplete compression
Persistent intraluminal filling defect with color flow
    Doppler imaging
Absent/decreased transmitted cardiac pulsatility
Abnormal response to respiratory maneuvers
Large collateral veins

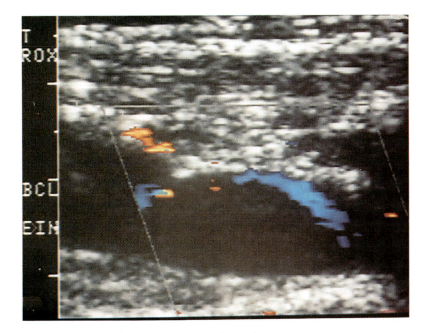

FIG. 30-11. Acute subclavian vein thrombosis. Transverse color flow Doppler ultrasonogram of the subclavian vein shows extensive hypoechoic thrombus with minimal peripheral flow remaining.

confirm the normal inferior superficial relationship of the vein with the adjacent artery. This will avoid the pitfall of confusing well-developed collateral vessels for a patent subclavian vein in patients with chronic venous occlusion. The axillary and upper arm veins can also be evaluated with transverse compression or color flow Doppler ultrasound. The extent of the examination into the arm depends on the clinical indication, but typically it is continued through the bifurcation of the axillary vein.

Findings. The normal and abnormal findings in the upper extremity veins mirror those seen in the lower extremity veins. Patients with venous thrombosis have incomplete collapse of the vein with compression. Thrombus or an intraluminal filling defect is visible in the color column of the vein with color flow Doppler ultrasound (Fig. 30-11 on page 957). Absent or decreased cardiac pulsatility with duplex spectral analysis and abnormal response to an inspiratory sniff are also helpful. Abundant, well-developed collateral vessels are common because of long-standing venous occlusion.

Accuracy. The accuracy of ultrasound versus venography in patients with acute DVT of the upper extremity has not been studied as extensively as in the lower extremity. The available literature shows sensitivity ranging from 78% to 100% and specificities of 92% to 100%.[20-22] The lower accuracy in the upper extremity compared with that in the lower extremity is a result of the greater number of technical challenges facing the examiner.

REFERENCES

Lower Extremity Veins

1. Sandler DA, Martin JF. Autopsy proven pulmonary embolism in hospital patients: are we detecting enough deep vein thrombosis? *J Roy Soc Med* 1989;82:203-205.
2. Salzman EW. Venous thrombosis made easy (editorial). *N Engl J Med* 1986;314:847-848.
3. Haeger K. Problems of acute deep venous thrombosis. I. The interpretation of signs and symptoms. *Angiology* 1969;20:219-223.
4. Barnes RW, Wu KK, Hoak JC. Fallibility of the clinical diagnosis of venous thrombosis. *JAMA* 1975;234:605-607.
5. Lewis BD, James EM, Welch TJ et al. Diagnosis of acute deep venous thrombosis of the lower extremities: prospective evaluation of color Doppler flow imaging versus venography. *Radiology* 1994;192:651-655.
6. Rose SC, Zwiebel WJ, Nelson BD et al. Symptomatic lower extremity deep venous thrombosis: accuracy, limitations, and role of color duplex flow imaging in diagnosis. *Radiology* 1990;175:639-644.
7. Polak JF, Culter SS, O'Leary DH. Deep veins of the calf: assessment with color Doppler flow imaging. *Radiology* 1989;171:481-485.
8. Atri M, Herba MJ, Reinhold C et al. Accuracy of sonography in the evaluation of calf deep vein thrombosis in both postoperative surveillance and symptomatic patients. *AJR* 1996;166:1361-1367.
9. Pezzullo JA, Perkins AB, Cronan JJ. Symptomatic deep vein thrombosis: diagnosis with limited compression US. *Radiology* 1996;198:67-70.
10. Frederick MG, Hertzberg BS, Kliewer MA et al. Can the US examination for lower extremity deep venous thrombosis be abbreviated? A prospective study of 755 examinations. *Radiology* 1996;199:45-47.
11. Cronan JJ. Venous thromboembolic disease: the role of US. *Radiology* 1993;186:619-630.
12. Weinmann EE, Salzman EW. Deep-vein thrombosis. *N Engl J Med* 1994;331:1630-1641.
13. Cronan JJ, Leen V. Recurrent deep venous thrombosis: limitations of US. *Radiology* 1989;170:739-742.
14. Baxter GM, Duffy P, MacKechnie S. Colour Doppler ultrasound of the post-phlebitic limb: sounding a cautionary note. *Clin Radiol* 1991;43:301-304.

Upper Extremity Veins

15. Bonnet F, Loriferne JF, Texier JP et al. Evaluation of Doppler examination for diagnosis of catheter-related deep vein thrombosis. *Intensive Care Med* 1989;15:238-240.
16. McDonough JJ, Altemeier WA. Subclavian venous thrombosis secondary to indwelling catheters. *Surg Gynecol Obstet* 1971;133:397-400.
17. Horattas MC, Wright DJ, Fenton AH et al. Changing concepts of deep venous thrombosis of the upper extremity—report of a series and review of the literature. *Surgery* 1988;104:561-567.
18. Becker DM, Philbrick JT, Walker FB IV. Axillary and subclavian venous thrombosis. Prognosis and treatment. *Arch Intern Med* 1991;151:1934-1943.
19. Monreal M, Lafoz E, Ruiz J et al. Upper-extremity deep venous thrombosis and pulmonary embolism. A prospective study. *Chest* 1991;99:280-283.
20. Knudson GJ, Wiedmeyer DA, Erickson SJ et al. Color Doppler sonographic imaging in the assessment of upper-extremity deep venous thrombosis. *AJR* 1990;154:399-403.
21. Baxter GM, Kincaid W, Jeffrey RF et al. Comparison of colour Doppler ultrasound with venography in the diagnosis of axillary and subclavian vein thrombosis. *Br J Radiol* 1991;64:777-781.
22. Morton MJ, James EM, Welch TJ et al. Duplex and color Doppler imaging in the evaluation of upper extremity and thoracic inlet deep venous thrombosis (exhibit). *AJR* 1994;162(suppl):192.

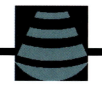

Index